Veterans and Agent Orange

Update 2012

Committee to Review the Health Effects in
Vietnam Veterans of Exposure to Herbicides
(Ninth Biennial Update)

Board on the Health of Select Populations

INSTITUTE OF MEDICINE
OF THE NATIONAL ACADEMIES

THE NATIONAL ACADEMIES PRESS
Washington, D.C.
www.nap.edu

THE NATIONAL ACADEMIES PRESS 500 Fifth Street, NW Washington, DC 20001

NOTICE: The project that is the subject of this report was approved by the Governing Board of the National Research Council, whose members are drawn from the councils of the National Academy of Sciences, the National Academy of Engineering, and the Institute of Medicine. The members of the committee responsible for the report were chosen for their special competences and with regard for appropriate balance.

This study was supported by Contract/Grant No. VA241-P-2024 between the National Academy of Sciences and the US Department of Veterans Affairs. Any opinions, findings, conclusions, or recommendations expressed in this publication are those of the author(s) and do not necessarily reflect the views of the organizations or agencies that provided support for the project.

International Standard Book Number-13: 978-0-309-28886-6
International Standard Book Number-10: 0-309-28886-X

Additional copies of this report are available for sale from the National Academies Press, 500 Fifth Street, NW, Keck 360, Washington, DC 20001; (800) 624-6242 or (202) 334-3313; http://www.nap.edu.

For more information about the Institute of Medicine, visit the IOM home page at: **www.iom.edu.**

Printed in the United States of America

The serpent has been a symbol of long life, healing, and knowledge among almost all cultures and religions since the beginning of recorded history. The serpent adopted as a logotype by the Institute of Medicine is a relief carving from ancient Greece, now held by the Staatliche Museen in Berlin.

Suggested citation: IOM (Institute of Medicine). 2014. *Veterans and Agent Orange: Update 2012.* Washington, DC: The National Academies Press.

"Knowing is not enough; we must apply.
Willing is not enough; we must do."
—Goethe

INSTITUTE OF MEDICINE
OF THE NATIONAL ACADEMIES

Advising the Nation. Improving Health.

THE NATIONAL ACADEMIES

Advisers to the Nation on Science, Engineering, and Medicine

The **National Academy of Sciences** is a private, nonprofit, self-perpetuating society of distinguished scholars engaged in scientific and engineering research, dedicated to the furtherance of science and technology and to their use for the general welfare. Upon the authority of the charter granted to it by the Congress in 1863, the Academy has a mandate that requires it to advise the federal government on scientific and technical matters. Dr. Ralph J. Cicerone is president of the National Academy of Sciences.

The **National Academy of Engineering** was established in 1964, under the charter of the National Academy of Sciences, as a parallel organization of outstanding engineers. It is autonomous in its administration and in the selection of its members, sharing with the National Academy of Sciences the responsibility for advising the federal government. The National Academy of Engineering also sponsors engineering programs aimed at meeting national needs, encourages education and research, and recognizes the superior achievements of engineers. Dr. C. D. Mote, Jr. is president of the National Academy of Engineering.

The **Institute of Medicine** was established in 1970 by the National Academy of Sciences to secure the services of eminent members of appropriate professions in the examination of policy matters pertaining to the health of the public. The Institute acts under the responsibility given to the National Academy of Sciences by its congressional charter to be an adviser to the federal government and, upon its own initiative, to identify issues of medical care, research, and education. Dr. Harvey V. Fineberg is president of the Institute of Medicine.

The **National Research Council** was organized by the National Academy of Sciences in 1916 to associate the broad community of science and technology with the Academy's purposes of furthering knowledge and advising the federal government. Functioning in accordance with general policies determined by the Academy, the Council has become the principal operating agency of both the National Academy of Sciences and the National Academy of Engineering in providing services to the government, the public, and the scientific and engineering communities. The Council is administered jointly by both Academies and the Institute of Medicine. Dr. Ralph J. Cicerone and Dr. C. D. Mote, Jr., are chair and vice chair, respectively, of the National Research Council.

www.national-academies.org

COMMITTEE TO REVIEW THE HEALTH EFFECTS IN VIETNAM VETERANS OF EXPOSURE TO HERBICIDES (NINTH BIENNIAL UPDATE)

MARY K. WALKER (*Chair*), Professor, Department of Pharmaceutical Sciences, University of New Mexico, Albuquerque

REBECCA A. BETENSKY, Professor, Department of Biostatistics, Harvard School of Public Health, Boston, Massachusetts

MICHAEL J. CARVAN III, Shaw Associate Professor, School of Freshwater Sciences, University of Wisconsin–Milwaukee

SCOTT DAVIS, Professor and Chair, Department of Epidemiology, School of Public Health, University of Washington, Seattle

NAIHUA DUAN, Professor, Department of Biostatistics, Columbia University Medical Center, New York, New York

STEPHANIE M. ENGEL, Associate Professor, Department of Epidemiology, Gillings School of Global Public Health, University of North Carolina at Chapel Hill

JENNIFER R. GRANDIS, Professor and Vice Chair for Research, Department of Otolaryngology and Pharmacology, University of Pittsburgh, Pennsylvania

KARL KELSEY, Professor, Epidemiology and Pathology and Laboratory Medicine, Brown University, Providence, Rhode Island

STEPHEN B. KRITCHEVSKY, Director, J. Paul Sticht Center on Aging, Wake Forest University Baptist Medical Center, Winston-Salem, North Carolina

JAMES R. OLSON, Professor, Department of Pharmacology and Toxicology, School of Medicine and Biomedical Sciences, University at Buffalo, New York

GAIL S. PRINS, Professor, Department of Urology, University of Illinois, Chicago

HELEN H. SUH, Associate Professor, Department of Health Sciences, Bouve School of Health Sciences, Northeastern University, Boston, Massachusetts

MARC WEISSKOPF, Associate Professor, Department of Environmental and Occupational Epidemiology, Harvard School of Public Health, Boston, Massachusetts

LORI A. WHITE, Associate Professor, Department of Biochemistry and Microbiology, School of Environmental and Biological Sciences, Rutgers University, New Brunswick, New Jersey

LUOPING ZHANG, Professor, School of Public Health, University of Califorina, Berkeley

Study Staff

MARY BURR PAXTON, Study Director
JENNIFER A. COHEN, Program Officer
TIA S. CARTER, Senior Program Assistant (through March 2013)
ANDREA COHEN, Financial Associate
FREDERICK (RICK) ERDTMANN, Director, Board on the Health of Select Populations
NORMAN GROSSBLATT, Senior Editor

Reviewers

This report has been reviewed in draft form by individuals chosen for their diverse perspectives and technical expertise, in accordance with procedures approved by the National Research Council's Report Review Committee. The purpose of the independent review is to provide candid and critical comments that will assist the institution in making its published report as sound as possible and to ensure that the report meets institutional standards of objectivity, evidence, and responsiveness to the study charge. The review comments and draft manuscript remain confidential to protect the integrity of the deliberative process. We thank the following for their review of the report:

Linda S. Birnbaum, National Institute of Environmental Health Sciences
Margit L. Bleecker, Center for Occupational and Environmental Neurology
Kim Boekelheide, Brown University
Norman E. Breslow, University of Washington
James Brophy, McGill University
David L. Eaton, University of Washington
Edward Elton George, Massachusetts General Hospital
Elaine S. Jaffe, National Cancer Institute
David W. Kennedy, University of Pennsylvania Health System
Kevin Kip, University of South Florida, College of Nursing
Roderick J.A. Little, University of Michigan
John Meeker, University of Michigan School of Public Health
Murray A. Mittleman, Harvard School of Public Health
Rosemary Polomano, University of Pennsylvania School of Nursing

Noel R. Rose, Johns Hopkins University School of Medicine
Hugh H. Tilson, University of North Carolina at Chapel Hill

Although the reviewers listed above have provided many constructive comments and suggestions, they were not asked to endorse the conclusions or recommendations, nor did they see the final draft of the report before its release. The review of the report was overseen by **Kristine M. Gebbie**, Flinders University School of Nursing and Midwifery, Adelaide, South Australia. Appointed by the Institute of Medicine, she was responsible for making certain that an independent examination of the report was carried out in accordance with institutional procedures and that all review comments were carefully considered. Responsibility for the final content of this report rests entirely with the authoring committee and the institution.

Preface

This update focuses on the relevant scientific studies published from October 1, 2010, through September 30, 2012, that is, after the literature considered in *Update 2010*. To accomplish the review, the Institute of Medicine (IOM) established a committee of 15 members representing a wide array of expertise to evaluate the newest scientific evidence and to consider it in light of the studies reviewed in *Veterans and Agent Orange* (*VAO*), *Update 1996*, *Update 1998*, *Update 2000*, *Update 2002*, *Update 2004*, *Update 2006*, *Update 2008*, and *Update 2010*. A link to the experience and expertise of previous committees was provided by recruiting eight members from committees responsible for earlier updates. All committee members were selected because they are experts in their fields, have no conflicts of interest with regard to the matter under study, and have taken no public positions concerning the potential health effects of herbicides in Vietnam veterans or related aspects of herbicide or 2,3,7,8-tetrachlorodibenzo-*p*-dioxin (TCDD) exposure. Biographic sketches of committee members and staff appear in Appendix D.

In this second decade of evaluation, the committee sought the most accurate information and advice from the widest possible array of knowledgeable sources for consideration. To be consistent with National Academies' procedures, the committee met in a series of closed sessions in which members could freely examine, characterize, and weigh the strengths and limitations of the evidence. The committee also convened five open meetings—in September, November, and December 2012 and in January and March 2013—to provide an opportunity for veterans and veterans service organizations, researchers, policy makers, and other interested parties to present their concerns, review their research, and exchange information directly with committee members. The oral presentations and written statements submitted to the committee are listed in Appendix A. The committee thanks the persons who provided valuable insights into the health problems experienced by Vietnam veterans.

The committee is grateful to Mary Paxton, who skillfully served as study director for this project. It also acknowledges the excellent work of IOM staff members Jennifer Cohen, Tia Carter, and Frederick (Rick) Erdtmann. Thanks are also extended to Andrea Cohen, who handled the finances for the project; Norman Grossblatt, who provided editorial skills; and William McLeod and Daniel Bearss, who conducted database searches.

The committee benefited from the assistance of several scientists and researchers who generously lent their time and expertise to give committee members insight into particular issues, provide copies of newly released research, or answer queries about their work. Lisa Cassis, a professor and chair at the University of Kentucky, discussed her research on metabolic and vascular disease. Han Kang, who recently retired as the principal investigator and director of the Environmental Epidemiology Service at the US Department of Veterans Affairs (VA), provided the committee with insight into VA's research programs (past and present), focusing on US Vietnam veterans. Dr. Kang was again helpful, as was Brenda Eskenazi who is the chair of epidemiology at the University of California, Berkeley, in responding to the committee's requests for additional information concerning birth weight in their published studies. Andy Olshan, the chair of epidemiology at the University of North Carolina, and Kim Boekelheide, a professor of medical science at Brown University, joined the committee via conference call to discuss issues related to paternally mediated effects.

Mary K. Walker, PhD, FAHA, *Chair*
Committee to Review the Health Effects in Vietnam Veterans of Exposure to Herbicides (Ninth Biennial Update)

Contents

Figures and Tables

FIGURES

TABLES

Summary

From 1962 to 1971, the US military sprayed herbicides over Vietnam to strip the thick jungle canopy that could conceal opposition forces, to destroy crops that those forces might depend on, and to clear tall grasses and bushes from the perimeters of US base camps and outlying fire-support bases. Mixtures of 2,4-dichlorophenoxyacetic acid (2,4-D), 2,4,5-trichlorophenoxyacetic acid (2,4,5-T), picloram, and cacodylic acid made up the bulk of the herbicides sprayed. The herbicide mixtures used were named according to the colors of identification bands painted on the storage drums; the main chemical mixture sprayed was Agent Orange, a 50:50 mixture of 2,4-D and 2,4,5-T. At the time of the spraying, 2,3,7,8-tetrachlorodibenzo-*p*-dioxin (TCDD), the most toxic form of dioxin, was an unintended contaminant generated during the production of 2,4,5-T and so was present in Agent Orange and some other formulations sprayed in Vietnam. It is important to remember that Agent Orange is not synonymous with TCDD or dioxin.

Complaints from returning Vietnam veterans about their own health and that of their children, combined with emerging toxicologic evidence of adverse effects of phenoxy herbicides and TCDD from animal studies and some positive findings from epidemiologic studies, resulted in sustained controversy. In 1991, because of continuing uncertainty about long-term health effects of the sprayed herbicides in Vietnam veterans, Congress passed Public Law (PL) 102-4, the Agent Orange Act of 1991. That legislation directed the Secretary of Veterans Affairs to ask the National Academy of Sciences (NAS) to perform a comprehensive evaluation of scientific and medical information regarding the health effects of exposure to Agent Orange, other herbicides used in Vietnam, and the various components of those herbicides, including TCDD. The legislation also instructed the Secretary to ask NAS to conduct updates every 2 years for 10 years from the date of the first report to review newly available literature and draw conclusions from the overall evidence.

In response to the first request, the Institute of Medicine (IOM) convened a committee, whose conclusions IOM published in 1994 in *Veterans and Agent Orange: Health Effects of Herbicides Used in Vietnam* (*VAO*). The work of later committees resulted in the publication of biennial updates (*Update 1996*, *Update 1998*, *Update 2000*, *Update 2002*, and *Update 2004*) and of focused reports on the scientific evidence regarding type 2 diabetes, acute myeloid leukemia in children, and the latent period for respiratory cancer.

Enacted in 2002, PL 107-103, the Veterans Education and Benefits Expansion Act of 2001, mandated that the *VAO* biennial updates continue through 2014. *Update 2006*, *Update 2008*, and *Update 2010* were published under that legislation. The current update presents this committee's review of peer-reviewed scientific reports concerning associations between health outcomes and exposure to TCDD and other chemicals in the herbicides used in Vietnam that were published in October 2010–September 2012 and the committee's integration of this information with the previously established evidence database.

CHARGE TO THE COMMITTEE

In accordance with PL 102-4 and PL 107-103, the Committee to Review the Health Effects in Vietnam Veterans of Exposure to Herbicides (Ninth Biennial Update) was asked to "determine (to the extent that available scientific data permit meaningful determinations)" the following regarding associations between specific health outcomes and exposure to TCDD and other chemicals in herbicides used by the military in Vietnam:

> A) whether a statistical association with herbicide exposure exists, taking into account the strength of the scientific evidence and the appropriateness of the statistical and epidemiological methods used to detect the association;
> B) the increased risk of disease among those exposed to herbicides during service in the Republic of Vietnam during the Vietnam era; and
> C) whether there exists a plausible biological mechanism or other evidence of a causal relationship between herbicide exposure and the disease. [PL 102-4, Section 3 (d)]

Judicial history and the congressional mandate, quoted above, dictated that the committee's statement of task is framed in terms of "association" between exposure and health outcomes. This and all prior committees fully recognized that an association does not establish a causal relationship and that the rigor of the evidentiary database needed to support a finding of statistical association is weaker than that needed to establish causality. Nonetheless, any positive evidence supporting a causal relationship would enhance the conviction that an observed statistical association is reliable. Such scientific evidence, of course, would include any information assembled in relation to plausible biologic mechanisms as directed in Article C. In accord with its charge, the committee examined outcome measures commonly used to evaluate statistical associations while assessing the adequacy of control for bias and confounding and the likelihood that an observed association could be explained by chance. The committee also assessed evidence of biologic plausibility derived from laboratory findings in cell culture or animal models. In particular, associations found to have multiple supportive lines of evidence were interpreted as having stronger scientific support for reflecting causal effects.

In conducting its study, the present committee operated independently of the Department of Veterans Affairs (VA) and other government agencies. The committee was not asked to make and did not make judgments regarding specific cases in which individual Vietnam veterans have claimed injury from herbicide exposure. This report provides scientific information for the Secretary of Veterans Affairs to consider as VA exercises its responsibilities to Vietnam veterans. The committee was not charged to focus on broader issues, such as the potential costs of compensation for veterans or policies regarding such compensation.

COMMITTEE'S APPROACH TO ITS CHARGE

Following the pattern established by prior VAO committees, the present committee concentrated its review on epidemiologic studies to fulfill its charge of assessing whether specific human health effects are associated with exposure to at least one of the herbicides sprayed in Vietnam or to TCDD. The committee also considered controlled laboratory investigations that provided information on whether scientifically relevant association between the chemicals of interest and a given effect is biologically plausible.

The VAO committees began their evaluation presuming neither the presence nor the absence of association for any particular health outcome. Over the sequence of reviews, evidence of various degrees of association, lack of association, or persistent indeterminacy with respect to a wide array of disease states has accrued. For many conditions, however, particularly ones that are very uncommon, any association with the chemicals of interest has remained unaddressed in the medical research literature; for these (unless the condition is logically subsumed under a broader disease category that has been evaluated), the committee remains neutral, abiding by the maxim that "absence of evidence is not evidence of absence."

In accord with Congress's mandated presumption of herbicide exposure of all Vietnam veterans, VAO committees have treated Vietnam-veteran status as a proxy for some herbicide exposure when no more specific exposure information is available. To obtain information potentially relevant to the evaluation of health effects related to herbicide exposure in addition to that available from studies of Vietnam veterans, the committee reviewed studies of other groups potentially exposed to the constituents of the herbicide mixtures used in Vietnam (2,4-D, 2,4,5-T, TCDD, cacodylic acid, and picloram). In addition to retrieving articles identified on the basis of keywords specifying the chemicals and chemical classes of interest, literature searches for the earliest reports in the VAO series had been structured to retrieve all studies of several occupational groups, including chemical, agricultural, pulp and paper, sawmill, and forestry workers. To the extent that studies of those workforces were recovered in new searches directed at particular agents of exposure, they were incorporated into the database. Some occupational and environmental cohorts that received exceptionally high exposures—such as the International Agency for Research on Cancer (IARC) and Seveso cohorts discussed in this report—are now well characterized and are producing a stream of informative results. The Agricultural Health Study (AHS), a continuing prospective cohort study of agricultural populations with specific information on the chemicals of interest, is also steadily contributing new findings to the database. The Vietnam veterans themselves are advancing in age and, when studied, are capable of providing substantial information on chronic health conditions directly; however, the intensity of research on this target population has waned in recent years. As the information in the database on populations that had established exposures to the chemicals of interest has grown, the committee has come to depend less on data from studies that yielded nonspecific exposure information and has been able to focus more on findings of studies that had refined exposure specificity.

As in *Update 2010*, the results tables in this report are grouped by study population rather than by the update in which the studies were originally reviewed. That change was made to emphasize and clarify the relationship among successive publications that have provided insight into the health responses of particular exposed populations that have been studied for many years. Studies of cohorts have been ordered in a given table to reflect the hierarchic nature of many of the study populations—for example, workers in the Dow Chemical Company plant in Midland, Michigan, are one of several cohorts composing the National Institute for Occupational Safety and Health (NIOSH) cohort, which in turn is one of the many international cohorts making up the IARC cohort—and the citations indicating the source of particular results have been moved to the last column of the table. To allow for the possibility that a case-control study may investigate the relationship of a health outcome to both occupational and environmental factors and in recognition of the difference between this protocol and that of cohort and cross-sectional studies, case-control studies have been gathered into a separate section in the results tables. Finally, the exposure of interest in each study population has been explicitly noted in the tables to facilitate judgments about when consistency might be expected between populations that experience the same exposure.

The original legislation, PL 102-4, did not provide a list of specific diseases and conditions suspected of being associated with herbicide exposure. Such a list was developed on the basis of diseases and conditions that had been mentioned in the scientific literature or in other documents identified through the original *VAO*'s extensive literature searches. The *VAO* list has been augmented in response to developments in the literature, requests by VA, and concerns of Vietnam veterans.

The information that the present committee reviewed was identified through a comprehensive search of relevant databases, including databases covering epidemiologic, biologic, medical, toxicologic, chemical, historical, and regulatory information. More than 6,800 potentially relevant citations were identified during searches of literature published between the date of the literature cut-off for *Update 2010* and the current update deadline, September 30, 2010–September 30, 2012. After screening of the citation abstracts for relevance, about 1,100 were retained for closer consideration. Ultimately, about 60 papers on epidemiologic studies and several score of toxicologic studies and exposure evaluations ultimately contributed new information to this review. Additional information came from veterans and other interested people who testified at public hearings and offered written submissions.

To determine whether there is a scientifically relevant association between exposure and a health outcome, epidemiologists estimate the magnitude of an appropriate measure (such as the relative risk or the odds ratio) that describes the relationship between exposure and disease in a defined population or group. In evaluating the strength of the evidence linking herbicide exposure with a particular outcome, the committee considered whether such estimates of risk might not reflect a causal association (because of confounding, chance, or bias related to errors in selection and measurement) or might accurately represent true associations; although they are not required, data supporting biologic plausibility strengthen confidence that an association is not spurious. It has been the practice of all VAO committees to evaluate all studies according to the same criteria and then to weigh findings of similar strength and validity equivalently, whether or not the study subjects are Vietnam veterans, when drawing conclusions. The committee recognizes that an absolute conclusion about the absence of association might never be attained because, as is generally the case in science, studies of health outcomes after herbicide exposure cannot demonstrate that a purported outcome is impossible, only that it is statistically improbable.

EVIDENCE REVIEWED BY THE COMMITTEE

The sections below summarize new epidemiologic information evaluated in this update and integrated with that previously assembled. The epidemiologic studies have been divided, both here and in the health-outcome chapters, into four categories—Vietnam-veteran, occupational, environmental, and case-control—depending on the population addressed and the study design.

Vietnam-Veterans Studies

Notably few studies concerning the health of Vietnam veterans were identified as having been published since the three evaluated in *Update 2010*, and almost all addressed psychological endpoints, which are not within the scope of this report. There were no new studies of Vietnam-veteran cohorts and only a single, largely uninformative case-control study on Korean veterans with cardiac disease, which assessed hypertension and hyperlipidemia in terms of whether or not they had served in Vietnam.

Occupational Studies

The committee reviewed several occupational studies published since *Update 2010*. Researchers reported on cancer mortality in pentachlorophenol (PCP) workers who are part of the NIOSH cohort and cancer incidence in a NIOSH subcohort of chemical workers in a Dow plant in Michigan. Plasma dioxin concentrations and cause-specific mortality were investigated in German production workers in a plant included in the IARC cohort in Hamburg, Germany, and three new studies of IARC subcohorts in the Netherlands reported on cancer mortality, ischemic heart disease, humoral immunity, atopic disease, and immune suppression in herbicide workers. An examination of pesticide appliers and gliomas in participants in the Upper Midwest Health Study was reviewed, and eight recent reports from the AHS examined cancer incidence, body-mass index, amyotrophic lateral sclerosis, and mortality in private pesticide applicators (farmers), their spouses, and commercial pesticide applicators in Iowa and North Carolina.

Environmental Studies

Several new studies of the effects of environmental exposure to the chemicals of interest have been published since *Update 2010*. Cancer incidence and reproductive factors were investigated in people who lived near the site of the industrial accident in Seveso, Italy. Five new studies published by the Prospective Investigations of the Vasculature in Uppsala Seniors (PIVUS) group reported on stroke, atherosclerosis, diabetes, and obesity. Several new studies from Taiwan examined hypertension, cardiovascular disease, and insulin resistance in people who lived in the vicinity of a closed PCP factory. Hypertension and bone mineral density and environmental exposures were investigated via the National Health and Nutrition Examination Survey, and diabetes and hypertension were examined in the Anniston (Alabama) Community Health Survey. Reproductive outcomes—including birth weight, onset of puberty, infant growth, immune function, leukemia, and congenital cryptorchidism—were studied in mother–infant pairs exposed to TCDD and other chemicals that have dioxin-like biologic activity in Japan, Finland, the Netherlands, the United States, and Vietnam.

Case-Control Studies

New case-control studies examined the possible association of occupational exposures with prostate cancer, lymphoid neoplasms, myelodysplastic syndromes, and Parkinson disease. Additional new case-control studies examined environmental exposures to the chemicals of interest and breast cancer, melanoma, non-Hodgkin lymphoma, endometriosis, menstrual cycles, and Parkinson disease. And a large Canadian study published papers investigating both categories of exposure as related to several cancers.

THE COMMITTEE'S CONCLUSIONS

Health Outcomes

In *Update 2012*, the committee has elected to change the categorization of one health outcome listed in Table S-1. **The committee voted unanimously to move *stroke* to the "limited and suggestive" category** because of new evidence showing a statistically significant association in the well-designed PIVUS study; evidence of an overall increase in stroke and cerebrovascular disease associated with exposure to the chemicals of interest in environmental, occupational, and Vietnam-veteran populations in the most relevant of previously considered studies; demonstrated biological plausibility from human and animal studies; and the strong connection between stroke and hypertension, cardiovascular disease, and diabetes (three conditions already in the limited and suggestive category). The published data did not permit the committee to distinguish hemorrhagic from ischemic stroke, but given that only a small percentage of strokes are of the hemorrhagic type in Western populations, this was not seen to be an impediment. That single change in the classifications made in previous updates is in boldface in Table S-1.

This conclusion and the decision not to modify any other findings from earlier VAO committees were made after the present committee weighed the strengths and limitations of the epidemiologic evidence reviewed in this report and in previous VAO reports. Although the studies published since *Update 2010* are the subject of detailed evaluation in this report, the committee drew its conclusions in the context of the entire body of literature. The contribution of recent publications to the evidence database was substantial, but the committee did not weigh them more heavily merely because they were new. Epidemiologic methods and analytic capabilities have improved, but many of the recent studies were par-

TABLE S-1 Summary of *Ninth Biennial Update* of Findings on Vietnam-Veterans, Occupational, and Environmental Studies Regarding Scientifically Relevant Associations[a] Between Exposure to Herbicides and Specific Health Outcomes[b]

Sufficient Evidence of an Association

Epidemiologic evidence is sufficient to conclude that there is a positive association. That is, a positive association has been observed between exposure to herbicides and the outcome in studies in which chance, bias, and confounding could be ruled out with reasonable confidence.[c] For example, if several small studies that are free of bias and confounding show an association that is consistent in magnitude and direction, there could be sufficient evidence of an association. There is sufficient evidence of an association between exposure to the chemicals of interest and the following health outcomes:

Soft-tissue sarcoma (including heart)
* Non-Hodgkin lymphoma
* Chronic lymphocytic leukemia (including hairy cell leukemia and other chronic B-cell leukemias)
* Hodgkin lymphoma
Chloracne

Limited or Suggestive Evidence of an Association

Epidemiologic evidence suggests an association between exposure to herbicides and the outcome, but a firm conclusion is limited because chance, bias, and confounding could not be ruled out with confidence.[b] For example, a well-conducted study with strong findings in accord with less compelling results from studies of populations with similar exposures could constitute such evidence. There is limited or suggestive evidence of an association between exposure to the chemicals of interest and the following health outcomes:

Laryngeal cancer
Cancer of the lung, bronchus, or trachea
Prostate cancer
* Multiple myeloma
* AL amyloidosis
Early-onset peripheral neuropathy
Parkinson disease
Porphyria cutanea tarda
Hypertension
Ischemic heart disease
Stroke (category change from *Update 2010*)
Type 2 diabetes (mellitus)
Spina bifida in offspring of exposed people

Inadequate or Insufficient Evidence to Determine an Association

The available epidemiologic studies are of insufficient quality, consistency, or statistical power to permit a conclusion regarding the presence or absence of an association. For example, studies fail to control for confounding, have inadequate exposure assessment, or fail to address latency. There is inadequate or insufficient evidence to determine association between exposure to the chemicals of interest and the following health outcomes that were explicitly reviewed:

Cancers of the oral cavity (including lips and tongue), pharynx (including tonsils), or nasal cavity (including ears and sinuses)
Cancers of the pleura, mediastinum, and other unspecified sites in the respiratory system and intrathoracic organs

TABLE S-1 Continued

Esophageal cancer
Stomach cancer
Colorectal cancer (including small intestine and anus)
Hepatobiliary cancers (liver, gallbladder, and bile ducts)
Pancreatic cancer
Bone and joint cancer
Melanoma
Nonmelanoma skin cancer (basal-cell and squamous-cell)
Breast cancer
Cancers of reproductive organs (cervix, uterus, ovary, testes, and penis; excluding prostate)
Urinary bladder cancer
Renal cancer (kidney and renal pelvis)
Cancers of brain and nervous system (including eye)
Endocrine cancers (thyroid, thymus, and other endocrine organs)
Leukemia (other than chronic B-cell leukemias, including chronic lymphocytic leukemia and hairy cell leukemia)
Cancers at other and unspecified sites
Infertility
Spontaneous abortion (other than after paternal exposure to TCDD, which appears *not* to be associated)
Neonatal or infant death and stillbirth in offspring of exposed people
Low birth weight in offspring of exposed people
Birth defects (other than spina bifida) in offspring of exposed people
Childhood cancer (including acute myeloid leukemia) in offspring of exposed people
Neurobehavioral disorders (cognitive and neuropsychiatric)
Neurodegenerative diseases, excluding Parkinson disease
Chronic peripheral nervous system disorders
Hearing loss
Respiratory disorders (wheeze or asthma, chronic obstructive pulmonary disease, and farmer's lung)
Gastrointestinal, metabolic, and digestive disorders (changes in hepatic enzymes, lipid abnormalities, and ulcers)
Immune system disorders (immune suppression, allergy, and autoimmunity)
Circulatory disorders (other than hypertension, ischemic heart disease, and stroke)
Endometriosis
Disruption of thyroid homeostasis
Eye problems
Bone conditions

This committee used a classification that spans the full array of cancers. However, reviews for nonmalignant conditions were conducted only if they were found to have been the subjects of epidemiologic investigation or at the request of the Department of Veterans Affairs. *By default, any health outcome on which no epidemiologic information has been found falls into this category.*

Limited or Suggestive Evidence of *No* Association

Several adequate studies, which cover the full range of human exposure, are consistent in not showing a positive association between any magnitude of exposure to a component of the

continued

TABLE S-1 Continued

herbicides of interest and the outcome. A conclusion of "no association" is inevitably limited to the conditions, exposures, and length of observation covered by the available studies. *In addition, the possibility of a very small increase in risk at the exposure studied can never be excluded.* There is limited or suggestive evidence of *no* association between exposure to the herbicide component of interest and the following health outcome:

Spontaneous abortion after paternal exposure to TCDD

[a]This change in wording was made to emphasize the scientific nature of the VAO task and procedures and reflects no change in the present committee's criteria from those used in previous updates.

[b]*Herbicides* indicates the following chemicals of interest: 2,4-dichlorophenoxyacetic acid (2,4-D), 2,4,5-trichlorophenoxyacetic acid (2,4,5-T) and its contaminant 2,3,7,8-tetrachlorodibenzo-*p*-dioxin (TCDD or dioxin), cacodylic acid, and picloram. The evidence regarding association was drawn from occupational, environmental, and veteran studies in which people were exposed to the herbicides used in Vietnam, to their components, or to their contaminants.

[c]Evidence of an association is strengthened by experimental data supporting biologic plausibility, but its absence would not detract from the epidemiologic evidence.

*The committee notes the consistency of these findings with the biologic understanding of the clonal derivation of lymphohematopoietic cancers that is the basis of the World Health Organization classification system.

ticularly useful for this committee's purpose also because they produced results in terms of serum TCDD concentrations or the amount of exposure to dioxin-like chemicals. Of course, observations on the health of our population of primary concern, Vietnam veterans, are increasingly informative as they age.

Table S-1 defines four categories of association and gives criteria for assigning health outcomes to them. (Although the committee for this update did not modify the criteria used by previous VAO committees for assigning categories of association to health outcomes, it has inserted "scientifically relevant" before "association" in the title of Table S-1 to clarify that the strength of evidence evaluated, based on the quality of the scientific studies reviewed, was a fundamental component of the committee's deliberations to address the imprecisely defined legislative target of "statistical association.")

On the basis of its evaluation of case-control studies and studies of veteran, occupational, and environmentally exposed populations, the committee allocated particular health outcomes to categories of relative certainty of association with exposure to the herbicides that were used in Vietnam or to any of their components or contaminants (with no intention of specifying particular chemicals). The committee notes that experimental data related to biologic plausibility of conditions statistically associated with exposure to Agent Orange have gradually emerged since the beginning of this series of VAO reports and that these findings can inform decisions about how to categorize the degree of association of individual conditions; Table S-1 includes a footnote to this effect.

As mandated by PL 102-4, the distinctions among categories are based on statistical association, not on strict causality. The committee was directed to review the scientific data, not to recommend VA policy; therefore, conclusions reported in Table S-1 are not intended to imply or suggest policy decisions. The conclusions are related to associations between exposure and outcomes in human populations, not to the likelihood that any individual's health problem is associated with or caused by the herbicides in question.

Risk in Vietnam Veterans

There have been numerous health studies of Vietnam veterans, but most have been hampered by relatively poor measures of exposure to herbicides or TCDD and by other methodologic problems. In light of those problems, many conclusions regarding associations between exposure to the chemicals of interest and disease have been based on studies of people exposed in various occupational and environmental settings rather than on studies of Vietnam veterans, although more recent studies of health consequences in the maturing veterans themselves have generated more informative findings than originally available to VAO committees. The committee believes that there is sufficient evidence to reach general or qualitative conclusions about associations between herbicide exposure and health outcomes, but the lack of adequate exposure data on Vietnam veterans themselves makes it difficult to estimate the degree of increased risk of disease in Vietnam veterans as a group or individually. Without information on the extent of herbicide exposure of Vietnam veterans and quantitative information about the dose–time–response relationship for each health outcome in humans, estimation of the risks experienced by veterans exposed to the chemicals of interest during the Vietnam War is not possible.

Because of those limitations, only general assertions can be made about risks to Vietnam veterans, depending on the category of association into which a given health outcome has been placed. If there were "limited or suggestive evidence of *no* association" between herbicide exposure and a health outcome, the evidence would suggest that no increased risk of the outcome in Vietnam veterans was attributable to exposure to the chemicals of interest (at least given the conditions, exposures, and lengths of observation covered by the studies reviewed). Even qualitative estimates are not possible when there is "inadequate or insufficient" evidence of an association. For outcomes categorized as having "sufficient" or "limited or suggestive" evidence of an association with herbicide exposure, the lack of exposure information on Vietnam veterans prevents calculation of precise risk estimates.

The information needed for assigning risk estimates continues to be absent despite concerted efforts to model the exposure of the troops in Vietnam, to measure serum TCDD concentrations of individual veterans, and to model the dynamics of retention and clearance of TCDD in the human body. Accordingly, several successive VAO committees have stated as a general conclusion that, at least for the present, it was not possible to derive quantitative estimates of any increased risks of various adverse health effects that Vietnam veterans may have experienced in association with exposure to the herbicides sprayed in Vietnam. Given the amount of time that has passed since the Vietnam era, the present committee agreed with the assessment of previous committees that the necessary information to perform such estimation for Vietnam veterans is extremely unlikely ever to become available.

COMMITTEE RECOMMENDATIONS

IOM has been asked to make recommendations concerning the need, if any, for additional scientific studies to resolve continuing scientific uncertainties about the health effects of the herbicides used in Vietnam and their contaminants. Although advances have been made over the last several years in understanding the health effects of exposure to the herbicides used in Vietnam and to TCDD and in elucidating the mechanisms that underlie the effects, there are still subjects on which increased knowledge could be very useful.

This committee recommends that VA query its own medical databases more actively to identify potential associations between Vietnam service and specific health outcomes, particularly outcomes that are so common or so specific that they are infrequently addressed in epidemiology studies. Moreover, if a perceived conflict of interest exists in surveying its own databases, it is recommended that an external advisory group be formed to determine the best mechanism for mining the information so that these medical databases can be available for external study.

The committee for *Update 2008* concluded that it was possible that epigenetic changes arising from exposure to the herbicides sprayed in Vietnam might cause paternally mediated effects in offspring, and such potential would most likely be attributable to the TCDD contaminant in Agent Orange. There is a growing body of evidence that TCDD—and arsenicals—can induce epigenetic changes in animal models, but there remain extremely limited data on the risk that paternal exposure to xenobiotics in general, and the VAO chemicals of interest in particular, will result in adverse effects on their offspring. Consequently, this committee continues to recommend that laboratory research be conducted to characterize TCDD's potential for inducing epigenetic modifications.

The committee also recommends development of epidemiologic protocols to address the logistical challenge of determining whether adverse effects are being manifested in the adult children and grandchildren of Vietnam veterans as a result of male veterans' exposure. The best cohorts for revealing potential associations would be those on which there is well-characterized exposure information. Another alternative would be to adopt a case-control approach and explore whether information about Vietnam exposure or specific herbicide exposure could be ascertained in any of the many birth cohorts that have been established in the last several decades. To home in on a paternal effect, however, it will be necessary to establish that the mothers did not have the opportunity for exposure to the chemicals of interest above background levels.

As in previous years, this committee recommends the pursuit of additional research in toxicology. The development of animal models of neurologic outcomes and of various chronic health conditions and their progression would be useful for understanding the possible contributions of the chemicals of interest to compromising the health of aging Vietnam veterans. Specifically, determining the mechanism by which dioxin-like chemicals induce B-cell cancers and how such exposure alters the susceptibility to obesity and components of metabolic syndrome would fill important knowledge gaps. Health problems such as metabolic syndrome, chronic obstructive pulmonary disease (COPD), and measurement of biomarkers of immune or inflammatory disease merit study in human populations.

The committee notes that the earlier investment in studying several exposed populations has produced useful findings; the NIOSH, Seveso, Air Force Health Study (AFHS), and Army Chemical Corps (ACC) cohorts all merit continuing followup or more comprehensive analysis. Longitudinal analyses of cancer, cardiovascular, and reproductive outcomes represented in the complete database assembled in the course of the AFHS are especially important. The committee is encouraged that VA has reinitiated the National Vietnam Veterans Longitudinal Study and has launched the Army Chemical Corps Vietnam-Era Veterans Health study to investigate the relationship of herbicide exposure during the Vietnam War with hypertension and COPD in ACC veterans.

Several of the committee's recommendations are similar to those offered in previous updates because little activity has been seen in several critical topics. Proposals for studies that would use data and biologic samples from the AFHS have only recently been approved, and published results from these investigations are still several years off. Meanwhile, critical integrative analyses, such as longitudinal evaluation of the cancer data, have not yet been made public, and the unique potential of this resource has languished. It is the committee's conviction that work needs to be undertaken promptly to resolve questions regarding several health outcomes, among them COPD, tonsil cancer, melanoma, Alzheimer disease, and paternally transmitted effects in offspring. Creative analysis of VA's own data resources and further work on cohorts that have already been established may well be the most effective way to address those outcomes and to gain a better understanding of the role of herbicide exposure in development of stroke, prostate cancer, and Parkinson disease in Vietnam veterans.

1

Introduction

The Agent Orange Act of 1991—Public Law (PL) 102-4, enacted February 6, 1991, and codified as Section 1116 of Title 38 of the United States Code—directed the Secretary of Veterans Affairs to ask the National Academy of Sciences (NAS) to conduct an independent comprehensive review and evaluation of scientific and medical information regarding the health effects of exposure to herbicides used during military operations in Vietnam. The herbicides picloram and cacodylic acid were to be addressed, as were chemicals in various formulations that contain the herbicides 2,4-dichlorophenoxyacetic acid (2,4-D) and 2,4,5-trichlorophenoxyacetic acid (2,4,5-T). 2,4,5-T contained the contaminant 2,3,7,8-tetrachlorodibenzo-*p*-dioxin, referred to in this report as TCDD to represent a single—and the most toxic—congener of the tetrachlorodibenzo-*p*-dioxins (tetraCDDs), also commonly referred to as dioxin. It should be noted that TCDD and Agent Orange are not the same. NAS also was asked to recommend, as appropriate, additional studies to resolve continuing scientific uncertainties and to comment on particular programs mandated in the law. The legislation called for biennial reviews of newly available information for a period of 10 years; the period was extended to 2014 by the Veterans Education and Benefits Expansion Act of 2001 (PL 107-103).

In response to the request from the Department of Veterans Affairs (VA), the Institute of Medicine (IOM) of the National Academies convened the Committee to Review the Health Effects in Vietnam Veterans of Exposure to Herbicides. The results of the original committee's work were published in 1994 as *Veterans and Agent Orange: Health Effects of Herbicides Used in Vietnam*, hereafter referred to as *VAO* (IOM, 1994). Successor committees formed to fulfill the requirement for updated reviews produced *Veterans and Agent Orange: Update 1996* (IOM,

1996), *Update 1998* (IOM, 1999), *Update 2000* (IOM, 2001), *Update 2002* (IOM, 2003a), *Update 2004* (IOM, 2005a), *Update 2006* (IOM, 2007), *Update 2008* (IOM, 2009), and *Update 2010* (IOM, 2011).

In 1999, VA asked the IOM to convene a committee to conduct an interim review of type 2 diabetes associated with exposure to any of the chemicals of interest (COIs); that effort resulted in the report *Veterans and Agent Orange: Herbicide/Dioxin Exposure and Type 2 Diabetes*, hereafter referred to as *Type 2 Diabetes* (IOM, 2000). In 2001, VA asked the IOM to convene a committee to conduct an interim review of childhood acute myelogenous leukemia (AML, now preferably referred to as acute myeloid leukemia) associated with parental exposure to any of the COIs; the committee's review of the literature, including literature available since the review for *Update 2000*, was published as *Veterans and Agent Orange: Herbicide/Dioxin Exposure and Acute Myelogenous Leukemia in the Children of Vietnam Veterans*, hereafter referred to as *Acute Myelogenous Leukemia* (IOM, 2002). In PL 107-103, passed in 2001, Congress directed the Secretary of Veterans Affairs to ask NAS to review "available scientific literature on the effects of exposure to an herbicide agent containing dioxin on the development of respiratory cancers in humans" and to address "whether it is possible to identify a period of time after exposure to herbicides after which a presumption of service-connection" of the disease would not be warranted; the result of that effort was *Veterans and Agent Orange: Length of Presumptive Period for Association Between Exposure and Respiratory Cancer*, hereafter referred to as *Respiratory Cancer* (IOM, 2004).

In conducting their work, the committees responsible for those reports operated independently of VA and other government agencies. They were not asked to and did not make judgments regarding specific cases in which individual Vietnam veterans have claimed injury from herbicide exposure. The reports were intended to provide scientific information for the Secretary of Veterans Affairs to consider as VA exercises its responsibilities to Vietnam veterans. This VAO update and all previous VAO reports are freely accessible online at the National Academies Press's website (http://www.nap.edu).

CHARGE TO THE COMMITTEE

In accordance with PL 102-4, the committee was asked to "determine (to the extent that available scientific data permit meaningful determinations)" the following regarding associations between specific health outcomes and exposure to TCDD and other chemicals in the herbicides used by the military in Vietnam:

A) whether a statistical association with herbicide exposure exists, taking into account the strength of the scientific evidence and the appropriateness of the statistical and epidemiological methods used to detect the association;

B) the increased risk of the disease among those exposed to herbicides during service in the Republic of Vietnam during the Vietnam era; and
C) whether there exists a plausible biological mechanism or other evidence of a causal relationship between herbicide exposure and the disease. [PL 102-4, Section 3 (d)]

The committee notes that as a consequence of congressional and judicial history, both its congressional mandate and the statement of task are phrased with the target of evaluation being "association" between exposure and health outcomes, although biologic mechanism and causal relationship are also mentioned as part of the evaluation in Article C. As used technically and as thoroughly addressed in a report on decision making (IOM, 2008) and in the section "Evaluation of the Evidence" in Chapter 2 of *Update 2010* (IOM, 2011), the criteria for causation do not themselves constitute a set checklist, but they are somewhat more stringent than those for association. The unique mandate of VAO committees to evaluate association rather than causation means that the approach delineated in the IOM report on decision making (IOM, 2008) is not entirely applicable here. The rigor of the evidentiary database needed to support a finding of statistical association is weaker than that to support causality; however, positive findings on any of the indicators for causality would strengthen a conviction that an observed statistical association was reliable. In accord with its charge, the committee examined a variety of indicators appropriate for the task, including factors commonly used to evaluate statistical associations—such as the adequacy of control for bias and confounding and the likelihood that an observed association could be explained by chance—and it assessed evidence concerning biologic plausibility derived from laboratory findings in cell culture or animal models. The full array of indicators examined was used to categorize the strength of the evidence. In particular, associations that manifested multiple indicators were interpreted as having stronger scientific support. Table 1-1 presents the starting point for this committee's deliberations, namely, the cumulative findings of VAO committees through *Update 2010* derived using this approach. (The current committee has not modified the criteria used by previous VAO committees to assign categories of association to particular health outcomes but will henceforth state the object of its evaluation to be "scientifically relevant association" in order to clarify that the strength of evidence evaluated, based on the quality of the scientific studies reviewed, was a fundamental component of the committee's deliberations to address the imprecisely defined legislative target of "statistical association.")

Following delivery of the committee's charge by a VA representative at the first meeting, the open session continued with brief presentations by other members of the public. It has been the practice of VAO committees to conduct open sessions, not only to gather additional information from people who have particular expertise on points that arise during deliberations but also especially to hear from individual Vietnam veterans and others concerned about aspects of

TABLE 1-1 Summary from *Update 2010* (*Eighth Biennial Update*) of Findings of Veterans, Occupational, and Environmental Studies Regarding Associations[a] Between Exposure to Herbicides and Specific Health Outcomes[b]

Sufficient Evidence of an Association

Epidemiologic evidence is sufficient to conclude that there is a positive association. That is, a positive association has been observed between exposure to herbicides and the outcome in studies in which chance, bias, and confounding could be ruled out with reasonable confidence.[c] For example, if several small studies that are free of bias and confounding show an association that is consistent in magnitude and direction, there could be sufficient evidence of an association. There is sufficient evidence of an association between exposure to the chemicals of interest and the following health outcomes:

Soft-tissue sarcoma (including heart)
* Non-Hodgkin lymphoma
* Chronic lymphocytic leukemia (including hairy cell leukemia and other chronic B-cell leukemias)
* Hodgkin lymphoma
Chloracne

Limited or Suggestive Evidence of an Association

Epidemiologic evidence suggests an association between exposure to herbicides and the outcome, but a firm conclusion is limited because chance, bias, and confounding could not be ruled out with confidence.[b] For example, a well-conducted study with strong findings in accord with less compelling results from studies of populations with similar exposures could constitute such evidence. There is limited or suggestive evidence of an association between exposure to the chemicals of interest and the following health outcomes:

Laryngeal cancer
Cancer of the lung, bronchus, or trachea
Prostate cancer
* Multiple myeloma
* AL amyloidosis
Early-onset peripheral neuropathy (category clarification from *Update 2008*)
Parkinson disease
Porphyria cutanea tarda
Hypertension
Ischemic heart disease
Type 2 diabetes (mellitus)
Spina bifida in offspring of exposed people

Inadequate or Insufficient Evidence to Determine an Association

The available epidemiologic studies are of insufficient quality, consistency, or statistical power to permit a conclusion regarding the presence or absence of an association. For example, studies fail to control for confounding, have inadequate exposure assessment, or fail to address latency. There is inadequate or insufficient evidence to determine association between exposure to the chemicals of interest and the following health outcomes that were explicitly reviewed:

Cancers of the oral cavity (including lips and tongue), pharynx (including tonsils), or nasal cavity (including ears and sinuses)
Cancers of the pleura, mediastinum, and other unspecified sites in the respiratory system and intrathoracic organs

continued

TABLE 1-1 Continued

Esophageal cancer
Stomach cancer
Colorectal cancer (including small intestine and anus)
Hepatobiliary cancers (liver, gallbladder, and bile ducts)
Pancreatic cancer
Bone and joint cancer
Melanoma
Nonmelanoma skin cancer (basal cell and squamous cell)
Breast cancer
Cancers of reproductive organs (cervix, uterus, ovary, testes, and penis; excluding prostate)
Urinary bladder cancer
Renal cancer (kidney and renal pelvis)
Cancers of brain and nervous system (including eye)
Endocrine cancers (thyroid, thymus, and other endocrine organs)
Leukemia (other than all chronic B-cell leukemias, including chronic lymphocytic leukemia and hairy cell leukemia)
Cancers at other and unspecified sites
Infertility
Spontaneous abortion (other than after paternal exposure to TCDD, which appears *not* to be associated)
Neonatal or infant death and stillbirth in offspring of exposed people
Low birth weight in offspring of exposed people
Birth defects (other than spina bifida) in offspring of exposed people
Childhood cancer (including acute myeloid leukemia) in offspring of exposed people
Neurobehavioral disorders (cognitive and neuropsychiatric)
Neurodegenerative diseases, excluding Parkinson disease
Chronic peripheral nervous system disorders
Hearing loss (newly addressed health outcome)
Respiratory disorders (wheeze or asthma, chronic obstructive pulmonary disease, and farmer's lung)
Gastrointestinal, metabolic, and digestive disorders (changes in hepatic enzymes, lipid abnormalities, and ulcers)
Immune system disorders (immune suppression, allergy, and autoimmunity)
Circulatory disorders (other than hypertension and ischemic heart disease)
Endometriosis
Effects on thyroid homeostasis
Eye problems (newly addressed health outcome)
Bone conditions (newly addressed health outcome)

This committee used a classification that spans the full array of cancers. However, reviews for nonmalignant conditions were conducted only if they were found to have been the subjects of epidemiologic investigation or at the request of the Department of Veterans Affairs. *By default, any health outcome on which no epidemiologic information has been found falls into this category.*

Limited or Suggestive Evidence of *No* Association

Several adequate studies, which cover the full range of human exposure, are consistent in not showing a positive association between any magnitude of exposure to a component of the herbicides of interest and the outcome. A conclusion of "no association" is inevitably limited to the conditions, exposures, and length of observation covered by the available studies. *In addition, the*

TABLE 1-1 Continued

possibility of a very small increase in risk at the exposure studied can never be excluded. There is limited or suggestive evidence of *no* association between exposure to the herbicide component of interest and the following health outcomes:

Spontaneous abortion after paternal exposure to TCDD

[a]This table is the product of the committee for *Update 2010*; the current committee has decided to add "scientifically relevant" before "association" in its own work product to emphasize the scientific nature of the VAO task and procedures without implying any change in the present committee's criteria from those used in previous updates.

[b]*Herbicides* indicates the following chemicals of interest: 2,4-dichlorophenoxyacetic acid (2,4-D), 2,4,5-trichlorophenoxyacetic acid (2,4,5-T) and its contaminant 2,3,7,8-tetrachlorodibenzo-*p*-dioxin (TCDD or dioxin), cacodylic acid, and picloram. The evidence regarding association was drawn from occupational, environmental, and veteran studies in which people were exposed to the herbicides used in Vietnam, to their components, or to their contaminants.

[c]Evidence for an association is strengthened by experimental data supporting biologic plausibility, but its absence would not detract from the epidemiologic evidence.

*The committee notes the consistency of these findings with the biologic understanding of the clonal derivation of lymphohematopoietic cancers that is the basis of the World Health Organization classification system.

their health experience that may be service-related. Open sessions were held during the first four of the committee's five meetings, and the agendas and the issues raised are presented in Appendix A. The comments and information provided by the public were used to identify information gaps in the literature regarding specific health outcomes of concern to Vietnam veterans.

Chapter 2 provides details of the committee's approach to its charge and the methods that it used in reaching conclusions.

CONCLUSIONS OF PREVIOUS VETERANS AND AGENT ORANGE REPORTS

Health Outcomes

VAO, *Update 1996*, *Update 1998*, *Update 2000*, *Update 2002*, *Update 2004*, *Type 2 Diabetes*, *Acute Myelogenous Leukemia*, *Respiratory Cancer*, *Update 2006*, *Update 2008*, and *Update 2010* contain detailed reviews of the scientific studies evaluated by the committees and their implications for cancer, reproductive and developmental effects, neurologic disorders, and other health effects.

The original VAO committee addressed the statutory mandate to evaluate the association between herbicide exposure and individual health conditions by assigning each of the health outcomes under study to one of four categories on the basis of the epidemiologic evidence reviewed. The categories were adapted from the ones used by the International Agency for Research on Cancer in evaluating evidence of the carcinogenicity of various substances (IARC, 1977). Successor VAO committees adopted the same categories.

The question of whether the committee should be considering statistical association rather than causality has been controversial. In legal proceedings that predated passage of the legislation that mandated the VAO series of reviews, *Nehmer v United States Veterans Administration* (712 F. Supp. 1404, 1989) found that:

> the legislative history, and prior VA and congressional practice, support our finding that Congress intended that the Administrator predicate service connection upon a finding of a significant statistical association between dioxin exposure and various diseases. We hold that the VA erred by requiring proof of a causal relationship.

The committee believes that the categorization of strength of evidence as shown in Table 1-1 is consistent with that court ruling. In particular, the ruling does not preclude the consideration of the factors usually assessed in determining a causal relationship (Hill, 1965; IOM, 2008) as indicators of the strength of scientific evidence of an association. In accord with the court ruling, the committee was not seeking proof of a causal relationship, but any information that supports a causal relationship, such as a plausible biologic mechanism as specified in Article C of the charge to the committee, would also lend credence to the reliability of an observed association. Understanding of causal relationships is the ultimate objective of science, whereas the committee's goal of assessing statistical association is an intermediate (less well-defined) point along a continuum between no association and causality.

The categories, the criteria for assigning a particular health outcome to a category, and the health outcomes that have been assigned to the categories in past updates are discussed below. Table 1-1 summarizes the conclusions of *Update 2010* regarding associations between health outcomes and exposure to the herbicides used in Vietnam or to any of their components or contaminants. That integration of the literature through September 2010 served as the starting point for the current committee's deliberations. It should be noted that the categories of association concern the occurrence of health outcomes in human *populations* in relation to chemical exposure; they do not address the likelihood that any *individual's* health problem is associated with or caused by the chemicals in question.

Health Outcomes with Sufficient Evidence of an Association

In this category, a positive association between herbicides and the outcome must be observed in epidemiologic studies in which chance, bias, and confounding can be ruled out with reasonable confidence. The committee regarded evidence from several studies that satisfactorily addressed bias and confounding and that show an association that is consistent in magnitude and direction as sufficient evidence of an association. Experimental data supporting biologic plausibility strengthen evidence of an association but are not a prerequisite.

The original VAO committee found sufficient evidence of an association between exposure to herbicides and three cancers—soft-tissue sarcoma, non-Hodgkin lymphoma, and Hodgkin lymphoma—and two other health outcomes, chloracne and porphyria cutanea tarda (PCT). After reviewing all the literature available in 1995, the committee responsible for *Update 1996* concluded that the statistical evidence still supported that classification for the three cancers and chloracne but that the evidence of an association with PCT warranted its being placed in the category of limited or suggestive evidence of an association with exposure. No changes were made in this category in *Update 1998* or *Update 2000*.

As the committee responsible for *Update 2002* began its work, VA requested that it evaluate whether chronic lymphocytic leukemia (CLL) should be considered separately from other leukemias. That committee concluded that CLL could be considered separately and, on the basis of the epidemiologic literature and the etiology of the disease, placed CLL in the "sufficient" category. In response to a request from VA, the committee for *Update 2008* affirmed that hairy-cell leukemia belonged in the category of sufficient evidence of an association with the related conditions CLL and chronic B-cell lymphomas.

Health Outcomes with Limited or Suggestive Evidence of an Association

In this category, the evidence must suggest an association between exposure to herbicides and the outcome considered, but the evidence can be limited by the inability to rule out chance, bias, or confounding confidently. The coherence of the full body of epidemiologic information, in light of biologic plausibility, is considered when the committee reaches a judgment about association for a given outcome. Because the VAO series has four herbicides and TCDD as agents of concern whose profiles of toxicity are not expected to be uniform, apparent inconsistencies can be expected among study populations that have experienced different exposures. Even for a single exposure, a spectrum of results would be expected, depending on the power of the studies and other design factors.

The committee responsible for *VAO* found limited or suggestive evidence of an association between exposure to herbicides and three categories of cancer: respiratory cancer (after individual evaluations of laryngeal cancer and of cancers of the trachea, lung, or bronchus), prostate cancer, and multiple myeloma (MM). The *Update 1996* committee added three health outcomes to the list: PCT, acute and subacute peripheral neuropathy (indicated as early-onset transient peripheral neuropathy after *Update 2004* and then respecified as simply early-onset peripheral neuropathy after *Update 2010*), and spina bifida in children of veterans. Transient peripheral neuropathies had not been addressed in *VAO*, because they are not amenable to epidemiologic study. In response to a VA request, however, the

Update 1996 committee reviewed those neuropathies and based its determination on case histories. A combination of a 1995 analysis of birth defects among the offspring of veterans who served in Operation Ranch Hand and results of earlier studies of neural-tube defects in the children of Vietnam veterans (published by the Centers for Disease Control and Prevention) led the *Update 1996* committee to distinguish spina bifida from other reproductive outcomes and to place it in the "limited or suggestive evidence" category. No changes were made in this category in *Update 1998*.

After the publication of *Update 1998*, the committee responsible for *Type 2 Diabetes*, on the basis of its evaluation of newly available scientific evidence and the cumulative findings of research reviewed in previous VAO reports, concluded that there was limited or suggestive evidence of an association between exposure to the herbicides used in Vietnam or the contaminant TCDD and type 2 diabetes (mellitus). The evidence reviewed in *Update 2000* supported that finding.

The committee responsible for *Update 2000* reviewed the material in earlier reports and the newly published literature and determined that there was limited or suggestive evidence of an association between exposure to herbicides used in Vietnam or the contaminant TCDD and AML in the children of Vietnam veterans. After release of *Update 2000*, researchers in one of the studies that it reviewed discovered an error in the published data. The committee for *Update 2000* was reconvened to re-evaluate the previously reviewed and new literature regarding AML, and it produced *Acute Myelogenous Leukemia*, which reclassified AML in children from "limited or suggestive evidence of an association" to "inadequate or insufficient evidence to determine an association."

After reviewing the data reviewed in previous VAO reports and recently published scientific literature, the committee responsible for *Update 2006* determined that there was limited or suggestive evidence of an association between exposure to the herbicides used in Vietnam or the contaminant TCDD and hypertension. AL amyloidosis was also moved to the category of "limited or suggestive evidence of an association" primarily on the basis of its close biologic relationship with MM.

With a bit more consistent epidemiologic data augmented by increased understanding of mechanisms arising from new toxicologic research, the committee for *Update 2008* was able to resolve the *Update 2006* committee's lack of consensus and moved ischemic heart disease into this category, joining hypertension, another cardiovascular condition. New studies of Parkinson disease that yielded findings of an association with the specific herbicides of interest were deemed to move the evidence to the category of limited or suggestive.

Health Outcomes with Inadequate or Insufficient Evidence to Determine an Association

By default, any health outcome is in this category before enough reliable scientific data accumulate to promote it to the category of sufficient evidence or limited or suggestive evidence of an association or to move it to the category of limited or suggestive evidence of *no* association. In this category, available studies may have inconsistent findings or be of insufficient quality or statistical power to support a conclusion regarding the presence of an association. Such studies might have failed to control for confounding or might have had inadequate assessment of exposure.

The cancers and other health effects so categorized in *Update 2010* are listed in Table 1-1, but several health effects have been moved into or out of this category since the original *VAO* committee reviewed the evidence then available. Skin cancer was moved into this category in *Update 1996* when inclusion of new evidence no longer supported its classification as a condition with limited or suggestive evidence of *no* association. Similarly, the *Update 1998* committee moved urinary bladder cancer from the category of limited or suggestive evidence of *no* association to this category; although there was no evidence that exposure to herbicides or TCDD is related to urinary bladder cancer, newly available evidence weakened the evidence of *no* association. The committee for *Update 2000* had partitioned AML in the offspring of Vietnam veterans from other childhood cancers and put it into the category of suggestive evidence; but a separate review, as reported in *Acute Myelogenous Leukemia*, found errors in the published information and returned it to this category with other childhood cancers. In *Update 2002*, CLL was moved from this category to join Hodgkin and non-Hodgkin lymphomas in the category of sufficient evidence of an association.

The committee responsible for *Update 2006* removed several cancers (of the brain, stomach, colon, rectum, and pancreas) from the category of limited or suggestive evidence of *no* association into this category partly because of some changes in evidence since they were originally placed in the "*no* association" category but primarily because that committee had concerns about the lack of information on all five COIs and each of these cancers.

Health Outcomes with Limited or Suggestive Evidence of *No* Association

The original *VAO* committee defined this category for health outcomes for which several adequate studies covering the "full range of human exposure" were consistent in showing *no* association with exposure to herbicides at any concentration and had relatively narrow confidence intervals. A conclusion of "*no* association" is inevitably limited to the conditions, exposures, and observation periods covered by the available studies, and the possibility of a small increase in risk related to the magnitude of exposure studied can never be excluded. However, a change in classification from inadequate or insufficient evidence of an association to limited or suggestive evidence of *no* association would require new studies that correct for the methodologic problems of previous studies and that have samples large enough to limit the possible study results attributable to chance.

The original *VAO* committee found a sufficient number and variety of well-designed studies to conclude that there was limited or suggestive evidence of *no* association between the exposures of interest and a small group of cancers: gastrointestinal tumors (colon, rectum, stomach, and pancreas), skin cancers, brain tumors, and urinary bladder cancer. The *Update 1996* committee removed skin cancers and the *Update 1998* committee removed urinary bladder cancer from this category because the evidence no longer supported a conclusion of *no* association. The *Update 2002* committee concluded that there was adequate evidence to determine that spontaneous abortion is *not* associated with paternal exposure specifically to TCDD; the evidence on this outcome was deemed inadequate for drawing a conclusion about an association with maternal exposure to any of the COIs or with paternal exposure to any of the COIs other than TCDD. No changes in this category were made in *Update 2000* or *Update 2004*. The *Update 2006* committee removed brain cancer and several digestive cancers from this category because of concern that the overall paucity of information on picloram and cacodylic acid made it inappropriate for those outcomes to remain in this category. This left the finding of evidence of *no* association between paternal exposure to TCDD and spontaneous abortion as the sole entry in this category.

Determining Increased Risk in Vietnam Veterans

The second part of the committee's charge is to determine, to the extent permitted by available scientific data, the increased risk of disease among people exposed to herbicides or the contaminant TCDD during service in Vietnam. Previous reports pointed out that most of the many health studies of Vietnam veterans were hampered by relatively poor measures of exposure to herbicides or TCDD and by other methodologic problems. Most of the evidence on which the findings regarding associations are based, therefore, comes from studies of people exposed to TCDD or herbicides in occupational and environmental settings rather than from studies of Vietnam veterans. The committees that produced *VAO* and the updates found that the body of evidence was sufficient for reaching conclusions about statistical associations between herbicide exposures and health outcomes but that the lack of adequate data on Vietnam veterans themselves complicated consideration of the second part of the charge.

The evidence of herbicide exposure among various groups studied suggests that although some had documented high exposures (such as participants in Operation Ranch Hand and Army Chemical Corps personnel), most Vietnam veterans had lower exposures to herbicides and TCDD than did the subjects of many occupational and environmental studies (see Figure 1-1 from Pirkle et al., 1995). Individual veterans who had very high exposures to herbicides, however, could have risks approaching those described in the occupational and environmental studies.

Estimating the magnitude of risk of each particular health outcome among herbicide-exposed Vietnam veterans requires quantitative information about the

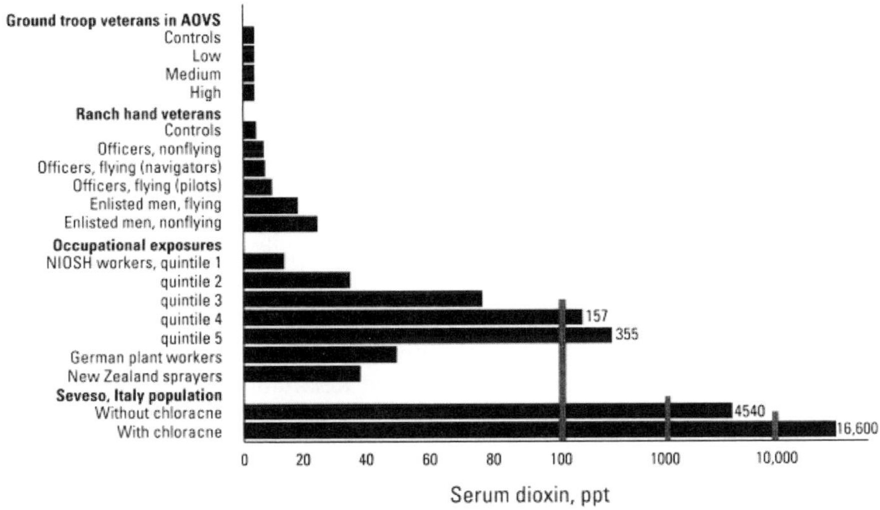

FIGURE 1-1 Comparison of TCDD exposures in various populations.
SOURCE: Pirkle et al., 2005.

dose–time–response relationship for the health outcome in humans, information on the extent of herbicide exposure among Vietnam veterans, and estimates of individual exposure. Committees responsible for *VAO* and the updates have concluded that in general it is impossible to quantify the risk to veterans posed by their exposure to herbicides in Vietnam. Statements to that effect were made for each health outcome in *VAO* (IOM, 1994) and in every update through *Update 2004*. The committee responsible for *Update 2006* chose to eliminate the repetitive restatements in favor of the following general conclusion: "At least for the present, it is not possible to derive quantitative estimates of the increase in risk of various adverse health effects that Vietnam veterans may have experienced in association with exposure to the herbicides sprayed in Vietnam." The committee responsible for later updates and the current committee have opted to retain the modification in the formatting of the health outcomes sections.

After decades of research, the challenge of estimating the magnitude of potential risk posed by exposure to the COIs remains intractable. The requisite information is still absent despite concerted efforts to reconstruct likely exposure by modeling on the basis of records of troop movements and spraying missions (Stellman and Stellman, 2003, 2004; Stellman et al., 2003a,b), to extrapolate from agricultural models of drift associated with spraying (Ginevan et al., 2009a; Teske et al., 2002), to measure serum TCDD in individual veterans (Kang et al., 2006; Michalek et al., 1995), and to model the pharmacokinetics of TCDD clearance (Aylward et al., 2005a,b; Cheng et al., 2006b; Emond et al., 2004, 2005, 2006). There is still uncertainty about the specific agents that may be responsible for a particular health effect. Even if one accepts an individual veteran's serum TCDD concentration as the optimal surrogate for overall exposure to Agent Orange and the other herbicide mixtures sprayed in Vietnam, not only is the measurement nontrivial but the hurdle of accounting for biologic clearance and extrapolating to the proper time frame remains. The committee therefore believes that it is very unlikely that additional information or more sophisticated methods are going to become available that would permit any sort of quantitative assessment of Vietnam veterans' increased risks of particular adverse health outcomes attributable to exposure to the chemicals associated with herbicide spraying in Vietnam.

Existence of a Plausible Biologic Mechanism or Other Evidence of a Causal Relationship

Toxicologic data form the basis of the committee's response to the third part of its charge—to determine whether there is a plausible biologic mechanism or other evidence of a causal relationship between herbicide exposure and a health effect. A separate chapter summarizes toxicologic findings on the chemicals of concern. In *VAO* and updates before *Update 2008*, a considerable amount of detail had been provided about individual newly published toxicology studies; the current committee concurs with the decision made by the previous two committees that it is more informative for the general reader to provide integrated toxicologic profiles for the COIs by interpreting the underlying experimental findings. When there are specific toxicologic findings pertinent to a particular health outcome, they are discussed in the chapter reviewing the epidemiologic literature on that condition. The current committee has continued the endeavor to refine this approach to make the chapter on toxicologic information more accessible to lay readers and more illuminating about its relevance to epidemiologic findings.

In *VAO* and updates before *Update 2006*, this topic has been discussed in the conclusions section for each health outcome after a statement of the committee's judgment about the adequacy of the epidemiologic evidence of an association of that outcome with exposure to the COIs. As *Update 2006* noted, the degree of biologic plausibility itself influences whether the committee perceives positive findings to be indicative of a pattern or the product of statistical fluctuations. To provide the reader with a more logical sequence, the committee responsible for *Update 2006* placed the biologic-plausibility sections between the presentation of new epidemiologic evidence and the synthesis of all the evidence; this in turn led to the ultimate statement of the committee's conclusion. The later committees have supported that change and have continued to arrange the sections in that fashion.

ORGANIZATION OF THIS REPORT

The remainder of this report is organized in 13 chapters. Chapter 2 briefly describes the considerations that guided the committee's review and evaluation of the scientific evidence. Chapter 3 addresses exposure-assessment issues. Chapter 4 summarizes the toxicology data on the effects of 2,4-D, 2,4,5-T and its contaminant TCDD, cacodylic acid, and picloram; the data contribute to the consideration of the biologic plausibility of health effects in human populations. Chapter 5 of *Update 2010*, which had two roles with respect to the epidemiologic information that constitutes the core of the committee's deliberations has been separated into two chapters corresponding to those roles. First, the new Chapter 5 characterizes the relevant new epidemiologic literature published in this update period, indicating the study design, exposure measures, health outcomes reported on, and population studied. A new feature in this update is the placement of a summary of the finding of each health outcome chapter at its beginning. The second role is now addressed in Chapter 6, which provides a cumulative overview of the study populations that have generated findings (in some instances, in the form of dozens of separate publications) reviewed in the VAO report series. In addition to showing where the new literature fits into this compendium of publications on Vietnam veterans, occupational cohorts, environmentally exposed groups, and case-control study populations, it includes description and critical appraisal of the design, exposure assessment, and analysis approaches used.

The committee's evaluation of the epidemiologic literature and its conclusions regarding associations between particular health outcomes that might be manifested long after exposure to the COIs are presented in the several chapters that follow. In *Update 2010*, three short-term responses presumptively associated with herbicide exposure (early-onset peripheral neuropathy, chloracne, and PCT) were moved from the body of the report to Appendix B because they develop shortly after exposure but are unlikely to arise for the first time decades after exposed people left Vietnam.

Chapter 7 addresses immunologic effects and discusses the reasons for what might be perceived as a discrepancy between a clear demonstration of immunotoxicity in animal studies and a paucity of epidemiologic studies that had such findings. Its placement reflects the committee's belief that immunologic changes may constitute an intermediary mechanism in the generation of more distinct clinical conditions discussed in the following chapters. Chapter 8 discusses issues related to the possible overall carcinogenic potential of the COIs, particularly TCDD, and then assesses the available epidemiologic evidence on specific types of cancer, which are regarded as individual disease states that might be found to be service-related.

In this update, what had been one chapter on reproductive and developmental effects has been partitioned into two chapters. The first, Chapter 9, addresses reproductive problems that may have been manifested in the veterans themselves: reduced fertility, pregnancy loss, or gestational issues (low birth weight or preterm delivery). The second, Chapter 10, focuses on problems that might be manifested later in the lives of veterans' children or even in later generations.

Chapter 11 addresses neurologic disorders. Chapter 12 deals with a set of conditions related to cardiovascular and metabolic effects. Chapter 13 now contains the residual "other health outcomes": respiratory disorders, gastrointestinal problems, thyroid homeostasis and other endocrine disorders, eye problems, and bone conditions.

A summary of the committee's findings and its research recommendations are presented in Chapter 14.

REFERENCES[1]

Aylward LL, Brunet RC, Carrier G, Hays SM, Cushing CA, Needham LL, Patterson DG Jr, Gerthoux PM, Brambilla P, Mocarelli P. 2005a. Concentration-dependent TCDD elimination kinetics in humans: Toxicokinetic modeling for moderately to highly exposed adults from Seveso, Italy, and Vienna, Austria, and impact on dose estimates for the NIOSH cohort. *Journal of Exposure Analysis and Environmental Epidemiology* 15(1):51–65.

Aylward LL, Brunet RC, Starr TB, Carrier G, Delzell E, Cheng H, Beall C. 2005b. Exposure reconstruction for the TCDD-exposed NIOSH cohort using a concentration- and age-dependent model of elimination. *Risk Analysis* 25(4):945–956.

Cheng H, Aylward L, Beall C, Starr TB, Brunet RC, Carrier G, Delzell E. 2006b. TCDD exposure-response analysis and risk assessment. *Risk Analysis* 26(4):1059–1071.

Emond C, Birnbaum LS, DeVito MJ. 2004. Physiologically based pharmacokinetic model for developmental exposures to TCDD in the rat. *Toxicological Sciences* 80(1):115–133.

Emond C, Michalek JE, Birnbaum LS, DeVito MJ. 2005. Comparison of the use of physiologically based pharmacokinetic model and a classical pharmacokinetic model for dioxin exposure assessments. *Environmental Health Perspectives* 113(12):1666–1668.

Emond C, Birnbaum LS, DeVito MJ. 2006. Use of a physiologically based pharmacokinetic model for rats to study the influence of body fat mass and induction of CYP1A2 on the pharmacokinetics of TCDD. *Environmental Health Perspectives* 114(9):1394–1400.

Ginevan ME, Ross JH, Watkins DK. 2009a. Assessing exposure to allied ground troops in the Vietnam War: A comparison of AgDRIFT and Exposure Opportunity Index models. *Journal of Exposure Science and Environmental Epidemiology* 19:187–200.

Hill AB. 1965. The environment and disease: Association or causation? *Proceedings of the Royal Society of Medicine* 58:295–300.

IARC (International Agency for Research on Cancer). 1977. *Some Fumigants, the Herbicides 2,4-D and 2,4,5-T, Chlorinated Dibenzodioxins and Miscellaneous Industrial Chemicals.* IARC Monographs on the Evaluation of the Carcinogenic Risk of Chemicals to Man, Vol. 15. Lyon, France: World Health Organization, IARC.

IOM (Institute of Medicine). 1994. *Veterans and Agent Orange: Health Effects of Herbicides Used in Vietnam.* Washington, DC: National Academy Press.

IOM. 1996. *Veterans and Agent Orange: Update 1996.* Washington, DC: National Academy Press.

IOM. 1999. *Veterans and Agent Orange: Update 1998.* Washington, DC: National Academy Press.

IOM. 2000. *Veterans and Agent Orange: Herbicide/Dioxin Exposure and Type 2 Diabetes.* Washington, DC: National Academy Press.

IOM. 2001. *Veterans and Agent Orange: Update 2000.* Washington, DC: National Academy Press.

IOM. 2002. *Veterans and Agent Orange: Herbicide/Dioxin Exposure and Acute Myelogenous Leukemia in the Children of Vietnam Veterans.* Washington, DC: The National Academies Press.

[1]Throughout this report, the same alphabetic indicator after year of publication is used consistently for a given reference when there are multiple citations by the same first author in a given year. The convention of assigning the alphabetic indicators in order of citation in a given chapter is not followed.

IOM. 2003. *Veterans and Agent Orange: Update 2002.* Washington, DC: The National Academies Press.

IOM. 2004. *Veterans and Agent Orange: Length of Presumptive Period for Association Between Exposure and Respiratory Cancer.* Washington, DC: The National Academies Press.

IOM. 2005a. *Veterans and Agent Orange: Update 2004.* Washington, DC: The National Academies Press.

IOM. 2005b. *Gulf War and Health: Volume 3—Fuel, Combustion Products, and Propellants.* Washington, DC: The National Academies Press.

IOM. 2007. *Veterans and Agent Orange: Update 2006.* Washington, DC: The National Academies Press.

IOM. 2008. *Improving the Presumptive Disability Decision-making Process for Veterans.* Washington, DC: The National Academies Press.

IOM. 2009. *Veterans and Agent Orange: Update 2008.* Washington, DC: The National Academies Press.

IOM. 2011. *Veterans and Agent Orange: Update 2010.* Washington, DC: The National Academies Press.

Kang HK, Dalager NA, Needham LL, Patterson DG, Lees PSJ, Yates K, Matanoski GM. 2006. Health status of Army Chemical Corps Vietnam veterans who sprayed defoliant in Vietnam. *American Journal of Industrial Medicine* 49(11):875–884.

Michalek J, Wolfe W, Miner J, Papa T, Pirkle J. 1995. Indices of TCDD exposure and TCDD body burden in veterans of Operation Ranch Hand. *Journal of Exposure Analysis and Environmental Epidemiology* 5(2):209–223.

Pirkle JL, Sampson EJ, Needham LL, Pattterson DG, Ashley DL. 1995. Using biological monitoring to assess human exposure to priority toxicants. *Environmental Health Perspectives* 103(Suppl 3):45–48.

Stellman JM, Stellman SD. 2003. *Contractor's Final Report: Characterizing Exposure of Veterans to Agent Orange and Other Herbicides in Vietnam.* Submitted to the National Academy of Sciences, Institute of Medicine in fulfillment of Subcontract VA-5124-98-0019, June 30, 2003.

Stellman SD, Stellman JM. 2004. Exposure opportunity models for Agent Orange, dioxin, and other military herbicides used in Vietnam, 1961–1971. *Journal of Exposure Analysis and Environmental Epidemiology* 14(4):354–362.

Stellman J, Stellman S, Christians R, Weber T, Tomasallo C. 2003a. The extent and patterns of usage of Agent Orange and other herbicides in Vietnam. *Nature* 422:681–687.

Stellman J, Stellman S, Weber T, Tomasallo C, Stellman A, Christian R Jr. 2003b. A geographic information system for characterizing exposure to Agent Orange and other herbicides in Vietnam. *Environmental Health Perspectives* 111(3):321–328.

Teske ME, Bird SL, Esterly DM, Curbishley TB, Ray ST, Perry SG. 2002. AgDRIFT®: A model for estimating near-field spray drift from aerial applications. *Environmental Toxicology and Chemistry* 21(3):659–671.

2

Evaluating the Evidence

This chapter outlines the approach used by the Committee to Review the Health Effects in Vietnam Veterans of Exposure to Herbicides (Ninth Biennial Update) and its predecessors to evaluate the available scientific evidence. A more complete description is found in Chapter 5 of *Veterans and Agent Orange: Health Effects of Herbicides Used in Vietnam*, hereafter referred to as *VAO* (IOM, 1994).

CHOICE OF HEALTH OUTCOMES

As discussed in Chapter 1, the committee was charged with summarizing the strength of the scientific evidence of associations between exposure to various herbicides and contaminants during service in the Vietnam War and individual diseases or other health outcomes. Public Law 102-4, which mandated the committee's work, however, did not specify particular health outcomes suspected of being associated with herbicide exposure. Such a list of outcomes was developed on the basis of diseases and conditions addressed in the scientific literature identified through the original *VAO* committee's extensive literature searches. The list has been amended in the VAO updates in response to new publications, to requests from the Department of Veterans Affairs (VA) and various veterans' service organizations, and to concerns of Vietnam veterans and their families. Comments received at public hearings and in written submissions from veterans and other interested persons have been valuable in identifying issues to be pursued in greater depth in the scientific literature.

The VAO committees began their evaluation by presuming neither the presence nor the absence of an association between exposure and any particular health outcome. Over the series of reviews, evidence of various degrees of association, lack of association, or persistent indeterminacy with respect to a wide array of disease states has accrued. For many conditions, however, particularly uncommon ones, associations with the chemicals of interest (COIs) have remained unaddressed in the medical research literature; for these, the committee remains neutral on the basis of the understanding that "absence of evidence is not evidence of absence."

IDENTIFICATION OF RELEVANT LITERATURE

Study Populations Considered

Mixtures of 2,4-dichlorophenoxyacetic acid (2,4-D), 2,4,5-trichlorophenoxyacetic acid (2,4,5-T), picloram, and cacodylic acid made up the bulk of the herbicides sprayed in Vietnam. At the time of the spraying, 2,3,7,8-tetrachlorodibenzo-*p*-dioxin (TCDD, a form of dioxin) was an unintended contaminant in the production of 2,4,5-T and so was present in Agent Pink, Agent Green, Agent Purple, Agent Orange, and Agent Orange II, which all contained 2,4,5-T. It is important to note that TCDD and Agent Orange are not the same. Databases have been searched for the names of those compounds, their synonyms and abbreviations, and their Chemical Abstracts Service (CAS) numbers. The evidence indicates that a single protein, the aryl hydrocarbon receptor (AHR), mediates essentially all the toxicity of TCDD, so *aryl hydrocarbon receptor* also was used as a keyword.

One of the herbicides used in Vietnam was cacodylic acid, or dimethylarsinic acid of valence 5 (DMA^V), an organic form of arsenic. In addition to being synthesized as a herbicide, DMA^V is a metabolite of inorganic arsenic exposure in humans. DMA^V was long thought to be a biologically inactive metabolite, but evidence suggests that methylated forms, such as MMA^{III} (Aposhian et al., 2000) and perhaps DMA^{III} and DMA^V (Cohen et al., 2006), can be responsible for some of the adverse effects of inorganic arsenic. VAO committees have carefully reconsidered that evidence repeatedly but have continued to conclude that it does not support a conclusion that exposure to DMA^V would be expected to result in the same adverse health effects as would exposure to toxic concentrations of inorganic arsenic. Therefore, as in prior VAO reports, the literature on the health effects of inorganic arsenic was not considered here. Further details on the effects of inorganic arsenic can be found in *Arsenic in Drinking Water* (NRC, 1999) and *Arsenic in Drinking Water: 2001 Update* (NRC, 2001). For cacodylic acid and picloram, the search terms were the chemical names, synonyms, and CAS numbers of the herbicides.

This report concentrates on the evidence published after the completion of work on *Veterans and Agent Orange: Update 2010* (IOM, 2011). Relevant new contributions to the literature made during the period October 1, 2010–September 30, 2012, were sought. The information that the committee used was compiled through a comprehensive electronic search of public and commercial databases—biologic, medical, toxicologic, chemical, historical, and regulatory—that provide citations of the scientific literature. In addition, the reference lists of some review and research articles, books, and reports were examined for potentially relevant articles. As noted above, the terms used in the search strategy included the chemical names, synonyms, and CAS numbers of the specific COIs—2,4-D, 2,4,5-T, TCDD, cacocylic acid, and picloram (see Figure 2-1 for chemical structures and CAS numbers)—and the more generic terms involved with this project: *Vietnam veteran*, *Agent Orange*, *aryl hydrocarbon receptor*, *dioxin*, *herbicide*, and *phenoxy*. Results on other specific phenoxy herbicides are also of interest: 2-methyl-4-chlorophenoxyacetic acid (MCPA) and 2-(2-methyl-4-chlorophenoxy) propionic acid (MCPP or Mecoprop) are structurally similar to 2,4-D, while 2-(2,4,5-trichlorophenoxy) propionic acid (2,4,5-TP or Silvex) have structures analogous to 2,4,5-T (see Figure 2-1); although the benzoate herbicide dicamba (2-methoxy-3,6-dichlorobenzoic acid) is not always categorized with the phenoxy herbicides, it has structural similarities with this class, and measures of its association with various adverse health outcomes have been factored into the evidence. Because some polychlorinated biphenyls (PCBs) and polychlorodibenzofurans (PCDFs) have dioxin-like biologic activity, studies of populations exposed to PCBs or PCDFs were reviewed when results were presented in terms of toxic equivalents (TEQs). Findings related only to exposure to the diverse chemical families of pesticides were considered too nonspecific for inclusion in the evidence database that was used to draw conclusions about associations. (An ancillary analysis conducted during preparation of *Update 2008* determined that the term *pesticide* did not identify any relevant citations that were not picked up by more specific terms, so it was eliminated from the searches conducted since this reduced considerably the number of extraneous hits to be culled.)

(With the structural representation at hand in Figure 2-1, one can readily see the basis of an assertion heard repeatedly from individual Vietnam veterans that "benzene is contained in TCDD." Indeed, the two rings at the ends of the three-ring structure constituting the basic structure of dioxin compounds, to which chlorine molecules or other chemical radicals can be attached, do have the molecular structure of a single benzene molecule, and "dibenzo-dioxin" in TCDD's chemical name does mean the molecule is a benzene-substituted dioxane. The benzene ring structure is a basic building block of a vast number of organic compounds, both industrial [such as polyaromatic hydrocarbons, the phenoxy herbicides, picloram, and PCBs] and natural [such as estradiol, a hormone present in both men and women]. However, the biologically active compound benzene does not emerge from dioxin, whose three-ring structure is extremely stable and resistant to metabolism.)

Phenoxy Herbicides

2,4-D [94-75-7]

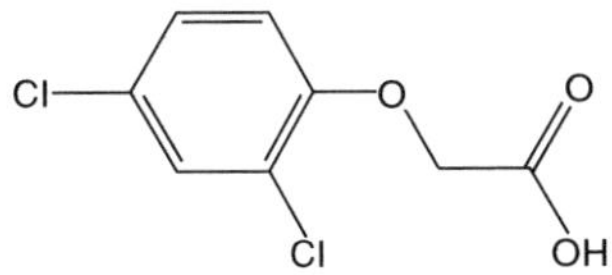

2,4,5-T [93-76-5]

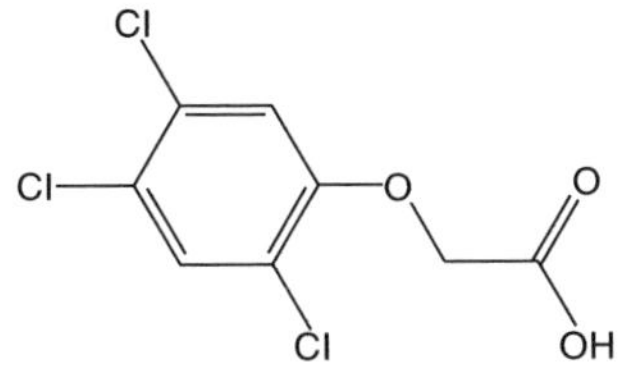

MCPA [94-74-6]

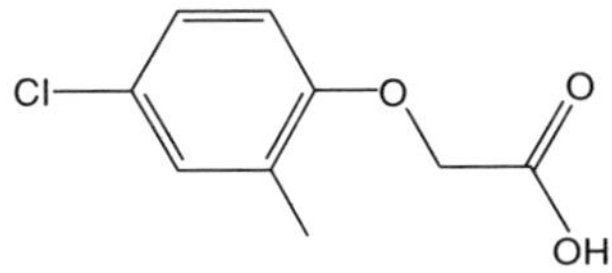

Silvex [93-72-1]

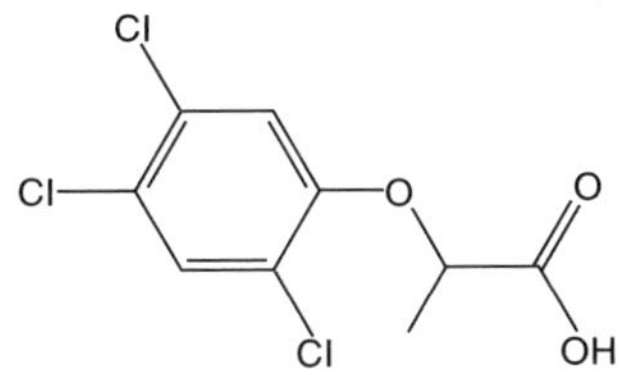

MCPP [93-65-2]

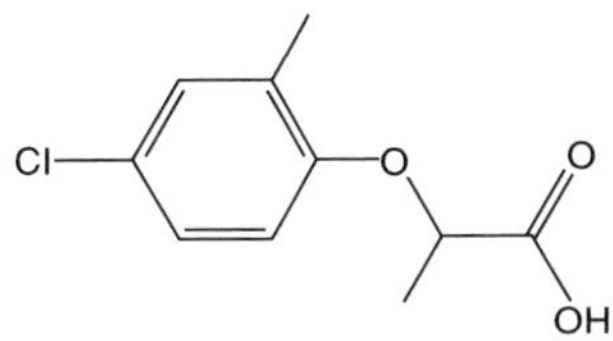

Dicamba [1918-00-9]

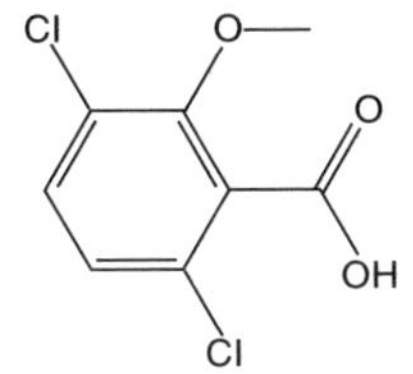

2,3,7,8-TCDD [1746-01-6]

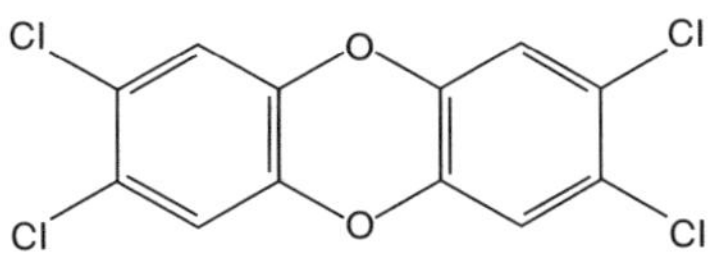

Picloram [1918-02-1]

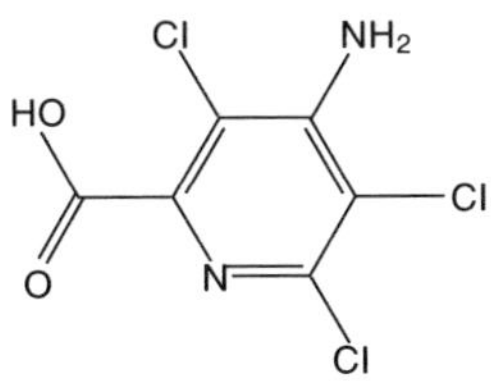

Cacodylic Acid [75-60-5]

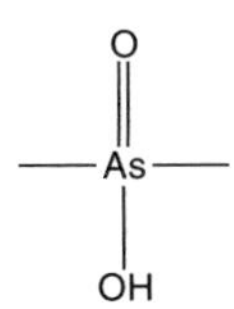

FIGURE 2-1 Chemical structures and CAS numbers for specific chemicals of interest.

Study Populations Considered

Because they are the target population of the charge to the VAO committees, studies of Vietnam veterans (serving in any of the armed forces, American or otherwise) have always been accorded considerable weight in the committees' deliberations, whether or not estimation of exposure to herbicide-related substances has been attempted. Characterization of exposure in studies of the veterans was extremely uncommon at the time of the original *VAO* report, and the Vietnam veterans' own ages were still below the ages at which many chronic illnesses are manifested. Consequently, the original committee made extensive efforts to consider several groups known or thought to have potentially higher and better-characterized exposure to TCDD or phenoxy herbicides than Vietnam veterans themselves—both occupational exposure (for example, chemical-production, paper and pulp, sawmill, tannery, waste-incinerator, railroad, agricultural, and forestry workers) and environmental exposure (for example, residents of Seveso, Times Beach, Quail Run, and Vietnam).

Successive committees have been able to concentrate more on studies that explicitly addressed the exposures specified by the charge. Some occupational and environmental cohorts that received exceptionally high exposures (such as the International Agency for Research on Cancer [IARC] and Seveso cohorts) are now well characterized and producing a stream of informative results. The Agricultural Health Study, a continuing prospective cohort study of agricultural populations with specific information on the COIs, is also now contributing a steady stream of information to the database. Most important, the Vietnam veterans themselves are advancing in age and when studied are capable of directly providing substantial information on chronic health conditions and, in some study populations, information related to serum TCDD concentrations. The committee for *Update 2006* decided that exhaustive searches on job titles, occupations, or industries to identify additional study populations that had possible, but not specifically characterized, exposure to the COIs were no longer an efficient means of augmenting the evidence database in that they are more likely to yield citations with information about a health outcome at the expense of considerable uncertainty about exposure.

The previous and current committees followed the *Update 2006* committee's practice of more circumscribed searching. As the information in the database on populations that had established exposure to the COIs has grown, VAO committees have become less dependent on data from studies that had nonspecific exposure information and have been able to focus more on findings of studies that had refined exposure specificity. In recognition of the more pivotal role that findings drawn directly from Vietnam veterans were able to play in its decisions, the committee for *Update 2008* reordered its consideration of populations. For each health outcome, studies of Vietnam veterans, the target population of the VAO series, are addressed first and then occupational and environmental studies.

The committee's exact criteria concerning exposure specificity are presented at the end of Chapter 3.

It is well accepted that any TCDD or herbicide effect may be diluted somewhat in studies of Vietnam veterans because some of the veterans may not have been exposed or may have been exposed only at low concentrations. The problem is exacerbated in studies in which exposure is defined in terms of occupation (even on the basis of a full job history). Exploratory studies based on linking to a one-time statement of occupation (for example, on a death certificate or in a census) are thought to be of little use even when a job–exposure matrix is used to "convert" standardized job codes to specific exposures. Not only is there uncertainty about whether all members of the sample have been exposed to one of the COIs unless detailed personal monitoring and industrial-hygiene work have been performed; for most occupational categories, there is also considerable certainty that the workers were exposed to many other potentially toxic agents. Thus, such studies may well minimize the effects of exposure to TCDD or the herbicides of interest while yielding misleading indications of health problems resulting from other exposures.

Processing of Identified Publications

The search strategy was devised to ensure that abstracts of all potentially relevant articles were subjected to closer screening, but it also resulted in the identification of a large number of nonrelevant studies. The searches produced in excess of 6,900 "hits," including some studies that were identified more than once. It was evident from the abstracts of most of the cited articles that they did not address health effects in association with exposure to the COIs; for example, many of the cited studies investigated the efficacy of herbicides in killing weeds. All studies that discussed health effects were considered if the search-related information (title, abstract, and keywords) indicated that any of the herbicides of interest (or any of their components) may have been investigated. For each of the more than 700 potentially relevant citations ultimately identified, a copy of the entire article was obtained online and reviewed more thoroughly by the committee for inclusion in its report. For the present update, very few documents of interest had to be retrieved as hard copies from library sources.

In large part, included reports are peer-reviewed journal articles, but generally available and formally published government studies (particularly those investigating health effects in Vietnam veterans) are also included under the presumption that they have been carefully reviewed. In practice, the articles are generally in English, but VAO committees have obtained translations for crucial ones that were not in English, as in the case of reports of a study of Korean veterans of the Vietnam War (Kim HA et al., 2003; Kim JS et al., 2003) when *Update 2004* was produced.

TCDD, the 2,3,7,8-chlorinated congener of dioxin, is the most potent of the polychlorinated dibenzo-*p*-dioxins (PCDDs), dibenzofurans, and biphenyls, so it is presumed to be the most problematic of the dioxin-like chemicals contaminating the phenoxy herbicides used in Vietnam. However, our concern is not limited to that congener. In nonlaboratory settings—for example, epidemiologic studies—exposures occur not only to TCDD but also to mixtures of dioxins, dibenzofurans, and PCBs, which vary in their degree of chlorination. The concept of toxic equivalency has been developed primarily to permit overarching estimation of oral exposure and risk from environmentally persistent chemicals that have structural similarities to PCDDs and PCDFs that bind the AHR, induce the same spectrum of effects, and bioaccumulate in the food chain (van den Berg et al., 2006). A toxicity equivalency factor (TEF) is an estimate of the dioxin-like potency of an individual congener relative to the toxicity of TCDD. TEQs are often used to estimate the cumulative toxic potency of mixtures as the sum of TEFs weighted by the concentrations of the corresponding congeners in the mixture; this total is denoted as the mixture's TEQ in terms of dioxin-like activity. That approach is often taken in epidemiologic studies that focus on PCBs. Many epidemiologic studies of PCBs have been recovered in VAO literature searches although they were not specifically sought. Because dioxin-like and non–dioxin-like PCB congeners are found together in environmental mixtures and are known to mediate toxicity by various mechanisms, the relative contribution of dioxin-like PCBs to an individual health outcome can be difficult to determine. Therefore, evidence from epidemiologic studies of PCB exposure has been retained only for reported results on specific dioxin-like congeners or in terms of TEQs. While all studies reporting TEQs based on PCBs were reviewed, those studies that reported TEQs based only on mono-ortho PCBs (which are PCBs 105, 114, 118, 123, 156, 157, 167, and 189) were given very limited consideration since mono-ortho PCBs typically contribute less than 10% to total TEQs, based on the World Health Organization (WHO) revised TEFs of 2005 (La Rocca et al., 2008; van den Berg et al., 2006).

The committee for *Update 2008* investigated what pesticides are used in greenhouses and determined that greenhouse workers are not likely to be exposed to herbicides, particularly those of interest for VAO committee deliberations (Czarnota, 2004; Neal, 2006; University of Connecticut, 2006). Results on such populations (Abell et al., 2000, on fertility; Hansen et al., 1992, on cancer in female workers) were retroactively excluded from the evidence database considered in *Update 2008*, and no new citations of studies of such workers have been retained. Further consultation (e-mail in Public Access File, November 12, 2012) with Helle Raun Andersen, an Associate Professor at the University of Southern Denmark and a researcher on a series of epidemiologic studies of reproductive effects among greenhouse workers, confirmed the lack of herbicide exposure among such workers for the current committee.

Integration of New Information

More than 60 articles on epidemiologic studies and several dozen toxicology studies contributed new information to the present update. New evidence on each health outcome was reviewed in detail. The committee's conclusions, however, are based on the accumulated evidence, not just on recently published studies. In a considerable number of instances over the course of the VAO reports, single study populations have generated multiple entries for a given health outcome. Before *Update 2010*, the procedure had been to enter new results into the summary results tables in groups corresponding to successive updates, so it has been difficult to recognize which findings are based on the experience of the same set of people.

The current committee has continued the revisions begun by the committee for *Update 2010* in formatting the tables of cumulative results on health outcomes in an effort to make the interrelationships more evident for its own deliberations and for the reader. The goal of focusing on an integrated picture of how a health outcome was manifested in a given study population has been enhanced by moving the citations to the far right of the findings to put less emphasis on individual publications. The reported findings on a given condition from a particular study population have been gathered and presented in reverse chronologic order so that the most mature set of statistics appears first. In many instances, that will represent the most informative set of data—the set that has the greatest power to demonstrate an adverse effect in the population in question. For some health problems, particularly those common in old age, the toxic effect associated with an external factor may be to manifest a disease sooner. In such situations, the evidence of an association with an exposure may consist of a wave of diagnoses in younger people, and the prevalence will equalize with that in the control group as the populations age. The committee therefore decided that it could not retain only the most recent findings when considering the experience of a given study population.

The cohorts themselves have been ordered in the tables to reflect the overarching cohorts of which they are subgroups. The exposure of interest in each cohort is explicitly noted in the tables to facilitate judgments about when consistency might be expected among populations that experience the same exposure. That should minimize misapprehensions that there are inconsistencies if two excellent studies of groups exposed to different COIs have incongruent findings.

Primary findings are the components of the evidence that the committee endeavors to integrate in drawing its conclusions. Reanalyses (without the incorporation of additional information), pooled analyses, reviews, and so on, may be discussed in conjunction with primary results or in synthesis sections on a given health outcome, but they themselves are not part of the evidence dataset.

COMMITTEE'S APPROACH

The committee's general approach to the evaluation of scientific evidence corresponds closely to the approach developed by the original *VAO* committee as delineated in detail in Chapter 5 of *VAO*. The committee had three specific tasks: to determine whether there is a statistical association between exposure to the herbicides used in Vietnam and health outcomes; to determine the increase in risk of effects among Vietnam veterans; and to determine whether plausible biologic mechanisms provide support for a causal relationship with a given health outcome.

Statistical Association

The issues in determining whether a statistical association exists are detailed in Chapter 5 of *VAO*. Since that first committee, the primary relevant evidence for consideration has come from epidemiologic studies—investigations in which large groups of people are studied to identify an association between exposure to a chemical of interest and the occurrence of particular health outcomes. The current committee has not modified the criteria used by previous VAO committees to assign categories of association to particular health outcomes but will henceforth state the object of its evaluation to be "scientifically relevant association" in order to clarify that the strength of evidence evaluated, based on the quality of the scientific studies reviewed, was a fundamental component of the committee's deliberations to address the imprecisely defined legislative target of "statistical association."

Epidemiologists estimate associations between exposure and outcome in a specific population or group in terms of relative risk by using such measures as standardized mortality ratio, odds ratio, rate ratio, or hazard ratio. Those measures indicate the magnitude of a difference in the rate of an outcome between two populations. For example, if the rate in an exposed population is twice the rate in a nonexposed population, the relative risk is 2. Similarly, if the odds of a health outcome are 1:20 in an exposed population but 1:100 in a nonexposed population, the odds ratio is 5. In this report, both *relative risk* (also called *risk ratio*) and *odds ratio* are used to represent the association between exposure and adverse outcome. Both measures are often reported in prospective cohort studies. Case-control studies usually report odds ratios, and they cannot report relative risk because the base rate in the control group is usually not available in these studies. However, it is possible for case-control studies to provide estimates of relative risk if ancillary information on the base rate is available (Hsieh et al., 1985; Langholz, 2010). For rare diseases with low rates in both the exposed group and the control group, odds are approximately identical with risk, so an odds ratio is approximately identical with a relative risk. That is,

$$odds = risk/(1 - risk),$$

so that when *risk* is close to zero, (1 − *risk*) is close to 1; therefore, *odds* will be close to *risk*. An estimated relative risk or odds ratio greater than 1 indicates a positive association; it is more likely that the outcome will be seen in exposed people than in nonexposed people. A relative risk or odds ratio between zero and 1 indicates a negative or inverse association; the outcome is less likely in exposed people. A relative risk or odds ratio of 1 suggests the absence of association, which is usually the null hypothesis to be tested. A statistically significant association is one that would be unlikely to occur by chance—that is, if the null hypothesis is true. (Chapters 7–13 contain tables of results abstracted from the studies that provide evidence on individual health outcomes. Because the distinction between *risk* and *odds* is of little consequence in the deliberations of VAO committees, the column labeled "Estimated Risk" presents findings without specifying the precise nature of the reported statistic.)

Determining whether an estimated association between an exposure and an outcome represents a real relationship requires careful scrutiny because there can be more than one explanation for an estimate. *Bias* is a distortion of the measure of association that results from flawed selection in the assembly of the study population or from error in measurement of studied characteristics. *Confounding* is a distortion of the measure of association that results from failure to recognize or account for some factor related both to exposure and to outcome. *Chance* is the degree to which an estimated association might vary randomly among different samples of the population studied. The width of a *confidence interval* is used to quantify the likely statistical variability of an exposure–disease association, but it does not incorporate quantification of distortions that may arise from the systematic problems mentioned above. Even when a relative risk or standardized mortality ratio substantially exceeds 1, a conclusion regarding increased risk must be qualified when the confidence interval is wide. In drawing conclusions, the committee examined the most thoroughly adjusted quantitative estimates of association, judged whether adjustment for any crucial confounders was lacking, and evaluated the potential influences of bias and chance. In integrating the findings of various studies, the committee considered the degree of statistical significance associated with every estimated risk (a reflection of the magnitude of the observed effect and the power of the study designs) and took note of whether dose-response relationships were evident with increasing exposure rather than simply tallying the "significant" and "nonsignificant" outcomes as dichotomous items of evidence. The committee also considered whether controlled laboratory investigations provide information consistent with the COIs being associated with a given effect and perhaps causally linked to it.

In pursuing the question of statistical association, the committee recognized that an absolute conclusion about the absence of association is unattainable. As in science generally, studies of health effects associated with herbicide exposure cannot demonstrate that a purported effect is impossible or could never occur but only that it is statistically improbable. Any instrument of observation, even an excellent epidemiologic study, is limited in its resolving power. In a strict technical sense, therefore, the absence of an association between even one chemical and a health outcome cannot be proved. Convincingly demonstrating the lack of a particular effect of all five of the COIs simultaneously would be a daunting effort, especially in light of the paucity of information concerning picloram and cacodylic acid. The present committee therefore endorses the decision by the committee for *Update 2006* to reclassify several types of cancer that had been classified since *VAO* (1994) as having "suggestive evidence of *no* association" with "exposure to herbicides."

Interaction or synergism among the COIs or with other agents is another theoretical concern. The committee was not charged with attributing effects to specific COIs, and joint effects among them should be adequately identified by the committee's approach. The combinations of the chemicals with other agents that might be problematic are virtually infinite. Real-life experience, as investigated with epidemiologic studies, effectively integrates any results of exposure to a target substance with results of all other possibly detrimental or mitigating exposures that a population might have. It may not be possible to partition contributions of the COIs from those of all other factors quantitatively, but, to the extent that the possibility of confounding influences can be appraised, the committee will have achieved its objective.

Increased Risk in Vietnam Veterans

When all the available epidemiologic evidence has been evaluated, it is presumed that Vietnam veterans are at increased risk for a specific health outcome if there is evidence of a positive association between one or more of the COIs and the outcome. The best measure of potency for the quantification of risk to veterans would be the rate of the outcome in exposed Vietnam veterans compared with the rate in nonexposed veterans, adjusted for the degree to which any other factors that differ between exposed and nonexposed veterans might influence those rates. Conley and Heerwig (2012) have noted, however, that elements of bias may have been involved in the selection of service members for deployment. A dose–response relationship established in another human population suitably adjusted for such factors would be similarly suitable.

It is difficult to quantify risk when exposures of a population have not been measured accurately. Recent serum TCDD concentrations are available only for subgroups enrolled in the Air Force Health Study (AFHS) (the Operation Ranch Hand veterans and Southeast Asia comparison subjects) and from VA's study of deployed and nondeployed members of the Army Chemical Corps. Pharmacokinetic models, with their own set of assumptions, must be applied to extrapolate from contemporary readings to obtain presumably accurate estimates of original exposure of Vietnam-era veterans. The absence of reliable measures of exposure of Vietnam veterans to the COIs limits the committee's ability to quantify risks of specific diseases in this population.

Although serum TCDD measurements in only a small portion of Vietnam-era veterans are available, the observed distributions of these most reliable measures of exposure make it clear that they cannot be used as a standard for partitioning veterans into discrete exposure groups, such as service on Vietnamese soil, service in the Blue Water Navy, and service elsewhere in Southeast Asia. For example, many TCDD values observed in the comparison group from the AFHS exceeded US background concentrations and overlapped considerably with those of the Operation Ranch Hand subjects.

As explained in Chapter 1, the committee for *Update 2006* decided to make a general statement about its continuing inability to address that aspect of its charge quantitatively rather than to reiterate a disclaimer in the concluding section for every health outcome, and the present committee has retained that approach.

Plausible Biologic Mechanisms

Chapter 4, "Information Related to Biologic Plausibility," previously called "Toxicology," details the experimental basis of assessment of biologic plausibility or the extent to which an observed statistical association in epidemiologic studies is consistent with other biologic or medical knowledge. Does the observation of a particular health effect make sense on the basis of what is known about how the chemicals in question act at the tissue, cellular, or molecular level? The relationship between a particular exposure and a specific human health outcome is addressed in the context of research on the effects of the chemicals on biologic systems and of evidence from animal studies.

Chapter 4 presents an integrated toxicity profile of each of the COIs without providing detailed commentary on each possibly relevant toxicology article published in the update period. Experimental information pertinent to a particular health outcome is now presented immediately after the epidemiologic evidence on that outcome in the "Biologic Plausibility" sections on individual health outcomes (Chapters 7–13).

A positive statistical association between an exposure and an outcome does not necessarily mean that the exposure is the cause of the outcome. Data from toxicology studies may support or conflict with a hypothesis that a specific chemical can contribute to the occurrence of a particular disease. Many toxicology studies are conducted with laboratory animals so that variables, including the amount and duration of exposure, can be controlled precisely. Studies that use isolated cells in culture also can elucidate how a chemical alters cellular processes. The objectives of those toxicology studies are to determine what toxic effects are observed at different exposure levels and to identify the mechanisms by which the effects are produced. Ultimately, the results of the toxicology studies should be consistent with what is known about the human disease process if they are to support a conclusion that the development of the disease was influenced by an exposure.

Animal studies and in vitro studies with human cells and cell lines do provide links that are important for understanding underlying biochemical mechanisms associated with toxicity induced by xenobiotics (exogenous chemicals). In some cases, however, toxic effects that are not detected in humans are observed in animal studies. Many potential factors may contribute to differences between results of controlled animal studies and effects observed in humans. The following are among the most important:

- **Physiologic differences.** Laboratory animals are not miniature humans. Depending on the biologic process under investigation, a particular test species may match the human system more closely and so be a better experimental model.
- **Magnitude of exposure.** Often the TCDD exposure used for animal studies has been many orders of magnitude higher than Vietnam veterans are likely to have received during military service.
- **Duration of exposure.** Although TCDD is a persistent organic pollutant, animal studies seldom examine chronic low-level exposure that occurs over a period of years or even many months.
- **Timing of exposure.** It is well known that many organ systems are highly susceptible to xenobiotic exposure during critical stages of development, such as gestation; the response of some systems (such as the immune system) may also depend on the timing of exposure to antigens relative to the timing of exposure to xenobiotics such as TCDD.
- **The route of exposure.** Route of exposure by which an exogenous agent enters an organism may influence the nature of any toxic response elicited. The outcomes of animal studies may be perturbed by the delivery of treatment doses by "unnatural" routes of exposure such as a bolus by gavage or intraperitoneal injection, but route of exposure does not seem to be a major reason why results of epidemiology studies may not agree with the findings of controlled studies for the COIs considered in the VAO series.
- **Other genetic susceptibilities.** The etiologies of most diseases in humans and in animals are likely to be influenced by numerous genes and to involve complex gene–environment interactions, and preliminary evidence suggests that TCDD can induce epigenetic modifications of an organism's DNA that may alter future expression of the genome.
- **Sex differences.** There are well-known differences between male and female animals in susceptibility to xenobiotic exposures, some of which are modified by sex steroids.

- **Prior and recurring exposures to multiple sources.** Humans are exposed to xenobiotics from multiple sources throughout their lifetime.
- **Complex mixtures.** Most xenobiotic exposures occur in complex mixtures; the makeup of these mixtures can influence the ultimate toxic effects heavily. In addition to dietary modulation of response to other exposures of both humans and animals, human metabolism is perturbed by dietary supplements, prescription and over-the-counter pharmaceuticals, and other factors (such as cigarette-smoking and ambient pollution).
- **Stress.** Stress—of known or unknown origin—is a well-known modifier of human disease responses (such as immune responses); stress is an ever-present variable that is difficult to assess or control for in epidemiologic studies because there is substantial individual variation in response to it (Cohen et al., 2007).

The absence of evidence of biologic plausibility from toxicology studies, however, does not rule out the possibility of a biologic relationship. In fact, cases in which the epidemiologic evidence is strong but toxicologic support is lacking often drive new toxicology research.

As noted in *VAO*, not only is information on biologic plausibility one of the primary elements in the oft-cited list of factors that have rather imprecisely become known as the Bradford Hill (1965) "criteria" for causality (discussed in more detail at the end of this chapter); insights about biologic processes also inform whether an observed pattern of statistical association might be interpreted as the product of more than error, bias, confounding, and chance. The committee used toxicologic information in that fashion and placed the information before its synthesis and conclusion to provide readers with a more coherent argument for its ultimate conclusion about the adequacy of the available evidence to support the existence of a particular association.

EVALUATION OF THE EVIDENCE

Scientifically relevant associations between exposures to the COIs and specific health outcomes are determined through an analysis of available epidemiologic studies that is informed by an understanding of the toxicology of the chemicals and their exposure pathways. In reaching conclusions, VAO committees consider the nature of the exposures, the nature of the health outcomes, the populations exposed, and the quality of the evidence examined. Some specific issues that this and prior committees have considered are addressed below.

Human Studies

The committee reviewed studies of Vietnam veterans and of other populations that might have been exposed to the COIs. The other populations factored into the committee's evaluation included cohorts of workers in chemical production and agriculture and populations residing near sites of environmental contamination. The committee believes that studies of such nonveteran subjects can help in the assessment of whether the COIs are associated with particular health outcomes. As noted above in describing the literature search, studies of nonveteran subjects were identified because one of the COIs was specified by the original researchers as presenting a possible toxic exposure rather than on the basis of occupational definitions. Some of the studies provide stronger evidence about health outcomes than do studies of veterans because exposures were measured sooner after occurrence and were more thoroughly characterized than has been the case in most studies of veterans. Furthermore, in the studies of workers in chemical-production plants, the magnitude and duration of exposure to the chemicals were generally greater, so the likelihood that any possible health consequence would be manifested was greater. The studies were often large enough to examine health risks among groups of people that had different levels of exposure, so dose–response relationships could be investigated. The general practice of VAO committees has been to evaluate all studies, whether or not their subjects were Vietnam veterans, according to the same criteria in determining the strength and validity of findings. Because studies of Vietnam veterans address the very population of concern to the legislation that mandated the present review, demonstrations of increased incidence of particular health outcomes among them are of unquestionable pertinence in drawing conclusions.

The committee has concluded that it would be inappropriate to use quantitative techniques, such as meta-analysis, to combine individual study results into a single summary measure of statistical association. The committee reached that conclusion because of the many differences among studies in definitions of exposure, health outcomes considered, criteria for defining study populations, correction for confounding factors, and degree of detail in reporting results. The appropriate use of meta-analysis requires more methodologic consistency among studies, especially in the definition of exposure, than is present in the literature that the committee reviewed (Egger et al., 2002; Petitti, 2000). A detailed discussion of the results of individual studies in appropriate categories (Vietnam-veteran, occupational, or environmental exposure; and exposure to Agent Orange or equivalent dioxin-contaminated phenoxy herbicides, to dioxin, to phenoxy herbicides without dioxin contamination, to cacodylic acid, or to picloram) with a thorough examination of each study's strengths and weaknesses is fully informative without making unfounded assumptions of homogeneity.

In general, VAO committees have not considered case reports, case series, or other published studies that lacked control or comparison groups. An exception has been made, however, for early-onset peripheral neuropathy; individual case reports were reviewed because the rapid appearance and frequently transient nature of the condition impose methodologic constraints that might have precluded the application of standard epidemiologic techniques.

Because any effect of Agent Orange in individuals or groups of veterans is evaluated in terms of disease or medical outcome, attention to disease classification was important to the committee in assembling pertinent data from various investigations related to a particular outcome before integrating the information. The researchers who conducted the studies that the committee reviewed faced the same challenge in interpreting the available documentation when assigning diagnostic labels to given subjects and then grouping the labels for analysis.

Pathologists, clinicians, and epidemiologists use several classification systems, including the *International Classification of Diseases* (ICD): the *International Classification of Diseases, Ninth Revision* (ICD-9), *Clinical Modification* (ICD-9-CM), and the *International Classification of Diseases for Oncology,* all developed under the auspices of the WHO. The 10th revision of ICD (ICD-10) is currently used to classify mortality information. Most of the subjects investigated in the studies cited in the VAO updates were diagnosed under earlier systems, and most of the articles report results in accordance with ICD-9 if they use ICD codes at all, so VAO committees have retained the use of ICD-9. ICD codes are a hierarchic system for indicating type of disease and site. For example, ICD-9 162 specifies cancers of the lung, trachea, or bronchus; 162.2, cancer of a main bronchus; 162.3, cancer of an upper lobe; 162.4, cancer of a middle lobe; and 162.5, cancer of a lower lobe.

For a patient to receive a correct cancer diagnosis, careful staging of the extent of disease is necessary, and a biopsy of the tissue must be analyzed with microscopy, often with special immunohistochemical stains, to confirm a clinical impression. Many of the epidemiologic studies reviewed by VAO committees have not used the ICD approach to classification of disease and have relied instead on clinical impression alone. Death-certificate diagnoses are notoriously inaccurate if the certificates are completed by medical officers who are not familiar with the decedents' medical history (Smith Sehdev and Hutchins, 2001). Self-reported diagnoses, which are obtained from survey questionnaires, often are partially or completely inaccurate; for instance, a patient may report having been treated for stomach cancer although the correct diagnosis was gastric adenocarcinoma, gastric lymphoma, pancreatic cancer, large bowel cancer, or peritoneal cancer.

Many epidemiologic studies report disease outcome by organ system. For instance, the term *digestive system* may be used for conditions that are benign or malignant and that affect the esophagus, stomach, liver, pancreas, small bowel, large bowel, or rectum. Therefore, if a report indicated that a cohort has an increased incidence of digestive system cancer, it would be unclear whether the association was attributable to excess cases of esophageal, gastric, hepatic, pancreatic, or intestinal cancers or to some combination thereof. Such generalization is complicated by the fact that the cause of cancer may differ between anatomic sites. For instance, there are strong associations between *Helicobacter pylori* infection and gastric cancer, between smoking and squamous cell carcinoma of the esophagus, and between chronic hepatitis B infection and hepatic cancer. Furthermore, a single site may experience a carcinogenic response to multiple agents.

The committee recognizes that outcome misclassification is a possibility when recording of a diagnosis with a specific ICD code is used as the means of entering an observation into an analysis, but this system has been refined over many decades and is virtually universally used and understood, in addition to being exhaustive and explicit. Therefore, this and previous VAO committees have opted to use the ICD system as an organizing tool. Although the groupings of cancer sites for which conclusions about association have been presented may correspond more closely with National Institute for Occupational Safety and Health or National Cancer Institute Surveillance Epidemiology and End Results categories (see Appendix C), the underlying ICD codes provide the most exactitude. In this report, ICD codes appear almost exclusively in the introductory sections of health-outcome discussions (particularly for cancers) to specify precisely what outcome the committee is addressing and, when possible, in the results table to indicate exactly what the primary researchers believed that they were investigating. (See Appendix C for cancer groupings with corresponding ICD-9 and ICD-10 codes.)

Rare diseases, such as hairy-cell leukemia and tonsil cancer, are difficult to study because it is hard to accumulate enough cases to permit analysis. Often, the result is that observed cases are included in a broader, less specific category. Thus, epidemiologic data may not be available for assessing whether a particular rare disease is associated with Agent Orange exposure. In some instances, such as chronic lymphocytic leukemia and AL amyloidosis, VAO committees have reached conclusions on the basis of the data available and the etiology of the disease. Through systematic application of the hierarchic nature of the ICD coding system, committees intend to draw, for every type of cancer, an explicit conclusion about the adequacy of available evidence to support an association between herbicide exposure and that type of cancer. For nonmalignant conditions, however, the diversity of disease processes involved makes the use of broad ICD ranges less useful, but, because VAO committees could not possibly address every rare nonmalignant disease, they do not draw explicit conclusions about diseases that are not discussed. Thus, the category of "inadequate or insufficient evidence to determine an association" is the default or starting point for any health outcome; if a condition or outcome is not addressed specifically, it will be in this category.

The committee is aware of the concerns of some veterans about the role of herbicide exposure in the occurrence of multiple health outcomes, such as multiple cancers, in a given person. Little research has been done to address whether the rate of concurrence is greater than would be expected by chance. Simultaneous analysis of multiple health outcomes could potentially provide more insight into whether the chemicals of interest cause multiple health effects, into competing risks among various health outcomes, and into the interactive effects of health outcomes; but addressing health conditions individually has remained challenging.

VAO committees wanted to be clear in indicating what evidence is factored into their conclusions. The practice in the VAO reports has been to augment the results table for a given health outcome with any additional publications considered in the current update in the categories of Vietnam-veteran, occupational, or environmental studies. Inclusion of sequential sets of results from followups of a study population has the potential to create the appearance of a greater weight of evidence than is warranted, so *Update 2006* and *Update 2008* used italicized citations in results tables to indicate that results had been superseded. The committee for *Update 2010* did not want to convey the notion that earlier findings were of no importance. In an effort to get a comprehensive and comprehensible picture of the history of each study population, the committee for *Update 2010* decided to abandon the sequential entries by update that had been used in the results tables since *Update 1996*. The format adopted in the last update for the results tables is a refinement of the cohort-based approach that was introduced in *Update 2006* for cardiovascular diseases. To facilitate the reader's locating the discussion of the characteristics of particular study populations and the attributes of the publications based on them, the order of studies in the results tables corresponds to their presentation in Chapter 6. The main categorization of veteran, occupational, and environmental cohort studies and case-control studies has been retained in both instances. In an effort to provide a coherent picture of the occurrence over time of a specific health outcome in a given study population, the current committee has shifted its emphasis away from individual publications by moving the citation that was the source of a particular finding to the right-most column in the results tables.

An issue related to evidence evaluation that was of concern for the *Update 2006* committee was the evidence category of "*no* association." That committee determined that a conclusion of *no* association would require substantive evidence of such a lack of effect of each of the chemicals of interest. Given the paucity of available information on cacodylic acid and picloram, that conclusion would seem suspect even if substantial evidence uniformly supported a finding of *no* association both with exposure to the phenoxy herbicides and with exposure to TCDD. Later committees have concurred in that determination and adopted a similar approach to the placement of health outcomes in this category.

Exposure Assessment

Much of the evidence that VAO committees have considered has been drawn from studies of populations that were not in Vietnam during the period when Agent Orange and other herbicides were used as defoliants. The most informative of those studies were well-documented investigations of occupational exposures to TCDD or specific herbicides, such as 2,4-D and 2,4,5-T. In many other studies, TCDD exposure was combined with exposures to an array of "dioxin-like" compounds, and the herbicides were often analyzed as members of a functional class; this is less informative for the committee's purpose than individual results on a specific compound. In the real-world situations investigated in epidemiologic studies, exposure to multiple possibly toxic chemicals is the rule rather than the exception; for example, farmers and other agricultural populations are likely to be exposed to insecticides, fungicides, and herbicides. In such studies, the committee looked for evidence of health effects that are associated with the specific compounds in the defoliants used in Vietnam and sought consideration of and adjustment for other possibly confounding exposures.

The quality of exposure information in the scientific literature reviewed by this and previous VAO committees varies widely. Some studies relied on interviews or questionnaires to determine the extent and frequency of exposure. Such self-reported information generally carries less weight than would more objective measures of exposure. The strength of questionnaire-based information as evidence of exposure is enhanced to the extent that the information can be corroborated or validated by other sources. Written records of chemical purchase or production can provide one type of objective information. Even more useful are scientific measurements of exposure. In some occupational studies, for example, workers wear air-sampling instruments that measure the concentration of a contaminant in each worker's breathing zone. Measurement of chemicals or their products in such biologic specimens, as blood and urine can provide reliable indications of exposure for specific periods. Studies that categorize exposure from well-documented environmental sources of contaminants can be useful in the identification of exposed populations, but their results may be inaccurate if people with different magnitudes of exposure are assigned to the same general category of exposure. Studies that explore environmental exposure and disease frequency in regional populations (such as states and counties) are known as ecologic studies. Most ecologic studies are considered preliminary or "hypothesis-generating" studies because they lack information on exposure and disease on an individual basis and are unable to address potential confounding factors.

Chapter 3 of this update addresses issues of exposure estimation in more detail. The agent of interest may be assessed with various degrees of specificity. For instance, any of the four herbicides in question could be individually measured, and phenoxy herbicides would be a useful broader category for 2,4,5-T and 2,4-D; but a report of findings in terms simply of "herbicides" is only on the margin of being informative, and results stated in terms of "pesticides" are too vague to be useful. For a given chemical of interest, the measure of exposure may be increasingly imprecise—for example, concentrations in target tissue, serum concentrations, cumulative exposure, possible exposure, and so on down to merely a report of service in a job or industry category. Those approaches can address complexities in specificity, duration, and intensity of exposure with various degrees of success. All may provide some information about association with a chemical of interest, but this committee has determined that investigation of associations between an exposure of concern and most health outcomes has reached the stage where some characterizations of exposure are too nonspecific to promote insight. For health outcomes with little evidence, a somewhat looser criterion would apply so that no possible signal of an association would be overlooked.

Animal and Mechanistic Studies

Animal models used as surrogates for the study of a human disease must reproduce, with some degree of fidelity, the manifestations of the disease in humans. However, a given effect of an exposure in an animal species does not necessarily establish its occurrence in humans, nor does an apparent absence of a particular effect in animals mean the effect could not occur in humans. In addition to possible species differences, many factors affect the ability to extrapolate from results of animal studies to health effects in humans. Animals used in experimental studies are most often exposed to purified chemicals, not to mixtures. Even if herbicide formulations or mixtures are used, the conditions of exposure might not realistically reproduce human exposures that occur in the field. Furthermore, Vietnam veterans were exposed to other agents—such as tobacco smoke, insecticides, therapeutics, drugs, diesel fumes, and alcohol—that may increase or decrease the ability of chemicals in herbicides to produce a particular adverse health outcome. Few, if any, studies either in humans or in experimental animals have examined those interactions.

As discussed in Chapter 4, TCDD is thought to be responsible for many of the toxic effects of the herbicides used in Vietnam. Attempts to establish correlations in the effects of TCDD between experimental systems and humans are particularly problematic because of known species-, sex-, and outcome-specific differences in susceptibility to TCDD toxicity. Some data indicate that humans might be more resistant than are other species to TCDD's toxic effects (Ema et al., 1994; Moriguchi et al., 2003); other data suggest that, for some outcomes, human sensitivity could be the same as or greater than that of some experimental animals (DeVito et al., 1995). Differences in vulnerability may also be affected by variations in the rate at which TCDD is eliminated from the body (see Chapter 4 for details on the toxicokinetics of TCDD). Although degree of susceptibility is generally thought to be an inherent biological response, it can be influenced by life stage, past history, co-exposures, etc.

It is important to account for TCDD's mode of action in considering species and strain differences. There is a consensus that most of the toxic effects of TCDD involve interaction with the AHR, a protein that binds TCDD and some other aromatic hydrocarbons with high affinity, although it is now recognized that the AHR performs actions other than just that of a transcriptional enhancer, such as having a role in rapid signal transduction. Formation of an active complex that involves the intracellular receptor, the ligand (the TCDD molecule), and other proteins is followed by interaction of the activated complex with specific sites on DNA. That interaction can alter the expression of genes involved in the regulation of cellular processes. The development of mice that lack the AHR has helped to establish a definitive association between the AHR and TCDD-mediated toxicity. The affinity of TCDD for the AHR is species- and strain-specific, and responses to binding of the receptor vary among cell types and developmental stages. In addition, genetic differences in the properties of the AHR are known in human populations, as they are in laboratory animals, so some people would be at intrinsically greater or less risk for the toxic effects of TCDD.

Although studying AHR biology in transformed human cell lines minimizes the inherent error associated with species extrapolations, caution must be exercised because it is still not clear to what extent toxicity is affected by the transformation itself or by the conditions under which cell lines are cultured in vitro. Furthermore, humans have AHR with differing affinities for dioxin, so a single transformed human cell line will not accurately reflect the responses observed in the entire human population.

Publication Bias

Some studies are more likely to be published than others. That is the concept of publication bias, which has been documented in biomedical research (Song et al., 2000; Stern and Simes, 1997). Most commonly, bias can be introduced when studies whose hypotheses are supported by statistically significant results or that are otherwise deemed favorable by their authors are selectively submitted for publication. In addition, papers with "interesting findings" may be of more interest to journal editors and reviewers and thus be more likely to be accepted for publication after submission. Conversely, "negative" studies, in which the hypotheses being tested are not supported by the study findings, often go unpublished. Investigators employed by industry may be inhibited from submitting findings that have potential legal or economic ramifications.

Thus, conclusions about associations between exposure and outcome that are based solely on published results could be subject to bias. Despite that, the committee does not believe that its conclusions have been unduly affected by publication bias, for two reasons: the extensive publicity surrounding the possibility of health effects associated with the herbicides used in Vietnam has created considerable pressure to publish all findings on the subject, and the many published studies assembled and reviewed contain among their results the full range of possible statistical associations, from convincingly negative through indeterminate to strongly positive.

Role of Judgment

This committee's process of reaching conclusions about statistical associations involved more than a formulaic application of quantitative procedures to the assembled evidence. First, the committee had to assess the relevance and validity of individual reports. Then, it had to evaluate the possible influences of measurement error, selection bias, confounding, and chance on the reported results. Next, the committee integrated all the evidence within and among diverse fields of research. Finally, the conclusions drawn were based on consensus within the committee. Those aspects of the committee's review required thoughtful consideration of alternative approaches at several points and could not be accomplished by adherence to a narrowly prescribed formula.

The realized approach, as described here, has been determined to a large extent by the nature of the exposures, of the health outcomes, and of the resulting evidence available for examination; therefore, it has evolved in the course of the work of this and previous VAO committees. The quantitative and qualitative procedures underlying the present review have been made as explicit as possible, but ultimately the conclusions about association expressed in this report are based on the committee's collective judgment. The committee has endeavored to express its judgments as clearly and precisely as the data allowed.

In delivering the charge to the committee for *Update 2010*, VA's representative requested that the committee delineate, for health outcomes found to have some evidence supporting statistical association, how well each of the factors that make up the so-called Bradford Hill criteria for causality (Hill, 1965) has been satisfied. It was thought that having a scientific perspective on the extent to which those factors, in addition to biologic plausibility, were met would facilitate the Secretary of Veterans Affairs in making a policy decision concerning a presumptive relationship of any new health outcome to exposure to the herbicides used by the military in Vietnam.

The committee for *Update 2010* was uniformly and strongly of the opinion that execution of a checklist of the Hill criteria would not be an appropriate approach for fulfilling its charge, and the current committee is in complete agreement with the decision of the previous committee. The list of issues that Hill discussed are not a definitive set of factors to be addressed in evaluating whether a collection of evidence supports causality. The nine aspects of a statistical association noted by Hill (1965)—strength, consistency, specificity, temporality, biologic gradient, plausibility, coherence, experiment, and analogy—to contribute to a finding of causality vary in the importance that might be assigned to them, but none is sufficient, and only temporality (that the cause precedes the effect) is necessary. Philosophers of science have established that a set of sufficient criteria for causality does not exist (Rothman and Greenland, 1998). Citing Weed and Gorelick (1996) and Holman et al. (2001), Rothman et al. (2008) noted that "epidemiologists have *not* agreed on a set of causal criteria or on how to apply them [emphasis in orginal]. . . . The typical use of causal criteria is to make a case for a position for or against causality that has been arrived at by other, unstated means." The establishment of causality is not an absolute or discrete (or necessarily permanent) state. The Hill criteria have often been used as a point of reference in addressing the subject of causation in evaluating possible environmental harms, but even in theoretical and optimal circumstances scientists have not derived a definitive algorithm for establishing causality. The extent to which a relationship is judged to be causal entails many *subjective* elements involving the universe of information considered and the weight accorded to each evidentiary component considered. Furthermore, with regard to chronic diseases, causality is rarely limited to a single factor.

For those reasons, the committee for *Update 2010* did not adopt the suggestion to perform what would be in effect a checklist approach to distilling evidence concerning underlying causality for any observed statistical association between a human health effect and exposure to the components of the herbicides sprayed in Vietnam. The current committee also interprets its charge to be to summarize the scientific evidence for consideration by the Secretary, whose role is to make the policy decision of whether a contribution of herbicide exposure to the occurrence of an adverse health effect is likely enough to merit recognition as a presumptive condition.

REFERENCES[1]

Abell A, Juul S, Bonde JP. 2000. Time to pregnancy among female greenhouse workers. *Scandinavian Journal of Work, Environment and Health* 26(2):131–136.

Aposhian HV, Gurzau ES, Le XC, Gurzau A, Healy SM, Lu X, Ma M, Yip L, Zakharyan RA, Maiorino RM, Dart RC, Tircus MG, Gonzalez-Ramirez D, Morgan DL, Avram D, Aposhian MM. 2000. Occurrence of monomethylarsonous acid in urine of humans exposed to inorganic arsenic. *Chemical Research in Toxicology* 13(8):693–697.

Cohen S, Janicki-Deverts D, Miller GE. 2007. Psychological stress and disease. *Journal of the American Medical Association* 298(14):1685–1687.

Cohen SM, Arnold LL, Eldan M, Lewis AS, Beck BD. 2006. Methylated arsenicals: The implications of metabolism and carcinogenicity studies in rodents to human risk assessment. *Critical Reviews in Toxicology* 36(2):99–133.

Conley D, Heerwig J. 2012. The long-term effects of military conscription on mortality: Estimates from the Vietnam-era draft lottery. *Demography* 49:841–855.

Czarnota MA. 2004. *Weed Control in Greenhouses: Bulletin 1246.* University of Georgia, College of Agricultural and Environmental Sciences, Cooperative Extension.

DeVito MJ, Birnbaum LS, Farland WH, Gasiewicz TA. 1995. Comparisons of estimated human body burdens of dioxin-like chemicals and TCDD body burdens in experimentally exposed animals. *Environmental Health Perspectives* 103(9):820–831.

Egger M, Ebrahim S, Smith GD. 2002. Where now for meta-analysis? *International Journal of Epidemiology* 31(1):1–5.

Ema M, Ohe N, Suzuki M, Mimura J, Sogawa K, Ikawa S, Fujii-Kuriyama Y. 1994. Dioxin binding activities of polymorphic forms of mouse and human arylhydrocarbon receptors. *Journal of Biological Chemistry* 269(44):27337–27343.

Hansen ES, Hasle H, Lander F. 1992. A cohort study on cancer incidence among Danish gardeners. *American Journal of Industrial Medicine* 21(5):651–660.

Hill AB. 1965. The environment and disease: Association or causation? *Proceedings of the Royal Society of Medicine* 58:295–300.

[1]Throughout this report, the same alphabetic indicator after year of publication is used consistently for a given reference when there are multiple citations by the same first author in a given year. The convention of assigning the alphabetic indicators in order of citation in a given chapter is not followed.

Holman DJ, Arnold-Reed DE, de Klerk N, McComb C, English D. 2001. A psychometric experiment in casual inference to estimate evidential weights used by epidemiologists. *Epidemiology* 12(2):246–255.

Hsieh DA, Manski CF, McFadden D. 1985. Estimation of response probabilities from augmented retrospective observations. *Journal of the American Statistical Association* 80(391):651–662.

IOM (Institute of Medicine). 1994. *Veterans and Agent Orange: Health Effects of Herbicides Used in Vietnam.* Washington, DC: National Academy Press.

IOM. 2011. *Veterans and Agent Orange: Update 2010.* Washington, DC: The National Academies Press.

Kim HA, Kim EM, Park YC, Yu JY, Hong SK, Jeon SH, Park KL, Hur SJ, Heo Y. 2003. Immunotoxicological effects of Agent Orange exposure to the Vietnam War Korean veterans. *Industrial Health* 41(3):158–166.

Kim JS, Lim HS, Cho SI, Cheong HK, Lim MK. 2003. Impact of Agent Orange exposure among Korean Vietnam veterans. *Industrial Health* 41(3):149–157.

La Rocca C, Alivernini S, Badiali M, Cornoldi A, Iacovella N, Silvestroni L, Spera G, Turrio-Baldassarri L. 2008. TEQs and body burden for PCDDs, PCDFs, and dioxin-like PCBs in human adipose tissue. *Chemosphere* 73(1):92–96.

Langholz B. 2010. Case-control studies = odds ratios: Blame the retrospective model. *Epidemiology* 21(1):10–12.

Moriguchi T, Motohashi H, Hosoya T, Nakajima O, Takahashi S, Ohsako S, Aoki Y, Nishimura N, Tohyama C, Fujii-Kuriyama Y, Yamamoto M. 2003. Distinct response to dioxin in an arylhydrocarbon receptor (AHR)-humanized mouse. *Proceedings of the National Academy of Sciences of the United States of America* 100(10):5652–5657.

Neal NC. 2006. *Greenhouse Weed Control: Horticultural Information Leaflet 570.* North Carolina State University.

NRC (National Research Council). 1999. *Arsenic in Drinking Water.* Washington, DC: National Academy Press.

NRC. 2001. *Arsenic in Drinking Water: 2001 Update.* Washington, DC: National Academy Press.

Petitti DB. 2000. *Meta-Analysis, Decision Analysis, and Cost-Effectiveness Analysis: Methods for Quantitative Synthesis in Medicine.* New York: Oxford Press.

Rothman KJ, Greenland S. 1998. *Modern Epidemiology* (2nd edition). Philadelphia, PA: Lippincott Williams & Wilkins.

Rothman KJ, Greenland S, Lash TL. 2008. *Modern Epidemiology* (3rd edition). Philadelphia, PA: Lippincott Williams & Wilkins.

Smith Sehdev AE, Hutchins GM. 2001. Problems with proper completion and accuracy of the cause-of-death statement. *Archives of Internal Medicine* 161(2):277–284.

Song F, Eastwood AJ, Gilbody S, Duley L, Sutton AJ. 2000. Publication and related biases. *Health Technology Assessment* 4(10):1–115.

Stern JM, Simes RJ. 1997. Publication bias: Evidence of delayed publication in a cohort study of clinical research projects. *British Medical Journal* 315(7109):640–645.

University of Connecticut. 2006. *Greenhouse Weed Control.* University of Connecticut, Storrs, Cooperative Extension System.

van den Berg M, Birnbaum L, Denison MS, De Vito M, Farland W, Feeley M, Fiedler H, Hakansson H, Hanberg A, Haws L, Rose M, Safe S, Schrenk D, Tohyama C, Tritscher A, Tuomisto J, Tysklind M, Walker N, Peterson R. 2006. The 2005 World Health Organization re-evaluation of human and mammalian toxic equivalency factors for dioxins and dioxin-like compounds. *Toxicological Sciences* 93(2):223–241.

Weed DL, Gorelick LS. 1996. The practice of casual inference in cancer epidemiology. *Cancer Epidemiology, Biomarkers and Prevention* 5:303–311.

3

Exposure to the Herbicides Used in Vietnam

Assessment of human exposure continues to be a key element in addressing two of the charges that guide the work of this committee. This chapter first presents background information on the military use of herbicides in Vietnam from 1961 to 1971 with a review of our knowledge of exposures of those who served in Vietnam and of the Vietnamese population to the herbicides and to the contaminant 2,3,7,8-tetrachlorodibenzo-*p*-dioxin, which is referred to in this report as TCDD (and commonly referred to as dioxin) and is the most toxic congener of the tetrachlorodibenzo-*p*-dioxins. It then reviews several key methodologic issues in human population studies: disease latency, possible misclassification based on exposure, and exposure specificity required for scientific evaluation of study results. Further discussion is presented to underscore the difficulties of assessing exposure in the complex environment that characterized Vietnam during the period of interest and to describe two modeling approaches that address exposure of ground troops to Agent Orange and that lead to different conclusions.

Exposure of human populations can be assessed in a number of ways, including use of historical information, questionnaires and interviews, measurements in environmental media, and measurements in biologic specimens. Researchers often rely on a mixture of qualitative and quantitative information to derive such estimates (Armstrong et al., 1994; Checkoway et al., 2004). The most basic approach compares members of a presumably exposed group with the general population or with a nonexposed group; this method of classification offers simplicity and ease of interpretation. A more refined method assigns each study subject to an exposure category—such as high, medium, or low exposure—and calculates disease risk for each group separately and compares it with the risk for a reference or nonexposed group; this method can identify the presence or absence of an exposure–response trend. In some cases, more detailed information is available for quantitative exposure estimates that can be used to construct what are sometimes called exposure metrics. The metrics integrate quantitative estimates of exposure intensity (such as chemical concentration in air or extent of skin contact) with exposure duration to produce an estimate of cumulative exposure. Exposure also can be assessed by measuring chemicals and their metabolites in human tissues. Such biologic markers of exposure integrate absorption from all exposure routes, but their interpretation requires knowledge of pharmacokinetic processes. All those exposure-assessment approaches have been used in studies of Vietnam veterans.

MILITARY USE OF HERBICIDES IN VIETNAM

Military use of herbicides in Vietnam took place from 1962 through 1971. Tests conducted in the United States and elsewhere designed to evaluate defoliation efficacy were used to select specific herbicides (IOM, 1994; Young and Newton, 2004). Four compounds were used in the herbicide formulations in Vietnam: 2,4-dichlorophenoxyacetic acid (2,4-D), 2,4,5-trichlorophenoxyacetic acid (2,4,5-T), 4-amino-3,5,6-trichloropicolinic acid (picloram), and dimethylarsinic acid (cacodylic acid). The chemical structures of those compounds are presented in Chapter 2 (see Figure 2-1). The herbicides were used to defoliate inland hardwood forests, coastal mangrove forests, cultivated lands, and zones around military bases. In 1974, a National Resource Council committee estimated the amount of herbicides sprayed from helicopters and other aircraft by using records gathered from August 1965 through February 1971 (NRC, 1974). That committee calculated that about 18 million gallons (about 69 million liters) of herbicide was sprayed over about 3.6 million acres (about 1.5 million hectares) in Vietnam in that period. The amount of herbicides sprayed on the ground to defoliate the perimeters of base camps and fire bases and the amount sprayed by Navy boats along riverbanks were not estimated.

A revised analysis of spray activities and exposure potential of troops emerged from a study overseen by a committee of the Institute of Medicine (IOM, 1997, 2003a,b). That work yielded new estimates of the amounts of military herbicides used in Vietnam from 1961 through 1971 (Stellman et al., 2003a). The investigators reanalyzed the original data sources that were used to develop herbicide-use estimates in the 1970s and identified errors that inappropriately removed spraying missions from the dataset. They also added new data on spraying missions that took place before 1965. Finally, a comparison of procurement records with spraying records found errors that suggested that additional spraying had taken place but gone unrecorded at the time. The new analyses led to revision of estimates of the amounts of the agents applied, as indicated in Table 3-1. The new research effort estimated that about 77 million liters were applied, about 9 million liters more than the previous estimate.

TABLE 3-1 Military Use of Herbicides in Vietnam (1961–1971)

Code Name	Chemical Constituents[a]	Concentration of Active Ingredient[a]	Years Used[a]	Amount Sprayed: *VAO* Estimate[b]	Amount Sprayed: Revised Estimate[a]
Pink	60% *n*-butyl ester, 40% isobutyl ester of 2,4,5-T	961–1,081 g/L acid equivalent	1961, 1965	464,817 L (122,792 gal)	50,312 L sprayed; 413,852 L additional on procurement records
Green	*n*-butyl ester of 2,4,5-T	—	1961, 1965	31,071 L (8,208 gal)	31,026 L on procurement records
Purple	50% *n*-butyl ester of 2,4-D, 30% *n*-butyl ester of 2,4,5-T, 20% isobutyl ester of 2,4,5-T	1,033 g/L acid equivalent	1962–1965	548,883 L (145,000 gal)	1,892,733 L
Orange	50% *n*-butyl ester of 2,4-D, 50% *n*-butyl ester of 2,4,5-T	1,033 g/L acid equivalent	1965–1970	42,629,013 L (11,261,429 gal)	45,677,937 L (could include Agent Orange II)
Orange II	50% *n*-butyl ester of 2,4-D, 50% isooctyl ester of 2,4,5-T	910 g/L acid equivalent	After 1968	—	Unknown; at least 3,591,000 L shipped
White	Acid weight basis: 21.2% triisopropanolamine salts of 2,4-D, 5.7% picloram	By acid weight, 240 g/L 2,4-D, 65 g/L picloram	1966–1971	19,860,108 L (5,246,502 gal)	20,556,525 L
Blue powder	Cacodylic acid (dimethylarsinic acid) sodium cacodylate	Acid, 65% active ingredient; salt, 70% active ingredient	1962–1964	—	25,650 L
Blue aqueous solution	21% sodium cacodylate + cacodylic acid to yield at least 26% total acid equivalent by weight	Acid weight, 360 g/L	1964–1971	4,255,952 L (1,124,307 gal)	4,715,731 L
Total, all formulations	—	—	—	67,789,844 L (17,908,238 gal)	76,954,766 L (including procured)

[a]Based on Stellman et al., 2003a.
[b]Based on data from MRI, 1967; NRC, 1974; Young and Reggiani, 1988.

Herbicides were identified by the color of a band on 55-gallon shipping containers and were called Agent Pink, Agent Green, Agent Purple, Agent Orange, Agent White, and Agent Blue. Agent Green and Agent Pink were used in 1961 and 1965, and Agent Purple in 1962–1965. Agent Orange was used in 1965–1970, and a slightly different formulation (Agent Orange II) probably was used after 1968. Agent White was used in 1966–1971. Agent Blue was used in powder form in 1962–1964 and as a liquid in 1964–1971. Agent Pink, Agent Green, Agent Purple, Agent Orange, and Agent Orange II all contained 2,4,5-T and were contaminated to some extent with TCDD. Agent White contained 2,4-D and picloram. Agent Blue (powder and liquid) contained cacodylic acid. The chlorinated phenoxy acids 2,4-D and 2,4,5-T persist in soil for only a few weeks; picloram is much more stable, persisting in soil for years; and cacodylic acid is nonvolatile and stable in sunlight (NRC, 1974). More details on the herbicides used are presented in the initial IOM report, *Veterans and Agent Orange: Health Effects of Herbicides Used in Vietnam*, referred to as *VAO* (IOM, 1994).

TCDD IN HERBICIDES USED IN VIETNAM

TCDD is formed during the manufacture of 2,4,5-T in the following manner: trichlorophenol (2,4,5-TCP), the precursor for its synthesis, is formed by the reaction of tetrachlorobenzene and sodium hydroxide (see Figure 3-1a); 2,4,5-T is formed when 2,4,5-TCP reacts with chloroacetic acid (see Figure 3-1b); small amounts of TCDD are formed as a byproduct of the intended main reaction (see Figure 3-1b) when a molecule of 2,4,5-TCP reacts with the tetrachlorobenzene stock (see Figure 3-1c) instead of with chloroacetic acid. In each step in the reaction, a chlorine atom is replaced with an oxygen atom, and this leads to the final TCDD molecule (NRC, 1974). In the class of compounds known as polychlorinated dibenzo-*p*-dioxins (PCDDs), 75 congeners can occur, depending on the number and placement of the chlorine atoms. Cochrane et al. (1982) noted that TCDD had been found in pre-1970 samples of 2,4,5-TCP. Other PCDDs—2,7-dichloro-dibenzo-*p*-dioxin and 1,3,6,8-tetrachloro-dibenzo-*p*-dioxin—were measured in the same samples. The concentration of TCDD in any given lot of 2,4,5-T depended on the manufacturing process (FAO/UNEP, 2009; Young et al., 1976).

The manufacture of 2,4-D is a different process: its synthesis is based on dichlorophenol, a molecule formed from the reaction of phenol with chlorine (NZIC, 2009). Neither tetrachlorobenzene nor trichlorophenol is formed during this reaction, so TCDD is not normally a byproduct of the manufacturing process. However, other, less toxic PCDDs have been detected in pre-1970 commercial-grade 2,4-D (Cochrane et al., 1982; Rappe et al., 1978; Tosine, 1983). Cochrane et al. (1982) found multiple PCDDs in isooctyl ester, mixed butyl ester, and dimethylamine salt samples of 2,4-D. It has also been noted that cross-contam-

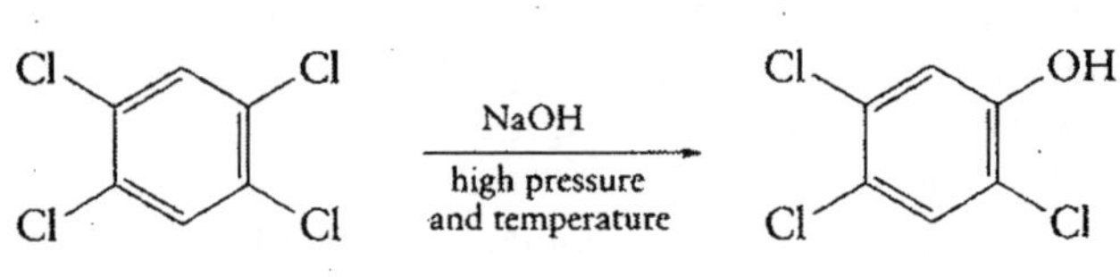

a. Trichlorophenol, the precursor for the synthesis of 2,4,5-T, is formed by the reaction of tetrachlorobenzene and sodium hydroxide (NaOH).

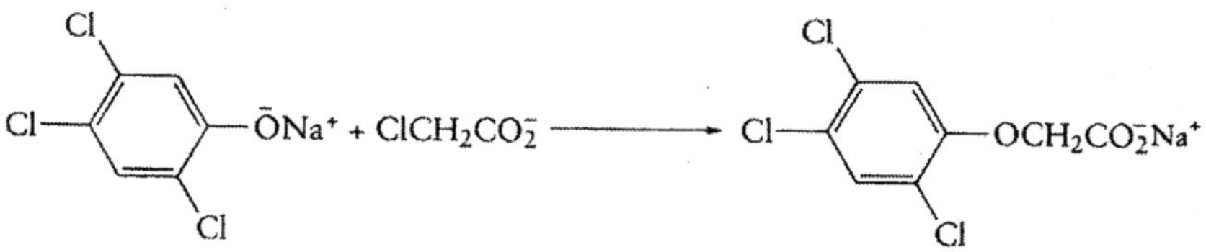

b. The herbicide 2,4,5-T is formed when a reactive form of trichlorophenol (2,4,5-trichlorophenoxide) reacts with chloroacetic acid.

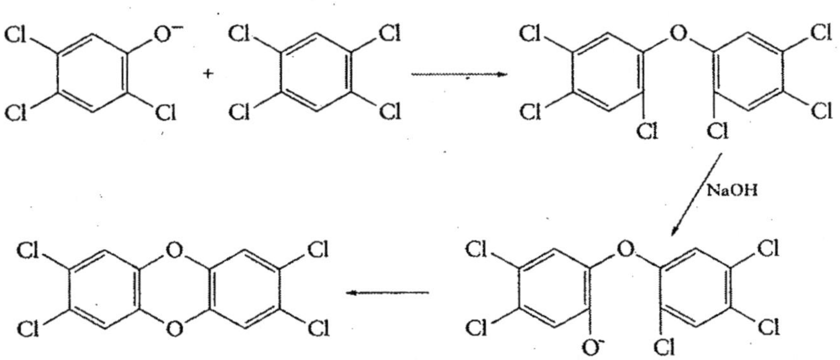

c. TCDD is formed when a molecule of trichlorophenol reacts with its own precursor, tetrachlorobenzene. Two intermediate steps are shown in this diagram. At each step, an oxygen–carbon bond forms as a chlorine atom is released. This reaction does not occur in the synthesis of 2,4-D because precursors with adjacent chlorines are not used in its production.

FIGURE 3-1 TCDD formation during 2,4,5-T production.

ination of 2,4-D with 2,3,7,8-TCDD occurred in the operations of at least one major manufacturer (Lilienfeld and Gallo, 1989).

TCDD concentrations in individual herbicide shipments were not recorded but were known to vary from batch to batch and between manufacturers. TCDD concentrations in stocks of Agent Orange remaining after the conflict, which either had been returned from South Vietnam or had been procured but not shipped, ranged from less than 0.05 ppm to almost 50 ppm and averaged 2–3 ppm in two sets of samples (NRC, 1974; Young et al., 1978). Comparable manufacturing standards for the domestic use of 2,4,5-T in 1974 required that TCDD not be present at over 0.05 ppm (NRC, 1974).

Data from Young and Gough were originally used to estimate the amount of TCDD in the various herbicide formulations (Gough, 1986; Young, 1992; Young et al., 1978). Young et al. (1978) estimated that Agent Green, Agent Pink, and Agent Purple—used early in the program (through 1965)—contained 16 times the mean TCDD content of the formulations used in 1965–1970, and mean TCDD concentrations in Agent Pink and Agent Green were estimated at 66 ppm. Gough (1986) estimated that about 167 kg of TCDD was sprayed in Vietnam over a 6-year period.

Later analysis by researchers at Columbia University benefited from access to military spray records that had not been available earlier and has resulted in substantial revisions of the estimates (Stellman et al., 2003a). The investigators were able to incorporate newly found data on spraying in the early period of the war (1961–1965) and to document that larger volumes of TCDD-containing herbicides were used in Vietnam than had been estimated previously. They also found the earlier estimates of TCDD contamination in the herbicide formulations to be low, noting that the original estimates were based on samples at the lower end of the distribution of concentration. They concluded that the mean TCDD concentration in Agent Orange was closer to 13 ppm than to the earlier estimate of 3 ppm. They therefore proposed 366 kg of TCDD as a plausible estimate of the total amount of TCDD applied in Vietnam during 1961–1971.

EXPOSURE OF VIETNAM VETERANS

Determination of exposures of US military personnel who served in Vietnam has been perhaps the greatest challenge in the study of health effects associated with herbicides and TCDD. Some military personnel stationed in cities or on large bases may have received little or no herbicide exposure, whereas troops who moved through defoliated areas soon after treatment may have been exposed through soil contact, drinking water, or bathing. Reliable estimates of the magnitude and duration of such exposures are not possible in most cases, given the lack of contemporaneous chemical measurements, the lack of a full understanding of the movement and behavior of the defoliants in the environment, and the lack of records of individual behaviors and locations. Consequently, most studies have focused on populations that had well-defined tasks that brought them into contact with the agents. It is believed that the subjects of those studies, primarily Air Force personnel involved in fixed-wing aircraft spraying activities (often referred to as Operation Ranch Hand) and members of the US Army Chemical Corps (ACC), may have had among the highest exposures. As described below, exposures of ground troops are difficult to define, so this group has not been studied as intensively. In accord with Congress's mandated presumption of herbicide exposure of all Vietnam veterans, VAO committees have treated Vietnam-veteran status as a proxy for some herbicide exposure when more specific exposure information is not available.

Exposure of Herbicide Handlers

Military personnel who came into direct contact with the herbicidal chemicals through mixing, loading, spraying, and clean-up activities had relatively high exposures to them. The US Environmental Protection Agency refers to such personnel as pesticide handlers and provides special guidance for preventing or minimizing their exposure during those activities in its worker-protection standard for pesticides (EPA, 1992). The number of US military personnel who handled herbicides directly is not known precisely, but two groups have been identified as high-risk subpopulations among veterans: Air Force personnel involved in Operation Ranch Hand and members of the ACC who used hand-operated equipment and helicopters to conduct smaller-scale operations, including defoliation around special-forces camps; clearing the perimeters of airfields, depots, and other bases; and small-scale crop destruction (NRC, 1980; Thomas and Kang, 1990; Warren, 1968). Additional units and individuals handled or sprayed herbicides around bases or lines of communication; for example, Navy river patrols were reported to have used herbicides to clear inland waterways, and engineering personnel used herbicides to remove underbrush and dense growth in constructing fire-support bases. The latter groups have not been the subject of epidemiologic studies. The herbicides used in Vietnam were not considered to present an important human health hazard at the time, so few precautions were taken to prevent exposure of personnel (GAO, 1978, 1979); that is, military personnel did not typically use chemical-protective gloves, coveralls, or protective aprons, so substantial skin exposure almost certainly occurred in these populations in addition to exposure by inhalation and incidental ingestion (such as by hand-to-mouth contact).

The Air Force personnel who participated in Operation Ranch Hand were the first Vietnam-veteran population to receive special attention with regard to herbicide exposure. In the Air Force Health Study (AFHS), job and work history, biomarkers, and health outcomes of members of this Operation Ranch Hand cohort were contrasted with Air Force personnel who had served elsewhere in Southeast Asia during the Vietnam era. The AFHS began in 1979 (IOM, 2006).

The exposure index initially proposed relied on military spray records for the TCDD-containing herbicides (Agent Orange, Agent Purple, Agent Pink, and Agent Green); these records also helped to identify the members of the cohort. The subjects were further characterized by military occupation, and exposure in the cohort and the comparison group was evaluated through measurement of TCDD in blood (serum) samples drawn in 1987 or later. A general increase in serum TCDD was detected in people whose jobs involved more frequent handling of herbicides, but there was no clear demarcation between the distributions of serum TCDD concentrations in the Operation Ranch Hand subjects and those in the comparison group (AFHS, 1991). Several methods for estimating herbicide exposure of members of the cohort were developed on the basis of questionnaires and focused on such factors as number of days of skin exposure, percentage of skin area exposed, and the concentration of TCDD in the different herbicidal formulations (Michalek et al., 1995). Most recent analyses of the AFHS data have relied on serum TCDD concentration as the primary exposure metric for epidemiologic classification (Kern et al., 2004; Michalek et al., 2001, 2003; Pavuk et al., 2003). IOM has issued a comprehensive review of the AFHS with recommendations for the use of the extensive data collected in the project (IOM, 2006).

Members of the ACC performed herbicide-spraying operations on the ground and by helicopter and were thereby involved in the direct handling and distribution of Agent Orange and other herbicides in Vietnam. They were not identified for detailed study of health effects related to herbicide exposure until the late 1980s (Thomas and Kang, 1990). An initial feasibility study recruited Vietnam veterans and nondeployed Vietnam-era veterans from within the ACC (Kang et al., 2001). Blood samples collected from 50 Vietnam veterans in 1996 showed an association between reporting of spraying herbicides and higher serum TCDD concentrations; this finding was confirmed in a followup study of a larger fraction of the cohort (Kang et al., 2006).

Other veteran populations may also have been involved in handling Agent Orange although probably to a small degree. As discussed in Young (2009), for example, the Department of Defense (DOD) in 1971 initiated Operation PACER IVY, which was responsible for removing stocks of Agent Orange from Vietnam to Johnston Island in the central Pacific Ocean. Operation PACER IVY was the responsibility of the 7th Air Force with assistance from Operation Ranch Hand units and the ACC. PACER IVY procedures included identification of unused herbicides, transport of the identified herbicides to a central location in Vietnam for relabeling, and, for about half of the barrels, re-drumming before shipment. Potential Agent Orange hot spots included central PACER IVY locations, such as Du Nang, Bien Hoa, and to a small extent Phu Cat and Nha Trang airbases (Young, 2006). Although this is not certain, exposures of Allied troops from PACER IVY may have been low given that most of the relabeling, repackaging, and handling of Agent Orange during PACER IVY was overseen and conducted by Chinese contractors, local Vietnamese, and the Vietnamese military. However, spills of Agent Orange in the de-drumming and storage areas that contaminated surrounding soils and asphalt were noted (Young, 2009), and suggested sources of exposure. Other possible points of contamination for Vietnam-era veterans include defoliation tests conducted in South Vietnam as part of Project AGILE; ports in New Orleans, Louisiana; Baltimore, Maryland; Seattle, Washington; Mobile, Alabama; and Gulfport, Michigan, which served as embarkation points for shipping of Agent Orange to Vietnam; storage locations on Johnston Island, where contamination could have occurred from re-drumming and maintenance of drums that contained Agent Orange; and at-sea incineration of Agent Orange as part of Operation PACER HO (Young, 2009). Because the Army of the Republic of Vietnam (ARVN) was responsible for handling, transport, and storage of Agent Orange from the time it was delivered to Vietnam until loading onto Operation Ranch Hand aircraft, Agent Orange exposures of Allied troops during these procedures may have been negligible.

Exposure of Ground Troops

In light of the widespread use of herbicides in Vietnam for many years, it is reasonable to assume that many military personnel were inadvertently exposed to the chemicals of concern. In surveys of Vietnam veterans who were not part of the Operation Ranch Hand or ACC groups, 25–55% believed that they had been exposed to herbicides (CDC, 1989a). That view has been supported by government reports (GAO, 1979) and reiterated by veterans and their representatives in testimony to the VAO committees over the last several years.

In contrast with those reports and veteran testimony, Young and colleagues provide evidence in a series of papers that is consistent with minimal exposures to herbicides (Young et al., 2004a,b). They used data from unpublished military records and environmental-fate studies to argue that ground troops had little direct contact with herbicide sprays and that TCDD residues in Vietnam had low bioavailability, respectively. They also argued that direct exposures of ground troops were relatively low because herbicide-spraying missions were carefully planned, and spraying occurred only when friendly forces were not in the target area.

To resolve the issue, numerous attempts were made in the 1980s to characterize herbicide exposures of people who served as ground troops in Vietnam (CDC, 1988; Erickson et al., 1984; NRC, 1982; Stellman and Stellman, 1986; Stellman et al., 1988). The efforts combined self-reports of contact with herbicides or military service records with aerial-spray data to produce an "exposure opportunity index" (EOI). For example, Erickson et al. (1984) created five exposure categories based on military records to examine the risks of birth defects among the offspring of veterans. Those studies were conducted carefully and provided reasonable estimates based on available data, but no means of testing the validity of the estimates were available at the time.

The search for a validation method led to the development of exposure biomarkers in veterans. Initial studies measured concentrations of dioxin in adipose tissue of veterans (Gross et al., 1984; Schecter et al., 1987). A study sponsored by the New Jersey Agent Orange Commission was the first to link dioxin concentrations in adipose tissue to dioxin concentrations in blood (Kahn et al., 1988). At the same time, the Centers for Disease Control (now the Centers for Disease Control and Prevention) undertook what came to be called the Agent Orange Validation Study, measuring TCDD in the serum portion of blood from a relatively large sample of Vietnam veterans and other Vietnam-era veterans (CDC, 1989b). The study did not find a statistically significant difference in mean serum TCDD concentrations between the groups: mean values in each group were about 4 parts per trillion (ppt), and only two Vietnam veterans had concentrations greater than 20 ppt (CDC, 1988). A review of a preliminary report of the work by an advisory panel established through the IOM concluded that the long lag between exposure and the serum measurements (about 20 years) called into question the accuracy of exposure classification based on serum concentrations. The panel concluded that estimates based on troop locations and herbicide-spraying activities might be more reliable indicators of exposure than serum measurements (IOM, 1987).

The report of the first VAO committee (IOM, 1994) proposed further work on exposure reconstruction and development of a model that could be used to categorize exposures of ground troops. The committee cautioned that serum TCDD measurements should not be regarded as a "gold standard" of exposure, that is, as a fully accurate measure of herbicide exposure. Efforts to develop exposure-reconstruction models for US Vietnam veterans are discussed later in this chapter.

One other effort to reconstruct exposure has been reported by researchers in the Republic of Korea who developed an exposure index for Korean military personnel who served in Vietnam (Kim et al., 2001, 2003). The exposure index was based on herbicide-spray patterns in military regions in which Korean personnel served during 1964–1973, time–location data on the military units stationed in Vietnam, and an exposure score derived from self-reported activities during service. The researchers were not successful in an attempt to validate their exposure index with serum dioxin measurements.

Exposure of Personnel Who Had Offshore Vietnam Service

US Navy riverine units are known to have used herbicides while patrolling inland waterways (IOM, 1994), and it is generally acknowledged that estuarine waters became contaminated with herbicides and dioxin as a result of shoreline spraying and runoff from spraying on land, particularly in heavily sprayed areas that experienced frequent flooding. Thus, military personnel who did not serve on land could have been among those exposed to the chemicals during the Vietnam conflict. In recent years, there has been concern about dioxin exposure among personnel who served offshore but within the territorial limits of the Republic of

Vietnam. It has been hypothesized that in addition to possibly experiencing drift from herbicide-spray missions, personnel on these ships that converted seawater by distillation may have been exposed via drinking water. Those concerns were heightened by findings from an Australian study (Muller et al., 2002) that showed that TCDD could be enriched in a simulation of the potable-water distillation process that was used on the US Navy and Royal Australian Navy ships during the Vietnam War era. The National Academies convened the Blue Water Navy Vietnam Veterans and Agent Orange Exposure Committee to address that specific issue; its report (IOM, 2011) found that information to determine the extent of exposure experienced by Blue Water Navy personnel was inadequate, but that there were possible routes of exposure.

EXPOSURE OF THE VIETNAMESE POPULATION

As summarized by Constable and Hatch (1985), Vietnamese researchers have made a number of attempts to characterize the herbicide exposure of residents of Vietnam in the process of trying to assess adverse reproductive outcomes. Some compared residents of the South with residents of the unsprayed North, and others endeavored to compare South Vietnamese people who lived in sprayed and unsprayed villages as determined by observed defoliation. For evaluating reproductive outcomes, pregnancy outcomes of North Vietnamese women married to veterans who had served in South Vietnam were compared with those of women whose husbands had not. In some cases, records of herbicide spraying have been used to refine exposure measurements. In assessing infant mortality, Dai et al. (1990) considered village residents to have been exposed if a herbicide mission had passed within 10 km of the village center and classified exposure further by length of residence in a sprayed area and the number of times that the area reportedly had been sprayed.

A small number of studies have provided information on TCDD concentrations in Vietnamese civilians who were exposed during the war (Schecter et al., 1986, 2002, 2006). Dwernychuk et al. (2002) emphasized the need to evaluate dioxin contamination around former air bases in Vietnam. They collected environmental and food samples, human blood, and breast milk from residents of the Aluoi Valley of central Vietnam. The investigators identified locations where relatively high dioxin concentrations remained in soil or water systems. Soil dioxin concentrations were particularly high around former airfields and military bases where herbicides were handled. Fish harvested from ponds in those areas were found to contain high dioxin concentrations. More recently, Dwernychuk (2005) elaborated on the importance of "hot spots" as important locations for future studies and argued that herbicide use at former US military installations was the most likely cause of the hot spots. The Bien Hoa Air Base, considered a hot spot because of the use of chemical defoliants around the base, was the focus of a study that examined dioxin contamination in soils in Vietnam (Mai et al.,

2007). The study found high soil concentrations but did not involve estimation of the exposure of people who lived in the vicinity of the bases.

Several publications have reported environmental concentrations and body burdens of dioxins in various areas throughout Vietnam (Brodsky et al., 2009; Feshin et al., 2008; Hatfield Consultants, 2009a,b,c; Nhu et al., 2009; Saito et al., 2010; Tai et al., 2011). Like previous publications, that by Tai et al. (2011) reported that dioxin concentrations in breast milk were related to the residence location of the mothers, with levels and total toxic equivalents (TEQs) highest in areas where herbicides were stored and sprayed during the war. PCDD and PCDF TEQ, for example, were about three times higher in the sprayed areas and four times higher in the hot spots than in unsprayed areas. However, dioxin concentrations in breast milk, even in women who lived in sprayed areas or hot spots, were lower than those documented in previous publications. The differences were attributed to the fact that the study characterized dioxin in the general population compared with the highly exposed populations of previous studies. Nevertheless, the findings of Tai et al. (2011) were consistent with earlier findings that showed pervasive exposure to dioxins more than a half-century after the Vietnam War.

Additional studies have addressed dioxin uptake in other contaminated environments. For example, Tohyama et al. (2011) assessed the exposure of 138 people, including 66 children 3–15 years old, who lived on dioxin-contaminated soil (concentrations up to 6,800 ppt) in Tokyo, Japan, focusing on people who were suspected of being exposed to the contaminated soil. For those at least 16 years old, the blood dioxin concentrations did not vary with the estimated level of contamination and were higher (10 ± 0.54 pg TEQ/g lipid) than those observed in American Vietnam-era veterans, which averaged 4 ppt in both the deployed and the nondeployed groups (CDC, 1988). For the children, however, the mean concentrations were 13 (± 1.9) and 6.6 (± 0.65) pg TEQ/g lipid (equivalent to ppt) for the 3- to 6-year-olds and the 7- to 15-year-olds, respectively, and those who were fed only breast milk had higher concentrations than did those fed a combination of breast milk and formula or only formula. The range observed in the youngest age group (0.94–46 pg TEQ/g lipid) bracketed the readings for all 138 subjects.

Demond et al. (2012) noted the results of the University of Michigan Dioxin Exposure Study of 946 residents of the countries surrounding the Dow facilities (Demond et al., 2008, Garabrant et al., 2009) and reviewed other studies that measured concentrations in human serum arising from exposure to dioxin-contaminated soil. Their overall conclusion was that serum TCDD concentrations did not directly reflect the degree of soil contamination; consumption of animal products raised on the contaminated soil, however, was related to increases in serum TEQs.

The above studies are not directly relevant to the present committee's task, but they may prove useful in future epidemiologic studies of the Vietnamese population and in the development of risk-mitigation policies.

MODELS FOR CHARACTERIZING HERBICIDE EXPOSURE[1]

The IOM, following up on the recommendations contained in the original *VAO* report (IOM, 1994), issued a request for proposals seeking individuals and organizations to develop historical exposure-reconstruction approaches suitable for epidemiologic studies of herbicide exposure of US veterans during the Vietnam War (IOM, 1997). The request resulted in the project Characterizing Exposure of Veterans to Agent Orange and Other Herbicides in Vietnam. The project was carried out under contract by a team of researchers in Columbia University's Mailman School of Public Health. The Columbia University project integrated various sources of information concerning spray activities and information on locations of military units assigned to Vietnam, all compiled into a database, to generate individualized estimates of the exposure potential of troops serving in Vietnam (Stellman and Stellman, 2003)

"Mobility-factor" analysis, a new concept for studying troop movement, was developed for use in reconstructing herbicide-exposure histories. The analysis is a three-part classification system for characterizing the location and movement of military units in Vietnam. It comprises a mobility designation (stable or mobile), a distance designation (usually in kilometers) to indicate how far a unit might travel in a day, and a notation of the modes of travel available to the unit (by air, by water, or on the ground by truck, tank, or armored personnel carrier). A mobility factor was assigned to every unit that served in Vietnam.

The data were combined into a geographic information system (GIS) for Vietnam. Herbicide-spraying records were integrated into the GIS and linked with data on military-unit locations to derive individual exposure-opportunity scores. The results are the subject of reports by the contractor (Stellman and Stellman, 2003) and the Committee on the Assessment of Wartime Exposure to Herbicides in Vietnam (IOM, 2003a,b). A summary of the findings on the extent and pattern of herbicide spraying (Stellman et al., 2003a), a description of the GIS for characterizing exposure to Agent Orange and other herbicides in Vietnam (Stellman et al., 2003b), and an explanation of the exposure-opportunity models based on that work (Stellman and Stellman, 2004) have been published in peer-reviewed journals. The publications have argued that it is feasible to conduct epidemiologic investigations of veterans who served as ground troops during the Vietnam War. The IOM later issued a report that examined the feasibility of using the Agent Orange Reconstruction Model developed by Columbia University (IOM, 2008). The report concluded that "despite the shortcomings of

[1]Since initial publication of this update and release of its findings, the IOM received a letter from Ginevan et al. (2013) following up on their earlier correspondence (Ross and Ginevan, 2012) and raising concerns about the discussion of the Stellmans' EOI model and associated critiques. Their letters, as well as one from Stellman and Stellman (2013), are available in the Public Access File for this project. This ongoing dispute about modeling of Vietnam veterans' exposure to herbicides played no role in the conclusions reached by the committee for this update.

the exposure assessment model in its current form and the inherent limitations in the approach, the committee agreed that the model holds promise for supporting informative epidemiologic studies of herbicides and health among Vietnam veterans and that it should be used to conduct studies."

A pair of industry-sponsored papers that used a mathematical model of herbicide dispersion and deposition from aerial spraying concluded that actual ground deposition of Agent Orange was many orders of magnitude lower than that predicted by previous exposure estimations proposed for use in evaluating ground-troop health effects (Ginevan et al., 2009a,b). The new papers first undertook a quantitative evaluation of the Stellman EOI model (Stellman and Stellman, 2004; Stellman et al., 2003a,b) recommended for possible use in an epidemiologic evaluation of ground troops by IOM (2008). The new evaluation revealed frequent and substantial inconsistencies in the calculated EOI that were based in part on the use of a central equation "contrary to a large body of pesticide exposure assessment practice," the general imprecision of spray-flight path records, the use of 1.2-km^2 exposure cells in the model, and "unknown computational errors" in the model. The analyses demonstrated unexpected and unexplained 1,000-fold differences in model output for sample flight paths that appear to be in all respects equivalent. The authors proposed the use of the AgDRIFT Tier III model as a more accurate and appropriate estimator of potential exposures for ground troops. That model uses a combination of standard Lagrangian and Gaussian techniques in combination with empirically derived information, such as aerosol penetration through a forest canopy, to estimate ground-level exposure. The AgDRIFT Tier III model is purportedly validated and used by the US Forest Service to plan aerial application of various agents to forests. The AgDRIFT model predicts a much smaller area under the spray path and Agent Orange concentrations lower by several orders of magnitude than the EOI estimates for the same set of sample flight paths. That effect is particularly pronounced at points distant from the spray path; the AgDRIFT model predicts Agent Orange exposures up to 20 orders of magnitude lower than the EOI model at a point 4 km away from the flight-path centerline. Finally, the authors pointed out that the use of any exposure model for ground troops will be severely limited by the imprecision of spatial and temporal measures of troop movements.

Stellman and Stellman (2013) provided the committee with a letter submitted to the editor of the *Journal of Exposure Science and Environmental Epidemiology* in response to the critique of their model in Ginevan et al. (2009b); they also provided supplemental material. In their letter, Stellman and Stellman, the senior authors of the EOI model, question the validity of most, if not all, of the Ginevan et al. (2009a,b) findings, citing serious errors regarding the paper's use of "incorrect data and its fundamentally incorrect and negative interpretations." The Stellmans, for example, noted several key errors in Ginevan's reporting of "E4 scores," which were used as the basis of much of the Ginevan et al. critique of the EOI model. Stellman and Stellman found that Ginevan et al. used in their analysis raw E4 scores, instead of the log-transformed E4 scores as used by the Stellmans. As a result, variability in the EOI on the flight line as reported by Ginevan et al. was artificially high; the Stellmans' reports that a log-transform of the E4 scores produces reasonable values that vary within 10% around the mean for each mission. Furthermore, the Stellmans' state that use of raw E4 scores leads to a host of other incorrect assertions and theories, such as "their use of an incorrect score of 60,791 for one point, when the true score is zero in our [the EOI] system."

Given the lack of data to validate either model and the lack of an impartial evaluation of both models by a third party, it is not possible for the committee to ascertain the accuracy and precision of estimates from either model or the claims of either Stellman and Stellman (2013) or Ginevan et al. (2009a,b). It should also be noted that because the intent and outcomes of the two models differ substantially, model results and interpretation are likely to differ. The Stellman and Stellman model, for example, predicts potential exposure to troops on the basis of military data on spray history and troop locations. The AgDRIFT Tier III model, in contrast, predicts ground concentrations and their spatial dispersion; by design, the AgDRIFT model does not consider troop-location data. Many studies have shown that the agreement and correlation between pollutant exposures and concentrations can be poor, so it is not surprising that the results and interpretation of two models differ substantially, especially given command directives that prohibited spraying when Allied troops were on the ground. The command directives suggest that the opportunity for Vietnam veterans to be exposed would be lowest in areas under the spray path, where concentrations would be highest.

Since *Update 2010*, Young and Cecil (2011) have published a review that states that few, if any, ground-troop veterans were exposed to Agent Orange on the basis of arguments made earlier (Young et al., 2004a,b). They also state that the EOI model is flawed, given deficiencies in model assumptions concerning spray operations and areas; information not considered by the model, such as meteorologic characteristics; and command directives that prohibited spraying when Allied troops were on the ground in the areas to be sprayed.

The issue of Allied troop presence during spraying is one of the central issues in the debate regarding the use of the EOI model. The EOI model relied on actual military data on spray history and troop locations, which, as pointed out both by Stellman and Stellman (2004) and Young (2009), are limited in their spatial and temporal resolution and accuracy. The accuracy of the records with regard to missions flown, mission locations, number of gallons sprayed, among other important information, was examined by MITRE Corporation (Heizer, 1971). MITRE reported that about 2% of the records were missing data, 6% of the records had serious transcription or measurement errors, and 23% of records that had complete data were off by 50% in the reported distance sprayed (Young, 2009). However, the overall quality of the data was found to be good and could be improved with adjustments, as performed by Stellman (2003a,b) and others (ESG, 1985; NRC, 1974). Whether the adjustments improved the quality of the military data is not known, but Young (2009) has criticized methods used to adjust the records.

Nevertheless, the committee cannot dismiss EOI model findings solely on the basis that command directives prohibited spraying, given that the EOI model is based on actual military data. Inasmuch as the AgDRIFT and EOI models focus on different outcomes, however, the committee does not recommend that one model be used instead of the other for the purposes of epidemiologic studies, nor does it advocate or discourage use of either the AgDRIFT or the EOI model in epidemiologic studies. If either model is used in epidemiologic studies to predict exposure, results should be interpreted in light of the model limitations noted.

The controversy surrounding the use of the EOI and AgDRIFT models points to the difficulties inherent in assessing Agent Orange exposures of Vietnam veterans. For Operation Ranch Hand and ACC cohorts, exposure assessment is the most straightforward of all assessments of Vietnam veterans in that their exposures to Agent Orange originate predominantly from one source and one exposure route. Nevertheless, attempts to quantify their exposures, even at the level of serum biomarkers of exposure, have been less than satisfactory. For ground troops, who make up the largest group of concern, exposure assessment is considerably more complex; multiple, dispersed sources of Agent Orange exposure over multiple possible routes occurred over an extended period long ago. As a result, few studies have characterized exposure beyond "in-theater" vs "not-in-theater" comparisons. Considerable work, however, has been done by National Academies committees and others to develop exposure assessments for ground troops based on numbers, patterns, and timing of aerial spray missions combined with troop-location information. Aerial spraying has been the focus of much of the committee's efforts given that 95% of Agent Orange used during the Vietnam War was applied by aerial spraying (Stellman et al., 2003a,b).

Regardless, it is important to note that sole emphasis on aerial spraying as an exposure source should be reconsidered. To ascribe a health effect to an exposure in an epidemiologic study accurately, one must account for *all* sources and routes of exposure—a concept now popularly termed total exposure assessment. In the Vietnam theater, there were undoubtedly multiple sources and routes of TCDD exposure of ground troops other than being directly under an aerial-spray mission. The relative magnitudes of those sources and whether the aerial spray route predominated are unknown and now probably unknowable. For instance, troops in the field commonly collected drinking water from streams. Some of those streams are still highly polluted with TCDD. Although the ultimate source of the TCDD in the streams may have been aerial spraying, the concentration of TCDD in the water would not necessarily correlate with spray-mission exposure estimates and could conceivably far exceed the "direct exposure" estimates, depending on the terrain, rainfall, timing of water collection, and other unknown factors. The dynamic nature of TCDD released into the environment is largely unknown quantitatively, so an exposure assessment that accounts for all sources of TCDD exposure is impossible. In addition, an assessment of total exposure must include an understanding of coexposures that could confound TCDD exposure analyses or otherwise directly account for an observed health effect. Studies have not factored coexposures into health risk estimates.

METHODOLOGIC ISSUES IN EXPOSURE ASSESSMENT

Analyses of Vietnam-veteran studies have been an important source of information for understanding associations between the herbicides used in Vietnam and specific health outcomes, but, as discussed in Chapter 2, the committee has extended its review of the scientific literature to other populations whose exposure could be estimated with greater accuracy. Those populations are discussed in detail in Chapter 5. We focus here on several key methodologic issues that complicate development of accurate estimates of exposure of the Vietnam-veteran population and the other study populations discussed in this report: the latent period between exposure and disease, exposure misclassification, and exposure specificity.

Latency

The temporal relationship between exposure and disease is complex and often difficult to define in studies of human populations. Many diseases do not appear immediately after exposure. Cancer, for example, might not appear for many years after exposure. The time between a defined exposure period and the occurrence of disease is often referred to as a latent period (IOM, 2004). Exposures can be brief (sometimes referred to as acute exposures) or protracted (sometimes referred to as chronic exposures). At one extreme, an exposure can be the result of a single event, as in an accidental poisoning. At the other extreme, a person exposed to a chemical that is stored in the body may continue to experience "internal exposure" for years even if exposure from the environment has ceased. The definition of the proper time frame for duration of exposure constitutes a challenge to exposure scientists.

Misclassification

Exposure misclassification in epidemiologic studies can affect estimates of risk. A typical situation is in a case-control study in which the reported measurement of exposure of either group or both groups can be misclassified. The simplest situation to consider is one in which the exposure is classified into just two levels, for example, "ever exposed" vs "never exposed." If the probability of exposure misclassification is the same in cases and controls (that is, nondifferential), it can be shown that the estimated association between disease and exposure is biased toward the null value; in other words, one would expect the true association to be stronger than the observed association. However, if the probability of misclassification is different between cases and controls, bias in the estimated association can occur in either direction, and the true association might be stronger or weaker than the observed association.

The situation in which exposure is classified into more than two levels is somewhat more complicated. Dosemeci et al. (1990) have demonstrated that in that situation the slope of a dose–response trend is not necessarily attenuated toward the null value even if the probability of misclassification is the same in the two groups of subjects being compared; the observed trend in disease risk among the several levels of exposure may be either an overestimate or an underestimate of the true trend. Greenland and Gustafson (2006) have discussed the effect of exposure misclassification on the statistical significance of the result, demonstrating that if one adjusts for exposure misclassification when the exposure is represented as binary (for example, ever exposed vs never exposed), the resulting association is not necessarily more significant than in the unadjusted estimate. That result remains true even though the observed magnitude of the association (for example, the relative risk) might be increased.

Specificity

Incorporation of findings of studies of persons exposed to components of the herbicides sprayed in Vietnam requires some decisions about their relative contributions to the VAO project's evidentiary database. Only a few herbicidal chemicals were used as defoliants during the Vietnam conflict: esters and salts of 2,4-D and 2,4,5-T, cacodylic acid, and picloram in various formulations. Many scientific studies reviewed by the committee report exposures to broad categories of chemicals rather than to those specific chemicals. The categories are presented in Tables 3-2 and 3-3 with their relevance to the committee's charge. The information in these tables has helped to guide the committee's evaluation of epidemiologic studies. Earlier VAO committees did not address the issue of exposure specificity in exactly this manner. The committee for *VAO* and the first several updates gave more weight to results that were based on job title (for example, "farmer" with no additional information) than have the committees for the last four updates, but they entirely excluded findings from the Yusho and Yucheng polychlorinated dibenzofuran and biphenyl (PCDF and PCB) poisonings, whereas recent committees have considered studies that analyzed for dioxin-like PCDF and PCB congeners and expressed the results in terms of TEQs. Nonetheless, those studies that report TEQs based only on mono-ortho PCBs (which are PCBs 105, 114, 118, 123, 156, 157, 167, and 189) were given very limited consideration since mono-ortho PCBs typically contribute less than 10% to total TEQs, based on the World Health Organization revised TEFs of 2005 (La Rocca et al., 2008; van den Berg et al., 2006).

Many studies have examined the relationship between exposure to "pesti-

TABLE 3-2 Current Committee Guidance for the Classification of Exposure Information in Epidemiologic Studies That Focus on the Use of Pesticides or Herbicides, and Relevance of the Information to the Committee's Charge to Evaluate Exposures to 2,4-D and 2,4,5-T (Phenoxy Herbicides), Cacodylic Acid, and Picloram

Specificity of Exposure Reported in Study	Additional Information	Relevance to Committee's Charge
Pesticides	COIs were not used, or there was no additional information	Not relevant
	COIs were used	Limited relevance
Herbicides	COIs were not used	Not relevant
	There was no additional information	Limited relevance
	COIs were used	Relevant
Phenoxy herbicides	—	Highly relevant
2,4-D or 2,4,5-T	—	Highly relevant
Cacodylic acid[a]	—	Highly relevant
Picloram	—	Highly relevant

NOTE: 2,4-D, 2,4-dichlorophenoxyacetic acid; 2,4,5-T, 2,4,5-trichlorophenoxyacetic acid; COI, chemical of interest.

[a]None of the epidemiologic studies reviewed by the committee to date has specified exposure to cacodylic acid.

cides" and adverse health outcomes, and others have used the category of "herbicides" without identifying specific chemicals. A careful reading of a scientific report often reveals that none of the chemicals of interest (COIs) (that is, those used in Vietnam, as delineated above) contributed to the exposures of the study population, so such studies could be excluded from consideration. But in many cases, the situation is more ambiguous. For example, reports that define exposure in the broad category of "pesticides," with no further information, have little relevance to the committee's charge to determine associations between exposures to herbicides used in Vietnam and adverse health outcomes. Reports that define exposure in the more restricted category of "herbicides" are of greater relevance but are of little value unless it is clear from additional information that exposure to one or more of the herbicides used in Vietnam occurred in the study population—for example, if a published report indicates that the COIs were among the pesticides or herbicides used by the study population, the lead author of the report has been contacted and has indicated that the COIs were among the chemicals used, the COIs are used commonly for the crops identified in the study, or the COIs are used commonly for a specific purpose, such as removal of weeds and shrubs along highways.

TABLE 3-3 Current Committee Guidance for the Classification of Exposure Information in Epidemiologic Studies That Focus on Exposure to Dioxin-Like Chemicals and Relevance of the Information to the Committee's Charge

Specificity of Exposure Reported in Study	Additional Information	Relevance to Committee's Charge
Dioxin-like chemicals	Exposure to PCBs or polychlorinated dibenzofuran (PCDFs)	Limited relevance
Dioxin-like chemicals	Results expressed in terms of (total) toxic equivalent (TEQs) or concentrations of individual congeners recognized as having dioxin-like activity[a]	Highly relevant
TCDD or mixture of PCDDs	Established on the basis of environmental sampling or work histories	Highly relevant
TCDD or mixture of PCDDs	Concentrations in tissues of a subset of participants (preferably soon after exposure)	Very highly relevant
TCDD or mixture of PCDDs	Concentrations in tissues of individual participants (preferably soon after exposure)	Most informative

NOTE: PCB, polychlorinated biphenyl; PCDD, polychlorinated dibenzo-*p*-dioxin (highly chlorinated, if four or more chlorines); PCDF, polychlorinated dibenzofurans; TCDD, 2,3,7,8-tetrachlorodibenzo-*p*-dioxin; TEQ, toxicity equivalent.

[a]The values of toxic equivalency factors for individual dioxin-like chemicals, which are weighted by concentration and summed to derive TEQs, are presented in Table 4-2.

Among the various chemical classes of herbicides that have been identified in published studies reviewed by the committee, phenoxy herbicides, particularly 2,4-D and 2,4,5-T, are directly relevant to the exposures experienced by US military forces in Vietnam. On the basis of the assumption that compounds with similar chemical structure may have analogous biologic activity, information on the effects of other chemicals in the phenoxy herbicide class—such as Silvex, 2-methyl-4-chlorophenoxyacetic acid, 2-(2-methyl-4-chlorophenoxy) propionic acid (Mecoprop), and dicamba—has been factored into the committee's deliberations with somewhat less weight. The very few epidemiologic findings on exposure to picloram or cacodylic acid have been regarded as highly relevant. The committee has decided to include many studies that report on unspecified herbicides in the health-effects sections, and their results have been entered into the health-outcome–specific tables; however, these studies tend to contribute little to the evidence considered by the committee. The many studies that provide chemical-specific exposure information are believed to be far more informative for the committee's purposes.

A similar issue arises in the evaluation of studies that document exposure to dioxin-like compounds. Most "dioxin" studies reviewed by the committee have focused on TCDD, but TCDD is only one of a number of PCDDs. The committee recognizes that in real-world conditions exposure to TCDD virtually never occurs in isolation and that there are hundreds of similar compounds to which humans might be exposed, including other PCDDs, polychlorinated dibenzofurans (PCDFs), and PCBs. Exposure to TCDD is almost always accompanied by exposure to one or more of the other compounds. The literature on the other compounds, particularly PCBs, has not been reviewed systematically by the committee unless TCDD was identified as an important component of the exposure or the risks of health effects were expressed in terms of TEQs, which are the sums of toxicity equivalence factors for individual dioxin-like compounds as measured by activity with the aryl hydrocarbon receptor (AHR). The committee took that approach for two reasons. First, exposure of Vietnam veterans to substantial amounts of the other chemicals, relative to exposure to TCDD, has not been documented. Second, the most important mechanism for TCDD toxicity involves its ability to bind to and activate the AHR. Many of the other chemicals act by different or multiple mechanisms, so it is difficult to attribute toxic effects after such exposures specifically to TCDD. Furthermore, people's environmental exposures to dioxin-like chemicals and their non–dioxin-like counterparts are to mixtures of components that tend to correlate, so it is not surprising that specific chemicals measured in a person's serum also tend to correlate; this means that it will be difficult for epidemiologic studies to attribute any observed association to a particular chemical configuration (Longnecker and Michalek, 2000). Analyses in terms of TEQs circumvent that problem to some extent.

REFERENCES[2]

AFHS (Air Force Health Study). 1991. *An Epidemiologic Investigation of Health Effects in Air Force Personnel Following Exposure to Herbicides. Serum Dioxin Analysis of 1987 Examination Results.* Air Force Health Study. Brooks AFB, TX: USAF School of Aerospace Medicine. 9 vols.

Armstrong BK, White E, Saracci R. 1994. *Principles of Exposure Assessment in Epidemiology.* New York: Oxford University Press.

Brodsky ES, Shelepchikov AA, Feshin DB, Roumak VS, Umnova NV, Kuznetsov AN, Sau TK, Truong NX, Pavlov DS. 2009. The current level of dioxin pollution in the area of large-scale spraying of Agent Orange in Vietnam. *Doklady Biological Sciences* 429:526–530.

CDC (Centers for Disease Control). 1988. Serum 2,3,7,8-tetrachlorodibenzo-*p*-dioxin levels in US Army Vietnam era veterans. *Journal of the American Medical Association* 260:1249–1254.

CDC. 1989a. *Health Status of Vietnam Veterans.* Vietnam Experience Study. Atlanta: US Department of Health and Human Services. Vols. I–V, Supplements A–C.

CDC. 1989b. *Comparison of Serum Levels of 2,3,7,8-Tetrachlorodibenzo-*p*-Dioxin with Indirect Estimates of Agent Orange Exposure Among Vietnam Veterans: Final Report.* Centers for Disease Control. Atlanta: US Department of Health and Human Services.

Checkoway H, Pearce NE, Kriebel D. 2004. *Research Methods in Occupational Epidemiology* (2nd Edition). New York: Oxford University Press.

[2]Throughout this report, the same alphabetic indicator after year of publication is used consistently for a given reference when there are multiple citations by the same first author in a given year. The convention of assigning the alphabetic indicators in order of citation in a given chapter is not followed.

Cochrane WP, Sirgh J, Miles W, Wakeford B, Scott J. 1982. Analysis of technical and formulated products of 2,4-dichlorophenoxyacetic acid for the presence of chlorinated dibenzo-*p*-dioxins. In: Hutzinger O, Frei RW, Merian E, Pocchiari F, eds. *Chlorinated Dioxins and Related Compounds: Impact on the Environment.* Oxford: Pergamon Press, pp. 209–213.

Constable JD, Hatch MC. 1985. Reproductive effects of herbicide exposure in Vietnam: Recent studies by the Vietnamese and others. *Teratogenesis, Carcinogenesis, and Mutagenesis* 5:231–250.

Dai LC, Phuong NTN, Thom LH, Thuy TT, Van NTT, Cam LH, Chi HTK, Thuy LB. 1990. A comparison of infant mortality rates between two Vietnamese villages sprayed by defoliants in wartime and one unsprayed village. *Chemosphere* 20:1005–1012.

Demond A, Adriaens P, Towey T, Chang SC, Hong B, Chen Q, Chang CW, Franzblau A, Garabrant D, Gillespie B, Hedgeman E, Knutson K, Lee CY, Lepkowski J, Olson K, Ward B, Zwica L, Luksemburg W, Maier M. 2008. Statistical comparison of residential soil concentrations of PCDDs, PCDFs, and PCBs from two communities in Michigan. *Environmental Science and Technology* 42:5441–5448.

Demond A, Franzblau A, Garabrant D, Jiang X, Adriaens P, Chen Q, Gillespie B, Hao W, Hong B, Jolliet O, Lepkowski J. 2012. Human exposure from dioxins in soil. *Environmental Science and Technology* 46(3):1296–1302.

Dosemeci M, Wacholder S, Lubin JH. 1990. Does nondifferential misclassification of exposure always bias a true effect toward the null value? *American Journal of Epidemiology* 132(4):746–748.

Dwernychuk LW. 2005. Dioxin hot spots in Vietnam. *Chemosphere* 60(7):998–999.

Dwernychuk LW, Cau HD, Hatfield CT, Boivin TG, Hung TM, Dung PT, Thai ND. 2002. Dioxin reservoirs in southern Viet Nam–A legacy of Agent Orange. *Chemosphere* 47(2):117–137.

EPA (US Environmental Protection Agency). 1992. *Worker Protection Standard.* Washington, DC: US Environmental Protection Agency.

Erickson JD, Mulinare J, Mcclain PW. 1984. Vietnam veterans' risks for fathering babies with birth defects. *Journal of the American Medical Association* 252:903–912.

ESG (Environmental Support Group). 1985. *Services HERBS Tape—A Record of Helicopter and Ground Spraying Missions, Aborts, Leaks, and Incidents.* NTIS Document ADA 229879, Springfield, VA.

FAO/UNEP (Food and Agriculture Organization, United Nations Environment Programme). 2009. *2,4,5-T and Its Salts and Esters. Decision Guidance Documents.* Secretariat for the Rotterdam Convention on the Prior Informed Consent Procedure for Certain Hazardous Chemicals and Pesticides in International Trade. Joint FAO/UNEP Programme for the Operation of the Prior Informed Consent. Accessed March 9, 2009, at http://www.pic.int/en/DGDs/2,4,5-TEN.doc.

Feshin DB, Shelepchikov AA, Brodskii ES, Kalinkevich GA, Mir-Kadyrova EY, Rumak VS, Pavlov DS. 2008. Current levels of PCDDs and PCDFs in the placenta and breast milk of the population of Vietnam. *Doklady Biological Sciences* 423:443–446.

GAO (General Accounting Office). 1978. *Use of Agent Orange in Vietnam.* Washington, DC: GAO. CED-78-158.

GAO. 1979. *US Ground Troops in South Vietnam Were in Areas Sprayed with Herbicide Orange.* Report by the Comptroller General of the United States. Washington, DC: GAO. FPCD 80-23.

Garabrant D, Franzblau A, Lepkowski J, Gillespie B, Adriaens P, Demond A, Hedgeman E, Knutson K, Zwica L, Olson K, Towey T, Chen Q, Hong B, Chang CW, Lee SY, Ward B, LaDronka K, Luksemburg W, Maier M. 2009. The University of Michigan dioxin exposure study: Predictors of human serum dioxin concentrations in Midland and Saginaw, Michigan. *Environmental Health Perspectives* 117:818–824.

Ginevan ME, Ross JH, Watkins DK. 2009a. Assessing exposure to allied ground troops in the Vietnam War: A comparison of AgDRIFT and exposure opportunity index models. *Journal of Exposure Science and Environmental Epidemiology* 19(2):187–200.

Ginevan ME, Watkins DK, Ross JH, O'Boyle RA. 2009b. Assessing exposure to allied ground troops in the Vietnam War: A quantitative evaluation of the Stellman exposure opportunity index model. *Chemosphere* 75(11):1512–1518.

Ginevan ME, Watkins DK, Ross JH. 2013. *Comments to the IOM Committee Regarding the* Veterans and Agent Orange: Update 2012 *Draft Report*. In Public Access File for the Committee to Review the Health Effects in Vietnam Veterans of Exposure to Herbicides: Ninth Biennial Update (received December 23, 2013).

Gough M. 1986. *Dioxin, Agent Orange: The Facts.* New York: Plenum Press.

Greenland P, Gustafson S. 2006. The performance of random coefficient regression in accounting for residual confounding. *Biometrics* 62(3):760–768.

Gross ML, Lay JO, Lippstreu D, Lyon PA, Kangas N, Harless RL, Taylor SE. 1984. 2,3,7,8-tetrachlorodibenzo-*p*-dioxin levels in adipose tissue of Vietnam veterans. *Environmental Research* 33:261.

Hatfield Consultants. 2009a. *Comprehensive Assessment of Dioxin Contamination in Da Nang Airport, Vietnam: Environmental Levels, Human Exposure and Options for Mitigating Impacts–Final Report.* North Vancouver, British Columbia, Canada: Ford Foundation Special Initiative on Agent Orange/Dioxin.

Hatfield Consultants. 2009b. Appendices. North Vancouver, British Columbia, Canada: Ford Foundation Special Initiative on Agent Orange/Dioxin.

Hatfield Consultants. 2009c. *Comprehensive Assessment of Dioxin Contamination in Da Nang Airport, Vietnam: Environmental Levels, Human Exposure and Options for Mitigating Impacts—Final Summary of Findings.* North Vancouver, British Columbia, Canada: Ford Foundation Special Initiative on Agent Orange/Dioxin.

Heizer JR. 1971. *Data Quality Analysis of the HERB 01 Data File.* MITRE Technical Report, MTR-5105. Prepared for the Defense Communications Agency. McLean, VA: MITRE.

IOM (Institute of Medicine). 1987. *Review of Comparison of Serum Levels of 2,3,7,8-TCDD with Indirect Estimates of Agent Orange Exposure in Vietnam Veterans.* Fifth Letter Report. Washington DC: National Academy Press.

IOM. 1994. *Veterans and Agent Orange: Health Effects of Herbicides Used in Vietnam.* Washington, DC: National Academy Press.

IOM. 1997. *Characterizing Exposure of Veterans to Agent Orange and Other Herbicides Used in Vietnam: Scientific Considerations Regarding a Request for Proposals for Research.* Washington, DC: National Academy Press.

IOM. 2003a. *Characterizing Exposure of Veterans to Agent Orange and Other Herbicides Used in Vietnam: Interim Findings and Recommendations.* Washington, DC: The National Academies Press.

IOM. 2003b. *Characterizing Exposure of Veterans to Agent Orange and Other Herbicides Used in Vietnam: Final Report.* Washington, DC: The National Academies Press.

IOM. 2004. *Veterans and Agent Orange: Length of Presumptive Period for Association Between Exposure and Respiratory Cancer.* Washington, DC: The National Academies Press.

IOM. 2006. *Disposition of the Air Force Health Study.* Washington, DC: The National Academies Press.

IOM. 2008. *The Utility of Proximity-Based Herbicide Exposure Assessment in Epidemiologic Studies of Vietnam Veterans.* Washington DC: The National Academies Press.

IOM. 2011. *Blue Water Navy Vietnam Veterans and Agent Orange Exposure.* Washington DC: The National Academies Press.

Kahn PC, Gochfeld M, Nygren M, Hansson M, Rappe C, Velez H, Ghent-Guenther T, Wilson WP. 1988. Dioxins and dibenzofurans in blood and adipose tissue of Agent Orange-exposed Vietnam veterans and matched controls. *Journal of the American Medical Association* 259:1661–1667.

Kang HK, Dalager NA, Needham LL, Patterson DG, Matanoski GM, Kanchanaraksa S, Lees PSJ. 2001. US Army Chemical Corps Vietnam Veterans Health Study: Preliminary results. *Chemosphere* 43:943–949.

Kang HK, Dalager NA, Needham LL, Patterson DG, Lees PSJ, Yates K, Matanoski GM. 2006. Health status of Army Chemical Corps Vietnam veterans who sprayed defoliant in Vietnam. *American Journal of Industrial Medicine* 49(11):875–884.

Kern PA, Said S, Jackson WG Jr, Michalek JE. 2004. Insulin sensitivity following agent orange exposure in Vietnam veterans with high blood levels of 2,3,7,8-tetrachlorodibenzo-*p*-dioxin. *Journal of Clinical Endocrinology and Metabolism* 89(9):4665–4672.

Kim JS, Kang HK, Lim HS, Cheong HK, Lim MK. 2001. A study on the correlation between categorizations of the individual exposure levels to Agent Orange and serum dioxin levels among the Korean Vietnam veterans. *Korean Journal of Preventive Medicine* 34(1):80–88.

Kim JS, Lim HS, Cho SI, Cheong HK, Lim MK. 2003. Impact of Agent Orange exposure among Korean Vietnam veterans. *Industrial Health* 41:149–157.

La Rocca C, Alivernini S, Badiali M, Cornoldi A, Iacovella N, Silvestroni L, Spera G, Turrio-Baldassarri L. 2008. TEQs and body burden for PCDDs, PCDFs, and dioxin-like PCBs in human adipose tissue. *Chemosphere* 73(1):92–96.

Lilienfeld DE, Gallo MA. 1989. 2,4-D, 2,4,5-T and 2,3,7,8-TCDD: An overview. *Epidemiological Review* 11:28–58.

Longnecker MP, Michalek JE. 2000. Serum dioxin level in relation to diabetes mellitus among Air Force veterans with background levels of exposure. *Epidemiology* 11(1):44–48.

Mai TA, Doan TV, Tarradellas J, de Alencastro LF, Grandjean D. 2007. Dioxin contamination in soils in Southern Vietnam. *Chemosphere* 67(9):1802–1807.

Michalek JE, Wolfe WH, Miner JC, Papa TM, Pirkle JL. 1995. Indices of TCDD exposure and TCDD body burden in veterans of Operation Ranch Hand. *Journal of Exposure Analysis and Environmental Epidemiology* 5(2):209–223.

Michalek JE, Akhtar FZ, Longnecker MP, Burton JE. 2001. Relation of serum 2,3,7,8-tetrachlorodibenzo-*p*-dioxin (TCDD) level to hematological examination results in veterans of Operation Ranch Hand. *Archives of Environmental Health* 56(5):396–405.

Michalek JE, Ketchum NS, Tripathi RC. 2003. Diabetes mellitus and 2,3,7,8-tetrachlorodibenzo-*p*-dioxin elimination in veterans of Operation Ranch Hand. *Journal of Toxicology and Environmental Health, Part A* 66(3):211–221.

MRI (Midwest Research Institute). 1967. *Assessment of Ecological Effects of Extensive or Repeated Use of Herbicides.* MRI Project No. 3103-B. Kansas City, MO: MRI. NTIS AD-824-314.

Muller JF, Gaus C, Bundred K, Alberts V, Moore MR, Horsley K. 2002. *Co-distillation of Agent Orange and Other Persistent Organic Pollutants in Evaporative Water Distillation.* Funded by the Australian Department of Veterans' Affairs.

Nhu DD, Kido T, Naganuma R, Sawano N, Tawara K, Nishijo M, Nakagawa H, Hung NN, Thom LTH. 2009. A GIS study of dioxin contamination in a Vietnamese region sprayed with herbicide. *Environmental Health and Preventive Medicine* 14(6):353–360.

NRC (National Research Council). 1974. *The Effects of Herbicides in South Vietnam.* Washington, DC: National Academy Press.

NRC. 1980. *Review of US Air Force Protocol: Epidemiological Investigation of Health Effects in Air Force Personnel Following Exposure to Herbicide Orange.* Washington, DC: National Academy Press.

NRC. 1982. *The Effects of Exposure to Agent Orange on Ground Troops in Vietnam: A Report of the Subcommittee Appointed to Review a Protocol.* Washington, DC: National Academy Press.

NZIC (New Zealand Institute of Chemistry). 2009. *The production of phenoxy herbicides.* New Zealand Institute of Chemistry. Accessed March 9, 2009, at http://nzic.org.nz/ChemProcesses/production/index.html.

Pavuk M, Schecter AJ, Akhtar FZ, Michalek JE. 2003. Serum 2,3,7,8-tetrachlorodibenzo-*p*-dioxin (TCDD) levels and thyroid function in Air Force veterans of the Vietnam War. *Annals of Epidemiology* 13(5):335–343.

Rappe C, Buser HR, Bosshardt HP. 1978. Identification and quantitation of polychlorinated dibenzo-*p*-dioxins (PCDDs) and dibenzofurans (PCDFs) in 2,4,5-T ester formulations and herbicide orange. *Chemosphere* 5:431–438.

Ross J, Ginevan M. 2012. *Comments to the IOM Committee Regarding Discussions of Exposure Evaluation and Modeling in Two Recent IOM Reports.* In Public Access File for the Committee to Review the Health Effects in Vietnam Veterans of Exposure to Herbicides: Ninth Biennial Update (received October 24, 2012).

Saito K, Nhu DD, Suzuki H, Kido T, Naganuma R, Sakakibara C, Tawara K, Nishijo M, Nakagawa H, Kusama K, Dung PT, Thom LH, Hung NN. 2010. Association between dioxin concentrations in breast milk and food group intake in Vietnam. *Environmental Health and Preventive Medicine* 15(1):48–56.

Schecter A, Ryan JJ, Constable JD. 1986. Chlorinated dibenzo-*p*-dioxin and dibenzofuran levels in human adipose tissue and milk samples from the north and south of Vietnam. *Chemosphere* 15:1613–1620.

Schecter A, Constable JD, Arghestani S, Tong H, Gross ML. 1987. Elevated levels 2,3,7,8-tetrachlorodibenzodioxin in adipose tissue of certain US veterans of the Vietnam war. *Chemosphere* 16:1997–2002.

Schecter A, Pavuk M, Constable JD, Dai LC, Papke O. 2002. A follow-up: High level of dioxin contamination in Vietnamese from Agent Orange, three decades after the end of spraying [letter]. *Journal of Occupational and Environmental Medicine* 44(3):218–220.

Schecter A, Quynh HT, Papke O, Tung KC, Constable JD. 2006. Agent Orange, dioxins, and other chemicals of concern in Vietnam: Update 2006. *Journal of Occupational and Environmental Medicine* 48(4):408–413.

Stellman JM, Stellman SD. 2003. *Contractor's Final Report: Characterizing Exposure of Veterans to Agent Orange and Other Herbicides in Vietnam.* Submitted to the National Academy of Sciences, Institute of Medicine in fulfillment of Subcontract VA-5124-98-0019, June 30, 2003.

Stellman JM, Stellman SD. 2013. Letter submitted to the editor of *Journal of Exposure Science and Environmental Epidemiology* concerning Ginevan et al. (2009b) and supplementary materials. In Public Access File for the Committee to Review the Health Effects in Vietnam Veterans of Exposure to Herbicides: Ninth Biennial Update (received January 7, 2013).

Stellman JM, Stellman SD, Christian R, Weber T, Tomasallo C. 2003a. The extent and patterns of usage of Agent Orange and other herbicides in Vietnam. *Nature* 422:681–687.

Stellman JM, Stellman SD, Weber T, Tomasallo C, Stellman AB, Christian R. 2003b. A geographic information system for characterizing exposure to Agent Orange and other herbicides in Vietnam. *Environmental Health Perspectives* 111:321–328.

Stellman SD, Stellman JM. 1986. Estimation of exposure to Agent Orange and other defoliants among American troops in Vietnam: A methodological approach. *American Journal of Industrial Medicine* 9:305–321.

Stellman SD, Stellman JM. 2004. Exposure opportunity models for Agent Orange, dioxin, and other military herbicides used in Vietnam, 1961–1971. *Journal of Exposure Analysis and Environmental Epidemiology* 14:354–362.

Stellman SD, Mager-Stellman J, Sommer JF Jr. 1988. Combat and herbicide exposures in Vietnam among a sample of American Legionnaires. *Environmental Research* 47:112–128.

Tai PT, Nishijo M, Kido T, Nakagawa H, Maruzeni S, Naganuma R, Anh NT, Morikawa Y, Luong HV, Anh TH, Hung NN, Tawara K, Nishijo H. 2011. Dioxin concentrations in breast milk of Vietnamese nursing mothers: A survey four decades after herbicide spraying. *Environmental Science and Technology* 45(15):6625–6632.

Thomas TL, Kang HK. 1990. Mortality and morbidity among Army Chemical Corps Vietnam veterans: A preliminary report. *American Journal of Industrial Medicine* 18:665–673.

Tohyama C, Uchiyama I, Hoshi S, Hijiya M, Miyata H, Nagai M, Nakai S, Yauchi M, Ohkubo S. 2011. Polychlorinated dioxins, furans, and biphenyls in blood of children and adults living in a dioxin-contaminated area in Tokyo. *Environmental Health Perspectives* 16(1):6–15.

Tosine H. 1983. Dioxins: A Canadian perspective. In: *Chlorinated Dioxins and Dibenzofurans in the Total Environment*, Choudhary G, Keith LH, Rappe C, eds. Woburn, MA: Butterworth Publishers, pp. 3–14.

van den Berg M, Birnbaum LS, Denison M, De Vito M, Farland W, Feeley M, Fiedler H, Hakansson H, Hanberg A, Haws L, Rose M, Safe S, Schrenk D, Tohyama C, Tritscher A, Tuomisto J, Tysklind M, Walker N, Peterson RE. 2006. The 2005 World Health Organization reevaluation of human and mammalian Toxic Equivalency Factors for dioxins and dioxin-like compounds. *Toxicological Sciences* 93(2):223–241.

Warren WF. 1968. *A Review of the Herbicide Program in South Vietnam.* San Francisco: Scientific Advisory Group. Working Paper No. 10-68. NTIS AD-779–797.

Young AL. 1992. *The Military Use of Herbicides in Vietnam.* Presentation to the Institute of Medicine Committee to Review the Health Effects in Vietnam Veterans of Exposure to Herbicides. December 8, 1992. Washington, DC.

Young AL. 2006. *The History of the US Department of Defense Programs for the Testing, Evaluation, and Storage of Tactical Herbicides.* Submitted to US Army Research Center, Triangle Park, North Carolina (Contract # DAAD19-02-D-0001).

Young AL. 2009. *The History, Use, Disposition and Environmental Fate of Agent Orange.* New York: Springer Science and Business Media, LLC.

Young AL, Cecil PF. 2011. Agent Orange exposure and attributed health effects in Vietnam veterans. *Military Medicine* 176(7):29–34.

Young AL, Newton M. 2004. Long overlooked historical information on Agent Orange and TCDD following massive applications of 2,4,5-T-containing herbicides, Eglin Air Force Base, Florida. *Environmental Science and Pollution Research* 11(4):209–221.

Young AL, Reggiani GM, eds. 1988. *Agent Orange and Its Associated Dioxin: Assessment of a Controversy.* Amsterdam: Elsevier.

Young AL, Thalken CE, Arnold EL, Cupello JM, Cockerham LG. 1976. *Fate of 2,3,7,8 tetrachlorodibenzo-*p*-dioxin (TCDD) in the Environment: Summary and Decontamination Recommendations.* Colorado Springs: US Air Force Academy. USAFA TR 76 18.

Young AL, Calcagni JA, Thalken CE, Tremblay JW. 1978. *The Toxicology, Environmental Fate, and Human Risk of Herbicide Orange and Its Associated Dioxin.* Brooks AFB, TX: Air Force Occupational and Environmental Health Lab. USAF OEHL TR 78 92.

Young AL, Cecil PF Sr, Guilmartin JF Jr. 2004a. Assessing possible exposures of ground troops to Agent Orange during the Vietnam War: The use of contemporary military records. *Environmental Science and Pollution Research* 11(6):349–358.

Young AL, Giesy JP, Jones P, Newton M, Guilmartin JF Jr, Cecil PF Sr. 2004b. Assessment of potential exposure to Agent Orange and its associated TCDD. *Environmental Science and Pollution Research* 11(6):347–348.

4

Information Related to Biologic Plausibility

The committee reviewed all relevant experimental studies of 2,4-dichlorophenoxyacetic acid (2,4-D), 2,4,5-trichlorophenoxyacetic acid (2,4,5-T), 4-amino-3,5,6-trichloropicolinic acid (picloram), dimethylarsinic acid (DMA, also called cacodylic acid), and 2,3,7,8-tetrachlorodibenzo-*p*-dioxin (TCDD) that have been published since *Update 2010* (IOM, 2011) and has incorporated the findings into this chapter when it is appropriate and into the biologic-plausibility sections of Chapters 7–13 when they are of consequence for particular health outcomes. For each substance, this chapter includes a review of toxicokinetic properties, a brief summary of the toxic outcomes investigated in animal experiments, and a discussion of underlying mechanisms of action as illuminated by in vitro studies. The final section of this chapter presents two newly emerging subjects of molecular and biologic science that provide novel insight into potential mechanisms of xenobiotic-induced disease and that may increase the biologic plausibility of toxic actions of the herbicides sprayed in Vietnam.

Establishment of biologic plausibility through laboratory studies strengthens the evidence of a cause–effect relationship between herbicide exposure and health effects reported in epidemiologic studies and thus supports the existence of the less stringent relationship of association, which is the target of this committee's work. Experimental studies of laboratory animals or cultured cells allow observation of effects of herbicide exposure under highly controlled conditions, which is difficult or impossible to achieve in epidemiologic studies. Such conditions include genetic differences between people, and frequency and magnitude of exposure, exposure to other chemicals, and pre-existing health conditions, all of which can be controlled in a laboratory animal study.

Once a chemical contacts the body, it becomes subject to the processes of absorption, distribution, metabolism, and excretion. The combination of those four biologic processes determines the concentration of the chemicals in the body and how long each organ is exposed to it and thus influences its toxic or pharmacologic activity.

Absorption of a substance in an organism normally takes place by uptake into the bloodstream from mucous surfaces, such as the intestinal walls of the digestive tract during ingestion. Low solubility, chemical instability in the stomach, and inability to permeate the intestinal wall can all reduce the extent to which a substance is absorbed after being ingested. The solubility of a chemical in fat and its hydrophobicity influence the pathways by which it is absorbed, its relative potential to be metabolized (structurally transformed), and ultimately whether it persists in the body or is excreted. Absorption is a critical determinant of a chemical's bioavailability, that is, the fraction of it that reaches the systemic circulation. In addition to ingestion, routes of exposure experienced by humans are inhalation (entry via the airways) and dermal exposure (entry via the skin). Animal studies may involve additional routes of exposure that are not ordinarily encountered by humans, such as intravenous or intraperitoneal injection, in which a chemical is injected into the bloodstream or abdominal cavity, respectively.

Distribution refers to the movement of a substance from the site of entry to the tissues and organs where it may have its ultimate effect or be sequestered. Distribution takes place most commonly via the bloodstream.

Metabolism is the breaking down that all substances begin to experience as soon as they enter the body. For many foreign substances, the breakdown to carbon dioxide and water is not complete and is more precisely referred to as biotransformation. Most of this process takes place in the liver by the action of enzymes, including cytochrome P450s, which catalyze the oxidative metabolism of many chemicals. As metabolism occurs, the parent chemical is converted to new chemicals called metabolites, which are often more water-soluble (polar) and thus more readily excreted. When the resulting metabolites are pharmacologically or toxicologically inert, metabolism has deactivated the administered dose of the parent chemical and thus reduced its effects on the body. Metabolism may activate a chemical to a metabolite that is more potent or more toxic than it is.

Excretion is the removal of substances or their metabolites from the body, most commonly in urine or feces, whereas elimination applies to the disappearance of the parent molecule from the bloodstream. The rate of excretion of a chemical from the body is often limited by the rate of metabolism of the parent chemical into more water-soluble, readily excreted metabolites. Elimination is often incomplete, especially in the case of chemicals that resist biotransformation, and incomplete excretion results in the accumulation of foreign substances that can adversely affect biologic functions. Elimination is first-order when its rate is directly proportional to the amount of chemical then in the body, which would also mean that the chemical's half-life is independent of dose.

The routes and rates of absorption, distribution, biotransformation or metabolism, and excretion of a toxic substance collectively are termed toxicokinetics (or pharmacokinetics for chemicals used as pharmaceutical agents). Those processes determine the amount of a particular substance or metabolite that reaches specific organs or cells and that persists in the body. Understanding the toxicokinetics of a chemical is useful for valid reconstruction of exposure of humans, but it is most important for assessing the risk of effects from exposure to a chemical by determining the concentration of the active chemical in target tissues. The principles involved in toxicokinetics are similar among chemicals, although the degree to which different processes influence distribution depends on the structure and other inherent properties of the chemicals. Thus, the lipophilicity or hydrophobicity of a chemical and its structure influence the pathways by which it is metabolized and whether it persists in the body or is excreted. The degree to which different toxicokinetic processes influence the toxic potential of a chemical depends on metabolic pathways, which often differ among species. For that reason, attempts at extrapolation from experimental animal studies to human exposures must be done extremely carefully.

Many chemicals were used by the US armed forces in Vietnam. The nature of the substances themselves was discussed in more detail in Chapter 6 of the original *Veterans and Agent Orange: Health Effects of Herbicides Used in Vietnam* (*VAO*) report (IOM, 1994). Four herbicides documented in military records were of particular concern and are examined here: 2,4-D, 2,4,5-T, picloram, and cacodylic acid. This chapter also examines TCDD, the most toxic congener of the tetrachlorodibenzo-*p*-dioxins (tetraCDDs), also commonly referred to as dioxin—which is a contaminant of 2,4,5-T—because its potential toxicity is of concern. Considerably more information is available on TCDD than on the herbicides themselves. Other contaminants present in 2,4-D and 2,4,5-T are of less concern. Except as noted, the laboratory studies of the chemicals of concern used pure compounds or formulations; the epidemiologic studies discussed in later chapters often tracked exposures to mixtures.

PICLORAM

Chemistry

Picloram (Chemical Abstracts Service Number [CAS No.] 1918-02-1; see chemical structure in Figure 4-1) was used with 2,4-D in the herbicide formulation Agent White, which was sprayed in Vietnam. It is also used commonly in Australia in a formulation that has the trade name Tordon 75D®. Tordon 75D contains several chemicals, including 2,4-D, picloram, a surfactant diethyleneglycolmonoethyl ether, and a silicone defoamer. A number of studies of picloram used such mixtures as Tordon formulations or other mixtures of 2,4-D and picloram that are similar to Agent White.

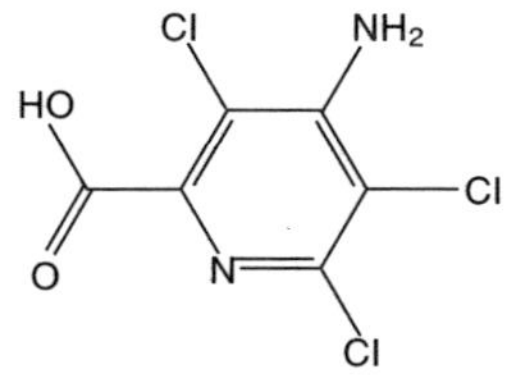

4-amino-3,5,6-trichloropicolinic acid

FIGURE 4-1 Structure of picloram.

Toxicokinetics

The original *VAO* committee reviewed studies of the toxicokinetics of picloram. Studies of animals showed rapid absorption through the gastrointestinal tract and rapid elimination of picloram as the unaltered parent chemical in urine. Nolan et al. (1984) examined the toxicokinetics of picloram in six healthy male volunteers who were given single oral doses of 0.5 or 5.0 mg/kg and a dermal dose of 2.0 mg/kg. Picloram was rapidly absorbed in the oral study and rapidly excreted unchanged in urine. More than 75% of the dose was excreted within 6 hours, and the remainder with an average half-life of 27 hours. On the basis of the quantity of picloram excreted in urine in the skin study, the authors noted that only 0.2% of the picloram applied to the skin was absorbed. Because of its rapid excretion, picloram has low potential to accumulate in humans.

In general, the literature on picloram toxicity continues to be sparse. Studies of humans and animals indicate that picloram is rapidly eliminated as the parent chemical. Studies of animals indicate that picloram is sparingly toxic at high doses.

Toxicity Profile

The original *VAO* committee reviewed studies of the carcinogenicity, genotoxicity, acute toxicity, chronic systemic toxicity, reproductive and developmental toxicity, and immunotoxicity of picloram. In general, there is some evidence on cancer in some rodent models but not in other species (NCI, 1978). Because of some concern that contaminants in the picloram (in particular, hexachlorobenzene) might be responsible for the carcinogenicity, picloram itself has not been established as a chemical carcinogen.

Studies conducted by the Environmental Protection Agency (EPA) (1988c) yielded no evidence that picloram is a genotoxic agent. Picloram is considered a mild irritant; it has produced erythema in rabbits only at high doses. The available information on the acute toxicity of picloram is paltry. Some neurologic effects—including hyperactivity, ataxia, and tremors—were reported in pregnant rats exposed to picloram at 750 or 1,000 mg/kg (Thompson et al., 1972).

Chronic Systemic Toxicity

Several studies have reported various effects of technical-grade picloram on the livers of rats. In the carcinogenicity bioassay conducted by Stott et al. (1990), treatment-related hepatomegaly, hepatocellular swelling, and altered tinctorial properties in the central regions of the liver lobules were noted in the groups exposed at 60 and 200 mg/kg per day. Males and females exposed at the 200 mg/kg dose had higher liver weights than controls. The no-observed-effect level (NOEL) was 20 mg/kg per day, and the lowest observed-effect level was 60 mg/kg per day for histologic changes in centrilobular hepatocellular tissues. According to the EPA (1988c), hexachlorobenzene (a contaminant of technical grade picloram at 197 ppm) was probably not responsible for the hepatic effects. Gorzinski and colleagues (1987) also reported a dose-related increase in liver weights, hepatocellular hypertrophy, and changes in centrilobular tinctorial properties in male and female F344 rats exposed to picloram at 150 mg/kg per day and higher in the diet for 13 weeks. In a 90-day study, cloudy swelling in the liver cells and bile duct epithelium occurred in male and female F344 rats given 0.3% or 1.0% technical picloram in the diet (EPA, 1988c). Hepatic effects have also been reported in dogs exposed to picloram: increased liver weights were reported in beagles that received 35 mg/kg per day or more in the diet for 6 months (EPA, 1988c). No other effects of chronic exposure to picloram have been reported.

Reproductive and Developmental Toxicity

The reproductive toxicity of picloram was evaluated in a two-generation study; however, few animals were evaluated, and no toxicity was detected at the highest dose tested, 150 mg/kg per day (EPA, 1988c). Some developmental toxicity was produced in rabbits exposed to picloram by gavage at 400 mg/kg per day on days 6–18 of gestation. Fetal abnormalities were forelimb flexure, fused ribs, hypoplastic tail, and omphalocele, each occurring in a single litter (John-Greene et al., 1985). Some maternal toxicity was observed at that dose, however, and EPA concluded on the basis of the sporadic findings that the malformations were not treatment-related (EPA, 1988c). No teratogenic effects were produced in the offspring of rats given picloram by gavage at up to 1,000 mg/kg per day on days 6–15 of gestation, but the occurrence of bilateral accessory ribs was significantly increased (Thompson et al., 1972).

Immunotoxicity

Studies of the potential immunotoxicity of picloram included dermal sensitization in humans and rodent immunoassays. In one study, 53 volunteers received nine 24-hour applications of 0.5 mL of a 2% potassium picloram solution on the skin of both upper arms. Each volunteer received challenge doses 17–24 days later. The formulation of picloram (its potassium salt) was not a skin sensitizer or an irritant (EPA, 1988c). In a similar study, a 5% solution of picloram (M-2439, Tordon 101 formulation) produced slight dermal irritation and a sensitization response in six of the 69 volunteers exposed. When the individual components of M-2439—picloram, triisopropanolamine (TIPA) salt, and 2,4-D TIPA salt—were tested separately, no sensitization reaction occurred (EPA, 1988c). Tordon K+, but not technical-grade picloram, was also found to be a skin sensitizer in guinea pigs (EPA, 1988c). CD1 mice exposed to Tordon 202C (94% 2,4-D and 6% picloram) had no consistent adverse effects on antibody responses (Blakley, 1997), but the lack of a consistent response may be due to the fact that CD1 mice are outbred.

Mechanisms

No well-characterized mechanisms of toxicity for picloram are known.

CACODYLIC ACID

Chemistry

Arsenic (As) is a naturally occurring element that exists in a trivalent form (As^{+3} or As^{III}) and a pentavalent form (As^{+5} or As^{V}). See Figure 4-2 for chemical structures of selected arsenic-containing compounds—sodium arsenite, which contains As^{III}, is generally considered to be the most toxic of these arsenic compounds. Arsenic is commonly present in drinking-water sources that are associated with volcanic soils and can reach high concentrations (over 50 ppb). Numerous human health effects have been attributed to drinking-water exposure, particularly bladder, skin, and lung cancers and vascular diseases.

Arsenic exists in both inorganic and organic (methylated) forms and is readily metabolized in humans and other species. Inorganic arsenic can be converted to organic forms. Although organic forms can be converted into inorganic forms by microorganisms in the soil, there is no evidence that this can occur in humans or other vertebrate species (Cohen et al., 2006). The arsenic in cacodylic acid (CAS No. 75-60-5) has a valence of +5. Cacodylic acid (also known as dimethylarsinic acid [DMA^{V}] by its more standard chemical name), disodium methanearsonate, and monosodium methanearsonate are herbicides that EPA approved for use in the United States, where they are occasionally applied on golf courses and large open spaces. Cacodylic acid was the form of arsenic used in Agent Blue, one of the mixtures used for defoliation in Vietnam; DMA^{V} made up about 30% of Agent Blue. Agent Blue was chemically and toxicologically unrelated to Agent Orange, which consisted of phenoxy herbicides contaminated with dioxin-like compounds. As shown in Figure 4-3, DMA^{III} and DMA^{V}, as well as monomethyl arsonous acid (MMA^{III}) and monomethyl arsonic acid (MMA^{V}), are metabolic

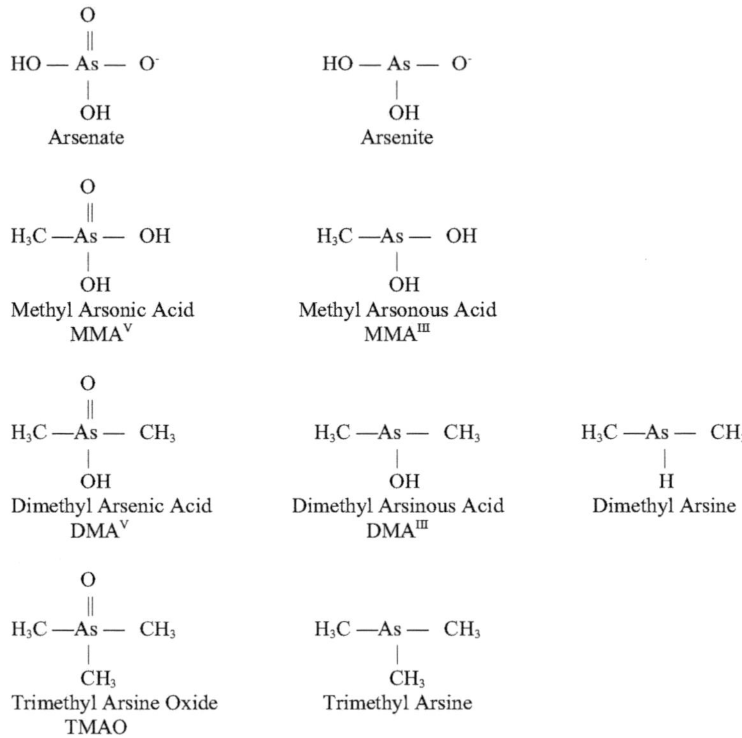

FIGURE 4-2 Structures of selected arsenic-containing compounds.

products of exposure to inorganic arsenic. Methylation of inorganic arsenic used to be considered a detoxification process associated with increased excretion (Vahter and Concha, 2001). However, some of the methylated metabolic intermediates, especially MMA^{III}, have been found to be more toxic than the parent sodium arsenite (Aposhian et al., 2000). The methylation pathway of inorganic arsenic results in the formation of DMA^{V} and DMA^{III}.

The committee contemplated the relevance of animal data collected after exposure to inorganic arsenic, leading to DMA^{V} being formed endogenously, vs data collected after direct exposure to exogenous DMA^{V}, which is the form of arsenic and manner of potential exposure applicable to Vietnam veterans. It has not been established—nor can it be inferred—that the observed effects of exposure to inorganic arsenic are caused by endogenous formation of DMA^{V}. Furthermore, results of recent studies suggest that there is an increased incidence of cancer in people who generate less DMA^{V} endogenously (Huang SK et al., 2008), which would imply that complete methylation of inorganic arsenic to DMA^{V} is associated with reduced risk of inorganic arsenic–induced adverse health outcomes

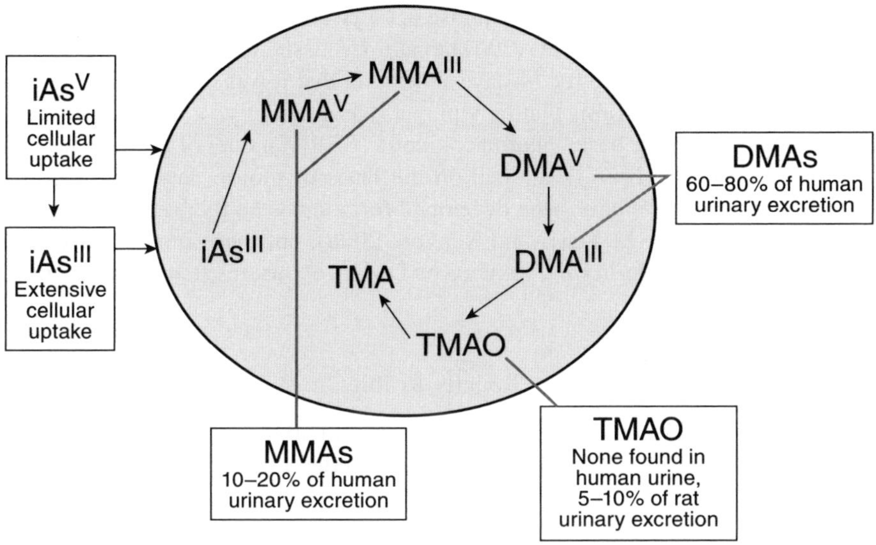

FIGURE 4-3 General pathways of arsenic metabolism after exposure to inorganic arsenic (iAs).
SOURCE: Adapted with permission from Cohen et al., 2006.

(Hall and Gamble, 2012). Finally, because there is no evidence that DMA is demethylated to inorganic arsenic in humans or other animals (Cohen et al., 2006), the committee chose not to consider the literature on inorganic arsenic for this report. The reader is referred to *Arsenic in Drinking Water* (NRC, 1999a) and *Arsenic in Drinking Water: 2001 Update* (NRC, 2001). The committee considered and reviewed only those toxicologic studies in which animals were directly exposed to DMA^V.

Toxicokinetics

The metabolism and disposition of DMA^V has recently been reviewed (Cohen et al., 2006; Suzuki et al., 2010). In general, it is rapidly excreted mostly unchanged in the urine of most animal species after systemic exposure. However, rats differ from most other mammals (including humans) in that a larger percentage (10%) of DMA^V binds to hemoglobin in red blood cells, and that leads to a considerably longer half-life in blood (Cui et al., 2004; Suzuki et al., 2004). The binding of DMA^V to hemoglobin is 10 times higher in rats than in humans (Lu et al., 2004). Chronic exposure of normal rat hepatocytes to DMA^V resulted in decreased uptake and increased excretion, so that over time they developed resistance to its cytotoxic effects (Kojima et al., 2006); the tolerance was mediated by induction of glutathione-*S*-transferase activity and of multiple-drug–resistant protein expression. Adair et al. (2007) examined tissue distribution of DMA in rats after dietary exposure for 14 days and found that it was extensively metabolized to trimethylated forms that may play a role in toxicity.

A physiologically based pharmacokinetic (PBPK) model of intravenous and ingested DMA^V has been developed on the basis of mouse data (Evans et al., 2008). Similar models have been developed for humans on the basis of exposure to inorganic arsenic (El-Masri and Kenyon, 2008), but these models have limited utility for considering the toxicity of DMA^V exposures that are relevant to Vietnam veterans.

Toxicity Profile

This section discusses the toxicity associated with organic forms of arsenic, most notably DMA^V because it is the active ingredient in Agent Blue. The toxicity of inorganic arsenic is not considered relevant to veteran exposures to Agent Blue.

Neurotoxicity

Kruger et al. (2006) found that DMA^{III} and DMA^V significantly attenuated neuronal ion currents through *N*-methyl-D–aspartate receptor ion channels whereas only DMA^V inhibited ion currents through α-amino-3-hydroxy-5-methylisoxazole-4-propionic acid receptors. The data suggest that those methylated forms of arsenic may have neurotoxic potential.

Immunotoxicity

Previous studies have shown that a low concentration of DMA^V (10^{-7} M) could increase proliferation of human peripheral blood monocytes after their stimulation with phytohemagglutinin whereas it took a high concentration (10^{-4} M) to inhibit release of interferon-γ. This suggested that various immunomodulatory effects of DMA^V have their own concentration specificity (Di Giampaolo et al., 2004).

Skin Toxicity

In a recent evaluation of effects of topical exposure of pregnant mice to DMA (valence not stated) on the skin of the dams and offspring (Kim et al., 2012), no effects were observed in offspring, but exposure increased skin thickness in the area of application and altered expression of apoptosis-related genes (Bcl-2, Bad, caspase-12). The results suggested that transient DMA exposure can be a skin irritant and produce dermatitis.

Genotoxicity and Carcinogenicity

DMA^{III} and DMA^{V} are genotoxic and increase oxidative stress and cause DNA damage. Gómez et al. (2005) demonstrated that DMA^{III} induced a dose-related increase in DNA damage and oxidative stress in Jurkat cells. DMA^{III} was considerably more potent than DMA^{V} in inducing DNA damage in Chinese hamster ovary cells (Dopp et al., 2004), and this was associated with a greater uptake of DMA^{III} into the cells. An additional study showed that DMA^{V} is poorly membrane-permeable, but when forced into cells by electroporation it can induce DNA damage (Dopp et al., 2005). Similarly, analysis of arsenical dimethylated metabolites in human bladder cancer cells found dimethylmonothioarsinic acid ($DMMTA^{V}$) and DMA^{III} to be the most toxic and DMA^{V} to be less toxic in terms of DNA damage (Naranmandura et al., 2011). DNA damage from $DMMTA^{V}$ was shown to be related to accumulation of reactive oxygen species and down-regulation of p53 and p21 (DNA repair proteins); these processes were mediated in part through intracellular conversion to DMA^{V} and DMA^{III} (Naranmandura et al., 2011). Thus, although extracellular DMA^{V} has little toxic effect in cells because of its low uptake, intracellular DMA^{V} can be highly toxic. Gene-expression profiling of bladder urothelium after chronic exposure to DMA^{V} in drinking water showed significant increases in genes that regulate oxidative stress (Sen et al., 2005), whereas hepatic gene-expression profiling showed that DMA^{V} exposure induced changes consistent with oxidative stress (Xie et al., 2004). In vivo, DMA^{V}-induced proliferation of the urinary bladder epithelium could be attenuated with the antioxidant *N*-acetylcysteine (Wei et al., 2005).

DMA^{III} and DMA^{V} are carcinogenic. Cancer has been induced in the urinary bladder, kidneys, liver, thyroid glands, and lungs of laboratory animals exposed to high concentrations of DMA. In a 2-year bioassay, rats fed 40 or 100 ppm DMA^{V} developed epithelial carcinomas and papillomas in the urinary bladder and nonneoplastic changes in the kidneys (Arnold et al., 2006). Similarly, Wang et al. (2009) found that exposure of F344 rats to DMA^{V} in drinking water at 1, 4, 40, or 100 ppm resulted in a change in the urinary bladder epithelium, but there were no changes in DNA repair capacity. In another study, Cohen et al. (2007a) exposed F344 rats to DMA^{V} in the diet for 2 years and found an increase in bladder tumors in those receiving 100 ppm; they postulated that trimethylated forms of arsenic may be responsible for bladder cancer in rats. Direct bladder exposure of rats to 90 mg/kg DMA^{V} induced infiltration and proliferation of urothelial epithelium mediated through oxidative stress pathways and extracellular signal-regulated kinase signaling (Takahashi et al., 2011). It is noteworthy that co-treatment with an antioxidant, N-acetylcysteine, worsened the DMA^{V}-induced bladder injury, rather than ameliorating it as expected. In the mouse lung, DMA^{V} acted as a tumor initiator (Yamanaka et al., 2009) and as a tumor promoter (Mizoi et al., 2005). DMA^{V} can also act as a complete carcinogen, inducing lung tumors in susceptible strains of mice, including those with deficient DNA-repair activity (Hayashi et al., 1998; Kinoshita et al., 2007). Yamanaka et al. (2009) suggest that DMA^{III} can act as a tumor promoter through the formation of a DMA^{III} radical after reduction of DMA^{V}. Recent studies have also found that oral exposure of adult mice to 200 ppm DMA^{V} in addition to fetal arsenic exposure can act as a promoter of renal and hepatocellular carcinoma, markedly increasing tumor incidence beyond that produced by fetal arsenic exposure alone (Tokar et al., 2012). Those findings emphasize how multiple life events can contribute to an adverse health outcome in which adult DMA^{V} exposure triggered an otherwise dormant disease.

Mechanisms

Oxidative stress is a common theme that runs through the literature on the mechanisms of action of arsenic, particularly with regard to cancer in animals, although some studies have suggested that methylated arsenicals (MMA^{III} and DMA^{III}) can induce mutations in mammalian cells at concentrations below those required to produce oxidative stress after in vitro exposure (Klein et al., 2008). Recent studies have shown that mice that are deficient in enzymes associated with repair of oxidative DNA damage are highly susceptible to induction of tumors, particularly lung tumors, by DMA^{V} (Kinoshita et al., 2007). The chemical reaction of arsenicals with thiol groups in sensitive target tissues, such as red blood cells and kidneys, may also be a mechanism of action of organic arsenicals (Naranmandura and Suzuki, 2008).

The variation in the susceptibility of various animal species to tumor formation caused by inorganic and organic arsenic is thought to depend heavily on differences in metabolism and distribution. Thus, genetic differences may play an important role. Numerous investigators are examining potential human susceptibility factors and gene polymorphisms that may increase a person's risk of cancer and other diseases induced by arsenicals (Aposhian and Aposhian, 2006; Hernandez et al., 2008; Huang SK et al., 2008; Huang YK et al., 2008; McCarty et al., 2007; Meza et al., 2007; Steinmaus et al., 2007, 2010), but it is not yet possible to identify polymorphisms that may contribute to a person's susceptibility to DMA-induced cancer or tissue injury.

PHENOXY HERBICIDES 2,4-DICHLOROPHENOXY ACID AND 2,4,5-TRICHLOROPHENOXYACETIC ACID

Chemistry

2,4-D (CAS No. 94-75-7) is an odorless and, when pure, white crystalline powder (Figure 4-4); it may appear yellow when phenolic impurities are present. The melting point of 2,4-D is 138°C, and the free acid is corrosive to metals. It is soluble in water and in a variety of organic solvents (such as acetone, alcohols, ketones, ether, and toluene). 2,4,5-T (CAS No. 93-76-5) is an odorless, white

2,4-D [94-75-7] **2,4,5-T** [93-76-5]

FIGURE 4-4 Structures of 2,4-D and 2,4,5-T.

to light-tan solid with a melting point of 158°C. 2,4,5-T is noncorrosive and is soluble in alcohol and water. It reacts with organic and inorganic bases to form salts and with alcohols to form esters.

Uses of 2,4-D and 2,4,5-T

2,4-D has been used commercially in the United States since World War II to control the growth of broadleaf plants and weeds on range lands, lawns, golf courses, forests, roadways, parks, and agricultural land; it remains a widely used herbicide approved for use by the European Union and EPA. Formulations include 2,4-D amine and alkali salts and esters, which are mobile in soil and readily absorbed through the leaves and roots of many plants. Like 2,4-D, 2,4,5-T was developed and marketed as a herbicide during World War II. However, the registration for 2,4,5-T was canceled by EPA in 1978 when it became clear that it was contaminated with TCDD during the manufacturing process. It is recognized that the production of 2,4-D also involves the generation of some dioxin contaminants, even some with dioxin-like activity, but the fraction of TCDD is comparatively very small, as illustrated in Chapter 4.

The herbicidal properties of 2,4-D and 2,4,5-T are related to their ability to mimic the plant growth hormone indole acetic acid. They are selective herbicides in that they affect the growth of only broadleaf dicots (which include most weeds) and do not affect monocots, such as wheat, corn, and rice.

Toxicokinetics

Several studies have examined the absorption, distribution, metabolism, and excretion of 2,4-D and 2,4,5-T in animals and humans. Data on both compounds are consistent among species and support the conclusion that absorption of oral or inhaled doses is rapid and complete. Absorption through the skin is much lower but may be increased with the use of sunscreens or alcohol (Brand et al., 2002; Pont et al., 2004). After absorption, 2,4-D and 2,4,5-T are distributed widely in the body but are eliminated quickly, predominantly in unmetabolized form in urine (Sauerhoff et al., 1977), but 2,4,5-trichlorophenol and 2,4-dichlorophenol have been identified as trace metabolites in urine. The half-life of single doses of 2,4-D or 2,4,5-T in humans has been estimated to be about 18–23 hours (Gehring et al., 1973; Kohli et al., 1974; Sauerhoff et al., 1977; WHO, 1984). Hines et al. (2003) found that concentrations of 2,4-D and its metabolites in the urine of herbicide applicators were consistent with 2,4-D urinary half-life estimates of 13–40 hours in humans.

Toxicity Profile

The toxicity database on 2,4-D is extensive (http://toxnet.nlm.nih.gov/ search on "2,4-D;" accessed April 23, 2013), whereas the available data on the toxicity of purified 2,4,5-T, independent of its contamination by TCDD, are sparse. TCDD is much more toxic than 2,4,5-T, and much of the toxicity attributed to 2,4,5-T in early studies was later shown to be caused by the TCDD contaminant. The following summary therefore focuses on 2,4-D toxicity, and information on pure 2,4,5-T is added when it is available.

After a single oral dose, 2,4-D is considered to produce moderate acute toxicity with an LD_{50} (dose lethal to 50% of exposed animals) of 375 mg/kg in rats, 370 mg/kg in mice, and from less than 320 to 1,000 mg/kg in guinea pigs. Rats and rabbits have dermal LD_{50}s of 1,500 mg/kg and 1,400 mg/kg, respectively. 2,4,5-T itself also produces moderate acute toxicity, with oral LD_{50}s of 389 mg/kg in mice and 500 mg/kg in rats. Death from acute poisoning with 2,4-D or 2,4,5-T has been attributed to the ability of the chemicals to uncouple oxidative phosphorylation, a vital process used by almost all cells in the body as the primary means of generating energy. After exposure to high doses, death due to multiple organ failure can occur rapidly. Studies in rats, cats, and dogs indicate that the central nervous system is the principal target organ for acute 2,4-D toxicity in mammals and suggest that the primary site of action is the cerebral cortex or the reticular formation (Arnold et al., 1991; Dési et al., 1962a,b). Neurotoxicity in humans is the predominant effect of acute inhalation and oral exposure to 2,4-D; symptoms include stiffness of arms and legs, incoordination, lethargy, anorexia, stupor, and coma. 2,4-D is also an irritant of the gastrointestinal tract, causing nausea, vomiting, and diarrhea.

Chronic exposure to 2,4-D at relatively high concentrations has been shown to produce a variety of toxic effects, including hepatic and renal toxicity, neurotoxicity, and hematologic changes. A NOEL of 2,4-D of 1 mg/kg was identified for renal toxicity in rats (Hazleton Laboratories America, 1987). Exposure to 2,4-D was associated with reduced survival and decreased growth rates of offspring of mothers fed high doses during pregnancy that were associated with maternal toxicity. However, even at high exposures, 2,4-D did not affect fertility and did not produce teratogenic effects in the offspring (Charles et al., 2001; Munro et al., 1992). A recent study suggests that chronic exposure of adult male rats to 2,4-D results in a reduction in the weight of the testes, prostate, epidydimes, and seminal vesicles and a reduction in sperm density (Joshi et al., 2012). The purity of 2,4,5-T has been shown to influence its reproductive toxicity: TCDD contamination increases its fetotoxic effects and induces teratogenic effects. Immunotoxicity of 2,4-D has been reported in a small number of studies. At high doses that produced clinical toxicity, suppression of the antibody response was observed, whereas other measures of immune function were normal. The immunotoxicity of 2,4,5-T has not been evaluated in laboratory animals.

The carcinogenicity of 2,4-D and 2,4,5-T has been studied in rats, mice, and dogs after exposure in their food, direct placement in their stomachs, or exposure of their skin. All the studies had negative results except one that found an increased incidence of brain tumors in male rats—but not female rats—that received the highest dose of 2,4-D. The occurrence of malignant lymphoma in dogs kept as pets was reported to be higher when owners reported that they used 2,4-D on their lawns than when they did not (Hayes et al., 1991, 1995), but detailed reanalysis did not confirm this finding (Kaneene and Miller, 1999). A controlled study that used dogs exposed to 2,4-D in the laboratory had negative results. Timchalk (2004) suggested that dogs are not relevant for comparative evaluation of human health risk attributable to 2,4-D exposure because they excrete 2,4-D less efficiently than rats or humans do. 2,4-D is not metabolized to reactive intermediates capable of interacting with DNA, and the evidence supports the conclusion that 2,4-D is not a genotoxic carcinogen. However, a recent study shows that lymphocytes from smokers show genotoxic damage after exposure to 2,4-D, whereas lymphocytes from nonsmokers do not (Sandal and Yilmaz, 2011); this suggests that although 2,4-D may not be a carcinogen, it may influence the activity of known carcinogens.

2,3,7,8-TETRACHLORODIBENZO-*P*-DIOXIN

Chemistry

TCDDs are polychlorinated dibenzo-*p*-dioxins that have a triple-ring structure consisting of two benzene rings connected by an oxygenated ring with four attached chlorine atoms; in the case of the dioxin congener of greatest concern, 2,3,7,8-TCDD (commonly called simply TCDD), the chlorine atoms are attached at the 2, 3, 7, and 8 positions of the benzene rings (see Figure 4-5). The chemical properties of TCDD include a molecular weight of 322, a melting point of 305–306°C, a boiling point of 445.5°C, and a log octanol–water partition coefficient of 6.8 (National Toxicology Program substance profile). It is very lipophilic, or fat soluble, is virtually insoluble in water (19.3 ng/L), and is soluble in organic solvents, such as benzene and acetone. It has been suggested that volatilization of dioxin from water may be an important mechanism of transfer from the aqueous

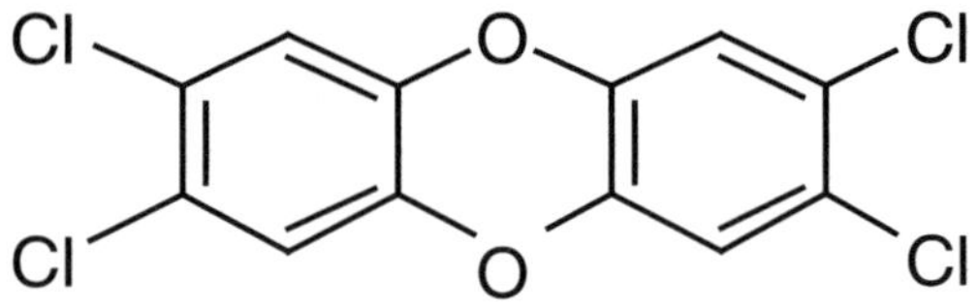

2,3,7,8-tetrachlorodibenzo-*p*-dioxin

FIGURE 4-5 Chemical structure of TCDD.

to the atmospheric phase (EPA, 2004); however, because of its very low water solubility, most TCDD is bound to sediments and particulate matter.

Toxicokinetics

The absorption, distribution, biotransformation, and excretion of TCDD have been extensively studied in humans and a number of other animal models in the last 25 years. Given the plethora of data, this section highlights and summarizes only key findings. A more exhaustive review may be found at http://www.epa.gov/ncea/pdfs/dioxin/nas-review.

TCDD is absorbed into the body rapidly but is eliminated slowly. Because it is very lipophilic, resistant to biotransformation, and slowly eliminated, the concentration of TCDD in the lipid fraction of blood serum is thought to be in dynamic equilibrium with that in the lipid fraction in other tissue compartments. Thus, the lipid-adjusted blood serum concentration of TCDD is used to estimate total body burdens; at high TCDD concentrations, however, the liver sequesters some of the dioxin, so lipid adjustment that ignores the hepatic fraction would underestimate the total body burden. Exposure of humans to TCDD is thought to occur primarily via the mouth, skin, and lungs. In laboratory animals, oral administration of TCDD has been shown to result in absorption of 50–93% of the administered dose (Nolan et al., 1979; Rose et al., 1976). Similarly, a study performed in a 42-year-old man found that 87% of the oral dose was absorbed (Poiger and Schlatter, 1986). Dermal absorption appears to be dose-dependent: lower absorption occurs at higher doses (Banks and Birnbaum, 1991). Studies performed in vitro with tissues isolated from humans indicate that human skin may be more resistant to absorption (Weber et al., 1991). The varied and complex environmental matrices make environmental exposures difficult to quantify. Animal studies have demonstrated that the presence of soil or lipophilic agents dramatically reduces dermal absorption of TCDD: application in an activated carbon–water paste essentially eliminates absorption in contrast with absorption of pure compound dissolved in solvents. Oral bioavailability of TCDD and related compounds also depends on the matrix: contaminated breast milk and food products have much higher bioavailability than soil-bound or sediment-bound TCDD, and activated carbon essentially blocks oral bioavailability (Olson, 2012).

After ingestion and gastrointestinal absorption, TCDD associates primarily with the lipoprotein fraction of the blood and later partitions into the cellular membranes and tissues (Henderson and Patterson, 1988). TCDD is distributed to all compartments of the body; the amounts differ from organ to organ, but most studies indicate that the primary disposition of TCDD is in the liver and adipose tissues. For example, in a human volunteer, it was found that 135 days after ingestion 90% of TCDD was in fat (Poiger and Schlatter, 1986), and TCDD persists in adipose tissue in the rhesus monkey (Bowman et al., 1989). The disposition and elimination of TCDD depend on the tissue examined, the time that has elapsed since exposure, total exposure, and other factors. For example, the concentration of cytochrome P450 1A2 (CYP1A2) (Poland et al., 1989) in the liver is increased by TCDD. Direct binding of TCDD to CYP1A2 is thought to result in sequestration of TCDD in the liver and to inhibit its distribution to other tissues. The importance of CYP1A2 concentrations for the toxic actions of TCDD has also been demonstrated in several laboratory situations; for instance, CYP1A2-knockout mice were more susceptible than wild-type mice to TCDD immunotoxicity (Smialowicz et al., 2008), and maternal hepatic CYP1A2 was found to sequester TCDD and protect mouse fetuses against TCDD-induced teratogenesis (Dragin et al., 2006). In addition, distribution of TCDD is age-dependent, as shown by studies in which young animals displayed the highest concentration of TCDD in the liver and older animals the highest concentrations in kidneys, skin, and muscle (Pegram et al., 1995). Finally, the rate of elimination of TCDD, particularly after low exposures, depends heavily on the amount of adipose tissue mass (Aylward et al., 2005a; Emond et al., 2005, 2006).

In laboratory animals, TCDD is metabolized slowly. It is eliminated primarily in feces as both the parent chemical and its more polar metabolites. However, elimination appears to be dose-dependent: at low doses, about 35% of the administered dose of TCDD was detected in the feces; at higher doses, about 46% was observed (Diliberto et al., 2001). The dose-dependent occurrence of TCDD metabolites in the feces is thought to be due to increased expression of metabolizing enzymes at higher doses and to hepatic sequestration, which makes dioxins more available for metabolism. A measure of elimination is half-life, which is defined as the time required for the plasma concentration or the amount of a chemical in the body to be reduced by half. The half-life of TCDD in humans varies with body-mass index (BMI), age, sex, and concentration in the body and has been found to vary from 0.4 to more than 10 years (see Table 4-1).

Milbrath et al. (2009) conducted a comprehensive review of studies that reported the congener-specific elimination rates of TCDD and related compounds and analyzed the relationships between the apparent half-lives of the compounds as a function of age, body fat, smoking status, and breastfeeding. In infants (under 2 years old), the compounds have a reported half-life of 0.4 year (Leung et al.,

TABLE 4-1 Estimates of TCDD Half-Life in Humans and Animals

Reference	Half-Life[a]	Confidence Interval	Comment
Human studies:			
Leung et al., 2006	0.4 year		Breastfed infants, 0–1 year after exposure
Aylward et al., 2005a	< 3 years		Toxicokenetic model estimates for exposures > 10,000 pg/g of serum lipid
	> 10 years		< 50 pg/g of serum lipid
Emond et al., 2005			PBPK model based on 10
	Weeks		Operation Ranch Hand veterans
	> 10 years		40,000 pg/g of serum lipid
			138 pg/g of serum lipid
Flesch-Janys et al., 1996	7.2 years		Adult males, Boehringer cohort
Geusau et al., 2002			0–3 years after exposure:
	1.7 years[b]		Adult female 1, 144,000 pg/g of serum lipid
	3.4 years[b]		Adult female 2, 26,000 pg/g of serum lipid
Kumagai and Koda, 2005			Adult male, incinerator workers,
	1.1–2.3 years		0–1.3 years after exposure
Michalek et al., 2002	0.34 year[b]		Adult males, Seveso cohort, 0–3 months after exposure
	6.9 years		3–16 years after exposure
	9.8 years		Adult females, Seveso cohort, 3–16 years after exposure
	7.5 years		Adult males, Operation Ranch Hand veterans, 9–33 years after exposure
Needham et al., 1994	7.8 years	7.2–9.7 years	Adults, Seveso cohort
Pirkle et al., 1989	7.1 years	5.8–9.6 years	Adult males, Operation Ranch Hand veterans, 9–23 years after exposure
Milbrath et al., 2009	7.2 years		Reference half-life for 48.7-year-old
Sorg et al., 2009	15.4 months		Victor Yushchenko: TCDD at 108,000 ppt lipid
Animal studies:			*Monkeys*
Neubert et al., 1990	73.7 days	60.9–93.8 days	single injection
			Mice
DeVito and Birnbaum, 1995	15 days		female B6C3F1
Gasiewicz et al., 1983	11 days[c]		C5BL/6J
	24.4 days[c]		DBA/2J
	12.6 days[c]		B6D2F1/J
Koshakji et al., 1984	20 days		male ICR/Ha Swiss
			Rats

TABLE 4-1 Continued

Reference	Half-Life[a]	Confidence Interval	Comment
Emond et al., 2006			Inducible elimination PBPK model estimates,
	10 days		10^3 µg/kg acute treatment
	75 days		10^{-3} µg/kg acute treatment
Hurst et al., 1998	8 days		Long-Evans, excretion from liver
Pohjanvirta and Tuomisto, 1990	21.9 days		male Han/Wistar, resistant strain
Viluksela et al., 1996	20.2 days		Long-Evans, TurkuAB strain
	28.9 days[d]		Long-Evans, Charles River strain
Weber et al., 1993	16.3 ± 3.0 days		male Sprague-Dawley

[a]Half-lives of TCDD in humans based on measurement of TCDD in serum samples.

[b]Shorter half-lives measured in humans during first months after exposure or in severely contaminated persons consistent with nonlinear elimination predicted by physiologically based pharmacokinetic (PBPK) models (for example, Carrier et al., 1995). Greater half-life in females attributed to greater BMI index.

[c]Total cumulative excretion of ^{3}H-TCDD-derived radioactivity.

[d]Attributed to differences in dilution due to different growth rates.

2006), and in adults, a half-life of 7.2 years (Milbrath et al., 2009). As people age, the growth results in a dilution effect and shorter half-lives. Aging also results in an increase in and redistribution of body fat and lipophilic chemicals that alter their rate of elimination (Van der Molen et al., 1996). Human studies of the Operation Ranch Hand cohort have consistently found a similar relationship between increasing half-life of TCDD and increasing BMI (Michalek and Tripathi, 1999; Michalek et al., 1992, 1996). Smoking and breastfeeding are associated with promoting elimination of TCDD and, in the case of breastfeeding, exposing infants through breast milk. Polycyclic aromatic hydrocarbons (PAHs) in cigarette smoke are capable of inducing CYP1A1, 1A2, and 1B1, which in turn may increase the rate of metabolism and later elimination of TCDD. A 30% decrease in TCDD half-life has been associated with smoking (Flesch-Janys et al., 1996).

Special Case of the Poisoning of Victor Yushchenko

In 2004, Victor Yushchenko, a candidate for the presidency of the Ukraine, was poisoned with TCDD. It led to severe chloracne and a blood serum TCDD concentration of 108,000 ppt (pg/g lipid wt), which is about 50,000 times as great as that in the general population at the time. The incident provided an opportunity to assess the toxicokinetics of TCDD after what was apparently a single large exposure. Serum and fat analysis of TCDD supports the first-order elimination half-life of 15.4 months in Yushchenko, and the similar decay curves confirmed that TCDD was in equilibrium between serum lipids and subcutaneous fat (Sorg et al., 2009). That is much shorter than the 7.2-year reference half-life reported by Milbrath et al. (2009) and supports the dose-dependent elimination of TCDD, which is associated with induction of potential TCDD-metabolizing enzymes (CYP1A1, 1A2, and 1B1) in very high TCDD exposures. Two metabolites of TCDD (2,3,7-trichloro-8-hydroxydibenzo-*p*-dioxin and 1,3,7,8-tetrachloro-2-hydroxydibenzo-*p*-dioxin) were detected in feces, serum, and urine but not in fat and skin. Over a 12-month period, about 38% of the TCDD-derived material was eliminated as metabolites (95% in feces, 5% in urine) and 62% as parent chemical. The metabolite:TCDD ratio in the blood serum was about one-fiftieth of that in the feces; this supports the conclusion that the metabolites were not originally ingested with TCDD. The very slow metabolism of TCDD has been previously reported in laboratory animal models (Gasiewicz et al., 1983; Olson, 1986; Olson et al., 1980; Poiger and Schlatter, 1979), but this is the first report of metabolism in humans. It is also noteworthy that the structures of the human metabolites are the same as previously reported in the rat and dog (Poiger et al., 1982; Sawahata et al., 1982).

In light of the variables discussed above and the effect of differences in physiologic states and metabolic processes, which can affect the mobilization of lipids and possibly of compounds stored in them, complex PBPK models have been developed to integrate exposure dose with organ mass, blood flow, metabolism, and lipid content to predict the movement of toxicants into and out of each organ. A number of recent modeling studies have been performed in an effort to understand the relevance of animal experimental studies to exposures that occur in human populations (Aylward et al., 2005a,b; Beaudouin et al., 2010; Emond et al., 2005).

Toxicity Profile

Effects on Tissues and Organs of Laboratory Animals

The effects of TCDD in laboratory animals have been observed in a number of species (rats, mice, guinea pigs, hamsters, monkeys, cows, and rabbits) after the administration of a variety of doses and after periods that represent acute exposures (less than 24 hours), subchronic exposures (1 day–3 months), and chronic exposure (more than 3 months). Some differences have been observed between species, particularly with respect to degree of sensitivity, but in general the effects observed are qualitatively similar. Relatively high exposures of TCDD affect a variety of organs and result in organ dysfunction and death. Animal species vary widely in lethal toxicity of TCDD; the oral LD_{50} of the chemical varies from 1 μg/kg (in guinea pigs) to 5,000 μg/kg (in hamsters). There is up to a 5,000-fold interspecies variability in the acute lethal potency of TCDD in mature guinea pigs, rats, and hamsters. The developing fetus, however, is especially vulnerable to TCDD exposure, and there is only about a 10-fold variability in fetal lethal potency among these species (Kransler et al., 2007; Peterson et al., 1993; Poland and Knutson, 1982). A characteristic of TCDD exposure is a wasting syndrome that includes loss of adipose and muscle tissue and severe weight loss, but the specific mechanisms of lethality remain unknown. In most rodents, exposure to TCDD leads to hepatic enlargement, the presence of hepatic lesions, and impaired hepatic function. The thymus is also sensitive. Finally, in both humans and nonhuman primates, TCDD exposure results in chloracne and associated dermatologic changes. As will be discussed in more detail in Chapters 6–13, studies performed in animal models have indicated that exposure to TCDD adversely affects the heart, the skin, and the immune, endocrine, and reproductive systems and increases the incidence of cancers of the liver, skin, thyroid, adrenal cortex, hard palate, nasal turbinates, tongue, and respiratory and lymphatic systems (ATSDR, 1998; Barouki et al., 2012; Birnbaum, 1994; Huff et al., 1994; Knerr and Schrenk, 2006). When TCDD has been administered to pregnant animals, birth defects—such as cleft palate, malformations of the reproductive organs of male and female progeny, and abnormalities in the cardiovascular, pulmonary, and nervous systems—have been observed.

Effects on Enzymes, Hormones, and Receptors in Laboratory Animals and Cultured Cells

In addition to adversely affecting the ability of specific organs to fulfill their normal physiologic roles, TCDD has been found to alter the function and expression of essential proteins, particularly a number of enzymes. The metabolism of foreign chemicals often changes their biologic properties, increasing their polarity (water solubility) and thus promoting the elimination of the metabolites. The enzymes that are most affected by TCDD are ones that act on or metabolize xenobiotics and hormones. Among the enzymes affected by TCDD, the best-studied is CYP1A1, which metabolizes xenobiotics. In laboratory animals, exposure to TCDD commonly results in an increase in CYP1A1 in most tissues; CYP1A1 therefore is often used as a marker of TCDD exposure. Related enzymes, which are also increased with TCDD exposure, include CYP1B1 and CYP1A2, which with CYP1A1 are capable of biotransforming some procarcinogens to potentially mutagenic and carcinogenic metabolites.

Other enzymes that are affected by TCDD metabolize hormones, such as thyroid hormones, retinoic acid, testosterone, estrogens, and adrenal steroids. Those hormones transmit their signals by interacting with specific proteins called receptors and in this manner initiate a chain of events in many tissues of the body. For example, binding of the primary female sex hormone, estrogen, to the estrogen receptor promotes the formation of breasts and the thickening of the endometrium and regulates the menstrual cycle. Exposure to TCDD can increase the metabolism of estrogen and thus lead to a decrease in the amount of estrogen available for binding and activating the estrogen receptor. The ultimate effect of TCDD is an interference with all the bodily functions that are regulated by estrogens. Similarly, the actions of TCDD on the adrenal steroids can adversely affect their ability to regulate glucose tolerance, insulin sensitivity, lipid metabolism, obesity, vascular function, and cardiac remodeling. In addition to changing the amount of hormone present, TCDD has been found to interfere with the ability of receptors to fulfill their role in transmitting hormone signals. Animal models have shown that exposure to TCDD can increase the amounts of enzymes in the body and interfere with the ability of hormones to activate their specific hormone receptors. Those actions of TCDD on enzymes and hormone receptors are thought to underlie, in part, observed developmental and reproductive effects and cancers that are hormone-responsive.

Effects on Paths of Cellular Differentiation

The broad spectrum of TCDD effects on hormone and growth factor systems, cytokines, and other signal-transducer pathways indicates that TCDD is an extremely powerful growth dysregulator (Birnbaum, 1994). Research performed primarily in cultured cells has shown that TCDD can affect the ability of cells to undergo such processes as proliferation, differentiation, and apoptosis. During the proliferative process, cells grow and divide. When cells are differentiating, they are undergoing a change from less specialized to more specialized. Cellular differentiation is essential for an organism to mature from a fetal to an adult state. In the adult, proper differentiation is required for normal functions of the body, for example, in maintaining a normally responsive immune system. Processes of controlled cell death, such as apoptosis, are similarly important during development of the fetus and are necessary for normal physiologic functions in the adult. Apoptosis is a way for the body to eliminate damaged or unnecessary cells. The ability of a cell to undergo proliferation, differentiation, and apoptosis is tightly controlled by an intricate network of signaling molecules that allows the body to maintain the appropriate size and number of all the specialized cells that form the fabric of complex tissues and organs. Disruption of that network that alters the delicate balance of cell fate can have severe consequences, including impairment of the function of the organ because of the absence of specialized cells. Alternatively, the presence of an excess of some kinds of cells can result in the formation and development of tumors. Thus, the ability of TCDD to disrupt the normal course of a specific cell to proliferate, differentiate, or undergo apoptosis is thought to underlie (at least in part) its adverse effects on the immune system and the developing fetus and its ability to promote the formation of some cancers.

Mechanisms

TCDD binds and activates the aryl hydrocarbon receptor (AHR) in the cells of virtually every tissue in the body. The ability of TCDD to bind to the AHR with high affinity is considered to be necessary—but not sufficient—to produce the wide array of adverse effects associated with TCDD exposure. The pathologic responses associated with exposure to TCDD are thought to be due to binding to and activation of the AHR and later alterations in the expression of TCDD-regulated genes and to altered signaling of biologic pathways that interact with the AHR signal-transduction mechanism (Poland and Knutson, 1982; Safe, 1990; Schmidt and Bradfield, 1996; Whitlock, 1990).

The AHR functions as a ligand-activated nuclear transcription factor. On binding of agonists (ligands), such as TCDD, the AHR forms a heterodimer with a structurally related protein called AHR nuclear translocator (ARNT). The dimeric complex binds to core DNA sequences called xenobiotic-responsive elements (XREs) or dioxin-responsive elements (DREs) in the promotor region of responsive genes and enhances the transcription of those genes. Many of the AHR-regulated genes encode drug-metabolizing enzymes, such as CYP1A1, CYP1A2, CYP1B1, and a variety of phase II conjugating enzymes. Although the up-regulation of these enzymes is a sensitive biomarker of exposure to TCDD and in part contributes mechanistically to some of the adverse effects of TCDD, the tissue-, species-, time-, and dose-specific modulation (increase or decrease) of many genes is thought to contribute to the wide array of toxic responses to TCDD exposure (Black et al., 2012; Boverhof et al., 2006; Ovando et al., 2006, 2010; Perdew, 2008; Puga et al., 2009).

AHR Signaling Pathways

The primary and most intensely studied pathway by which TCDD elicits biologic responses is depicted in Figure 4-6. In the absence of bound ligand, the inactive AHR is retained in the cytoplasm of the cell in a complex consisting of two molecules of the heat-shock protein hsp90, one molecule of prostaglandin E synthase 3 (p23) (Kazlauskas et al., 1999), and one molecule of the immunophilin-like protein hepatitis B virus X-associated protein 2 (XAP2) (Petrulis et al., 2003), previously identified as either AHR-interacting protein (AIP; Ma and Whitlock, 1997) or AHR-associated protein 9 (ARA9; Carver and Bradfield, 1997). The hsp90 dimer–p23 complex plays multiple roles in the protection of the AHR from proteolysis, maintaining it in a conformation that makes it accessible to ligand binding at the same time that it prevents the premature binding of ARNT (Carver et al., 1994; Pongratz et al., 1992; Whitelaw et al., 1993). XAP2 interacts with the carboxyl terminus of hsp90 and with the AHR nuclear-localization signal (NLS), a short amino acid domain that targets the receptor for interaction with

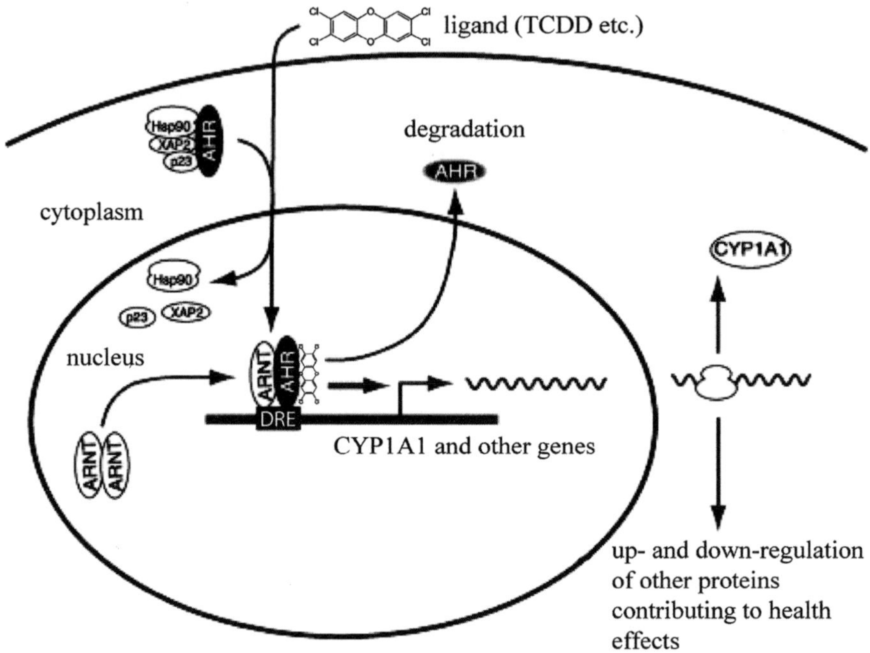

FIGURE 4-6 Mechanism of gene induction and repression after AHR activation by TCDD.

nuclear-transport proteins. Binding of XAP2 blocks such interaction, preventing the inappropriate trafficking of the receptor into the nucleus (Petrulis et al., 2003).

Binding of ligand (such as TCDD) induces the release of XAP2 and the exposure of the NLS and leads to the binding of nuclear-import proteins and translocation of the cytosolic complex into the nucleus (Davarinos and Pollenz, 1999; Song and Pollenz, 2002). Once in the nucleus, hsp90, p23, and XAP2 dissociate from the AHR, and this allows the binding of ARNT (Hoffman et al., 1991; Probst et al., 1993). The activated AHR–ARNT heterodimeric complex is then capable of directly or indirectly interacting with DNA by binding to recognition sequences in the regulatory region of responsive genes (Dolwick et al., 1993; Probst et al., 1993).

The canonical DNA recognition motif of the AHR–ARNT complex is referred to as the AHR-responsive element (AHRE, also referred to as the DRE or the XRE, for dioxin- or xenobiotic-responsive element, respectively). This element is found in the promoter region of AHR-responsive genes and contains the core sequence 5′-GCGTG-3′ (Shen and Whitlock, 1992), which is part of a more extensive consensus-binding sequence, 5′-T/GNGCGTGA/CG/CA-3′ (Lusska et al., 1993; Yao and Denison, 1992). The AHR–ARNT complex binds to the AHRE core sequence in such a manner that ARNT binds to 5′-GTG-3′ and AHR binds to 5′-TC/TGC-3′ (Bacsi et al., 1995; Swanson et al., 1995). A second type of element, termed AHRE-II, 5′-CATG(N6)C[T/A]TG-3′, has been shown to be capable of acting indirectly with the AHR–ARNT complex (Boutros et al., 2004; Sogawa et al., 2004). The end result of the process is the recruitment of the transcriptional machinery associated with RNA polymerase II and the initiation of differential changes in the expression of the genes bearing the AHR–ARNT recognition motif. Many of the genes code for proteins responsible for detoxification reactions directed at the elimination of the ligand. Research suggests that post-translational modifications in histone proteins may modify the response (Hestermann and Brown, 2003; Schnekenburger et al., 2007).

In addition to the widely accepted view that the actions of TCDD are mediated by binding of the activated AHR–ARNT dimer to AHREs on DNA, which results in altered gene expression (Figure 4-6), more recent studies suggest that a "nongenomic" pathway within the cytoplasm also contributes to the toxic effects of TCDD, as reviewed by Matsumura (2009). The TCDD-mediated activation of AHR within the cytoplasm does not involve binding to ARNT or DNA and appears to contribute to rapid inflammatory responses associated with TCDD (Sciullo et al., 2008). In several cell lines, activation of protein kinase C (PKC) and the later activation of the serine phosphorylated form of cytosolic phospholipase A2 (cPLA2) takes place within 15 min of TCDD exposure (Dong and Matsumura, 2008; Park et al., 2007). It is proposed that within the cytoplasm, TCDD-mediated activation of AHR leads to a rapid increase in intracellular Ca^{2+}, plus activation of cPLA2, protein kinases, and pro-inflammatory proteins, such as cyclooxygenase (COX-2) (Matsumura, 2009). This pathway and other alternative mechanisms of TCDD-mediated AHR activation have also been reviewed by Denison et al. (2011) and Perdew (2008).

AHR Physiology

The vertebrate AHR is presumed to have evolved from its counterpart in invertebrates, in which it serves a ligand-independent role in normal development processes. The ancestral function of the AHR appears to be the regulation of specific aspects of embryonic development, it having acquired the ability to bind xenobiotic compounds only during vertebrate evolution (Hahn, 2001). The invertebrate AHR also functions as a transcription factor and binds to the same dimerization partner (ARNT) and DNA-response elements as the vertebrate protein, but it does not respond to any of the environmental ligands recognized by the vertebrate receptor. Instead, it regulates diverse developmental processes that are independent of exogenous ligand exposure, such as neuronal differentiation during worm development in *Caenorhabditis elegans* (Huang et al., 2004; Qin and Powell-Coffman, 2004) or normal morphogenesis of legs, antennae, and bristles in *Drosophila melanogaster* (Adachi-Yamada et al., 2005; Céspedes et al., 2010). In developing vertebrates, the AHR seems to play a role in cellular proliferation and differentiation and, in keeping with this role in invertebrates, also has a developmental role in craniofacial, renal, and cardiovascular morphogenesis (Birnbaum et al., 1989; Fernandez-Salguero et al., 1997; Lahvis et al., 2005). Other potential functional roles of the AHR include reproduction, innate immunity, tumor suppression, and blood-pressure regulation (Fujii-Kuriyama and Kawajiri, 2010).

The clearest adaptive physiologic response to AHR activation is the induction of xenobiotic-metabolizing enzymes involved in detoxification of toxic ligands. Evidence of that response, which was described above, was first observed in conjunction with the induction of *Cyp1a1*, which resulted from exposure to PAHs or TCDD and was directly related to activation of the AHR signaling pathway (Israel and Whitlock, 1983, 1984). Because of the presence of the AHRE motif in their gene promoters, other metabolizing genes were tested and found to be induced by AHR ligands, and this led to the identification of a so-called AHR gene battery of phase I and phase II detoxification genes that code for the drug-metabolizing enzymes CYP1A1, CYP1A2, CYP1B1, NQO1, ALHD3A1, UGT1A2, and GSTA1 (Nebert et al., 2000). Presumably, vertebrates have evolved those enzymes to detect a wide array of foreign, potentially toxic chemicals, represented in the wide variety of substrates that the AHR is able to bind to and whose biotransformation and elimination it is able to facilitate.

A potential complication of the adaptive responses elicited by AHR activation is the induction of a toxic response. Toxicity may result from the adaptive response itself if the induction of metabolizing enzymes results in the production of toxic metabolites. For example, the PAH benzo[a]pyrene (B[a]P), an AHR ligand, induces its own metabolism and detoxification by the AHR-dependent signaling mechanism described earlier but paradoxically becomes bioactivated to a toxic metabolite in several tissues by metabolism that depends on CYP1A1 and CYP1B1 activity (Harrigan et al., 2004). A second potential source of AHR-mediated toxicity may be aberrant changes in global gene expression beyond those observed in the AHR gene battery. The global changes in gene expression may lead to deleterious changes in cellular processes and physiology. Microarray analysis has proved invaluable in understanding and characterizing that response (Boverhof et al., 2006; Martinez et al., 2002; Ovando et al., 2006, 2010; Puga et al., 2000, 2004; Takeda et al., 2012; Vezina et al., 2004).

It is clear that the AHR is an essential component of the toxicity of dioxin and of dioxin-like chemicals (DLCs). Homozygous deletion of the AHR in mice leads to a phenotype that is resistant to the toxic effects of TCDD and to the carcinogenic effects of B[a]P (Fernandez-Salguero et al., 1996; Lahvis and Bradfield, 1998; Schmidt et al., 1996). AHR knockout mice, however, have other phenotypic effects, including reduced liver size, hepatic fibrosis, and cardiovascular abnormalities. Hence, it is likely that dioxin has effects that are due to disruption of endogenous AHR functions and that are unrelated to the intrinsic toxicity of some of its ligands.

Definition of Dioxin-Like Compounds, Toxic Equivalence Factor, and Toxic Equivalents

TCDD has the highest affinity for the AHR, but many other chemicals have dioxin-like properties: they have similar chemical structures, have similar physiochemical properties, and cause a common battery of toxic responses because of their relatively high affinity for the AHR. Because of their hydrophobic nature and resistance to metabolism, these chemicals persist and bioaccumulate in fatty tissues of animals and humans. Although there are several hundred polychlorinated, polybrominated, and mixed polychlorinated-polybrominated dibenzo-*p*-dioxins, dibenzofurans, and biphenyls, only a relatively small number of congeners of these chemical classes display dioxin-like activity. Only 17 polychlorinated dibenzo-*p*-dioxins and polychlorinated dibenzofurans with chlorine at the 2, 3, 7, and 8 positions and a few of the coplanar polychlorinated biphenyls that are often measured in environmental samples are recognized as being DLCs.

In the context of risk assessment, these polychlorinated–polybrominated dibenzo-*p*-dioxin, polychlorinated dibenzofuran, and biphenyl DLCs are commonly found as complex mixtures when detected in environmental media and biologic tissues or when measured as environmental releases from specific sources. That complicates the human health risk assessment that may be associated with exposures to varied mixtures of DLCs. To address the problem, the concept of toxic equivalence has been adopted by the scientific community, and the toxic equivalence factor (TEF) has been developed and introduced to facilitate risk assessment of exposure to those chemical mixtures. On the most basic level, TEFs compare the potential toxicity of each DLC found in a mixture with the toxicity of TCDD, the most toxic member of the group. The procedure involves assigning individual TEFs to the DLCs on the basis of in vivo and in vitro potency relative to TCDD, which is assigned a TEF of 1.0. The DLCs have been assigned TEFs ranging from 0.00001 to 1.0 by the World Health Organization (WHO) (van den Berg et al., 2006, as summarized in Table 4-2). Interim TEF values have been established for brominated congeners by the most recent (2011) joint WHO-UNEP (UN Environment Programme) meeting to evaluate the WHO Toxicity Equivalency Factor scheme. The recommendation is to use the TEF of the corresponding chlorinated congener as an interim TEF value for brominated congeners for human risk assessment (van den Berg et al., 2013).

When several chemicals are present in a mixture, the toxicity of the mixture is estimated by multiplying the TEF of each DLC in the mixture by its mass concentration and summing the products to yield the TCDD toxic equivalents (TEQs) of the mixture. In that approach to assessing dioxin-like activity of a complex real-world mixture of DLCs, an environmental or biologic specimen

TABLE 4-2 World Health Organization Toxicity Equivalence Factors (TEFs) for Dioxin-Like Chemicals (Values Revised as of 2005)

Chemical	TEF
Chlorinated dibenzo-*p*-dioxins	
2,3,7,8-TCDD	1.0
1,2,3,7,8-PeCDD	1.0
1,2,3,4,7,8-HxCDD	0.1
1,2,3,6,7,8-HxCDD	0.1
1,2,3,7,8,9-HxCDD	0.1
1,2,3,4,6,7,8-HpCDD	0.01
OctoCDD	0.0003
Chlorinated dibenzofurans	
2,3,7,8-TCDF	0.1
1,2,3,7,8-PeCDF	0.03
2,3,4,7,8-PeCDF	0.3
1,2,3,4,7,8-HxCDF	0.1
1,2,3,6,7,8-HxCDF	0.1
1,2,3,7,8,9-HxCDF	0.1
2,3,4,7,8,9-HxCDF	0.1
1,2,3,4,6,7,8-HpCDF	0.01
1,2,3,4,7,8,9-HpCDF	0.01
OctoCDF	0.0003
Non-*ortho*-substituted PCBs	
PCB 77—3,3′,4,4′-tetraCB	0.0001
PCB 81—3,4,4′,5-tetraCB	0.0003
PCB 126—3,3′,4,4′,5-pentaCB	0.1
PCB 169—3,3′,4,4′,5,5′-hexaCB	0.03
Mono-*ortho*-substituted PCBs	
PCB 105—2,3,3′,4,4′-pentaCB	0.00003
PCB 114—2,3,4,4′,5-pentaCB	0.00003
PCB 118—2,3′,4,4′,5-pentaCB	0.00003
PCB 123—2′,3,4,4′,5-pentaCB	0.00003
PCB 156—2,3,3′,4,4′,5-hexaCB	0.00003
PCB 157—2,3,3′,4,4′,5′-hexaCB	0.00003
PCB 167—2,3′,4,4′,5,5′-hexaCB	0.00003
PCB 189—2,3,3′,4,4′,5,5′-heptaCB	0.00003

NOTE: CB, chlorinated biphenyl; CDD, chlorinated dibenzo-*p*-dioxin; CDF, chlorinated dibenzofuran; PCB, polychlorinated biphenyl; TEF, toxicity equivalency factor.
SOURCE: Adapted from: van den Berg et al. (2006).

with a 100-ppt (100-pg/g) TEQ is toxicologically equivalent to 100-ppt TCDD. There are two accepted specialized methods for assessing the DLCs in a complex biologic or environmental specimen: one involves analytic chemistry that quantifies specific DLCs (high-resolution gas chromatography–mass spectroscopy), and the other a reporter-gene biologic screen that assesses dioxin-like activity due to binding to the AHR in a transformed cell line (CALUX, EPA method 4435).

Epidemiologic studies discussed in this and other updates assess exposure by reporting the specific concentration of TCDD in a specimen or by expressing dioxin-like activity in a complex mixture in units of TEQs.

Carcinogenic Classification

EPA and the International Agency for Research on Cancer (IARC), a branch of WHO, have defined criteria to classify the potential carcinogenicity of chemicals on the basis of the weight of scientific evidence from animal, human, epidemiologic, mechanistic, and mode-of-action studies. EPA classified TCDD as a "probable human carcinogen" in 1985 and as "carcinogenic to humans" in a 2003 reassessment. In 1998, the IARC panel of experts concluded that the weight of scientific evidence supported the classification of dioxin as a class I carcinogen, that is, as "carcinogenic to humans." Four years later, the US National Toxicology Program upgraded its classification to "known to be a human carcinogen." In 2006, a panel of experts convened by the National Research Council to evaluate the EPA reassessment concluded that TCDD was "likely to be carcinogenic to humans;" this designation reflected the revised EPA *Guidelines for Carcinogen Risk Assessment* made public in 2005.

Genotoxicity

Genotoxicity describes a deleterious action that affects the integrity of a cell's DNA. Genotoxic substances are known to be potentially mutagenic or carcinogenic. Although TCDD is carcinogenic in humans and laboratory animals, it is generally classified as nongenotoxic and nonmutagenic (Wassom et al., 1977). There is no evidence of covalent binding of TCDD or its metabolites to DNA (Poland and Glover, 1979). TCDD does interact with DNA through a receptor-mediated pathway that involves the initial binding of TCDD to the AHR, binding of the activated receptor complex to DREs on DNA and later alterations in expression of TCDD-regulated genes, and altered signaling of biologic pathways that interact with the AHR signal-transduction mechanism (Poland and Knutson, 1982; Safe, 1990; Schmidt and Bradfield, 1996; Whitlock, 1990). TCDD, 2,4,5-T, and 2,4-D were not mutagenic in *Salmonella typhimurium* with or without the addition of liver metabolic-activation enzymes (Blevins, 1991; Mortelmans et al., 1984). TCDD-induced cytogenetic damage in laboratory mice showed no increase in the frequencies of sister-chromatid exchanges, chromosomal aberrations, or micronuclei in bone marrow cells of either C57Bl/6J or DBA/2J mice after administration of a single high dose of TCDD—up to 150 μg/kg (Meyne et al., 1985). TCDD did not alter the frequency or spectrum of mutations in male and female Big Blue transgenic rats (Thornton et al., 2001). There is one report of a positive result with TCDD in a test that measured induction of chromosomal deletions resulting from intrachromosomal recombination in mouse embryos in vivo (Schiestl et al., 1997).

In summary, the vast majority of studies did not detect mutagenic activity of TCDD in a variety of in vitro and in vivo short-term tests.

Other Toxic Outcomes

Chloracne is a signature effect of high exposure to TCDD and DLCs in some species and in humans who are sensitive.

There is an extensive body of evidence from experimental studies in animal-model systems that TCDD, other dioxins, and several DLCs are immunotoxic (Kerkvliet, 2009). Although the available evidence on dioxin immunotoxicity in humans is scant, mechanistic considerations support the notion that chemical alterations of immune function would cause adverse health outcomes because of the critical role that the immune system plays in general protection—fighting off infection and eliminating cancer cells at early stages. Because of those considerations, the chemicals are potential immunotoxicants.

Similarly, reproduction and embryonic development clearly are targets of TCDD, other dioxins, and DLCs; it is found consistently that the adverse effects are more prevalent during fetal development than in the adult. Although data on those effects in humans are practically nonexistent, some good data are now emerging on the developmental effects of DLCs in humans (Mocarelli et al., 2008). Human and animal studies have revealed other potential health outcomes, including cardiovascular disease, hepatic disease, thyroid dysfunction, lipid disorders, neurotoxicity, and metabolic disorders, such as diabetes.

A number of effects of TCDD exposure in vitro appear to be independent of AHR-mediated transcription and in at least one instance perhaps independent of AHR itself. Guo et al. (2004) showed that TCDD induced expression of transforming growth factor-α and other genes involved in extracellular matrix deposition in cells from mice that had homozygous ablation of the *Ahr* gene. Studies have shown that TCDD can mobilize calcium from intracellular sources and increase calcium imported from the culture medium (Puga et al., 1995). Mitochondrial oxidative stress has been shown to be induced when calcium is mobilized (Senft et al., 2002). Calcium mobilization by TCDD may have an important effect on signal-transduction mechanisms that control gene expression, inasmuch as several proto-oncogenes, such as *c-fos*, are activated by calcium changes.

Summary of Biologic Plausibility That TCDD Induces Adverse Effects in Humans

Mechanistic studies in vitro and in laboratory animals have characterized the biochemical pathways and types of biologic events that contribute to adverse effects of exposure to TCDD. For example, much evidence indicates that TCDD, acting via the AHR in partnership with ARNT, alters gene expression. Receptor binding may result in release of other cytoplasmic proteins that alter the expression or activity of other cell-regulatory proteins. Mechanistic studies also indicate that many other cellular-component proteins contribute to the gene-regulatory effect and that the response to TCDD exposure involves a complex interplay between genetic and environmental factors. Comparative data from animal and human cells in vitro and from tissues suggest a strong qualitative similarity among species in response to TCDD, and this further supports the applicability to humans of the generalized model of initial events in response to dioxin exposure. Several studies indicate, however, that there may be substantial quantitative differences in qualitatively similar responses among species, with humans generally being less sensitive than rodents.

Biochemical and biologic responses to TCDD exposure are considered adaptive or simply reflective of exposure and not adverse in themselves if they take place within the normal homeostatic ranges of an organism. However, they may exceed normal physiologic boundaries or constitute early events in a pathway that leads to damage in sensitive members of the population. In the latter case, the response is toxic and would be expected to cause an adverse health effect. Those generalizations set the ground rules for the concept of *biologic plausibility*, which relies on extrapolation from animal studies to human risks, and for the *precautionary principle*, which bases decision making on minimizing exposure if the precise nature or magnitude of the potential damage that a substance may cause in humans is uncertain.

LIMITATIONS OF EXTRAPOLATING RESULTS OF LABORATORY STUDIES TO HUMAN RESPONSES

In some instances, toxic responses identified in laboratory-animal and cell-culture studies are not detected in epidemiologic studies after human exposure to the same chemicals. Although animal and cell-culture studies provide important links to understanding of biochemical and molecular mechanisms associated with toxicity induced by xenobiotics, many factors must be considered in extrapolating their results to human disease and disease progression. The following are key factors that might limit the ability of laboratory studies to predict human responses completely and accurately.

- **Magnitude and duration of exposure.** In many instances, animal and cell-culture studies are conducted at higher exposures and for shorter durations than are typical in human exposures. For example, the concentrations of TCDD used in animal studies can be many times higher than in the TCDD exposures of Vietnam veterans during their military service. In addition, TCDD is a persistent organic pollutant, and this results in human exposure that occurs over a lifetime, whereas animal studies seldom examine chronic low-level exposure that occurs over a period of many months or years. Animal studies that establish a measurement of body burden over a specific period provide the best potential for extrapolation to humans.

- **Toxicokinetics.** The toxicokinetics—absorption, distribution, metabolism, and excretion—of xenobiotics can vary widely between laboratory animals and humans. As shown in Table 4-1, the biologic half-life of TCDD varies from 8–29 days in rats and mice to about 7 years in humans even though drug-metabolizing enzymes—including cytochrome P450 1A1, 1A2, and 1B1—are up-regulated or induced via TCDD-mediated activation of the AHR in both rat and human livers (Black et al., 2012).
- **Timing of exposure.** Many organ systems are more susceptible to xenobiotic exposure during critical stages of development, differentiation, or function—such as during gestation or in the face of another external challenge (for example, antigens, smoking, dietary salt, and fat)—than at other times. Therefore, the response of some systems (such as immune or cardiovascular systems) may depend on the timing of exposure relative to the other challenges.
- **Exposure composition.** Most animal and cell-culture studies involve exposure to single chemicals or a well-defined mixture, but most human exposures are to complex mixtures from multiple sources.
- **Difference in AHR affinity.** The binding affinity of AHR for TCDD differs between species (discussed in Okey et al., 2005). Many strains of mice used for toxicologic study harbor a high-affinity AHR allele (AHR^b) and exhibit greater sensitivity to hepatic CYP1A induction, immunosuppression, birth defects, and other responses than do strains that carry the low-affinity allele (AHR^d). That simple allelic difference in AHR affinity has not been observed in humans, and the TCDD-binding affinity of the AHR found in most humans more closely resembles the low-affinity mouse AHR^d allele. Nonetheless, Nebert et al. (2004) reported that some people have a TCDD-binding affinity that is 12 times higher than that in others. Thus, although humans are generally considered less sensitive on the basis of an AHR that has a low TCDD-binding affinity, this assumption may not apply to everyone.
- **Complex disease etiology.** The etiology of human diseases is highly influenced by genetics, environmental factors, and gene–environment interactions; these factors can be protective as well as deleterious. In addition to the chemical of interest, environmental factors commonly influencing human responses include diet, prescription and over-the-counter pharmaceuticals, cigarette smoking, alcohol consumption, and stress. Stress produced via known or unknown sources is a well-known modifier of human disease responses (for example, immune and cardiovascular responses). Furthermore, stress is an ever-present variable that is difficult to assess or

control for in epidemiologic studies because there is substantial individual variation in response to it (Cohen et al., 2007b). In contrast, laboratory studies are often conducted with inbred strains of animals under tightly controlled experimental conditions and thus may underestimate or overestimate the potential contribution of a single chemical exposure to disease development.

- **Sex differences.** There are well-known differences in susceptibility to xenobiotic exposures between male and female animals, some of which are modified by sex steroids. For example, female Sprague Dawley rats are significantly more responsive to the hepatotoxic (neoplastic and non-neoplastic) effects of TCDD than are males of the same strain (Kociba et al., 1978).

EPIGENETICS

Epigenetics is the term used to describe mechanisms that regulate gene expression and genomic stability and are independent of changes in DNA sequence and mitotically stable; that is, they will be replicated when a cell divides (Christensen and Marsit, 2011; Cortessis et al., 2012; Skinner et al., 2010). The epigenetic marks on DNA are maintained every time a cell divides and are needed to maintain the identity and function of the cell type.

The history of epigenetics began in the 1940s when Conrad Waddington coined the term *epigenetics* to describe gene–environment interactions that alter biologic traits (Waddington, 1940, 1953, 1956). It was not until the 1970s that the first molecular epigenetic factor was described: DNA methylation, the chemical addition of a methyl group to DNA (Holliday and Pugh, 1975). In the 1980s, the role of DNA methylation in modifying gene expression—turning genes on and off—was established (Chen and Riggs, 2005). In the 1990s, the chemical modification of histone proteins associated with DNA also was shown to modify gene expression, thus establishing a second molecular epigenetic mechanism (Turner, 1998). In the early 2000s, various small noncoding RNA molecules were shown to regulate DNA activity (Sato et al., 2011). Around 2005, the first mapping of genome-wide epigenetic marks (epigenomes) was conducted (Pokholok et al., 2005). The marks act together in an exquisitely choreographed fashion to control the cellular ability to interact with, process, and initiate events and to respond to the signals and needs of the individual and local tissue environment.

Today, the processes recognized as epigenetic mechanisms are DNA methylation (Chen and Riggs, 2005; Holliday and Pugh, 1975), histone modification (Turner, 1998), alterations in chromatin structure (Murr, 2010), and modulation of expression by some small RNA molecules (Valeri et al., 2009). DNA methylation is the addition of a methyl group onto specific nucleotides. In mammals, it occurs at cytosine nucleotides that are adjacent to guanine nucleotides. Methylation of DNA can alter the expression of the adjacent gene, particularly if it occurs in the promoter of the gene. Other modulations of DNA include hydroxymethylation (which is prominent in stem cells) and adenylation. Histones are the proteins that bind and form complex structures with DNA called nucleosomes. Chemical modifications of histones, such as methylation and acetylation, can alter histone structure and modify gene expression, particularly if the modification occurs in the promoter of the gene (Turner, 1998). The coiling or twisting of the DNA–histone complexes creates a structure called chromatin, and the structure of the chromatin can alter gene expression. The most recently recognized epigenetic factor consists of small noncoding RNA molecules that can associate with mRNA and regulate gene expression.

The interaction of all those epigenetic processes creates the epigenome, and the epigenome has a critical role in regulating gene expression independently of changes in DNA sequence (Christensen and Marsit, 2011; Cortessis et al., 2012; Skinner et al., 2010). The variation that is possible in the epigenome is startling: the histone proteins that control chromatin configurations have many dozens of possible modifications, and there are upwards of 50 million nucleotides in the DNA where methylation can occur and participate in regulating the cellular state. That implies that trillions of configurations of the epigenome are possible.

Environmental epigenetics involves the ability of environmental factors—such as nutrition, toxicants, and stress—to alter epigenetic programming. Thus, epigenetics provides a molecular mechanism by which environmental factors can influence disease etiology (Jirtle and Skinner, 2007; Szyf, 2007). The role of epigenetics in disease etiology has been shown for cancer and a number of other diseases (Christensen and Marsit, 2011; Cortessis et al., 2012; Skinner et al., 2010). In addition, exposure to environmental factors at critical times of development has the ability to alter epigenetic programming and to cause changes in gene expression (Skinner et al., 2010). Hence, immune responses, fetal development, and reproductive health are important examples of how epigenetic mechanisms play crucial roles in normal physiology.

New investigative tools and a more refined understanding of the epigenetic process have given rise to active research on the nature of the relationship between environmental exposure to epigenetically active agents and the occurrence of diverse disease states, including cancer, reproductive developmental conditions, and immune dysregulation. The committee sought to review data on the potential relationship of the exposures of interest with adverse epigenetic effects in the directly exposed veterans in an attempt to find evidence linking the exposures to disease processes that might have been mediated epigenetically. We also sought to review relevant data on female veterans and male veterans separately inasmuch as the epigenetic consequences of exposures could be different, particularly in the case of adverse reproductive outcomes.

A relevant example is that in vitro treatment of preimplantation embryos with TCDD alters the DNA methylation of imprinted genes (Wu et al., 2004). That in turn affects the functions and development of cells, tissues, and biologic systems.

It is well established that early-life exposures or environmental influences are associated with the onset of disease much later in life (Barker et al., 2010). Thus, an early developmental alteration in the epigenome provides a molecular mechanism whereby adult diseases can have a developmental basis.

Most epigenetic modifications occur in somatic cells and are not heritable, but do have the potential to generate effects in the exposed the individual. There is, however, the possibility of epigenetic transgenerational inheritance, which involves the ability of the environment to promote a permanent alteration in the germ line that is transmitted to later generations (Skinner et al., 2010). Manikkam et al. (2012) have shown that exposure of pregnant female rats to TCDD at critical times of development of the germ line (when epigenetic programming is being established) can lead to abnormalities in the third-generation offspring, including kidney disease and changes in the ovaries and sperm of the offspring. There are few data on possible male-mediated heritable effects of TCDD or other environmental compounds. The sparse data include results of studies of lead, a known developmental toxicant. Lead exposure can alter semen quality in males (Alexander et al., 1996) and has been shown to induce paternally mediated developmental toxicity in rats (Anjum et al., 2011); this demonstrates that male-mediated effects on reproduction can be induced by reproductive toxicants. However, there is a serious need for additional study of the question, particularly of the effects of the compounds of interest to this committee.

In summary, the ability of epigenetic mechanisms to regulate gene expression might underlie the ability of xenobiotic exposure to contribute to disease development and the potential for offspring to inherit effects of the disrupted epigenetic processes.

DEVELOPMENTAL IMMUNOTOXICITY

A second emerging field in biologic science that may provide insight into the mechanism of xenobiotic-induced disease is the disruption of the developing immune system by xenobiotic exposure, developmental immunotoxicity (DIT). The developing immune system is among the most sensitive physiologic targets of prenatal and childhood environmental insult. The sensitivity is due, in part, to the novel processes of gene rearrangement, somatic-cell selection, and immune-cell distribution that are required to produce a security system that can effectively protect not only the child but also the aging adult against external challenges without itself producing immune-mediated chronic disease. To produce that security system, the maturation of the immune system needs a critical series of steps that produce highly specialized immune cells that are capable of self vs nonself recognition and are tailored to the specialized functional environments of different tissues and organs (such as brain, lungs, skin, liver, gastrointestinal tract, and reproductive tract). A disruption of immune development can place the integrity of the organism at risk.

Among the known risk factors for DIT are such chemicals as heavy metals, some pesticides, industrial solvents such as trichloroethylene, and polychlorinated biphenyls. The adverse outcomes of DIT may become apparent soon after exposure or can emerge much later in life. Often, childhood or adult infections can trigger the appearance of DIT-associated immune problems that were established earlier in life (Dietert, 2009). DIT-induced alterations can also contribute to myriad health problems related to dysfunction or pathologic conditions in virtually any tissue or organ. Chemicals, drugs, infectious agents, and physical and emotional stressors can act synergistically and increase the risk of DIT. Not everyone is at identical risk for DIT. People who have particular genotypes may be at increased risk for specific chemical-induced DIT on the basis of heritable factors that affect metabolism or immune vulnerability.

The heightened sensitivity of the developing immune system is due to the existence of critical developmental windows of vulnerability during which environmental interference with key steps of immune maturation can change the entire course of immune development and result in later-life immune dysfunction and increased risk of disease. The events programmed for these critical developmental windows have several basic features:

- They are necessary, usually one-time events of early development, with no equivalents in adults.
- They lock in building blocks on which additional maturational events rely.
- If they do not occur both on time and efficiently, the ramifications are usually profound, prolonged, and irreversible.

Examples of critical windows of immune vulnerability and the chemicals that can cause disruptions have been described in several reviews (Dietert and Dietert, 2008; Dietert and Piepenbrink, 2006; Dietert et al., 2000; Holsapple et al., 2003; Landreth, 2002) and include

- The process of the seeding of immune cells in tissues where they grow into resident populations.
- The selection process of thymocytes in the thymus to distinguish nonself from self during the development of acquired immunity.
- The maturation of macrophage populations in the lung, in the brain, and elsewhere.
- The maturation of dendritic cells to provide balanced immune responses.
- The initial development, expansion, and seeding to the periphery of t-regulatory cell populations.

The increased sensitivity of the fetal, neonatal, and juvenile immune systems compared with the immune system of an adult can be manifested as a sensitivity to lower doses of chemical exposure than doses that affect the adult; a greater persistence of the immune problems that follow exposure than are seen in adults; a broader array of immune problems than are experienced by adults; and greater likelihood that a second later-life chemical exposure or environmental stressor will trigger an unexpected immune problem.

It is important to note that disruption of immune maturation is not the only route for DIT. Early-life chemical exposure may affect the status of genes (the epigenome) in such a way that their pattern of expression in later life is affected and thereby alters immune functional capacity. Such changes in gene status that affect immune status could occur in the exposed generation (for people exposed in utero or during childhood), or they could carry through one or more additional generations as a result of true epigenetic alterations.

REFERENCES[1]

Adachi-Yamada T, Harumoto T, Sakurai K, Ueda R, Saigo K, O'Connor MB, Nakato H. 2005. Wing-to-leg homeosis by spineless causes apoptosis regulated by fish-lips, a novel leucine-rich repeat transmembrane protein. *Molecular and Cellular Biology* 25(8):3140–3150.

Adair BM, Moore T, Conklin SD, Creed JT, Wolf DC, Thomas DJ. 2007. Tissue distribution and urinary excretion of dimethylated arsenic and its metabolites in dimethylarsinic acid-or arsenate-treated rats. *Toxicology and Applied Pharmacology* 222(2):235–242.

Alexander BH, Checkoway H, van Netten C, Muller CH, Ewers TG, Kaufman JD, Mueller BA, Vaughan TL, Faustman EM. 1996. Semen quality of men employed at a lead smelter. *Occupational and Environmental Medicine* 53:411–416.

Anjum MR, Sainath SB, Suneetha Y, Reddy PS. 2011. Lead acetate induced reproductive and paternal mediated developmental toxicity in rats. *Ecotoxicology and Environmental Safety* 74(4):793–799.

Aposhian HV, Aposhian MM. 2006. Arsenic toxicology: Five questions. *Chemical Research in Toxicolology* 19(1):1–15.

Aposhian HV, Gurzau ES, Le XC, Gurzau A, Healy SM, Lu X, Ma M, Yip L, Zakharyan RA, Maiorino RM, Dart RC, Tircus MG, Gonzalez-Ramirez D, Morgan DL, Avram D, Aposhian MM. 2000. Occurrence of monomethylarsonous acid in urine of humans exposed to inorganic arsenic. *Chemical Research in Toxicology* 13:393–397.

Arnold EK, Beasley VR, Parker AJ, Stedelin JR. 1991. 2,4-D toxicosis II: A pilot study of clinical pathologic and electroencephalographic effects and residues of 2,4-D in orally dosed dogs. *Veterinary and Human Toxicology* 33:446–449.

Arnold LL, Eldan M, Nyska A, van Gemert M, Cohen SM. 2006. Dimethylarsinic acid: Results of chronic toxicity/oncogenicity studies in F344 rats and in B6C3F1 mice. *Toxicology* 223(1-2):82–100.

ATSDR (Agency for Toxic Substances and Disease Registry). 1998. Toxicological profile for chlorinated dibenzo-*p*-dioxins. US Department of Health and Human Services, Public Health Service, Agency for Toxic Substances and Disease Registry.

[1]Throughout this report, the same alphabetic indicator after year of publication is used consistently for a given reference when there are multiple citations by the same first author in a given year. The convention of assigning the alphabetic indicators in order of citation in a given chapter is not followed.

Aylward LL, Brunet RC, Carrier G, Hays SM, Cushing CA, Needham LL, Patterson DG Jr, Gerthoux PM, Brambilla P, Mocarelli P. 2005a. Concentration-dependent TCDD elimination kinetics in humans: Toxicokinetic modeling for moderately to highly exposed adults from Seveso, Italy, and Vienna, Austria, and impact on dose estimates for the NIOSH cohort. *Journal of Exposure Analysis and Environment Epidemiology* 15(1):51–65.

Aylward LL, Brunet RC, Starr TB, Carrier G, Delzell E, Cheng H, Beall C. 2005b. Exposure reconstruction for the TCDD-exposed NIOSH cohort using a concentration- and age-dependent model of elimination. *Risk Analysis* 25(4):945–956.

Bacsi SG, Reisz-Porszasz S, Hankinson O. 1995. Orientation of the heterodimeric aryl hydrocarbon (dioxin) receptor complex on its asymmetric DNA recognition sequence. *Molecular Pharmacology* 47(3):432–438.

Banks YB, Birnbaum LS. 1991. Absorption of 2,3,7,8-tetrachlorodibenzo-*p*-dioxin (TCDD) after low dose dermal exposure. *Toxicology and Applied Pharmacology* 107(2):302–310.

Barker DJ, Gelow J, Thornburg K, Osmond C, Kajantie E, Eriksson JG. 2010. The early origins of chronic heart failure: Impaired placental growth and initiation of insulin resistance in childhood. *European Journal of Heart Failure* 12(8):819–825.

Barouki R, Aggerbeck M, Aggerbeck, Coumoul X. 2012. The aryl hydrocarbon receptor system. *Drug Metabolism and Drug Interactions* 27(1):3–8.

Beaudouin R, Micallef S, Brochot C. 2010. A stochastic whole-body physiologically based pharmacokinetic model to assess the impact of inter-individual variability on tissue dosimetry over the human lifespan. *Regulatory Toxicology and Pharmacology* 57(1):103–116.

Birnbaum LS. 1994. Evidence for the role of the Ah receptor in response to dioxin. *Progress in Clinical and Biological Research* 387:139–154.

Birnbaum L, Harris M, Stocking L, Clark A, Morrissey R. 1989. Retinoic acid and 2,3,7,8–tetrachlorodibenzo-*p*-dioxin selectively enhance teratogenesis in C57BL/6N mice. *Toxicology and Applied Pharmacology* 98:487–500.

Black MB, Budinsky RA, Dombkowski A, Cukovic D, LeCluyse EL, Ferguson SS, Thomas RS, Rowlands JC. 2012. Cross-species comparisons of transcriptomic alterations in human and rat primary hepatocytes exposed to 2,3,7,8-tetrachlorodibenzo-*p*-dioxin. *Toxicological Sciences* 127(1):199–215.

Blakley BR. 1997. Effect of Roundup and Tordon 202C herbicides on antibody production in mice. *Veterinary and Human Toxicology* 39(4):204–206.

Blevins RD. 1991. 2,3,7,8-tetrachlorodibenzodioxin in fish from the Pigeon River of eastern Tennessee, USA: Its toxicity and mutagenicity as revealed by the Ames Salmonella assay. *Archives of Environmental Contamination and Toxicology* 20:366–370.

Boutros P, Moffat ID, Franc MA, Tijet N, Tuomisto J, Pohjanvirta R, Okey AB. 2004. Dioxin-responsive AHRE–II gene battery: Identification by phylogenetic footprinting. *Biochemical and Biophysical Research Communications* 321(3):707–715.

Boverhof DR, Burgoon LD, Tashiro C, Sharratt B, Chittim B, Harkema JR, Mendrick DL, Zacharewski TR. 2006. Comparative toxicogenomic analysis of the hepatotoxic effects of TCDD in Sprague Dawley rats and C57BL/6 mice. *Toxicological Sciences* 94(2):398–416.

Bowman RE, Schantz SL, Weerasinghe NCA, Gross ML, Barsotti DA. 1989. Chronic dietary intake of 2,3,7,8-tetrachlorodibenzo-*p*-dioxin (TCDD) at 5 and 25 parts per trillion in the monkey: TCDD kinetics and dose–effect estimate of reproductive toxicity. *Chemosphere* 18:243–252.

Brand RM, Spalding M, Mueller C. 2002. Sunscreens can increase dermal penetration of 2,4-dichlorophenoxyacetic acid. *Journal of Toxicology–Clinical Toxicology* 40(7):827–832.

Carrier G, Brunet RC, Brodeur J. 1995. Modeling of the toxicokinetics of polychlorinated dibenzo-*p*-dioxins and dibenzofurans in mammalians, including humans. II. Kinetics of absorption and disposition of PCDDs/PCDFs. *Toxicology and Applied Pharmacology* 131(2):267–276.

Carver L, Bradfield C. 1997. Ligand-dependent interaction of the aryl hydrocarbon receptor with a novel immunophilin homolog in vivo. *Journal of Biological Chemistry* 272:11452–11456.

Carver L, Jackiw V, Bradfield C. 1994. The 90-kDa heat shock protein is essential for Ah receptor signaling in a yeast expression system. *Journal of Biological Chemistry* 269:30109–30112.

Céspedes MA, Galindo MI, Couso JP. 2010. Dioxin toxicity in vivo results from an increase in the dioxin-independent transcriptional activity of the aryl hydrocarbon receptor. *PLoS ONE* 5(11):e15382.

Charles JM, Hanley TR, Wilson RD, van Ravenzwaay B, Bus JS. 2001. Developmental toxicity studies in rats and rabbits on 2,4-dichlorophenoxyacetic acid and its forms. *Toxicological Sciences* 60:121–131.

Chen ZX, Riggs AD. 2005. Maintenance and regulation of DNA methylation patterns in mammals. *Biochemistry and Cell Biology* 83(4):438–448.

Christensen BC, Marsit CJ. 2011. Epigenomics in environmental health. *Frontiers in Genetics* 2:84.

Cohen SM, Arnold LL, Eldan M, Lewis AS, Beck BD. 2006. Methylated arsenicals: The implications of metabolism and carcinogenicity studies in rodents to human risk assessment. *Critical Reviews in Toxicology* 36(2):99–133.

Cohen SM, Ohnishi T, Arnold LL, Le XC. 2007a. Arsenic-induced bladder cancer in an animal model. *Toxicology and Applied Pharmacology* 222(3):258–263.

Cohen SM, Janicki-Deverts D, Miller GE. 2007b. Psychological stress and disease. *Journal of the American Medical Association* 298(14):1685–1687.

Cortessis VK, Thomas DC, Levine AJ, Breton CV, Mack TM, Siegmund KD, Haile RW, Laird PW. 2012. Environmental epigenetics: Prospects for studying epigenetic mediation of exposure–response relationships. *Human Genetics* 131:1565–1589.

Cui X, Kobayashi Y, Hayakawa T, Hirano S. 2004. Arsenic speciation in bile and urine following oral and intravenous exposure to inorganic and organic arsenics in rats. *Toxicological Sciences* 82(2):478–487.

Davarinos N, Pollenz R. 1999. Aryl hydrocarbon receptor imported into the nucleus following ligand binding is rapidly degraded via the cytosplasmic proteasome following nuclear export. *Journal of Biological Chemistry* 274:28708–28715.

Denison MS, Soshilov AA, He G, DeGroot DE, Zhao B. 2011. Exactly the same but different: Promiscuity and molecular mechanism of action of the aryl hydrocarbon (dioxin) receptor. *Toxicological Sciences* 124(1):1–22.

Dési I, Sos J, Nikolits I. 1962a. New evidence concerning the nervous site of action of a chemical herbicide causing professional intoxication. *Acta Physiologica Academiae Scientiarum Hungaricae* 22:73–80.

Dési I, Sos J, Olasz J, Sule F, Markus V. 1962b. Nervous system effects of a chemical herbicide. *Archives of Environmental Health* 4:95–102.

DeVito M, Birnbaum L. 1995. The importance of pharmacokinetics in determining the relative potency of 2,3,7,8-tetrachlorodibenzo-*p*-dioxin and 2,3,7,8-tetrachlorodibenzofuran. *Fundamental and Applied Toxicology* 24:145–148.

Dietert R. 2009. Distinguishing environmental causes of immune dysfunction from pediatric triggers of disease. *The Open Pediatric Medicine Journal* 3:38–44.

Dietert R, Dietert J. 2008. Potential for early-life immune insult including developmental immunotoxicity in autism and autism spectrum disorders: Focus on critical windows of immune vulnerability. *Journal of Toxicology and Environmental Health—Part B: Critical Reviews* 11(8):660–680.

Dietert R, Piepenbrink M. 2006. Perinatal immunotoxicity: Why adult exposure assessment fails to predict risk. *Environmental Health Perspectives* 114(4):477–483.

Dietert R, Etzel R, Chen D, Halonen M, Holladay S, Jarabek A, Landreth K, Peden D, Pinkerton K, Smailowicz R, Zoetis T. 2000. Workshop to identify critical windows of exposure for children's health: Immune and respiratory systems work group summary. *Environmental Health Perspectives* 108(Suppl 3):483–490.

Di Giampaolo L, Di Gioacchino M, Qiao N, Travaglini P, D'Intino A, Kouri M, Ponti J, Castellani ML, Reale M, Gabriele E, Boscolo P. 2004. "In vitro" effects of different arsenic compounds on PBMC (preliminary study). *Giornale Italiano di Medicina del Lavoro Ed Ergonomia* 26(3):183–186.

Diliberto JJ, DeVito MJ, Ross DG, Birnbaum LS. 2001. Subchronic exposure of [3H]-2,3,7,8-tetrachlorodibenzo-*p*-dioxin (TCDD) in female B6C3F1 mice: Relationship of steady-state levels to disposition and metabolism. *Toxicological Sciences* 61:241–255.

Dolwick KM, Swanson HI, Bradfield CA. 1993. In vitro analysis of Ah receptor domains involved in ligand-activated DNA recognition. *Proceedings of the National Academy of Sciences* 90:8566–8570.

Dong B, Matsumura F. 2008. Roles of cytosolic phospholipase A2 and Src kinase in the early action of 2,3,7,8-tetrachlorodibenzo-*p*-dioxin through a nongenomic pathway in MCF10A cells. *Molecular Pharmacology* 74:255–263.

Dopp E, Hartmann LM, Florea AM, von Recklinghausen U, Pieper R, Shokouhi B, Rettenmeier AW, Hirner AV, Obe G. 2004. Uptake of inorganic and organic derivatives of arsenic associated with induced cytotoxic and genotoxic effects in Chinese hamster ovary (CHO) cells. *Toxicology and Applied Pharmacology* 201(2):156–165.

Dopp E, Hartmann LM, von Recklinghausen U, Florea AM, Rabieh S, Zimmermann U, Shokouhi B, Yadav S, Hirner AV, Rettenmeier AW. 2005. Forced uptake of trivalent and pentavalent methylated and inorganic arsenic and its cyto-/genotoxicity in fibroblasts and hepatoma cells. *Toxicological Sciences* 87(1):46–56.

Dragin N, Dalton TP, Miller ML, Shertzer HG, Nebert DW. 2006. For dioxin-induced birth defects, mouse or human CYP1A2 in maternal liver protects whereas mouse CYP1A1 and CYP1B1 are inconsequential. *Journal of Biological Chemistry* 281(27):18591–18600.

El-Masri HA, Kenyon EM. 2008. Development of a human physiologically based pharmacokinetic (PBPK) model for inorganic arsenic and its mono-and di-methylated metabolites. *Journal of Pharmacokinetics and Pharmacodynamics* 35(1):31–68.

Emond C, Michalek JE, Birnbaum LS, DeVito MJ. 2005. Comparison of the use of physiologically based pharmacokinetic model and a classical pharmacokinetic model for dioxin exposure assessments. *Environmental Health Perspectives* 113(12):1666–1668.

Emond C, Birnbaum LS, DeVito MJ. 2006. Use of a physiologically based pharmacokinetic model for rats to study the influence of body fat mass and induction of CYP1A2 on the pharmacokinetics of TCDD. *Environmental Health Perspectives* 114(9):1394–1400.

EPA (US Environmental Protection Agency). 1988c. *Guidance for the Reregistration of Pesticide Products Containing Picloram as the Active Ingredient.* Washington, DC: EPA, Office of Pesticide Programs.

EPA. 2004. *Exposure and Human Health Reassessment of 2,3,7,8-Tetrachlorodibenzo-p-Dioxin (TCDD) and Related Compounds—National Academy Sciences (NAS) Review Draft.* Washington, DC. National Center for Environmental Assessment.

Evans BR, Karchner SI, Allan LL, Pollenz RS, Tanguay RL, Jenny MJ, Sherr DH, Hahn ME. 2008. Repression of aryl hydrocarbon receptor (AHR) signaling by AHR repressor: Role of DNA binding and competition for AHR nuclear translocator. *Molecular Pharmacology* 73(2):387–398.

Fernandez-Salguero PM, Hilbert DM, Rudikoff S, Ward JM, Gonzalez FJ. 1996. Aryl-hydrocarbon receptor-deficient mice are resistant to 2,3,7,8-tetrachlorodibenzo-*p*-dioxin-induced toxicity. *Toxicology and Applied Pharmacology* 140:173–179.

Fernandez-Salguero PM, Ward JM, Sundberg JP, Gonzalez FJ. 1997. Lesions of aryl-hydrocarbon receptor-deficient mice. *Veterinary Pathology* 34(6):605–614.

Flesch-Janys D, Becher H, Gurn P, Jung D, Konietzko J, Manz A, Papke O. 1996. Elimination of polychlorinated dibenzo-*p*-dioxins and dibenzofurans in occupationally exposed persons. *Journal of Toxicology and Environmental Health* 47(4):363–378.

Fujii-Kuriyama Y, Kawajiri K. 2010. Molecular mechanisms of the physiological functions of the aryl hydrocarbon (dioxin) receptor, a multifunctional regulator that senses and responds to environmental stimuli. *Proceedings of the Japan Academy—Series B: Physical and Biological Sciences* 86(1):40–53.

Gasiewicz T, Geiger L, Rucci G, Neal R. 1983. Distribution, excretion, and metabolism of 2,3,7,8-tetrachlorodibenzo-*p*-dioxin in C57BL/6J, DBA/2J, and B6D2F1/J mice. *Drug Metabolism and Disposition* 11:397–403.

Gehring PJ, Kramer CG, Schwetz BA, Rose JQ, Rowe VK. 1973. The fate of 2,4,5-trichlorophenoxyacetic acid (2,4,5–T) following oral administration to man. *Toxicology and Applied Pharmacology* 26:352–361.

Geusau A, Schmaldienst S, Derfler K, Päpke O, Abraham K. 2002. Severe 2,3,7,8-tetrachlorodibenzo-*p*-dioxin (TCDD) intoxication: Kinetics and trials to enhance elimination in two patients. *Archives of Toxicology* 76:316–325.

Gómez SE, Del Razo LM, Muñoz Sanchez JL. 2005. Induction of DNA damage by free radicals generated either by organic or inorganic arsenic (As^{III}, MMA^{III}, and DMA^{III}) in cultures of B and T lymphocytes. *Biological Trace Element Research* 108(1-3):115–126.

Gorzinski SJ, Johnson KA, Campbell RA, Landry TD. 1987. Dietary toxicity of picloram herbicide in rats. *Journal of Toxicology and Environmental Health* 20:367–377.

Guo J, Sartor M, Karyala S, Medvedovic M, Kann S, Puga A, Ryan P, Tomlinson CR. 2004. Expression of genes in the TGF-beta signaling pathway is significantly deregulated in smooth muscle cells from aorta of aryl hydrocarbon receptor knockout mice. *Toxicology and Applied Pharmacology* 194(1):79–89.

Hahn ME. 2001. Dioxin toxicology and the aryl hydrocarbon receptor: Insights from fish and other non-traditional models. *Marine Biotechnology (New York, NY)* 3(Suppl 1):S224–S238.

Hall MN, Gamble MV. 2012. Nutritional manipulation of one-carbon metabolism: Effects on arsenic methylation and toxicity. *Journal of Toxicology*, article ID 595307, 11 pp.

Harrigan JA, Vezina CM, McGarrigle BP, Ersing N, Box HC, Maccubbin AE, Olson JR. 2004. DNA adduct formation in precision-cut rat liver and lung slices exposed to benzo[a]pyrene. *Toxicological Sciences* 77(2):307–314.

Hayashi H, Kanisawa M, Yamanaka K, Ito T, Udaka N, Ohji H, Okudela K, Okada S, Kitamura H. 1998. Dimethylarsinic acid, a main metabolite of inorganic arsenics, has tumorigenicity and progression effects in the pulmonary tumors of A/J mice. *Cancer Letters* 125(1-2):83–88.

Hayes HM, Tarone RE, Cantor KP, Jessen CR, McCurnin DM, Richardson RC. 1991. Case-control study of canine malignant lymphoma: Positive association with dog owner's use of 2,4-D herbicides. *Journal of the National Cancer Institute* 83(17):1226–1231.

Hayes HM, Tarone RE, Cantor KP. 1995. On the association between canine malignant lymphoma and opportunity for exposure to 2,4-dichlorophenoxyacetic acid. *Environmental Research* 70(2):119–125.

Hazleton Laboratories America. 1987. *Oncogenicity Study in Mice with 2,4-Dichlorophenoxyacetic Acid (2,4-D). Final Report.* Prepared for the Industry Task Force on 2,4-D Research Data.

Henderson L, Patterson DJ. 1988. Distribution of 2,3,7,8-tetrachlorodibenzo-*p*-dioxin in human whole blood and its association with, and extractability from, lipoproteins. *Bulletin of Environmental Contamination and Toxicology* 40(4):604–611.

Hernandez A, Xamena N, Surralles J, Sekaran C, Tokunaga H, Quinteros D, Creus A, Marcos R. 2008. Role of the Met(287)Thr polymorphism in the AS3MT gene on the metabolic arsenic profile. *Mutation Research* 637(1-2):80–92.

Hestermann E, Brown M. 2003. Agonist and chemopreventative ligands induce differential transcriptional cofactor recruitment by aryl hydrocarbon receptor. *Molecular and Cellular Biology* 23(21):7920–7925.

Hines CJ, Deddens JA, Striley CA, Biagini RE, Shoemaker DA, Brown KK, Mackenzie BA, Hull RD. 2003. Biological monitoring for selected herbicide biomarkers in the urine of exposed custom applicators: Application of mixed-effect models. *Annals of Occupational Hygiene* 47(6):503–517.

Hoffman EC, Reyes H, Chu FF, Sander F, Conley LH, Brooks BA, Hankinson O. 1991. Cloning of a factor required for activity of the Ah (dioxin) receptor. *Science* 252:954–958.

Holliday R, Pugh JE. 1975. DNA modification mechanisms and gene activity during development. *Science* 187(4173):226–232.

Holsapple M, West L, Landreth K. 2003. Species comparison of anatomical and functional immune system development. *Birth Defects Research–Part B* 68:321–334.

Huang SK, Chiu AWH, Pu YS, Huang YK, Chung CJ, Tsai HJ, Yang MH, Chen CJ, Hsueh YM. 2008. Arsenic methylation capability, heme oxygenase-1 and NADPH quinone oxidoreductase-1 genetic polymorphisms and the stage and grade of urothelial carcinomas. *Urologia Internationalis* 80(4):405–412.

Huang X, Powell-Coffman JA, Jin Y. 2004. The AHR-1 aryl hydrocarbon receptor and its co-factor the AHA-1 aryl hydrocarbon receptor nuclear translocator specify GABAergic neuron cell fate in C. elegans. *Development* 131(4):819–828.

Huang YK, Pu YS, Chung CJ, Shiue HS, Yang MH, Chen CJ, Hsueh YM. 2008. Plasma folate level, urinary arsenic methylation profiles, and urothelial carcinoma susceptibility. *Food and Chemical Toxicology* 46(3):929–938.

Huff J, Lucier G, Tritscher A. 1994. Carcinogenicity of TCDD: Experimental, mechanistic, and epidemiologic evidence. *Annual Review of Pharmacology and Toxicology* 34:343–372.

Hurst CH, Abbott BD, DeVito MJ, Birnbaum LS. 1998. 2,3,7,8-tetrachlorodibenzo-*p*-dioxin in pregnant Long Evans rats: Disposition to maternal and embryo/fetal tissues. *Toxicological Sciences* 45(2):129–136.

IOM (Institute of Medicine). 1994. *Veterans and Agent Orange: Health Effects of Herbicides Used in Vietnam.* Washington, DC: National Academy Press.

IOM. 2011. *Veterans and Agent Orange: Update 2010.* Washington, DC: The National Academies Press.

Israel DI, Whitlock JP Jr. 1983. Induction of mRNA specific for cytochrome P1-450 in wild type and variant mouse hepatoma cells. *Journal of Biological Chemistry* 258:10390–10394.

Israel DI, Whitlock JP Jr. 1984. Regulation of cytochrome P1-450 gene transcription by 2,3,7,8-tetrachlorodibenzo-*p*-dioxin in wild type and variant mouse hepatoma cells. *Journal of Biological Chemistry* 259:5400–5402.

Jirtle RL, Skinner MK. 2007. Environmental epigenomics and disease susceptibility. *Nature Review Genetics* 8(4):253–262.

John-Greene JA, Ouellette JH, Jeffries TK, Johnson KA, Rao KS. 1985. Teratological evaluation of picloram potassium salt in rabbits. *Journal of Food and Chemical Toxicology* 23:753–756.

Joshi SC, Tibrewal P, Sharma A, Sharma P. 2012. Evaluation of toxic effects of 2,4-D (2,4-dichlorophenoxyacetic acid) on fertility and biochemical parameters of male reproductive system of albino rats. *International Journal of Pharmacy and Pharmaceutical Sciences* 4(3):338–342.

Kaneene JB, Miller R. 1999. Re-analysis of 2,4-D use and the occurrence of canine malignant lymphoma. *Veterinary and Human Toxicology* 41(3):164–170.

Kazlauskas A, Poellinger L, Pongratz I. 1999. Evidence that the co-chaperone p23 regulates ligand responsiveness of the dioxin (aryl hydrocarbon) receptor. *Journal of Biological Chemistry* 274:13519–13524.

Kerkvliet NI. 2009. AHR-mediated immunomodulation: The role of altered gene transcription. *Biochemical Pharmacology* 77:746–760.

Kim E, Kim M, Sung K, Hyun J, Jang J, Kim K. 2012. Effect of topical dimethylarsinic acid on the expression of apoptosis-related proteins in mouse skin. *Bulletin of Environmental Contamination and Toxicology* 88:672–677.

Kinoshita A, Wanibuchi H, Wei M, Yunoki T, Fukushima S. 2007. Elevation of 8-hydroxydeoxyguanosine and cell proliferation via generation of oxidative stress by organic arsenicals contributes to their carcinogenicity in the rat liver and bladder. *Toxicology and Applied Pharmacology* 221(3):295–305.

Klein OD, Kostiner DR, Weisiger K, Moffatt E, Lindeman N, Goodman S, Tuchman M, Packman S. 2008. Acute fatal presentation of ornithine transcarbamylase deficiency in a previously healthy male. *Hepatology International* 2(3):390–394.

Knerr S, Schrenk D. 2006. Carcinogenicity of 2,3,7,8-tetrachlorodibenzo-*p*-dioxin in experimental models. *Molecular Nutrition and Food Research* 50(10):897–907.

Kociba RJ, Keyes DG, Beyer JE, Carreon RM, Wade CE, Dittenber DA, Kalnins RP, Frauson LE, Park CN, Barnard SD, Hummel RA, Humiston CG. 1978. Results of a two-year chronic toxicity and oncogenicity study of 2,3,7,8-tetrachlorodibenzo-*p*-dioxin in rats. *Toxicology and Applied Pharmacology* 46(2):279–303.

Kohli JD, Khanna RN, Gupta BN, Dhar MM, Tandon JS, Sircar KP. 1974. Absorption and excretion of 2,4,5-trichlorophenoxy acetic acid in man. *Archives Internationales de Pharmacodynamie et de Therapie* 210:250–255.

Kojima C, Qu W, Waalkes MP, Himeno S, Sakurai T. 2006. Chronic exposure to methylated arsenicals stimulates arsenic excretion pathways and induces arsenic tolerance in rat liver cells. *Toxicological Sciences* 91(1):70–81.

Koshakji RP, Harbison RD, Bush MT. 1984. Studies on the metabolic fate of [14C] 2,3,7,8-tetrachlorodibenzo-*p*-dioxin (TCDD) in the mouse. *Toxicology and Applied Pharmacology* 73:69–77.

Kransler KM, McGarrigle BP, Olson JR. 2007. Comparative developmental toxicity of 2,3,7,8-tetrachlorodibenzo-*p*-dioxin in the hamster, rat and guinea pig. *Toxicology* 229:214–225.

Kruger K, Gruner J, Madeja M, Hartmann LM, Hirner AV, Binding N, Muhoff U. 2006. Blockade and enhancement of glutamate receptor responses in Xenopus oocytes by methylated arsenicals. *Archives of Toxicology* 80(8):492–501.

Kumagai S, Koda S. 2005. Polychlorinated dibenzo-*p*-dioxin and dibenzofuran concentrations in serum samples of workers at an infectious waste incineration plant in Japan. *Journal of Occupational and Environmental Hygiene* 2(2):120–125.

Lahvis G, Bradfield C. 1998. Ahr null alleles: Distinctive or different? *Biochemical Pharmacology* 56(7):781–787.

Lahvis GP, Pyzalski RW, Glover E, Pitot HC, McElwee MK, Bradfield CA. 2005. The aryl hydrocarbon receptor is required for developmental closure of the ductus venosus in the neonatal mouse. *Molecular Pharmacology* 67(3):714–720.

Landreth K. 2002. Critical windows in development of the rodent immune system. *Human and Experimental Toxicology* 21:493–498.

Leung HW, Kerger BD, Paustenbach DJ. 2006. Elimination half-lives of selected polychlorinated dibenzodioxins and dibenzofurans in breast-fed human infants. *Journal of Toxicology and Environmental Health–Part A* 69(6):437–443.

Lu M, Wang H, Li XF, Lu X, Cullen WR, Arnold LL, Cohen SM, Le XC. 2004. Evidence of hemoglobin binding to arsenic as a basis for the accumulation of arsenic in rat blood. *Chemical Research in Toxicology* 17(12):1733–1742.

Lusska A, Shen E, Whitlock JP Jr. 1993. Protein-DNA interactions at a dioxin-responsive enhancer. *Journal of Biological Chemistry* 268:6575–6580.

Ma Q, Whitlock J Jr. 1997. A novel cytoplasmic protein that interacts with the Ah receptor, contains tetratricopeptide repeat motifs, and augments the transcriptional response to 2,3,7,8-tetrachlorodibenzo-*p*-dioxin. *Journal of Biological Chemistry* 272(14):8878–8884.

Manikkam M, Guerrero-Bosagna C, Tracey R, Haque MM, Skinner MK. 2012. Transgenerational actions of environmental compounds on reproductive disease and identification of epigenetic biomarkers of ancestral exposures. *PLoS ONE* 7(2):e31901.

Martinez JM, Afshari CA, Bushel PR, Masuda A, Takahashi T, Walker NJ. 2002. Differential toxicogenomic responses to 2,3,7,8-tetrachlorodibenzo-*p*-dioxin in malignant and nonmalignant human airway epithelial cells. *Toxicological Sciences* 69(2):409–423.

Matsumura F. 2009. The significance of the nongenomic pathway in mediating inflammatory signaling of the dioxin-activated Ah receptor to cause toxic effects. *Biochemical Pharmacology* 77:608–626.

McCarty KM, Chen YC, Quamruzzaman Q, Rahman M, Mahiuddin G, Hsueh YM, Su L, Smith T, Ryan L, Christiani DC. 2007. Arsenic methylation, GSTT1, GSTM1, GSTP1 polymorphisms, and skin lesions. *Environmental Health Perspectives* 115(3):341–345.

Meyne J, Allison DC, Bose K, Jordan SW, Ridolpho PF, Smith J. 1985. Hepatotoxic doses of dioxin do not damage mouse bone marrow chromosomes. *Mutation Research* 157:63–69.

Meza M, Gandolfi AJ, Klimecki WT. 2007. Developmental and genetic modulation of arsenic biotransformation: A gene by environment interaction? *Toxicology and Applied Pharmacology* 222(3):381–387.

Michalek JE, Tripathi RC. 1999. Pharmacokinetics of TCDD in veterans of Operation Ranch Hand: 15-year follow-up. *Journal of Toxicology and Environmental Health* 57(6):369–378.

Michalek JE, Tripathi RC, Caudill SP, Pirkle JL. 1992. Investigation of TCDD half-life heterogenicity in veterans of Operation Ranch Hand. *Journal of Toxicology and Environmental Health* 35:29–38.

Michalek JE, Pirkle JL, Caudill SP, Tripathi RC, Patterson DG Jr, Needham LL. 1996. Pharmacokinetics of TCDD in veterans of Operation Ranch Hand: 10-year follow-up. *Journal of Toxicology and Environmental Health* 47:209–220.

Michalek JE, Pirkle JL, Needham LL, Patterson DG Jr, Caudill SP, Tripathi RC, Mocarelli P. 2002. Pharmacokinetics of 2,3,7,8-tetrachlorodibenzo-*p*-dioxin in Seveso adults and veterans of Operation Ranch Hand. *Journal of Exposure Analysis and Environmental Epidemiology* 12(1):44–53.

Milbrath MO, Wenger Y, Chang CW, Emond C, Garabrant D, Gillespie BW, Jolliet O. 2009. Apparent half-lives of dioxins, furans, and polychlorinated biphenyls as a function of age, body fat, smoking status, and breast-feeding. *Environmental Health Perspectives* 117(3):417–425.

Mizoi M, Takabayashi F, Nakano M, An Y, Sagesaka Y, Kato K, Okada S, Yamanaka K. 2005. The role of trivalent dimethylated arsenic in dimethylarsinic acid-promoted skin and lung tumorigenesis in mice: Tumor-promoting action through the induction of oxidative stress. *Toxicology Letters* 158(2):87–94.

Mocarelli P, Gerthoux PM, Patterson DG, Milani S, Limonta G, Bertona M, Signorini S, Tramacere P, Colombo L, Crespi C, Brambilla P, Sarto C, Carreri V, Sampson EJ, Terner WE, Needham LL. 2008. Dioxin exposure, from infancy through puberty, produces endocrine disruption and affects human semen quality. *Environmental Health Perspectives* 116(1):70–77.

Mortelmans K, Haworth S, Speck W, Zeiger E. 1984. Mutagenicity testing of Agent Orange components and related chemicals. *Toxicology and Applied Pharmacology* 75:137–146.

Munro IC, Carlo GL, Orr JC, Sund KG, Wilson RD, Kennepohl E, Lynch BS, Jablinske M, Lee NL. 1992. A comprehensive integrated review and evaluation of the scientific evidence relating to the safety of the herbicide 2,4-D. *American College of Toxicology* 11:559–664.

Murr R. 2010. Interplay between different epigenetic modifications and mechanisms. *Advances in Genetics* 70:101–141.

Naranmandura H, Suzuki KT. 2008. Formation of dimethylthioarsenicals in red blood cells. *Toxicology and Applied Pharmacology* 227(3):390–399.

Naranmandura H, Carew MW, Xu S, Lee J, Leslie EM, Weinfeld M, Le XC. 2011. Comparative toxicity of arsenic metabolites in human bladder cancer EJ-1 cells. *Chemical Research in Toxicology* 24:1586–1596.

NCI (National Cancer Institute). 1978. *Bioassay of Picloram for Possible Carcinogenicity. Report Series No. 23.* Bethesda, MD: NCI.

Nebert DW, Roe AL, Dieter MZ, Solis WA, Yang Y, Dalton TP. 2000. Role of the aromatic hydrocarbon receptor and [Ah] gene battery in the oxidative stress response, cell cycle control, and apoptosis. *Biochemical Pharmacology* 59(1):65–85.

Nebert DW, Dalton TP, Okey AB, Gonzalez FJ. 2004. Role of aryl hydrocarbon receptor-mediated induction of the CYP1 enzymes in environmental toxicity and cancer. *Journal of Biological Chemistry* 279(23):23847–23850.

Needham L, Gerthoux P, Patterson D, Brambilla P, Pirkle J, Tramacere P, Turner W, Beretta C, Sampson E, Mocarelli P. 1994. Half-life of 2,3,7,8-tetrachlorodibenzo-*p*-dioxin in serum of Seveso adults: Interim report. *Organohalogen Compounds* 21:81–85.

Neubert DW, Wiesmuller T, Abraham K, Krowke R, Hagenmaier H. 1990. Persistence of various polychlorinated dibenzo-*p*-dioxins and dibenzofurans (PCDDs and PCDFs) in hepatic and adipose tissue of marmoset monkeys. *Archives of Toxicology* 64:431–442.

Nolan RJ, Freshour NL, Kastl PE, Saunders JH. 1984. Pharmacokinetics of picloram in male volunteers. *Toxicology and Applied Pharmacology* 76(2):264–269.

Nolan R, Smith F, Hefner J. 1979. Elimination and tissue distribution of 2,3,7,8-tetrachlorodibenzo-*para*-dixion (TCDD) in female guinea-pigs following a single oral dose. *Toxicology and Applied Pharmacology* 48(1):A162.

NRC (National Research Council). 1999a. *Arsenic in Drinking Water.* Washington, DC: National Academy Press.

NRC. 2001. *Arsenic in Drinking Water: Update 2001.* Washington, DC: National Academy Press.

Okey AB, Franc MA, Moffat ID, Tijet N, Boutros PC, Korkalainen M, Tuomisto J, Pohjanvirta R. 2005. Toxicological implications of polymorphisms in receptors for xenobiotic chemicals: The case of the aryl hydrocarbon receptor. *Toxicology and Applied Pharmacology* 207(Suppl 2):43–51.

Olson JR. 2012. Pharmacokinetics of dioxins and related compounds. In: *Dioxins and Health*, Third Edition, A. Schecter, ed., John Wiley & Sons, Inc., pps 109–169.

Olson JR, Gasiewicz TA, Neal RA. 1980. Tissue distribution, excretion, and metabolism of 2,3,7,8-tetrachlorodibenzo-*p*-dioxin (TCDD) in the golden syrian hamster. *Toxicology and Applied Pharmacology* 56:78–85.

Olson LJ. 1986. The immune system and pesticides. *The Journal of Pesticide Reform* 6(2):20–25.

Ovando BJ, Vezina CM, McGarrigle BP, Olson JR. 2006. Hepatic gene downregulation following acute and subchronic exposure to 2,3,7,8-tetrachlorodibenzo-*p*-dioxin. *Toxicological Sciences* 94(2):428–438.

Ovando BJ, Ellison CA, Vezina CM, Olson JR. 2010. Toxicogenomic analysis of exposure to TCDD, PCB126 and PCB153: Identification of genomic biomarkers of exposure to AhR ligands. *BMC Genomics* 11:583–598.

Park S, Dong B, Matsumura F. 2007. Rapid activation of c-Src kinase by dioxin is mediated by the Cdc37-HSP90 complex as part of Ah receptor signaling in MCF10A cells. *Biochemistry* 46:899–908.

Pegram RA, Diliberto JJ, Moore TC, Gao P, Birnbaum LS. 1995. 2,3,7,8-tetrachlorodibenzo-*p*-dioxin (TCDD) distribution and cytochrome P4501A induction in young adult and senescent male mice. *Toxicology Letters* 76:119–126.

Perdew GH. 2008. Ah receptor binding to its cognate response element is required for dioxin-mediated toxicity. *Toxicological Sciences* 106(2):301–303.

Peterson RE, Theobald HM, Kimmel GL. 1993. Developmental and reproductive toxicity of dioxins and related compounds: Cross-species comparisons. *Critical Reviews in Toxicology* 23:283–335.

Petrulis J, Kusnadi A, Ramadoss P, Hollingshead B, Perdew G. 2003. The hsp90 co-chaperone XAP2 alters importin beta recognition of the bipartite nuclear localization signal of the Ah receptor and represses transcriptional activity. *Journal of Biological Chemistry* 278:2677–2685.

Pirkle J, Wolfe W, Patterson D, Needham L, Michalek J, Miner J, Peterson M, Phillips D. 1989. Estimates of the half-life of 2,3,7,8-tetrachlorodibenzo-*p*-dioxin in Vietnam veterans of Operation Ranch Hand. *Journal of Toxicology and Environmental Health* 27:165–171.

Pohjanvirta R, Tuomisto J. 1990. Remarkable residual alterations in responses to feeding regulatory challenges in Han/Wistar rats after recovery from the acute toxicity of 2,3,7,8-tetrachlorodibenzo-*p*-dioxin (TCDD). *Food and Chemical Toxicology* 28:677–686.

Poiger H, Schlatter C. 1979. Biological degradation of TCDD in rats. *Nature* 281(5733):706–707.

Poiger H, Schlatter C. 1986. Pharmacokinetics of 2,3,7,8-TCDD in man. *Chemosphere* 15:1489–1494.

Poiger H, Buser HR, Weber H, Zweifel U, Schlatter C. 1982. Structure elucidation of mammalian TCDD-metabolites. *Experientia* 38:484–486.

Pokholok DK, Harbison CT, Levine S, Cole M, Hannett NM, Lee TI, Bell GW, Walker K, Rolfe PA, Herbolsheimer E, Zeitlinger J, Lewitter F, Gifford DK, Young RA. 2005. Genome-wide map of nucleosome acetylation and methylation in yeast. *Cell* 122(4):517–527.

Poland A, Glover E. 1979. An estimate of the maximum in vivo covalent binding of 2,3,7,8-tetrachlorodibenzo-*p*-dioxin to rat liver protein, ribosomal RNA and DNA. *Cancer Research* 39(9):3341–3344.

Poland A, Knutson JC. 1982. 2,3,7,8-tetrachlorodibenzo-*p*-dioxin and related halogenated aromatic hydrocarbons: Examination of the mechanism of toxicity. *Annual Reviews of Pharmacology and Toxicology* 22:517–554.

Poland A, Teitelbaum P, Glover E. 1989. [125I]2-iodo-3,7,8-trichlorodibenzo-*p*-dioxin-binding species in mouse liver induced by agonists for the Ah receptor: Characterization and identification. *Molecular Pharmacology* 36(1):113–120.

Pongratz I, Mason GGF, Poellinger L. 1992. Dual roles of the 90-kDa heat shock protein hsp90 in modulating functional activities of the dioxin receptor. *Journal of Biological Chemistry* 267:13728–13734.

Pont AR, Charron AR, Brand RM. 2004. Active ingredients in sunscreens act as topical penetration enhancers for the herbicide 2,4-dichlorophenoxyacetic acid. *Toxicology and Applied Pharmacology* 195:348–354.

Probst MR, Reisz-Porszasz S, Agbunag RV, Ong MS, Hankinson O. 1993. Role of the aryl hydrocarbon receptor nuclear translocator protein in aryl hydrocarbon (dioxin) receptor action. *Molecular Pharmacology* 44:511–518.

Puga A, Bohm J, Hoffer A, Leikauf G, Shertzer H, Zhou S. 1995. Dioxin alters calcium homeostasis and the regulation of arachidonate metabolism in mouse hepatoma cells. *Proceeding of the 15th International Symposium on Chlorinated Dioxins and Related Compounds* 25:381–386.

Puga A, Maier A, Medvedovic M. 2000. The transcriptional signature of dioxin in human hepatoma HepG2 cells. *Biochemical Pharmacology* 60(8):1129–1142.

Puga A, Sartor MA, Huang MY, Kerzee JK, Wei YD, Tomlinson CR, Baxter CS, Medvedovic M. 2004. Gene expression profiles of mouse aorta and cultured vascular smooth muscle cells differ widely, yet show common responses to dioxin exposure. *Cardiovascular Toxicology* 4(4):385–404.

Puga A, Ma C, Marlowe J. 2009. The aryl hydrocarbon receptor cross-talks with multiple signal transduction pathways. *Biochemical Pharmacology* 77(4):713–722.

Qin H, Powell-Coffman JA. 2004. The Caenorhabditis elegans aryl hydrocarbon receptor, AHR-1, regulates neuronal development. *Developmental Biology* 270(1):64–75.

Rose JQ, Ransy JC, Wentzler TH, Hummel RA, Gehring PJ. 1976. The fate of 2,3,7,8-tetrachlorodibenzo-*p*-dioxin following single and repeated oral doses to the rat. *Toxicology and Applied Pharmacology* 36:209–226.

Safe SH. 1990. Polychlorinated biphenyls (PCBs), dibenzo-*p*-dioxins (PCDDs), dibenzofurans (PCDFs), and related compounds: Environmental and mechanistic considerations which support the development of toxic equivalency factors (TEFs). *Critical Reviews of Toxicology* 21:51–88.

Sandal S, Yilmaz B. 2011. Genotoxic effects of chlorpyrifos, cypermethrin, endosulfan and 2,4-D on human peripheral lymphocytes cultured from smokers and nonsmokers. *Environmental Toxicology* 26:433–442.

Sato F, Tsuchiya S, Meltzer SJ, Shimizu K. 2011. MicroRNAs and epigenetics. *FEBS Journal* 278:1598–1609.

Sauerhoff MW, Braun WH, Blau GE, Gehring PJ. 1977. The fate of 2,4-dichlorophenoxyacetic acid (2,4-D) following oral administration to man. *Toxicology* 8:3–11.

Sawahata T, Olson JR, Neal RA. 1982. Identification of metabolites of 2,3,7,8-tetrachlorodibenzo-*p*-dioxin (TCDD) formed on incubation with isolated rat hepatocytes. *Biochemical and Biophysical Research Communications* 105:341–346.

Schiestl R, Aubrecht J, Yap WY, Kandikonda S, Sidhom S. 1997. Polychlorinated biphenyls and 2,3,7,8-tetrachlorodibenzo-*p*-dioxin induce intrachromosomal recombination in vitro and in vivo. *Cancer Research* 57:4378–4383.

Schmidt JV, Bradfield CA. 1996. Ah receptor signaling pathways. *Annual Review of Cell Development–Biology* 12:55–89.

Schmidt JV, Su GH, Reddy JK, Simon MC, Bradfield CA. 1996. Characterization of a murine Ahr null allele: Involvement of the Ah receptor in hepatic growth and development. *Proceedings of the National Academy of Sciences* 93(13):6731–6736.

Schnekenburger M, Peng L, Puga A. 2007. HDAC1 bound to the Cyp1a1 promoter blocks histone acetylation associated with Ah receptor-mediated trans-activation. *Biochimica et Biophysica ACTA/General Subjects* 1769:569–578.

Sciullo EM, Vogel FA, Li W. 2008. Initial and extended inflammatory messages of the nongenomic signaling pathway of the TCDD-activated Ah receptor in U937 macrophages. *Archives of Biochemistry and Biophysics* 480(2):143–155.

Sen B, Wang A, Hester SD, Robertson JL, Wolf DC. 2005. Gene expression profiling of responses to dimethylarsinic acid in female F344 rat urothelium. *Toxicology* 215(3):214–226.

Senft AP, Dalton TP, Nebert DW, Genter MB, Puga A, Hutchinson RJ, Kerzee JK, Uno S, Shertzer HG. 2002. Mitochondrial reactive oxygen production is dependent on the aromatic hydrocarbon receptor. *Free Radical Biology and Medicine* 33(9):1268–1278.

Shen ES, Whitlock JP. 1992. Protein–DNA interactions at a dioxin responsive enhancer: Mutational analysis of the DNA binding site for the liganded Ah receptor. *Journal of Biological Chemistry* 267:6815–6819.

Skinner MK, Manikkam M, Guerrero-Bosagna C. 2010. Epigenetic transgenerational actions of environmental factors in disease etiology. *Trends Endocrinology and Metabolism* 21(4):214–222.

Smialowicz RJ, DeVito MJ, Williams WC, Birnbaum LS. 2008. Relative potency based on hepatic enzyme induction predicts immunosuppressive effects of a mixture of PCDDs/PCDFs and PCBs. *Toxicology and Applied Toxicology* 227:477–484.

Sogawa K, Numayama-Tsuruta K, Takahashi T, Matsushita N, Miura C, Nikawa J, Gotoh O, Kikuchi Y, Fujii-Kuriyama Y. 2004. A novel induction mechanism of the rat CYP1A2 gene mediated by Ah receptor–ARNT heterodimer. *Biochemical and Biophysical Research Communications* 318(3):746–755.

Song Z, Pollenz RS. 2002. Ligand-dependent and independent modulation of aryl hydrocarbon receptor localization, degradation, and gene regulation. *Molecular Pharmacology* 62(4):806–816.

Sorg O, Zennegg M, Schmid P, Fedosyuk R, Valikhnovskyi R, Gaide O, Kniazevych V, Saurat JH. 2009. 2,3,7,8-tetrachlorodibenzo-*p*-dioxin (TCDD) poisoning in Victor Yushchenko: Identification and measurement of TCDD metabolites. *Lancet* 374(9696):1179–1185.

Steinmaus C, Moore LE, Shipp M, Kalman D, Rey OA, Biggs ML, Hopenhayn C, Bates MN, Zheng S, Wiencke JK, Smith AH. 2007. Genetic polymorphisms in MTHFR 677 and 1298, GSTM1 and T1, and metabolism of arsenic. *Journal of Toxicology and Environmental Health–Part A* 70(2):159–170.

Steinmaus C, Yuan Y, Kalman D, Rey OA, Skibola CF, Dauphine D, Basu A, Porter KE, Hubbard A, Bates MN, Smith MT, Smith AH. 2010. Individual differences in arsenic metabolism and lung cancer in a case-control study in Cordoba, Argentina. *Toxicology and Applied Pharmacology* 247(2):138–145.

Stott WT, Johnson KA, Landry TD, Gorzinski SJ, Cieszlak FS. 1990. Chronic toxicity and oncogenicity of picloram in Fischer 344 rats. *Journal of Toxicology and Environmental Health* 30:91–104.

Suzuki KT, Katagiri A, Sakuma Y, Ogra Y, Ohmichi M. 2004. Distributions and chemical forms of arsenic after intravenous administration of dimethylarsinic and monomethylarsonic acids to rats. *Toxicology and Applied Pharmacology* 198(3):336–344.

Suzuki S, Arnold LL, Pennington KL, Chen B, Naranmandura H, Le XC, Cohen SM. 2010. Dietary administration of sodium arsenite to rats: Relations between dose and urinary concentrations of methylated and thio-metabolites and effects on the rat urinary bladder epithelium. *Toxicology and Applied Pharmacology* 244(2):99–105.

Swanson HI, Chan WK, Bradfield CA. 1995. DNA binding specificities and pairing rules of the Ah receptor, ARNT, and SIM proteins. *Journal of Biological Chemistry* 270(44):26292–26302.

Szyf M. 2007. The dynamic epigenome and its implications in toxicology. *Toxicological Sciences* 100(1):7–23.

Takahashi N, Yoshida T, Ohnuma A, Horiuchi H, Ishitsuka K, Kashimoto Y, Kuwahara M, Nakashima N, Harada T. 2011. The enhancing effect of the antioxidant N-acetylcysteine on urinary bladder injury induced by dimethylarsinic acid. *Toxicologic Pathology* 39:1107–1114.

Takeda T, Fujii M, Taura J, Ishii Y, Yamada H. 2012. Dioxin silences gonadotropin expression in perinatal pups by inducing histone deacetylases: A new insight into the mechanism for the imprinting of sexual immaturity by dioxin. *Journal of Biological Chemistry* 287(22):18440–18450.

Thompson DJ, Emerson JL, Strebing RJ, Gerbig CG, Robinson VB. 1972. Teratology and postnatal studies on 4-amino-3,5,6-trichloropicolinic acid (picloram) in the rat. *Food and Cosmetics Toxicology* 10:797–803.

Thornton AS, Oda Y, Stuart GR, Glickman BW, de Boer JG. 2001. Mutagenicity of TCDD in Big Blue transgenic rats. *Mutation Research* 478:45–50.

Timchalk C. 2004. Comparative inter-species pharmacokinetics of phenoxyacetic acid herbicides and related organic acids. Evidence that the dog is not a relevant species for evaluation of human health risk. *Toxicology* 200(1):1–19.

Tokar EJ, Diwan BA, Waalkes MP. 2012. Renal, hepatic, pulmonary and adrenal tumors induced by prenatal inorganic arsenic followed by dimethylarsinic acid in adulthood in CD1 mice. *Toxicology Letters* 209:179–185.

Turner BM. 1998. Histone acetylation as an epigenetic determinant of long-term transcriptional competence. *Cellular and Molecular Life Sciences* 54(1):21–31.

Vahter M, Concha G. 2001. Role of metabolism in arsenic toxicity. *Pharmacology and Toxicology* 89(1):1–5.

Valeri N, Vannini I, Fanini F, Calore F, Adair B, Fabbri M. 2009. Epigenetics, miRNAs, and human cancer: A new chapter in human gene regulation. *Mammalian Genome* 20:573–580.

van den Berg M, Birnbaum L, Denison MS, DeVito M, Farland W, Feeley M, Fiedler H, Hakansson H, Hanberg A, Haws L, Rose M, Safe S, Schrenk D, Tohyama C, Tritscher A, Tuomisto J, Tysklind M, Walker N, Peterson R. 2006. The 2005 World Health Organization re-evaluation of human and mammalian toxic equivalency factors for dioxins and dioxin-like compounds. *Toxicological Sciences* 93(2):223–241.

van den Berg M, Denison MS, Birnbaum L, DeVito M, Fiedler H, Falandysz J, Rose M, Schrenk D, Safe S, Tohyama C, Tritscher A, Tysklind M, Peterson RE. 2013. Polybrominated dibenzo-*p*-dioxins, dibenzofurans and biphenyls: Inclusion in the toxicity equivalency factor concept for dioxin-like compounds. *Toxicological Sciences* 133(2):197–208.

Van der Molen GW, Kooijman SALM, Slob W. 1996. A generic toxicokinetic model for persistent lipophilic compounds in humans: An application to TCDD. *Toxicological Sciences* 31(1):83–84.

Vezina CM, Walker NJ, Olson JR. 2004. Subchronic exposure to TCDD, PeCDF, PCB126, and PCB153: Effect on hepatic gene expression. *Environmental Health Perspectives* 112(16):1636–1644.

Viluksela M, Duong TV, Stahl BU, Li X, Tuomisto J, Rozman KK. 1996. Toxicokinetics of 2,3,7,8-tetrachlorodibenzo-*p*-dioxin (TCDD) in two substrains of male Long-Evans rats after intravenous injection. *Fundamental and Applied Toxicology* 31:184–191.

Waddington CH. 1940. *Organisers and Genes.* United Kingdon: Cambridge University Press.

Waddington CH. 1953. Gene assimilation of an acquired character. *Evolution* 7:118–126.

Waddington CH. 1956. *Principles of Embryology.* United Kingdom: George Allen and Unwin Ltd.

Wang A, Wolf DC, Sen B, Knapp GW, Holladay SD, Huckle WR, Caceci T, Robertson JL. 2009. Dimethylarsinic acid in drinking water changed the morphology of urinary bladder but not the expression of DNA repair genes of bladder transitional epithelium in f344 rats. *Toxicologic Pathology* 37(4):425–437.

Wassom JS, Huff JE, Loprieno N. 1977. A review of the genetic toxicology of chlorinated dibenzo-*p*-dioxins. *Mutation Research* 47:141–160.

Weber LW, Zesch A, Rozman K. 1991. Penetration, distribution and kinetics of 2,3,7,8-tetrachlorodibenzo-*p*-dioxin in human skin in vitro. *Archives of Toxicology* 65:421–428.

Weber LW, Ernst SW, Stahl BU, Rozman K. 1993. Tissue distribution and toxicokinetics of 2,3,7,8-tetrachlorodibenzo-*p*-dioxin in rats after intravenous injection. *Fundamental and Applied Toxicology* 21:523–534.

Wei M, Arnold L, Cano M, Cohen SM. 2005. Effects of co-administration of antioxidants and arsenicals on the rat urinary bladder epithelium. *Toxicological Sciences* 83(2):237–245.

Whitelaw M, Pongratz I, Wilhelmsson A, Gustafsson JA, Poellinger L. 1993. Ligand-dependent recruitment of the ARNT coregulatory determines DNA recognition by the dioxin receptor. *Molecular and Cellular Biology* 13:2504–2514.

Whitlock JP Jr. 1990. Genetic and molecular aspects of 2,3,7,8-tetrachlorodibenzo-*p*-dioxin action. *Annual Review of Pharmacology and Toxicology* 30:251–277.

WHO (World Health Organization). 1984. *2,4-Dichlorophenoxyacetic Acid (2,4-D).* Environmental Health Criteria 29. Geneva: WHO.

Wu Q, Ohsako S, Ishimura R, Suzuki JS, Tohyama C. 2004. Exposure of mouse preimplantation embryos to 2,3,7,8-tetrachlorodibenzo-*p*-dioxin (TCDD) alters the methylation status of imprinted genes H19 and Igf2. *Biology of Reproduction* 70(6):1790–1797.

Xie Y, Trouba KJ, Liu J, Waalkes MP, Germolec DR. 2004. Biokinetics and subchronic toxic effects of oral arsenite, arsenate, monomethylarsonic acid, and dimethylarsinic acid in v-Ha-ras transgenic (Tg.AC) mice. *Environmental Health Perspectives* 112(12):1255–1263.

Yamanaka K, Kato K, Mizoi M, An Y, Nakanao M, Hoshino M, Okada S. 2009. Dimethylarsine likely acts as a mouse-pulmonary tumor initiator via the production of dimethylarsine radical and/or its peroxy radical. *Life Sciences* 84(17-18):627–633.

Yao E, Denison M. 1992. DNA sequence determinants for binding of transformed Ah receptor to a dioxin-responsive enhancer. *Biochemistry* 31:5060–5067.

5

Epidemiologic Studies: Compendium of New Publications

The continuing effort to evaluate and integrate epidemiologic studies pertinent to possible health effects of the chemicals of interest (COIs)—2,4-dichlorophenoxyacetic acid (2,4-D), 2,4,5-trichlorophenoxyacetic acid (2,4,5-T) and its contaminant 2,3,7,8-tetrachlorodibenzo-*p*-dioxin (TCDD), 4-amino-3,5,6-trichloropicolinic acid (picloram), and dimethylarsinic acid (DMA or cacodylic acid)—has involved the review of thousands of publications over successive reports (the original retrospective report, eight updates prior to the current report, and three short reports on single issues, as delineated in the second and third paragraphs of Chapter 1). The search strategy used to identify these publications is described starting on the first page of Chapter 2, along with explanations of various refinements that have been employed since the initial volume in this series was prepared.

The first part of this chapter tabulates publications of primary epidemiologic research that appeared in the period from October 1, 2010 (the closing date for inclusion in *Update 2010* [IOM, 2011]), through September 30, 2012, as a compendium of new information on human health outcomes considered by the present committee. In this chapter and later chapters, epidemiologic studies are organized into categories according to the populations being studied (Vietnam veterans, occupational populations other than Vietnam veterans, and nonoccupational populations affected by environmental exposures) or by study design (case-control). The various study designs (most important, cohort, case-control, and cross-sectional) have strengths and weaknesses that influence their potential to contribute evidence considered in the health-outcomes chapters.

The second part of this chapter provides design information on populations that are the subject of multiple references in this and earlier Veterans and

Agent Orange (VAO) reviews—including new studies of populations that have been studied previously and studies of new populations that had multiple health outcomes—to avoid repeating design information in multiple health-outcomes chapters. (Design information on studies of new populations that involve single health outcomes is provided in the various health-outcomes chapters.) For presentation of the background information, the study populations are arranged into categories on the basis of whether they are composed of Vietnam veterans, occupationally exposed workers, or environmentally exposed individuals or were assembled according to a case-control approach focused on particular health outcomes.

In addition to reviewing studies involving exposures to the specific COIs listed previously, this and earlier VAO committees have considered studies that examined compounds chemically related to the herbicides used in Vietnam, such as 2-(2-methyl-4-chlorophenoxy) propionic acid, hexachlorophene, and chlorophenols, particularly 2,4,5-trichlorophenol. Some publications did not indicate the specific herbicides to which study participants were exposed or the magnitude of exposure; those limitations were considered when the committee weighed the relevance of each publication, as detailed in Chapter 2. The committee also considers studies of exposure to polychlorinated biphenyls and other dioxin-like compounds (DLCs) informative if their results were reported in terms of TCDD toxic equivalents (TEQs) or concentrations of specific congeners of DLCs. Available details of exposure assessment and use of the resulting data in analyses are discussed in Chapter 3, which follows the same sequence to categorize study populations.

NEW EPIDEMIOLOGIC PUBLICATIONS

The new epidemiologic publications reviewed by the committee for this update are listed in Tables 5-1, 5-2, and 5-3. The conditions listed in the "Health Outcomes Reported" columns are indicative of the chapters in which the new publications are considered. Note, however, that studies assessing the occurrence of various cancers after exposure scenarios temporally comparable with exposure during military service are discussed in Chapter 8, which addresses cancer outcomes as applicable to the veterans themselves. Studies of childhood cancers in relation to parental exposure to the COIs are discussed in Chapter 10, which addresses possible adverse effects in veterans' offspring. Cancer studies that consider *only* childhood exposure are not considered relevant to the committee's charge.

Publications Reporting a Single Health Outcome in New Populations

New publications reporting a single health outcome in populations not studied previously are listed in Table 5-1, with an indication of the outcomes. De-

TABLE 5-1 Publications Reporting a Single Health Outcome in New Populations

Citation	Study Design	Exposure Measure(s) Having Results	Health Outcome(s) Reported	Study Population
Studies of Vietnam Veterans				
None				
Occupational Studies				
Kamel et al., 2012	Case-control (nested)	Pesticides, herbicides, 2,4-D, 2,4,5-T, dicamba	ALS	AHS
Environmental Studies				
Buck Louis et al., 2011	Cross-sectional	anti-estrogenic PCBs (correspond to dl PCBs)	Menstrual cycles	Women without reproductive problems
Goncharov et al., 2011	Cross-sectional	PCB subsets (mono-ortho TEQ, estrogenic)	Hypertension	Anniston (AL) Community Health Survey
Kezios et al., 2012	Pregnancy cohort	dl PCB 118	Birth weight, gestational age	California Child Health and Development Studies, University of California, Berkeley
Leijs et al., 2012	Prospective cohort	Prenatal TEQs for dioxin/furans, dl PCBs	Sons' thyroid metabolism at puberty	Mother–baby pairs from Netherlands (followup on cohort of Ilsen et al., 1996)
Miyashita et al., 2011	Cohort	Total dioxins, furans, dl PCBs (non-*ortho* and mono-*ortho*) in maternal blood (3rd trimester)	Immune function in offspring (infections [otitis media], allergies [asthma, eczema, food allergies])	Hokkaido Study on Environment and Children's Health Japanese mothers and infants examined at birth and at 18 months of age
Nishijo et al., 2012	Birth cohort	TEQs PCDD/Fs in breast milk 1 mo after birth	Infant growth (birth, 1 mo, 4 mo), neurodevelopment	Mother–infant pairs from contaminated area of Vietnam

TABLE 5-1 Continued

Citation	Study Design	Exposure Measure(s) Having Results	Health Outcome(s) Reported	Study Population
Virtanen et al., 2012; Krysiak-Baltyn et al., 2012	Case-control (nested)	TEQs for dioxins, furans, PCBs in placenta, individual results on comprehensive list of dl-PCBs; in breast milk	Congenital cryptorchidism; Seeking pattern of congeners distinguishing cases with cryptorchidism form controls [results of interest in Virtanen et al., 2012]	Danish-Finnish Prospective Cohort: boys examined at birth and 3 months of age
Case-Control Studies				
Band et al., 2011	Case-control	2,4-D, MCPA, dicamba	Prostate cancer	British Columbia farmers
Bonefeld-Jorgensen et al., 2011	Case-control	Sum dl PCBs, AHR-TEQs	Breast cancer	Inuit women from Greenland sampled 2000–2003
Cai et al., 2011	Case-control	Dioxins, furans, all dl-PCBs, TEQ in peritoneal fluid and serum	Endometriosis	Japanese women undergoing diagnostic laparoscopy for infertility enrolled from October 2004 to March 2007
Gallagher et al., 2011	Case-control	dl PCBs 118, 156, total dl PCBs in serum	Melanoma	Study participants were recruited using a population-based British Columbia Cancer Registry
Lv et al., 2011	Case-control	Occupational exposure to herbicides [marginal]	MDS	Shanghai, China
Postuma et al., 2012	Case-control	Occupational herbicide exposure, non-occupational only as specific as "pesticides" [marginal]	REM sleep behavior disorder (prognostic sign of PD and dementia)	Cases drawn from seven centers

continued

TABLE 5-1 Continued

Citation	Study Design	Exposure Measure(s) Having Results	Health Outcome(s) Reported	Study Population
Rollison et al., 2011	Case-control	Pesticides, herbicides (case-control comparison shown for telomere length and then telomere length within MDS cases compared on basis of pesticide use) [marginal]	MDS (indirect evidence)	Newly diagnosed MDS cases in Florida
Rugbjerg et al., 2011	Case-control	Self-reported pesticide exposure (2,4-D & 2,4,5-T in "herbicides," "pesticides with known neurotoxicity" classes) [marginal]	PD	British Columbia PD cases and controls
Slater et al., 2011	Case-control	Household chemicals (specificity to level of "herbicides") [marginal]	Leukemia in infants	Infants diagnosed with acute leukemia at < 1 year of age at Children's Oncology Group institutions in US and Canada
Wong et al., 2010	Case-control	Primarily job title, but also "herbicides" [marginal]	NHL	Newly diagnosed patients in Shanghai
Zakerinia et al., 2012	Case-control	Pesticides [for individual types]; Herbicides for all lymphomas	Lymphoid neoplasms (HL, NHL, multiple myeloma, T-cell)	Diagnoses at Nemazee Hospital, Shiraz, Iran

NOTE: 2,4-D, 2,4-dichlorophenoxyacetic acid; 2,4,5-T, 2,4,5-trichlorophenoxyacetic acid; AHR, aryl hydrocarbon receptor; AHS, Agricultural Health Study; ALS, amyotrophic lateral sclerosis; dl, dioxin-like; HL, Hodgkin lymphoma; MCPA, 2-methyl-4-chlorophenoxyacetic acid; MDS, myelodysplastic syndrome; NHL, non-Hodgkin lymphoma; PCB, polychlorinated biphenyl; PCDD, polychlorinated dibenzo-*p*-dioxin; PCDF, polychlorinated dibenzofuran; REM, rapid eye movement; TEQ, total toxic equivalent.

scriptions and critiques of the designs of the studies are provided in the sections of the report that discuss the results related to particular health outcomes. The publications in this table are predominantly case-control studies, where the focus of the investigation is on a particular health outcome.

Publications Reporting Multiple Health Outcomes in New Populations

New publications reporting multiple health outcomes in populations not studied previously are listed in Table 5-2, with a list of outcomes that were investigated. Comprehensive discussions of the designs of the studies are presented in Chapter 6, organized according to the type of study population. The results, with comments related to their reliability or limitations, appear in the appropriate outcome-specific sections of Chapters 7–13.

New Publications on Previously Studied Populations

The new publications on previously studied populations are listed in Table 5-3. The new publications are reviewed in the context of the history of publications on the same populations to take into account the fact that they are not presenting entirely new evidence but rather enhancing a picture that has been emerging for many years.

A number of long-term studies of populations exposed to the COIs are of particular importance to the VAO project. The disease experiences of those populations are updated with the passage of time. Placing each new publication into its historical context helps the committee to combine the evidence from various publications appropriately and to take into consideration the interdependence of related publications. Such clusters of studies are useful in describing the course of a population's response to an exposure, and joint consideration of an entire body of research on a population may yield insight into relationships with potential confounding factors.

Many groups potentially exposed to the COIs have been monitored periodically, including the cohorts of the International Agency for Research on Cancer (IARC) and the National Institute for Occupational Safety and Health (NIOSH); residents of Seveso; and Operation Ranch Hand and Army Chemical Corps personnel. For the sake of completeness, the discussions of specific health outcomes and the associated cumulative-results tables in Chapters 7–13 include references to publications discussed in previous VAO reports and to new publications. In drawing its conclusions, the committee combined the evidence in new publications and the evidence synthesized in the most recent update (*Update 2010*), taking into account the interdependence of related publications.

Individual researchers who belong to research consortia that are evaluating cohorts in large multicenter studies (such as the IARC and NIOSH cohort studies) sometimes publish reports based on the subsets of study participants that they themselves are monitoring. The VAO committees take into consideration all reports that have been published, including those based on entire cohorts and those based on subcohorts. In drawing its conclusions, the committee factored in both types of studies, taking into consideration the interdependence among related studies. In particular, some subcohort studies have access to information

TABLE 5-2 Publications on Multiple Health Outcomes in New Study Populations

Citation	Study Design	Exposure Measures(s) Having Results	Health Outcome(s) Reported	Study Population
Studies of Vietnam Veterans				
Kim JB et al., 2012	Case-control	TCDD	HT, hyperlipidemia, clinical outcomes (rate and severity of major adverse coronary events)	Korean VV (50–70 yrs of age undergoing angiograms for acute coronary syndrome)
Occupational Studies				
None				
Environmental Studies				
Chang et al., 2011a	Cross-sectional	Serum PCDD/F TEQ	Insulin resistance	Taiwan, 1,449 non-diabetic residents around closed PCP factory
Chang et al., 2011b	Cross-sectional	Serum PCDD/F TEQ	CVD	Taiwan, 914 residents without CVD around closed PCP factory
Chang et al., 2012	Cross-sectional	Serum PCDD/F TEQ, also consideration of diet as source	Blood chemistries [Indirect evidence—more like biologic plausibility]	Taiwan, workers from closed PCP factory vs residents vs general population
Lee et al., 2010	Nested case-control	dl-PCBs 105, 118, 156, 157, 167 in serum	Diabetes	CARDIA cohort
Lee et al., 2011a	Nested case-control	dl-PCBs 105, 118, 156, 157, 167 in serum	Obesity, dyslipedemia, insulin resistance	CARDIA cohort participants; study subjects recruited at baseline in 1985–1986 and followed for 20 yrs
Lee et al. 2011b	Cross-sectional and prospective	dl-PCBs 105, 118, 156, 157, 189 in serum	Diabetes	PIVUS (men and women analyzed together)
Lee et al., 2012a	Cross-sectional and prospective	dl-PCBs 105, 118, 126, 156, 157, 169, 189 in serum	Abdominal obesity	PIVUS (men and women analyzed separately)

TABLE 5-2 Continued

Citation	Study Design	Exposure Measures(s) Having Results	Health Outcome(s) Reported	Study Population
Lee et al., 2012b	Cross-sectional and prospective	dl-PCBs 105, 118, 126, 156, 157, 169, 189 in serum	stroke	PIVUS (men and women analyzed separately)
Lind et al., 2012	Cross-sectional and prospective	Circulating POPs (dl PCBs 105, 118, 126, 156, 157, 169, 189)	Atherosclerosis (carotid artery plaques, intima-media thickness, gray scale of median)	PIVUS study
Rönn et al., 2011	Cross-sectional, prospective	dl-PCBs 105, 118, 123, 169, 156, 157, 189 in serum	Fat mass, obesity	PIVUS study participants; Uppsala elderly
Silverstone et al., 2012	Cross-sectional	PCB subsets (mono-ortho TEQ, estrogenic)	Diabetes	Anniston (Alabama) Community Health Survey
Stolevik et al., 2011	Prospective cohort	Prenatal exposure, TEQs for all dioxins, furans, dl PCBs (estimated from mothers' food frequency questionnaire)	Infection, eczema, wheeze	Birth cohort from Norwegian Mother and Child Cohort Study (MoBa)
Case-Control Studies				
Rocheleau et al., 2011	Case-control	maternal occupational herbicides expo, 1 mo before conception, 1st trimester, or 2nd–3rd trimester	Hypospadias	National Birth Defects Prevention Study (NBDPS)

NOTE: AO, Agent Orange; CARDIA, Coronary Artery Risk Development in Young Adults cohort; CVD, cardiovascular disease; dl, dioxin-like; HT, hypertension; NBDPS, National Birth Defects Prevention Study; PCB, polychlorinated biphenyl; PCDD, polychlorinated dibenzo-*p*-dioxin; PCDF, polychlorinated dibenzofuran; PCP, pentachlorophenol; PIVUS, Prospective Investigation of the Vasculature in Uppsala Seniors; POP, persistant organic pollutant; TCDD, 2,3,7,8-tetrachlorodibenzo-*p*-dioxin; TEQ, total toxic equivalent; VV, Vietnam veteran.

TABLE 5-3 Publications on Previously Studied Populations

Citation	Study Design	Exposure Measure(s) Having Results	Health Outcome(s) Reported	Study Population
Studies of Vietnam Veterans				
None				
Occupational Studies				
Andreotti et al., 2010	Cohort	Dicamba and BMI as factors for colon cancer [marginal]	Focus on BMI at enrollment and incidence of various cancers [not relevant] Colon cancer from interaction of dicamba and BMI	AHS (licensed pesticide applicators and spouses)
Boers et al., 2012	Cohort	Chlorophenoxy herbicides (plasma TCDD)	All cancers and specific (stomach, pancreas, trachea/bronchus/lung, melanoma, genital, prostate, bladder, kidney, NHL, leukemia), and IHD	Subcohort of IARC cohort (Netherlands) [followup to 2006 like Boers et al. (2010)]
Burns et al., 2011	Cohort	2,4-D	Cancer incidence (1985–2007) from all cancer and full spectrum individually	Subcohort of NIOSH (Dow Chemical, Midland, Michigan plant workers)
Kenborg et al., 2012	Cohort	Pesticide exposure mainly to herbicides (including phenoxys) [marginal]	Incidence PD and smoking-related cancers (lung, larynx, bladder)	Danish Union of Gardeners
Koutros et al., 2010a	Cohort	Pesticides [2,4-D known to be among most frequently used herbicides] [marginal]	Cancer incidence (extended through 2006) from all cancers and full spectrum individually	AHS (licensed pesticide applicators: private, commercial and spouses)

TABLE 5-3 Continued

Citation	Study Design	Exposure Measure(s) Having Results	Health Outcome(s) Reported	Study Population
Koutros et al., 2010b, 2011; Barry et al., 2011, 2012	Nested case-control	2,4,5-T; 2,4-D; 2,4,5-TP; dicamba	Prostate cancer incidence 1993–2003 [most complete dose response info in Koutros et al., 2011]	AHS (licensed pesticide applicators); interaction between pesticide use and SNPs (in metabolic DNA repair, and 8q24 genes) for prostate cancer risk
Manuwald et al., 2012	Cohort	Cumulative TCDD exposure estimated from tissue samples and job history	All cancers and full spectrum individually	German production workers at Hamburg plant (IARC)
Ruder and Yiin, 2011	Cohort	PCP (subgroups with and without exposure to TCDD in addition)	Mortality (to 2005) (full spectrum)	US PCP workers (NIOSH)
Saberi Hosnijeh et al., 2011	Cohort	2,4-D, 2,4,5-T, 2,4,5-TCP, MCPA, MCPP	Humoral immunity (C-4, associated with NHL), atopic disease (asthma)	Subcohort of IARC (Dutch phenoxy herbicide workers)
Saberi Hosnijeh et al., 2012	Cohort	2,4-D, 2,4,5-T, 2,4,5-TCP, MCPA, MCPP	Plasma cytokine concentrations (possible suppression of immunity)	Subcohort of IARC (Dutch phenoxy herbicide workers)
Waggoner et al., 2011	Cohort	Pesticides (2,4-D known to be among most frequently used herbicides) [marginal]	Mortality (1993–2007) (includes full spectrum of individual cancers; diabetes mellitus; and diseases of systems related to respiration, digestion, bone and connective tissue, heart and circulation)	AHS (licensed pesticide applicators and spouses)
Environmental Studies				
Cho et al., 2011	Cross-sectional	DLCs (PCB 126, hpCDD, OCDD)	Bone mineral density, fat mass	NHANES (1999–2004)

continued

TABLE 5-3 Continued

Citation	Study Design	Exposure Measure(s) Having Results	Health Outcome(s) Reported	Study Population
Humblet et al., 2011	Cohort	Dioxin, PCB concentrations in maternal blood (TEQs)	Pubertal onset	Mother–son pairs from Chapaevsk, Russia
Jones et al., 2011	Cross-sectional	Urinary arsenic	Hypertension	NHANES (2003–2008)
Lambertino et al., 2011	Cohort	Σdl PCBs	Uterine leiomyoma	Great Lakes Fish Consumption Study
Mocarelli et al., 2011	Cohort	Serum concentrations of TCDD	Sperm quality and reproductive hormones in offspring	Seveso; sons born (1977–1984) to dioxin-exposed mothers
Su et al., 2012	Cohort	TEQs for PCBs, PCDD/Fs	Reproductive development	Taiwanese Mother-and-Child Study; followup to 8 yrs of age
Tsukimori et al., 2012b	Cohort	Dioxin, furan, and PCB TEQs in maternal blood extrapolated back to delivery	Birth weight (by sex of infant)	Yusho mothers and children
Warner et al., 2011	Cohort	Serum concentrations of TCDD	Breast cancer	SWHS (Seveso women 0–40 yrs old at time of accident; followup through 2008)
Case-Control Studies				
Hohenadel et al., 2011	Case-control	Herbicides, phenoxys, 2,4-D alone and in combination with malathion	NHL	Cross-Canada Study of Pesticides and Health
Karunanayake et al., 2012	Case-control	≥ 10 hr/yr pesticide expo (2,4-D, Mecoprop, MCPA, Diclofomethyl, and dicamba)	Hodgkin Lymphoma	Cross-Canada Study of Pesticides and Health

TABLE 5-3 Continued

Citation	Study Design	Exposure Measure(s) Having Results	Health Outcome(s) Reported	Study Population
Pahwa et al., 2011	Case-control	Pesticide use (results on all phenoxys, 2,4-D, Mecoprop, MCPA, Diclofop-methyl)	STS	Cross-Canada Study of Pesticides and Health
Viel et al., 2011	Case-control	TEQs for dioxins, furans, and dl PCBs	NHL	NHL cases using population-based cancer registry, living in vicinity of a solid-waste incinerator in France
Yiin et al., 2012	Case-control	Quantified pesticide exposure (phenoxys, 2,4-D, dicamba)	Gliomas	UMHS (pesticide applicators)

NOTE: 2,4-D, 2,4-dichlorophenoxyacetic acid; 2,4,5-T, 2,4,5-trichlorophenoxyacetic acid; 2,4,5-TCP, 2,4,5-trichlorophenol; 2,4,5-TP, 2-(2,4,5-trichlorophenoxy) propionic acid; AHS, Agricultural Health Study; AML, acute myeloid leukemia; BMI, body mass index; CLL, chronic lymphocytic leukemia; CML, chronic myeloid leukemia; CNS, central nervous system; COI, chemical of interest; dl, dioxin-like; DLBCL, diffuse large B-cell lymphoma; DLC, dioxin-like compound; DNA, deoxyribonucleic acid; FL, follicular lymphoma; GI, gastrointestinal; HD, Hodgkin disease; hpCDD, heptachlorodibenzo-*p*-dioxin; IARC, International Agency for Research on Cancer; IHD, ischemic heart disease; MCL, mantle cell lymphoma; MCPA, 2-methyl-4-chlorophenoxyacetic acid; MM, multiple myeloma; MZL, marginal zone lymphoma; NHANES, National Health and Nutrition Examination Survey; NHL, non-Hodgkin lymphoma; NIOSH, National Institute of Occupational Safety and Health; OCDD, octachlorodibenzo-*p*-dioxin; PCB, polychlorinated biphenyl; PCDD, polychlorinated dibenzo-*p*-dioxin; PCDF, polychlorinated dibenzofuran; PCP, pentachlorophenol; SLL, small lymphocytic lymphoma; SNP, single-nucleotide polymorphism; STS, soft-tissue sarcoma; SWHS, Seveso Women's Health Study; TCDD, 2,3,7,8-tetrachlorodibenzo-*p*-dioxin; TEQ, total toxic equivalent; UMHS, Upper Midwest Health Study.

not available for the entire cohort, such as data on individual serum TCDD concentrations and personal information that can be used to adjust for confounders of concern. Furthermore, even when analyses based on an entire cohort would include data on a subcohort as a subset, reports on the subcohort might provide additional information on the consistency of the relationships among subcohorts, such as whether there are important subcohort-by-exposure interaction effects, when these issues were not considered in the full-cohort studies. As long as the structures of study populations are recognized, VAO committees have been less concerned about over-weighting unstable positive findings on small subgroups or giving "repeated consideration" to duplicative results than would be the case if a quantitative meta-analysis were being undertaken.

Many of the cohorts that have contributed to the cumulative findings of the VAO committees are no longer being followed; however, the cohorts' histories are briefly recapitulated in the body of this report. Additional background information can be found in earlier reports in this series. It is notable that the literature search for this update identified only a single epidemiology study of physical (not mental) health outcomes and the COIs in Vietnam veterans (Kim et al., 2012); the Vietnam veterans were Korean servicemen and the comparisons involving presumed herbicide exposure were designed in such a fashion that the study provided no usable information on any health outcome.

REFERENCES[1]

Andreotti G, Hou L, Beane Freeman LE, Mahajan R, Koutros S, Coble J, Lubin J, Blair A, Hoppin JA, Alavanja M. 2010. Body mass index, agricultural pesticide use, and cancer incidence in the Agricultural Health Study cohort. *Cancer Causes and Control* 21(11):1759–1775.

Band PR, Abanto Z, Bert J, Lang B, Fang R, Gallagher RP, Le ND. 2011. Prostate cancer risk and exposure to pesticides in British Columbia farmers. *Prostate* 71(2):168–183.

Barry KH, Koutros S, Berndt SI, Andreotti G, Hoppin JA, Sandler DP, Burdette LA, Yeager M, Freeman LEB, Lubin JH, Ma X, Zheng T, Alavanja MCR. 2011. Genetic variation in base excision repair pathway genes, pesticide exposure, and prostate cancer risk. *Environmental Health Perspectives* 119(12):1726–1732.

Barry KH, Koutros S, Andreotti G, Sandler DP, Burdette LA, Yeager M, Beane Freeman LE, Lubin JH, Ma X, Zheng T, Alavanja MCR, Berndt SI. 2012. Genetic variation in nucleotide excision repair pathway genes, pesticide exposure and prostate cancer risk. *Carcinogenesis* 33(2):331–337.

Boers D, Portengen L, Bueno de Mesquita HB, Heederik D, Vermeulen R. 2010. Cause-specific mortality of Dutch chlorophenoxy herbicide manufacturing workers. *Occupational and Environmental Medicine* 67(1):24–31.

Boers D, Portengen L, Turner WE, Bueno de Mesquita HB, Heederik D, Vermeulen R. 2012. Plasma dioxin levels and cause–specific mortality in an occupational cohort of workers exposed to chlorophenoxy herbicides, chlorophenols and contaminants. *Occupational and Environmental Medicine* 69(2):113–118.

Bonefeld-Jorgensen EC, Long M, Bossi R, Ayotte P, Asmund G, Kruger T, Ghisari M, Mulvad G, Kern P, Nzulumiki P, Dewailly E. 2011. Perfluorinated compounds are related to breast cancer risk in Greenlandic Inuit: A case control study. *Environmental Health: A Global Access Science Source* 10:88.

Buck Louis GM, Rios LI, McLain A, Cooney MA, Kostyniak PJ, Sundaram R. 2011. Persistent organochlorine pollutants and menstrual cycle characteristics. *Chemosphere* 85(11):1742–1748.

Burns C, Bodner K, Swaen G, Collins J, Beard K, Lee M. 2011. Cancer incidence of 2,4-D production workers. *International Journal of Environmental Research and Public Health* 8(9):3579–3590.

Cai LY, Izumi S, Suzuki T, Goya K, Nakamura E, Sugiyama T, Kobayashi H. 2011. Dioxins in ascites and serum of women with endometriosis: A pilot study. *Human Reproduction* 26(1):117–126.

Chang JW, Chen HL, Su HJ, Liao PC, Guo HR, Lee CC. 2011a. Simultaneous exposure of non-diabetics to high levels of dioxins and mercury increases their risk of insulin resistance. *Journal of Hazardous Materials* 185(2–3):749–755.

[1]Throughout this report, the same alphabetic indicator after year of publication is used consistently for a given reference when there are multiple citations by the same first author in a given year. The convention of assigning the alphabetic indicators in order of citation in a given chapter is not followed.

Chang JW, Chen HL, Chang CC, Su HJ, Liao PC, Lee CC. 2011b. Predicting the risk of cardiovascular disease in people exposed to moderate to high levels of dioxin. *Journal of Hazardous Materials* 198:317–322.

Chang JW, Chen HL, Su HJ, Liao PC, Lee CC. 2012. Biochemical study of retired pentachlorophenol workers with and without following dietary exposure to pcdd/fs. *Chemosphere* 88(7):813–819.

Cho MR, Shin JY, Hwang JH, Jacobs DR Jr, Kim SY, Lee DH. 2011. Associations of fat mass and lean mass with bone mineral density differ by levels of persistent organic pollutants: National Health and Nutrition Examination Survey 1999–2004. *Chemosphere* 82:1268–1276.

Gallagher RP, MacArthur AC, Lee TK, Weber JP, Leblanc A, Mark Elwood J, Borugian M, Abanto Z, Spinelli JJ. 2011. Plasma levels of polychlorinated biphenyls and risk of cutaneous malignant melanoma: A preliminary study. *International Journal of Cancer* 128(8):1872–1880.

Goncharov A, Pavuk M, Foushee HR, Carpenter DO. 2011. Blood pressure in relation to concentrations of PCB congeners and chlorinated pesticides. *Environmental Health Perspectives* 119(3):319–325.

Hohenadel K, Harris SA, McLaughlin JR, Spinelli JJ, Pahwa P, Dosman JA, Demers PA, Blair A. 2011. Exposure to multiple pesticides and risk of non-Hodgkin lymphoma in men from six Canadian provinces. *International Journal of Environmental Research and Public Health* 8(6):2320–2330.

Humblet O, Williams PL, Korrick SA, Sergeyev O, Emond C, Birnbaum LS, Burns JS, Altshul L, Patterson DG, Turner WE, Lee MM, Revich B, Hauser R. 2011. Dioxin and polychlorinated biphenyl concentrations in mother's serum and the timing of pubertal onset in sons. *Epidemiology* 22(6):827–835.

Ilsen A, Briet JM, Koppe JG, Pluim HJ, Oosting J. 1996. Signs of enhanced neuromotor maturation in children due to perinatal load with background levels of dioxins. Follow-up until age 2 years and 7 months. *Chemosphere* 33(7):1317–1326.

IOM (Institute of Medicine). 2011. *Veterans and Agent Orange: Update 2010.* Washington, DC: The National Academies Press.

Jones MR, Tellez-Plaza M, Sharrett AR, Guallar E, Navas-Acien A. 2011. Urine Arsenic and hypertension in US adults. The 2003–2008 National Health and Nutrition Examination Survey. *Epidemiology* 22:153–161.

Kamel F, Umbach DM, Bedlack RS, Richards M, Watson M, Alavanja MCR, Blair A, Hoppin JA, Schmidt S, Sandler DP. 2012. Pesticide exposure and amyotrophic lateral sclerosis. *NeuroToxicology* 33(3):457–462.

Karunanayake CP, Spinelli JJ, McLaughlin JR, Dosman JA, Pahwa P, McDuffie HH. 2012. Hodgkin lymphoma and pesticides exposure in men: A Canadian case-control study. *Journal of Agromedicine* 17(1):30–39.

Kenborg L, Lassen CF, Lander F, Olsen JH. 2012. Parkinson's disease among gardeners exposed to pesticides—A Danish cohort study. *Scandinavian Journal of Work, Environment and Health* 38(1):65–69.

Kezios KL, Liu X, Cirillio PM, Kalantzi OI, Wang Y, Petreas MX, Park JS, Bradwin G, Cohn BA, Factor-Litvak P. 2012. Prenatal polychlorinated biphenyl exposure is associated with decreased gestational length but not birth weight: Archived samples from the child health and development studies pregnancy cohort. *Environmental Health: A Global Access Science Source* 11(1):1–13.

Kim JB, Kang WY, Moon SG, Kim HJ, Kim KH, Kim YH, Hwang SH, Hwang SH, Kim W. 2012. Clinical outcome of veterans with acute coronary syndrome who had been exposed to Agent Orange. *Chonnam Medical Journal* 48(1):47–51.

Koutros S, Alavanja MCR, Lubin JH, Sandler DP, Hoppin JA, Lynch CF, Knott C, Blair A, Freeman LEB. 2010a. An update of cancer incidence in the Agricultural Health Study. *Journal of Occupational and Environmental Medicine* 52(11):1098–1105.

Koutros S, Beane Freeman LE, Berndt SI, Andreotti G, Lubin JH, Sandler DP, Hoppin JA, Yu K, Li Q, Burdette LA, Yuenger J, Yeager M, Alavanja MCR. 2010b. Pesticide use modifies the association between genetic variants on chromosome 8q24 and prostate cancer. *Cancer Research* 70(22):9224–9233.

Koutros S, Andreotti G, Berndt SI, Hughes Barry K, Lubin JH, Hoppin JA, Kamel F, Sandler DP, Burdette LA, Yuenger J, Yeager M, Alavanja MCR, Freeman LEB. 2011. Xenobiotic–metabolizing gene variants, pesticide use, and the risk of prostate cancer. *Pharmacogenetics and Genomics* 21(10):615–623.

Krysiak-Baltyn K, Toppari J, Skakkebaek NE, Jensen TS, Virtanen HE, Schramm KW, Shen H, Vartiainen T, Kiviranta H, Taboureau O, Audouze K, Brunak S, Main KM. 2012. Association between chemical pattern in breast milk and congenital cryptorchidism: Modelling of complex human exposures. *International Journal of Andrology* 35(3):294–302.

Lambertino A, Turyk M, Anderson H, Freels S, Persky V. 2011. Uterine leiomyomata in a cohort of Great Lakes sport fish consumers. *Environmental Research* 111(4):565–572.

Lee DH, Steffes MW, Sjödin A, Jones RS, Needham LL, Jacobs DR Jr. 2010. Low dose of some persistent organic pollutants predicts type 2 diabetes: A nested case-control study. *Environmental Health Perspectives* 118(9):1235–1242.

Lee DH, Steffes MW, Sjodin A, Jones RS, Needham LL, Jacobs DR Jr. 2011a. Low dose organochlorine pesticides and polychlorinated biphenyls predict obesity, dyslipidemia, and insulin resistance among people free of diabetes. *PLoS ONE* 6 (1):e15977.

Lee DH, Lind PM, Jacobs DR Jr, Salihovic S, van Bavel B, Lind L. 2011b. Polychlorinated biphenyls and organochlorine pesticides in plasma predict development of type 2 diabetes in the elderly: The prospective investigation of the vasculature in Uppsala seniors (PIVUS) study. *Diabetes Care* 34(8):1778–1784.

Lee DH, Lind L, Jacobs DR Jr, Salihovic S, van Bavel B, Lind PM. 2012a. Associations of persistent organic pollutants with abdominal obesity in the elderly: The prospective investigation of the vasculature in Uppsala seniors (PIVUS) study. *Environment International* 40:170–178.

Lee DH, Lind PM, Jacobs DR, Salihovic S, van Bavel B, Lind L. 2012b. Background exposure to persistent organic pollutants predicts stroke in the elderly. *Environment International* 47:115–120.

Leijs MM, Ten Tusscher GW, Olie K, Van Teunenbroek T, Van Aalderen WM, De Voogt P, Vulsma T, Bartonova A, Krayer Von Krauss M, Mosoiu C, Riojas-Rodriguez H, Calamandrei G, Koppe JG. 2012. Thyroid hormone metabolism and environmental chemical exposure. *Environmental Health: A Global Access Science Source* 11(Suppl 1):S10.

Lind PM, van Bavel B, Salihovic S, Lind L. 2012. Circulating levels of persistent organic pollutants (POPs) and carotid atherosclerosis in the elderly. *Environmental Health Perspectives* 120(1):38–43.

Lv L, Lin G, Gao X, Wu C, Dai J, Yang Y, Zou H, Sun H, Gu M, Chen X, Fu H, Bao L. 2011. Case-control study of risk factors of myelodysplastic syndromes according to World Health Organization classification in a Chinese population. *American Journal of Hematology* 86(2):163–169.

Manuwald U, Garrido MV, Berger J, Manz A, Baur X. 2012. Mortality study of chemical workers exposed to dioxins: Follow-up 23 years after chemical plant closure. *Occupational and Environmental Medicine* 69(9):636–642.

Miyashita C, Sasaki S, Saijo Y, Washino N, Okada E, Kobayashi S, Konishi K, Kajiwara J, Todaka T, Kishi R. 2011. Effects of prenatal exposure to dioxin-like compounds on allergies and infections during infancy. *Environmental Research* 111(4):551–558.

Mocarelli P, Gerthoux PM, Needham LL, Patterson DG Jr, Limonta G, Falbo R, Signorini S, Bertona M, Crespi C, Sarto C, Scott PK, Turner WE, Brambilla P. 2011. Perinatal exposure to low doses of dioxin can permanently impair human semen quality. *Environmental Health Perspectives* 119:713–718.

Nishijo M, Tai PT, Nakagawa H, Maruzeni S, Anh NTN, van Luong H, Anh TH, Honda R, Morikawa Y, Kido T, Nishijo H. 2012. Impact of perinatal dioxin exposure on infant growth: A cross-sectional and longitudinal studies in dioxin-contaminated areas in Vietnam. *PLoS ONE* 7(7):e40273.

Pahwa P, Karunanayake CP, Dosman JA, Spinelli JJ, McLaughlin JR. 2011. Soft-tissue sarcoma and pesticides exposure in men: Results of a Canadian case-control study. *Journal of Occupational and Environmental Medicine* 53(11):1279–1286.

Postuma RB, Montplaisir JY, Pelletier A, Dauvilliers Y, Oertel W, Iranzo A, Ferini–Strambi L, Arnulf I, Hogl B, Manni R, Miyamoto T, Mayer G, Stiasny-Kolster K, Puligheddu M, Ju Y, Jennum P, Sonka K, Santamaria J, Fantini ML, Zucconi M, Leu-Semenescu S, Frauscher B, Terzaghi M, Miyamoto M, Unger MM, De Cock VC, Wolfson C. 2012. Environmental risk factors for REM sleep behavior disorder: A multicenter case-control study. *Neurology* 79(5):428–434.

Rocheleau CM, Bertke SJ, Deddens JA, Ruder AM, Lawson CC, Waters MA, Hopf NB, Riggs MA, Whelan EA. 2011. Maternal exposure to polychlorinated biphenyls and the secondary sex ratio: An occupational cohort study. *Environmental Health* 10:20.

Rollison DE, Epling-Burnette PK, Park JY, Lee JH, Park H, Jonathan K, Cole AL, Painter JS, Guerrier M, Melendez-Santiago J, Fulp W, Komrokji R, Lancet J, List AF. 2011. Telomere length in myelodysplastic syndromes. *Leukemia and Lymphoma* 52(8):1528–1536.

Rönn M, Lind L, Bavel BV, Salihovic S, Michaelsson K, Lind PM. 2011. Circulating levels of persistent organic pollutants associate in divergent ways to fat mass measured by DXA in humans. *Chemosphere* 85(3):335–343.

Ruder AM, Yiin JH. 2011. Mortality of US pentachlorophenol production workers through 2005. *Chemosphere* 83(6):851–861.

Rugbjerg K, Anne Harris M, Shen H, Marion SA, Tsui JKC, Teschke K. 2011. Pesticide exposure and risk of Parkinson's disease—A population-based case-control study evaluating the potential for recall bias. *Scandinavian Journal of Work, Environment and Health* 37(5):427–436.

Saberi Hosnijeh F, Boers D, Portengen L, Bueno de Mesquita HB, Heederik D, Vermeulen R. 2011. Long-term effects on humoral immunity among workers exposed to 2,3,7,8-tetrachlorodibenzo-*p*-dioxin (TCDD). *Occupational and Environmental Medicine* 68(6):419–424.

Saberi Hosnijeh F, Boers D, Portengen L, Bueno de Mesquita HB, Heederik D, Vermeulen R. 2012. Plasma cytokine concentrations in workers exposed to 2,3,7,8-tetrachlorodibenzo-*p*-dioxin (TCDD). *Frontiers in Oncology* 2:37.

Silverstone AE, Rosenbaum PF, Weinstock RS, Bartell SM, Foushee HR, Shelton C, Pavuk M. 2012. Polychlorinated biphenyl (PCB) exposure and diabetes: Results from the Anniston community health survey. *Environmental Health Perspectives* 120(5):727–732.

Slater ME, Linabery AM, Spector LG, Johnson KJ, Hilden JM, Heerema NA, Robison LL, Ross JA. 2011. Maternal exposure to household chemicals and risk of infant leukemia: A report from the children's oncology group. *Cancer Causes and Control* 22(8):1197–1204.

Stolevik SB, Nygaard UC, Namork E, Haugen M, Kvalem HE, Meltzer HM, Alexander J, van Delft JHM, Loveren HV, Lovik M, Granum B. 2011. Prenatal exposure to polychlorinated biphenyls and dioxins is associated with increased risk of wheeze and infections in infants. *Food and Chemical Toxicology* 49(8):1843–1848.

Su PH, Huang PC, Lin CY, Ying TH, Chen JY, Wang SL. 2012. The effect of in utero exposure to dioxins and polychlorinated biphenyls on reproductive development in eight year-old children. *Environment International* 39(1):181–187.

Tsukimori K, Uchi H, Mitoma C, Yasukawa F, Chiba T, Todaka T, Kajiwara J, Yoshimura T, Hirata T, Fukushima K, Wake N, Furue M. 2012b. Maternal exposure to high levels of dioxins in relation to birth weight in women affected by Yusho disease. *Environment International* 38(1):79–86.

Viel JF, Floret N, Deconinck E, Focant JF, De Pauw E, Cahn JY. 2011. Increased risk of non–Hodgkin lymphoma and serum organochlorine concentrations among neighbors of a municipal solid waste incinerator. *Environment International* 37(2):449–453.

Virtanen HE, Koskenniemi JJ, Sundqvist E, Main KM, Kiviranta H, Tuomisto JT, Tuomisto J, Viluksela M, Vartiainen T, Skakkebaek NE, Toppari J. 2012. Associations between congenital cryptorchidism in newborn boys and levels of dioxins and PCBs in placenta. *International Journal of Andrology* 35(3):283–293.

Waggoner JK, Kullman GJ, Henneberger PK, Umbach DM, Blair A, Alavanja MCR, Kamel F, Lynch CF, Knott C, London SJ, Hines CJ, Thomas KW, Sandler DP, Lubin JH, Beane Freeman LE, Hoppin JA. 2011. Mortality in the Agricultural Health Study, 1993–2007. *American Journal of Epidemiology* 173(1):71–83.

Warner M, Mocarelli P, Samuels S, Needham L, Brambilla P, Eskenazi B. 2011. Dioxin exposure and cancer risk in the Seveso Women's Health Study. *Environmental Health Perspectives* 119(12):1700–1705.

Wong O, Harris F, Armstrong TW, Hua F. 2010. A hospital-based case-control study of non-Hodgkin lymphoid neoplasms in Shanghai: Analysis of environmental and occupational risk factors by subtypes of the WHO classification. *Chemico-Biological Interactions* 184:129–146.

Yiin JH, Ruder AM, Stewart PA, Waters MA, Carrean T, Butler MA, Calvert GM, Davis-King KE, Schulte PA, Mandel JS, Morton RF, Reding DJ, Rosenman KD. 2012. The Upper Midwest Health Study: A case-control study of pesticide applicators and risk of glioma. *Environmental Health: A Global Access Science Source* 11(1):13pp.

Zakerinia M, Namdari M, Amirghofran S. 2012. The relationship between exposure to pesticides and the occurrence of lymphoid neoplasm. *Iranian Red Crescent Medical Journal* 14(6):337–344.

6

Epidemiologic Studies: Background on Multiply Referenced Populations

This chapter presents study-design information on populations of Vietnam veterans, occupational cohorts, and environmentally exposed groups that have been reported on repeatedly, often for many health outcomes, and on case-control studies that have generated multiple publications relevant to the *Veterans and Agent Orange* (VAO) series. One-time reports on given study populations that addressed only single health outcomes are not discussed in this chapter.

In drawing its conclusions, the committee synthesized the evidence from studies that have gathered data and published results over an extended period of time, taking into account the interdependence among related studies. In particular, if new results are based on updating or adding subjects to previously studied populations or concern a subset of original study populations, this synthesis considers redundancy among studies while recognizing that separately reported information can impart new relevance to other data on a study population. The design information provided in this chapter links repeated studies and clarifies their interdependence.

This chapter also provides design information on studies involving multiple health outcomes to avoid repetition in the health-outcome chapters (Chapters 7–13). Some of the populations have been studied previously and reviewed in previous VAO publications (thus, these populations are multiply referenced both over time and among health outcomes), and others have not been addressed in other VAO publications. The procedures used to identify relevant literature on health effects in human populations in conjunction with exposure to the chemicals of interest (COIs) are provided in Chapter 2. Details of exposure assessment in individual studies are presented in the present chapter, whereas generic issues of exposure assessment are discussed in Chapter 3 with the special challenges involved in characterizing and reconstructing the herbicide exposures of Vietnam veterans.

The original *VAO* committee and the update committees up to that for *Update 2006* have been satisfied with exposure characterization as nonspecific as "usual occupation" on a death certificate or "current occupation" from a census. With the passage of time, exposure assessments in epidemiology studies have been increasingly exact in both specificity and amount, and this has led the members of the more recent updates to establish stricter criteria for accepting exposure as sufficiently specific for results to be added to the evidentiary database. The current committee now seeks results expressed in terms of the five chemicals of interest for this project or their analogues and regards classification based only on job title as inadequate; restriction by the investigators to "herbicide" exposure is considered specific enough only to provide supporting evidence. According to the policy established by the Agent Orange Act of 1991, studies of Vietnam veterans are presumed to involve relevant exposure, as are studies of workers at a particular plant during a period when it is known to have been producing phenoxy herbicides or other chemicals recognized as having been contaminated with TCDD.

In *Update 2010*, the committee undertook a major change in the formatting of the tables of cumulative results on the health outcomes that was aimed at making relationships among publications more evident for its own deliberations and for the reader. The prior practice had been to insert findings from new publications in the results tables at the beginning of the sections on veteran, occupational, and environmental studies and so to create bands of studies reviewed in individual updates. Now, however, the reported findings on a given condition from a particular study population described in any of the VAO reports are gathered and presented in reverse chronologic order to provide the full history of the study of each endpoint in each group studied. The current update has attempted to shift the focus further to the total picture presented by a study population by clustering related findings and shifting the citations that were the source of particular results to the far right of the results tables. For instance, all incidence findings on the Seveso cohort over the successive followup periods are grouped first, and they are followed by all the analogous mortality findings, even when that means separating various sorts of results from the same publication.

Within the three general types of exposure that cohorts or cross-sectional study populations may have experienced, the order of the study populations (Vietnam veterans, occupationally exposed workers, and environmentally exposed people) roughly reflects the degree of importance attributed to the information generated. In the present update, the occupational-study populations have been partitioned into those involved in the production of herbicides and other industrial products contaminated with TCDD and those involved in occupational use of the herbicides of interest, because of substantial differences in the nature and intensity of their exposures. Doing so entailed splitting the findings on sprayers cohorts from those on production workers in the large International Agency for Research on Cancer (IARC) cohort of phenoxy herbicide workers.

Studies of subgroups are presented after those on an overarching cohort. For example, when first reported (Saracci et al., 1991), the original IARC Cohort of Phenoxy Herbicide Workers was composed of 20 cohorts in 10 countries that had been studied separately. When mortality in those workers was followed up (Kogevinas et al., 1997), they were augmented with 16 additional cohorts—four German study populations and 12 groups of workers studied separately in US manufacturing facilities—which together make up the independently studied National Institute for Occupational Safety and Health (NIOSH) cohort. To simplify the location of underlying information on study populations, their discussion in this chapter follows the order in which their findings are presented in the results tables for each health outcome.

The section below on Vietnam veterans covers studies conducted in the United States by the Air Force, the Centers for Disease Control and Prevention (CDC), the Department of Veterans Affairs (VA), the American Legion, and individual states; it also covers studies of Australian and South Korean Vietnam veterans. The section "Occupational Studies" covers studies of workers other than Vietnam veterans exposed occupationally to the COIs, including production workers, agriculture and forestry workers (including herbicide and pesticide applicators), and paper and pulp workers. The section "Environmental Studies" covers studies of populations exposed to the COIs from nonoccupational sources, including the general population, such as the National Health and Nutrition Examination Survey cohort, and people who had usually high exposures because of industrial sources in their residential neighborhoods, such as residents of Seveso, Italy; southern Vietnam; suburban Taichung, Taiwan; Chapaevsk, Russia; and Times Beach, Missouri. This chapter ends with a section that addresses publications that are based on repeatedly mentioned case-control study populations; case-control studies that assessed Vietnam-veteran status, however, are included in the section on veteran studies, and nested case-control studies are presented in conjunction with the cohorts from which they were derived.

VIETNAM-VETERAN STUDIES

Studies of Vietnam veterans who might have been exposed to herbicides, including Agent Orange, have been conducted in the United States at the national and state levels and in Australia and Korea. Exposures have been estimated by various means, and health outcomes have been evaluated with reference to various comparison or control groups. This section is organized primarily by research sponsor because it is more conducive to a methodologic presentation of the studies. The specificity of exposure spans a wide range from individual exposures of Ranch Hand and Army Chemical Corps (ACC) personnel, as reflected in serum

2,3,7,8-tetrachlorodibenzo-*p*-dioxin (TCDD) measurements, to the use of service in Vietnam as a surrogate for TCDD exposure in some studies.

Several comparison groups have been used for veteran cohort studies: Vietnam veterans who were stationed in areas where herbicide-spraying missions were unlikely to have taken place; Vietnam-era veterans who were in the military at the time of the conflict but did not serve in Vietnam; veterans who served in other wars or conflicts, such as the Korean War and World War II; and various US populations (either state or national).

In all studies of Vietnam veterans (whether or not the study participants were American), the study participants are the target population of the committee's charge, and they are assumed to have had a higher probability of exposure to the COIs than people who did not serve in Vietnam, whether or not their individual exposures are characterized beyond the mere fact that they were deployed to Vietnam.

The publication period considered in the present update saw a number of publications concerning psychologic outcomes in American and Australian Vietnam veterans, but these conditions do not fall in the spectrum of physical responses included in the VAO statement of task (Campbell and Renshaw, 2012; Franzen et al., 2012; Gellis and Gehrman, 2011; Renshaw and Caska, 2012; Yesavage et al., 2012). Conley and Heerwig (2012) investigated whether eligibility for military conscription (although not necessarily being conscripted or actually deployed to Vietnam) might be associated with mortality in later life by using the draft lottery for 1950–1952 birth cohorts as a natural experiment. Mortality data were obtained from the National Center for Health Statistics multiple-cause-of-death file, 1989–2002; the date of birth was used to determine draft status so that mortality in draft-eligible and draft-ineligible people could be compared. That study provides valid estimates of the effects of the Vietnam-era draft, but there is no specific information on actual deployment or exposure to the COIs. Wilmoth et al. (2010) examined the association between veteran status and trajectories of health conditions, limitations on activities of daily living, and self-rated health in 12,631 male participants from the 1992–2006 waves of the Health and Retirement Study; they compared nonveterans and veterans, veterans with and without wartime service, and war-service veterans who served during World War II, Korea, Vietnam, and multiple wars. Again, there is no specific information on exposure to the COIs.

US Air Force Health Study

Although no new reports from the Air Force Health Study (AFHS) were identified in the current literature review, reports and findings from the study have provided important information that was incorporated into the previous VAO reports and continues to play an important role in the committee's assessment of the overall evidence for the current report. The data-gathering phase of this study is complete, but the committee remains interested in seeing additional publications that provide longitudinal analysis of the vast amount of information assembled and make use of the collection of preserved biologic samples.

Major defoliation activities in Vietnam were conducted by Air Force personnel as part of Operation Ranch Hand. Veterans who took part in the defoliation activities became the first subpopulation of Vietnam veterans to receive special attention with regard to Agent Orange and have become known as the Ranch Hand cohort within the AFHS. To determine whether exposure to herbicides, including Agent Orange, had adverse health effects, the Air Force made a commitment to Congress and the White House in 1979 to conduct an epidemiologic study of Ranch Hand personnel (AFHS, 1982). Results of biologic-marker studies of Ranch Hand personnel have been consistent with their being exposed, as a group, to TCDD. When the Ranch Hand cohort was classified by military occupation, a general increase in serum TCDD was detected in people whose jobs involved more frequent handling of herbicides (AFHS, 1991a).

The exposure index initially proposed in the AFHS relied on military records of spraying of TCDD-containing herbicides (Agent Orange, Agent Purple, Agent Pink, and Agent Green) as reported in the Herbicide Reporting System (HERBS) tapes for the period starting in July 1965 and on military procurement records and dissemination information for the period before July 1965. In 1991, the exposure index was compared with the results of the Ranch Hand serum-TCDD analysis. The exposure index and the TCDD body burden correlated weakly.

Michalek et al. (1995) developed several indexes of herbicide exposure of members of the Ranch Hand cohort and tried to relate them to the measurements of serum TCDD from 1987 to 1992. Self-administered questionnaires completed by veterans of Operation Ranch Hand were used to develop three indexes of herbicide or TCDD exposure: number of days of skin exposure; percentage of skin area exposed; and the product of the number of days of skin exposure, the percentage of skin exposed, and a factor for the concentration of TCDD in the herbicide. A fourth index, which used no information gathered from individual study participants, was calculated by multiplying the volume of herbicide sprayed during a person's tour of duty by the concentration of TCDD in herbicides sprayed in that period and then dividing the product by the number of crew members in each job specialty at the time.

Each of the four indexes tested was significantly related to serum TCDD, although the models explained only 19–27% of the variability in serum TCDD concentrations. Days of skin exposure had the highest correlation. Military job classification (non–Ranch Hand combat troops, Ranch Hand administrators, Ranch Hand flight engineers, and Ranch Hand ground crew), which is separate from the four indexes, explained 60% of the variability in serum TCDD. When the questionnaire-derived indexes were applied within each job classification, days of skin exposure added statistical significance, but not substantially, to the variability explained by job alone.

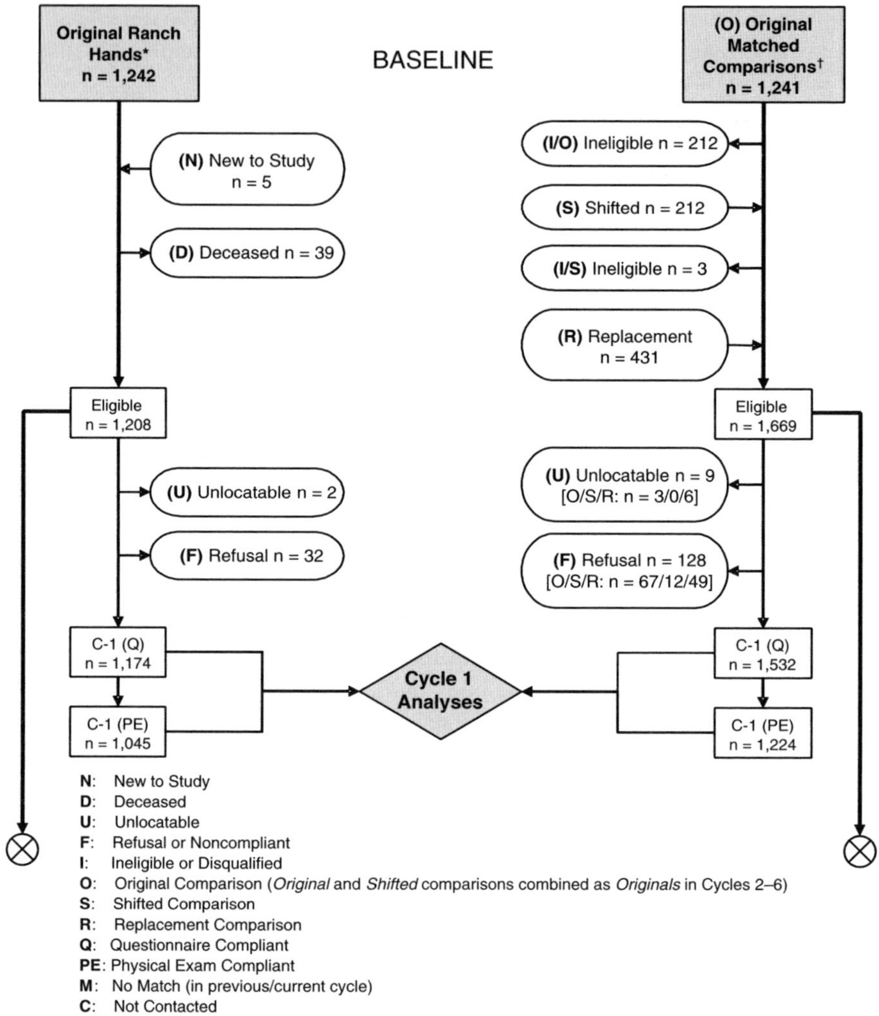

* Total does not reflect the 22 Ranch Hands known at the Baseline to have been killed in action.
† One Ranch Hand (Black officer) remained unmatched to a comparison.
‡ Numbers of eligible and participating Ranch Hands reflect AFHS reports (AFHS, 2000 & 2005) and not the numbers that would be expected—Cycle 5, PE: n = 869; Cycle 6, Eligible n = 1,042, PE: n = 776—from reported changes in the study population recorded in AFHS reports.

FIGURE 6-1 Flowchart of procedures followed and participant involvement in the Air Force Health Study.
NOTE: Flowchart numbers reflect what was known to AFHS investigators at any given cycle according to AFHS reports and do not reflect corrections made to earlier cycles due to the identification of misclassified subjects in later cycles. Identical study population counts vary on occasion within and across cycle reports. Thus, this reconstruction should

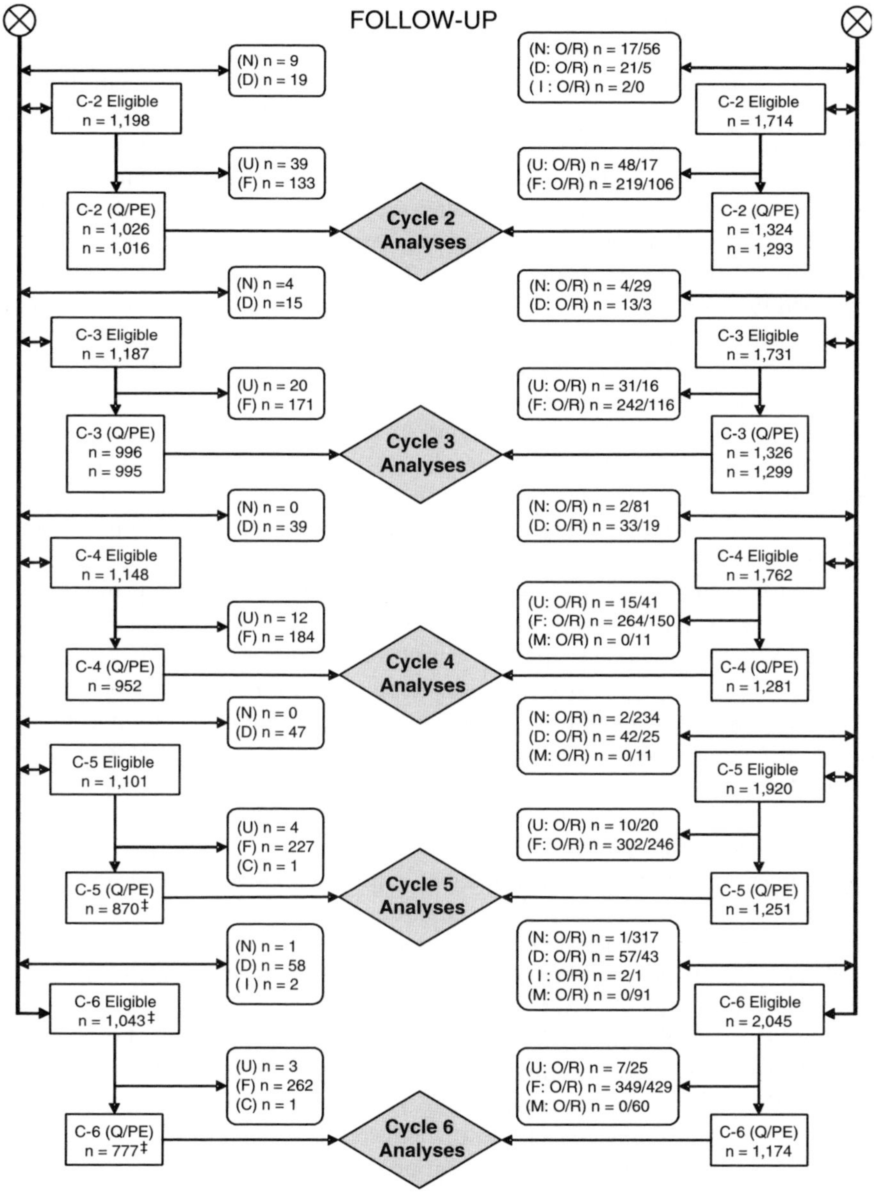

be considered a general overview of AFHS population dynamics. Eligibility in any cycle reflects eligibility in a previous cycle, and not compliance in a previous cycle, corrected for between-cycle newly identified or deceased subjects.
SOURCES: AFHS, 1984a, 1987, 1990, 1995, 2000, 2005; IOM, 2006.

As depicted in Figure 6-1, a retrospective matched-cohort study design was used to examine morbidity and mortality; followup was scheduled to continue until 2002. Records from the National Personnel Records Center and the US Air Force Human Resources Laboratory were searched and cross-referenced to identify all Ranch Hand personnel (AFHS, 1982; Michalek et al., 1990). A total of 1,269 participants were originally identified (AFHS, 1983). A control population of 24,971 C-130 crew members and support personnel assigned to duty in Southeast Asia (SEA) but not occupationally exposed to herbicides (AFHS, 1983) was selected from the same data sources. Control participants were individually matched for age, type of job (based on Air Force specialty code), and race (white or not white) to control for age-related, educational, socioeconomic-status, and race-related differences in development of chronic disease. To control for many potential confounders related to the physical and psychophysiologic effects of combat stress and the SEA environment, Ranch Hands were matched to control participants who performed similar combat or combat-related jobs (AFHS, 1982). Rank also was used as a surrogate of exposure. Alcohol use and smoking were included in the analysis when they were known risk factors for the outcome of interest.

Ten matches formed a control set for each exposed participant. For the mortality study, the intent was to follow each exposed participant and a random sample of half of each participant's control set for 20 years in a 1:5 matched design. The morbidity component of followup consisted of a 1:1 matched design; the first control was randomized to the mortality-ascertainment component of the study. If a control was noncompliant, another control from the matched "pool" was selected; controls who died were not replaced.

The baseline physical examination occurred in 1982, and examinations took place in 1985, 1987, 1992, 1997, and 2002. Morbidity was ascertained through questionnaires and physical examination, which emphasized dermatologic, neurobehavioral, hepatic, immunologic, reproductive, and neoplastic conditions. Some 1,208 Ranch Hands and 1,668 comparison participants were eligible for baseline examination. Initial questionnaire response rates were 97% for the exposed cohort and 93% for the nonexposed; baseline physical-examination responses were 87% and 76%, respectively (Wolfe et al., 1990). Deaths were identified and reviewed by using US Air Force Military Personnel Center records, the VA Beneficiary Identification Record Locator Subsystem (BIRLS), and the Internal Revenue Service database of active Social Security numbers. Death certificates were obtained from the appropriate health departments (Michalek et al., 1990).

Ranch Hands were divided into three categories on the basis of their potential exposure:

- *Low potential.* Pilots, copilots, and navigators. Exposure was primarily through preflight checks and spraying missions.

- *Moderate potential.* Crew chiefs, aircraft mechanics, and support personnel. Exposure could occur by contact during dedrumming and aircraft loading operations, onsite repair of aircraft, and repair of spray equipment.
- *High potential.* Spray-console operators and flight engineers. Exposure could occur during operation of spray equipment and through contact with herbicides in the aircraft.

Ostensibly, the AFHS was designed to answer exactly the question that the VAO project is asking, but the nature of the "exposed" (Ranch Hand veterans) and "comparison" (SEA veterans) groups and the evolving practices of VAO committees in endeavoring to fulfill the intention of their congressional mandate make interpretation less straightforward.

Results have been published for baseline morbidity (AFHS, 1984a), baseline mortality (AFHS, 1983), and for reproductive outcomes (AFHS, 1992; Michalek et al., 1998a; Wolfe et al., 1995). Mortality updates have been published for 1984–1986, 1989, and 1991 (AFHS, 1984b, 1985, 1986, 1989, 1991a). An interim technical report updated cause-specific mortality in Ranch Hands through 1993 (AFHS, 1996). Michalek et al. (1998b) and Ketchum and Michalek (2005) reported on 15-year and 20-year followup of postservice mortality, respectively, in veterans of Operation Ranch Hand, updating an earlier cause-specific mortality study by Michalek et al. (1990). Comparisons presented in the voluminous reports on the followup examinations of 1984, 1987, 1992, 1997, and 2002 (cited as AFHS, 1987, 1990, 1995, 2000, 2005) have been deemed not useful for the purposes of the VAO reviews because of the prevalence or cross-sectional nature of the data on only those in the cohort who were still alive and participated in a particular examination.

Blood samples for determination of serum TCDD concentrations were drawn at the periodic examinations conducted in 1982 from 36 Ranch Hands (Pirkle et al., 1989); in 1987 from 866 Ranch Hands (AFHS, 1991b); in 1992 from 455 Ranch Hands (AFHS, 1995); and in 1997 from 443 Ranch Hands (AFHS, 2000). For veterans whose TCDD was not measured in 1987 but was measured later, the later measurement was extrapolated to 1987 by using a first-order kinetics model with a constant half-life of 7.6 years. Analyses of the serum TCDD readings were included in the report on the 1987 followup examination (AFHS, 1991b), and other Ranch Hand publications have addressed the relationship between serum TCDD and reproductive hormones (Henriksen et al., 1996); diabetes mellitus, glucose, and insulin (Henriksen et al., 1997); skin disorders (Burton et al., 1998); infant death (Michalek et al., 1998a); sex ratios (Michalek et al., 1998c); skin cancer (Ketchum et al., 1999); insulin, fasting glucose, and sex-hormone–binding globulin (Michalek et al., 1999a); immunologic responses (Michalek et al., 1999b); diabetes mellitus (Longnecker and Michalek, 2000; Steenland et al., 2001); cognitive function (Barrett et al., 2001); hepatic abnormalities (Michalek et al., 2001a); peripheral neuropathy (Michalek et al., 2001b); hematologic results

(Michalek et al., 2001c); psychologic functioning (Barrett et al., 2003); correlations between diabetes and TCDD elimination (Michalek et al., 2003); thyroid function (Pavuk et al., 2003); cancer incidence (Akhtar et al., 2004; Pavuk et al., 2005); insulin sensitivity (Kern et al., 2004), prostate cancer (Pavuk et al., 2006); serum testosterone and risk of benign prostate hyperplasia (Gupta et al., 2006); and diabetes and cancer incidence (Michalek and Pavuk, 2008). All the VAO updates—*Veterans and Agent Orange: Herbicide/Dioxin Exposure and Type 2 Diabetes* (IOM, 2000), and *Veterans and Agent Orange: Length of Presumptive Period for Association Between Exposure and Respiratory Cancer* (IOM, 2004)—have discussed reports and papers that address the cohort in more detail.

The tendency of the AFHS researchers to use differing cutpoints and population definitions for analogous analyses suggests their a posteriori selection in a fashion that influences the results. For example, Michalek and Pavuk (2008) allude to the commonly held assumption that Agent Orange was more heavily contaminated earlier in the war as the motivation for making various temporal partitions in their analyses, but the choices were not consistent. For cancer, service in 1968 or before was considered to fall in the critical exposure period, whereas days of spraying were counted through 1967 and the variable for "days of spraying" was assigned the value "low" or "high" by partitioning the resulting distribution at 30 days. For diabetes, however, service in 1969 or before was regarded as being in the critical exposure period, and the variable "days of spraying" was split into "low" and "high" at 90 days or more, with no specification of the period over which the counting was done.

The AFHS is perceived by many to be the central piece of research for decision-making by the VAO committees, but it also has important limitations that all VAO committees have had to take into consideration. A recent Institute of Medicine (IOM) report, *Disposition of the Air Force Health Study* (IOM, 2006), which was undertaken by another IOM committee as the AFHS was approaching the end of its data-gathering phase, described the limitations of the AFHS effectively and was quoted in extensive detail in *Updates 2006* and *2008*. In summary, VAO committees have recognized the following features as the primary strengths and limitations of the AFHS:

- The AFHS is one of the most pertinent studies for the VAO reviews, with a study population that was directly exposed to the COIs in the Vietnam War theater.
- It can be argued that the AFHS population is not representative of the entire population of Vietnam veterans, so its findings might not be generalizable to all Vietnam veterans.
- The AFHS might be underpowered for detecting small effects, especially rare outcomes, because of its relatively small sample. Therefore, its findings are vulnerable to false negatives (failure to detect an important association). This also raises questions about the stability of positive findings;

this is somewhat less problematic if they are repeated over examination cycles, although the results of the examination cycles themselves are not fully independent repetitions.

- For AFHS analyses that used non-AFHS Vietnam veterans as the comparison group, the comparison group might also have been exposed to the COIs although the exposure was likely to be substantially higher in the AFHS group than in the comparison group. Therefore, the comparison is not an ideal "exposed vs unexposed" comparison but rather a "high exposure vs low exposure" comparison. The exposure in the comparison group might also make the study findings vulnerable to false negatives if the exposure differential between the AFHS group and the comparison group was not large enough to allow an association between exposure and outcome to be detected. However, that problem does not affect the validity of positive findings.

US Department of Veterans Affairs

VA Army Chemical Corps Cohort

The study of members of the US ACC was conducted by VA, whose other research efforts on Vietnam veterans are discussed together below. It is discussed immediately after the AFHS because of the importance that VAO committees have attributed to it. Like the Ranch Hand personnel, members of the ACC were involved directly in handling and distributing herbicides in Vietnam. Because the ACC personnel were expected to have been highly exposed to Agent Orange, VAO committees recommended study of this important group of Vietnam veterans (IOM, 1994) and later encouraged publication of its findings (IOM, 2004). The availability of serum TCDD concentrations in a subset of this cohort of Vietnam veterans has made its findings particularly useful in appraising possible associations with various health outcomes.

ACC troops performed chemical operations on the ground and by helicopter and were thereby involved in the direct handling and distribution of herbicides in Vietnam. The ACC population was belatedly identified for the study of health effects related to herbicide exposure (Thomas and Kang, 1990). In an extension, Dalager and Kang (1997) compared mortality in veterans of the ACC specialties, including Vietnam veterans and non-Vietnam veterans. Results of an initial feasibility study were reported by Kang et al. (2001). They recruited 565 veterans—284 Vietnam veterans and 281 non-Vietnam veterans—as controls. Blood samples were collected in 1996 from 50 Vietnam veterans and 50 control veterans, and 95 of the samples met CDC standards of quality assurance and quality. Comparison of the entire Vietnam cohort with the entire non-Vietnam cohort showed that the geometric mean TCDD concentrations did not differ significantly ($p = 0.6$). Of the 50 Vietnam veterans sampled, analysis of questionnaire responses indicated that those who reported spraying herbicides had higher TCDD concentrations than did those who reported no spraying activities. The authors concluded that Agent Orange exposure was a likely contributor to TCDD concentrations in Vietnam veterans who had a history of spraying herbicides.

Kang et al. (2006) reported findings of the main study. A health survey of 1,499 Vietnam veterans and 1,428 non-Vietnam veterans was administered by telephone. Exposure to herbicides was assessed by analyzing serum specimens from a sample of 897 veterans for dioxin. Veterans who reported spraying herbicides had significantly higher TCDD serum concentrations than did Vietnam veterans and other veterans who did not report herbicide spraying. The final analysis compared Vietnam-veteran sprayers with Vietnam-veteran nonsprayers in the entire study population.

Having determined the vital status of the ACC personnel through 2005, Cypel and Kang (2010) presented results on mortality from the following: cancers (oral and pharyngeal, digestive, respiratory, prostate, testicular, skin, brain, and lymphopoietic [leukemia]), diabetes, circulatory conditions (hypertension and cerebrovascular), respiratory conditions (pneumonia, influenza, and chronic obstructive pulmonary disease), and cirrhosis of the liver. The study compared 2,872 ACC personnel who served in Vietnam with 2,737 ACC personnel who did not serve in Vietnam, using survival analysis that controls for race, age at entry into followup, rank, and duration of military service. It also compared 662 ACC personnel who served in Vietnam and reported spraying herbicides with 811 who did not serve in Vietnam and did not report spraying, controlling for additional covariates obtained in the telephone survey—body-mass index (BMI) and smoking status. Mortality in both cohorts was also compared with the expected mortality in US males. Concerns were raised that the findings in Cypel and Kang (2010) regarding respiratory diseases were not adjusted for smoking status, probably an important confounding factor for respiratory diseases, in the analyses based on the entire ACC cohort that compared those who served in Vietnam with those who did not. (The subcohort analyses that compared sprayers with nonsprayers were adjusted for smoking status.)

The primary strengths and limitations of the ACC studies are similar to those of the AFHS. No new ACC studies were reported during the current review period.

VA Female US Vietnam-Veteran Cohort

Although estimates vary, 5,000–7,000 US women are believed to have served in Vietnam after volunteering for military service (Thomas et al., 1991). The vast majority of them served as combat nurses—mostly in the Army Nurse Corps—but some also served with the Women's Army Corps and the Air Force, Navy, and Marine Corps (Spoonster-Schwartz, 1987; Thomas et al., 1991).

In 1986, Public Law (PL) 99-972 was enacted. It required that an epidemiologic study be conducted to examine long-term adverse health effects on female Vietnam veterans as a result of their exposure to traumatic experiences, exposure to such herbicides as Agent Orange or other chemicals or medications, or any similar experience or exposure during such service. The first study that VA conducted to assess mortality in female Vietnam veterans was by Thomas et al. (1991). No comprehensive record of female personnel who served in Vietnam in 1964–1972 existed, so researchers gathered military service data from each branch of the armed forces to conduct the mortality study through December 31, 1987. Female Army and Navy personnel were identified from morning reports and muster rolls of hospitals and administrative support units where women were likely to have served. Military personnel were identified as female by their names, leaving open the possibility that some women may have been inadvertently excluded from the analysis. Women who served in the Air Force and Marine Corps were identified through military records. The combined roster of all female personnel from the military branches was considered by the researchers to be generally complete. A comparison group consisted of female veterans who were identified through the same process as the female Vietnam veterans but had not served in Vietnam during their military service. Demographic information and information on overseas tours of duty, unit assignments, jobs, and principal duties were abstracted from military records. Mortality information was obtained from VA's BIRLS, the Social Security Administration, the Internal Revenue Service, the National Death Index, and military personnel records. When women whose service in the military fell outside the period of interest, whose records were lacking data, or who served in SEA but not in Vietnam were excluded, the analysis included 132 deaths in 4,582 female Vietnam veterans and 232 deaths in 5,324 comparison veterans who served in the military during July 4, 1965–March 28, 1973. Cause-specific mortality was derived for Vietnam veterans and comparison veterans and compared with mortality in US women with adjustment for race, age, and calendar period. Dalager et al. (1995b) updated mortality in the original cohort until December 31, 1991, using the same study protocol as Thomas et al. (1991). After updating of mortality figures and adjustment of the existing cohort on the basis of new information about the study groups based on the inclusion criteria, 4,586 Vietnam veterans and 5,325 comparison veterans were included in the final analyses (Dalager et al. 1995b).

VA also published studies of pregnancy outcomes and gynecologic cancers—namely, neoplasms of the cervix, uterus, and ovary—in US female Vietnam veterans (Kang et al., 2000a,b). Army veterans were identified from a list obtained by the US Army and Joint Services Environmental Support Group; computerized lists were also provided by the Air Force, Navy, and Marine Corps. Military-service data were abstracted from personnel records. Of 5,230 eligible veterans, 4,390 whose permanent tour of duty included service in Vietnam were alive on January 1, 1992. From a pool of 6,657 potential control participants whose military units did not serve in Vietnam, 4,390 veterans who were alive on January 1,

1992, were randomly selected as controls. After exclusion of 250 veterans and 250 nonveterans who participated in a pilot study, an attempt was made to locate the remaining 4,140 veterans in each group. Various location strategies were used, and fewer than 5% (370) were not located; another 339 were deceased. A full telephone interview was conducted on 6,430; 775 refused (13% of Vietnam veterans and 17% of non-Vietnam veterans), and another 366 completed only a short written questionnaire. A questionnaire was administered on demographic background, general health, lifestyle, menstrual history, pregnancy history, pregnancy outcomes, and military experience, including nursing occupation and combat exposure. Information on pregnancy risks and complications—including smoking, infections, medications, exposure to X-rays, occupational history, and exposure to anesthetic gases, ethylene oxide, herbicides, and pesticides—was collected for each pregnancy. In Kang et al. (2000a), the first pregnancy after the beginning of Vietnam service was designated as the index pregnancy of each woman. For the comparison group, the first pregnancy after July 4, 1965, was used as the index pregnancy of each woman. Odds ratios were calculated for reproductive history and pregnancy outcomes. The study analyzed data on 3,392 Vietnam and 3,038 non-Vietnam veterans and on 1,665 Vietnam and 1,912 non-Vietnam veteran index pregnancies. In Kang et al. (2000b), a self-reported history of gynecologic cancers (defined by the authors as cancers of the breast, ovary, uterus, and cervix) was collected. The authors attempted to "retrieve hospital records on all reported cancers as far back as 30 years." Of records successfully found, 99% of the breast cancers and 90% of all cancers were confirmed. The authors did not provide data on validation of the three sites other than breast, but stated that Vietnam status was not associated with verification of the outcome.

After the publications by Kang et al. (2000a,b), Congress passed PL 106-419, which provides compensation for children of female Vietnam veterans who are born with birth defects unrelated to an existing familial disorder, to a birth-related injury, or to a fetal or neonatal infirmity with a well-established cause. Eighteen birth defects are covered by the legislation, including cleft lip or palate, congenital heart disease, hypospadias, neural-tube defects, and Williams syndrome. A complete list of covered birth defects can be found in Section 3.815 of the legislation.

Cypel and Kang (2008) conducted a mortality study of female Vietnam veterans and compared their mortality with that in a control group of women who were in military service but did not participate in the Vietnam War. Non-Vietnam veterans were selected randomly from among female veterans who never served in Vietnam and were matched to the Vietnam veterans according to rank and military occupation.

No reports on female Vietnam Veterans have been published since *Update 2008*.

VA Proportionate-Mortality Cohort

Among the earliest reports on Vietnam veterans was a proportionate-mortality study by Breslin et al. (1988). The participants were men who had served as ground troops in the US Army or Marine Corps at any time from July 4, 1965, through March 1, 1973. A list of 186,000 Vietnam-era veterans who served in the Army or Marine Corps and were reported deceased as of July 1, 1982, was assembled from VA's BIRLS; 75,617 names were randomly selected from the list for inclusion in the study. Information extracted from the selected military records included the places, dates, and branch of military service; date of birth; sex; race; military occupation specialty codes; education level; type of discharge; and confirmation of service in Vietnam. Additional information was extracted on veterans who served in SEA, including the first and last dates of service in SEA, the military unit, and the country where the veteran served. For the final sample of 52,253 Army and Marine Corps veterans, cause of death was ascertained from death certificates or Department of Defense Report of Casualty forms for 51,421 men, including 24,235 who served in Vietnam and 26,685 men who did not serve in SEA; 501 deaths were excluded from the final analyses because service in SEA was in a country other than Vietnam or the location of military service was unknown. Each veteran's cause of death was coded by a nosologist who used the 8th revision of the *International Classification of Diseases*.

On the basis of the proportionate-mortality study (Breslin et al., 1988), Burt et al. (1987) conducted a nested case-control study of non-Hodgkin lymphoma (NHL) with controls selected from among the cardiovascular-disease deaths. In a followup of the Breslin et al. study, Bullman et al. (1990) compared cause-specific proportionate mortality in 6,668 Army I Corps Vietnam veterans—veterans who served in the northernmost part of South Vietnam in a combat zone designated as Military Region I by the US military—with that in 27,917 Army Vietnam-era veterans who had not served in Vietnam. The study by Bullman et al. included the study population identified by Breslin et al. and an additional 9,555 Army Vietnam-era veterans whose deaths were identified after the BIRLS mortality data were extended through December 31, 1984. Similarly, Watanabe et al. (1991) updated the Vietnam-veteran mortality experience reported by Breslin et al. (1988) by extending the followup from January 1, 1982, to December 31, 1984. An additional 11,325 deceased Army and Marine Vietnam-era veterans were identified from the period and included in the study. The study population for Watanabe et al. consisted of 62,068 military veterans, of whom 29,646 served in Vietnam and 32,422 never served in SEA. Proportionate-mortality ratios were calculated for three referent groups: branch-specific (Army and Marine Corps) non-Vietnam veterans, all non-Vietnam veterans combined, and the US male population. A third followup proportionate-mortality study (Watanabe and Kang, 1996) used the veterans from Breslin et al. (1988) and Watanabe et al. (1991) and included an additional 9,040 randomly selected Vietnam-era veterans who died from July 1, 1984, through June 30, 1988. The final study included 70,630 veterans—33,833 who served in Vietnam and 36,797 who never served in SEA—and the analyses were performed with the same referent groups described previously (Watanabe et al., 1991).

Other VA Studies

VA also conducted studies that focused on specific health outcomes, using data from VA's Agent Orange Registry (AOR), a computer database containing health information on Vietnam veterans who voluntarily undergo examinations in a VA hospital. The AOR was set up in 1978 to monitor Vietnam veterans' health complaints or problems that could be related to Agent Orange exposure during military service in Vietnam. The examinations consist of an exposure history, a medical history, laboratory tests, and an examination of body systems most commonly affected by toxic chemicals. As of June 1, 2008, the registry contained information from 506,184 examinations (Agent Orange Review, 2008).

Using early data from the registry, Bullman et al. (1991) examined the risk of posttraumatic stress disorder (PTSD) in a case-control study of veterans who received AOR medical examinations during January 1983–December 1987. The final analyses include 374 PTSD cases and 373 controls whose military records were used to verify Vietnam service, Military Occupational Specialty Codes (MOSCs), primary duties, military branch, dates of Vietnam service, medals, awards, and disciplinary actions for each veteran. Similarly, Bullman et al. (1994) studied the risk of testicular cancer by using the AOR health records of veterans who received Agent Orange medical examinations during March 1982–January 1991. The final analyses in that study included 97 testicular-cancer cases and 311 controls. A surrogate metric for Agent Orange exposure was developed by using branch of service, combat MOSCs, geographic area of service in Vietnam, location of military units in relation to herbicide-spraying missions, and the length of time between spray missions and military operations in sprayed areas.

Watanabe and Kang (1995) compared postservice mortality in Vietnam veterans in the Marine Corps with that in Vietnam-era marines who did not serve in Vietnam. All study participants were on active duty during 1967–1969 and were followed from their discharge date or from the date of the US military withdrawal from Vietnam until their date of death or December 31, 1991, whichever came first. The final study population included 10,716 Vietnam and 9,346 non-Vietnam veteran marines.

Kang et al. (1991) conducted a case-control study that compared dioxin and dibenzofuran concentrations in the adipose tissue of 36 Vietnam veterans with those in 79 non-Vietnam veterans and a sample of US men born in 1936–1954. All tissue samples were archived specimens from the US Environmental Protection Agency National Human Adipose Tissue Survey and had been collected by hospitals and medical examiners from men who died from external causes or surgical procedures. Military service—branch of service, MOSC, and geographic service location in Vietnam, if applicable—was researched and verified with military records. Controls were matched by birth year and sample collection year (± 2 years), and the final analyses were adjusted by age and BMI.

Dalager et al. (1991) examined NHL in male Vietnam veterans in a hospital-based case-control study. Study participants were identified via inpatient discharge records from VA medical centers for fiscal years 1969–1985. Cases were identified as having a malignant lymphoma and a birth date during 1937–1954. Controls were identified from VA medical-center discharge records and were matched by hospital, discharge date, and birth date. The location and dates of each veteran's military service were verified by using military records. A surrogate Agent Orange exposure opportunity was also developed for each Vietnam veteran according to branch of service, combat experience, and geographic location of the military unit assignment. The final analysis included 201 cases and 358 controls. Another study by Dalager et al. (1995a) examined the association between Hodgkin lymphoma (HL) and Vietnam service. It used the same method as the 1991 Dalager et al. study; the analysis included 283 HL cases and 404 controls.

VA has evaluated specific health outcomes, including case-control studies of soft-tissue sarcoma (STS) (Kang et al., 1986, 1987), testicular cancer (Bullman et al., 1994), and lung cancer (Mahan et al., 1997). It also has conducted a study of self-reported physical health (Eisen et al., 1991) and PTSD (Goldberg et al., 1990) in monozygotic twins who served during the Vietnam era.

VA has examined other outcomes in Vietnam veterans: PTSD (Bullman et al., 1991; True et al., 1988), suicide and motor-vehicle crashes (Bullman and Kang, 1996; Farberow et al., 1990), and tobacco use (McKinney et al., 1997). The studies have been included for completeness, but the outcomes that they address are outside the purview of this committee. *VAO* and *Update 1998* discuss them in detail; most did not deal with exposure to Agent Orange, and exposure to "combat" was evaluated as the risk factor of interest.

US Centers for Disease Control and Prevention Studies

Surveys of US Vietnam veterans who were not part of the Operation Ranch Hand or ACC groups indicated that 25–55% believed that they were exposed to herbicides (CDC, 1989a; Erickson et al., 1984a,b; Stellman and Stellman, 1986). Several attempts have been made to estimate exposure of Vietnam veterans who were not part of the Ranch Hand or ACC groups. CDC has undertaken a series of studies to examine various health outcomes in Vietnam veterans as directed by Congress in the Veterans Health Programs Extension and Improvement Act of 1979 (PL 96-151) and the Veterans' Health Care, Training, and Small Business Loan Act of 1981 (PL 97-72).

CDC Birth-Defects Study

The first was a case-control interview study of birth defects in offspring of men who served in Vietnam (Erickson et al., 1984a,b). In 1983, the US government asked CDC to conduct a study of possible long-term health effects in Vietnam veterans exposed to Agent Orange. The CDC Agent Orange study (CDC, 1985) attempted to classify veterans' service-related exposures to herbicides. That involved determining the proximity of troops to Agent Orange spraying by using military records to track troop movement and the HERBS tapes to locate herbicide-spraying patterns. The CDC birth-defects study developed an exposure-opportunity index to score Agent Orange exposure (Erickson et al., 1984a,b).

CDC Agent Orange Validation Study

In 1987, CDC conducted the CDC Agent Orange Validation Study (AOVS) to test the validity of the various indirect methods used to estimate exposure of ground troops to Agent Orange in Vietnam. The study measured serum TCDD in a nonrandom sample of Vietnam veterans and in Vietnam-era veterans who did not serve in Vietnam (CDC, 1988a). Vietnam veterans were selected for the study on the basis of the number of Agent Orange hits that they were thought to have experienced given the number of days on which their company was within 2 km and 6 days of a recorded Agent Orange spraying event. Blood samples were obtained from 66% of 646 Vietnam veterans and from 49% of the eligible comparison group of 97 veterans. More than 94% of those whose serum was obtained had served in one of five battalions.

The median serum TCDD in Vietnam veterans in 1987 was 4 parts per trillion (ppt) (range, under 1 to 45 ppt). Only two veterans had concentrations above 20 ppt. The "low" exposure group consisted of 298 Vietnam veterans, the "medium" exposure group 157 veterans, and the "high" exposure group 191 veterans. The distribution of TCDD measurements was nearly identical with that in the control group of 97 non-Vietnam veterans. The CDC validation study concluded that study participants could not be distinguished from controls on the basis of serum TCDD. In addition, neither record-derived estimates of exposure nor self-reported exposure to herbicides could predict Vietnam veterans with currently high serum TCDD (CDC, 1988a, 1989a). The report concluded that it was unlikely that military records alone could be used to identify a large number of veterans who might have been heavily exposed to TCDD in Vietnam.

CDC Vietnam Experience Study

Using exposure estimates from the AOVS, CDC conducted the CDC Vietnam Experience Study (VES), a historical cohort study of the health experience of Vietnam veterans (CDC, 1989b). The study was divided into three parts: physical health, reproductive outcomes and child health, and psychosocial characteristics (CDC, 1987, 1988a,b,c, 1989b). Using VES data, CDC examined postservice mortality (through 1983) in a cohort of 9,324 US Army veterans who served in Vietnam and in 8,989 Vietnam-era Army veterans who served in Korea, Germany, or the United States (Boyle et al., 1987; CDC, 1987). Another study (O'Brien et al., 1991) combined the mortality and interview data to identify all veterans who had NHL. To evaluate whether self-reported assessment of exposure to herbicides influences the reporting of adverse health outcomes, CDC designed a study of VES participants (Decoufle et al., 1992). In a followup of CDC's VES cohort, Boehmer et al. (2004) reported findings on mortality during 1965–2000.

The serum TCDD measurements in Vietnam veterans also suggested that exposure to TCDD in Vietnam was substantially lower, *on the average*, than that of persons exposed as a result of the industrial explosion in Seveso or that of the heavily exposed occupational workers who have been the focus of many of the studies evaluated by the present committee. The assessment of *average* exposure does not preclude heavy exposure of subgroups of Vietnam veterans.

CDC Selected Cancers Study

CDC undertook the CDC Selected Cancers Study (CDC, 1990a) to investigate the effects of military service in Vietnam and of exposure to herbicides on the health of American veterans, specifically NHL (CDC, 1990b), STS and other sarcomas (CDC, 1990c), HL (CDC, 1990d), and nasal, nasopharyngeal, and primary liver cancers (CDC, 1990d).

CDC National Vietnam Veterans Readjustment Study

The CDC National Vietnam Veterans Readjustment Study (NVVRS) investigated primarily psychological outcomes. It is now being updated to become the National Vietnam Veterans Longitudinal Study. To date the only resulting publication (Currier and Holland, 2012) on a sample from the NVVRS addressed psychologic outcomes in association with combat trauma and bereavement.

Other US Vietnam-Veteran Studies

American Legion Study

The American Legion, a voluntary service organization for veterans, conducted a cohort study of the health and well-being of Vietnam veterans who were members. Studies examined physical health and reproductive outcomes, social–behavioral consequences, and PTSD in veterans who had served in SEA and elsewhere (Snow et al., 1988; Stellman JM et al., 1988; Stellman SD et al., 1988). No additional studies have been published on the cohort.

State Studies

Several states have conducted studies of Vietnam veterans, most of them unpublished in the scientific literature. *VAO* and *Update 1996* reviewed studies of veterans of Hawaii (Rellahan, 1985), Iowa (Wendt, 1985), Maine (Deprez et al., 1991), Massachusetts (Clapp, 1997; Clapp et al., 1991; Kogan and Clapp, 1985, 1988; Levy, 1988), Michigan (Visintainer et al., 1995), New Jersey (Fiedler and Gochfeld, 1992; Kahn et al., 1988, 1992a,b,c), New Mexico (Pollei et al., 1986), New York (Greenwald et al., 1984; Lawrence et al., 1985), Pennsylvania (Goun and Kuller, 1986), Texas (Newell, 1984), West Virginia (Holmes et al., 1986), and Wisconsin (Anderson et al., 1986a,b). Chamie et al. (2008) examined the association between Agent Orange and prostate cancer in all Vietnam-era veterans using the VA health system in northern California; the reliability of this study of about 13,000 men is limited by its reliance on self-reported exposure status and the exclusion of prostate cases diagnosed before 1998, when computerized records became available. No additional state studies have been published.

Additional studies have examined health outcomes that included spontaneous abortion (Aschengrau and Monson, 1989) and adverse outcomes late in pregnancy in spouses of Vietnam veterans (Aschengrau and Monson, 1990). After a published study indicated a potential association between testicular cancer in dogs and their service in Vietnam (Hayes et al., 1990), Tarone et al. (1991) conducted a case-control study of testicular cancer in male veterans. VAO summarized those studies, and no additional studies have been published on these study populations.

Australian Vietnam-Veteran Studies

Over many years the Australian government has commissioned studies to follow health outcomes in two sets of Australian veterans who served in Vietnam.

Australian Vietnam Veterans

The Australian Vietnam Veterans study population corresponds to the cohort defined by the "Nominal Roll of Vietnam Veterans," which lists Australians who served on land or in Vietnamese waters from May 23, 1962, to July 1, 1973, including military and some nonmilitary personnel of both sexes. People who served in all branches of service in the "defence forces" and "Citizen Military Forces" (such as diplomatic, medical, and entertainment personnel) were considered. The comprehensive studies, however, are limited to male members of the military and most of the analyses focus on men in the "defence forces"—the Army (41,084), the Navy (13,538), and the Air Force (4,570). Association of Vietnam service with cancer incidence (ADVA, 2005b) was sought by comparing diagnoses from 1982–2000 among male Vietnam veterans with those in the general population of Australia. The results in this report supersede those in the report of the Australian Department of Veterans' Affairs (CDVA, 1998a). Morbidity in all female Vietnam veterans had been studied in an earlier report (CDVA, 1998b). Additional case-control studies of the incidence of adrenal gland cancers, leukemia, and NHL were conducted in this population (AIHW, 1999, 2000, 2001).

A related report (ADVA, 2005a) considered the causes of death of men in all branches of service through 2001. The numbers of deaths were 4,045 in the Army, 1,435 in the Navy, and 686 in the Air Force. The mortality experience of military personnel serving in Vietnam was compared with that of the general population of Australia and reported by branch of service. The findings of this study supersede those in the report on mortality from 1980 to 1994 (CDVA, 1998a). There had been several earlier studies of mortality among Austalian Vietnam veterans (CIH, 1984a,b,c; Crane et al., 1997a,b; Evatt, 1985; Fett et al., 1987a,b; Forcier et al., 1987).

Australian Conscripted Army National Service

The Australian Conscripted Army National Service study population is a subset of the veterans considered in the overall Australian Vietnam Veterans study group. The 19,240 conscripted male Army veterans deployed to Vietnam ("National Service" veterans) were compared with their 24,729 non-deployed counterparts ("National Service non-veterans"). This comparison between contemporaries who had been sufficiently healthy to enter the service provided a means of adjusting for a possible "healthy-warrior" effect. The results on death and cancer in the Australian conscripted Army National Service veterans (ADVA, 2005c) supersede those of earlier internal comparisons of deployed and non-deployed Vietnam War–era National Service veterans (CIH, 1984a; Crane et al., 1997b; Fett et al., 1987a,b). Those government-sponsored studies of Australian Vietnam veterans did not characterize the veterans' exposure to the herbicides sprayed in Vietnam beyond the fact that they served on land or in Vietnamese waters during May 23, 1962–July 1, 1973. It is the convention of VAO committees to regard Vietnam veterans in general as being more likely to have received higher exposures to the COIs than the general public, but it would have been informative to validate that assumption by gathering biomarkers of exposure, such as serum measurements, in a sample of Australian Vietnam veterans.

Update 2000 had moved the occurrence of acute myeloid leukemia in offspring of Vietnam veterans to the limited or suggestive category of association primarily on the basis of findings reported by the Australian Institute of Health and Welfare (AIHW, 2000) but rescinded in a revised report (AIHW, 2001). The reversal of the conclusion on this matter by the committee for *Update 2000* is discussed in *Veterans and Agent Orange: Herbicide/Dioxin Esposure and Acute Myelogenous Leukemia in the Children of Vietnam Veterans* (IOM, 2002).

Sample of 1,000 Australian Vietnam Veterans

O'Toole et al. (1996a,b,c) studied a broad spectrum of health issues in a random sample of 1,000 Australian Vietnam veterans (both regular enlisted and conscripted Army National Service members) selected from Australia's comprehensive roster of 57,643 service members deployed to Vietnam. In wave 1, conducted in 1990–1993, 641 members of the sample were located and interviewed. In wave 2, conducted in 2005–2006, O'Toole et al. (2009) obtained responses from 450 (51.4% of those not known to have died); 391 responded to both waves. The Australian Bureau of Statistics National Health Survey was administered in both waves with collection of additional data on combat experience, PTSD, and general psychiatric status. The veterans' self-reported health status was compared with that of the general male Australian population gathered during the government's administration of the same survey in 1989–1990 and 2004–2005; it is not clear that this instrument was administered to the two groups under comparable conditions. The low response rates make the findings vulnerable to nonresponse bias, and the use of self-report measures of health conditions might be of low validity and subject to recall bias. The committee for *Update 2010* was skeptical about the reliability of the nearly uniform findings of statistically increased prevalence of nearly 50 health conditions. O'Toole et al. (2010) reported on the mortality in the sample through 2004 as related to previously gathered information on psychosocial factors that are not within the scope of VAO reviews. It is of interest, however, that they found that 11.7% of the veterans in the sample had died by the end of 2004.

Case-Control Study of Birth Defects in Australian Infants

The Australian government sponsored a case-control study of 8,517 infants with congenital anomalies born in 1966–1979 at 34 hospitals in New South Wales, Victoria, and the Australian Capital Territory matched by period of birth, mother's age, hospital, and means of hospital payment to live-born infants without diagnosed birth defects (Donovan et al., 1983, 1984; Evatt, 1985). The fathers of both groups were identified and their names compared to the roster of men who had served in the Australian Army in 1962–1972; additional means of verification were used to determine whether the child's father had been in the Army during this interval (329 cases and 338 controls) and also whether he had been deployed to Vietnam (127 cases and 123 controls). Adjusting for maternal age, infant sex, multiple births, and father's place of birth, conditional logistic regression was used to compare the Vietnam veterans (National Service or regular Army) to other era veterans and to all other fathers for all birth anomalies and for seven diagnostic groups.

Korean Vietnam-Veteran Studies

Study of TCDD Concentrations in Korean Vietnam Veterans

Military personnel of the Republic of Korea served in Vietnam during 1964–1973. Kim JS et al. (2001) attempted to use serum dioxin concentrations to validate an index for estimating group exposure. The study involved 720 veterans who served in Vietnam and 25 veterans who did not. The exposure index was based on Agent Orange spraying patterns in military regions in which Korean personnel served, time–location data on the military units stationed in Vietnam, and an exposure score derived from self-reported activities during service. A total of 13 pooled samples were submitted to CDC for serum dioxin analysis. One analytic sample was prepared from the pooled blood of the 25 veterans who did not serve in Vietnam. The remaining 12 samples were intended to correspond to 12 exposure categories; each was created by pooling blood samples from 60 veterans. The 12 exposure categories ultimately were reduced to four exposure groups, each representing a quartile of 180 Vietnam veterans but characterized by only three serum TCDD measurements.

The paper by Kim JS et al. (2001) reported highly significant Pearson correlation coefficients and results of multiple logistic-regression analysis. The statistical analyses apparently were based on the assignment of the pooled serum dioxin value to each person in the exposure group and thereby inflated the true sample size. The multiple regression analysis evaluated such variables as age, BMI, and consumption of tobacco or alcohol. In a later report on the same exposure groups and serum dioxin data, the authors corrected their analysis (Kim JS et al., 2003). A correlation was observed between serum dioxin concentrations and ordinal exposure categories, but the correlation was not statistically significant. The authors attributed the lack of statistical significance to the small sample, and they noted that the data exhibited a distinct monotonic upward trend; average serum dioxin concentrations, 0.3, 0.6, 0.62, 0.78, and 0.87 pg/g (lipid-adjusted) for exposure categories 0–4, respectively. The decision to pool blood samples from a large number of persons in each exposure set (Kim JS et al., 2001) greatly reduced the power of the validation study. Instead of 180 samples in each of the final exposure categories, the pooled analysis produced only three samples in each category. The lipid-adjusted serum TCDD concentrations in the 12 pooled samples from Vietnam veterans ranged from 0.25 to 1.2 pg/g, whereas the single sample from the non-Vietnam veterans contained 0.3 pg/g. The narrow range of results makes the biologic relevance of any differences questionable.

Thus, it appears that there was not a clear separation between Korean Vietnam veterans and non-Vietnam veterans. Furthermore, the range of mean values in the four Vietnam-veteran exposure categories was narrow, and all concentrations were relatively low (less than 1 pg/g). The relatively low serum dioxin concentrations observed in the 1990s in those people are the residual of substantially higher initial concentrations, as has been seen in other Vietnam-veteran groups. However, the concentrations reported in the Korean-veterans study are significantly lower than are those reported in American Vietnam veterans in the 1988 CDC AOVS, which was nonetheless unable to distinguish Vietnam veterans from non-Vietnam veterans on the basis of serum dioxin (CDC, 1988a). The Korean authors were able to construct plausible exposure categories based on military records and self-reporting, but they were unable to validate the categories with serum dioxin measurements.

Study of Role of Vietnam Service in Recovery of Koreans with Acute Coronary Syndrome

Kim JB et al. (2012) reported on the association between exposure to TCDD and recovery outcomes (HT, hyperlipidemia, and the rate and severity of major adverse coronary events) in men who presented with acute coronary syndrome (obstruction of coronary ateries and chest pain) during 2004–2009 at Gwangju Veterans Hospital. The age range was limited to 50–70 years to reflect the current age of Korean veterans of the Vietnam War. There were 251 patients: 121 were Vietnam veterans (assumed to have been exposed to TCDD), and 130 were not. Medical records were reviewed to determine a variety of cardiovascular recovery outcomes. T tests, chi-square tests, and logistic regression were used to determine whether measures of recovery differed between the acute coronary patients who had served in Vietnam and those who had not. The study findings are not informative about associations between TCDD and acute coronary syndrome itself, as the researchers allege.

Other Studies of Korean Vietnam Veterans

Epidemiologic studies have also looked at immunotoxicologic outcomes (Kim HA et al., 2003) and skin and general disease patterns (Mo et al., 2002) in Korean Vietnam veterans who were exposed to Agent Orange during the Vietnam War.

OCCUPATIONAL STUDIES

Several occupational groups in the United States and elsewhere have been exposed to the COIs. Exposure characterization varies widely in the metric used, the extent of detail, confounding by other exposures, and whether individual, surrogate, or group (ecologic) measures are used. Some studies use job titles as broad surrogates of exposure; others rely on disease-registry data.

The committee reviewed many epidemiologic studies of occupationally exposed groups for evidence of an association between exposure to TCDD or to the herbicides used in Vietnam—primarily the phenoxy herbicides 2,4-dichlorophenoxyacetic acid (2,4-D) and 2,4,5-trichlorophenoxyacetic acid (2,4,5-T)—and health risks. TCDD is an unwanted byproduct of 2,4,5-T production but not of 2,4-D production. Other contaminants, including other dioxins (such as 1,3,6,8-tetrachlorodibenzo-*p*-dioxin), have been reported at low concentrations in 2,4-D, but those identified do not have the toxicity of TCDD (ATSDR, 1998; Huston, 1972; Norström et al., 1979). In reviewing the studies, the committee considered two types of exposure separately: exposure to 2,4-D or 2,4,5-T and exposure to TCDD from 2,4,5-T or other sources. That separation is necessary because some health effects could be associated with exposure to 2,4-D or 2,4,5-T in the absence of substantial TCDD exposure. After recognition of the problem of dioxin contamination in phenoxy herbicides, production conditions were modified to minimize contamination, but use of the products most subject to containing specifically TCDD (2,4,5-T and Silvex) was banned. As a result, study participants exposed to phenoxy herbicides only after the late 1970s would not be assumed to have been at risk for exposure to TCDD.

The distinction is particularly important for workers in agriculture and forestry, including farmers and herbicide appliers, whose exposure is primarily the result of mixing, loading, and applying herbicides. In addition to those occupational groups, the committee considered studies of occupational exposure to dioxins, focusing on workers in chemical plants that produced phenoxy herbicides or chlorophenols, which tend to be contaminated with polychlorinated dibenzo-*p*-dioxins (PCDDs). Waste-incineration workers were also included in the occupation category because they can come into contact with dioxin-like compounds while handling byproducts of incineration. Other occupationally exposed groups included were pulp and paper workers exposed to dioxins through bleaching processes that use chlorinated compounds, and sawmill workers exposed to chlorinated dioxins that can be contaminants of chlorophenates used as wood preservatives.

Studies of Herbicide Production Workers

International Agency for Research on Cancer Phenoxy Herbicide Cohort

A multisite study by IARC involved 18,390 production workers and phenoxy herbicide sprayers working in 10 countries (Saracci et al., 1991). The full cohort was established by using the International Register of Workers Exposed to Phenoxy Herbicides and Their Contaminants. Twenty cohorts were combined for the analysis: one each in Australia, Austria, Canada, Finland, and Sweden; two each in Denmark, Italy, the Netherlands, and New Zealand; and seven in the United Kingdom. There were 12,492 production workers and 5,898 sprayers in the full cohort.

Questionnaires were constructed for workers who were manufacturing chlorophenoxy herbicides or chlorinated phenols and for herbicide sprayers; the questionnaires were completed with the assistance of industrial hygienists. Information from production records and job histories was examined when available. Workers were classified as exposed, probably exposed, with unknown exposure, or nonexposed. The exposed-workers group (13,482) consisted of all those known to have sprayed chlorophenoxy herbicides and all who worked in particular aspects of chemical production. Two subcohorts (totaling 416) had no job titles available but worked in chemical-production facilities that were likely to produce TCDD exposure, so they were deemed probably exposed. Workers with no exposure information (541) were classified as of unknown exposure. Nonexposed workers (3,951) were those who had never been employed in parts of factories that produced chlorophenoxy herbicides or chlorinated phenols and had never sprayed chlorophenoxy herbicides. Two nested case-control studies were undertaken with the IARC cohort to evaluate the relationship between STSs and lymphomas (Kogevinas et al., 1992, 1995). Kogevinas et al. (1993) presented the information available on the subcohort of 701 women who were occupationally exposed to chlorophenoxy herbicides, chlorophenols, and dioxins included in 11 of the cohorts in seven of the countries; nine deaths and 29 incident cancer cases were reported (too few to tabulate results).

An expanded and updated analysis of the IARC cohort with an emphasis on cancer mortality was published in 1997 (Kogevinas et al., 1997). The researchers added herbicide production workers in 12 plants in the United States (the NIOSH cohort) and four plants in Germany. The 21,863 male and female workers exposed to phenoxy herbicides or chlorophenols were classified in three categories of exposure to TCDD or higher-chlorinated dioxins: those exposed (13,831), those not exposed (7,553), and those with unknown exposure (479). Several exposure metrics were constructed for the cohort—years since first exposure, duration of exposure (in years), year of first exposure, and job title—but detailed methods were not described. The overall results were for mortality in 1939–1992, but for some of the subcohorts, followup had begun as late as 1975, and at the time of publication, mortality in some had been tracked only through 1983. For nonneoplastic causes of death, Vena et al. (1998) repeated the grouped statistics for all phenoxy-herbicide workers in the updated IARC cohort (as previously presented in Kogevinas et al., 1997) and provided results partitioned according to whether the workers had the potential for exposure to TCDD and more highly chlorinated dioxin contaminants .

No new studies of the IARC cohort have been published since *Update 1998*.

International Agency for Research on Cancer Subcohorts

In addition to the NIOSH cohort and its component subcohorts (discussed below), several of the subcohorts that make up the IARC cohort have generated independent reports that have been evaluated separately by VAO committees to garner additional insights, such as results associated with TCDD concentrations measured in some subjects: Austrian production workers (Jäger et al., 1998; Neuberger et al., 1998, 1999); British production workers (Coggon et al., 1986, 1991); Danish production workers (Lynge, 1985, 1993); Dutch production workers (Boers et al., 2010, 2012; Bueno de Mesquita et al., 1993; Hooiveld et al., 1998); German production workers (Becher et al., 1996; Flesch-Janys, 1997; Flesch-Janys et al., 1995; Manz et al., 1991); and New Zealand production workers (McBride et al. 2009a,b; Smith et al., 1981, 1982; 't Mannetje et al., 2005). Several of the component cohorts have not been the subject of any separate publications: Australian herbicide sprayers, Canadian herbicide sprayers, Finnish production workers, two cohorts of Italian production workers, and Swedish production workers. The international production-worker cohorts are discussed below in alphabetical order, followed by the NIOSH cohort and its subcohorts. The section on studies of herbicide-using workers, which follows discussion of all production-worker studies, includes consideration of the separate reports on the New Zealand herbicide sprayers.

Dutch production workers The two Dutch subcohorts of the IARC cohort consist of 2,106 male workers employed in two manufacturing factories producing and formulating chlorophenoxy herbicides: 2,4,5-T in factory A during 1955–1985 and 2-methyl-4-chlorophenoxyacetic acid (MCPA), 2-(2-methyl-4-chlorophenoxy)propionic acid (Mecoprop, MCPP); and 2,4-D in factory B during 1965–1986. Accordingly, members of both subcohorts had potential exposure to phenoxy herbicides, but only those in factory A could have been exposed to TCDD. The study populations were defined as all workers who worked in factory A during 1955–1985 or factory B during 1965–1986.

Hooiveld et al. (1998) updated the mortality experience (1955–1991) of production workers in the two Dutch chemical factories in the Netherlands with known exposure to dioxins: workers in herbicide production, nonexposed production workers, and workers known to have been exposed as a result of an accident that occurred in 1963. On the basis of an assumption of first-order TCDD elimination with an estimated half-life of 7.1 years, measured TCDD concentrations were extrapolated to the time of maximum TCDD exposure of a group of 47 workers. A regression model was then used to estimate, for each cohort member, the effect on estimated maximum TCDD exposure attributable to exposure as a result of the accident, duration of employment in the main production department, and time of first exposure (before or after 1970).

Boers et al. (2010) conducted updated analyses based on the third followup of the Dutch subcohorts of the IARC cohort, examining cause-specific mortality (cancer and noncancer) in 2,106 male workers employed in factories A and B. Both cohorts were followed through 2006, accumulating 65,087 person-years, with 567 deaths observed. Sample loss was minimal (< 1% lost to followup, < 5% emigrated). Death certificates obtained by linkage to Statistics Netherlands were used to ascertain cause-specific mortality, including various cancers, endocrine or blood diseases, nervous system, ischemic heart disease, other heart disease, cerebrovascular diseases, respiratory diseases, digestive diseases, and genitourinary diseases. Exposure to chlorophenoxy herbicides was determined on the basis of the type of work experience (such as production vs office) and involvement in the accident of 1963 in factory A (factory A: 539 exposed, 482 nonexposed; factory B: 411 exposed, 626 nonexposed). TCDD measures taken in 1993 support that exposure classification; the highest mean TCDD concentrations were found in workers involved in the 1963 accident (1,841.8 ppt) and those who worked in main production (608.2 ppt), whereas concentrations in nonexposed workers were much lower (7.6 ppt). Cox proportional-hazards models with attained age as the time scale were used to assess hazard ratios for exposed vs nonexposed workers. Exposure to phenoxy herbicides and dioxins was expected to be different between factory A and factory B, and the factories were therefore analyzed separately. Further nested case-control studies were conducted for the factory A cohort by using all cancer cases (112) and three controls per case matched on age and employment period; analysis used conditional logistic regression.

Since *Update 2010*, several new studies based on this cohort have been published. Boers et al. (2012) conducted more detailed dose–response analyses of the updated mortality data on the cohorts reported in Boers et al. (2010). From May 2007 to September 2008, blood was drawn for the determination of plasma TCDD concentrations in a systematically selected subsample of 187 workers (101 in factory A, 86 in factory B). Serum concentrations measured in the workers in factory B (geometric mean = 0.4 ppt) confirmed they had not experienced TCDD exposures above background. The combination of linear regression on the log-transformed serum results and work-history details was used to derive a model to predict current TCDD in the entire cohort, from which back-extrapolation predicted each person's concentration when he left employment in factory A or B. There were considerable individual differences from the previously assigned exposure groups, but overall the exposures predicted by the empirical model had a high rank correlation (Spearman's r = 0.79) with the exposure statuses used in previous analyses. A Cox proportional-hazards model was used to assess exposure–outcome relationships on the basis of the predicted exposures as a time-varying covariate. To allow for latency, a 1-year lag was used for noncancer endpoints and a 10-year lag for cancer outcomes. The log-linear TCDD model was applied to the workers in factory A only and to the entire cohort, including workers from factory B, who had been exposed only to phenoxy herbicides as confirmed by the serum samples from the 86 factory B subjects who had only background concentrations of TCDD.

Saberi Hosnijeh et al. (2011) examined the association between TCDD exposure and outcomes, including humoral immunity (serum immunoglobulin and complement factor concentrations) and atopic diseases (self-reported asthma, hay fever, eczema, and allergy) in a subsample of 153 workers, including 45 who had TCDD exposure in factory A, matched individually with a nonexposed comparison group consisting of 39 in factory A and 69 in factory B. TCDD exposure was characterized by using exposure status (exposed vs nonexposed), current serum concentration, and back-extrapolated serum concentration at the time of last exposure. Logarithmic transformation was used for TCDD and immune-marker concentrations. Statistical analyses were conducted with t tests, chi-square tests, and linear regression. Similarly, Saberi Hosnijeh et al. (2012) examined the association between TCDD exposure and serum cytokine concentrations in a subsample of workers in factory A (47 with high exposure, 38 with low exposure).

German production workers Becher et al. (1996) conducted an analysis of the four German cohorts added to the IARC cohort as of 1997: the Boehringer–Ingelheim cohort (also reported on in more detail by Manz et al., 1991 and later researchers); a cohort in the BASF Ludwigshafen plant that did not include those involved in a 1953 accident; and cohorts in a Bayer plant in Uerdingen and a Bayer plant in Dormagen. Preliminary information on the four cohorts had been published earlier (Becher et al., 1992). All the plants were involved in production of phenoxy herbicides or chlorophenols. Additional information is available only on the Boehringer–Ingelheim cohort, and the workers involved in the 1953 accident have been studied separately.

Boehringer–Ingelheim Cohort in Hamburg As first reported by Manz et al. (1991), workers in the Boehringer–Ingelheim plant in Hamburg had high potential for TCDD exposure because of production of trichlorophenol (TCP) and 2,4,5-T from 1951 to 1954 and from 1957 to 1984. The hiatus was motivated by a chloracne outbreak, and production recommenced when a process that resulted in less TCDD contamination became available. The cohort consisted of 1,184 men and 399 women, who had been employed for at least 3 months during 1952–1984. Vital status of all but 46 workers (2.9%) through 1989 was established; 313 deaths were observed in the men and 54 in the women. Detailed results were reported only for the men. Mortality from all causes did not differ from what would be predicted by rates for West Germany (standardized mortality ratio, [SMR] = 1.00, 95% confidence interval [CI] 0.89–1.12); compared with what was probably a more appropriate occupational cohort of Boehringer gas workers, however, mortality from all causes (only through 1985 because of limitations of available information) was significantly higher (SMR = 1.34, 95% CI 1.18–1.51). The risk of death from all cancers was marginally higher than the West German rates (SMR = 1.24, 95% CI 1.00–1.52) and more definitively so compared with the gas workers (SMR = 1.39, 95% CI 1.10–1.75).

Flesch-Janys et al. (1995) updated the cohort's vital staus through 1992 and added a quantitative exposure assessment based on blood or adipose-tissue measurements of PCDDs and polychlorinated dibenzofurans (PCDFs). The authors estimated maximum PCDD and PCDF exposure of 190 workers with a first-order kinetics model, half-lives with an elimination study of 48 workers in the cohort, and background concentrations in the German population. They then regressed the estimated maximum PCDD and PCDF exposures of the workers against the length of time that they worked in each production department in the plant. The working-time weights were then used with work histories of the remainder of the cohort to estimate PCDD and PCDF exposure of each person at the end of his or her employment. Those values were used to estimate TCDD doses in the population. (At this the stage of updating, the Hamburg cohort was discussed with three other German cohorts by Becher et al. [1996] and became a subcohort of the IARC phenoxy-herbicide cohort as updated by Kogevinas et al. [1997].)

Manuwald et al. (2012) updated the mortality experience of 1,191 men and 398 women in the Hamburg cohort. Subjects entered the cohort on the date of their first employment in the plant, and vital status was sought through 2007; loss to followup was only 3.2%. SMRs calculated relative to the population of Hamburg showed that death from all causes was slightly higher in men (698 deaths, SMR = 1.14, 95% CI 1.06–1.23); in the entire cohort, the increase in mortality was significant (SMR = 1.08, 95% CI 1.01–1.16), but not in women (180 deaths, SMR = 0.91, 95% CI 0.78–1.05). Similarly, mortality from all malignant neoplasms was slightly higher in men (226 cancer deaths, SMR = 1.14, 95% CI 1.06–1.23), and the increase in mortality was significant in the entire cohort (SMR = 1.33, 95% CI 1.18–1.49), but not in women (65 cancer deaths, SMR = 0.91, 95% CI 0.78–1.05). Individual cumulative exposure was estimated from work history on the basis of company records, and the intensity of TCDD exposure in workplaces was based on previous analyses of serum and fat-tissue dioxin concentrations. Cochran–Armitage trend tests on quartiles of cumulative exposure were conducted for deaths from all causes, all malignancies, breast cancer, cancers of digestive organs, respiratory cancers, and circulatory diseases.

BASF Ludwigshafen Plant Workers Involved in Accident Cleanup *(not in IARC cohort)* An accident on November 17, 1953, during the manufacture of TCP in a BASF plant in Germany resulted in extreme exposure of some workers to TCDD. *VAO*, *Update 1996*, *Update 1998*, and *Update 2000* summarized studies of those workers, including a mortality study of persons initially exposed or later involved in cleanup (Thiess et al., 1982), an update and expansion of that study (Zober et al., 1990), and a morbidity followup (Zober et al., 1994). In addition, Ott and Zober (1996) and Zober et al. (1997) examined cancer incidence and mortality in workers exposed to TCDD after the accident or during reactor cleanup, maintenance, or demolition. No new studies have been published on these workers since *Update 2000*.

New Zealand Production Workers

The mortality status of the New Zealand cohort that was incorporated into the original IARC cohort was followed up through 2000 by 't Mannetje et al. (2005).

The New Plymouth plant produced phenoxy herbicides from the "late" 1950s through the "mid-1980s." It is of interest to note that this plant also produced picloram, one of the COIs about which very little information is available. Complete employment records for 1969–1984 were available, so the study included anyone who had worked at least 1 month in that period—a cohort of 713 men and 100 women (the 1984 cohort).

Burns et al. (2010), Collins et al. (2009c), and McBride et al. (2009a,b) examined the New Zealand production-worker subcohort of the IARC cohort, which comprised employees who worked at the Dow AgroSciences (formerly Ivon Watkins-Dow) plant in New Plymouth that manufactured diverse agrochemical products, including phenoxy herbicides. McBride et al. (2009a) conducted expanded analyses and updated previous analyses of cause-specific mortality (from both cancer and other conditions). The cohort was inflated to 1,599 participants (referred to hereafter as the 1988 cohort), including a substantial number of people who had minimal opportunity for exposure, by extending the employment period for eligibility to November 1, 1988, and removing the requirement that employment lasted at least 1 month. McBride et al. (2009b) further expanded the cohort to 1,754 participants (the 2003 cohort) by further extending eligibility to anyone who worked at the site at any time until October 1, 2003. Both enlarged cohorts were followed through 2004. The New Zealand Health Information Service Mortality Collection was used to identify deaths (247 in both cohorts; there seem to have been no deaths in the increment of 155 workers who were in the 2003 cohort but not in the 1988 cohort). Exposure status was classified according to work experience. A subsample of the 1988 cohort participated in a serum-dioxin analysis (346, 70% exposed).

Collins et al. (2009c) described the group's serum TCDD concentrations overall, and Burns et al. (2010) performed analyses to determine what factors might predict serum TCDD: age, BMI, and employment history were found to be significant determinants. In particular, the exposed group had significantly ($p = 0.03$) higher concentrations (9.9 ppt) than did the nonexposed group (4.8 ppt); number of years since termination is associated significantly ($p = 0.002$) with lower TCDD; and serum TCDD is also associated significantly ($p < 0.0001$) with predicted cumulative TCDD exposure on the basis of area-under-the-curve in a pharmacokinetic model of the accumulation and elimination of dioxins. Both studies reported SMRs that were derived by using the Occupational Cohort Mortality Analysis Program with the New Zealand population as the reference population and adjusted for age, sex, and calendar age. For the 1988 cohort, SMRs were stratified by exposure status (ever exposed and never exposed) and by predicted cumulative exposure categories. For the 2003 cohort, SMRs were reported for the entire cohort and stratified by employment duration (less than 3 months and at least 3 months) and by latency (15 years and less than 15 years of latency). For the 1988 cohort, proportional-hazards survival analysis was also used to test the association between mortality and predicted cumulative exposure categories.

The New Zealand studies have several important limitations. The sample loss was substantial: 13% were lost to followup in both cohorts, and 8% of the 1988 cohort and 9% of the 2003 cohort emigrated. If sample loss was nonrandom, the study findings might be vulnerable to sample selection bias. In addition, the inclusion in the 2003 cohort of the employees hired as recently as 2003 is questionable. It appears that no deaths were observed in the increment between the 1988 cohort and the 2003 cohort (those hired since 1988), presumably because these participants are relatively young. The inclusion of the incremental participants might dilute the power of the study to detect effects of TCDD exposure on health outcomes that require a long latent period; participants who have not yet "matured" through the latent period might be contributing noise rather than signal to the analyses. The committee, therefore, did not give substantial weight to the dose–response findings of McBride et al. (2009b).

The serum concentrations of dioxins and furans observed in a subset of the workers in the Dow phenoxy-herbicide plant in New Zealand have been used in estimating individual exposure (Aylward et al., 2010; Collins et al., 2009c).

National Institute for Occupational Safety and Health Studies

NIOSH PCP Cohort Ruder and Yiin (2011) reported findings on mortality in 2,122 pentachlorophenol (PCP) production workers in four plants—Midland, Michigan; Sauget, Illinois; Tacoma, Washington; and Wichita, Kansas—in the NIOSH dioxin registry. For analytic purposes, the cohort was partitioned into a subcohort of 1,402 workers (PCP-only group) who were employed only in production of PCP, which has dioxin and furan contaminants that do not include the most toxic 2,3,7,8-TCDD congener, and a subcohort of 720 (PCP-plus-TCDD group) who also worked in TCP production and so did have exposure to TCDD). The cohort was followed through December 31, 2005. Exposure was specified both as exposure status (exposed vs not exposed, for cohort members vs reference population) and as cumulative duration of exposure stratified into four quartiles. Statistical analyses were based on SMRs with the US population as the reference, and standardized rate ratios were used to compare workers in cumulative duration categories.

NIOSH Cross-Sectional Medical Study Before the first publication of mortality results in the main cohort, the NIOSH Cross-Sectional Medical Study gathered comprehensive medical histories, conducted medical examinations, and measured the pulmonary function of workers employed in chemical-manufacturing at plants in Newark, New Jersey (1951–1969), and Verona, Missouri (1968–1972). Control participants were recruited from surrounding neighborhoods (Sweeney et al., 1989, 1993). The New Jersey plant manufactured 2,4,5-TCP and 2,4,5-T; the

Missouri plant manufactured 2,4,5-TCP, 2,4,5-T, and hexachlorophene. Specific health outcomes were evaluated in the members of this subcohort, including porphyria cutanea tarda (Calvert et al., 1994); effects on pulmonary function (Calvert et al., 1991); effects on hepatic and gastrointestinal function (Calvert et al., 1992); mood (Alderfer et al., 1992); effects on the peripheral nervous system (Sweeney et al., 1993); and effects on reproductive hormones (Egeland et al., 1994). Sweeney et al. (1996, 1997/1998) reviewed and updated noncancer outcomes, including effects on hepatic function, gastrointestinal disorders, chloracne, diabetes, and serum glucose, hormone, and lipid concentrations. The data gathered from the two plants were also examined for cardiovascular effects (Calvert et al., 1998); diabetes mellitus, thyroid function, and endocrine function (Calvert et al., 1999); immune characteristics (Halperin et al., 1998); and cancer incidence (Kayajanian, 2002). Halperin et al. (1995) investigated the relationship between serum TCDD concentrations and cytochrome P450 induction in 400 of the original 586 subjects in the cohort. Lawson et al. (2004) studied three birth outcomes—birth weight, preterm delivery, and birth defects—in offspring of the cohort members by comparing serum TCDD concentrations with those in a reference population. TCDD exposures at conception were estimated by using physiologically based pharmacokinetic modeling (Dankovic et al., 1995; Thomaseth and Salvan, 1998).

NIOSH TCDD Mortality Cohort Since 1978, an extensive set of data on chemical production workers potentially contaminated with TCDD in 1942–1984 has been compiled by NIOSH. More than 5,000 workers who were involved in production or maintenance in any of 12 companies were identified from personnel and payroll records; 172 additional workers identified previously by their employers as being exposed to TCDD were also included in the study cohort (Suskind and Hertzberg, 1984). The employees' possible exposure resulted from working with substances of which TCDD was a contaminant: 2,4,5-TCP, 2-(2,4,5-trichlorophenoxy) propionic acid (Silvex, 2,4,5-TP), 2-(2,4,5-trichlorophenoxy) ethyl 2,2-dichloropropionate (Erbon), *O,O*-dimethyl *O*-(2,4,5-trichlorophenyl) phosphorothioate (Ronnel®), and hexachlorophene. The 12 plants involved were large manufacturing sites of major chemical companies, so many of the participants were potentially exposed to many other compounds, some of which could be toxic and carcinogenic. The NIOSH cohort was added to the IARC cohort as of the 1997 publication by Kogevinas et al.

Exposure status was determined initially through a review of process operating conditions, employee duties, and analytic records of TCDD in industrial-hygiene samples, process streams, products, and waste (Fingerhut et al., 1991). Occupational exposure to TCDD-contaminated processes was confirmed by measuring serum TCDD in 253 cohort members. Duration of exposure, defined as the number of years worked in processes contaminated with TCDD, was used as the primary exposure metric in the study. The use of duration of exposure as a surrogate for cumulative exposure was based on a correlation (Pearson correlation efficient, 0.72) between log-transformed serum TCDD and number of years worked in TCDD-contaminated processes. Duration of exposure of individual workers was calculated from work records, and exposure-duration categories were created: less than 1 year, 1 to less than 5 years, 5 to less than 15 years, and 15 years and longer. In some cases, information on duration of exposure was not available, so a separate metric—duration of employment—was defined as the total time that each worker was employed at the study plant. Fingerhut et al. (1991) used the exposure measures in assessing mortality through 1987.

A followup study (Steenland et al., 1999) examined the association between TCDD exposure and cause of death through 1993; it examined specific health outcomes, including cancer (all and site-specific), respiratory disease, cardiovascular disease, and diabetes. The researchers used a more refined exposure assessment than that used in previous analyses; it excluded workers whose records were inadequate to determine duration of exposure, and this reduced the number of study participants to a subcohort of 3,538 workers (69% of the overall cohort). The exposure assessment for the subcohort was based on a job–exposure matrix (JEM) that assigned each remaining worker a quantitative exposure score for each year of work (Piacitelli and Marlow, 1997).

No new studies on the entire NIOSH cohort were published during the current review period.

Subcohorts of the NIOSH TCDD Mortality Cohort

Monsanto The NIOSH study cohort (Fingerhut et al., 1991) included employees of the Monsanto facility in Nitro, West Virginia, that produced 2,4,5-T in 1948–1969. Zack and Suskind (1980) examined the mortality experience of the 121 men who had chloracne associated with an unintentional release that occurred on March 8, 1949. Other studies considered mortality and other health outcomes in additional workers involved in numerous aspects of 2,4,5-T production at the Monsanto plant (Collins et al., 1993; Moses et al., 1984; Suskind and Hertzberg, 1984; Zack and Gaffey, 1983). The Monsanto studies were discussed in more detail in *VAO*. No additional studies on those participants alone have been published; they have since been followed as part of the NIOSH and IARC cohorts.

Dow 2,4-D Production Workers Since *Update 2010*, Burns et al. (2011) have reported on cancer incidence in 2,4-D production workers in the Dow Midland plant. The exposed cohort consisted of 1,316 men who worked in 2,4-D operations during 1945–1994 and were alive on January 1, 1985, when the Michigan statewide cancer registry was initiated. Exposure was considered both as a category (exposed [cohort members] vs not exposed [reference population]) and as a cumulative variable estimated as (job-specific exposure estimate) × (duration on the job) summed over all jobs held since 1945. Workers were stratified into three categories according to estimated cumulative exposure. The cohort was followed in 1985–2007. Cancer incidence was ascertained from the Michigan statewide cancer registry and data linked to Arizona and Ohio, states where cohort members might reside. Three nested cohorts were used for statistical analyses to address potential problems with data that were missing because of migration outside the three states with data linkage. Cohort 1 consisted of the entire exposed cohort (1,316 who had 25,267 person-years of followup). Cohort 2 required Michigan residency; followup was terminated when a person was known not to be a Michigan resident, either because company records showed a permanent non-Michigan address or a death certificate showed a state other than Michigan as the state of residency (1,256 who had 23,354 person-years). Cohort 3 had a more stringent residency requirement; followup was terminated when a person was no longer known to be a Michigan resident (1,108 who had 18,897 person-years). For Cohort 2, people of unknown residency status were assumed to remain Michigan residents and were included in the followup; for Cohort 3, such people were assumed to be nonresident and were excluded. Standardized incidence ratios (SIRs) were derived for all three cohorts with Michigan white males as the reference population; Fisher's exact confidence interval was used to characterize uncertainty. For Cohort, 2 additional analyses were conducted by using the NCI Surveillance, Epidemiology, and End Results (SEER) registry population and a regional population as the reference populations and by stratifying the cohort according to cumulative duration and cumulative exposure categories.

There are concerns that the study findings might be biased, for several reasons. First, the study cohort might be healthier than the general population being used as the reference population. Second, the lack of a latent period in the study design might lead to an attenuation effect on the risk estimates; this is similar to the Villeneuve and Steenland (2010) criticism of the Dow-Midland mortality study reported in Collins et al. (2009a). Third, Cohort 2, used as the researchers' focus of the study, might be vulnerable to an attenuation effect because of the uncertainty of residency status. For the present VAO review, the results on Cohort 3 are considered least subject to bias, and hence most reliable, although this smallest group is subject to the most variability; consistency in results among the three cohorts is considered confirmatory.

All Dow TCP-Exposed Workers TCP was produced in Dow's facility in Midland, Michigan, from 1942 to 1979, and 2,4,5-T was produced there from 1948 to 1982. The cohort of TCP workers who were potentially exposed specifically to TCDD is one of the eight cohorts in the NIOSH cohort of dioxin-exposed US workers that were entered into the IARC phenoxy herbicides cohort.

Collins et al. (2009a) updated the vital status through 2003 of 1,615 people who had worked with TCP or 2,4,5-T during 1942–1982; 58,743 person-years were accumulated, and 662 deaths were observed. SMRs for cause-specific mortality in the cohort—with and without the overlap of 196 people with the PCP cohort in Collins (2009b)—were calculated by using the US population as the reference population and using the Occupational Mortality Analysis Program.

Dow PCP Production Workers This set of people were engaged in the manufacture of PCP from 1937 to 1980 in the same plant where the TCP cohort worked. Unlike TCP, PCP did not contain TCDD, but it did contain other highly chlorinated dioxin congeners, and 20% of the PCP workers had suffered from chloracne. Those who had no TCDD exposure are not in IARC or NIOSH cohorts. This group is one of four cohorts included in NIOSH's PCP cohort (Fingerhut et al., 1984; Ruder and Yiin, 2011).

Dow has tracked a cohort of its manufacturing workers who were exposed to PCP (Ramlow et al., 1996). The exposure assessment evaluated the available industrial-hygiene and process data, including recollections from employees about processes and jobs, information about changes in processes and engineering controls, measurements from surface wipes, and exposure-monitoring data from area sampling and personal breathing zones. Jobs in the "flaking/prilling/packaging area" were determined to have higher potential exposure because of dermal exposure to airborne PCP; the industrial-hygiene data suggested a difference of about a factor of 3 between the areas of highest and lowest potential exposure. An estimated exposure-intensity score of 1–3 (from lowest to highest potential exposure intensity) was assigned to each job. Information concerning the use of personal protective equipment was deemed to be unreliable. For each participant, cumulative PCP and TCDD exposure indexes were calculated by multiplying the duration of each exposed job by its estimated exposure intensity and then summing across all exposed jobs.

Collins et al. (2009b) conducted a mortality study of the Dow PCP production workers with the accrual of years at risk starting at the beginning of 1940. The cohort was followed for "up to 64 years." Although the date of closure of the followup was not provided explicitly, it appears that the cohort was followed through 2003, as were the TCP workers (Collins et al., 2009a). The cohort consisted of 773 PCP workers; 27,035 person-years were accumulated, and 370 deaths were observed. SMRs for the PCP cohort (with and without the overlap of 196 people in the TCP cohort) were given for cause-specific mortality with the US population as the referent population. Proportional-hazards survival analysis was also used to assess the association between mortality and predicted cumulative exposure as total toxic equivalent (TEQ) to TCDD.

Dow TCDD-Exposed Production Workers Dow conducted a study of 204 workers engaged in the production of 2,4,5-T (Ott et al., 1980) and one of 61 TCP manufacturing workers who had chloracne (Cook et al., 1980). Industrial hygienists developed a JEM that ranked employee exposures as low, moderate, or high on the basis of available air-monitoring data and professional judgment. The matrix was merged with employee work histories to assign an estimate of exposure to each job. A cumulative dose was then developed for each of the 878 employees by multiplying the representative 8-hour time-weighted average (TWA) exposure value for each job by the number of years in the job and then adding the products for all jobs. A 2,4-D TWA of 0.05 mg/m^3 was used for low, 0.5 mg/m^3 for moderate, and 5 mg/m^3 for high exposure. The role of dermal exposure in the facilities does not appear to have been considered in the exposure estimates. It is not clear to what extent the use of air measurements alone can provide accurate classification of workers into low-, moderate-, and high-exposure groups. Biologic monitoring of 2,4-D apparently was not included in the study.

Bond et al. (1983) investigated potential exposure to TCDD and morbidity in the sets of workers reported on by Cook et al. (1980) and Ott et al. (1980). Potential TCDD exposure and reproductive outcomes were studied in the offspring of 930 men who worked with chlorophenol during 1939–1975 (Townsend et al., 1982). Dow employees who had a diagnosis of chloracne or who were classified as having chloracne on the basis of a clinical description were followed prospectively for mortality (Bond et al., 1987). There was a succession of mortality studies of workers involved in 2,4-D production in several of the plants (Bloemen et al., 1993; Bond et al., 1988; Burns et al., 2001), which also were conducted with the same exposure-assessment procedures.

Dow assembled a large cohort at the Midland, Michigan, plant (Bond et al., 1989a; Cook et al., 1986, 1987). Exposure to TCDD in the cohort was characterized on the basis of chloracne diagnosis (Bond et al., 1989b). Within the cohort, a subcohort study of women (Ott et al., 1987) and a case-control study of STS (Sobel et al., 1987) were conducted. The Dow cohorts have been followed as part of the NIOSH and IARC cohorts since 1991 and 1997, respectively.

Bodner et al. (2003) published a 10-year followup of the work of Cook et al. (1986), comparing the mortality experience of 2,187 male Dow workers who were potentially heavily exposed to dioxin before 1983 with that of the NIOSH and IARC cohorts. Dow researchers have published a study of serum dioxin concentrations measured in 2002 in former chlorophenol workers (Collins et al., 2006). Most of the workers in the study were included in the NIOSH and IARC cohorts. The authors used their data to estimate worker exposure at the time of exposure termination by using several pharmacokinetic models. They concluded that their findings were consistent with those of other studies that reported high serum dioxin concentrations in chlorophenol workers after occupational exposure.

Czech Worker Studies

Several studies of Czech workers have been reviewed by VAO committees. The original committee reviewed a 10-year followup study of 55 men in Czechoslovakia who were exposed to TCDD during the production of 2,4,5-T

(Pazderova-Vejlupková et al., 1981). The exposure occurred because of excessive temperature and pressure in the production process over an extended period (1965–1968) rather than as a consequence of a major release at a single time. More than 80 workers were affected, but the researchers provided little information about those who were not included in the study. Researchers observed several disorders in the workers, including chloracne, metabolic disturbances, abnormal results of glucose-tolerance tests, evidence of a mild hepatic lesion, nervous system focal damage, and psychologic disorders. In a 30-year followup, Pelclová et al. (2001, 2002) examined biochemical, neuropsychologic, neurologic, and lipid-metabolism abnormalities in the surviving Czech cohort. Previous VAO committees concluded that there were methodologic problems of selection bias; lack of control for confounding by educational achievement, tobacco use, or alcohol use; the use of self-reported symptoms; and the lack of an objective measure of exposure. In 2004, Pelclová and colleagues (2007) compared vascular function of 15 exposed workers with that of 14 healthy male health-care workers who had no history of occupational exposure to TCDD. Urban et al. (2007) evaluated the same set of workers, looking at over-all health effects. Further details on those studies were given in *Update 2006* and *Update 2008*.

Pelclová et al. (2009) reported on an update on the exposed cohort that was based on examination and testing of 11 participants in a followup visit in 2008, including internal and neurologic examination, eye fundus examination, TCDD in plasma, thyroid-stimulating hormone, testosterone and serum lipids, ultrasonography of the carotid artery, nerve-conduction study, electroencephalography, visual-evoked potential, Lanthony test of acquired visual impairment, single-photon emission computed tomography of the brain, neuropsychologic examination (eight consented), and carbohydrate-deficient transferrin, an index of long-term alcohol consumption. Mean TCDD concentration remained high (274.0 pg/g of blood lipids), with a wide dispersion (53–756 pg/g) among the 11 participants. Prevalences of health conditions were compared with those in the male population of comparable age. Paired t tests and F tests were used to test for changes in assessments obtained repeatedly during followup visits; Spearman's rank correlation coefficient was used to test the association between health outcomes (such as color-vision impairment) and risk factors (such as concentrations of TCDD and carbohydrate-deficient transferring). This study has important limitations. With a low retention rate (11 participants of the original cohort of 80), the study findings are vulnerable to nonresponse bias. No description of sample loss was given, even regarding the loss of four participants from the 2004 followup reported in Pelclová et al. (2007). The comparison with the prevalence in the male population of comparable age is important in the interpretation of the study findings, but no description of the comparison group is given beyond citations of its (presumed) sources.

Since *Update 2010*, Pelclová et al. (2011) have reported on further comparisons of markers of oxidative or nitrosative stress and inflammation in plasma, urine, and exhaled breath condensate of the 11 exposed workers studied previously in Pelclová et al. (2009) compared with 16 health-care workers (seven men, nine women). This study has similar limitations as in Pelclová et al. (2009). In particular, the mixed-sex comparison group might not be appropriate for the all-male cohort of exposed people.

Studies of Other Industrial Cohorts

Other Chemical Plants

Studies have reviewed health outcomes in UK chemical workers exposed to TCDD as a result of an industrial accident in 1968 (Jennings et al., 1988; May, 1982, 1983), 2,4-D production workers in the former Soviet Union (Bashirov, 1969), 2,4-D and 2,4,5-T production workers in the United States (Poland et al., 1971), white men employed at a US chemical plant that manufactured flavors and fragrances (Thomas, 1987), and US chemical workers engaged in the production of PCP, lower-chlorinated phenols, and esters of chlorophenoxy acids (Hryhorczuk et al., 1998). The long-term immunologic effects of TCDD were examined in 11 industrial workers involved in production and maintenance operations in a German chemical factory that produced 2,4,5-T (Tonn et al., 1996), and immunologic effects were studied in a cohort of workers formerly employed at a German pesticide-producing plant (Jung et al., 1998). *VAO*, *Update 1998*, and *Update 2000* detailed those studies. Garaj-Vrhovac and Zeljezić (2002) conducted a study of workers occupationally exposed to a complex mixture of pesticides (atrazine, alachlor, cyanazine, 2,4-D, and malathion) during their production.

Waste-Incineration Worker Studies

A study in Japan examined the association between serum-dioxin concentrations (TEQ values for PCDDs, PCDFs, and coplanar polychlorinated biphenyls) and oxidative DNA-damage markers in municipal-waste–incineration workers (Yoshida et al., 2006).

A Korean study evaluated immunologic and reproductive toxicity (DNA damage and sperm quality) in 31 waste-incineration workers and 84 control participants (Oh et al., 2005). Rather than measuring serum dioxin, both studies inferred dioxin exposure of individual workers on the basis of dioxin concentrations in air and estimated exposures to polycyclic aromatic hydrocarbons by analyzing two urinary metabolites: 1-hydroxypyrene and 2-naphthol.

No studies of waste-incineration workers relevant to the COIs have been published since *Update 2006*.

Paper and Pulp Cohorts

Workers in the paper and pulp industry can be exposed to TCDD and other dioxins that can be generated by the bleaching process during the production and treatment of paper and paper products. *VAO* described mortality studies of pulp and paper-mill workers potentially exposed to TCDD in five mills in Washington, Oregon, and California (Robinson et al., 1986) and in a New Hampshire mill (Henneberger et al., 1989); of vested members of the United Paperworkers International Union (Solet et al., 1989); and of cancer incidence in male papermill workers in Finland (Jappinen and Pukkala, 1991). Rix et al. (1998) studied cancer incidence through 1993 in 11,130 male and 3,232 female workers employed at three Danish paper mills anytime in 1943–1990.

IARC Paper and Pulp Cohort *Update 2006* reviewed a collaborative study of cancer mortality (McLean et al., 2006) led by IARC that was composed of cohorts in 11 countries and had followup through 1990 to 1996 (depending on the country). The pooled data included several cohorts that had been evaluated individually in *VAO* and earlier updates. For departments in each company, industrial-hygiene experts estimated exposure to 27 agents over time. The 60,468 pulp and paper industry workers employed during 1920–1996 were assigned to the "nonvolatile organochlorines" (potential contamination with TCDD assumed) group (58,162) and the "volatile organochlorines" group (60,468). It is unclear how the entire cohort was portioned into apparently overlapping groups for "volatile" and "nonvolatile" organochlorines and these populations were subdivided for analyses into sets that "ever" or "never" had exposure to the chemicals, the "never exposed."

Sawmill Workers Sawmills use PCP (which has some contamination with dioxins but not the TCDD congener) as a fungicide, so the exposures experienced are more like "herbicide-use" than those encountered in herbicide production or in pulp and paper processes. Workers in sawmills might have been exposed to pentachlorophenates, which are contaminated with higher-chlorinated PCDDs (Cl_6–Cl_8), or to tetrachlorophenates, which are less contaminated with higher-chlorinated PCDDs. Wood is dipped into those chemical preservatives and then cut and planed in the mills. Most exposure is dermal, but some exposure can occur by inhalation (Hertzmann et al., 1997; Teschke et al., 1994).

McLean et al. (2009) studied serum dioxin concentrations in 94 former sawmill workers in New Zealand who were classified as exposed (71) and nonexposed (23) according to their work history. In addition, the serum-dioxin test results on 23 former sawmill workers in Sawmill Workers Against Poisons (SWAP) were provided for the study. A semiquantitative estimate of exposure intensity was also developed by using a PCP exposure algorithm that incorporated the participants' job titles and specific work tasks: mixing of PCP solutions, cleaning sludge, and spraying. Serum concentrations of PCDDs and PCDFs were analyzed; the total TEQ was calculated by using the World Health Organization (WHO) toxic equivalence factors (TEFs) (van den Berg et al., 2006). Mean concentrations in exposed workers were higher than those in the nonexposed: 1,2,3,6,7,8-hexachlorodibenzodioxin, 1,2,3,4,6,7,8-heptachlorodibenzodioxin, and octachlorodibenzodioxin concentrations were 2–3 times higher and the WHO TEQs about 40% higher (13.67 pg/g vs 9.56 pg/g). The congener profiles in serum were consistent with those in PCP solutions, and dioxin concentrations increased with both employment duration and estimated exposure intensity. The averages in the SWAP members were 2–3 times those in the exposed study participants (37.74 pg/g).

Studies of Herbicide-Using Workers

Various methods have been used to estimate occupational exposure of agricultural workers to herbicides or TCDD. The simplest method derives data from death certificates, cancer registries, or hospital records (Burmeister, 1981), in which information on "usual occupation" is used to construe likely exposure to the COIs. Although such information is relatively easy to obtain, it does not provide information on duration or intensity of exposure, and it cannot even be used to determine whether a worker was exposed to a specific agent. In some studies of agricultural workers, examination of differences between occupational practices has allowed identification of subsets of workers who were likely to have had higher exposures (Hansen et al., 1992; Musicco et al., 1988; Ronco et al., 1992; Vineis et al., 1986; Wiklund, 1983; Wiklund and Holm, 1986; Wiklund et al., 1988a). In other studies, county of residence was used as a surrogate for exposure, and agricultural censuses of farm production and chemical use were relied on for characterizing exposure in individual counties (Blair and White, 1985; Cantor, 1982; Gordon and Shy, 1981), exposure was estimated on the basis of the number of years of employment in a specific occupation as a surrogate for exposure duration, or information on herbicide use at each farm was used as a surrogate of its operator's exposure (Morrison et al., 1992; Wigle et al., 1990). Still others used self-reported information on exposure that recounted direct handling of a herbicide, whether it was applied by tractor or hand-held sprayer, and what types of protective equipment or safety precautions were used (Hoar et al., 1986; Zahm et al., 1990). A set of studies validated self-reported information with written records, signed statements, or telephone interviews with co-workers or former employers (Carmelli et al., 1981; Woods and Polissar, 1989).

Forestry and other outdoor workers, such as highway-maintenance workers, are also likely to have been exposed to herbicides and other chemicals. Exposure of those groups has been classified by using approaches similar to those noted above for agricultural workers, for example, by using the number of years employed, job category, and occupational title.

American Herbicide-User Studies

Agricultural Health Study

The US Agricultural Health Study (AHS) is a prospective investigation of cohorts of private pesticide applicators (farmers), their spouses, and commercial pesticide applicators in Iowa and North Carolina, with a total of 89,658 participants, including 57,311 applicators (82% of those seeking licensing) and 32,347 spouses (75% of all spouses). The applicators are predominantly but not exclusively male, and the spouses are predominantly but not exclusively female. The AHS is sponsored by the National Cancer Institute (NCI), the Environmental Protection Agency, and the National Institute of Environmental Health Sciences. Enrollment in the study was offered to applicants for applicator certification in Iowa and North Carolina. The project's website (www.aghealth.org) provides many details about the study, including specification of which pesticides were the subject of information gathered from the enrollment forms and mailed questionnaires (Alavanja et al., 1994).

In phase I (1993–1997), the enrollment form for both commercial (8.6%) and private (largely farmers) applicators asked for the details of use of 22 pesticides (10 herbicides, including 2,4-D; nine insecticides; two fungicides; and one fumigant) and yes–no responses as to whether 28 other pesticides (eight herbicides, including 2,4,5-T and Silvex, 2,4,5-TP; 13 insecticides; four fungicides; and three fumigants) had ever been used.

A subset of 24,034 applicators also completed and mailed back a take-home questionnaire. The questionnaire asked for details about use of the 28 pesticides with yes–no information on the enrollment form and for yes–no responses as to whether 108 other pesticides (34 herbicides, including organic arsenic, which would cover cacodylic acid; 36 insecticides; 29 fungicides; and nine fumigants) had ever been "frequently" used. Dosemeci et al. (2002) published an algorithm designed to characterize personal exposures of that population. Weighting factors for key exposure variables were developed from the literature on pesticide exposure. This quantitative approach has the potential to improve the accuracy of exposure classification for the cohort but has not yet been used in published epidemiologic studies.

The response rate for the take-home questionnaire, 42%, is rather low. Although no pronounced differences in demographics, medical histories, or farming practices were found between those who completed and did not complete the questionnaire (Tarone et al., 1997), selection bias might compromise the validity of studies based on the questionnaire because of differences that might not have been captured in the enrollment form.

Phase II was a 5-year followup conducted in 1999–2003. Computer-assisted telephone interviews (CATIs) were completed by 60,138 participants. The interviews specified "pesticides" in general to include herbicides. They asked about specific pesticides on individual crops; for several crops, only if atrazine or 2,4-D was specified was a participant asked whether it had been used alone or as part of the manufacturer's mixture. A full pesticide list was not posted on the website with the followup questionnaire. In addition, dietary histories were completed by 35,164 respondents, and buccal-cell samples were gathered from 34,810 participants. The rate of response to the phase II survey—67% overall and 63% of the original cohort of 55,748 male applicators—is modest and leaves some room for selection bias to compromise the validity of studies based on the survey. In phase III (2005–2010), responses to an updated CATI were provided by 43,426 participants.

Numerous reports on the AHS cohort have been considered in earlier updates. All have developed pesticide-exposure estimates or exposure categories from self-administered questionnaires. Using various subsets of the study population, they have addressed a variety of health outcomes: doctor visits resulting from pesticide exposure (Alavanja et al., 1998), chemical predictors of wheeze (Hoppin et al., 2002), prostate cancer incidence (Alavanja et al., 2003, 2005), lung cancer incidence (Alavanja et al., 2004), reproductive effects (Farr et al., 2004, 2006), cancer risk in the 21,375 children of pesticide appliers born in 1975 or later (Flower et al., 2004), mortality (Blair et al., 2005a), morbidity (Alavanja et al., 2005; Blair et al., 2005b), rheumatoid arthritis (De Roos et al., 2005a), breast-cancer incidence (Engel et al., 2005), neurotoxicity of chronic exposure to modest amounts of pesticides (Kamel et al., 2005), and prevalence of wheeze (Hoppin et al., 2006a). Three additional publications have discussed pesticide-use patterns in the population (Hoppin, 2005, Hoppin et al., 2006b; Kirrane et al., 2004; Samanic et al., 2005). The AHS questionnaire collected detailed information regarding herbicide use; 2,4-D was the most commonly reported herbicide. Kamel et al. (2007a) evaluated questionnaire responses from more than 18,000 AHS participants, who listed a variety of neurologic symptoms, including memory and concentration problems. Another study by Kamel et al. (2007b) evaluated Parkinson disease (PD) in participants in the AHS. Lee WJ et al. (2007) analyzed incident colorectal cancers diagnosed in AHS participants in 1993–2005. Associations with self-reported exposures to 50 pesticides (including 2,4-D, 2,4,5-T, and 2,4,5-TP) were studied. Samanic et al. (2006) reported on the incidence of all cancers combined and selected individual cancers in male pesticide applicators in the AHS particularly with respect to reported exposures to the benzoic acid herbicide dicamba (3,6-dichloro-2-methoxybenzoic acid). Dicamba was used in combination with other herbicides, such as 2,4-D and Agent Orange. Montgomery et al. (2008) discussed the relationship between self-reported incident diabetes and pesticide and herbicide exposure in 31,787 licensed pesticide applicators and their spouses. Saldana et al. (2007) reported on the cross-sectional relationship between pesticide and herbicide exposure and a history of gestational diabetes in the wives of licensed applicators. Of 11,273 women asked about their pregnancies closest to enrollment, 506 (4.5%) reported gestational diabetes. Hoppin et al. (2006c) evaluated participants who experienced wheeze, Hoppin et al. (2007a) evaluated farmer's lung (hypersensitivity pneumonitis), Hoppin et al. (2007b) and Valcin et al. (2007) evaluated chronic bronchitis, and Hoppin et al. (2008) evaluated atopic and nonatopic asthma in women.

Andreotti et al. (2009) conducted a case-control analysis of pancreatic cancer in participants who completed the enrollment form (93 incident cases in 64 applicators and 29 spouses and 82,503 cancer-free controls). Ever use of 24 chemicals and intensity-weighted lifetime days—(lifetime exposure days) × (exposure intensity score)—of 13 chemicals were assessed. Risk estimates were calculated by using unconditional logistic regression for various exposures and controlling for age, smoking, and diabetes.

Hoppin et al. (2009) reported on pesticide use and 127 cases of allergic and 314 cases of nonallergic adult-onset asthma in 19,704 male private applicators at least 20 years old in the AHS who completed both the enrollment form and the take-home questionnaire, with full information on smoking, asthma history, age, BMI, and high pesticide-exposure events. The researchers excluded 487 female applicators with 19 cases of asthma because of the small sample. Logistic regression was used to evaluate the association between farming exposures and adult-onset asthma, allowing for separate associations with allergic and nonallergic asthma and adjusting for age, state (Iowa or North Carolina), smoking status (current, past, or never), and BMI. For each of 48 pesticides, exposure status was specified as ever use vs never use. Further exposure–response analyses were conducted with a three-level specification for exposure—never used, median use or less, and greater than median use—according to the distribution for intensity-adjusted days of use for the specific pesticide. As noted previously, the findings from this study might be vulnerable to selection bias because of the low response rate (42%) for the take-home survey.

Mills et al. (2009) reported on the association between lifetime use of 49 pesticides and the incidence of and mortality from myocardial infarction (MI) in the AHS cohort: 476 deaths in 54,069 male participants who completed the enrollment form, and 839 nonfatal events in 32,024 male participants who completed the phase II telephone interview. Deaths from MI, as either a primary or a contributing cause, were recorded from state and national death records starting at enrollment and going through December 31, 2006. The incidence of nonfatal MI was determined on the basis of a positive response on the 5-year followup questionnaire to the question "Has a doctor or other health professional ever told you that you had a heart attack (or myocardial infarction)?" First MIs that occurred after enrollment were counted as incident MIs. Separate analyses for mortality and incidence were conducted by using Cox regression and adjusting for state (Iowa or North Carolina), age, and smoking status (whether or not the participant had smoked 100 cigarettes in his or her lifetime). The incidence analysis also adjusted for BMI. The analyses were conducted for each pesticide specified as ever used and as lifetime days of exposure. As noted previously, the validity of the findings for the incidence analysis might be compromised because of the modest rate of response to the phase II survey—63% according to the committee's calculation (35,088 respondents of 55,748 in the original cohort), reported as 70% in Mills et al. (2009). In particular, for incidence analyses reported in Mills et al. (2009), this survey is vulnerable to selection bias because of left truncation, that is, missing participants who died before the survey.

Goldner et al. (2010) examined the association between organochlorine exposure and thyroid disease in 19,529 female spouses in the AHS. The analysis was limited to female spouses of private applicators who completed both the take-home survey in phase I (pesticide use) and the followup interview in phase II (thyroid disease) and had complete data on all covariates. Thyroid-disease status (none in 14,486, hyperthyroidism in 369, hypothyroidism in 1,114, and other in 560) was ascertained from self-reported history of physician diagnoses obtained during phase II interviews. Logistic regression was used to estimate the association between use of herbicides (including 2,4-D and 2,4,5-T) and insecticides and thyroid-disease status (with no disease as the reference group) with adjustment for education, age, smoking (never, past, or current), BMI, and hormone-replacement therapy (ever or never). As noted previously, the findings from this study might be vulnerable to selection bias because of the low overall rate of response to the combination of the take-home survey and the followup interview.

Dennis et al. (2010) reported on 150 cases of cutaneous melanoma diagnosed after enrollment in the AHS of pesticide applicators who completed both the enrollment form and the take-home questionnaire during phase I, excluding 24,704 who had a cancer diagnosis before enrollment. Cases were identified through linkage to cancer registries, state death registries, and the National Death Index with a cutoff date of December 31, 2005. Dichotomous measures (ever or never used) were used for arsenic pesticides (lead arsenate and inorganic and organic arsenic). Categorical measures (no, low, or high) based on intensity-weighted lifetime days of exposure were used for other chemicals, including 2,4-D, 2,4,5-T, and 2,4,5-TP. Unconditional logistic regression was used to estimate the association between melanoma and exposure with adjustment for age, sex, and other variables "as indicated" (apparently selection through an unspecified variable selection procedure), including sun exposure, tendency to burn, red hair, and BMI.

Thomas et al. (2010) reported on a monitoring study of 2,4-D and chlorpyrifos exposures in a sample of AHS participants. For 69 2,4-D applicators, geometric mean values were 7.8 and 25 mg/L in preapplication and postapplication urine, respectively ($p < 0.05$ for difference), and 0.37 mg/m^3 in personal air. The estimated amounts of dermal absorption through the hands (hand loading) and through total skin surface (body loading) were 0.39 mg and 2.9 mg of 2,4-D, respectively; the readings for individual applicators were correlated across these media. Glove use and the mode of application were found to be associated with the degree of exposure.

Slager et al. (2009) reported on current rhinitis in commercial pesticide applicators in the AHS (excluding private applicators, such as farmers). Of the 4,916 commercial pesticide applicators in the full AHS cohort, the 2,245 who had provided information on all the variates in the analysis model constituted the sample for this investigation. Current rhinitis was ascertained with the following question in the take-home questionnaire: "During the past 12 months have you had a stuffy, itchy, or runny nose?" Exposure to individual pesticides was specified both as a dichotomous measure (ever vs never in the preceding year) and as a categorical measure (days per year). Logistic regression was used to estimate the association between exposure and current rhinitis, with adjustment for age, education, and having grown up on a farm. As noted previously, the findings from this study might be vulnerable to selection bias because of the low rate of response to the take-home survey (46% by commercial applicators, slightly higher by the entire AHS cohort).

Crawford et al. (2008) reported on hearing loss in white male licensed pesticide applicators in the AHS, considering the hypothesis that some pesticides are neurotoxic and could potentially affect hearing. The study sample consisted of participants who completed the enrollment form and the take-home questionnaire during phase I and the followup telephone interview in phase II. Hearing loss was ascertained with the following question in the phase II interview: "Do you have trouble with your hearing in one or both ears (this is without a hearing aid)?" Potential cases of hearing loss attributable to a congenital condition or to infection or injury (determined by responses to survey questions) were excluded. The analysis also excluded participants who reported never using pesticides and excluded nonwhite and female respondents. Of 16,246 participants who completed all three surveys, 14,229 were retained in the final analysis sample. Logistic regression was used to estimate the associatons between exposure and hearing loss with adjustment for state, age, and exposures to noise, solvents, and metals. The overall low rate of response (less than 30%) to the combination of the three surveys raises concerns about the validity of the study findings. The authors argued that there were too few nonwhites and females (1.5% of eligible participants) for analysis. Although it might be reasonable to consider those participants to be too few to be analyzed as subgroups, it is unclear why they needed to be excluded from the main analysis. (Limited analysis for nonwhites is mentioned in the discussion.)

Although health outcome results in the whole cohort or entire subgroups are not fully relevant for the COIs and might be regarded as of marginal interest to more recent VAO committees, Blair et al. (2005b) have reported that 2,4-D is the pesticide most frequently used by the Iowa farmers and is often used by the rest of the applicators. Consequently, the results on relative rates of individual conditions seem comparable in exposure specificity with findings in production cohorts in which not all the workers included were necessarily exposed to the COIs and may have had additional toxic exposures. Therefore, the findings on mortality from enrollment through 2000 (Blair et al., 2005a) and on cancer incidence through 2002 (Alavanja et al., 2005) have been retained in the results tables for health outcomes. Accordingly, the committee for this update has added mortality findings through 2007 on various causes of death (Waggoner et al., 2011) and comparisons with state populations for cancer incidence updated through 2006 (Koutros et al., 2010a) to the health-outcomes results tables. Conventional SMRs and SIRs were calculated adjusted for age, calendar year, race, sex, and state. In an effort to compensate for the pronounced healthy-worker effect evident in the AHS cohorts, both Waggoner et al. (2011) and Koutros et al. (2010a) also calculated, in addition to conventional SMRs and SIRs, "relative" counterparts of these statistics—rSMR and rSIR, respectively. To obtain the relative rates, the standardized ratio for incidence or mortality was divided by the standardized ratio for all causes excluding it. Because even the usual SMRs and SIRs from these non-pesticide specific findings on the entire cohort are minimally informative, the committee opted not to consider the relative versions.

Waggoner et al. (2011) reported 4,880 deaths in the applicators (private and commercial) and 1,539 in the spouses, significantly fewer than expected for both (SMR = 0.54, 95% CI 0.52–0.55; and SMR = 0.52, 95% CI 0.50–0.5). Similarly, deaths from all types of cancer were significantly lower than the state rates in both applicators (SIR = 0.61, 95% CI 0.58–0.864) and spouses (SIR = 0.65, 95% CI 0.60–0.70). Koutros et al. (2010a) found 4,316 cancer cases in the private applicators, 219 in the commercial applicators, and 1,896 in the spouses. Findings on the commercial applicators were set aside, and the cancer incidence rates in both the private applicators (SIR = 0.85, 95% CI 0.83–0.88) and the spouses (SIR = 8.2, 95% CI 0.79–0.86) were again significantly lower than expected.

Several recent AHS publications (Andreotti et al., 2012; Barry et al., 2011, 2012; Koutros et al., 2010b, 2011) reported on a nested case-control substudy that examined the relationship of pesticide exposure (including herbicides of interest, such as 2,4-D and 2,4,5-T) and of genetic markers with the risk of prostate cancer. All men eligible for inclusion in the study were white applicators who had not had any cancer other than non-melanoma skin cancer before enrollment in the AHS and had provided a buccal-cell sample. Two controls matched on age to each case had to have been alive at the time of the case's diagnosis. The final study sample consisted of 776 prostate-cancer cases diagnosed in 1993–2004 and 1,444 controls. Although the primary focus of this substudy was on the interaction between pesticide exposure and genetic markers (how pesticide exposure modified the association between genetic markers and prostate cancer), some useful information about the association between exposure to particular pesticides and prostate cancer can still be gleaned as a by-product of the interaction analyses. Intensity-weighted lifetime exposure days are used in Andreotti et al. (2012) and Barry et al. (2011, 2012). Genotyping for an array of 26,512 single-nucleotide polymorphisms (SNPs) in 1,291 candidate genes was performed at the NCI's Core Genotype Facility. Unconditional logistic regression was used to estimate odds ratios and 95% confidence intervals for the associations between prostate cancer and the main effect for pesticide exposure, the main effect for genetic markers, and the interaction between pesticide exposure and genetic markers, adjusted for age and state. Only Koutros et al. (2011), who reported the findings for this substudy on 1,913 SNPs in 149 candidate genes known to play a role in the metabolism of xenobiotic substrates, also adjusted for family history of prostate cancer and provided main effects for exposure to individual pesticides and the incidence of prostate cancer. Koutros et al. (2010b) reported the findings on 211 SNPs in the 8q24 region known to be associated with prostate cancer. Andreotti et al. (2012) reported the findings on 220 SNPs in 59 genes involved in lipid metabolism. Barry et al. (2011) reported the findings on 394 SNPs in 31 base-excision repair genes involved in repairing oxidative DNA damage that are hypothesized to be possibly important for populations exposed to pesticides or other putative oxidative stress–inducing agents. Barry et al. (2012) reported findings on 324 SNPs in 27 necleotide excision repair (NER) genes thought to be important in repairing damages induced by putative prostate carcinogens. The false discovery rate (Benjamini and Hochberg, 1995) method is used to account for multiple comparisons involving a large number of pesticides and genetic markers.

Tanner et al. (2011) conducted a case-control study of PD in AHS participants. Suspect cases (170) were identified from self-reports and state mortality files and confirmed (115; 110 with pesticide data included in study) by a neurologist during home visits. Potential controls (644) were sampled randomly from the AHS cohort and frequency-matched about 3:1 to cases by age, sex, and state. Controls were confirmed (383; 358 with pesticide data included in study) by a neurologist or a neurologist-trained technician during home visits. CATIs were used to obtain detailed information on use, since the age of 14 years, of 31 selected pesticides expected to be possibly associated with PD (oxidative stressors and mitochondrial inhibitors), and key covariate information, including smoking and family history of PD. Participant characteristics were compared between cases and controls by using Fisher's exact test or Pearson's chi-square test for categorical variables and Wilcoxon's rank-sum test for continuous variables. Logistic regression was used for pesticides reported by at least 10 participants, controlling for potential confounding factors, including age, sex, state, and cigarette-smoking (ever or never).

Several recent AHS studies examined a variety of exposure issues. Blair et al. (2011) examined the effect of exposure misclassification, which is likely to occur when self-reported exposure assessment is used, on the relative risks estimated in the AHS and showed substantial attenuation toward the null. Similar results are likely for other studies that use self-reported exposure status. Coble et al. (2011) reported on an updated version of an estimation algorithm for pesticide exposure intensity, developed previously in Dosemeci et al. (2002) for the AHS, to incorporate new data obtained in two exposure-monitoring studies to modify the weighting factors used in the algorithm. Payne et al. (2012) conducted a Cox proportional-hazards regression to assess the risk posed by high pesticide exposure in the AHS cohort.

California United Farm Workers of America Study

Mills and Yang (2005) and Mills et al. (2005) analyzed lymphohematopoietic cancer and breast cancer, respectively, in nested case-control studies of Hispanic workers drawn from a cohort of 139,000 Californians who were members of the United Farm Workers of America (UFW). Estimates of exposure to specific pesticides, including 2,4-D, were developed through linkage of the union's job histories with the California Pesticide Use Reporting Database of the state's Department of Pesticide Regulation, which has records of all agricultural applications of pesticides in the state since 1970. Vital status and cancer incidence were ascertained through a probabilistic record linkage to the California Cancer Registry for the period 1988–2001. Mills and Yang (2007) conducted a nested case-control gastric cancer study embedded in the UFW cohort and identified cases of gastic cancer newly diagnosed in 1988–2003.

No reports relevant to the COIs have been published on the California UFW population since *Update 2008*.

Other US Studies of Agricultural Workers

Studies of proportionate mortality were conducted in Iowa farmers (Burmeister, 1981) and male and female farmers in 23 states (Blair et al., 1993). Mandel et al. (2005) reported results of urinary biomonitoring of farm families in Minnesota and South Carolina as a part of CropLife America's Farm Family Exposure Study. Curwin et al. (2005) measured 2,4-D concentrations in urine and hand-wipe samples to characterize exposures of farmers and nonfarmers in Iowa.

Studies in Other Countries

Australian Herbicide-User Studies

Fritschi et al. (2005) used CATIs and occupational histories reviewed by an industrial hygienist to estimate exposures to phenoxy herbicides in an Australian study.

Canadian Herbicide-User Studies

Ontario Farm Family Health Study The Ontario Farm Family Health Study (OFFHS) has produced several reports on exposure to phenoxyacetic acid herbicides, including 2,4-D. A study of male pesticide exposure and pregnancy outcome (Savitz et al., 1997) developed an exposure metric based on self-reports of mixing or application of crop herbicides, crop insecticides, and fungicides; livestock chemicals; yard herbicides; and building pesticides. Study participants were asked whether they participated in those activities during each month, and their exposure classifications were based on activities in 3-month periods. Exposure classification was refined with answers to questions about use of protective equipment and specificity of pesticide use.

A related study included analysis of 2,4-D residues in semen as a biologic marker of exposure (Arbuckle et al., 1999a). The study began with 773 potential participants, but only 215 eventually consented to participation. Of the 215, 97 provided semen and urine samples for 2,4-D analysis.

The OFFHS also examined pregnancy outcomes of stillbirth, gestational age, and birth weight (Savitz et al., 1997) and the effects of exposure to pesticides, including 2,4-D, on time to pregnancy (Curtis et al., 1999) and on the risk of spontaneous abortion (Arbuckle et al., 1999b, 2001). About 2,000 farm couples participated in the study. Exposure information was pooled from interviews with husbands and wives to construct a history of monthly agricultural and residential pesticide use. Exposure classification was based on a yes–no response for each month. Data on such variables as acreage sprayed and use of protective equipment were collected but were not available in all cases. Other studies have used herbicide biomonitoring in a subset of the population to evaluate the validity of self-reported predictors of exposure (Arbuckle et al., 2002). Assuming that the presence of 2,4-D in urine was an accurate measure of exposure and that the results of the questionnaire indicating 2,4-D use were more likely to be subject to exposure-classification error (that is, assuming that the questionnaire results were less accurate than the results of urinalysis), the questionnaire's prediction of exposure, compared with the urinary 2,4-D concentrations, had a sensitivity of 57% and a specificity of 86%. In multivariate models, pesticide formulation, protective clothing and gear, application equipment, handling practice, and personal-hygiene practice were valuable as predictors of urinary herbicide concentrations in the first 24 hours after application was initiated.

Urinary concentrations of 2,4-D and MCPA were measured in samples from farm applicators (Arbuckle et al., 2005) and from women who lived on Ontario farms (Arbuckle and Ritter, 2005). Indirect sources of herbicide exposure of farm families were evaluated through wipe sampling of surfaces and drinking-water samples (Arbuckle et al., 2006). Weselak et al. (2008) examined occupational exposures and birth defects in the offspring of OFFHS participants. Spouses completed questionnaires that requested the history of pesticide use on the farm. Pregnancies resulting in birth defects were reported by the female study participants. All birth defects were combined for study analyses, and exposure was examined by pesticide class, family, and active ingredient for two 3-month periods—before and after conception.

No reports on the OFFHS relevant to the COIs have been published since *Update 2008*.

Canadian Farm Operator Study The Canadian Farm Operator Study assembled a cohort of 156,242 male farmers from 1971 Canadian census data on the provinces of Manitoba, Saskatchewan, and Alberta and linked to the national mortality database to identify deaths occurring during June 1971–December 1987. The cohort was also matched to the Central Farm Registers for 1966, 1976, 1981, and 1986 to gather information on reported exposures and farm practices. Information on the amount of acreage on each farm sprayed in 1970 with herbicides (without product specificity) was used as surrogate for its operator's exposure in determining the risk of specific causes of death: NHL (Morrison et al., 1994; Wigle et al., 1990), prostate cancer (Morrison et al., 1993), brain cancer (Morrison et al., 1992), multiple myeloma (MM) (Semenciw et al., 1993), and leukemia (Semenciw et al., 1994). In the one-third sample that completed the census long form, people most likely to have been exposed (no employees or custom expenses reported) could be identified. The age at which years at risk began to accumulate for each person varied for the various causes of death assessed, and this resulted in different numbers of eligible subjects. No reports on relevant health outcomes have been published on participants in this study population since *Update 1996*.

Other Canadian Studies of Agricultural and Forestry Workers Faustini et al. (1996) evaluated the immune, neurobehavioral, and lung function of residents in an agricultural area of Saskatchewan, Canada, and focused on immunologic changes in 10 farmers who mixed and applied commercial formulations that contained chlorophenoxy herbicides. Studies have been conducted in forestry workers potentially exposed to the types of herbicides used in Vietnam. A cohort mortality study examined men employed by a Canadian public utility (Green, 1987, 1991). Senthilselvan et al. (1992) investigated asthma's relationship to pesticide use with self-reported data gathered in a cross-sectional servey completed by 1,939 of the 2,375 male farmers approached in Saskatchewan. Mortality and reproductive effects have been studied in British Columbia sawmill workers potentially exposed to chlorophenate wood preservatives used as fungicides (Dimich-Ward et al., 1996; Heacock et al., 1998; Hertzman et al., 1997); PCP, which would be a frequently used fungicide, is expected to have dioxin and furan contamination, but the 2,3,7,8-TCDD congener is unlikely to have been present.

Danish Herbicide-User Studies

Records of the Danish Union of General Workers for 10 trade unions of gardeners were used to identify 3,156 male members on May 1, 1975; similarly, 859 women were identified. The workers were known to be highly exposed to pesticides. Most of the women worked in greenhouses, where herbicides are not routinely used; for the men, however, exposure was mainly to herbicides, which included the phenoxy herbicides 2,4-D, 2,4,5-T, and MCPA. Matching of union records to the Danish Central Population Registry permitted establishment of the vital status of the entire cohort through 1984 for determination of person-years at risk; this provided for a latent period of 10–15 years by starting accumulation when people reached the age of 30 years. Using the Danish Cancer Registry, Hansen et al. (1992) determined cancer incidence in this cohort of Danish gardeners from 1975 to 1984 compared with the general Danish population and adjusted for age, sex, and calendar period.

Hansen et al. (2007) used analogous methods to extend the followup period for the men through 2001. The updated information was analyzed by using year of birth as a surrogate for intensity of exposure, with high exposure assumed for those born before 1915, low exposure for those born in 1934 or later, and intermediate exposure for those born in between.

Drawing from the same cohort of Danish gardeners and further stipulating that people were alive and living in Denmark at the beginning of 1977, Kenborg et al. (2012) established a cohort of 3,124 men who were monitored in the Danish Hospital Register for hospitalization for PD as a primary diagnosis during 1977–2008 and compared the results with the observed incidence of PD in all Danish men by calendar period and age group. Revisiting the Danish Cancer Registry, they also investigated the incidence of lung, larynx, and bladder cancers, which are recognized as smoking-related. The incidence of those cancers was compared by age and calendar period with the incidence in the general male Danish population, and the rates were used as a proxy for smoking frequency in the cohort. The birth cohorts defined by Hansen et al. (2007) were used again to stratify degree of exposure.

Ronco et al. (1992) studied mortality in Danish farmers. The utility of the findings was limited by their being largely unanalyzed products of linking the country's cancer registry with census records to garner information on recent occupation.

Dutch Herbicide-User Studies

A Dutch study of forestry workers exposed to 2,4,5-T investigated the prevalence of acne and hepatic dysfunction (van Houdt et al., 1983). No reports on forestry workers have been published since 2000.

Mortality from cancer and other causes in Dutch male herbicide applicators has been studied by Swaen et al. (1992, 2004).

Finnish Herbicide-User Studies

Asp et al. (1994) conducted a followup through 1989 on mortality and cancer morbidity in Finnish men who had applied 2,4-D and 2,4,5-T for at least 2 weeks in 1955–1971. This group of 1,971 was assembled in 1972 from records of the four Finnish employers primarily responsible for brush removal and assessed for mortality through 1980 (Riihimaki et al., 1982) and for cancer morbidity (Riihimaki et al., 1983) through 1978.

German Herbicide-User Studies

Barthel (1981) studied cancer incidence and overall mortality through 1970–1978 in 1,658 male agricultural plant-protection workers in the former German Democratic Republic who spent a portion of at least 5 years in 1948–1972 applying pesticides. Unlike most of the many pesticides thought to have contributed to the exposure of these workers, the phenoxy herbicides were available for use throughout this period. It was not known, however, which individuals used the the COIs, so exposure characterization was not as specific as current VAO committees require for results to be considered fully relevant. Among the cancers, only lung cancer had a large enough number of cases to permit analysis by the amount and time period of pesticide use.

Iceland Herbicide-User Studies

Using the national cancer and death registries, Zhong and Rafnsson (1996) determined cancer incidence from entry into a pesticide using occupation through 1993 for 2,449 mean and women in Iceland. A listing of the amount of specific pesticides sold for agricultural use in Iceland between 1976 and 1993 ranked was led by 2,4-D, but it was not characterized to which of these individual subjects had been exposed, so the results of this study do not constitute fully relevant evidence according to the criteria of recent VAO committees.

Italian Herbicide-User Studies

Ronco et al. (1992) also studied the incidence of specific types of cancer in Italian farmers. The utility of the findings was limited by their being the largely unanalyzed products of linking the country's cancer registry with census records to garner information on recent occupation.

Cancer mortality in a cohort of rice growers in the Novara Province of northern Italy was investigated by Gambini et al. (1997).

A cohort of male farmers in Italy's southern Piedmont region who were licensed to use agricultural pesticides in 1970–1974 was established. The use of phenoxy herbicides in the area was reported to be twice the national average. Corrao et al. (1989) evaluated cancer incidence in 25,945 on the basis of new diagnoses from hospital admissions in 1976–1983. In a continuation of that study, Torchio et al. (1994) reported on mortality through 1986 in the 23,401 who were residents of the Piedmont area at the time of registration; cause of death was abstracted from death certificates. The cohort was partitioned into people who lived near arable land, those who lived near woodlands, and those who lived near mixed-use land; separate results were reported for the first two groups. No reports on this cohort have been published since 1994.

New Zealand Herbicide-User Studies

A study evaluated cancer incidence in a group of New Zealand forestry workers (Reif et al., 1989). No reports on forestry workers have been published since 2000. 't Mannetje et al. (2005) evaluated a study population that included herbicide production workers and was a subcohort of the IARC cohort.

Norwegian Herbicide-User Studies

Kristensen et al. (1997) tested whether cancers or birth defects were increased in the offspring of Norwegian farmers who worked on farms with pesticide use documented by agricultural censuses.

South American Herbicide-User Studies

Lerda and Rizzi (1991) studied the incidence of sperm abnormalities in Argentinian farmers. The utility of the findings was limited by their being the largely unanalyzed products of linking each country's cancer registry with census records to garner information on recent occupation.

Swedish Herbicide-User Studies

The Swedish Cancer-Environment Register (CER) linked the cancer cases entered in the Swedish Cancer Registry with the records of people who responded to the 1960 and 1970 national censuses, which had obtained data on current occupation. The resulting database has been used in studies that evaluated cancer mortality and farm work (Wiklund, 1983); STS and malignant lymphoma in agricultural and forestry workers (Wiklund and Holm, 1986; Wiklund et al., 1988a); and the risk of NHL, HL, and MM in relation to occupational activities (Eriksson et al., 1992). No new studies using the Swedish CER that are relevant to the COIs have been published since the original *VAO* report.

Cancer mortality in Swedish railroad workers has been studied (Axelson and Sundell, 1974; Axelson et al., 1980). Another study examined mortality and cancer incidence in a cohort of Swedish lumberjacks (Thörn et al., 2000). Cancer in Swedish pesticide and herbicide applicators has been studied repeatedly (Dich and Wiklund, 1998; Wiklund et al., 1987, 1988b, 1989a,b).

Other Studies of Workers Using Herbicides

Other studies of the agricultural use of pesticides have not provided specific information on exposure to 2,4-D, TCDD, or other compounds relevant to Vietnam veterans' exposure (Bell et al., 2001a,b; Chiu et al., 2004; Duell et al., 2001; Garry et al., 2003; Gorell et al., 2004; Hanke et al., 2003; van Wijngaarden et al., 2003).

A series of papers from a workshop focused on methods of assessing pesticide exposure in farmworker populations (Arcury et al., 2006; Barr et al., 2006a,b; Hoppin et al., 2006b; Quandt et al., 2006). They provide a helpful review of current methodologic issues in exposure science for those populations but do not address the COIs directly.

ENVIRONMENTAL STUDIES

Industrial accidents have led to the evaluation of long-term health effects in neighboring nonworker populations of exposure to fairly high concentrations of the COIs. Effects on residents around normally performing industrial operations, such as waste incinerators, and even on people exposed only to "background" concentrations have also been studied. Because the systematic followup studies that have been conducted on the Seveso population and the numerous analyses of the large database generated by the continuing US National Health and Nutrition Examination Survey (NHANES) have contributed so prominently to the evidence base considered by VAO committees, this section opens with discussions of these two study populations. Other environmental studies follow alphabetically by country.

People's environmental exposures to dioxin-like chemicals and their non–dioxin-like counterparts are to mixtures of components that tend to correlate, so it is not surprising that specific chemicals measured in a person's serum also tend to correlate; this collinearity means that it will be difficult for epidemiologic studies to attribute any observed association to a particular chemical configuration (Longnecker and Michalek, 2000). Analyses in terms of TEQs circumvent that problem to some extent.

Seveso, Italy

A large industrial accident that resulted in environmental exposure to TCDD was caused by an uncontrolled reaction during TCP production in Seveso, Italy, on July 10, 1976. The degree of TCDD contamination in the soil has been used extensively as a means of imputing exposures of members of the population. Three areas were defined on the basis of soil sampling: Zone A (556 people), the most heavily contaminated, from which all residents were permanently evacuated within 20 days; Zone B (3,920), an area of lower contamination that all children and women in the first trimester of pregnancy were urged to avoid during daytime; and Zone R (26,227), a region with some contamination in which consumption of local crops was prohibited (Bertazzi et al., 1989a,b). The sample sizes differ among followup studies, presumably because of migration; the sample sizes given above were reported in Bertazzi et al. (1989b).

Cohort of Entire Exposed Population

Data on serum TCDD concentrations in Zone A residents have been presented by Mocarelli et al. (1990, 1991) and by CDC (1988d). In the 10 who had severe chloracne, TCDD concentrations were 828–56,000 ppt of lipid weight. In 10 without chloracne, TCDD concentrations were 1,770–10,400 ppt. TCDD was undetectable in all control participants but one. The highest of the concentrations exceeded any that had been estimated at the time for TCDD-exposed workers on the basis of backward extrapolation and a half-life of 7 years. Data on nearby soil concentrations, number of days that a person stayed in Zone A, and whether local food was consumed were considered in evaluating TCDD. That none of those data correlated with serum TCDD suggested strongly that the important exposure was from fallout on the day of the accident. The presence and degree of chloracne did correlate with TCDD. Adults seemed much less likely than children to develop chloracne after acute exposure, but surveillance bias could have affected that finding. Recent updates (Bertazzi et al., 1998, 2001) have not changed the exposure-assessment approach.

A number of studies of the Seveso population have used lipid-adjusted serum TCDD concentrations as the primary exposure metric (Baccarelli et al., 2002; Eskenazi et al., 2002a,b, 2003a, 2004; Landi et al., 2003). Fattore et al. (2003) measured current air concentrations of PCDDs in Zones A and B and compared them with measurements in a control area near Milan. The authors concluded that release from PCDD-contaminated soil did not add appreciably to air concentrations in the Seveso study area. Finally, Weiss et al. (2003) collected breast milk from 12 mothers in Seveso to compare TCDD concentrations with those in a control population near Milan. The investigators reported that the TCDD concentrations in human milk from mothers in Seveso were twice as high as those in controls. The authors concluded that breastfed children in the Seveso area were likely to have higher body burdens of TCDD than children in other areas.

Several cohort studies have been conducted on the basis of the exposure categories. Seveso residents have had long-term followup of their health outcomes, especially cancer. Bertazzi and colleagues conducted 10-year mortality followup studies of adults and children who were 1–19 years old at the time of the accident (Bertazzi et al., 1989a,b, 1992), 15-year followup studies (Bertazzi et al., 1997, 1998), and a 20-year followup study (Bertazzi et al., 2001). Pesatori et al. (1998) also conducted a 15-year followup study to update noncancer mortality. Consonni et al. (2008) reported on the 25-year followup (through 2001) vital status of residents ("present") in the Seveso area and reference territory at the time of the Seveso accident and of immigrants and newborns ("non-present") in the 10 years thereafter. Cause-specific mortality was determined for each zone, compared with that in the comparison cohort and adjusted for presence at the accident, sex, period, age, and time since the Seveso accident.

In addition to a 2-year prospective controlled study of workers potentially exposed to TCDD during cleanup of the most highly contaminated areas after the accident (Assennato et al., 1989a), studies have examined specific health effects associated with TCDD exposure in Seveso residents—chloracne, birth defects, and spontaneous abortion—and crude birth and death rates (Bisanti et al., 1980); the distribution of chloracne in Seveso children (Caramaschi et al., 1981); chemicals in the blood and urine of children who had chloracne (Mocarelli et al. 1986); chloracne and peripheral nervous system conditions (Barbieri et al., 1988); dermatologic and laboratory tests in a group of the children who had chloracne and in a group of controls (Assennato et al., 1989b); health status and TCDD concentrations in chloracne cases and noncases recruited previously by Landi et al. (1997, 1998) and followed by Baccarelli et al. (2005a); hepatic-enzyme–associated conditions (Ideo et al., 1982, 1985); abnormal pregnancy outcomes (Mastroiacovo et al., 1988); cytogenetic abnormalities in maternal and fetal tissues (Tenchini et al., 1983); neurologic disorders (Boeri et al., 1978; Filippini et al., 1981); cancer (Bertazzi et al., 1993; Pesatori et al., 1992, 1993); sex ratio of offspring who were born in Zone A (Mocarelli et al., 1996); immunologic effects (Baccarelli et al., 2002); aryl hydrocarbon receptor–dependent (AHR-dependent) pathway and toxic effects of TCDD in humans (Baccarelli et al., 2004); effects of TCDD-mediated alterations in the AHR-dependent pathway in people who lived in Zones A and B (Landi et al., 2003); and NHL-related t(14;18) translocation prevalence and frequency in dioxin-exposed healthy people in Seveso (Baccarelli et al., 2006). Baccarelli et al. (2005b) reviewed statistical strategies for handling nondetectable readings or readings near the detection limit in dioxin-measurement datasets. They recommended that a distribution-based multiple-imputation method be used to analyze environmental data when substantial proportions of observations have nondetectable readings.

Baccarelli et al. (2008) reported on crude sex ratios, birth weight, and neonatal thyroid function for all births in 1994–2005 to women who were less than 18 years old at the time of the Seveso accident. Mocarelli et al. (2008) investigated TCDD's effects on reproductive hormones and sperm quality in a comparison of 135 young men exposed to TCDD by the 1976 Seveso accident with 184 age-matched healthy men who lived outside the contamination zones. Both groups were divided into three categories that reflected their ages at the time of the Seveso accident: infancy to prepuberty (1–9 years), puberty (10–17 years), and adulthood (18–26 years).

Pesatori et al. (2008) investigated the incidence of pituitary tumors in the Seveso population (804 in Zone A, 5,941 in Zone B, and 38,624 in Zone R) compared with the reference population in the surrounding, noncontaminated area (232,745). The hospital discharge-registration system of the Lombardy Region (where the study area is) was used to identify incident cases of pituitary adenoma during 1976–1996. All relevant medical records were reviewed to confirm the diagnosis for each case. Risk ratios and 95% confidence intervals were estimated by using Poisson regression and adjusting for age, sex, and calendar period and an assumed 10-year latent period for dioxin effects. Pesatori et al. (2009) reported on cancer incidence in a 20-year followup of the Seveso cohort covering the period 1977–1996. The study included all participants 0–74 years old who lived in the study area (723 in Zone A, 4,821 in Zone B, 31,643 in Zone R, and 181,574 in the reference zone) at the time of the accident. Participants who moved outside the study area were traced with a success rate of over 99% (Consonni et al., 2008). Emigration was homogeneous among zones and ranged from 4.7% to 6.7%. The difference in exposure among zones was corroborated by soil TCDD measurements, serum concentrations of TCDD, and TEQs. In the absence of a regionwide cancer registry, incident cancer cases were ascertained from the 120-hospital network of the Lombardy region, where the study area is. Original medical records were examined to identify true cases, to retrieve diagnoses as accurately as possible, and to determine the dates of occurrence. The study covered malignant tumors at any site and benign tumors of liver, bladder, and central nervous system first diagnosed after the date of the accident. For cohort members who were not hospitalized or who emigrated outside Lombardy, cancer cases were identified solely from death certificates, so nonfatal incident cases were missed. Risk ratios and 95% confidence intervals for Zones A, B, and R vs the reference zone were derived by using Poisson regression and adjusting for sex, age, and period.

Since *Update 2010*, Mocarelli et al. (2011) have reported on the sperm quality and hormone concentrations of sons born from March 1977 to January 1984 to women exposed to dioxin in Seveso (78 invited, 39 participated) compared with men of similar age and socioeconomic status whose mothers did not live in the dioxin-contaminated areas and were recruited from healthy volunteer permanent blood donors (123 invited, 58 participated). The exposed group was exposed both in utero (39) and parinatally through breastfeeding (21). Mothers' serum TCDD concentrations were measured by using serum samples collected in 1976–1977 and kept frozen since and extrapolated to the time of conception. The outcome measures included sperm concentration, total count, progressive motility, and total motility count based on semen samples and follicle-stimulating hormone concentration based on fasting blood sample. A general linear model was used to analyze sperm and hormone data—including exposure group, lactation class, and group × lactation interaction—adjusted for age, days in abstinence, smoking, chemical exposures, BMI, alcohol use, education level, and employment status. Scale transformations were taken on the outcome measures to achieve approximate normal distribution and homoscedasticity. Although the study was carefully designed and implemented, the low response rate raises concerns about possible selection bias.

Seveso Women's Health Study

The Seveso Women's Health Study (SWHS) was undertaken to evaluate the association between individual serum TCDD concentrations and reproductive effects in women who resided in Seveso at the time of the 1976 accident. From a pool of 1,271 eligible women who were between infancy and 40 years old at the time of the accident, who had resided in Zone A or B, and for whom adequate serum remained from the samples collected shortly after the explosion, 981 were enrolled in the study group in 1996–1998. The fairly adequate 80% participation rate resulted from 17 women being lost to followup, 21 having died, 12 being seriously ill, and almost 250 refusing. All the women were interviewed by a nurse blinded as to their exposure status, and a subset received gynecologic examinations. Medical records of those who reported ever having received a diagnosis of cancer were obtained and subjected to blind review by a pathologist. The stored samples were used for new TCDD analyses with improved analytic techniques that became available in recent years.

As an initial step in the SWHS, Eskenazi et al. (2001) tested the validity of exposure classification by zone. Investigators measured serum TCDD in samples collected in 1976–1980 from 601 residents (97 in Zone A and 504 in Zone B). A questionnaire that the women completed in 1996–1998 included age, chloracne history, animal mortality in the vicinity, consumption of homegrown food, and location at the time of the explosion. Participants did not know their TCDD concentrations at the time of the interview, but most knew their zones of residence. Interviewers and TCDD analysts were blinded to participants' zones of residence. Zone of residence explained 24% of the variability in serum TCDD. Addition of the questionnaire data improved the regression model, explaining 42% of the variability. Those findings demonstrate a significant association between zone of residence and serum TCDD, but much of the variability in TCDD concentration is still unexplained by the models. Warner et al. (2005) compared a chemical-activated luciferase-gene expression bioassay with an isotope-dilution high-resolution gas-chromatography–high-resolution mass-spectrometry assay to measure PCDDs, PCDFs, and polychlorinated biphenyls (PCBs) in serum of 78 women who resided near Seveso to determine average total dioxin-like chemical TEQs; similar results were obtained with the two methods.

The women enrolled in the SWHS were assessed for cancer incidence during the 20 years after the accident (Warner et al., 2002). A pathologist blinded as to exposure status reviewed medical records of the 21 women who reported in their initial interview (conducted between March 1996 and July1998) ever having received a cancer diagnosis; 15 of these diagnoses were for breast cancer, so analysis was limited to all cancers and to this cancer type. The remaining six cancers consisted of three cases of thyroid cancer, a melanoma, a kidney cancer, and an unspecified tumor. For each woman, the earliest post-accident blood samples with at least 0.5 mL remaining were analyzed for TCDD. The resulting readings were back-extrapolated to the time of the 1976 explosion, assuming a 9-year half-life, as derived from data obtained on Vietnam veterans in the AFHS (Pirkle et al., 1989). Cox estimation of hazard ratios (HRs) was conducted by using those values and the women's ages at diagnosis or when they were interviewed for the controls, and a test for trend was conducted over four exposure categories with partitions at 10, 20, and 44 TCDD ppt; the results for both tests were marginally significant for breast cancer ($p = 0.05$ and $p = 0.07$, respectively) and slightly weaker for all cancers. A broad spectrum of possible confounders was assessed, but they had to be tested individually in the model. The small number of cases observed was a consequence of the cohort's being relatively small (981) and young at the time of interview (72% less than 50 years old).

Warner et al. (2011) added more than 10 years of observation on cancer incidence in the women in the SWHS, updating the borderline significant results for breast cancer published earlier (Warner et al., 2002) to cover the period from the 1976 explosion through 2009. Of the 981 women participating in the earlier study, 833 were located, alive, and willing to participate. They all were reinterviewed, provided clinical measurements, and allowed access to medical records for confirmation; a subset was given bone-density tests. The average age was now 50.8 years. In the update, an additional 45 cancers had been diagnosed, making the total 66 cases, of which 33 were breast cancers. Thyroid cancer was the next most prevalent, with seven cases, and the 15 other types of cancer observed had at most three cases. After adjustment for age at the time of the accident and for marital status, the risk of any cancer in association with lipid-adjusted, log-transformed serum TCDD concentrations at the time of the accident was distinctly elevated (HR = 1.86; 95% CI 1.29–2.52). It was a small cohort, so the analyses that could be conducted were curtailed, but the availability of serum TCDD concentrations measured from blood samples gathered fairly soon after the single-substance accident (which minimizes uncertainty about what exposure had been experienced and reduces the need for back-extrapolation) contributes substantially to the value of the results.

A series of studies have examined associations between serum TCDD and a variety of endpoints related to female reproductive functioning: menstrual cycle (Eskenazi et al., 2002a); endometriosis (Eskenazi et al., 2002b); pregnancy outcome (Eskenazi et al., 2003a); age at exposure to the accident (Eskenazi et al., 2004); age at menarche and age at menopause (Eskenazi et al., 2005); and age at menarche in women who were premenarcheal at the time of the explosion (Warner et al., 2004). Eskenazi et al. (2007) and Warner et al. (2007) examined the incidence of fibroids and ovarian function, respectively, in SWHS participants. Eskanazi et al. (2007) excluded women who had received a diagnosis of fibroids before 1976, leaving a total of 956 women for analysis. Fibroids were ascertained in 634 women by self-report, medical records, and ultrasonography. Analyses were adjusted for confounding by parity, family history of fibroids, age at menarche, current BMI, smoking, alcohol consumption, and education. Warner et al. (2007) studied menstrual function in SWHS participants who were 20–40 years old and not taking oral contraceptives; the evaluations included ultrasonography (96 women), serum hormone concentrations (87 women), and the occurrence of ovulation (203 women).

Eskenazi et al. (2010) examined the relationship between serum TCDD around the time of the accident and time to pregnancy (TTP) in 472 SWHS participants who had attempted pregnancy since the accident. In addition to other eligibility criteria for SWHS, participants were eligible for the study if they were no more than 40 years old at the time of the accident. Nine women were excluded because of fertility-related problems, leaving 463 eligible women in the analysis sample. The main analysis was restricted to the 278 women who delivered live births that were not the results of contraceptive failure. Alternative analyses included various subsamples excluded in the main analysis. TTP for the first postaccident pregnancy was determined from responses in interviews conducted in 1996–1998 to the question "How many months did it take to become pregnant? In other words, for how many months had you been having sexual intercourse without doing anything to prevent pregnancy?" Women whose TTP was 12 months or more were classified as infertile. Initial serum TCDD concentrations at the time of the accident were measured in stored samples from 444 participants (431 collected in 1976–1977 and 13 collected in 1978–1981). For 19 participants with insufficient stored samples, new samples were collected in 1996 or 1997. For the 27 women with detectable post-1977 TCDD measurements, TCDD was back-extrapolated to 1976 by using the Filser model (Kreuzer et al., 1997). Initial serum TCDD concentrations were extrapolated to the time when each woman initiated her attempt to become pregnant; Kreuzer et al. (1997) used a toxicokinetic model for women 16 years old or younger at the time of the accident, and Pirkle et al. (1989) used a first-order kinetic model that assumed a 9-year half-life. The association between serum TCDD and TTP was assessed by using a Cox proportional-hazards model to estimate the fecundability odds ratios (ORs) and 95% confidence intervals. The association between serum TCDD and infertility was assessed by using multiple logistic regression. Both models were adjusted for maternal age, maternal smoking in the year before conception, parity, menstrual-cycle irregularity, oral-contraceptive use in the year before attempt, paternal age near the time of conception, and history of reproductive and endocrine conditions, including pelvic infection and thyroid or urogenital problems. A variety of sensitivity analyses were conducted to investigate the consistency of study findings and to check for possible bias. Initial serum TCDD and extrapolated serum TCDD were specified as continuous variables on the logarithmic scale and as categorical variables.

US Environmental Studies

National Health and Nutrition Examination Survey

In the early 1960s, the CDC National Center for Health Statistics began the NHANES program as a means of monitoring and assessing the health and nutritional status of people of all ages living in the United States. In 1999, the survey became a continuous program that has a changing focus on a variety of health and nutrition measurements to meet emerging needs. A rich variety of data—demographic and socioeconomic data; dietary information; medical, dental, and physiologic assessments; and serum concentrations of persistent organic pollutants (POPs), including specific congeners of dioxins, furans, and PCBs—are collected through in-person interviews, health examinations, and blood samples obtained from a nationally representative sample of adults and children in the noninstitutionalized US population. Information obtained from NHANES data is used to determine prevalences of diseases, to assess nutritional status, and to establish national standards of height, weight, and blood pressure. Researchers also conduct analyses of the NHANES data for epidemiologic studies and health-science research on serum concentrations of various compounds in association with various health outcomes.

NHANES data from 1999–2002 were used to evaluate cardiovascular disease (Ha et al., 2007) and hypertension (Everett et al., 2008a,b). Lee DH et al. (2006, 2007a,b,c) used data from the same years to evaluate several health outcomes, including diabetes, the metabolic syndrome, insulin resistance, and arthritis. Turyk et al. (2007) analyzed NHANES data from 1999–2002 and 2001–2002 to evaluate associations with thyroid-hormone concentrations. Since *Update 2008*, several new publications have used NHANES data in reporting on associations between the COIs and various health outcomes.

Lee et al. (2008) examined the associations between serum concentrations of POPs and the prevalence of peripheral neuropathy and poor glycemic control (A1C ≥ 7.0%) in NHANES 1999–2002 participants who were at least 40 years old and had diabetes or impaired fasting glucose. Peripheral neuropathy is ascertained on the basis of one or more insensate sites on the foot. Diabetes is ascertained on the basis of high plasma glucose (≥ 126 mg/dL fasting or ≥ 200 mg/dL nonfasting) or on the basis of whether a person is taking insulin or an oral anti-diabetes agent. Although 49 POPs were measured, analysis was restricted to 25, of which at least 60% of study participants had detectable concentrations: three PCDDs, four PCDFs, five dioxin-like PCBs, seven non–dioxin-like PCBs, and six organochlorine (OC) pesticides. Logistic regression was used to determine the OR between each outcome (peripheral neuropathy or poor glycemic control) and each exposure to POP subclass with adjustment for age, sex, race or ethnicity, poverty, duration of diabetes, hypertension (yes or no), BMI, cigarette-smoking (never, former, or current), cotinine concentration, alcohol consumption, leisure-time physical activity (vigorous, moderate, or none), and A1C (neuropathy only). For each POP subclass, a cumulative measure was derived by summing the rank scores among individual chemicals that belonged to the subclass; the cumulative measure was then categorized into tertiles. Additional analyses were conducted for individual compounds by using the correlation coefficient between the rank score for each chemical and each outcome with adjustment for the same covariates listed above.

Ha et al. (2009) examined the association between serum concentrations of POPs and the prevalence of newly diagnosed hypertension in NHANES 1999–2002 adult participants 40 years old or older. After exclusion of 444 patients known to be hypertensive irrespective of antihypertensive medication, 165 diabetic patients, and 49 subjects whose blood-pressure values were missing, the final sample size was 524. Participants were considered to have hypertension if their systolic blood pressure was 140 mm Hg or higher or if their diastolic blood pressure was 90 mm Hg or higher. The analysis was restricted to 21 POPs of which at least 60% of study participants had detectable concentrations: three PCDDs, three PCDFs, five dioxin-like PCBs, six non–dioxin-like PCBs, and four OC pesticides. The discrepancy from Lee et al. (2008) in the number of POPs detected is probably due to the difference in the samples used. For each POP, participants whose serum concentrations were below the limit of detection were regarded as the reference group; participants who had detectable concentrations were categorized into quartiles. A cumulative measure for each POP subclass was derived by summing the category numbers (0 for nondetectable, 1 for detectable below the first quartile, and so on up to 4 for above the third quartile) of individual chemicals belonging to the subclass. The summary values were again categorized into quartiles. Logistic regression was used to derive adjusted ORs, which were stratified by sex and adjusted for age, race or ethnicity, poverty–income ratio, BMI, cigarette-smoking (never, former, or current), cotinine, alcohol consumption, and leisure-time physical activity (vigorous, moderate, or none).

Schreinemachers (2010) examined the association in healthy adults between exposure to 2,4-D, as indicated by its presence in urine, and biomarkers that are linked to the pathogenesis of acute MI and type 2 diabetes, namely, serum high-density lipoprotein (HDL), triglycerides, total cholesterol minus HDL, insulin, C-peptide, plasma glucose, and thyroid-stimulating hormone. Study participants, 20–59 years old, were selected from a subset of the NHANES III (1988–1994) sample. The study sample is regarded as a convenient sample rather than a representative sample of the US population because volunteers were recruited without a formal statistical sampling procedure. Among 1,338 candidate participants for the study, 375 were excluded because data on urinary 2,4-D were missing, and 236 were excluded on the basis of study exclusion criteria: history of congestive heart failure, heart attack, diabetes, thyroid disease, lupus, or cancer; a white blood cell count over 12×10^9 per liter, C-reactive protein over 10 mg/dL, or glycosylated hemoglobin (HbA1c) over 8%. Among the remaining 727 study participants, urinary 2,4-D was detectable in 102 (14%), with concentrations of 1–28 mg/dL. The outcome variables were compared between participants with and without detectable urinary 2,4-D by using Wilcoxon's rank-sum test. Further analysis was conducted with linear regression, and the outcome variables were transformed to a logarithmic scale. The linear-regression models included the following explanatory variables: 2,4-D (binary), HDL (continuous, log-transformed, and included in all models except when HDL itself was the dependent variable), urinary creatinine (continuous and log-transformed), sex, age, BMI, race or ethnicity, and smoking (none, past, and active). Alcohol consumption, education, household income, and hours of fasting before a blood sample was drawn were also checked for their effects on the regression coefficient for urinary 2,4-D. The analyses were conducted on the final study sample of 727 and on two subsamples that were expected to be more susceptible: participants who had HbA1c above the median (5.1%) of the total sample and participants who had thyroxine at or below the median (8.5 µg/dL) of the total sample.

Since *Update 2010*, several new NHANES studies have been published. Cho et al. (2011) reported on the associations between bone mineral density (BMD) and exposures to POPs, including OC pesticides, assessed from serum samples from NHANES participants in 1999–2004 (2,769 for OC pesticide analyses and 2,565 for POP analyses). The study also examined whether the POP levels modified the association between BMD and fat mass or lean mass. All analyses were stratified by sex and age group (cutoff 50 years). General linear models were used to derive adjusted means, adjusted for age, race or ethnicity, poverty–income ratio, fat mass, lean mass, height, smoking, physical activity, and postmenopausal hormone intake.

Elobeid et al. (2010) examined the association between POPs and obesity—BMI and waist circumference (WC)—in NHANES 1999–2002 participants (2,464 for BMI analysis and 2,448 for WC). Regression models were used to assess the association between the obesity measures and POPs, adjusted for sex, ethnicity, age, and age squared. An additional model for WC also adjusts for BMI.

Jones et al. (2011) examined the association between urinary arsenic and hypertension and blood pressure in NHANES 2003–2008 participants (4,167). Logistic-regression and linear-regression models were used for hypertension and blood pressure, respectively, adjusted for age, sex, race or ethnicity, urinary creatinine, education, BMI, and serum cotinine; models for blood pressure also adjusted for antihypertensive medication. All analyses accounted for the complex sample design for NHANES.

Anniston, Alabama, Community Health Survey In 2003, the Agency for Toxic Substances and Disease Registry (ATSDR) funded a study of the health effects of environmental exposures on the residents of Anniston, Alabama. Anniston housed a plant that produced PCBs from 1929 to 1971; it had been owned and operated by Monsanto since 1935. Residents of Anniston were known to have high concentrations of PCBs although these have not been found to be associated with employment in the plant or consumption of local fish and produce. PCBs have spread in Anniston via air, soil, and water movement. Before the ATSDR study, there had been minimal study of the health effects of PCBs on Anniston residents. Residents were recruited into the study through a stratified random sampling of housing units across the city weighted by proximity to the plant and by race. Of the 1,110 who agreed to be interviewed, 772 had blood drawn for biochemical and PCB analyses and had blood pressure measured. Of the 758 subjects who provided sufficient data to be retained in the study, 364 were taking antihypertensive medications and 394 were not.

Two methods were considered for PCB analysis: wet-weight values and lipid-standardized values. The latter are thought to be more prone to bias, but both were considered. Having two approaches makes comparisons between studies difficult. Another issue was the problem of PCB values that were below the level of detection (LOD). They amount to left-censored covariates in a regression model. They were dealt with by crude imputation of the LOD divided by the square root of 2 (Goncharov et al., 2010; Silverstone et al., 2012) or by 2 (Goncharov et al., 2011). This is highly biased, and alternative methods (such as multiple imputation) would have been preferable. It is also potentially problematic that the studies took different approaches.

Goncharov et al. (2010) studied the association between all PCBs and blood pressure. After adjustment for age there was a significant association between PCB concentrations and risk of hypertension. When people on antihypertensive medications were included in the models, the associations between PCB concentrations and risk of hypertension were diluted; this could be due to an effect of the medications on PCB metabolism.

Goncharov et al. (2011) extended the 2010 report by considering the effect of PCBs on the entire range of continuous blood pressure and by investigating 5 PCB groups and 33 individual PCB congeners. Only the 394 people who were not on antihypertensive medications were included in this study. The study found that serum PCB concentration is associated with blood pressure even in the normotensive range. Furthermore, the relationship was found to be strongest for ortho-substituted PCB congeners that have two or more chlorines and with some that have some dioxin-like activity. The overall concentrations of PCBs are higher in the Anniston population than in the US population overall.

Silverstone et al. (2012) examined the association between PCB exposure and diabetes in the Anniston study. Diabetes was present in 27% of 774 participants; 75% of the 27 were taking glycemic control medications. People who had prediabetes were identified and were excluded from some regression analyses because they were intermediate between the diabetic and normoglycemic groups. There was a nonmonotonic increase in the prevalence of diabetes with high PCB congener concentrations, but some of the groups (for example, by age) were small. Women had a consistently higher likelihood of diabetes in each subset of

PCBs (except the estrogenic subset). The findings suggest a low-dose PCB effect inasmuch as the ORs increased in the second quintile of PCB exposure and remained high. Advantages of this study are its adjustment for family history of diabetes and exclusion of people who had prediabetes. Lipid metabolism in people who have diabetes may affect the metabolism of PCBs.

Center for the Health Assessment of Mothers and Children of Salinas Cohort Castorina et al. (2010) compared metabolites of current-use pesticides and other precursor compounds in 538 women in the Center for the Health Assessment of Mothers and Children of Salinas (CHAMACOS) cohort with those in 342 pregnant women in NHANES 1999–2002. CHAMACOS (Eskenazi et al., 2003b) is a longitudinal birth-cohort study investigating the effect of in utero and postnatal environmental exposures on the health of children who live in the Salinas Valley of Monterey County, California. The study enrolled 601 pregnant women from September 1999 to November 2000 in six prenatal clinics in the largely agricultural Salinas area. Women were eligible if they were no more than 20 weeks into gestation, were at least 18 years old, were qualified to receive poverty-based government health insurance, and planned to continue receiving prenatal care in a participating clinic. Personal interviews were conducted during which information on demographics, household characteristics, health, and occupations of CHAMACOS participants was collected. Two interviews were conducted shortly after enrollment (mean, 13 weeks of gestation; SD, 5.2 weeks) and later in the second trimester (mean, 26 weeks of gestation; SD, 2.6 weeks) by bilingual (English and Spanish), bicultural study staff. At each prenatal interview, spot urine samples were collected from CHAMACOS participants and analyzed for metabolites, including organophosphorus, OC chemicals, pyrethroid pesticides, herbicides, and ethylene bisdithiocarbamate fungicides. Adequate urine samples with valid creatinine concentrations were collected from 538 (90%) of the 601 participants at the first sampling point and 481 (80%) at the second. In addition, pesticide-use data were extracted from the California-pesticide use reporting dataset and geocoded into square-mile units. NHANES reported concentrations of current-use pesticide metabolites measured in spot urine collected from representative samples of the US population stratified by age, sex, and racial or ethnic group (Barr et al., 2005; CDC, 2004). The NHANES comparison group consisted of 342 pregnant women 15–50 years old, a subset of the 3,048 US residents 6–59 years old who had metabolite concentrations measured in urine samples during NHANES testing in 1999 and 2002. The public-release versions of the NHANES data-sets, including demographic information and metabolite data, were used for the analyses. No sample weights were applied to the NHANES data. Descriptive analyses were conducted on the CHAMACOS and NHANES cohorts. Metabolite concentrations were compared between the two cohorts with a Wilcoxon rank-sum test and quantile regression at the 95th percentile adjusted for demographic variables, including age, current smoking (yes or no), ethnicity, and socioeconomic status. Analysis of variance was used to compare differences in detection frequency.

Coronary Artery Risk Development in Young Adults Study Lee et al. (2010) reported on the association between low-dose POPs and type 2 diabetes in the Coronary Artery Risk Development in Young Adults (CARDIA) cohort. Serum samples were collected at year 2 (1987–1988) and were later used to measure POPs. This was a nested case-control study in which subjects were required to be free of diabetes at years 0 and 2. From 1988 to 2006, 116 received a diagnosis of diabetes; 90 were randomly selected as cases. Controls were randomly selected from those who had not received a diagnosis of diabetes. Cases and controls were frequency-matched on BMI strata. The authors analyzed summary measures of POPs. The second summary measure selected POPs on the basis of their effect in the current study; this invalidates standard inference. The authors asserted that summary measures are useful because appropriate controls are those with globally low concentrations of POPs. Other limitations are the single measure of POPs and the age of the samples at analysis (18 years). The authors stated that the study was underpowered and that extensive statistical testing was performed.

Lee et al. (2011a) further investigated the 90 controls selected for the nested case-control study reported in Lee et al. (2010). This investigation is concerned with associations between exposure to POPs and obesity, dyslipidemia, and insulin resistance in people who are free of diabetes. Multiple comparisons are of concern, as is the small sample size.

Great Lakes Fish Consumption Study The Great Lakes Fish Consumption Study was initiated in early 1992. Bloom et al. (2006) measured serum dioxin in New York sport fishermen as part of a study of thyroid function. A methodologic study by Petreas et al. (2004) found generally high correlations between concentrations of dioxins and related chemicals in breast and abdominal fat in the same woman; this suggested that they could be used interchangeably in epidemiologic studies. The same study, however, also found that adjusting concentrations according to lipid content rather than weight of the fat samples is important because of the presence of nonlipid components in the samples.

In 2001–2005, 1,788 of the 4,200 people who had participated in the original study were contacted and asked for updated information on health, reproductive history, and fish consumption. Blood samples gathered from 515 of them were analyzed for serum concentrations of various POPs, including a number of PCBs. Turyk et al. (2009) investigated whether the serum results were related to self-reported diabetes. Lambertino et al. (2011) studied the self-reported occurrences of uterine leiomyomas (benign fibroid tumors) in 580 women using the serum results from the 197 women who had provided blood samples. The exposure measure for the category “dioxin-like PCBs” consisted of the summed concentrations of only the mono-ortho PCBs 118 and 167. Because results were based solely on mono-ortho PCBs, which typically contribute only a small percentage to total TEQs, the findings of these publications cannot be considered conclusive.

Pensacola, Florida Karouna-Renier et al. (2007) examined health effects related to dioxins and furans in soil at a Superfund site in Pensacola, Florida, that was contaminated by operations at a wood-treating company that operated from 1942 to 1982. In 2001, the study collected health and exposure histories and measured serum concentrations of 17 PCDD and PCDF congeners in 47 potentially exposed people who were selected nonsystematically from among former workers, their families, and residents. Logistic regression was used to predict the prevalence of health outcomes from TEQs with adjustment for age, race, sex, BMI, tobacco and alcohol use, and worker status.

Times Beach and Quail Run Cohorts

Several reports have provided information on environmental exposure to TCDD in the Times Beach area of Missouri (Andrews et al., 1989; Patterson et al., 1986), one of the incidents that heightened concerns about the health effects of dioxin. In 1971, TCDD-contaminated sludge from a hexachlorophene-production facility was mixed with waste oil and sprayed in various areas for dust control. Soil contamination in some samples exceeded 100 parts per billion. Among the Missouri sites with the highest soil TCDD concentrations was the Quail Run mobile-home park. Residents were considered exposed if they had lived in the park for at least 6 months during the time when contamination occurred (Hoffman et al., 1986).

Of 51 exposed participants, 87% had adipose-tissue TCDD concentrations below 200 ppt; however, TCDD concentrations in seven of the 51 were 250–750 ppt. In 128 nonexposed control participants, adipose-tissue TCDD ranged from undetectable to 20 ppt (median, 6 ppt). On the basis of a 7-year half-life, it is calculated that two study participants would have had adipose-tissue TCDD near 3,000 ppt at the time of their last exposure (Andrews et al., 1989).

Several studies evaluated health effects potentially attributable to exposure (Evans et al., 1988; Hoffman et al., 1986; Stehr et al., 1986; Stehr-Green et al., 1987; Stockbauer et al., 1988; Webb et al., 1987). Those studies were reviewed in *VAO*; no further work on the cohorts has been published.

Danish Environmental Studies

Halldorsson et al. (2009) studied the association between consumption of fatty fish, as a source of environmental exposure to dioxins and dioxin-like chemicals, and birthweight and development in 100 healthy pregnant women 25–35 years old selected from the Danish National Birth Cohort, which includes 101,046 women (Olsen et al., 2001). The 9,815 eligible women were stratified according to the frequency of fatty-fish intake (low, zero meals per month; medium, one to three; and high, over three); 34, 33, and 33 were randomly sampled in three strata, respectively. Four standardized CATIs (at gestation weeks 12 and 30 and at 6 and 18 months postpartum) were used to collect information on parental lifestyle and health. Participants received a food-frequency questionnaire in week 25 of gestation, and two maternal blood samples were collected during routine visits to a general practitioner. The blood samples were analyzed for CALUX-TEQs in picograms per gram of lipid. Birth outcomes (weight, length, and head circumference) based on measurements taken by the midwives who attended the births were extracted from the Danish National Birth Registry. Developmental milestones (such as sitting without support and crawling) were obtained from the telephone interviews conducted when the children were 5.7–7 months old. A total-development scale was derived by summing the indicators of the 13 milestones. Linear mixed models (with the multiple plasma samples specified as an individual-level random effect) were used to estimate the association between CALUX-TEQ and birth weight with adjustment for gestational age, infant sex, and maternal smoking. Logistic regression was used for the association between CALUX-TEQ (dichotomized into high and low relative to the sample median) and infant development milestones with adjustment for gestational age, duration of breastfeeding, infant age at interview, and maternal fish intake. Spearman rank correlation was used for the association between CALUX-TEQ and the total-development scale.

Finnish Environmental Studies

Turunen et al. (2008) studied mortality in 6,410 fishermen and their 4,260 wives in Finland in comparison with national mortality figures (standardized by sex, age, and period), assuming that the difference in mortality reflects the high consumption of contaminated fish by fishermen and their wives. A small subsample (88 fishermen and 94 wives) participated in a substudy of fish consumption and life habit and provided blood samples that were analyzed for nutrients and environmental contaminants, including dioxins and PCBs. The substudy found higher fish consumption and higher serum dioxins and PCBs in fishermen and their wives than in the general population studied in the 2000 health survey. However, the validity of the findings of the mortality study is limited by various types of confounding, including possible health benefits of fish consumption by fishermen and their wives and a possible healthy-worker effect in the cases of fishermen.

French Environmental Studies

Viel et al. (2000) reported on an investigation of apparent clusters of cases of STS and NHL in the vicinity of a municipal solid-waste incinerator (MSWI) in

Doubs, France. The presumptive source of TCDD in the region is an MSWI in the Besançon electoral ward in western Doubs. Dioxin emissions from the incinerator were measured in international TEQ units at 16.3 ng/m^3, far in excess of the European Union (EU) standard of 0.1 ng/m^3. TCDD concentrations in cow's milk measured on three farms near the incinerator were well below the EU guideline of 6 ng/kg of fat, but the concentrations were highest on the farm closest to the incinerator. Floret et al. (2003) examined the same population and investigated rates of NHL in Besançon, France. Cases were identified from a cancer registry of people who had a diagnosis of NHL in 1980–1995. Viel et al. (2008a) examined the same population and reported a case-control study conducted in 434 women who had breast cancer compared with 2,170 community controls selected according to the proximity of their residence to emissions from the waste incinerator.

Viel et al. (2008b) expanded the previous work and studied the association between NHL and dioxin exposure from MSWIs in four French administrative departments (Isère, Bas-Rhin, Haut-Rhin, and Tarn), which were covered by a population-based cancer registry. (The study did not include the area of previous studies, Doubs, which is a separate administrative department.) The study was conducted with geostatistical analysis at the level of block groups and compared exposures and outcomes in the 2,270 block groups in the area. The block groups had an average surface area of 9.45 km^2. The cases considered for this study were in people 15 years old and older who had received a diagnosis of NHL during the period 1990–1999 and were living in the study area at the time of their diagnosis. Anonymous data were extracted from cancer registries on date of birth, sex, date of diagnosis, address at the time of diagnosis, and cancer category. The block group for each case was geocoded by using the residential address.

A second-generation Gaussian atmospheric-dispersion model (ADMS 3) was used to derive "immission" estimates (defined by the researchers as "the amount of pollutant reaching a particular location as a result of—and in contrast to—the emission coming out the chimney") for dioxins, metals, and dusts in the area near each of 13 MSWIs operating in the study area. That involved a receptor grid of 200 m that was based on emission estimates for the MSWI, plant characteristics (chimney height and diameter, emission temperature, particle size, and density), topography indicators (roughness and relief), local meteorologic conditions, and so on. For each of the 2,270 block groups, the median of all immission estimates for receptors in the block group was used as the immission for the block group. For block groups under the plumes of multiple MSWIs, the sum of the immission estimates was used. A cumulative ground-level dioxin concentration estimate was derived for each block group by using the immission estimates transformed to account for the number of years that the plant had operated and the degradation rate in the soil. Poisson regression was applied at the block-group level to assess the association between observed number of NHL cases in each block group and the dioxin concentration (with a square-root transformation) estimated for the block group and adjusted for population density, urbanization, socioeconomic level, airborne traffic pollution, and industrial pollution.

Since *Update 2010*, Viel et al. (2011) have reported a new case-control study of NHL in a study area consisting of three electoral wards (170,000 people) that contained the Besançon MSWI. Cases (53 eligible, 34 participated) were identified from the local university hospital. Controls (34) were matched 1:1, randomly selected from blood donors living in the area matched on sex, age (± 5 years), and date of blood draw (± 1 year); 5 refusals were replaced. A wide spectrum of OCs was measured in a fasting blood sample drawn from each participant. Exact logistic-regression models were used to assess the association between NHL and exposure measures.

Cordier et al. (2004, 2010) studied the risk of birth defects attributable to environmental dioxins released from MSWIs in the Rhône-Alpes region (Lyon and surrounding areas) in southern France. The studies partially overlapped the areas studied by Viel et al. (2008b): all three studies included the administrative department of Isère.

Cordier et al. (2004) conducted a geostatistical analysis at the level of communities (official municipalities), studying 2,872 communities, each with fewer than 50,000 residents. Birth defects during the study period, 1988–1997, were identified from a population-based birth-defects registry (the French Central-East Registry). There were 70 MSWIs that operated in the study region for at least a year during the study period. Immission scores were derived by using a Gaussian plume model (POLAIR) for dioxin concentrations in kilometer grids within 10 km of the plants and using plant emission estimates, chimney heights, and local meteorologic data. For each community, the immission score at the geographic point with the highest population density was used as the contemporaneous exposure index for the community. (That is a bit different from the usual practice of using the population centroid for the community.) In addition, a cumulative exposure index was derived by multiplying the contemporaneous exposure index by the number of years that the plant was in operation. A total of 194 communities were classified as exposed, and the remaining 2,678 communities as nonexposed. In the exposed communities, only births after the start of the MSWI were considered in the analysis. Poisson regression was used to derive the relative risk of congenital malformations with adjustment for year of birth, maternal age, department of birth, population density, average family income, and (when available) local road traffic.

Cordier et al. (2010) examined the same population with a case-control study in 2001–2003, comparing 304 infants who had urinary tract birth defects with a random sample of 226 population controls that were frequency-matched for infant sex and year and district of birth. Of 353 cases identified in the birth-defects registry, 304 were located, and 187 were interviewed. The modest response rate (53% of all cases, although the authors claimed a higher response rate of 62%, excluding 49 cases not located) may compromise the validity of the study findings. The controls were recruited through CATIs that attempted to reach 3,000 telephone numbers in the region presumed to belong to families with children; this resulted in 226 control participants after 1,989 ineligible candidates were excluded. Exposure estimates for dioxins, furans, and metals in areas near each MSWI (in 100-m grids) were derived by using Gaussian modeling software (ADMS 3) that took into account emissions, plant characteristics (chimney height and diameter, emission temperature and speed, and distribution between gaseous and particulate phases), and local meteorologic conditions. Participants were classified as exposed or nonexposed; those exposed were further classified into above or below the median. Multiple logistic regression was used to estimate the association between dioxin exposure and urinary tract birth defects, with adjustment for stratification variables (child's sex and year and district of birth). Potential confounders were selected by using backward selection, including community characteristics (population density, deprivation score, and industrial dioxin sources besides MSWIs), maternal age, parental geographic origin, educational level, employment status during pregnancy, treatment for chronic disease during the first trimester, folic acid supplementation, history of urinary tract birth defects in first-degree relatives, parity, obesity, tobacco and alcohol use during pregnancy, and environmental tobacco-smoke exposure.

Japanese Environmental Studies

From 2002 to 2006, Ueruma et al. (2008a,b) assembled a stratified sample of 1,374 Japanese 15–73 years old (627 men and 747 women) who represented urban, farming, and fishing areas of the entire country. The participants completed questionnaires on occupational, medical, smoking, and residential histories and height and weight. They also provided blood samples that were analyzed with isotope-dilution high-resolution gas chromatography–mass spectrometry for PCDDs, PCDFs, and dioxin-like PCBs. Ueruma et al. (2008a) investigated the relationship of those chemicals with the prevalence of diabetes, defined as self-reported physician-diagnosed diabetes or occurrence of plasma HbA1c greater than 6.1% as a predictor of fasting plasma glucose above 126 mg/dL. Ueruma et al. (2008b) presented summary statistics on the serum concentrations of the individual chemicals in the blood of the study participants and on their distributions with respect to various demographic characteristics; they also provided the results of log-transformed correlation analyses of all PCDDs and PCDFs combined, of all dioxin-like PCBs, and of total TEQ with total cholesterol, high-density lipoprotein, and triglycerides.

Uemura et al. (2009) conducted further studies of the same cohort and examined the association of body burdens of dioxins and related chemicals with the prevalence of metabolic syndrome, assessed by using a modification of the National Cholesterol Education Program Adult Treatment Panel III definition (NCEP, 2002) to accommodate differences between Asian and Caucasian populations (Ko et al., 2005; Tan et al., 2004). In particular, participants were classified as having metabolic syndrome if they satisfied three or more of the following five criteria: BMI of at least 25 kg/m^2 (rather than abdominal waist circumference), serum triglycerides of at least 150 mg/dL, serum HDL under 40 mg/dL in men or under 50 mg/dL in women, systolic blood pressure of at least 130 mm Hg or diastolic blood pressure of at least 85 mm Hg or self-reported history of physician-diagnosed hypertension, and HbA1c of at least 5.6% (rather than fasting serum glucose) or self-reported history of physician-diagnosed diabetes. Logistic regression was used to assess the associations between exposures (TEQs for PCDDs, PCDFs, and dioxin-like PCBs and total TEQs) and the prevalence of metabolic syndrome, both adjusted and not adjusted for age, sex, smoking and drinking habits, regional block, residential area, and survey year. The analysis was conducted with and without prevalent diabetes cases. Further analyses were conducted for the adjusted associations of the TEQs with the five components of metabolic syndrome and the adjusted associations of the concentrations of the 16 selected congeners of which more than 75% of the subjects had detectable concentrations with the prevalence of metabolic syndrome.

Yusho Disease Group

Tsukimori et al. (2012) reported on the association between mother's dioxin exposure and children's birthweight in Japanese women affected by Yosho disease after an accidental exposure to rice oil contaminated with PCBs, PCDFs, and PCDDs in western Japan in 1968 that affected over 1,900 people. Of 737 affected women officially registered with the Study Group for Yusho, 206 reported having given birth after the Yusho incident. Of them, 101 (with 190 eligible births) had their dioxin concentrations measured and participated in the mother–child study. Maternal serum concentrations of contaminants were assessed, converted into TEQs, and extrapolated to the time of delivery. Multiple linear-regression models were used to examine the association between birth weight and maternal serum contaminant concentrations, log-transformed to account for their lognormal distributions. The models adjusted for potential confounders for birth weight, including maternal age, parity, maternal smoking during pregnancy, gestation age at delivery, infant sex, duration of breast feeding, number of births, and frequency of seafood consumption.

Norwegian Environmental Studies

Stolevik et al. (2011) reported on prenatal exposure to PCBs and increased risk of wheeze, eczema, and infections in newborns in the birth subcohort of the Norwegian Mother and Child Cohort Study. Maternal exposure to PCBs was determined from a validated food-frequency questionnaire that covered the first 4 months of pregnancy and that was adapted to include rarely eaten foods that are known to have high concentrations of PCBs and dioxins. Pregnant women were invited to enter the study in 2007–2008. Outcomes were determined through a questionnaire sent to the mothers at 1 year. Confounders in the statistical analyses were taken from the questionnaires filled out by the mothers during pregnancy and 6 months after birth. They included previous breastfeeding, parity, history of atopy, age, smoking, education, BMI, child's sex, and others. Logistic regression with backward selection was used to fit multivariate models. There is concern about selection bias because of the low participation rate (38.5%).

Russian Environmental Studies

Chapaevsk

Several studies in the Samara region of Russia have identified the Middle Volga Chemical Plant (also known as SZVH or Khimprom) in Chapaevsk, about 950 km southeast of Moscow, as a major source of TCDD pollution (Revazova et al., 2001; Revich et al., 2001). From 1967 to 1987, the plant produced γ-hexachlorocyclohexane (lindane) and its derivatives, and many of the workers experienced chloracne. Since then, it has produced various chlorinated products. Dioxins were detected in the small number of air, soil, drinking-water, and cow's-milk samples gathered in the region, but no description of how these media were sampled was given. When Revich et al. (2001) compared them with measurements from four other Russian cities that had industrial facilities, the TCDD concentrations observed in Chapaevsk exceeded all reported maximums. Revich et al. (2001) presented rudimentary comparisons of cancer incidence and mortality and reproductive outcomes with regional and national rates; residence in the city of Chapaevsk was used as a surrogate for exposure, and no attempt was made to create exposure categories based on factors that might have influenced the degree of TCDD exposure. The analyses of chromosomal aberrations and other cytologic indicators of genetic damage did partition the women studied into three groups on the basis of worker status or distance of residence from the factory (Revazova et al., 2001).

Chapaevsk Children's Study

Later research efforts on Chapaevsk residents have focused on quantifying serum concentrations of dioxins and TEQs associated with furans and PCBs. Akhmedkhanov et al. (2002) reported on a convenience sample of 24 volunteers. A cohort of 499 peripubertal boys (8–9 years old in 2003–2005) and their mothers has been established as the Russian Children's Study for assessing the effect of in utero and childhood exposure on development. The information generated by this study will be relevant to VAO reports only in conjunction with effects in offspring after maternal exposure to the extent that the consequences of gestational and childhood exposure can be distinguished. To date, however, published findings have not involved health outcomes but have been limited to detailed characterizations of serum concentrations in the boys (Burns et al., 2009, 2011) and their mothers (Humblet et al., 2010).

Swedish Environmental Studies

Prospective Investigation of the Vasculature in Uppsala Seniors (PIVUS)

The PIVUS study recruited participants, within 2 months after their 70th birthdays, randomly from the registry of residents of the community of Uppsala, Sweden, from April 2001 to June 2004. The primary aim was to investigate cardiovascular disease in an elderly population with adjustment for sex. Of the 2,025 subjects who were invited to participate, 1,016 were included, for a participation rate of about 50%; 50% were female. All participants answered a questionnaire about medical history, medication, diet, and smoking habits. The burden of POPs, including several dioxin-like PCBs, was assessed from blood serum or plasma.

Salihovic et al. (2012a) reported on circulating concentrations of POPs in 992 participants with valid measurements. They found significant sex differences in the concentrations of 17 of 21 POPs; women had higher concentrations of five of them. Appropriate adjustment for multiple comparisons (via Holm's method) was applied. Salihovic et al. (2012b) investigated a new method for extraction of POPs from human blood in the PIVUS study and found it to be robust.

Lee et al. (2011b) reported on the association between POPs and type 2 diabetes in the subjects of the PIVUS study. Of the 1,016 evaluated at baseline, 81% returned 5 years later at age 75. The cross-sectional study (baseline) included 989, and 725 were in the prospective analysis. The additional value of POPs on top of standard risk factors was evaluated with the C-statistic and the net reclassification index and the improved discrimination index. The cross-sectional analyses could not account for any measure of duration of exposure. The results are limited by the small number of incident diabetes cases (36), the multiple testing, and the correlation of POPs (and the ensuing difficulty of interpretation of association with diabetes).

Ronn et al. (2011) reported on associations of POPs with fat mass in the PIVUS study. Multiple imputation was used to handle missing dietary assessments. A strength of the study is its use of DXA screening to measure fat. There was considerable multiple testing without adjustment. The findings are limited by the cross-sectional design and the limited age of participants inasmuch as age could affect the findings in several ways; the published paper could report on only one subset of findings for this age group.

Lee et al. (2012a) reported on associations of POPs with abdominal obesity in the PIVUS study. Abdominal obesity was treated as a binary variable. The authors note concerns with residual confounding due to diet and physical activity. Furthermore, greater food consumption may lead to obesity and increased concentrations of chemicals. There could be alterations in pharmacodynamics of POPs because of health disorders, which themselves may influence obesity.

Lee et al. (2012b) reported on associations of POPS with stroke in the PIVUS study. Only hospital-treated strokes were considered. Ischemic and hemorrhagic strokes were not distinguished. There were 35 incident strokes during the 5 years of followup. Sex might be an important effect modifier, but the sample was too small to assess this. The POPs in this study may not be causally related to stroke but rather their concentrations may be correlated with other, causal POPs. The study was not able to use time of stroke in a survival analysis, which would have been a more powerful analysis.

Lind et al. (2012) reported on associations of POPs with carotid atherosclerosis in the PIVUS study. Ordinal logistic regression was used to model the ordinal outcome of number of involved arteries. A Bonferroni adjustment for multiple testing was applied.

Taiwanese Environmental Studies

Taiwan Residents Around Closed PCP Factory

Chang et al. (2010) reported on exposure to PCDDs and PCDFs and hypertension in metabolic syndrome in 1,490 nondiabetic Taiwanese who lived near a highly dioxin-contaminated area. This was a cross-sectional study (2005–2007) that accrued subjects from a health center near a deserted PCP factory. The sample constituted about 80% of the invited residents of the community. Univariate analyses of association with several components of metabolic syndrome were conducted, as was principal component factor analysis to identify a set of uncorrelated factors from among components of metabolic syndrome. Multiple regression models were fitted for each component. In addition, an analysis of association between each congener and the prevalence of metabolic syndrome was conducted. The authors list the following limitations of the study: unknown age at first exposure to PCDDs and PCDFs and unknown duration of exposure, a cross-sectional design that evaluates current association, adjustment for obesity as one element of metabolic syndrome, rather than BMI, and some arbitrary choices inherent in factor analysis. In summary, the large size of this study is a strength, but the unknown age and duration of exposure are clear weaknesses.

Chang et al. (2011a) reported on the same cross-sectional study, restricted to 1,449 non-diabetic residents (the slight decrease in sample size from the 2010 study is due to slightly different starting population sizes and to a difference of 19 diabetics people between the studies). The study aimed to investigate the joint effects of exposure to dioxins and mercury on pancreatic endocrine function. People who lived near the deserted factory were exposed both to PCDDs and PCDFs and to mercury from eating contaminated seafood from the reservoir near the factory. In multiple-regression models, the authors did not include PCDDs and PCDFs and mercury simultaneously but rather included each singly. They reported the correlation of PCDDs and PCDFs and mercury to be 0.14 ($p < 0.001$), which is low, so it is not apparent why they did not fit models that included both simultaneously and perhaps even with an interaction term to assess the magnitude of the contribution of each contaminant. They did, however, fit a model that included all combinations of tertiles of exposure to each. Again, a major limitation of this study is the absence of information on onset and duration of exposure. Furthermore, the authors note that the homeostasis model for insulin-resistance assessment is not the gold standard and that repeated testing may be needed for assessment in older people. The study did not address co-contamination with mercury.

Chang et al. (2011b) reported on the same cross-sectional study with enrollment extended to December 2009 and restricted to 914 residents who did not have cardiovascular disease (CVD) and who were 30–45 years old. The study aimed to investigate associations between PCDD and PCDF exposure and continuous measures of CVD within 10 years as measured by the Framingham risk score, a formula for combining established risk factors into a single number. Mercury concentrations were not adjusted for in the models, although seafood consumption was. One limitation is the use of the Framingham score; other factors are associated with risk but not included in the score (such as socioeconomic position, genetics, and imaging biomarkers). As in all the publications on this cohort, this one is limited by the lack of information about onset and duration of exposure.

Chang et al. (2012) reported on the same cross-sectional study during 2006–2009, with enrollment restricted to 1,167 residents who had fasted before blood sampling and were more than 50 years old. The study aimed to investigate the biochemical profiles of those exposed to PCDDs and PCDFs. Na-PCP, a widely used pesticide, had been used in the production process at the abandoned factory. After the factory shut down, a large quantity was improperly stored and released into the environment. Some of the retired workers moved away from the area and were not exposed by eating seafood, whereas others remained and were exposed, alongside other local residents. Thus, there were three exposure groups of retired Na-PCP workers: those who still lived locally (23), those who lived locally but did not knowingly eat polluted fish (37), and those who moved away (96). There were three control groups that did not include any Na-PCP workers: local residents who had eaten polluted fish (345), local residents who had not eaten polluted fish (666), and "background participants" in Taiwan's general population (645). The first two of the control groups made up the 1,167 in the study population. Limitations of the study include unknown PCDD and PCDF concentrations in retired workers who moved away or when exposure ceased. There may be important unmeasured confounders related to which workers moved away and which ones did not.

Taiwanese Mother-and-Child Studies

A prospective study of healthy Tiawanese mothers and their children recruited during the mothers' pregnancy is under way to study the associations between exposures to PCDDs, PCDFs, and PCBs and health outcomes (Chao et al., 2004, 2007; Su et al., 2010, 2012; Wang et al., 2004, 2005). The study enrolled pregnant women who had no clinical complications, were 25–35 years old, and delivered in the period between December 1, 2000–November 30, 2001, in a medical center in suburban Taichung in central Taiwan, where a solid-waste incinerator is. Participants completed a questionnaire concerning maternal age, occupation, disease history, cigarette-smoking, alcohol consumption, dietary habits, and baby's stature. Biologic samples (including placenta, umbilical cord blood, mother's venous blood, and breast milk) were collected for analysis of PCDDs, PCDFs, and PCBs. A total of 610 women were enrolled (80% of those invited). The placenta was collected from and the questionnaire completed by 430 participants. Of those, 250 provided sufficient venous blood for the chemical analyses. Of the 250, 175 provided adequate breast milk samples. Wang et al. (2004) reported on PCDDs, PCDFs, and PCBs in the biologic samples and correlations among specimens. Chao et al. (2004) reported on PCDDs, PCDFs, and PCBs in breast milk and the cumulative dose derived for infants exclusively breastfed vs those fed formula.

Wang et al. (2005) examined the association between in utero exposure to PCDDs, PCDFs, and PCBs and thyroid and growth hormones in the newborns. Hormone concentrations were compared between infants with high vs low dioxin/PCB TEQ (above vs below the median) and between females (62) and males (57) by using a two-sample t test or the Mann-Whitney U test (when the distribution deviated significantly from the normal distribution assumed for the t test). Spearman's correlation was used to evaluate the association between hormone concentrations and PCDD, PCDF, and PCB concentrations. Further analyses were carried out with stepwise multivariate regression analysis to adjust for age and other covariates selected through the stepwise selection procedure. Wang et al. (2006) examined the association between PCDDs, PCDFs, and PCBs measured in the placenta samples and estrogens and metabolites measured in mothers' blood samples by using Pearson correlations, linear and quadratic regressions, and multivariate regression analyses.

Su et al. (2010) reported on 2-year and 5-year followups of the mother–child pairs of Wang et al. (2005). Children's anthropomorphic measures were obtained, including height, weight, BMI, head circumference, chest girth, bone age, and the ratio between bone age and chronologic age. Thyroid, sex-hormone, and growth-factor concentrations were measured in venous blood samples obtained from children whose mothers' serum PCDD and PCDF TEQs were available. The anthropomorphic measures and thyroid, sex-hormone, and growth-factor concentrations were compared by sex (29 and 14 males at years 2 and 5, respectively, and 41 and 27 females at years 2 and 5) and pooled across sexes; those who had high vs low in utero PCDD and PCDF concentrations (≥ 15 vs < 15 pg-TEQ/g of lipid) were compared with a two-sample t test or (when not normally distributed) a Wilcoxon rank-sum test. Further analyses were conducted with multiple regression and stepwise selection for detecting factors that might affect growth or hormone concentrations.

Since *Update 2010*, Su et al. (2012) reported on the 8-year followup of the same cohort in a subset of 23 boys and 33 girls, substantially more than the numbers examined in the 5-year followup. In addition to anthropomorphic measures used in previous waves, reproductive development (breast, genital, and armpit stages) were assessed.

Vietnamese Environmental Studies

Various epidemiologic studies have been conducted in the Vietnamese population exposed to the spraying that occurred during the Vietnam War. In a review paper, Constable and Hatch (1985) summarized the unpublished results of studies conducted by researchers in Vietnam. They also examined nine reports that focused primarily on reproductive outcomes (Can et al., 1983a,b; Huong and Phuong, 1983; Khoa, 1983; Lang et al., 1983a,b; Nguyen, 1983; Phuong and Huong, 1983; Trung and Chien, 1983). Vietnamese researchers later published results of four additional studies: two on reproductive abnormalities (Phuong et al., 1989a,b), one on mortality (Dai et al., 1990), and one on hepatocellular carcinoma (Cordier et al., 1993). Ngo et al. (2006) published a meta-analysis that addressed an association between exposure to Agent Orange and birth defects and covered some reports reviewed previously by Constable and Hatch (1985), some new Vietnam studies, and studies on US and Australian veterans who served in Vietnam.

The committee has been interested in recent assessments of contaminant concentrations in Vietnam attributable to storage, distribution, and spraying of herbicides by the US military during the Vietnam War, but none has explored associations between the measured concentrations measured and health outcomes.

Dioxins and PCBs were among OC chemicals measured by Schecter et al. (2003) in food samples gathered in 2002 around Bien Hoa City, Vietnam, about 32 km north of Ho Chi Minh City (formerly Saigon). Bien Hoa City is known as a dioxin "hot spot," with a substantial leak of more than 5,000 gal of Agent Orange at the nearby Bien Hoa air base about 30 years before the study. Marked increases in TCDD concentrations and TEQs were found in ducks, chickens, and fish, but not in pork or beef. The study concluded that food appeared to be responsible for the increase in TCDD in residents of Bien Hoa City even though the original Agent Orange contamination occurred 30–40 years before sampling.

Hansen et al. (2009) studied maternal serum concentrations of OC chemicals (including dioxin-like PCBs 118, 126, 156, and 169) at the time of delivery in women from two communities in southern Vietnam: Nha Trang, a coastal city about 450 km northeast of Ho Chih Minh City, and Dien Khanh, a rural district about 10 km inland from Nha Trang. Of 246 women who delivered infants in May–July 2005, 94 in Nha Trang and 95 in Dien Khanh met the study's residence requirements, agreed to participate, and provided blood specimens. Mean concentrations of the ordinarily prevalent non–dioxin-like PCB 153 were 0.15 µg/L in Nha Trang and 0.10 µg/L in Dien Khanh; other PCB congeners were low in both communities. Age and parity were the most important predictors of plasma concentrations of all chemicals, whereas community of residence was also predictive for PCB 153. Correlations with the health status of mothers or children were not reported.

Nhu et al. (2009) examined the correlations of dioxin concentrations in soil, sediment, and breast milk in an area in Vietnam that had been sprayed with herbicide during the war, Cam Chinh commune in Quang Tri province, and a control site that was not sprayed, Cam Phuc commune in Ha Tinh province. Soil and sediment samples were taken randomly throughout Cam Chinh commune and analyzed for PCDDs and PCDFs. Spatial distribution of PCDDs and PCDFs was estimated by using lognormal kriging (Saito and Goovaerts, 2000). Breast-milk samples were taken from lactating mothers 20–40 years old who lived in two communes (86 in Cam Chinh commune and 71 in Cam Phuc commune) in September 2002–July 2003. The participants were also interviewed to collect information on personal habits, such as smoking, alcohol drinking, contraceptive-drug use, history of pesticide contact, disease history, number of pregnancies, age at each pregnancy, and reason for pregnancy failure, if applicable. The mean dioxin concentrations in soil and breast milk in the sprayed area were significantly higher than were those in the nonsprayed area. There were no significant correlations between the estimated dioxin concentrations in soil obtained with the kriging method and those in breast milk. Again, no results were presented with respect to the health status of mothers or infants.

Other Environmental Studies

Additional outcomes of environmental exposure to the COIs were studied: NHL in Yorkshire, England (Cartwright et al., 1988); adverse health effects after an electric-transformer fire in Binghamton, New York (Fitzgerald et al., 1989); lymphomas and STSs in Italy (Vineis et al., 1991); cancer in Finland (Lampi et al., 1992); early-onset Parkinson disease in Oregon and Washington (Butterfield et al., 1993); neuropsychologic effects in Germany (Peper et al., 1993); mortality and cancer incidence in two cohorts of Swedish fishermen whose primary exposure route was assumed to be diet (Svensson et al., 1995); immunologic effects of prenatal and postnatal exposure to PCB or TCDD in Dutch infants from birth to the age of 18 months (Weisglas-Kuperus et al., 1995); effects of inhalation exposure to TCDD and related chemicals in wood preservatives on cell-mediated immunity in German day-care center employees (Wolf and Karmaus, 1995); skin cancer in Alberta, Canada (Gallagher et al., 1996); immunologic effects in hobby fishermen in the Frierfjord in southeastern Norway (Lovik et al., 1996); HL, NHL, MM, and acute myeloid leukemia in various regions of Italy (Masala et al., 1996); NHL, HL, and chronic lymphocytic leukemia in a rural Michigan community (Waterhouse et al., 1996); cancer mortality in four northern wheat-producing US states (Schreinemachers, 2000); mortality and incinerator dioxin emissions in municipalities in Japan (Fukuda et al., 2003); prevalence of hypertension in Taiwanese who lived near municipal-waste incinerators (Chen HL et al., 2006); and adverse pregnancy outcomes in Japan on the basis of maternal residence at the time of birth (Tango et al., 2004).

Combustion records in the Zeeburg area of Amsterdam in the Netherlands were used as a surrogate for exposure to dioxins in a study of orofacial clefts (ten Tusscher et al., 2000). Location downwind or upwind of an incineration source was used to define exposed and reference groups for the study. A study of STS in the general population was conducted in and around the city of Mantua in northern Italy (Costani et al., 2000). Several industrial facilities are in Mantua, and residential proximity to them was presumed to result in increased TCDD exposure, but TCDD was not measured in the environment or in human tissues.

A study of dioxin exposure pathways in Belgium focused on longtime residents of the vicinity of two municipal-waste incinerators (Fierens et al., 2003a). Residents near a rural incinerator had significantly higher serum dioxin concentrations than did a control group (38 vs 24 TEQ pg/g of lipid). Concentrations in people who lived near the incinerators increased proportionally with intake of local-animal fat. A second study (Fierens et al., 2003b) measured dioxin body burden in 257 people who had been environmentally exposed to determine whether dioxin and PCB exposures were associated with type 2 diabetes and endometriosis. No difference in body burden was found between women who had endometriosis and women in a control group, but the risk of type 2 diabetes was significantly higher in those who had higher body burdens of dioxin-like chemicals and of PCBs. Another study of the correlation between dioxin-like chemicals in Italian and Belgian women and the risk of endometriosis used measurements of TCDD and other dioxins in blood (De Felip et al., 2004). There was no difference in body burden between women who had endometriosis and a control group, but serum-dioxin concentrations were substantially higher in the Belgian controls than in a similar group in Italy (45 vs 18 TEQ pg/g of lipid, respectively).

CASE-CONTROL STUDIES

Cross-Canada Study of Pesticides and Health (Rare Tumors Study)

After a pilot study done for the Canadian government, McDuffie et al. (2001) initiated a full population-based case-control study of men in six Canadian provinces that addressed several fairly uncommon malignancies—HL, NHL, MM, and STS—and the relationship of their occurrence with exposure to pesticides (both occupationally and domestically). A target number of cases of each cancer type was preset for each province; cases newly diagnosed starting on September 1, 1991, were gathered from the provincial cancer registries or hospital records in Quebec until the end of 1994 or until the target number was reached. Physician consent was obtained, diagnoses were confirmed with pathology reports and preserved tissues, and consent forms and questionnaires were sent to the cases. The controls were men at least 19 years old identified in the health-insurance records of Alberta, Saskatchewan, Manitoba, and Quebec; telephone listings for Ontario; and voter lists in British Columbia. The controls were selected randomly to obtain a stratified age distribution matching that of the cases. They, too, were sent consent forms and questionnaires. People who had died were dropped from the study, as were people who had Kaposi sarcoma or were HIV-positive. All 1,506 controls that responded were used in comparisons for each of four cancer groups: 316 HL cases, 517 NHL cases, 342 MM cases, and 357 STS cases.

The postal questionnaire gathered standard demographic information, personal and family medical histories, employment history, smoking behavior, and basic data on pesticide exposure. The pilot study had tested the reliability of self-reported pesticide use by comparison with purchase records. Any subject who reported at least 10 hours of pesticide exposure per year was asked to complete a telephone questionnaire on the details of pesticide exposure; in addition, 15% of the remaining subjects were randomly selected to answer the telephone survey. Conditional logistic regression stratified on age and province and adjusted for all covariates found to be associated with the outcome at the 0.05 level of significance was used to estimate ORs for specific active ingredients, including dicamba and the phenoxy herbicides 2,4-D, Mecoprop, MCPA, and diclofopmethyl. Dose–response relationships were investigated for cumulative categories of time spent in mixing or applying particular products.

A series of publications have addressed the relationship between each of the cancers and various risk factors. Those pertaining to herbicides overall or to the particular ones of interest are as follows:

- HL—Karunanayake et al., 2012; Pahwa et al., 2003
- NHL—Hohenadel et al., 2011; McDuffie et al., 2001
- MM—Pahwa et al., 2003, 2012
- STS—Pahwa et al., 2003, 2011

A number of other publications arising from that dataset have addressed topics somewhat more tangential to the interests of the VAO reports. For instance, McDuffie et al. (2005) and Pahwa et al. (2006) considered the possible interaction of exposure to insect repellents, particularly *N,N*-diethyl-*m*-toluamide (DEET) and phenoxy herbicides, in the genesis of the malignancies in question. McDuffie et al. (2009) examined family histories of cancer in first-degree relatives of the study participants (1,528 cases and 1,506 controls) to assess the interacton between family history and pesticide exposure. Hohenadel et al. (2011) investigated how various combinations of pesticide exposures influenced the occurrence of NHL. Ghosh et al. (2011) investigated the association of occupational exposures other than to pesticides with the occurrence of MM.

Children's Oncology Group Study (US)

In two related case-control studies, Chen Z et al. reported on exposure to pesticides (including herbicides) and the risk of childhood germ-cell tumors. One focused on parental occupational exposures (Chen Z et al., 2005) and the other on parental exposures to residential pesticides and chemicals (Chen Z et al., 2006), but they are based on the same overall case-control study.

No reports from the Children's Oncology Group have been published since *Update 2008*.

National Birth Defects Prevention Study (10 US centers, 1997–2003 births)

Rocheleau et al. (2011) reports on the association between maternal occupational pesticide exposure and risk of hypospadias in the National Birth Defects Prevention Study. This was a case-control study with 647 cases of hypospadias and 1,496 controls with estimated delivery dates of October 1997–December 2002. Mothers were interviewed about job status, which was then formally coded. Typical pesticide ratings were assigned to the job codes. Duration and confidence in exposure were used to refine them. Complete case analysis was conducted, with some sensitivity analysis around missingness (creation of a missing category). Most exposure was to insecticides only or to all three types (insecticides, herbicides, and fungicides). The analysis did not include fetuses that died with hypospadias. Multiple comparisons are a concern. There was generally a low level of pesticide exposure in the study population. Other exposures of the population (for example, in agricultural workers) could cause the outcome in question.

Upper Midwest Health Study

The Upper Midwest Health Study (UMHS) was initiated by NIOSH as a population-based case-control study of cancer risk in a nonmetropolitan Midwestern US population. Several reports from the study were reviewed in previous updates. Chiu et al. (2004) and Lee et al. (2004a) conducted pooled (combined) analyses of two earlier case-control studies of NHL carried out by the UMHS in Iowa and Minnesota (Cantor et al., 1992) and Nebraska (Zahm et al., 1990). Chiu et al. (2004) examined the association of NHL with agricultural pesticide use and familial cancer, and Lee WJ et al. (2004a, 2006) looked at NHL in asthmatic people who reported pesticide exposure. Data from Nebraska (Chiu et al., 2006, based on Zahm et al., 1990, 1993) were used to identify whether there was a higher risk of subtypes of NHL. Specifically, tissue samples were analyzed according to the presence of a specific chromosomal translocation (t[14;18][q32;q21]); only 172 of 385 cases were included.

Two studies focused on pesticide use and the risk of adenocarcinomas of the stomach and esophagus (Lee et al., 2004b) and the risk of gliomas (Lee et al., 2005). Cases were white Nebraska residents over 21 years old who were identified from the Nebraska Cancer Registry and matched to controls drawn from an earlier study by Zahm et al. (1990).

Researchers evaluated farm pesticide exposure in men (Ruder et al., 2004) and women (Carreon et al., 2005) in Iowa, Michigan, Minnesota, and Wisconsin in relation to gliomas as part of the UMHS. Ruder et al. (2006) reported a followup of Ruder et al. (2004) that evaluated gliomas in UMHS participants. The new analyses provided no evidence of greater use of pesticides in cases than in controls, and there was no breakdown by specific agents.

Ruder et al. (2009) reported another followup, which had similar findings and no breakdown by specific agents.

Since *Update 2010*, Yiin et al. (2012) has reported findings from new analyses of the UMHS sample that incorporated more detailed exposure information that was not used in previous analyses, including years of use and estimated cumulative exposures to categories of pesticides, including phenoxy herbicides, and use of specific agents, including 2,4-D and dicamba.

Other Case-Control Studies

Numerous case-control studies have been reviewed in previous updates. In 1977, case-series reports in Sweden (Hardell, 1977, 1979) of a potential connection between exposure to phenoxyacetic acids and STS prompted several case-control investigations (Eriksson et al., 1979, 1981, 1990; Hardell, 1981; Hardell and Eriksson, 1988; Hardell and Sandstrom, 1979; Wingren et al., 1990). After the initial STS reports (Hardell, 1977, 1979), case-control studies of other cancer outcomes were conducted in Sweden: of HL and NHL (Hardell and Bengtsson, 1983; Hardell et al., 1980, 1981; Persson et al., 1989, 1993), of NHL (Hardell and Eriksson, 1999; Olsson and Brandt, 1988), of nasal and nasopharyngeal carcinomas (Hardell et al., 1982), of gastric cancer (Ekström et al., 1999), and of primary or unspecified liver cancer (Hardell et al., 1984). To address criticism regarding potential observer bias in some of the case-control series, Hardell (1981) conducted another case-control study of colon cancer. Hardell et al. (1994) also examined the relationship between occupational exposure to phenoxyacetic acids and chlorophenols and various characteristics related to NHL—including histopathologic measures, stage, and anatomic location—on the basis of the NHL cases in a previous study (Hardell et al., 1981).

Prompted by the Swedish studies (Hardell, 1977, 1979), Smith and Pearce (1986) and Smith et al. (1983, 1984) conducted a set of case-control studies to evaluate the association between phenoxy herbicide and chlorophenol exposure and STS incidence and mortality in New Zealand. An expanded case series was collected, and additional case-control studies of exposure to phenoxy herbicides or chlorophenols and the risks of malignant lymphoma, NHL, and MM were conducted (Pearce et al., 1985, 1986a,b, 1987).

Geographic patterns of increased leukemia mortality in white men in the central part of the United States prompted a study of leukemia mortality in Nebraska farmers (Blair and Thomas, 1979). Additional case-control studies of leukemia were later conducted in Nebraska (Blair and White, 1985); in Iowa (Burmeister et al., 1982) on the basis of the cohort study of Burmeister (1981); and in Iowa and Minnesota (Brown et al., 1990). Another study investigated leukemia in association with NHL and 2,4-D in eastern Nebraska (Zahm et al., 1990).

Case-control studies have been conducted in various US populations for associations of herbicides with other cancers, including NHL (Cantor, 1982; Cantor et al., 1992; Hartge et al., 2005; Tatham et al., 1997; Zahm et al., 1993); MM (Boffetta et al., 1989; Brown et al., 1993; Morris et al., 1986); gastric cancer, prostate cancer, NHL, and MM (Burmeister et al., 1983); STS, HL, and NHL (Hoar et al., 1986); NHL and HL (Dubrow et al., 1988); and STS and NHL (Woods and Polissar, 1989; Woods et al., 1987). In a subset of participants in the Hartge et al. (2005) study, De Roos et al. (2005b) studied associations between overall TEQs of PCBs, furans, and dioxins but not TCDD alone.

Other case-control studies conducted outside the United States have addressed various cancers: STS and other cancers in the 15 regional cancer registries that constitute the National Cancer Register in England in connection with the chemicals of interest (COIs) (Balarajan and Acheson, 1984); ovarian cancer in the Piedmont region of Italy (Donna et al., 1984); STS in rice weeders in northern Italy (Vineis et al., 1986); mortality from esophageal cancer, pancreatic cancer, cutaneous melanoma, renal cancer, and brain cancer in three English counties (Magnani et al., 1987); brain gliomas in two hospitals in Milan, Italy (Musicco et al., 1988); lymphoid cancer in Milan, Italy (LaVecchia et al., 1989); primary lung cancer in pesticide users in Saskatchewan (McDuffie et al., 1990); STS and malignant lymphomas in the Victorian Cancer Registry of Australia (Smith and Christophers, 1992); oral-cancer risk in occupationally exposed workers in Sweden (Schildt et al., 1999); and renal-cell carcinoma in the Denmark Cancer Registry (Mellemgaard et al., 1994). Nanni et al. (1996) conducted a population-based case-control study—based on the work of Amadori et al. (1995)—of occupational and chemical risk factors for lymphocytic leukemia and NHL in northeastern Italy.

Noncancer health outcomes also have been investigated in case-control studies: spontaneous abortion (Carmelli et al., 1981); congenital malformations (García et al., 1998); immunosuppression and later decreased host resistance to infection in AIDS patients who had Kaposi sarcoma (Hardell et al., 1987); mortality in US Department of Agriculture extension agents (Alavanja et al., 1988) and conservationists (Alavanja et al., 1989); PD associated with occupational risk factors (Semchuk et al., 1993); birth defects in offspring of agriculture workers (Nurminen et al., 1994); mortality from neurodegenerative diseases associated with occupational risk factors (Schulte et al., 1996); PD associated with various rural factors, including exposure to herbicides and wood preservatives (Seidler et al., 1996); spina bifida in offspring associated with paternal occupation (Blatter et al., 1997); PD associated with occupational and environmental risk factors (Liou et al., 1997); and mortality from neurodegenerative diseases, including Alzheimer disease and presenile dementia, PD, and motor neuron disease associated with occupational factors (Park et al., 2005). Those studies have been discussed in detail in previous updates.

Orsi et al. (2009) have studied the association between occupational exposures to pesticides and lymphoid neoplasms by using a hospital-based case-control study in the main hospitals of six French cities (Brest, Caen, Nantes, Lille, Toulouse, and Bordeaux) from September 2000 to December 2004. Cases were eligible if they were male, were 20–75 years old, were residing in the hospital's catchment area (the administrative department where the hospital is or a neighboring department), lacked a history of immunosuppression or of taking immunosuppressant drugs, and had recently received a diagnosis of any lymphoid neoplasm except acute lymphoid leukemia. The diagnoses were classified by using the World Health Organization third edition of the *International Classification of Diseases for Oncology* codes and confirmed cytologically or histologically by a panel of pathologists and hematologists. Among 513 eligible incident cases, 491 (96%) participated: 87 with HL, 244 with NHL, 56 with MMs, and 104 with lymphoproliferative syndrome (LPS). The controls were male patients from the same hospitals who had no prior history of lymphoid neoplasm (LN), were residing in the hospital's catchment area, and were not admitted to the hospital for conditions directly related to occupation, smoking, or alcohol abuse. The controls were individually matched with the cases by hospital and age (± 3 years). Among 501 eligible controls, 456 (91%) participated. Participants were given a self-administered questionnaire, had a face-to-face interview, and had a reinterview by an occupational hygienist and an agronomist when needed to collect socioeconomic and lifestyle information, personal and family medical history, residential and occupational histories, and detailed information on occupational and nonoccupational exposure to herbicides and pesticides. Dichotomous exposure measures (ever or never exposed) were constructed for each category (insecticides, fungicides, and herbicides) and for each chemical family (such as OC chemicals and phenoxy herbicides). Unconditional logistic regression was used to estimate the ORs and confidence intervals for each outcome (all LN, NHL, HL, LPS, and MM) and chemical exposure with adjustment for age, hospital, and socioeconomic category (white collar or blue collar). Logistic regression was used for NHL subtypes (diffuse large B-cell lymphoma, follicular lymphoma, and other NHL) and LPS (chronic lymphocytic leukemia and hairy-cell leukemia).

Spinelli et al. (2007) conducted a population-based case-control study of histologically confirmed NHL in men and women 20–79 years old who lived in the greater metropolitan areas of Vancouver and Victoria, British Columbia, during 2000–2004. Population controls, frequency-matched to cases by 5-year age groups and area, were identified from the client registry of the provincial health care system. A random subset of controls was included in the analyses. The analyses were based on concentrations of OC and related chemicals in serum obtained from controls at the time of interview and from cases before chemotherapy. NHL patients who lost weight rapidly were excluded. Ng et al. (2010) examined the single-nucleotide polymorphisms (SNPs) in the aryl hydrocarbon receptor (AHR) gene that were genotyped for the same study cohorts (422 NHL cases and 459 controls) to measure the association between individual SNPs, haplotypes, and risk of NHL. Gene–environment interaction analyses were conducted for OC chemicals and AHR SNPs by using logistic regression.

Hartge et al. (2005) conducted a case-control study that used four NCI SEER registries (Detroit, Iowa, Los Angeles County, and Seattle) for associations of herbicides with NHL. In a subset of participants in the Hartge et al. study, De Roos et al. (2005b) studied associations between NHL and overall TEQs of PCBs, furans, and dioxins but not TCDD alone. Colt et al. (2009) studied whether the relationship between OC exposure and NHL is modified by immune-gene variation in the SEER study participants (1,172 cases and 513 controls). The study genotyped 61 polymorphisms in 36 immune genes and examined three exposures measured in plasma and dust: to PCB 180, to OC pesticides (TEQ), and to α-chlordane. Unconditional logistic regression was used to estimate the exposure–outcome association with stratification by genotype and adjustment for sex, age, race, education, and study region.

Firestone et al. (2005) reported on a population-based case-control study of incident PD cases in Washington state (250 cases and 388 controls). PD cases were identified in 1992–2002 at the Group Health Cooperative (GHC, a large managed-care organization) or the University of Washington. Control participants were sampled randomly from GHC enrollees who had no history of PD or other progressive neurologic disorder and were frequency-matched to cases by age, sex, GHC clinic location, and year of GHC enrollment. Participants were interviewed to obtain information on demographics, medical and occupational history, occupational and home-based pesticide use, drinking-water source, residential history, and smoking history. Both occupational exposures and residential exposures were reported. No specific COIs were reported beyond the broad category "herbicide." Unconditional logistic regression was used to estimate the association between PD and exposure, with adjustment for age, sex, and smoking.

Firestone et al. (2010) provided an expanded update (404 cases and 526 controls) that extended the same recruitment protocol through 2006. The participation rates were good among eligible cases (70%) and modest among eligible controls (60%); this left some room for selection bias due to nonresponse. Only occupational exposures were reported. Exposures to specific chemicals were reported, including 2,4-D (nine exposed cases and 12 exposed controls).

REFERENCES[1]

ADVA (Australia, Department of Veterans' Affairs). 2005a. *The Third Australian Vietnam Veterans Mortality Study 2005.* Canberra: Department of Veterans' Affairs.

ADVA. 2005b. *Cancer Incidence in Australian Vietnam Veteran Study 2005.* Canberra: Department of Veterans' Affairs.

ADVA. 2005c. *Australian National Service Vietnam Veterans: Mortality and Cancer Incidence 2005.* Canberra: Department of Veterans' Affairs.

AFHS (Air Force Health Study). 1982. *An Epidemiologic Investigation of Health Effects in Air Force Personnel Following Exposure to Herbicides: Study Protocol, Initial Report.* Brooks AFB, TX: USAF School of Aerospace Medicine. SAM-TR-82-44.

AFHS. 1983. *An Epidemiologic Investigation of Health Effects in Air Force Personnel Following Exposure to Herbicides. Baseline Mortality Study Results.* Brooks AFB, TX: USAF School of Aerospace Medicine. NTIS AD-A130-793.

AFHS. 1984a. *An Epidemiologic Investigation of Health Effects in Air Force Personnel Following Exposure to Herbicides. Baseline Morbidity Study Results.* Brooks AFB, TX: USAF School of Aerospace Medicine. NTIS AD-A138-340.

AFHS. 1984b. *An Epidemiologic Investigation of Health Effects in Air Force Personnel Following Exposure to Herbicides. Mortality Update: 1984.* Brooks AFB, TX: USAF School of Aerospace Medicine. NTIS AD-A162-687.

AFHS. 1985. *An Epidemiologic Investigation of Health Effects in Air Force Personnel Following Exposure to Herbicides. Mortality Update: 1985.* Brooks AFB, TX: USAF School of Aerospace Medicine. NTIS AD-A163-237.

AFHS. 1986. *An Epidemiologic Investigation of Health Effects in Air Force Personnel Following Exposure to Herbicides. Mortality Update: 1986.* Brooks AFB, TX: USAF School of Aerospace Medicine. USAFSAM-TR-86-43.

AFHS. 1987. *An Epidemiologic Investigation of Health Effects in Air Force Personnel Following Exposure to Herbicides. First Follow-up Examination Results.* Brooks AFB, TX: USAF School of Aerospace Medicine. USAFSAM-TR-87-27.

AFHS. 1989. *An Epidemiologic Investigation of Health Effects in Air Force Personnel Following Exposure to Herbicides. Mortality Update: 1989.* Brooks AFB, TX: USAF School of Aerospace Medicine. USAFSAM-TR-89-9.

AFHS. 1990. *An Epidemiologic Investigation of Health Effects in Air Force Personnel Following Exposure to Herbicides.* Brooks AFB, TX: USAF School of Aerospace Medicine. USAFSAM-TR-90-2.

AFHS. 1991a. *An Epidemiologic Investigation of Health Effects in Air Force Personnel Following Exposure to Herbicides. Mortality Update: 1991.* Brooks AFB, TX: Armstrong Laboratory. AL-TR-1991-0132.

[1]Throughout this report, the same alphabetic indicator after year of publication is used consistently for a given reference when there are multiple citations by the same first author in a given year. The convention of assigning the alphabetic indicators in order of citation in a given chapter is not followed.

AFHS. 1991b. *An Epidemiologic Investigation of Health Effects in Air Force Personnel Following Exposure to Herbicides. Serum Dioxin Analysis of 1987 Examination Results.* Brooks AFB, TX: USAF School of Aerospace Medicine. NTIS AD-A237-516.

AFHS. 1992. *An Epidemiologic Investigation of Health Effects in Air Force Personnel Following Exposure to Herbicides. Reproductive Outcomes.* Brooks AFB, TX: Armstrong Laboratory. AL-TR-1992-0090.

AFHS. 1995. *An Epidemiologic Investigation of Health Effects in Air Force Personnel Following Exposure to Herbicides. 1992 Follow-up Examination Results.* Brooks AFB, TX: Epidemiologic Research Division; Armstrong Laboratory. AL-TR-920107.

AFHS. 1996. *An Epidemiologic Investigation of Health Effects in Air Force Personnel Following Exposure to Herbicides. Mortality Update 1996.* Brooks AFB, TX: Epidemiologic Research Division; Armstrong Laboratory. AL/AO-TR-1996-0068.

AFHS. 2000. *An Epidemiologic Investigation of Health Effects in Air Force Personnel Following Exposure to Herbicides. 1997 Follow-up Examination Results.* Brooks AFB, TX: Epidemiologic Research Division. Armstrong Laboratory. AFRL-HE-BR-TR-2000-02.

AFHS. 2005. *An Epidemiologic Investigation of Health Effects in Air Force Personnel Following Exposure to Herbicides. 2002 Follow-up Examination Results.* Brooks AFB, TX: Epidemiologic Research Division. Armstrong Laboratory. AFRL-HE-BR-SR-2005-0003.

Agent Orange Review. 2008. IOM announces new Vietnam veterans and Agent Orange committee to prepare *2008 Update. Department of Veterans Affairs* 20(2):1–8.

AIHW (Australian Institute of Health and Welfare). 1999. *Morbidity of Vietnam Veterans: A Study of the Health of Australia's Vietnam Veteran Community: Volume 3: Validation Study.* Canberra: AIHW.

AIHW. 2000. *Morbidity of Vietnam Veterans. Adrenal Gland Cancer, Leukaemia and non-Hodgkin's Lymphoma: Supplementary Report No. 2.* (AIHW cat. No. PHE 28). Canberra: AIHW.

AIHW. 2001. *Morbidity of Vietnam Veterans. Adrenal Gland Cancer, Leukaemia and non-Hodgkin's Lymphoma: Supplementary Report No. 2.* Revised edition (AIHW cat. No. PHE 34). Canberra: AIHW.

Akhmedkhanov A, Revich B, Adibi JJ, Zeilert V, Masten SA, Patterson DG Jr, Needham LL, Toniolo P. 2002. Characterization of dioxin exposure in residents of Chapaevsk, Russia. *Journal of Exposure Analysis and Environmental Epidemiology* 12(6):409–417.

Akhtar FZ, Garabrant DH, Ketchum NS, Michalek JE. 2004. Cancer in US Air Force veterans of the Vietnam war. *Journal of Occupational and Environmental Medicine* 46(2):123–136.

Alavanja MC, Blair A, Merkle S, Teske J, Eaton B. 1988. Mortality among agricultural extension agents. *American Journal of Industrial Medicine* 14:167–176.

Alavanja MC, Merkle S, Teske J, Eaton B, Reed B. 1989. Mortality among forest and soil conservationists. *Archives of Environmental Health* 44:94–101.

Alavanja MC, Akland G, Baird D, Blair A, Bond A, Dosemeci M, Kamel F, Lewis R, Lubin J, Lynch C, et al. 1994. Cancer and non-cancer risk to women in agriculture and pest control: The Agricultural Health Study. *Journal of Occupational Medicine* 36(11):1247–1250.

Alavanja MC, Sandler DP, Mcdonnell CJ, Lynch CF, Pennybacker M, Zahm SH, Lubin J, Mage D, Steen WC, Wintersteen W, Blair A. 1998. Factors associated with self-reported, pesticide-related visits to health care providers in the Agricultural Health Study. *Environmental Health Perspectives* 106(7):415–420.

Alavanja MC, Samanic C, Dosemeci M, Lubin J, Tarone R, Lynch CF, Knott C, Thomas K, Hoppin JA, Barker J, Coble J, Sandler DP, Blair A. 2003. Use of agricultural pesticides and prostate cancer risk in the Agricultural Health Study cohort. *American Journal of Epidemiology* 157(9):800–814.

Alavanja MC, Hoppin JA, Kamel F. 2004. Health effects of chronic pesticide exposure: Cancer and neurotoxicity. *Annual Review of Public Health* 25:155–197.

Alavanja MC, Sandler DP, Lynch CF, Knott C, Lubin JH, Tarone R, Thomas K, Dosemeci M, Barker J, Hoppin JA, Blair A. 2005. Cancer incidence in the Agricultural Health Study. *Scandinavian Journal of Work, Environment and Health* 31(Suppl 1):39–45.

Alderfer R, Sweeney M, Fingerhut M, Hornung R, Wille K, Fidler A. 1992. Measures of depressed mood in workers exposed to 2,3,7,8-tetrachlorodibenzo-*p*-dioxin (TCDD). *Chemosphere* 25:247–250.

Amadori D, Nanni O, Falcini F, Saragoni A, Tison V, Callea A, Scarpi E, Ricci M, Riva N, Buiatti E. 1995. Chronic lymphocytic leukemias and non-Hodgkin's lymphomas by histological type in farming-animal breeding workers: A population case-control study based on job titles. *Occupational and Environmental Medicine* 52(6):374–379.

Anderson HA, Hanrahan LP, Jensen M, Laurin D, Yick WY, Wiegman P. 1986a. *Wisconsin Vietnam Veteran Mortality Study: Proportionate Mortality Ratio Study Results.* Madison: Wisconsin Division of Health.

Anderson HA, Hanrahan LP, Jensen M, Laurin D, Yick WY, Wiegman P. 1986b. *Wisconsin Vietnam Veteran Mortality Study: Final Report.* Madison: Wisconsin Division of Health.

Andreotti G, Freeman LEB, Hou L, Coble J, Rusiecki J, Hoppin JA, Silverman DT, Alavanja MCR. 2009. Agricultural pesticide use and pancreatic cancer risk in the Agricultural Health Study cohort. *International Journal of Cancer* 124(10):2495–2500.

Andreotti G, Koutros S, Berndt SI, Barry KH, Hou L, Hoppin JA, Sandler DP, Lubin JH, Burdette LA, Yuenger J, Yeager M, Freeman LEB, Alavanja MCR. 2012. The interaction between pesticide use and genetic variants involved in lipid metabolism on prostate cancer risk. *Journal of Cancer Epidemiology* 2012:11 pps.

Andrews JS Jr, Garrett WA, Patterson DG Jr, Needham LL, Roberts DW, Bagby JR, Anderson JE, Hoffman RE, Schramm W. 1989. 2,3,7,8-Tetrachlorodibenzo-*p*-dioxin levels in adipose tissue of persons with no known exposure and in exposed persons. *Chemosphere* 18(1-6):499–506.

Arbuckle TE, Ritter L. 2005. Phenoxyacetic acid herbicide exposure for women on Ontario farms. *Journal of Toxicology and Environmental Health Part A* 68(15):1359–1370.

Arbuckle TE, Schrader SM, Cole D, Hall JC, Bancej CM, Turner LA, Claman P. 1999a. 2,4-Dichlorophenoxyacetic acid (2,4-D) residues in semen of Ontario farmers. *Reproductive Toxicology* 13(6):421–429.

Arbuckle TE, Savitz DA, Mery LS, Curtis KM. 1999b. Exposure to phenoxy herbicides and the risk of spontaneous abortion. *Epidemiology* 10:752–760.

Arbuckle TE, Lin Z, Mery LS. 2001. An exploratory analysis of the effect of pesticide exposure on the risk of spontaneous abortion in an Ontario farm population. *Environmental Health Perspectives* 109(8):851–857.

Arbuckle TE, Burnett R, Cole D, Teschke K, Dosemeci M, Bancej C, Zhang J. 2002. Predictors of herbicide exposure in farm applicators. *International Archives of Occupational and Environmental Health* 75:406–414.

Arbuckle TE, Cole DC, Ritter L, Ripley BD. 2005. Biomonitoring of herbicides in Ontario farm applicators. *Scandinavian Journal of Work, Environment and Health* 31(Suppl 1):90–97.

Arbuckle TE, Bruce D, Ritter L, Hall JC. 2006. Indirect sources of herbicide exposure for families on Ontario farms. *Journal of Exposure Science and Environmental Epidemiology* 16(1):98–104.

Arcury TA, Quandt SA, Barr DB, Hoppin JA, McCauley L, Grzywacz JG, Robson MG. 2006. Farmworker exposure to pesticides: Methodologic issues for the collection of comparable data. *Environmental Health Perspectives* 114(6):923–928.

Aschengrau A, Monson RR. 1989. Paternal military service in Vietnam and risk of spontaneous abortion. *Journal of Occupational Medicine* 31:618–623.

Aschengrau A, Monson RR. 1990. Paternal military service in Vietnam and the risk of late adverse pregnancy outcomes. *American Journal of Public Health* 80:1218–1224.

Asp S, Riihimaki V, Hernberg S, Pukkala E. 1994. Mortality and cancer morbidity of Finnish chlorophenoxy herbicide applicators: An 18-year prospective follow-up. *American Journal of Industrial Medicine* 26:243–253.

Assennato G, Cannatelli P, Emmett E, Ghezzi I, Merlo F. 1989a. Medical monitoring of dioxin clean-up workers. *American Industrial Hygiene Association Journal* 50:586–592.

Assennato G, Cervino D, Emmett E, Longo G, Merlo F. 1989b. Follow-up of subjects who developed chloracne following TCDD exposure at Seveso. *American Journal of Industrial Medicine* 16:119–125.

ATSDR (Agency for Toxic Substances and Disease Registry). 1998. *Toxicological Profile for Chlorinated Dibenzo-*p*-dioxins (CDDs).* Atlanta, GA: Centers for Disease Control.

Axelson O, Sundell L. 1974. Herbicide exposure, mortality and tumor incidence. An epidemiological investigation on Swedish railroad workers. *Scandinavian Journal of Work, Environment and Health* 11:21–28.

Axelson O, Sundell L, Andersson K, Edling C, Hogstedt C, Kling H. 1980. Herbicide exposure and tumor mortality: An updated epidemiologic investigation on Swedish railroad workers. *Scandinavian Journal of Work, Environment and Health* 6:73–79.

Aylward LL, Bodner KM, Collins JJ, Wilken M, McBride D, Burns CJ, Hays SM, Humphry N. 2010. TCDD exposure estimation for workers at a New Zealand 2,4,5-T manufacturing facility based on serum sampling data. *Journal of Exposure Science and Environmental Epidemiology* 20(5):417–426.

Baccarelli A, Mocarelli P, Patterson DG Jr, Bonzini M, Pesatori A, Caporaso N, Landi MT. 2002. Immunologic effects of dioxin: New results from Seveso and comparison with other studies. *Environmental Health Perspectives* 110(12):1169–1173.

Baccarelli A, Pesatori AC, Masten SA, Patterson DG Jr, Needham LL, Mocarelli P, Caporaso NE, Consonni D, Grassman JA, Bertazzi PA, Landi MT. 2004. Aryl-hydrocarbon receptor-dependent pathways and toxic effects of TCDD in humans: A population-based study in Seveso, Italy. *Toxicology Letters* 149(1-3):287–293.

Baccarelli A, Pesatori AC, Consonni D, Mocarelli P, Patterson DG Jr, Caporaso NE, Bertazzi PA, Landi MT. 2005a. Health status and plasma dioxin levels in chloracne cases 20 years after the Seveso, Italy accident. *British Journal of Dermatology* 152(3):459–465.

Baccarelli A, Pfeiffer R, Consonni D, Pesatori AC, Bonzini M, Patterson DG Jr, Bertazzi PA, Landi MT. 2005b. Handling of dioxin measurement data in the presence of non-detectable values: Overview of available methods and their application in the Seveso chloracne study. *Chemosphere* 60(7):898–906.

Baccarelli A, Hirt C, Pesatori AC, Consonni D, Patterson DG Jr, Bertazzi PA, Dölken G, Landi MT. 2006. t(14;18) translocations in lymphocytes of healthy dioxin-exposed individuals from Seveso, Italy. *Carcinogenesis* 27(10):2001–2007.

Baccarelli A, Giacomini SM, Corbetta C, Landi MT, Bonzini M, Consonni D, Grillo P, Patterson DG Jr, Pesatori AC, Bertazzi PA. 2008. Neonatal thyroid function in Seveso 25 years after maternal exposure to dioxin. *PLoS Medicine* 5(7):1133–1142.

Balarajan R, Acheson ED. 1984. Soft tissue sarcomas in agriculture and forestry workers. *Journal of Epidemiology and Community Health* 38:113–116.

Barbieri S, Pirovano C, Scarlato G, Tarchini P, Zappa A, Maranzana M. 1988. Long-term effects of 2,3,7,8-tetrachlorodibenzo-*p*-dioxin on the peripheral nervous system. Clinical and neurophysiological controlled study on subjects with chloracne from the Seveso area. *Neuroepidemiology* 7:29–37.

Barr DB, Allen R, Olsson AO, Bravo R, Caltabiano LM, Montesano A, Nguyen J, Udunka S, Walden D, Walker RD, Weerasekera G, Whitehead RD Jr, Schober SE, Needham LL. 2005. Concentrations of selective metabolites of organophosphorus pesticides in the United States population. *Environmental Research* 99(3):314–326.

Barr DB, Landsittel D, Nishioka M, Thomas K, Curwin B, Raymer J, Donnelly KC, McCauley L, Ryan PB. 2006a. A survey of laboratory and statistical issues related to farmworker exposure studies. *Environmental Health Perspectives* 114(6):961–968.

Barr DB, Thomas K, Curwin B, Landsittel D, Raymer J, Lu C, Donnelly KC, Acquavella J. 2006b. Biomonitoring of exposure in farmworker studies. *Environmental Health Perspectives* 114(6):936–942.

Barrett DH, Morris RD, Akhtar FZ, Michalek JE. 2001. Serum dioxin and cognitive functioning among veterans of Operation Ranch Hand. *Neurotoxicology* 22:491–502.

Barrett DH, Morris RD, Jackson WG Jr, Stat M, Michalek JE. 2003. Serum dioxin and psychological functioning in US Air Force veterans of the Vietnam War. *Military Medicine* 168:153–159.

Barry KH, Koutros S, Berndt SI, Andreotti G, Hoppin JA, Sandler DP, Burdette LA, Yeager M, Freeman LEB, Lubin JH, Ma X, Zheng T, Alavanja MCR. 2011. Genetic variation in base excision repair pathway genes, pesticide exposure, and prostate cancer risk. *Environmental Health Perspectives* 119(12):1726–1732.

Barry KH, Koutros S, Andreotti G, Sandler DP, Burdette LA, Yeager M, Beane Freeman LE, Lubin JH, Ma X, Zheng T, Alavanja MCR, Berndt SI. 2012. Genetic variation in nucleotide excision repair pathway genes, pesticide exposure and prostate cancer risk. *Carcinogenesis* 33(2):331–337.

Barthel E. 1981. Increased risk of lung cancer in pesticide-exposed male agricultural workers. *Journal of Toxicology and Environmental Health* 8:1027–1040.

Bashirov AA. 1969. The health of workers involved in the production of amine and butyl 2,4-D herbicides. *Vrachebnoye Delo* 10:92–95.

Becher H, Wahrendorf J, Angerer R. 1992. A cohort study on persons exposed to phenoxy acid herbicides and their contaminants in Germany—Design and first results. *Chemosphere* 25(7-10):100–101.

Becher H, Flesch-Janys D, Kauppinen T, Kogevinas M, Steindorf K, Manz A, Wahrendorf J. 1996. Cancer mortality in German male workers exposed to phenoxy herbicides and dioxins. *Cancer Causes and Control* 7(3):312–321.

Bell EM, Hertz-Picciotto I, Beaumont JJ. 2001a. Case–cohort analysis of agricultural pesticide applications near maternal residence and selected causes of fetal death. *American Journal of Epidemiology* 154(8):702–710.

Bell EM, Hertz-Picciotto I, Beaumont JJ. 2001b. A case-control study of pesticides and fetal death due to congenital anomalies. *Epidemiology* 12(2):148–156.

Benjamini Y, Hochberg Y. 1995. Controlling the false discovery rate: A practical and powerful approach to multiple testing. *Journal of the Royal Statistical Society, Series B* 57(1):289–300.

Bertazzi PA, Zocchetti C, Pesatori AC, Guercilena S, Sanarico M, Radice L. 1989a. Mortality in an area contaminated by TCDD following an industrial incident. *Medicina Del Lavoro* 80:316–329.

Bertazzi PA, Zocchetti C, Pesatori AC, Guercilena S, Sanarico M, Radice L. 1989b. Ten-year mortality study of the population involved in the Seveso incident in 1976. *American Journal of Epidemiology* 129:1187–1200.

Bertazzi PA, Zocchetti C, Pesatori AC, Guercilena S, Consonni D, Tironi A, Landi MT. 1992. Mortality of a young population after accidental exposure to 2,3,7,8-tetrachlorodibenzodioxin. *International Journal of Epidemiology* 21:118–123.

Bertazzi PA, Pesatori AC, Consonni D, Tironi A, Landi MT, Zocchetti C. 1993. Cancer incidence in a population accidentally exposed to 2,3,7,8-tetrachlorodibenzo-*para*-dioxin. *Epidemiology* 4:398–406.

Bertazzi PA, Zochetti C, Guercilena S, Consonni D, Tironi A, Landi MT, Pesatori AC. 1997. Dioxin exposure and cancer risk: A 15-year mortality study after the "Seveso accident." *Epidemiology* 8(6):646–652.

Bertazzi PA, Bernucci I, Brambilla G, Consonni D, Pesatori AC. 1998. The Seveso studies on early and long-term effects of dioxin exposure: A review. *Environmental Health Perspectives* 106(Suppl 2):625–633.

Bertazzi PA, Consonni D, Bachetti S, Rubagotti M, Baccarelli A, Zocchetti C, Pesatori AC. 2001. Health effects of dioxin exposure: A 20-year mortality study. *American Journal of Epidemiology* 153(11):1031–1044.

Bisanti L, Bonetti F, Caramaschi F, Del Corno G, Favaretti C, Giambelluca SE, Marni E, Montesarchio E, Puccinelli V, Remotti G, Volpato C, Zambrelli E, Fara GM. 1980. Experiences from the accident of Seveso. *Acta Morphologica Academiae Scientarum Hungaricae* 28:139–157.

Blair A, Thomas TL. 1979. Leukemia among Nebraska farmers: A death certificate study. *American Journal of Epidemiology* 110:264–273.

Blair A, White DW. 1985. Leukemia cell types and agricultural practices in Nebraska. *Archives of Environmental Health* 40:211–214.

Blair A, Mustafa D, Heineman EF. 1993. Cancer and other causes of death among male and female farmers from twenty-three states. *American Journal of Industrial Medicine* 23:729–742.

Blair A, Sandler DP, Tarone R, Lubin J, Thomas K, Hoppin JA, Samanic C, Coble J, Kamel F, Knott C, Dosemeci M, Zahm SH, Lynch CF, Rothman N, Alavanja MC. 2005a. Mortality among participants in the Agricultural Health Study. *Annals of Epidemiology* 15(4):279–285.

Blair A, Sandler D, Thomas K, Hoppin JA, Kamel F, Cobel J, Lee WJ, Rusiecki J, Knott C, Dosemeci M, Lynch CF, Lubin J, Alavanja M. 2005b. Disease and injury among participants in the Agricultural Health Study. *Journal of Agricultural Safety and Health* 11(2):141–150.

Blair A, Thomas K, Coble J, Sandler DP, Hines CJ, Lynch CF, Knott C, Purdue MP, Zahm SH, Alavanja MC, Dosemeci M, Kamel F, Hoppin JA, Freeman LB, Lubin JH. 2011. Impact of pesticide exposure misclassification on estimates of relative risks in the Agricultural Health Study. *Occupational and Environmental Medicine* 68(7):537–541.

Blatter BM, Hermens R, Bakker M, Roeleveld N, Verbeek AL, Zielhuis GA. 1997. Paternal occupational exposure around conception and spina bifida in offspring. *American Journal of Industrial Medicine* 32(3):283–291.

Bloemen LJ, Mandel JS, Bond GG, Pollock AF, Vitek RP, Cook RR. 1993. An update of mortality among chemical workers potentially exposed to the herbicide 2,4-dichlorophenoxyacetic acid and its derivatives. *Journal of Occupational Medicine* 35:1208–1212.

Bloom M, Vena J, Olson J, Moysich K. 2006. Chronic exposure to dioxin-like compounds and thyroid function among New York anglers. *Environmental Toxicology and Pharmacology* 21(3):260–267.

Bodner KM, Collins JJ, Bloemen LJ, Carson ML. 2003. Cancer risk for chemical workers exposed to 2,3,7,8-tetrachlorodibenzo-*p*-dioxin. *Occupational and Environmental Medicine* 60:672–675.

Boehmer TK, Flanders WD, McGeehin MA, Boyle C, Barrett DH. 2004. Postservice mortality in Vietnam veterans: 30-year follow-up. *Archives of Internal Medicine* 164(17):1908–1916.

Boeri R, Bordo B, Crenna P, Filippini G, Massetto M, Zecchini A. 1978. Preliminary results of a neurological investigation of the population exposed to TCDD in the Seveso region. *Rivista di Patologia Nervosa e Mentale* 99:111–128.

Boers D, Portengen L, Bueno de Mesquita HB, Heederik D, Vermeulen R. 2010. Cause-specific mortality of Dutch chlorophenoxy herbicide manufacturing workers. *Occupational and Environmental Medicine* 67(1):24–31.

Boers D, Portengen L, Turner WE, Bueno de Mesquita HB, Heederik D, Vermeulen R. 2012. Plasma dioxin levels and cause-specific mortality in an occupational cohort of workers exposed to chlorophenoxy herbicides, chlorophenols and contaminants. *Occupational and Environmental Medicine* 69(2):113–118.

Boffetta P, Stellman SD, Garfinkel L. 1989. A case-control study of multiple myeloma nested in the American Cancer Society prospective study. *International Journal of Cancer* 43:554–559.

Bond GG, Ott MG, Brenner FE, Cook RR. 1983. Medical and morbidity surveillance findings among employees potentially exposed to TCDD. *British Journal of Industrial Medicine* 40:318–324.

Bond GG, Cook RR, Brenner FE, McLaren EA. 1987. Evaluation of mortality patterns among chemical workers with chloracne. *Chemosphere* 16:2117–2121.

Bond GG, Wetterstroem NH, Roush GJ, McLaren EA, Lipps TE, Cook RR. 1988. Cause specific mortality among employees engaged in the manufacture, formulation, or packaging of 2,4-dichlorophenoxyacetic acid and related salts. *British Journal of Industrial Medicine* 45:98–105.

Bond GG, McLaren EA, Lipps TE, Cook RR. 1989a. Update of mortality among chemical workers with potential exposure to the higher chlorinated dioxins. *Journal of Occupational Medicine* 31:121–123.

Bond GG, McLaren EA, Brenner FE, Cook RR. 1989b. Incidence of chloracne among chemical workers potentially exposed to chlorinated dioxins. *Journal of Occupational Medicine* 31:771–774.

Boyle C, Decoufle P, Delaney RJ, DeStefano F, Flock ML, Hunter MI, Joesoef MR, Karon JM, Kirk ML, Layde PM, McGee DL, Moyer LA, Pollock DA, Rhodes P, Scally MJ, Worth RM. 1987. *Postservice Mortality Among Vietnam Veterans.* Atlanta, GA: Centers for Disease Control. CEH 86-0076.

Breslin P, Kang H, Lee Y, Burt V, Shepard BM. 1988. Proportionate mortality study of US Army and US Marine Corps veterans of the Vietnam War. *Journal of Occupational Medicine* 30:412–419.

Brown LM, Blair A, Gibson R, Everett GD, Cantor KP, Schuman LM, Burmeister LF, Van Lier SF, Dick F. 1990. Pesticide exposures and other agricultural risk factors for leukemia among men in Iowa and Minnesota. *Cancer Research* 50:6585–6591.

Brown LM, Burmeister LF, Everett GD, Blair A. 1993. Pesticide exposures and multiple myeloma in Iowa men. *Cancer Causes and Control* 4:153–156.

Bueno de Mesquita HB, Doornbos G, van der Kuip DA, Kogevinas M, Winkelmann R. 1993. Occupational exposure to phenoxy herbicides and chlorophenols and cancer mortality in the Netherlands. *American Journal of Industrial Medicine* 23:289–300.

Bullman TA, Kang HK. 1996. The risk of suicide among wounded Vietnam veterans. *American Journal of Public Health* 86(5):662–667.

Bullman TA, Kang HK, Watanabe KK. 1990. Proportionate mortality among US Army Vietnam veterans who served in Military Region I. *American Journal of Epidemiology* 132:670–674.

Bullman TA, Kang H, Thomas TL. 1991. Posttraumatic stress disorder among Vietnam veterans on the Agent Orange Registry: A case-control analysis. *Annals of Epidemiology* 1:505–512.

Bullman TA, Watanabe KK, Kang HK. 1994. Risk of testicular cancer associated with surrogate measures of Agent Orange exposure among Vietnam veterans on the Agent Orange Registry. *Annals of Epidemiology* 4:11–16.

Burmeister LF. 1981. Cancer mortality in Iowa farmers: 1971–1978. *Journal of the National Cancer Institute* 66:461–464.

Burmeister LF, Van Lier SF, Isacson P. 1982. Leukemia and farm practices in Iowa. *American Journal of Epidemiology* 115:720–728.

Burmeister LF, Everett GD, Van Lier SF, Isacson P. 1983. Selected cancer mortality and farm practices in Iowa. *American Journal of Epidemiology* 118:72–77.

Burns CJ, Beard KK, Cartmill JB. 2001. Mortality in chemical workers potentially exposed to 2,4-dichlorophenoxyacetic acid (2,4-D) 1945–1994: An update. *Occupational and Environmental Medicine* 58:24–30.

Burns CJ, Collins JJ, Humphry N, Bodner KM, Aylward LL, McBride D. 2010. Correlates of serum dioxin to self-reported exposure factors. *Environmental Research* 110(2):131–136.

Burns CJ, Bodner K, Swaen G, Collins J, Beard K, Lee M. 2011. Cancer incidence of 2,4-D production workers. *International Journal of Environmental Research and Public Health* 8(9):3579–3590.

Burns JS, Williams PL, Sergeyev O, Korrick S, Lee MM, Revich B, Altshul L, Patterson DG Jr, Turner WE, Needham LL, Saharov I, Hauser R. 2009. Predictors of serum dioxins and PCBS among peripubertal Russian boys. *Environmental Health Perspectives* 117(10):1593–1599.

Burns JS, Williams PL, Sergeyev O, Korrick S, Lee MM, Revich B, Altshul L, Del Prato JT, Humblet O, Patterson DG, Turner WE, Needham LL, Starovoytov M, Hauser R. 2011. Serum dioxins and polychlorinated biphenyls are associated with growth among Russian boys. *Pediatrics* 127(1): e59–e68.

Burt VL, Breslin PP, Kang HK, Lee Y. 1987. *Non-Hodgkin's lymphoma in Vietnam veterans.* Washington, DC: Department of Medicine and Surgery, Veterans Administration.

Burton JE, Michalek JE, Rahe AJ. 1998. Serum dioxin, chloracne, and acne in veterans of Operation Ranch Hand. *Archives of Environmental Health* 53(3):199–204.

Butterfield PG, Valanis BG, Spencer PS, Lindeman CA, Nutt JG. 1993. Environmental antecedents of young-onset Parkinson's disease. *Neurology* 43:1150–1158.

Calvert GM, Sweeney MH, Morris JA, Fingerhut MA, Hornung RW, Halperin WE. 1991. Evaluation of chronic bronchitis, chronic obstructive pulmonary disease, and ventilatory function among workers exposed to 2,3,7,8-tetrachlorodibenzo-*p*-dioxin. *American Review of Respiratory Disease* 144:1302–1306.

Calvert GM, Hornung RW, Sweeney MH, Fingerhut MA, Halperin WE. 1992. Hepatic and gastrointestinal effects in an occupational cohort exposed to 2,3,7,8-tetrachlorodibenzo-*para*-dioxin. *Journal of the American Medical Association* 267:2209–2214.

Calvert GM, Sweeney MH, Fingerhut MA, Hornung RW, Halperin WE. 1994. Evaluation of porphyria cutanea tarda in US workers exposed to 2,3,7,8-tetrachlorodibenzo-*p*-dioxin. *American Journal of Industrial Medicine* 25:559–571.

Calvert GM, Wall DK, Sweeney MH, Fingerhut MA. 1998. Evaluation of cardiovascular outcomes among US workers exposed to 2,3,7,8-tetrachlorodibenzo-*p*-dioxin. *Environmental Health Perspectives* 106(Suppl 2):635–643.

Calvert GM, Sweeney MH, Deddens J, Wall DK. 1999. Evaluation of diabetes mellitus, serum glucose, and thyroid function among United States workers exposed to 2,3,7,8-tetrachlorodibenzo-*p*-dioxin. *Occupational and Environmental Medicine* 56(4):270–276.

Campbell SB, Renshaw KD. 2012. Distress in spouses of Vietnam veterans: Associations with communication about deployment experiences. *Journal of Family Psychology* 26(1):18–25.

Can N, Xiem NT, Tong NK, Duong DB. 1983a. A case-control survey of congenital defects in My Van District, Hai Hung Province. Summarized in: Constable JD, Hatch MC. *Reproductive Effects of Herbicide Exposure in Vietnam: Recent Studies by the Vietnamese and Others.* As cited in Constable and Hatch, 1985.

Can N, Xiem NT, Tong NK, Duong DB. 1983b. An epidemiologic survey of pregnancies in Viet Nam. Summarized in: Constable JD, Hatch MC. *Reproductive Effects of Herbicide Exposure in Vietnam: Recent Studies by the Vietnamese and Others.* As cited in Constable and Hatch, 1985.

Cantor KP. 1982. Farming and mortality from non-Hodgkin's lymphoma: A case-control study. *International Journal of Cancer* 29:239–247.

Cantor KP, Blair A, Everett G, Gibson R, Burmeister LF, Brown LM, Schuman L, Dick FR. 1992. Pesticides and other agricultural risk factors for non-Hodgkin's lymphoma among men in Iowa and Minnesota. *Cancer Research* 52:2447–2455.

Caramaschi F, Del Corno G, Favaretti C, Giambelluca SE, Montesarchio E, Fara GM. 1981. Chloracne following environmental contamination by TCDD in Seveso, Italy. *International Journal of Epidemiology* 10:135–143.

Carmelli D, Hofherr L, Tomsic J, Morgan RW. 1981. *A Case-Control Study of the Relationship Between Exposure to 2,4-D and Spontaneous Abortions in Humans.* SRI International. Prepared for the National Forest Products Association and the US Department of Agriculture, Forest Service.

Carreon T, Butler MA, Ruder AM, Waters MA, Davis-King KE, Calvert GM, Schulte PA, Connally B, Ward EM, Sanderson WT, Heineman EF, Mandel JS, Morton RF, Reding DJ, Rosenman KD, Talaska G, Cancer B. 2005. Gliomas and farm pesticide exposure in women: The Upper Midwest Health Study. *Environmental Health Perspectives* 113(5):546–551.

Cartwright RA, McKinney PA, O'Brien C, Richards IDG, Roberts B, Lauder I, Darwin CM, Bernard SM, Bird CC. 1988. Non-Hodgkin's lymphoma: Case-control epidemiological study in Yorkshire. *Leukemia Research* 12:81–88.

Castorina R, Bradman A, Fenster L, Barr DB, Bravo R, Vedar MG, Harnly ME, McKone TE, Eisen EA, Eskenazi B. 2010. Comparison of current-use pesticide and other toxicant urinary metabolite levels among pregnant women in the CHAMACOS cohort and NHANES. *Environmental Health Perspectives* 118(6):856–863.

CDC (Centers for Disease Control and Prevention). 1985. *Exposure Assessment for the Agent Orange Study. Interim Report Number 2.* Atlanta, GA: Center for Environmental Health.

CDC. 1987. Postservice mortality among Vietnam veterans. *Journal of the American Medical Association* 257:790–795.

CDC. 1988a. Health status of Vietnam veterans. II. Physical health. *Journal of the American Medical Association* 259:2708–2714.

CDC. 1988b. Health status of Vietnam veterans. I. Psychosocial characteristics. *Journal of the American Medical Association* 259:2701–2707.

CDC. 1988c. Health status of Vietnam veterans. III. Reproductive outcomes and child health. *Journal of the American Medical Association* 259:2715–2717.

CDC. 1988d. Preliminary report: 2,3,7,8-tetrachlorodibenzo-*p*-dioxin exposure in humans—Seveso, Italy. *Morbidity and Mortality Weekly Report* 37:733–736.

CDC. 1989a. *Comparison of Serum Levels of 2,3,7,8-Tetrachlorodibenzo-*p*-dioxin with Indirect Estimates of Agent Orange Exposure Among Vietnam Veterans: Final Report.* Atlanta, GA: US Department of Health and Human Services.

CDC. 1989b. *Health Status of Vietnam Veterans: Vietnam Experience Study. Vols. I–V, Supplements A–C.* Atlanta, GA: US Department of Health and Human Services.

CDC. 1990a. *The Association of Selected Cancers with Service in the US Military in Vietnam: Final Report.* Atlanta, GA: US Department of Health and Human Services.

CDC. 1990b. The association of selected cancers with service in the US military in Vietnam. I. Non-Hodgkin's lymphoma. *Archives of Internal Medicine* 150:2473–2483.

CDC. 1990c. The association of selected cancers with service in the US military in Vietnam. II. Soft-tissue and other sarcomas. *Archives of Internal Medicine* 150:2485–2492.

CDC. 1990d. The association of selected cancers with service in the US military in Vietnam. III. Hodgkin's disease, nasal cancer, nasopharyngeal cancer, and primary liver cancer. *Archives of Internal Medicine* 150:2495–2505.

CDC. 2004. 2001–2002 National Health and Nutrition Examination Survey (NHANES). http://www.cdc.gov/nchs/nhanes/nhanes2001–2002/nhanes01_02.htm (accessed April 1, 2011).

CDVA (Commonwealth Department of Veterans' Affairs). 1998a. *Morbidity of Vietnam Veterans: A Study of the Health of Australia's Vietnam Veteran Community. Volume 1: Male Vietnam Veterans Survey and Community Comparison Outcomes.* Canberra, Australia: Department of Veterans' Affairs.

CDVA. 1998b. *Morbidity of Vietnam Veterans: A Study of the Health of Australia's Vietnam Veteran Community. Volume 2: Female Vietnam Veterans Survey and Community Comparison Outcomes.* Canberra, Australia: Department of Veterans' Affairs.

Chamie K, DeVere White R, Lee D, Ok J, Ellison L. 2008. Agent Orange exposure, Vietnam War veterans, and the risk of prostate cancer. *Cancer* 113(9):2464–2470.

Chang JW, Chen HL, Su HJ, Liao PC, Guo HR, Lee CC. 2010. Dioxin exposure and insulin resistance in Taiwanese living near a highly contaminated area. *Epidemiology* 21(1):56–61.

Chang JW, Chen HL, Su HJ, Liao PC, Guo HR, Lee CC. 2011a. Simultaneous exposure of non-diabetics to high levels of dioxins and mercury increases their risk of insulin resistance. *Journal of Hazardous Materials* 185(2–3):749–755.

Chang JW, Chen HL, Chang CC, Su HJ, Liao PC, Lee CC. 2011b. Predicting the risk of cardiovascular disease in people exposed to moderate to high levels of dioxin. *Journal of Hazardous Materials* 198:317–322.

Chang JW, Chen HL, Su HJ, Liao PC, Lee CC. 2012. Biochemical study of retired pentachlorophenol workers with and without following dietary exposure to PCDD/FS. *Chemosphere* 88(7):813–819.

Chao HR, Wang SL, Lee CC, Yu HY, Lu YK, Päpke O. 2004. Level of polychlorinated dibenzo-*p*-dioxins, dibenzofurans and biphenyls (PCDD/Fs, PCBs) in human milk and the input to infant body burden. *Food and Chemical Toxicology* 42:1299–1308.

Chao HR, Wang SL, Lin LY, Lee WJ, Päpke O. 2007. Placental transfer of polychlorinated dibenzo-*p*-dioxins, dibenzofurans, and biphenyls in Taiwanese mothers in relation to menstrual cycle characteristics. *Food Chemical Toxicology* 45:259–265.

Chen HL, Su HJ, Guo YL, Liao PC, Hung CF, Lee CC. 2006. Biochemistry examinations and health disorder evaluation of Tiawanese living near incinerators and with low serum PCDD/Fs levels. *Science of the Total Environment* 366:538–548.

Chen Z, Stewart PA, Davies S, Giller R, Krailo M, Davis M, Robison L, Shu XO. 2005. Parental occupational exposure to pesticides and childhood germ-cell tumors. *American Journal of Epidemiology* 162(9):858–867.

Chen Z, Robison L, Giller R, Krailo M, Davis M, Davies S, Shu XO. 2006. Environmental exposure to residential pesticides, chemicals, dusts, fumes, and metals, and risk of childhood germ cell tumors. *International Journal of Hygiene and Environmental Health* 209(1):31–40.

Chiu BC, Weisenburger DD, Zahm SH, Cantor KP, Gapstur SM, Holmes F, Burmeister LF, Blair A. 2004. Agricultural pesticide use, familial cancer, and risk of non-Hodgkin lymphoma. *Cancer Epidemiology, Biomarkers and Prevention* 13(4):525–531.

Chiu BC, Dave BJ, Blair A, Gapstur SM, Zahm SH, Weisenburger DD. 2006. Agricultural pesticide use and risk of t(14;18)-defined subtypes of non-Hodgkin lymphoma. *Blood* 108(4):1363–1369.

Cho MR, Shin JY, Hwang JH, Jacobs DR Jr, Kim SY, Lee DH. 2011. Associations of fat mass and lean mass with bone mineral density differ by levels of persistent organic pollutants: National Health and Nutrition Examination Survey 1999–2004. *Chemosphere* 82:1268–1276.

CIH (Commonwealth Institute of Health). 1984a. Australian Veterans Health Studies. *Mortality Report. Part I. A Retrospective Cohort Study of Mortality Among Australian National Servicemen of the Vietnam Conflict Era, and An Executive Summary of the Mortality Report.* Canberra, Australia: Australian Government Publishing Service.

CIH. 1984b. *Australian Veterans Health Studies. The Mortality Report. Part II. Factors Influencing Mortality Rates of Australian National Servicemen of the Vietnam Conflict Era.* Canberra, Australia: Australian Government Publishing Service.

CIH. 1984c. *Australian Veterans Health Studies. The Mortality Report. Part III. The Relationship Between Aspects of Vietnam Service and Subsequent Mortality Among Australian National Servicemen of the Vietnam Conflict Era.* Canberra, Australia: Australian Government Publishing Service.

Clapp RW. 1997. Update of cancer surveillance of veterans in Massachusetts, USA. *International Journal of Epidemiology* 26(3):679–681.

Clapp RW, Cupples LA, Colton T, Ozonoff DM. 1991. Cancer surveillance of veterans in Massachusetts, 1982–1988. *International Journal of Epidemiology* 20:7–12.

Coble J, Thomas KW, Hines CJ, Hoppin JA, Dosemeci M, Curwin B, Lubin JH, Beane Freeman LE, Blair A, Sandler DP, Alavanja MC. 2011. An updated algorithm for estimation of pesticide exposure intensity in the Agricultural Health Study. *International Journal of Environmental Research and Public Health* 8(12):4608–4622.

Coggon D, Pannett B, Winter PD, Acheson ED, Bonsall J. 1986. Mortality of workers exposed to 2-methyl-4-chlorophenoxyacetic acid. *Scandinavian Journal of Work, Environment and Health* 12:448–454.

Coggon D, Pannett B, Winter P. 1991. Mortality and incidence of cancer at four factories making phenoxy herbicides. *British Journal of Industrial Medicine* 48:173–178.

Collins JJ, Strauss ME, Levinskas GJ, Conner PR. 1993. The mortality experience of workers exposed to 2,3,7,8-tetrachlorodibenzo-*p*-dioxin in a trichlorophenol process accident. *Epidemiology* 4:7–13.

Collins JJ, Budinsky RA, Burns CJ, Lamparski LL, Carson ML, Martin GD, Wilken M. 2006. Serum dioxin levels in former chlorophenol workers. *Journal of Exposure Science and Environmental Epidemiology* 16(1):76–84.

Collins JJ, Bodner K, Aylward LL, Wilken M, Bodner CM. 2009a. Mortality rates among trichlorophenol workers with exposure to 2,3,7,8-tetrachlorodibenzo-*p*-dioxin. *American Journal of Epidemiology* 170(4):501–506.

Collins JJ, Bodner K, Aylward LL, Wilken M, Swaen G, Budinsky R, Rowlands C, Bodnar CM. 2009b. Mortality rates among workers exposed to dioxins in the manufacture of pentachlorophenol. *Journal of Occupational and Environmental Medicine* 51(10):1212–1219.

Collins JJ, Wilken M, McBride D, Humphry NF, Herbison P, Burns CJ, Bodner K. 2009c. Serum concentrations of chlorinated dibenzo-*p*-dioxins and dibenzofurans among former New Zealand trichlorophenol workers. *Chemosphere* 76(11):1550–1556.

Colt JS, Rothman N, Severson RK, Hartge P, Cerhan JR, Chatterjee N, Cozen W, Morton LM, De Roos AJ, Davis S, Chanock S, Wang SS. 2009. Organochlorine exposure, immune gene variation, and risk of non-Hodgkin lymphoma. *Blood* 113(9):1899–1905.

Conley D, Heerwig J. 2012. The long-term effects of military conscription on mortality: Estimates from the Vietnam-era draft lottery. *Demography* 49:841–855.

Consonni D, Pesatori AC, Zocchetti C, Sindaco R, D'Oro LC, Rubagotti M, Bertazzi PA. 2008. Mortality in a population exposed to dioxin after the Seveso, Italy, accident in 1976: 25 years of follow-up. *American Journal of Epidemiology* 167(7):847–858.

Constable JD, Hatch MC. 1985. Reproductive effects of herbicide exposure in Vietnam: Recent studies by the Vietnamese and others. *Teratogenesis, Carcinogenesis, and Mutagenesis* 5:231–250.

Cook RR, Townsend JC, Ott MG, Silverstein LG. 1980. Mortality experience of employees exposed to 2,3,7,8-tetrachlorodibenzo-*p*-dioxin (TCDD). *Journal of Occupational Medicine* 22:530–532.

Cook RR, Bond GG, Olson RA. 1986. Evaluation of the mortality experience of workers exposed to the chlorinated dioxins. *Chemosphere* 15:1769–1776.

Cook RR, Bond GG, Olson RA, Ott MG. 1987. Update of the mortality experience of workers exposed to chlorinated dioxins. *Chemosphere* 16:2111–2116.

Cordier S, Le TB, Verger P, Bard D, Le CD, Larouze B, Dazza MC, Hoang TQ, Abenhaim L. 1993. Viral infections and chemical exposures as risk factors for hepatocellular carcinoma in Vietnam. *International Journal of Cancer* 55:196–201.

Cordier S, Chevrier C, Robert-Gnansia E, Lorente C, Brula P, Hours M. 2004. Risk of congenital anomalies in the vicinity of municipal solid waste incinerators. *Occupational and Environmental Medicine* 61(1):8–15.

Cordier S, Lehebel A, Amar E, Anzivino-Viricel L, Hours M, Monfort C, Chevrier C, Chiron M, Robert-Gnansia E. 2010. Maternal residence near municipal waste incinerators and the risk of urinary tract birth defects. *Occupational and Environmental Medicine* 67(7):493–499.

Corrao G, Caller M, Carle F, Russo R, Bosia S, Piccioni P. 1989. Cancer risk in a cohort of licensed pesticide users. *Scandinavian Journal of Work, Environment and Health* 15:203–209.

Costani G, Rabitti P, Mambrini A, Bai E, Berrino F. 2000. Soft tissue sarcomas in the general population living near a chemical plant in northern Italy. *Tumori* 86:381–383.

Crane PJ, Barnard DL, Horsley KW, Adena MA. 1997a. *Mortality of Vietnam Veterans: The Veteran Cohort Study. A Report of the 1996 Retrospective Cohort Study of Australian Vietnam Veterans.* Canberra, Australia: Department of Veterans Affairs.

Crane PJ, Barnard DL, Horsley KW, Adena MA. 1997b. *Mortality of National Service Vietnam Veterans: A Report of the 1996 Retrospective Cohort Study of Australian Vietnam Veterans.* Canberra, Australia: Department of Veterans Affairs.

Crawford JM, Hoppin JA, Alavanja MCR, Blair A, Sandler DP, Kamel F. 2008. Hearing loss among licensed pesticide applicators in the Agricultural Health Study. *Journal of Occupational and Environmental Medicine* 50(7):817–826.

Currier JM, Holland JM. 2012. Examining the role of combat loss among Vietnam War veterans. *Journal of Traumatic Loss* 25:102–105.

Curtis K, Savitz D, Weinberg C, Arbuckle T. 1999. The effect of pesticide exposure on time to pregnancy. *Epidemiology* 10(2):112–117. [Comment in *Epidemiology* 1999. 10(3):470.]

Curwin BD, Hein MJ, Sanderson WT, Barr DB, Heederik D, Reynolds SJ, Ward EM, Alavanja MC. 2005. Urinary and hand wipe pesticide levels among farmers and nonfarmers in Iowa. *Journal of Exposure Analysis and Environmental Epidemiology* 15(6):500–508.

Cypel Y, Kang H. 2008. Mortality patterns among women Vietnam-era veterans: Results of a retrospective cohort study. *Annals of Epidemiology* 18(3):244–252.

Cypel Y, Kang H. 2010. Mortality patterns of Army Chemical Corps veterans who were occupationally exposed to herbicides in Vietnam. *Annals of Epidemiology* 20(5):339–346.

Dai LC, Phuong NTN, Thom LH, Thuy TT, Van NTT, Cam LH, Chi HTK, Thuy LB. 1990. A comparison of infant mortality rates between two Vietnamese villages sprayed by defoliants in wartime and one unsprayed village. *Chemosphere* 20:1005–1012.

Dalager NA, Kang HK. 1997. Mortality among Army Chemical Corps Vietnam veterans. *American Journal of Industrial Medicine* 31(6):719–726.

Dalager NA, Kang HK, Burt VL, Weatherbee L. 1991. Non-Hodgkin's lymphoma among Vietnam veterans. *Journal of Occupational Medicine* 33:774–779.

Dalager NA, Kang HK, Burt VL, Weatherbee L. 1995a. Hodgkin's disease and Vietnam service. *Annals of Epidemiology* 5(5):400–406.

Dalager NA, Kang HK, Thomas TL. 1995b. Cancer mortality patterns among women who served in the military: The Vietnam experience. *Journal of Occupational and Environmental Medicine* 37:298–305.

Dankovic DA, Andersen ME, Salvan A, Stayner LT. 1995. A simplified PBPK model describing the kinetics of TCDD in humans (abstract). *Toxicologist* 15:272.

De Felip E, Porpora MG, di Domenico A, Ingelido AM, Cardelli M, Cosmi EV, Donnez J. 2004. Dioxin-like compounds and endometriosis: A study on Italian and Belgian women of reproductive age. *Toxicology Letters* 150(2):203–209.

De Roos AJ, Hartge P, Lubin JH, Colt JS, Davis S, Cerhan JR, Severson RK, Cozen W, Patterson DG Jr, Needham LL, Rothman N. 2005a. Persistent organochlorine chemicals in plasma and risk of non-Hodgkin's lymphoma. *Cancer Research* 65(23):11214–11226.

De Roos AJ, Cooper GS, Alavanja MC, Sandler DP. 2005b. Rheumatoid arthritis among women in the Agricultural Health Study: Risk associated with farming activities and exposures. *Annals of Epidemiology* 15(10):762–770.

Decoufle P, Holmgreen P, Boyle CA, Stroup NE. 1992. Self-reported health status of Vietnam veterans in relation to perceived exposure to herbicides and combat. *American Journal of Epidemiology* 135:312–323.

Dennis LK, Lynch CF, Sandler DP, Alavanja M. 2010. Pesticide use and cutaneous melanoma in pesticide applicators in the Agricultural Health Study. *Environmental Health Perspectives* 118(6):812–817.

Deprez RD, Carvette ME, Agger MS. 1991. *The Health and Medical Status of Maine Veterans: A Report to the Bureau of Veterans Services, Commission of Vietnam and Atomic Veterans.* Portland, ME: Public Health Resource Group.

Dich J, Wiklund K. 1998. Prostate cancer in pesticide applicators in Swedish agriculture. *Prostate* 34(2):100–112.

Dimich-Ward H, Hertzman C, Teschke K, Hershler R, Marion SA, Ostry A, Kelly S. 1996. Reproductive effects of paternal exposure to chlorophenate wood preservatives in the sawmill industry. *Scandinavian Journal of Work, Environment and Health* 22(4):267–273.

Donna A, Betta PG, Robutti F, Crosignani P, Berrino F, Bellingeri D. 1984. Ovarian mesothelial tumors and herbicides: A case-control study. *Carcinogenesis* 5:941–942.

Donovan JW, Adena MA, Rose G, Battistutta D. 1983. *Case-Control Study of Congenital Anomalies and Vietnam Service: Birth Defects Study. Report to the Minister for Veterans' Affairs.* Canberra, Australia: Australian Government Publishing Service.

Donovan JW, MacLennan R, Adena M. 1984. Vietnam service and the risk of congenital anomalies: A case-control study. *Medical Journal of Australia* 140:394–397.

Dosemeci M, Alavanja MC, Rowland AS, Mage D, Zahm SH, Rothman N, Lubin JH, Hoppin JA, Sandler DP, Blair A. 2002. A quantitative approach for estimating exposure to pesticides in the Agricultural Health Study. *Annals of Occupational Hygiene* 46(2):245–260.

Dubrow R, Paulson JO, Indian RW. 1988. Farming and malignant lymphoma in Hancock County, Ohio. *British Journal of Industrial Medicine* 45:25–28.

Duell EJ, Millikan RC, Savitz DA, Schell MJ, Newman B, Tse CKJ, Sandler DP. 2001. Reproducibility of reported farming activities and pesticide use among breast cancer cases and controls: A comparison of two modes of data collection. *Association of Emergency Physicians* 11(3):178–185.

Egeland GM, Sweeney MH, Fingerhut MA, Wille KK, Schnorr TM, Halperin WE. 1994. Total serum testosterone and gonadotropins in workers exposed to dioxin. *American Journal of Epidemiology* 139:272–281.

Eisen S, Goldberg J, True WR, Henderson WG. 1991. A co-twin control study of the effects of the Vietnam War on the self-reported physical health of veterans. *American Journal of Epidemiology* 134:49–58.

Ekström AM, Eriksson M, Hansson LE, Lindgren A, Signorello LB, Nyren O, Hardell L. 1999. Occupational exposures and risk of gastric cancer in a population-based case-control study. *Cancer Research* 59(23):5932–5937.

Elobeid MA, Padilla MA, Brock DW, Ruden DM, Allison DB. 2010. Endocrine disruptors and obesity: An examination of selected persistent organic pollutants in the NHANES 1999–2002 data. *International Journal of Environmental Research and Public Health* 7:2988–3005.

Engel LS, Hill DA, Hoppin JA, Lubin JH, Lynch CF, Pierce J, Samanic C, Sandler DP, Blair A, Alavanja MC. 2005. Pesticide use and breast cancer risk among farmers' wives in the Agricultural Health Study. *American Journal of Epidemiology* 161(2):121–135.

Erickson JD, Mulinare J, McClain PW, Fitch TG, James LM, McClearn AB, Adams MJ Jr. 1984a. *Vietnam Veterans' Risks for Fathering Babies with Birth Defects.* Atlanta, GA: US Department of Health and Human Services, Centers for Disease Control.

Erickson JD, Mulinare J, McClain PW, Fitch TG, James LM, McClearn AB, Adams MJ Jr. 1984b. Vietnam veterans' risks for fathering babies with birth defects. *Journal of the American Medical Association* 252:903–912.

Eriksson M, Hardell L, Berg NO, Moller T, Axelson O. 1979. Case-control study on malignant mesenchymal tumor of the soft tissue and exposure to chemical substances. *Lakartidningen* 76:3872–3875 [in Swedish].

Eriksson M, Hardell L, Berg NO, Moller T, Axelson O. 1981. Soft-tissue sarcomas and exposure to chemical substances: A case–referent study. *British Journal of Industrial Medicine* 38:27–33.

Eriksson M, Hardell L, Adami HO. 1990. Exposure to dioxins as a risk factor for soft tissue sarcoma: A population-based case-control study. *Journal of the National Cancer Institute* 82:486–490.

Eriksson M, Hardell L, Malker H, Weiner J. 1992. Malignant lymphoproliferative diseases in occupations with potential exposure to phenoxyacetic acids or dioxins: A register-based study. *American Journal of Industrial Medicine* 22:305–312.

Eskenazi B, Mocarelli P, Warner M, Samuels S, Needham L, Patterson D, Brambilla P, Gerthoux PM, Turner W, Casalini S, Cazzaniga M, Chee WY. 2001. Seveso Women's Health Study: Does zone of residence predict individual TCDD exposure? *Chemosphere* 43(4-7):937–942.

Eskenazi B, Warner M, Mocarelli P, Samuels S, Needham LL, Patterson DG Jr, Lippman S, Vercellini P, Gerthoux PM, Brambilla P, Olive D. 2002a. Serum dioxin concentrations and menstrual cycle characteristics. *American Journal of Epidemiology* 156(4):383–392.

Eskenazi B, Mocarelli P, Warner M, Samuels S, Vercellini P, Olive D, Needham LL, Patterson DG Jr, Brambilla P, Gavoni N, Casalini S, Panazza S, Turner W, Gerthoux PM. 2002b. Serum dioxin concentrations and endometriosis: A cohort study. *Environmental Health Perspectives* 110(7):629–634.

Eskenazi B, Mocarelli P, Warner M, Chee WY, Gerthoux PM, Samuels S, Needham LL, Patterson DG Jr. 2003a. Maternal serum dioxin levels and birth outcomes in women of Seveso, Italy. *Environmental Health Perspectives* 111(7):947–953.

Eskenazi B, Bradman A, Gladstone EA, Jaramillo S, Birch K, Holland N. 2003b. CHAMACOS, a longitudinal birth cohort study: Lessons from the fields. *Journal of Children's Health* 1(1):3–27.

Eskenazi B, Mocarelli P, Warner M, Needham LL, Patterson DG Jr, Samuels S, Turner W, Gerthoux PM, Brambilla P. 2004. Relationship of serum TCDD concentrations and age at exposure of female residents of Seveso, Italy. *Environmental Health Perspectives* 112(1):22–27.

Eskenazi B, Warner M, Marks AR, Samuels S, Gerthoux PM, Vercellini P, Olive DL, Needham L, Patterson D Jr, Mocarelli P. 2005. Serum dioxin concentrations and age at menopause. *Environmental Health Perspectives* 113(7):858–862.

Eskenazi B, Warner M, Samuels S, Young J, Gerthoux PM, Needham L, Patterson D, Olive D, Gavoni N, Vercellini P, Mocarelli P. 2007. Serum dioxin concentrations and risk of uterine leiomyoma in the Seveso Women's Health Study. *American Journal of Epidemiology* 166(1):79–87.

Eskenazi B, Warner M, Marks AR, Samuels S, Needham L, Brambilla P, Mocarelli P. 2010. Serum dioxin concentrations and time to pregnancy. *Epidemiology* 21(2):224–231.

Evans RG, Webb KB, Knutsen AP, Roodman ST, Roberts DW, Bagby JR, Garrett WA Jr, Andrews JS Jr. 1988. A medical follow-up of the health effects of long-term exposure to 2,3,7,8-tetrachlorodibenzo-*p*-dioxin. *Archives of Environmental Health* 43:273–278.

Evatt P. 1985. *Royal Commission on the Use and Effect of Chemical Agents on Australian Personnel in Vietnam, Final Report.* Canberra, Australia: Australian Government Publishing Service.

Everett CJ, Mainous AG 3rd, Frithsen IL, Player MS, Matheson EM. 2008a. Association of polychlorinated biphenyls with hypertension in the 1999–2002 National Health and Nutrition Examination Survey. *Environmental Research* 108(1):94–97.

Everett CJ, Mainous AG 3rd, Frithsen IL, Player MS, Matheson EM. 2008b. Commentary on association of polychlorinated biphenyls with hypertension. *Environmental Research* 108(3):428–429.

Farberow NL, Kang H, Bullman T. 1990. Combat experience and postservice psychosocial status as predictors of suicide in Vietnam veterans. *Journal of Nervous and Mental Disease* 178:32–37.

Farr SL, Cooper GS, Cai J, Savitz DA, Sandler DP. 2004. Pesticide use and menstrual cycle characteristics among premenopausal women in the Agricultural Health Study. *American Journal of Epidemiology* 160(12):1194–1204.

Farr SL, Cai J, Savitz DA, Sandler DP, Hoppin JA, Cooper GS. 2006. Pesticide exposure and timing of menopause: The Agricultural Health Study. *American Journal of Epidemiology* 163(8):731–742.

Fattore E, Di Guardo A, Mariani G, Guzzi A, Benfenati E, Fanelli R. 2003. Polychlorinated dibenzo-*p*-dioxins and dibenzofurans in the air of Seveso, Italy, 26 years after the explosion. *Environmental Science and Technology* 37(8):1503–1508.

Faustini A, Settimi L, Pacifici R, Fano V, Zuccaro P, Forastiere F. 1996. Immunological changes among farmers exposed to phenoxy herbicides: Preliminary observations. *Occupational and Environmental Medicine* 53(9):583–585.

Fett MJ, Adena MA, Cobbin DM, Dunn M. 1987a. Mortality among Australian conscripts of the Vietnam conflict era. I. Death from all causes. *American Journal of Epidemiology* 126:869–877.

Fett MJ, Nairn JR, Cobbin DM, Adena MA. 1987b. Mortality among Australian conscripts of the Vietnam conflict era. II. Causes of death. *American Journal of Epidemiology* 125:878–884.

Fiedler N, Gochfeld M. 1992. *Neurobehavioral Correlates of Herbicide Exposure in Vietnam Veterans.* New Jersey Agent Orange Commission.

Fierens S, Mairesse H, Heilier JF, De Burbure C, Focant JF, Eppe G, De Pauw E, Bernard A. 2003a. Dioxin/polychlorinated biphenyl body burden, diabetes and endometriosis: Findings in a population-based study in Belgium. *Biomarkers* 8(6):529–534.

Fierens S, Mairesse H, Hermans C, Bernard A, Eppe G, Focant JF, De Pauw E. 2003b. Dioxin accumulation in residents around incinerators. *Journal of Toxicology and Environmental Health Part A* 66(14):1287–1293.

Filippini G, Bordo B, Crenna P, Massetto N, Musicco M, Boeri R. 1981. Relationship between clinical and electrophysiological findings and indicators of heavy exposure to 2,3,7,8-tetrachlorodibenzodioxin. *Scandinavian Journal of Work, Environment and Health* 7:257–262.

Fingerhut MA, Halperin WE, Honchar PA, Smith AB, Groth DH, Russell WO. 1984. An evaluation of reports of dioxin exposure and soft tissue sarcoma pathology among chemical workers in the United States. *Scandinavian Journal of Work, Environment and Health* 10(5):299–303.

Fingerhut MA, Halperin WE, Marlow DA, Piacitelli LA, Honchar PA, Sweeney MH, Greife AL, Dill PA, Steenland K, Suruda AJ. 1991. Cancer mortality in workers exposed to 2,3,7,8-tetrachlorodibenzo-*p*-dioxin. *New England Journal of Medicine* 324:212–218.

Firestone JA, Smith-Weller T, Franklin G, Swanson P, Longstreth WT Jr, Checkoway H. 2005. Pesticides and risk of Parkinson disease: A population-based case-control study. *Archives of Neurology* 62:91–95.

Firestone JA, Lundin JI, Powers KM, Smith-Weller T, Franklin GM, Swanson PD, Longstreth WT Jr, Checkoway H. 2010. Occupational factors and risk of Parkinson's disease: A population-based case-control study. *American Journal of Industrial Medicine* 53(3):217–223.

Fitzgerald EF, Weinstein AL, Youngblood LG, Standfast SJ, Melius JM. 1989. Health effects three years after potential exposure to the toxic contaminants of an electrical transformer fire. *Archives of Environmental Health* 44:214–221.

Flesch-Janys D. 1997. Analyses of exposure to polychlorinated dibenzo-*p*-dioxins, furans, and hexachlorocyclohexane and different health outcomes in a cohort of former herbicide-producing workers in Hamburg, Germany. *Teratogenesis, Carcinogenesis and Mutagenesis* 17(4-5):257–264.

Flesch-Janys D, Berger J, Gurn P, Manz A, Nagel S, Waltsgott H, Dwyer JH. 1995. Exposure to polychlorinated dioxins and furans (PCDD/F) and mortality in a cohort of workers from a herbicide-producing plant in Hamburg, Federal Republic of Germany. *American Journal of Epidemiology* 142(11):1165–1175.

Floret N, Mauny F, Challier B, Arveux P, Cahn JY, Viel JF. 2003. Dioxin emissions from a solid waste incinerator and risk of non-Hodgkin lymphoma. *Epidemiology* 14(4):392–398.

Flower KB, Hoppin JA, Lynch CF, Blair A, Knott C, Shore DL, Sandler DP. 2004. Cancer risk and parental pesticide application in children of Agricultural Health Study participants. *Environmental Health Perspectives* 112(5):631–635.

Forcier L, Hudson HM, Cobbin DM, Jones MP, Adena MA, Fett MJ. 1987. Mortality of Australian veterans of the Vietnam conflict and the period and location of their Vietnam service. *Military Medicine* 152:9–15.

Franzen PL, Woodward SH, Bootzin RR, Germain A, Colrain IM. 2012. K-complexes are not preferentially evoked to combat sounds in combat-exposed Vietnam veterans with and without posttraumatic stress disorder. *International Journal of Psychophysiology* 83:393–398.

Fritschi L, Benke G, Hughes AM, Kricker A, Turner J, Vajdic CM, Grulich A, Milliken S, Kaldor J, Armstrong BK. 2005. Occupational exposure to pesticides and risk of non-Hodgkin's lymphoma. *American Journal of Epidemiology* 162(9):849–857.

Fukuda Y, Nakamura K, Takano T. 2003. Dioxins released from incineration plants and mortality from major diseases: An analysis of statistical data by municipalities. *Journal of Medical and Dental Sciences* 50:249–255.

Gallagher RP, Bajdik CD, Fincham S, Hill GB, Keefe AR, Coldman A, McLean DI. 1996. Chemical exposures, medical history, and risk of squamous and basal cell carcinoma of the skin. *Cancer Epidemiology, Biomarkers and Prevention* 5(6):419–424.

Gambini GF, Mantovani C, Pira E, Piolatto PG, Negri E. 1997. Cancer mortality among rice growers in Novara Province, northern Italy. *American Journal of Industrial Medicine* 31(4):435–441.

Garaj-Vrhovac V, Zeljezić D. 2002. Assessment of genome damage in a population of Croatian workers employed in pesticide production by chromosomal aberration analyis, micronucleus assay and Comet assay. *Journal of Applied Toxicology* 22(4):249–255.

García AM, Benavides FG, Fletcher T, Orts E. 1998. Paternal exposure to pesticides and congenital malformations. *Scandinavian Journal of Work, Environment and Health* 24(6):473–480.

Garry VF, Holland SE, Erickson LL, Burroughs BL. 2003. Male reproductive hormones and thyroid function in pesticide applicators in the Red River Valley of Minnesota. *Journal of Toxicology and Environmental Health* 66:965–986.

Gellis LA, Gehrman PR. 2011. Cognitive behavioral treatment for insomnia in veterans with long-standing posttraumatic stress disorder: A pilot study. *Journal of Aggression, Maltreatment and Trauma* 20:904–916.

Ghosh S, McLaughlin JR, Spinelli JJ, Dosman JA, McDuffie HH, Pahwa P. 2011. Multiple myeloma and occupational exposures: A population-based case-control study. *Journal of Occupational and Environmental Medicine* 53(6):641–646.

Goldberg J, True WR, Eisen SA, Henderson WG. 1990. A twin study of the effects of the Vietnam War on posttraumatic stress disorder. *Journal of the American Medical Association* 263:1227–1232.

Goldner WS, Sandler DP, Yu F, Hoppin JA, Kamel F, Levan TD. 2010. Pesticide use and thyroid disease among women in the Agricultural Health Study. *American Journal of Epidemiology* 171(4):455–464.

Goncharov A, Bloom M, Pavuk M, Birman I, Carpenter DO. 2010. Blood pressure and hypertension in relation to levels of serum polychlorinated biphenyls in residents of Anniston, Alabama. *Journal of Hypertension* 28:2053–2060.

Goncharov A, Pavuk M, Foushee HR, Carpenter DO. 2011. Blood pressure in relation to concentrations of PCB congeners and chlorinated pesticides. *Environmental Health Perspectives* 119(3):319–325.

Gordon JE, Shy CM. 1981. Agricultural chemical use and congenital cleft lip and/or palate. *Archives of Environmental Health* 36:213–221.

Gorell JM, Peterson EL, Rybicki BA, Johnson CC. 2004. Multiple risk factors for Parkinson's disease. *Journal of the Neurological Sciences* 217:169–174.

Goun BD, Kuller LH. 1986. *Final Report: A Case-Control Mortality Study on the Association of Soft Tissue Sarcomas, Non-Hodgkin's Lymphomas, and Other Selected Cancers and Vietnam Military Service in Pennsylvania Males.* Pittsburgh, PA: University of Pittsburgh.

Green LM. 1987. Suicide and exposure to phenoxy acid herbicides. *Scandinavian Journal of Work, Environment and Health* 13(5):460.

Green LM. 1991. A cohort mortality study of forestry workers exposed to phenoxy acid herbicides. *British Journal of Industrial Medicine* 48:234–238.

Greenwald P, Kovasznay B, Collins DN, Therriault G. 1984. Sarcomas of soft tissues after Vietnam service. *Journal of the National Cancer Institute* 73:1107–1109.

Gupta A, Ketchum N, Roehrborn CG, Schecter A, Aragaki CC, Michalek JE. 2006. Serum dioxin, testosterone, and subsequent risk of benign prostatic hyperplasia: A prospective cohort study of Air Force veterans. *Environmental Health Perspectives* 114(11):1649–1654.

Ha MH, Lee DH, Jacobs DR Jr. 2007. Association between serum concentrations of persistent organic pollutants and self-reported cardiovascular disease prevalence: Results from the National Health and Nutrition Examination Survey, 1999–2002. *Environmental Health Perspectives* 115(8):1204–1209.

Ha MH, Lee DH, Son HK, Park SK, Jacobs DR. 2009. Association between serum concentrations of persistent organic pollutants and prevalence of newly diagnosed hypertension: Results from the National Health and Nutrition Examination Survey 1999–2002. *Journal of Human Hypertension* 23(4):274–286.

Halldorsson TI, Thorsdottir I, Meltzer HM, Strom M, Olsen SF. 2009. Dioxin-like activity in plasma among Danish pregnant women: Dietary predictors, birth weight and infant development. *Environmental Research* 109(1):22–28.

Halperin W, Kalow W, Sweeney MH, Tang BK, Fingerhut M, Timpkins B, Wille K. 1995. Induction of P-450 in workers exposed to dioxin. *Occupational and Environmental Medicine* 52(2):86–91.

Halperin W, Vogt R, Sweeney MH, Shopp G, Fingerhut M, Petersen M. 1998. Immunological markers among workers exposed to 2,3,7,8-tetrachlorodibenzo-*p*-dioxin. *Occupational and Environmental Medicine* 55(11):742–749.

Hanke W, Romitti P, Fuortes L, Sobala W, Mikulski M. 2003. The use of pesticides in a Polish rural population and its effect on birth weight. *International Archives of Occupational and Environmental Health* 76:614–620.

Hansen ES, Hasle H, Lander F. 1992. A cohort study on cancer incidence among Danish gardeners. *American Journal of Industrial Medicine* 21:651–660.

Hansen ES, Lander F, Lauritsen JM. 2007. Time trends in cancer risk and pesticide exposure, a long-term follow-up of Danish gardeners. *Scandinavian Journal of Work, Environment and Health* 33(6):465–469.

Hansen S, Odland JO, Phi DT, Nieboer E, Sandanger TM. 2009. Maternal levels of organochlorines in two communities in southern Vietnam. *Science of the Total Environment* 408(2):225–232.

Hardell L. 1977. Malignant mesenchymal tumors and exposure to phenoxy acids: A clinical observation. *Lakartidningen* 74:2753–2754 [in Swedish].

Hardell L. 1979. Malignant lymphoma of histiocytic type and exposure to phenoxyacetic acids or chlorophenols. *Lancet* 1(8106):55–56.

Hardell L. 1981. Relation of soft-tissue sarcoma, malignant lymphoma and colon cancer to phenoxy acids, chlorophenols and other agents. *Scandinavian Journal of Work, Environment and Health* 7:119–130.

Hardell L, Sandstrom A. 1979. Case-control study: Soft-tissue sarcomas and exposure to phenoxyacetic acids or chlorophenols. *British Journal of Cancer* 39:711–717.

Hardell L, Bengtsson NO. 1983. Epidemiological study of socioeconomic factors and clinical findings in Hodgkin's disease, and reanalysis of previous data regarding chemical exposure. *British Journal of Cancer* 48:217–225.

Hardell L, Eriksson M. 1988. The association between soft tissue sarcomas and exposure to phenoxyacetic acids: A new case-referent study. *Cancer* 62:652–656.

Hardell L, Eriksson M. 1999. A case-control study of non-Hodgkin lymphoma and exposure to pesticides. *Cancer* 85(6):1353–1360.

Hardell L, Eriksson M, Lenner P. 1980. Malignant lymphoma and exposure to chemical substances, especially organic solvents, chlorophenols and phenoxy acids. *Lakartidningen* 77:208–210.

Hardell L, Eriksson M, Lenner P, Lundgren E. 1981. Malignant lymphoma and exposure to chemicals, especially organic solvents, chlorophenols and phenoxy acids: A case-control study. *British Journal of Cancer* 43:169–176.

Hardell L, Johansson B, Axelson O. 1982. Epidemiological study of nasal and nasopharyngeal cancer and their relation to phenoxy acid or chlorophenol exposure. *American Journal of Industrial Medicine* 3:247–257.

Hardell L, Bengtsson NO, Jonsson U, Eriksson S, Larsson LG. 1984. Aetiological aspects on primary liver cancer with special regard to alcohol, organic solvents and acute intermittent porphyria: An epidemiological investigation. *British Journal of Cancer* 50:389–397.

Hardell L, Moss A, Osmond D, Volberding P. 1987. Exposure to hair dyes and polychlorinated dibenzo-*p*-dioxins in AIDS patients with Kaposi sarcoma: An epidemiological investigation. *Cancer Detection and Prevention* (Suppl 1):567–570.

Hardell L, Eriksson M, Degerman A. 1994. Exposure to phenoxyacetic acids, chlorophenols, or organic solvents in relation to histopathology, stage, and anatomical localization of non-Hodgkin's lymphoma. *Cancer Research* 54:2386–2389.

Hartge P, Colt JS, Severson RK, Cerhan JR, Cozen W, Camann D, Zahm SH, Davis S. 2005. Residential herbicide use and risk of non-Hodgkin lymphoma. *Cancer Epidemiology, Biomarkers and Prevention* 14(4):934–937.

Hayes HM, Tarone RE, Casey HW, Huxsoll DL. 1990. Excess of seminomas observed in Vietnam service US military working dogs. *Journal of the National Cancer Institute* 82:1042–1046.

Heacock H, Hogg R, Marion SA, Hershler R, Teschke K, Dimich-Ward H, Demers P, Kelly S, Ostry A, Hertzman C. 1998. Fertility among a cohort of male sawmill workers exposed to chlorophenate fungicides. *Epidemiology* 9(1):56–60.

Henneberger PK, Ferris BG Jr, Monson RR. 1989. Mortality among pulp and paper workers in Berlin, New Hampshire. *British Journal of Industrial Medicine* 46:658–664.

Henriksen GL, Michalek JE, Swaby JA, Rahe AJ. 1996. Serum dioxin, testosterone, and gonadotropins in veterans of Operation Ranch Hand. *Epidemiology* 7(4):352–357.

Henriksen GL, Ketchum NS, Michalek JE, Swaby JA. 1997. Serum dioxin and diabetes mellitus in veterans of Operation Ranch Hand. *Epidemiology* 8(3):252–258.

Hertzman C, Teschke K, Ostry A, Hershler R, Dimich-Ward H, Kelly S, Spinelli JJ, Gallagher RP, McBride M, Marion SA. 1997. Mortality and cancer incidence among sawmill workers exposed to chlorophenate wood preservatives. *American Journal of Public Health* 87(1):71–79.

Hoar SK, Blair A, Holmes FF, Boysen CD, Robel RJ, Hoover R, Fraumeni JF. 1986. Agricultural herbicide use and risk of lymphoma and soft-tissue sarcoma. *Journal of the American Medical Association* 256:1141–1147.

Hoffman RE, Stehr-Green PA, Webb KB, Evans RG, Knutsen AP, Schramm WF, Staake JL, Gibson BB, Steinberg KK. 1986. Health effects of long-term exposure to 2,3,7,8-tetrachlorodibenzo-*p*-dioxin. *Journal of the American Medical Association* 255:2031–2038.

Hohenadel K, Harris SA, McLaughlin JR, Spinelli JJ, Pahwa P, Dosman JA, Demers PA, Blair A. 2011. Exposure to multiple pesticides and risk of non-Hodgkin lymphoma in men from six Canadian provinces. *International Journal of Environmental Research and Public Health* 8(6):2320–2330.

Holmes AP, Bailey C, Baron RC, Bosanac E, Brough J, Conroy C, Haddy L. 1986. *West Virginia Department of Health Vietnam-Era Veterans Mortality Study, Preliminary Report.* Charleston: West Virginia Health Department.

Hooiveld M, Heederik DJ, Kogevinas M, Boffetta P, Needham LL, Patterson DG Jr, Bueno de Mesquita HB. 1998. Second follow-up of a Dutch cohort occupationally exposed to phenoxy herbicides, chlorophenols, and contaminants. *American Journal of Epidemiology* 147(9):891–901.

Hoppin JA. 2005. Integrating exposure measurements into epidemiologic studies in agriculture. *Scandinavian Journal of Work, Environment and Health* 31(Suppl 1):115–117.

Hoppin JA, Umbach DM, London SJ, Alavanja CR, Sandler DP. 2002. Chemical predictors of wheeze among farmer pesticide applicators in the Agricultural Health Study. *American Journal of Critical Care Medicine* 165:683–689.

Hoppin JA, Umbach DM, London SJ, Lynch CF, Alavanja MC, Sandler DP. 2006a. Pesticides associated with wheeze among commercial pesticide applicators in the Agricultural Health Study. *American Journal of Epidemiology* 163(12):1129–1137.

Hoppin JA, Adgate JL, Eberhart M, Nishioka M, Ryan PB. 2006b. Environmental exposure assessment of pesticides in farmworker homes. *Environmental Health Perspectives* 114(6):929–935.

Hoppin JA, Umbach DM, London SJ, Lynch CF, Alavanja MC, Sandler DP. 2006c. Pesticides and adult respiratory outcomes in the Agricultural Health Study. *Annals of the New York Academy of Sciences* 1076:343–354.

Hoppin JA, Umbach DM, Kullman GJ, Henneberger PK, London SJ, Alavanja MC, Sandler DP. 2007a. Pesticides and other agricultural factors associated with self-reported farmer's lung among farm residents in the Agricultural Health Study. *Occupational and Environmental Medicine* 64(5):334–341.

Hoppin JA, Valcin M, Henneberger PK, Kullman GJ, Limbach DM, London SJ, Alavanja MCR, Sandler DP. 2007b. Pesticide use and chronic bronchitis among farmers in the Agricultural Health Study. *American Journal of Industrial Medicine* 50(12):969–979.

Hoppin JA, Umbach DM, London SJ, Henneberger PK, Kullman GJ, Alavanja MC, Sandler DP. 2008. Pesticides and atopic and nonatopic asthma among farm women in the Agricultural Health Study. *American Journal of Respiratory and Critical Care Medicine* 177(1):11–18.

Hoppin JA, Umbach DM, London SJ, Henneberger PK, Kullman GJ, Coble J, Alavanja MCR, Beane Freeman LE, Sandler DP. 2009. Pesticide use and adult-onset asthma among male farmers in the Agricultural Health Study. *European Respiratory Journal* 34(6):1296–1303.

Hryhorczuk DO, Wallace WH, Persky V, Furner S, Webster JR Jr, Oleske D, Haselhorst B, Ellefson R, Zugerman C. 1998. A morbidity study of former pentachlorophenol-production workers. *Environmental Health Perspectives* 106(7):401–408.

Humblet O, Williams PL, Korrick SA, Sergeyev O, Emond C, Birnbaum LS, Burns JS, Altshul L, Patterson DG Jr, Turner WE, Lee MM, Revich B, Hauser R. 2010. Predictors of serum dioxin, furan, and PCB concentrations among women from Chapaevsk, Russia. *Environmental Science and Technology* 44(14):5633–5640.

Huong LD, Phuong NTN. 1983. The state of abnormal pregnancies and congenital malformations at the Gyneco-Obstetrical Hospital of Ho Chi Minh City (formerly Tu Du Hospital). Summarized in: Constable JD, Hatch MC. *Reproductive Effects of Herbicide Exposure in Vietnam: Recent Studies by the Vietnamese and Others.* As cited in Constable and Hatch, 1985.

Huston BL. 1972. Identification of three neutral contaminants in production grade 2,4-D. *Journal of Agricultural and Food Chemistry* 20(3):724–727.

Ideo G, Bellati G, Bellobuono A, Mocarelli P, Marocchi A, Brambilla P. 1982. Increased urinary *d*-glucaric acid excretion by children living in an area polluted with tetrachlorodibenzo-*para*-dioxin (TCDD). *Clinica Chimica Acta* 120:273–283.

Ideo G, Bellati G, Bellobuono A, Bissanti L. 1985. Urinary *d*-glucaric acid excretion in the Seveso area, polluted by tetrachlorodibenzo-*p*-dioxin (TCDD): Five years of experience. *Environmental Health Perspectives* 60:151–157.

IOM (Institute of Medicine). 1994. *Veterans and Agent Orange: Health Effects of Herbicides Used in Vietnam.* Washington, DC: National Academy Press.

IOM. 2000. *Veterans and Agent Orange: Herbicide/Dioxin Exposure and Type 2 Diabetes.* Washington, DC: National Academy Press.

IOM. 2002. *Veterans and Agent Orange: Herbicide/Dioxin Exposure and Acute Myelogenous Leukemia in the Children of Vietnam Veterans.* Washington, DC: The National Academies Press.

IOM. 2004. *Veterans and Agent Orange: Length of Presumptive Period for Association Between Exposure and Respiratory Cancer.* Washington, DC: The National Academies Press.

IOM. 2006. *Disposition of the Air Force Health Study.* Washington, DC: The National Academies Press.

Jäger R, Neuberger M, Rappe C, Kundi M, Pigler B, Smith AG. 1998. Chloracne and other symptoms 23 years after dioxin-exposure. *Atemwegs-Und Lungenkrankheiten* 24(Suppl 1):S101–S104.

Jappinen P, Pukkala E. 1991. Cancer incidence among pulp and paper workers exposed to organic chlorinated compounds formed during chlorine pulp bleaching. *Scandinavian Journal of Work, Environment and Health* 17:356–359.

Jennings AM, Wild G, Ward JD, Ward AM. 1988. Immunological abnormalities 17 years after accidental exposure to 2,3,7,8-tetrachlorodibenzo-*p*-dioxin. *British Journal of Industrial Medicine* 45:701–704.

Jones MR, Tellez-Plaza M, Sharrett AR, Guallar E, Navas-Acien A. 2011. Urine arsenic and hypertension in US adults. The 2003–2008 National Health and Nutrition Examination Survey. *Epidemiology* 22:153–161.

Jung D, Berg PA, Edler L, Ehrenthal W, Fenner D, Flesch-Janys D, Huber C, Klein R, Koitka C, Lucier G, Manz A, Muttray A, Needham L, Päpke O, Pietsch M, Portier C, Patterson D, Prellwitz W, Rose DM, Thews A, Konietzko J. 1998. Immunological findings in formerly exposed workers to 2,3,7,8-tetrachlorodibenzo-*p*-dioxin (TCDD) and related compounds in pesticide production. *Arbeitsmedizin Sozialmedizin Umweltmedizin* (Suppl 24):38–43.

Kahn PC, Gochfeld M, Nygren M, Hansson M, Rappe C, Velez H, Ghent-Guenther T, Wilson WP. 1988. Dioxins and dibenzofurans in blood and adipose tissue of Agent Orange-exposed Vietnam veterans and matched controls. *Journal of the American Medical Association* 259:1661–1667.

Kahn PC, Gochfeld M, Lewis WW. 1992a. *Dibenzodioxin and Dibenzofuran Congener Levels in Four Groups of Vietnam Veterans Who Did Not Handle Agent Orange*. New Jersey Agent Orange Commission.

Kahn PC, Gochfeld M, Lewis WW. 1992b. *Immune Status and Herbicide Exposure in the New Jersey Pointman I Project*. New Jersey Agent Orange Commission.

Kahn PC, Gochfeld M, Lewis WW. 1992c. *Semen Analysis in Vietnam Veterans with Respect to Presumed Herbicide Exposure*. New Jersey Agent Orange Commission.

Kamel F, Engel LS, Gladen BC, Hoppin JA, Alavanja MC, Sandler DP. 2005. Neurologic symptoms in licensed private pesticide applicators in the Agricultural Health Study. *Environmental Health Perspectives* 113(7):877–882.

Kamel F, Engel LS, Gladen BC, Hoppin JA, Alavanja MC, Sandler DP. 2007a. Neurologic symptoms in licensed pesticide applicators in the Agricultural Health Study. *Human and Experimental Toxicology* 26(3):243–250.

Kamel F, Tanner C, Umbach D, Hoppin J, Alavanja M, Blair A, Comyns K, Goldman S, Korell M, Langston J, Ross G, Sandler D. 2007b. Pesticide exposure and self-reported Parkinson's disease in the Agricultural Health Study. *American Journal of Epidemiology* 165(4):364–374.

Kang HK, Weatherbee L, Breslin PP, Lee Y, Shepard BM. 1986. Soft tissue sarcomas and military service in Vietnam: A case comparison group analysis of hospital patients. *Journal of Occupational Medicine* 28:1215–1218.

Kang HK, Enzinger FM, Breslin P, Feil M, Lee Y, Shepard B. 1987. Soft tissue sarcoma and military service in Vietnam: A case-control study. *Journal of the National Cancer Institute* 79:693–699 [published erratum appears in *Journal of the National Cancer Institute* 79:1173].

Kang HK, Watanabe KK, Breen J, Remmers J, Conomos MG, Stanley J, Flicker M. 1991. Dioxins and dibenzofurans in adipose tissue of US Vietnam veterans and controls. *American Journal of Public Health* 81(3):344–348.

Kang HK, Mahan CM, Lee KY, Magee CA, Mather SH, Matanoski G. 2000a. Pregnancy outcomes among US women Vietnam veterans. *American Journal Industrial Medicine* 38(4):447–454.

Kang HK, Mahan CM, Lee KY, Magee CA, Selvin S. 2000b. Prevalence of gynecologic cancers among female Vietnam veterans. *Journal of Occupational and Environmental Medicine* 42:1121–1127.

Kang HK, Dalager NA, Needham LL, Patterson DG, Matanoski GM, Kanchanaraksa S, Lees PSJ. 2001. US Army Chemical Corps Vietnam veterans health study: Preliminary results. *Chemosphere* 43:943–949.

Kang HK, Dalager NA, Needham LL, Patterson DG, Lees PSJ, Yates K, Matanoski GM. 2006. Health status of Army Chemical Corps Vietnam veterans who sprayed defoliant in Vietnam. *American Journal of Industrial Medicine* 49(11):875–884.

Karouna-Renier NK, Rao KR, Lanza JJ, Davis DA, Wilson PA. 2007. Serum profiles of PCDDs and PCDFs, in individuals near the Escambia Wood Treatment Company Superfund Site in Pensacola, FL. *Chemosphere* 69:1312–1319.

Karunanayake CP, Spinelli JJ, McLaughlin JR, Dosman JA, Pahwa P, McDuffie HH. 2012. Hodgkin lymphoma and pesticides exposure in men: A Canadian case-control study. *Journal of Agromedicine* 17(1):30–39.

Kayajanian GM. 2002. The J-shaped dioxin dose response curve. *Ecotoxicology and Environmental Safety* 51:1–4.

Kenborg L, Lassen CF, Lander F, Olsen JH. 2012. Parkinson's disease among gardeners exposed to pesticides—A Danish cohort study. *Scandinavian Journal of Work, Environment and Health* 38(1):65–69.

Kern PA, Said S, Jackson WG Jr, Michalek JE. 2004. Insulin sensitivity following agent orange exposure in Vietnam veterans with high blood levels of 2,3,7,8-tetrachlorodibenzo-*p*-dioxin. *Journal of Clinical Endocrinology and Metabolism* 89(9):4665–4672.

Ketchum NS, Michalek JE. 2005. Postservice mortality of Air Force veterans occupationally exposed to herbicides during the Vietnam War: 20-year follow-up results. *Military Medicine* 170(5):406–413.

Ketchum NS, Michalek JE, Burton JE. 1999. Serum dioxin and cancer in veterans of Operation Ranch Hand. *American Journal of Epidemiology* 149(7):630–639.

Khoa ND. 1983. Some biologic parameters collected on the groups of people in an area affected by chemicals. Summarized in: Constable JD, Hatch MC. *Reproductive effects of herbicide exposure in Vietnam: Recent studies by the Vietnamese and others.* As cited in Constable and Hatch, 1985.

Kim HA, Kim EM, Park YC, Yu JY, Hong SK, Jeon SH, Park KL, Hur SJ, Heo Y. 2003. Immunotoxicological effects of Agent Orange exposure to the Vietnam War Korean veterans. *Industrial Health* 41:158–166.

Kim JB, Kang WY, Moon SG, Kim HJ, Kim KH, Kim YH, Hwang SH, Hwang SH, Kim W. 2012. Clinical outcome of veterans with acute coronary syndrome who had been exposed to Agent Orange. *Chonnam Medical Journal* 48(1):47–51.

Kim JS, Kang HK, Lim HS, Cheong HK, Lim MK. 2001. A study on the correlation between categorizations of the individual exposure levels to Agent Orange and serum dioxin levels among the Korean Vietnam veterans. *Korean Journal of Preventative Medicine* 34(1):80–88.

Kim JS, Lim HS, Cho SI, Cheong HK, Lim MK. 2003. Impact of Agent Orange exposure among Korean Vietnam veterans. *Industrial Health* 41:149–157.

Kirrane EF, Hoppin JA, Umbach DM, Samanic C, Sandler DP. 2004. Patterns of pesticide use and their determinants among wives of farmer pesticide applicators in the Agricultural Health Study. *Journal of Occupational and Environmental Medicine* 46(8):856–865.

Ko GT, Cockram CS, Chow CC, Yeung V, Chan WB, So WY, et al. 2005. High prevalence of metabolic syndrome in Hong Kong Chinese—Comparison of three diagnostic criteria. *Diabetes Research and Clinical Practice* 69:160–168.

Kogan MD, Clapp RW. 1985. *Mortality Among Vietnam Veterans in Massachusetts, 1972–1983.* Boston, MA: Massachusetts Office of the Commissioner of Veterans Services, Agent Orange Program.

Kogan MD, Clapp RW. 1988. Soft tissue sarcoma mortality among Vietnam veterans in Massachusetts, 1972–1983. *International Journal of Epidemiology* 17:39–43.

Kogevinas M, Saracci R, Bertazzi PA, Bueno de Mesquita BH, Coggon D, Green LM, Kauppinen T, Littorin M, Lynge E, Mathews JD, Neuberger M, Osman J, Pearce N, Winkelmann R. 1992. Cancer mortality from soft-tissue sarcoma and malignant lymphomas in an international cohort of workers exposed to chlorophenoxy herbicides and chlorophenols. *Chemosphere* 25:1071–1076.

Kogevinas M, Saracci R, Winkelmann R, Johnson ES, Bertazzi PA, Bueno de Mesquita BH, Kauppinen T, Littorin M, Lynge E, Neuberger M. 1993. Cancer incidence and mortality in women occupationally exposed to chlorophenoxy herbicides, chlorophenols, and dioxins. *Cancer Causes and Control* 4:547–553.

Kogevinas M, Kauppinen T, Winkelmann R, Becher H, Bertazzi PA, Bas B, Coggon D, Green L, Johnson E, Littorin M, Lynge E, Marlow DA, Mathews JD, Neuberger M, Benn T, Pannett B, Pearce N, Saracci R. 1995. Soft tissue sarcoma and non-Hodgkin's lymphoma in workers exposed to phenoxy herbicides, chlorophenols and dioxins: Two nested case-control studies. *Epidemiology* 6:396–402.

Kogevinas M, Becher H, Benn T, Bertazzi PA, Boffetta P, Bueno de Mesquita HB, Coggon D, Colin D, Flesch-Janys D, Fingerhut M, Green L, Kauppinen T, Littorin M, Lynge E, Mathews JD, Neuberger M, Pearce N, Saracci R. 1997. Cancer mortality in workers exposed to phenoxy herbicides, chlorophenols, and dioxins. An expanded and updated international cohort study. *American Journal of Epidemiology* 145(12):1061–1075.

Koutros S, Alavanja MCR, Lubin JH, Sandler DP, Hoppin JA, Lynch CF, Knott C, Blair A, Freeman LEB. 2010a. An update of cancer incidence in the Agricultural Health Study. *Journal of Occupational and Environmental Medicine* 52(11):1098–1105.

Koutros S, Beane Freeman LE, Berndt SI, Andreotti G, Lubin JH, Sandler DP, Hoppin JA, Yu K, Li Q, Burdette LA, Yuenger J, Yeager M, Alavanja MCR. 2010b. Pesticide use modifies the association between genetic variants on chromosome 8q24 and prostate cancer. *Cancer Research* 70(22):9224–9233.

Koutros S, Andreotti G, Berndt SI, Hughes Barry K, Lubin JH, Hoppin JA, Kamel F, Sandler DP, Burdette LA, Yuenger J, Yeager M, Alavanja MCR, Freeman LEB. 2011. Xenobiotic-metabolizing gene variants, pesticide use, and the risk of prostate cancer. *Pharmacogenetics and Genomics* 21(10):615–623.

Kristensen P, Irgens LM, Andersen A, Bye AS, Sundheim L. 1997. Birth defects among offspring of Norwegian farmers, 1967–1991. *Epidemiology* 8(5):537–544.

Kreuzer PE, Csanady GA, Baur C, Kessler W, Päpke O, Greim H, Filser JG. 1997. 2,3,7,8-Tetrachlorodibenzo-*p*-dioxin (TCDD) and congeners in infants. A toxicokinetic model of human lifetime body burden by TCDD with special emphasis on its uptake by nutrition. *Archives of Toxicology* 71(6):383–400.

Lambertino A, Turyk M, Anderson H, Freels S, Persky V. 2011. Uterine leiomyomata in a cohort of Great Lakes sport fish consumers. *Environmental Research* 111(4):565–572.

Lampi P, Hakulinen T, Luostarinen T, Pukkala E, Teppo L. 1992. Cancer incidence following chlorophenol exposure in a community in southern Finland. *Archives of Environmental Health* 47:167–175.

Landi MT, Needham LL, Lucier G, Mocarelli P, Bertazzi PA, Caporaso N. 1997. Concentrations of dioxin 20 years after Seveso. *Lancet* 349(9068):1811.

Landi MT, Consonni D, Patterson DG Jr, Needham LL, Lucier G, Brambilla P, Cazzaniga MA, Mocarelli P, Pesatori AC, Bertazzi PA, Caporaso NE. 1998. 2,3,7,8-Tetrachlorodibenzo-*p*-dioxin plasma levels in Seveso 20 years after the accident. *Environmental Health Perspectives* 106(5):273–277.

Landi MT, Bertazzi PA, Baccarelli A, Consonni D, Masten S, Lucier G, Mocarelli P, Needham L, Caporaso N, Grassman J. 2003. TCDD-mediated alterations in the AhR-dependent pathway in Seveso, Italy, 20 years after the accident. *Carcinogenesis* 24(4):673–680.

Lang TD, Tung TT, Van DD. 1983a. Mutagenic effects on the first generation after exposure to "Orange Agent." Summarized in: Constable JD, Hatch MC. *Reproductive effects of herbicide exposure in Vietnam: Recent studies by the Vietnamese and others.* As cited in Constable and Hatch, 1985.

Lang TD, Van DD, Dwyer JH, Flamenbuam C, Dwyer KM, Fantini D. 1983b. Self-reports of exposure to herbicides and health problems: A preliminary analysis of survey data from the families of 432 veterans in northern Vietnam. Summarized in: Constable JD, Hatch MC. *Reproductive effects of herbicide exposure in Vietnam: Recent studies by the Vietnamese and others.* As cited in Constable and Hatch, 1985.

LaVecchia C, Negri E, D'Avanzo B, Franceschi S. 1989. Occupation and lymphoid neoplasms. *British Journal of Cancer* 60:385–388.

Lawrence CE, Reilly AA, Quickenton P, Greenwald P, Page WF, Kuntz AJ. 1985. Mortality patterns of New York State Vietnam veterans. *American Journal of Public Health* 75:277–279.

Lawson CC, Schnorr TM, Whelan EA, Deddens JA, Dankovic DA, Piacitelli LA, Sweeney MH, Connally LB. 2004. Paternal occupational exposure to 2,3,7,8-tetrachlorodibenzo-*p*-dioxin and birth outcomes of offspring: Birth weight, preterm delivery, and birth defects. *Environmental Health Perspectives* 112(14):1403–1408.

Lee DH, Lee IK, Song K, Steffes M, Toscano W, Baker BA, Jacobs DR Jr. 2006. A strong dose-response relation between serum concentrations of persistent organic pollutants and diabetes: Results from the National Health and Examination Survey 1999–2002. *Diabetes Care* 29(7):1638–1644.

Lee DH, Steffes M, Jacobs DR Jr. 2007a. Positive associations of serum concentration of polychlorinated biphenyls or organochlorine pesticides with self-reported arthritis, especially rheumatoid type, in women. *Environmental Health Perspectives* 115(6):883–888.

Lee DH, Lee IK, Jin SH, Steffes M, Jacobs DR Jr. 2007b. Association between serum concentrations of persistent organic pollutants and insulin resistance among nondiabetic adults: Results from the National Health and Nutrition Examination Survey 1999–2002. *Diabetes Care* 30(3):622–628.

Lee DH, Lee IK, Porta M, Steffes M, Jacobs DR Jr. 2007c. Relationship between serum concentrations of persistent organic pollutants and the prevalence of metabolic syndrome among non-diabetic adults: Results from the National Health and Nutrition Examination Survey 1999–2002. *Diabetologia* 50(9):1841–1851.

Lee DH, Jacobs DR Jr, Steffes M. 2008. Association of organochlorine pesticides with peripheral neuropathy in patients with diabetes or impaired fasting glucose. *Diabetes* 57(11):3108–3111.

Lee DH, Steffes MW, Sjödin A, Jones RS, Needham LL, Jacobs DR Jr. 2010. Low dose of some persistent organic pollutants predicts type 2 diabetes: A nested case-control study. *Environmental Health Perspectives* 118(9):1235–1242.

Lee DH, Steffes MW, Sjodin A, Jones RS, Needham LL, Jacobs DR Jr. 2011a. Low dose organochlorine pesticides and polychlorinated biphenyls predict obesity, dyslipidemia, and insulin resistance among people free of diabetes. *PLoS ONE* 6 (1):e15977.

Lee DH, Lind PM, Jacobs DR Jr, Salihovic S, van Bavel B, Lind L. 2011b. Polychlorinated biphenyls and organochlorine pesticides in plasma predict development of type 2 diabetes in the elderly: The prospective investigation of the vasculature in Uppsala seniors (PIVUS) study. *Diabetes Care* 34(8):1778–1784.

Lee DH, Lind L, Jacobs DR Jr, Salihovic S, van Bavel B, Lind PM. 2012a. Associations of persistent organic pollutants with abdominal obesity in the elderly: The prospective investigation of the vasculature in Uppsala seniors (PIVUS) study. *Environment International* 40:170–178.

Lee DH, Lind PM, Jacobs DR, Salihovic S, van Bavel B, Lind L. 2012b. Background exposure to persistent organic pollutants predicts stroke in the elderly. *Environment International* 47:115–120.

Lee WJ, Cantor KP, Berzofsky JA, Zahm SH, Blair A. 2004a. Non-Hodgkin's lymphoma among asthmatics exposed to pesticides. *International Journal of Cancer* 111(2):298–302.

Lee WJ, Lijinsky W, Heineman EF, Markin RS, Weisenburger DD, Ward MH. 2004b. Agricultural pesticide use and adenocarcinomas of the stomach and oesophagus. *Occupational and Environmental Medicine* 61(9):743–749.

Lee WJ, Colt JS, Heineman EF, McComb R, Weisenburger DD, Lijinsky W, Ward MH. 2005. Agricultural pesticide use and risk of glioma in Nebraska, United States. *Occupational and Environmental Medicine* 62(11):786–792.

Lee WJ, Purdue MP, Stewart P, Schenk M, De Roos AJ, Cerhan JR, Severson RK, Cozen W, Hartge P, Blair A. 2006. Asthma history, occupational exposure to pesticides and the risk of non-Hodgkin's lymphoma. *International Journal of Cancer* 118(12):3174–3176.

Lee WJ, Sandler DP, Blair A, Samanic C, Cross AJ, Alavanja MC. 2007. Pesticide use and colorectal cancer risk in the Agricultural Health Study. *International Journal of Cancer* 121(2):339–346.

Lerda D, Rizzi R. 1991. Study of reproductive function in persons occupationally exposed to 2,4-dichlorophenoxyacetic acid (2,4-D). *Mutation Research* 262:47–50.

Levy CJ. 1988. Agent Orange exposure and posttraumatic stress disorder. *Journal of Nervous and Mental Disorders* 176:242–245.

Lind PM, van Bavel B, Salihovic S, Lind L. 2012. Circulating levels of persistent organic pollutants (POPs) and carotid atherosclerosis in the elderly. *Environmental Health Perspectives* 120(1):38–43.

Liou HH, Tsai MC, Chen CJ, Jeng JS, Chang YC, Chen SY, Chen RC. 1997. Environmental risk factors and Parkinson's disease: A case-control study in Taiwan. *Neurology* 48(6):1583–1588.

Longnecker MP, Michalek JE. 2000. Serum dioxin level in relation to diabetes mellitus among Air Force veterans with background levels of exposure. *Epidemiology* 11(1):44–48.

Lovik M, Johansen HR, Gaarder PI, Becher G, Aaberge IS, Gdynia W, Alexander J. 1996. Halogenated organic compounds and the human immune system: Preliminary report on a study in hobby fishermen. *Archives of Toxicology Supplement* 18:15–20.

Lynge E. 1985. A follow-up study of cancer incidence among workers in manufacture of phenoxy herbicides in Denmark. *British Journal of Cancer* 52:259–270.

Lynge E. 1993. Cancer in phenoxy herbicide manufacturing workers in Denmark, 1947–87—An update. *Cancer Causes and Control* 4:261–272.

Magnani C, Coggon D, Osmond C, Acheson ED. 1987. Occupation and five cancers: A case-control study using death certificates. *British Journal of Industrial Medicine* 44(11):769–776.

Mahan CM, Bullman TA, Kang HK, Selvin S. 1997. A case-control study of lung cancer among Vietnam veterans. *Journal of Occupational and Environmental Medicine* 39(8):740–747.

Mandel JS, Alexander BH, Baker BA, Acquavella JF, Chapman P, Honeycutt R. 2005. Biomonitoring for farm families in the Farm Family Exposure Study. *Scandinavian Journal of Work, Environment and Health* 31(Suppl 1):98–104.

Manuwald U, Garrido MV, Berger J, Manz A, Baur X. 2012. Mortality study of chemical workers exposed to dioxins: Follow-up 23 years after chemical plant closure. *Occupational and Environmental Medicine* 69(9):636–642.

Manz A, Berger J, Dwyer JH, Flesch-Janys D, Nagel S, Waltsgott H. 1991. Cancer mortality among workers in chemical plant contaminated with dioxin. *Lancet* 338:959–964.

Masala G, Di Lollo S, Picoco C, Crosignani P, Demicheli V, Fontana A, Funto I, Miligi L, Nanni O, Papucci A, Ramazzotti V, Rodella S, Stagnaro E, Tumino R, Vigano C, Vindigni C, Seniori Costantini A, Vineis P. 1996. Incidence rates of leukemias, lymphomas and myelomas in Italy: Geographic distribution and NHL histotypes. *International Journal of Cancer* 68(2):156–159.

Mastroiacovo P, Spagnolo A, Marni E, Meazza L, Bertollini R, Segni G, Borgna-Pignatti C. 1988. Birth defects in the Seveso area after TCDD contamination. *Journal of the American Medical Association* 259:1668–1672 [published erratum appears in the *Journal of the American Medical Association* 260:792].

May G. 1982. Tetrachlorodibenzodioxin: A survey of subjects ten years after exposure. *British Journal of Industrial Medicine* 39:128–135.

May G. 1983. TCDD: A study of subjects 10 and 14 years after exposure. *Chemosphere* 12:771–778.

McBride DI, Collins JJ, Humphry NF, Herbison P, Bodner KM, Aylward LL, Burns CJ, Wilken M. 2009a. Mortality in workers exposed to 2,3,7,8-tetrachlorodibenzo-*p*-dioxin at a trichlorophenol plant in New Zealand. *Journal of Occupational and Environmental Medicine* 51(9):1049–1056.

McBride DI, Burns CJ, Herbison GP, Humphry NF, Bodner K, Collins JJ. 2009b. Mortality in employees at a New Zealand agrochemical manufacturing site. *Occupational Medicine* 59(4):255–263.

McDuffie HH, Klaassen DJ, Dosman JA. 1990. Is pesticide use related to the risk of primary lung cancer in Saskatchewan? *Journal of Occupational Medicine* 32(10):996–1002.

McDuffie HH, Pahwa P, McLaughlin JR, Spinelli JJ, Fincham S, Dosman JA, Robson D, Skinnider LF, Choi NW. 2001. Non-Hodgkin's lymphoma and specific pesticide exposures in men: Cross–Canada study of pesticides and health. *Cancer Epidemiology, Biomarkers and Prevention* 10(11):1155–1163.

McDuffie HH, Pahwa P, Robson D, Dosman JA, Fincham S, Spinelli JJ, McLaughlin JR. 2005. Insect repellents, phenoxyherbicide exposure, and non-Hodgkin's lymphoma. *Journal of Occupational and Environmental Medicine* 47(8):806–816.

McDuffie HH, Pahwa P, Karunanayake CP, Spinelli JJ, Dosman JA. 2009. Clustering of cancer among families of cases with Hodgkin lymphoma (HL), multiple myeloma (MM), non-Hodgkin's lymphoma (NHL), soft tissue sarcoma (STS) and control subjects. *BMC Cancer* 9(70).

McKinney WP, McIntire DD, Carmody TJ, Joseph A. 1997. Comparing the smoking behavior of veterans and nonveterans. *Public Health Reports* 112(3):212–217.

McLean D, Pearce N, Langseth H, Jäppinen P, Szadkowska-Stanczyk I, Person B, Wild P, Kishi R, Lynge E, Henneberger P, Sala M, Teschke K, Kauppinen T, Colin D, Kogevinas M, Boffetta P. 2006. Cancer mortality in workers exposed to organochlorine compounds in the pulp and paper industry: An international collaborative study. *Environmental Health Perspectives* 114(7):1007–1012.

McLean D, Eng A, Walls C, Dryson E, Harawira J, Cheng S, Wong KC, 't Mannetje A, Gray M, Shoemack P, Smith A, Pearce N. 2009. Serum dioxin levels in former New Zealand sawmill workers twenty years after exposure to pentachlorophenol (PCP) ceased. *Chemosphere* 74(7):962–967.

Mellemgaard A, Engholm G, McLaughlin JK, Olsen JH. 1994. Occupational risk factors for renal-cell carcinoma in Denmark. *Scandinavian Journal of Work, Environment and Health* 20:160–165.

Michalek JE, Pavuk M. 2008. Diabetes and cancer in veterans of Operation Ranch Hand after adjustment for calendar period, days of sprayings, and time spent in Southeast Asia. *Journal of Occupational and Environmental Medicine* 50(3):330–340.

Michalek JE, Wolfe WH, Miner JC. 1990. Health status of Air Force veterans occupationally exposed to herbicides in Vietnam. II. Mortality. *Journal of the American Medical Association* 264:1832–1836.

Michalek JE, Wolfe WH, Miner JC, Papa TM, Pirkle JL. 1995. Indices of TCDD exposure and TCDD body burden in veterans of Operation Ranch Hand. *Journal of Exposure Analysis and Environmental Epidemiology* 5(2):209–223.

Michalek JE, Rahe AJ, Boyle CA. 1998a. Paternal dioxin, preterm birth, intrauterine growth retardation, and infant death. *Epidemiology* 9(2):161–167.

Michalek JE, Ketchum NS, Akhtar FZ. 1998b. Postservice mortality of US Air Force veterans occupationally exposed to herbicides in Vietnam: 15-year follow-up. *American Journal of Epidemiology* 148(8):786–792.

Michalek JE, Rahe AJ, Boyle CA. 1998c. Paternal dioxin and the sex of children fathered by veterans of Operation Ranch Hand. *Epidemiology* 9(4):474–475.

Michalek JE, Akhtar FZ, Kiel JL. 1999a. Serum dioxin, insulin, fasting glucose, and sex hormone-binding globulin in veterans of Operation Ranch Hand. *Journal of Clinical Endocrinology and Metabolism* 84(5):1540–1543.

Michalek JE, Ketchum NS, Check IJ. 1999b. Serum dioxin and immunologic response in veterans of Operation Ranch Hand. *American Journal of Epidemiology* 149(11):1038–1046.

Michalek JE, Ketchum N, Longnecker MP. 2001a. Serum dioxin and hepatic abnormalities in veterans of Operation Ranch Hand. *Annals of Epidemiology* 11(5):304–311.

Michalek JE, Akhtar FZ, Arezzo JC, Garabrant DH, Albers JW. 2001b. Serum dioxin and peripheral neuropathy in veterans of Operation Ranch Hand. *Neurotoxicology* 22:479–490.

Michalek JE, Akhtar FZ, Longnecker MP, Burton JE. 2001c. Relation of serum 2,3,7,8-tetrachlorodibenzo-*p*-dioxin (TCDD) level to hematological examination results in veterans of Operation Ranch Hand. *Archives of Environmental Health* 56(5):396–405.

Michalek JE, Ketchum NS, Tripathi RC. 2003. Diabetes mellitus and 2,3,7,8-tetrachlorodibenzo-*p*-dioxin elimination in veterans of Operation Ranch Hand. *Journal of Toxicology and Environmental Health, Part A*, 66:211–221.

Mills PK, Yang R. 2005. Breast cancer risk in Hispanic agricultural workers in California. *International Journal of Occupational and Environmental Health* 11(2):123–131.

Mills PK, Yang RC. 2007. Agricultural exposures and gastric cancer risk in Hispanic farm workers in California. *Environmental Research* 104(2):282–289.

Mills PK, Yang R, Riordan D. 2005. Lymphohematopoietic cancers in the United Farm Workers of America (UFW), 1988–2001. *Cancer Causes and Control* 16(7):823–830.

Mills KT, Blair A, Freeman LEB, Sandler DP, Hoppin JA. 2009. Pesticides and myocardial infarction incidence and mortality among male pesticide applicators in the Agricultural Health Study. *American Journal of Epidemiology* 170(7):892–900.

Mo HJ, Park HJ, Kim JH, Lee JY, Cho BK. 2002. A study about the skin and general disease patterns of the Vietnam veterans exposed to dioxin. *Korean Journal of Dermatology* 40(6):634–638.

Mocarelli P, Marocchi A, Brambilla P, Gerthoux P, Young DS, Mantel N. 1986. Clinical laboratory manifestations of exposure to dioxin in children. A six-year study of the effects of an environmental disaster near Seveso, Italy. *Journal of the American Medical Association* 256:2687–2695.

Mocarelli P, Patterson DG Jr, Marocchi A, Needham LL. 1990. Pilot study (phase II) for determining polychlorinated dibenzo-*p*-dioxin (PCDD) and polychlorinated dibenzofuran (PCDF) levels in serum of Seveso, Italy residents collected at the time of exposure: Future plans. *Chemosphere* 20:967–974.

Mocarelli P, Needham LL, Marocchi A, Patterson DG Jr, Brambilla P, Gerthoux PM, Meazza L, Carreri V. 1991. Serum concentrations of 2,3,7,8-tetrachlorodibenzo-*p*-dioxin and test results from selected residents of Seveso, Italy. *Journal of Toxicology and Environmental Health* 32:357–366.

Mocarelli P, Brambilla P, Gerthoux PM, Patterson DG Jr, Needham LL. 1996. Change in sex ratio with exposure to dioxin. *Lancet* 348(9024):409.

Mocarelli P, Gerthoux PM, Patterson DG Jr, Milani S, Limonta G, Bertona M, Signorini S, Tramacere P, Colombo L, Crespi C, Brambilla P, Sarto C, Carreri V, Sampson EJ, Turner WE, Needham LL. 2008. Dioxin exposure, from infancy through puberty, produces endocrine disruption and affects human semen quality. *Environmental Health Perspectives* 116(1):70–77.

Mocarelli P, Gerthoux PM, Needham LL, Patterson DG Jr, Limonta G, Falbo R, Signorini S, Bertona M, Crespi C, Sarto C, Scott PK, Turner WE, Brambilla P. 2011. Perinatal exposure to low doses of dioxin can permanently impair human semen quality. *Environmental Health Perspectives* 119:713–718.

Montgomery MP, Kamel F, Saldana TM, Alavanja MC, Sandler DP. 2008. Incident diabetes and pesticide exposure among licensed pesticide applicators: Agricultural Health Study, 1993–2003. *American Journal of Epidemiology* 167(10):1235–1246.

Morris PD, Koepsell TD, Daling JR, Taylor JW, Lyon JL, Swanson GM, Child M, Weiss NS. 1986. Toxic substance exposure and multiple myeloma: A case-control study. *Journal of the National Cancer Institute* 76:987–994.

Morrison H, Semenciw RM, Morison D, Magwood S, Mao Y. 1992. Brain cancer and farming in western Canada. *Neuroepidemiology* 11:267–276.

Morrison H, Savitz D, Semenciw RM, Hulka B, Mao Y, Morison D, Wigle D. 1993. Farming and prostate cancer mortality. *American Journal of Epidemiology* 137:270–280.

Morrison HI, Semenciw RM, Wilkins K, Mao Y, Wigle DT. 1994. Non-Hodgkin's lymphoma and agricultural practices in the prairie provinces of Canada. *Scandinavian Journal of Work, Environment and Health* 20:42–47.

Moses M, Lilis R, Crow KD, Thornton J, Fischbein A, Anderson HA, Selikoff IJ. 1984. Health status of workers with past exposure to 2,3,7,8-tetrachlorodibenzo-*p*-dioxin in the manufacture of 2,4,5-trichlorophenoxyacetic acid: Comparison of findings with and without chloracne. *American Journal of Industrial Medicine* 5:161–182.

Musicco M, Sant M, Molinari S, Filippini G, Gatta G, Berrino F. 1988. A case-control study of brain gliomas and occupational exposure to chemical carcinogens: The risks to farmers. *American Journal of Epidemiology* 128:778–785.

Nanni O, Amadori D, Lugaresi C, Falcini F, Scarpi E, Saragoni A, Buiatti E. 1996. Chronic lymphocytic leukæmias and non-Hodgkin's lymphomas by histological type in farming-animal breeding workers: A population case-control study based on a priori exposure matrices. *Occupational and Environmental Medicine* 53(10):652–657.

NCEP (National Cholesterol Education Program). 2002. Third report of the National Cholesterol Education Program (NCEP) Expert Panel on Detection, Evaluation, and Treatment of High Blood Cholesterol in Adults (Adult Treatment Panel III) final report. Circulation 106:3143–3421.

Neuberger M, Kundi M, Jäger R. 1998. Chloracne and morbidity after dioxin exposure (preliminary results). *Toxicology Letters* 96/97:347–350.

Neuberger M, Rappe C, Bergek S, Cai H, Hansson M, Jager R, Kundi M, Lim CK, Wingfors H, Smith AG. 1999. Persistent health effects of dioxin contamination in herbicide production. *Environmental Research* 81(3):206–214.

Newell GR. 1984. *Development and Preliminary Results of Pilot Clinical Studies. Report of the Agent Orange Advisory Committee to the Texas Department of Health.* University of Texas System Cancer Center.

Ng C, Janoo-Gilani R, Sipahimalani P, Gallagher R, Gascoyne R, Connors J, Weber J, Lai A, Leach S, Le N, Brooks-Wilson A, Spinelli J. 2010. Interaction between organochlorines and the AHR gene, and risk of non-Hodgkin lymphoma. *Cancer Causes and Control* 21:11–22.

Ngo AD, Taylor R, Roberts CL, Nguyen TV. 2006. Association between Agent Orange and birth defects: Systematic review and meta-analysis. *International Journal of Epidemiology* 35:1220–1230.

Nguyen HD. 1983. Pregnancies at the Polyclinic of Tay Ninh Province. Summarized in: Constable JD, Hatch MC. *Reproductive effects of herbicide exposure in Vietnam: Recent studies by the Vietnamese and others.* As cited in Constable and Hatch, 1985.

Nhu DD, Kido T, Naganuma R, Sawano N, Tawara K, Nishijo M, Nakagawa H, Hung NN, Thom LTH. 2009. A GIS study of dioxin contamination in a Vietnamese region sprayed with herbicide. *Environmental Health and Preventive Medicine* 14(6):353–360.

Norström A, Rappe C, Lindahl R, Buser HR. 1979. Analysis of some older Scandinavian formulations of 2,4-dichlorophenoxy acetic acid for contents of chlorinated dibenzo-*p*-dioxins and dibenzofurans. *Scandanavian Journal of Work, Environment and Health* 5:375–378.

Nurminen T, Rantala K, Kurppa K, Holmberg PC. 1994. Agricultural work during pregnancy and selected structural malformations in Finland. *Epidemiology* 1:23–30.

O'Brien TR, Decoufle P, Boyle CA. 1991. Non-Hodgkin's lymphoma in a cohort of Vietnam veterans. *American Journal of Public Health* 81:758–760.

Oh E, Lee E, Im H, Kang HS, Jung WW, Won NH, Kim EM, Sul D. 2005. Evaluation of immuno- and reproductive toxicities and association between immunotoxicological and genotoxicological parameters in waste incineration workers. *Toxicology* 2(1):65–80.

Olsen J, Melbye M, Olsen SF, Sorenson TI, Aaby P, Anderson AM, Taxbol D, Hansen KD, Juhl M, Schow TB, Sorensen HT, Andresen J, Mortensen EL, Olesen AW, Sondergaard C. 2001. The Danish National Birth Cohort—Its background, structure and aim. *Scandinavian Journal of Work, Environment and Health* 29:300–307.

Olsson H, Brandt L. 1988. Risk of non-Hodgkin's lymphoma among men occupationally exposed to organic solvents. *Scandinavian Journal of Work, Environment and Health* 14:246–251.

Orsi L, Delabre L, Monnerau A, Delva P, Berthou C, Fenaux P, Marti G, Soubeyran P, Huguet F, Mipied N, Leporrier M, Hemon D, Troussard X, Clavel J. 2009. Occupational exposure to pesticides and lymphoid neoplasms among men: Results of a French case-control study. *Occupational and Environmental Medicine* 66(5):291–298.

O'Toole BI, Marshall RP, Grayson DA, Schureck RJ, Dobson M, Ffrench M, Pulvertaft B, Meldrum L, Bolton J, Vennard J. 1996a. The Australian Vietnam Veterans Health Study: I. Study design and response bias. *International Journal of Epidemiology* 25(2):307–318.

O'Toole BI, Marshall RP, Grayson DA, Schureck RJ, Dobson M, Ffrench M, Pulvertaft B, Meldrum L, Bolton J, Vennard J. 1996b. The Australian Vietnam Veterans Health Study: II. Self-reported health of veterans compared with the Australian population. *International Journal of Epidemiology* 25(2):319–330.

O'Toole BI, Marshall RP, Grayson DA, Schureck RJ, Dobson M, Ffrench M, Pulvertaft B, Meldrum L, Bolton J, Vennard J. 1996c. The Australian Vietnam Veterans Health Study: III. Psychological health of Australian Vietnam veterans and its relationship to combat. *International Journal of Epidemiology* 25(2):331–340.

O'Toole BI, Catts SV, Outram S, Pierse KR, Cockburn J. 2009. The physical and mental health of Australian Vietnam veterans 3 decades after the war and its relation to military service, combat, and post-traumatic stress disorder. *American Journal of Epidemiology* 170(3):318–330.

O'Toole BI, Catts SV, Outram S, Pierse KR, Cockburn J. 2010. Factors associated with civilian mortality in Australian Vietnam Veterans three decades after the war. *Military Medicine* 175(2):88–95.

Ott MG, Zober A. 1996. Cause specific mortality and cancer incidence among employees exposed to 2,3,7,8-TCDD after a 1953 reactor accident. *Occupational and Environmental Medicine* 53(9):606–612.

Ott MG, Holder BB, Olson RD. 1980. A mortality analysis of employees engaged in the manufacture of 2,4,5-trichlorophenoxyacetic acid. *Journal of Occupational Medicine* 22:47–50.

Ott MG, Olson RA, Cook RR, Bond GG. 1987. Cohort mortality study of chemical workers with potential exposure to the higher chlorinated dioxins. *Journal of Occupational Medicine* 29:422–429.

Pahwa P, McDuffie HH, Dosman JA, Robson D, McLaughlin JR, Spinelli JJ, Fincham S. 2003. Exposure to animals and selected risk factors among Canadian farm residents with Hodgkin's disease, multiple myeloma, or soft tissue sarcoma. *Journal of Occupational and Environmental Medicine* 45(8):857–868.

Pahwa P, McDuffie HH, Dosman JA, McLaughlin JR, Spinelli JJ, Robson D, Fincham S. 2006. Hodgkin lymphoma, multiple myeloma, soft tissue sarcomas, insect repellents, and phenoxyherbicides. *Journal of Occupational and Environmental Medicine* 48(3):264–274.

Pahwa P, Karunanayake CP, Dosman JA, Spinelli JJ, McLaughlin JR. 2011. Soft-tissue sarcoma and pesticides exposure in men: Results of a Canadian case-control study. *Journal of Occupational and Environmental Medicine* 53(11):1279–1286.

Pahwa P, Karunanayake CP, Dosman JA, Spinelli JJ, McDuffie HH, McLaughlin JR. 2012. Multiple myeloma and exposure to pesticides: A Canadian case-control study. *Journal of Agromedicine* 17:40–50.

Park RM, Schulte PA, Bowman JD, Walker JT, Bondy SC, Yost MG, Touchstone JA, Dosemeci M. 2005. Potential occupational risks for neurodegenerative diseases. *American Journal of Industrial Medicine* 48(1):63–77.

Patterson DG Jr, Hoffman RE, Needham LL, Roberts DW, Bagby JR, Pinkle JL, Falk H, Sampson EJ, Houk VN. 1986. 2,3,7,8-Tetrachlorodibenzo-*p*-dioxin levels in adipose tissue of exposed and control persons in Missouri. *Journal of the American Medical Association* 256(19):2683–2686.

Pavuk M, Schecter AJ, Akhtar FZ, Michalek JE. 2003. Serum 2,3,7,8-tetrachlorodibenzo-*p*-dioxin (TCDD) levels and thyroid function in Air Force veterans of the Vietnam War. *Annals of Epidemiology* 13(5):335–343.

Pavuk M, Michalek JE, Schecter A, Ketchum NS, Akhtar FZ, Fox KA. 2005. Did TCDD exposure or service in Southeast Asia increase the risk of cancer in Air Force Vietnam veterans who did not spray Agent Orange? *Journal of Occupational and Environmental Medicine* 47(4):335–342.

Pavuk M, Michalek JE, Ketchum NS. 2006. Prostate cancer in US Air Force veterans of the Vietnam War. *Journal of Exposure Science and Environmental Epidemiology* 16(2):184–190.

Payne K, Andreotti G, Bell E, Blair A, Coble J, Alavanja M. 2012. Determinants of high pesticide exposure events in the Agricultural Health Cohort Study from enrollment (1993–1997) through phase II (1999–2003). *Journal of Agricultural Safety and Health* 18(3):167–179.

Pazderova-Vejlupková J, Lukás E, Němcova M, Pícková J, Jirásek L. 1981. The development and prognosis of chronic intoxication by tetrachlorodibenzo-*p*-dioxin in men. *Archives of Environmental Health* 36:5–11.

Pearce NE, Smith AH, Fisher DO. 1985. Malignant lymphoma and multiple myeloma linked with agricultural occupations in a New Zealand cancer registry-based study. *American Journal of Epidemiology* 121:225–237.

Pearce NE, Smith AH, Howard JK, Sheppard RA, Giles HJ, Teague CA. 1986a. Case-control study of multiple myeloma and farming. *British Journal of Cancer* 54:493–500.

Pearce NE, Smith AH, Howard JK, Sheppard RA, Giles HJ, Teague CA. 1986b. Non-Hodgkin's lymphoma and exposure to phenoxyherbicides, chlorophenols, fencing work, and meat works employment: A case-control study. *British Journal of Industrial Medicine* 43:75–83.

Pearce NE, Sheppard RA, Smith AH, Teague CA. 1987. Non-Hodgkin's lymphoma and farming: An expanded case-control study. *International Journal of Cancer* 39:155–161.

Pelclová D, Fenclová Z, Dlasková Z, Urban P, Lukáš E, Procházka B, Rappe C. 2001. Biochemical, neuropsychological, and neurological abnormalities following 2,3,7,8-tetrachlorodibenzo-*p*-dioxin (TCDD) exposure. *Archives of Environmental Health* 56:493–500.

Pelclová D, Fenclová Z, Preiss J, Procházka B, Spácil J, Dubská Z, Okrouhlík B, Lukáš E, Urban P. 2002. Lipid metabolism and neuropsychological follow-up study of workers exposed to 2,3,7,8-tetrachlorodibenzo-*p*-dioxin. *International Archives of Occupational and Environmental Health* 75(Suppl l):S60–S66.

Pelclová D, Prazny M, Skrha J, Fenclová Z, Kalousova M, Urban P, Navratil T, Senholdova Z, Smerhovsky Z. 2007. 2,3,7,8-TCDD exposure, endothelial dysfunction and impaired microvascular reactivity. *Human and Experimental Toxicology* 26(9):705–713.

Pelclová D, Fenclová Z, Urban P, Ridzon P, Preiss J, Kupka K, Malik J, Dubska Z, Navratil T. 2009. Chronic health impairment due to 2,3,7,8-tetrachlorodibenzo-*p*-dioxin exposure. *Neuroendocrinology Letters* 30(Suppl 1):219–224.

Pelclová D, Navratil T, Fenclová Z, Vlckova S, Kupka K, Urban P, Ridzon P, Zikan V, Landova L, Syslova K, Kuzma M, Kacer P. 2011. Increased oxidative/nitrosative stress markers measured non-invasively in patients with high 2,3,7,8-tetrachloro-dibenzo-*p*-dioxin plasma level. Neuro Endocrinology Letters 32(Suppl 1):71–76.

Peper M, Klett M, Frentzel-Beyme R, Heller WD. 1993. Neuropsychological effects of chronic exposure to environmental dioxins and furans. *Environmental Research* 60:124–135.

Persson B, Dahlander AM, Fredriksson M, Brage HN, Ohlson CG, Axelson O. 1989. Malignant lymphomas and occupational exposures. *British Journal of Industrial Medicine* 46:516–520.

Persson B, Fredriksson M, Olsen K, Boeryd B, Axelson O. 1993. Some occupational exposures as risk factors for malignant lymphomas. *Cancer* 72:1773–1778.

Pesatori AC, Consonni D, Tironi A, Landi MT, Zocchetti C, Bertazzi PA. 1992. Cancer morbidity in the Seveso area, 1976–1986. *Chemosphere* 25:209–212.

Pesatori AC, Consonni D, Tironi A, Zocchetti C, Fini A, Bertazzi PA. 1993. Cancer in a young population in a dioxin-contaminated area. *International Journal of Epidemiology* 22:1010–1013.

Pesatori AC, Zocchetti C, Guercilena S, Consonni D, Turrini D, Bertazzi PA. 1998. Dioxin exposure and nonmalignant health effects: A mortality study. *Occupational and Environmental Medicine* 55(2):126–131.

Pesatori AC, Baccarelli A, Consonni D, Lania A, Beck-Peccoz P, Bertazzi PA, Spada A. 2008. Aryl hydrocarbon receptor-interacting protein and pituitary adenomas: A population-based study on subjects exposed to dioxin after the Seveso, Italy, accident. *European Journal of Endocrinology* 159(6):699–703.

Pesatori AC, Consonni D, Rubagotti M, Grillo P, Bertazzi PA. 2009. Cancer incidence in the population exposed to dioxin after the "Seveso accident": Twenty years of follow-up. *Environmental Health* 8:1 of 11.

Petreas M, Smith D, Hurley S, Jeffrey SS, Gilliss D, Reynolds P. 2004. Distribution of persistent, lipid-soluble chemicals in breast and abdominal adipose tissues: Lessons learned from a breast cancer study. *Cancer Epidemiology, Biomarkers and Prevention* 13(3):416–424.

Phuong NTN, Huong LTD. 1983. The effects of toxic chemicals on the pregnancy of the women living at two localities in the South of Vietnam. Summarized in: Constable JD, Hatch MC. *Reproductive Effects of Herbicide Exposure in Vietnam: Recent Studies by the Vietnamese and Others.* As cited in Constable and Hatch, 1985.

Phuong NTN, Thuy TT, Phuong PK. 1989a. An estimate of differences among women giving birth to deformed babies and among those with hydatidiform mole seen at the Ob-Gyn hospital of Ho Chi Minh City in the south of Vietnam. *Chemosphere* 18:801–803.

Phuong NTN, Thuy TT, Phuong PK. 1989b. An estimate of reproductive abnormalities in women inhabiting herbicide sprayed and non-herbicide sprayed areas in the south of Vietnam, 1952–1981. *Chemosphere* 18:843–846.

Piacitelli LA, Marlow DA. 1997. NIOSH 2,3,7,8-tetrachlorodibenzo-*p*-dioxin exposure matrix. *Organohalogen Compounds* 33:510–514.

Pirkle JL, Wolfe WH, Patterson DG, Needham LL, Michalek JE, Miner JC, Peterson MR, Phillips DL. 1989. Estimates of the half-life of 2,3,7,8-tetrachlorodibenzo-*p*-dioxin in Vietnam veterans of Operation Ranch Hand. *Journal of Toxicology and Environmental Health* 27:165–171.

Poland AP, Smith D, Metter G, Possick P. 1971. A health survey of workers in a 2,4-D and 2,4,5-T plant with special attention to chloracne, porphyria cutanea tarda, and psychologic parameters. *Archives of Environmental Health* 22:316–327.

Pollei S, Mettler FA Jr, Kelsey CA, Walters MR, White RE. 1986. Follow-up chest radiographs in Vietnam veterans: Are they useful? *Radiology* 161:101–102.

Quandt SA, Hernandez-Valero MA, Grzywacz JG, Hovey JD, Gonzales M, Arcury TA. 2006. Workplace, household, and personal predictors of pesticide exposure for farmworkers. *Environmental Health Perspectives* 114(6):943–952.

Ramlow JM, Spadacene NW, Hoag SR, Stafford BA, Cartmill JB, Lerner PJ. 1996. Mortality in a cohort of pentachlorophenol manufacturing workers, 1940–1989. *American Journal of Industrial Medicine* 30(2):180–194.

Reif JS, Pearce N, Fraser J. 1989. Occupational risks of brain cancer: A New Zealand cancer registry-based study. *Journal of Occupational Medicine* 31(10):863–867.

Rellahan WL. 1985. *Aspects of the Health of Hawaii's Vietnam-Era Veterans.* Honolulu: Hawaii State Department of Health, Research, and Statistics Office.

Renshaw KD, Caska CM. 2012. Relationship distress in partners of combat veterans: The role of partners' perceptions of posttraumatic stress symptoms. *Behavior Therapy* 43:416–426.

Revazova J, Yurchenko V, Katosova L, Platonova V, Sycheva L, Khripach L, Ingel F, Tsutsman T, Zhurkov V. 2001. Cytogenetic investigation of women exposed to different levels of dioxins in Chapaevsk town. *Chemosphere* 43:999–1004.

Revich B, Aksel E, Ushakova T, Ivanova I, Zhuchenko N, Klyuev N, Brodsky B, Sotskov Y. 2001. Dioxin exposure and public health in Chapaevsk, Russia. *Chemosphere* 43:951–966.

Riihimaki V, Asp S, Hernberg S. 1982. Mortality of 2,4-dichlorophenoxyacetic acid and 2,4,5-trichlorophenoxyacetic acid herbicide applicators in Finland: First report of an ongoing prospective cohort study. *Scandinavian Journal of Work, Environment and Health* 8:37–42.

Riihimaki V, Asp S, Pukkala E, Hernberg S. 1983. Mortality and cancer morbidity among chlorinated phenoxyacid applicators in Finland. *Chemosphere* 12:779–784.

Rix BA, Villadsen E, Engholm G, Lynge E. 1998. Hodgkin's disease, pharyngeal cancer, and soft tissue sarcomas in Danish paper mill workers. *Journal of Occupational and Environmental Medicine* 40(1):55–62.

Robinson CF, Waxweiler RJ, Fowler DP. 1986. Mortality among production workers in pulp and paper mills. *Scandinavian Journal of Work, Environment and Health* 12:552–560.

Rocheleau CM, Bertke SJ, Deddens JA, Ruder AM, Lawson CC, Waters MA, Hopf NB, Riggs MA, Whelan EA. 2011. Maternal exposure to polychlorinated biphenyls and the secondary sex ratio: An occupational cohort study. *Environmental Health* 10:20.

Ronco G, Costa G, Lynge E. 1992. Cancer risk among Danish and Italian farmers. *British Journal of Industrial Medicine* 49:220–225.

Ronn M, Lind L, Bavel BV, Salihovic S, Michaelsson K, Lind PM. 2011. Circulating levels of persistent organic pollutants associate in divergent ways to fat mass measured by DXA in humans. *Chemosphere* 85(3):335–343.

Ruder AM, Yiin JH. 2011. Mortality of US pentachlorophenol production workers through 2005. *Chemosphere* 83(6):851–861.

Ruder AM, Waters MA, Butler MA, Carreon T, Calvert GM, Davis-King KE, Schulte PA, Sanderson WT, Ward EM, Connally LB, Heineman EF, Mandel JS, Morton RF, Reding DJ, Rosenman KD, Talaska G. 2004. Gliomas and farm pesticide exposure in men: The Upper Midwest Health Study. *Archives of Environmental Health* 59(12):650–657.

Ruder AM, Waters MA, Carreon T, Butler MA, Davis-King KE, Calvert GM, Schulte PA, Ward EM, Connally LB, Lu J, Wall D, Zivkovich Z, Heineman EF, Mandel JS, Morton RF, Reding DJ, Rosenman KD, The Brain Cancer Collaborative Study Group. 2006. The Upper Midwest Health Study: A case-control study of primary intracranial gliomas in farm and rural residents. *Journal of Agricultural Safety and Health* 12(4):255–274.

Ruder AM, Carreon T, Butler MA, Calvert GM, Davis-King KE, Waters MA, Schulte PA, Mandel JS, Morton RF, Reding DJ, Rosenman KD. 2009. Exposure to farm crops, livestock, and farm tasks and risk of glioma. *American Journal of Epidemiology* 169(12):1479–1491.

Saberi Hosnijeh F, Boers D, Portengen L, Bueno de Mesquita HB, Heederik D, Vermeulen R. 2011. Long-term effects on humoral immunity among workers exposed to 2,3,7,8-tetrachlorodibenzo-*p*-dioxin (TCDD). *Occupational and Environmental Medicine* 68(6):419–424.

Saberi Hosnijeh F, Boers D, Portengen L, Bueno de Mesquita HB, Heederik D, Vermeulen R. 2012. Plasma cytokine concentrations in workers exposed to 2,3,7,8-tetrachlorodibenzo-*p*-dioxin (TCDD). *Frontiers in Oncology* 2:37.

Saito H, Goovaerts P. 2000. Geostatistical interpolation of positively skewed and censored data in a dioxin contaminated site. *Environmental Science and Technology* 34:4228–4235.

Saldana TM, Basso O, Hoppin JA, Baird DD, Knott C, Blair A, Alavanja MC, Sandler DP. 2007. Pesticide exposure and self-reported gestational diabetes mellitus in the Agricultural Health Study. *Diabetes Care* 30(3):529–534.

Salihovic S, Lampa E, Lindström G, Lind L, Lind PM, van Bavel B. 2012a. Circulating levels of persistent organic pollutants (POPs) among elderly men and women from Sweden: Results from the Prospective Investigation of the Vasculature in Uppsala Seniors (PIVUS). *Environment International* 44:59–67.

Salihovic S, Mattioli L, Lindström G, Lind L, Lind PM, van Bavel B. 2012b. A rapid method for screening of the Stockholm Convention POPs in small amounts of human plasma using SPE and HRGC/HRMS. *Chemosphere* 86:747–753.

Samanic C, Hoppin JA, Lubin JH, Blair A, Alavanja MC. 2005. Factor analysis of pesticide use patterns among pesticide applicators in the Agricultural Health Study. *Journal of Exposure Analysis and Environmental Epidemiology* 15(3):225–233.

Samanic C, Rusiecki J, Dosemeci M, Hou L, Hoppin JA, Sandler DP, Lubin J, Blair A, Alavanja MC. 2006. Cancer incidence among pesticide applicators exposed to dicamba in the Agricultural Health Study. *Environmental Health Perspectives* 114(10):1521–1526.

Saracci R, Kogevinas M, Bertazzi PA, Bueno de Mesquita BH, Coggon D, Green LM, Kauppinen T, L'Abbe KA, Littorin M, Lynge E, Mathews JD, Neuberger M, Osman J, Pearce N, Winkelmann R. 1991. Cancer mortality in workers exposed to chlorophenoxy herbicides and chlorophenols. *Lancet* 338:1027–1032.

Savitz DA, Arbuckle T, Kaczor D, Curtis K. 1997. Male pesticide exposure and pregnancy outcome. *American Journal of Epidemiology* 146(12):1025–1036.

Schecter A, Quynh HT, Pavuk M, Päpke O, Malisch R, Constable JD. 2003. Food as a source of dioxin exposure in the residents of Bien Hoa City, Vietnam. *Journal of Occupational and Environmental Medicine* 45:781–788.

Schildt EB, Eriksson M, Hardell L, Magnuson A. 1999. Occupational exposures as risk factors for oral cancer evaluated in a Swedish case-control study. *Oncology Reports* 6(2):317–320.

Schreinemachers DM. 2000. Cancer mortality in four northern wheat-producing states. *Environmental Health Perspectives* 108(9):873–881.

Schreinemachers DM. 2010. Perturbation of lipids and glucose metabolism associated with previous 2,4-D exposure: A cross-sectional study of NHANES III data, 1988–1994. *Environmental Health* 9:11.

Schulte PA, Burnett CA, Boeniger MF, Johnson J. 1996. Neurodegenerative diseases: Occupational occurrence and potential risk factors, 1982 through 1991. *American Journal of Public Health* 86(9):1281–1288.

Seidler A, Hellenbrand W, Robra BP, Vieregge P, Nischan P, Joerg J, Oertel WH, Ulm G, Schneider E. 1996. Possible environmental, occupational, and other etiologic factors for Parkinson's disease: A case-control study in Germany. *Neurology* 46(5):1275–1284.

Semchuk KM, Love EJ, Lee RG. 1993. Parkinson's disease: A test of the multifactorial etiologic hypothesis. *Neurology* 43:1173–1180.

Semenciw RM, Morrison HI, Riedel D, Wilkins K, Ritter L, Mao Y. 1993. Multiple myeloma mortality and agricultural practices in the prairie provinces of Canada. *Journal of Occupational Medicine* 35:557–561.

Semenciw RM, Morrison HI, Morison D, Mao Y. 1994. Leukemia mortality and farming in the prairie provinces of Canada. *Canadian Journal of Public Health* 85:208–211.

Senthilselvan A, McDuffie HH, Dosman JA. 1992. Association of asthma with use of pesticides: Results of a cross-sectional survey of farmers. *American Review of Respiratory Disease* 146:884–887.

Silverstone AE, Rosenbaum PF, Weinstock RS, Bartell SM, Foushee HR, Shelton C, Pavuk M. 2012. Polychlorinated biphenyl (PCB) exposure and diabetes: Results from the Anniston community health survey. *Environmental Health Perspectives* 120(5):727–732.

Slager RE, Poole JA, LeVan TD, Sandler DP, Alavanja MCR, Hoppin JA. 2009. Rhinitis associated with pesticide exposure among commercial pesticide applicators in the Agricultural Health Study. *Occupational and Environmental Medicine* 66(11):718–724.

Smith AH, Pearce NE. 1986. Update on soft tissue sarcoma and phenoxyherbicides in New Zealand. *Chemosphere* 15:1795–1798.

Smith AH, Matheson DP, Fisher DO, Chapman CJ. 1981. Preliminary report of reproductive outcomes among pesticide applicators using 2,4,5-T. *New Zealand Medical Journal* 93:177–179.

Smith AH, Fisher DO, Pearce N, Chapman CJ. 1982. Congenital defects and miscarriages among New Zealand 2,4,5-T sprayers. *Archives of Environmental Health* 37:197–200.

Smith AH, Fisher DO, Giles HJ, Pearce N. 1983. The New Zealand soft tissue sarcoma case-control study: Interview findings concerning phenoxyacetic acid exposure. *Chemosphere* 12:565–571.

Smith AH, Pearce NE, Fisher DO, Giles HJ, Teague CA, Howard JK. 1984. Soft tissue sarcoma and exposure to phenoxyherbicides and chlorophenols in New Zealand. *Journal of the National Cancer Institute* 73:1111–1117.

Smith JG, Christophers AJ. 1992. Phenoxy herbicides and chlorophenols: A case-control study on soft tissue sarcoma and malignant lymphoma. *British Journal of Cancer* 65:442–448.

Snow BR, Stellman JM, Stellman SD, Sommer JF. 1988. Post-traumatic stress disorder among American Legionnaires in relation to combat experience in Vietnam: Associated and contributing factors. *Environmental Research* 47:175–192.

Sobel W, Bond GG, Skowronski BJ, Brownson PJ, Cook RR. 1987. A soft tissue sarcoma case-control study in a large multi-chemical manufacturing facility. *Chemosphere* 16:2095–2099.

Solet D, Zoloth SR, Sullivan C, Jewett J, Michaels DM. 1989. Patterns of mortality in pulp and paper workers. *Journal of Occupational Medicine* 31:627–630.

Spinelli JJ, Ng CH, Weber JP, Connors JM, Gascoyne RD, Lai AS, Brooks-Wilson AR, Le ND, Berry BR, Gallagher RP. 2007. Organochlorines and risk of non-Hodgkin lymphoma. *International Journal of Cancer* 121(12):2767–2775.

Spoonster-Schwartz L. 1987. Women and the Vietnam experience. *Journal of Nursing Scholarship* 19(4):168–173.

Steenland K, Piacitelli L, Deddens J, Fingerhut M, Chang LI. 1999. Cancer, heart disease, and diabetes in workers exposed to 2,3,7,8-tetrachlorodibenzo-*p*-dioxin. *Journal of the National Cancer Institute* 91(9):779–786.

Steenland K, Calvert G, Ketchum N, Michalek J. 2001. Dioxin and diabetes mellitus: An analysis of the combined NIOSH and Ranch Hand data. *Occupational and Environmental Medicine* 58:641–648.

Stehr PA, Stein G, Webb K, Schramm W, Gedney WB, Donnell HD, Ayres S, Falk H, Sampson E, Smith SJ. 1986. A pilot epidemiologic study of possible health effects associated with 2,3,7,8-tetrachlorodibenzo-*p*-dioxin contaminations in Missouri. *Archives of Environmental Health* 41:16–22.

Stehr-Green P, Hoffman R, Webb K, Evans RG, Knusten A, Schramm W, Staake J, Gibson B, Steinberg K. 1987. Health effects of long-term exposure to 2,3,7,8-tetrachlorodibenzo-*p*-dioxin. *Chemosphere* 16:2089–2094.

Stellman JM, Stellman SD, Sommer JF. 1988. Social and behavioral consequences of the Vietnam experience among American Legionnaires. *Environmental Research* 47:129–149.

Stellman SD, Stellman JM. 1986. Estimation of exposure to Agent Orange and other defoliants among American troops in Vietnam: A methodological approach. *American Journal of Industrial Medicine* 9:305–321.

Stellman SD, Stellman JM, Sommer JF Jr. 1988. Health and reproductive outcomes among American Legionnaires in relation to combat and herbicide exposure in Vietnam. *Environmental Research* 47:150–174.

Stockbauer JW, Hoffman RE, Schramm WF, Edmonds LD. 1988. Reproductive outcomes of mothers with potential exposure to 2,3,7,8-tetrachlorodibenzo-*p*-dioxin. *American Journal of Epidemiology* 128:410–419.

Stolevik SB, Nygaard UC, Namork E, Haugen M, Kvalem HE, Meltzer HM, Alexander J, van Delft JHM, Loveren HV, Lovik M, Granum B. 2011. Prenatal exposure to polychlorinated biphenyls and dioxins is associated with increased risk of wheeze and infections in infants. *Food and Chemical Toxicology* 49(8):1843–1848.

Su PH, Chen JY, Chen JW, Wang SL. 2010. Growth and thyroid function in children with in utero exposure to dioxin: A 5-year follow-up study. *Pediatric Research* 67(2):205–210.

Su PH, Huang PC, Lin CY, Ying TH, Chen JY, Wang SL. 2012. The effect of in utero exposure to dioxins and polychlorinated biphenyls on reproductive development in eight year-old children. *Environment International* 39(1):181–187.

Suskind RR, Hertzberg VS. 1984. Human health effects of 2,4,5-T and its toxic contaminants. *Journal of the American Medical Association* 251:2372–2380.

Svensson BG, Mikoczy Z, Stromberg U, Hagmar L. 1995. Mortality and cancer incidence among Swedish fishermen with a high dietary intake of persistent organochlorine compounds. *Scandinavian Journal of Work, Environment and Health* 21(2):106–115.

Swaen GMH, van Vliet C, Slangen JJM, Sturmans F. 1992. Cancer mortality among licensed herbicide applicators. *Scandinavian Journal of Work, Environment and Health* 18:201–204.

Swaen GMH, van Amelsvoort LGPM, Slangen JJM, Mohren DCL. 2004. Cancer mortality in a cohort of licensed herbicide applicators. *International Archives of Occupational and Environmental Health* 77:293–295.

Sweeney MH, Fingerhut MA, Connally LB, Halperin WE, Moody PL, Marlow DA. 1989. Progress of the NIOSH cross-sectional study of workers occupationally exposed to chemicals contaminated with 2,3,7,8-TCDD. *Chemosphere* 19:973–977.

Sweeney MH, Fingerhut MA, Arezzo JC, Hornung RW, Connally LB. 1993. Peripheral neuropathy after occupational exposure to 2,3,7,8-tetrachlorodibenzo-*p*-dioxin (TCDD). *American Journal of Industrial Medicine* 23:845–858.

Sweeney MH, Calvert G, Egeland GA, Fingerhut MA, Halperin WE, Piacitelli LA. 1996. *Review and update of the results of the NIOSH medical study of workers exposed to chemicals contaminated with 2,3,7,8-tetrachlorodibenzodioxin.* Presented at the symposium Dioxin Exposure and Human Health—An Update, Berlin, June 17.

Sweeney MH, Calvert GM, Egeland GA, Fingerhut MA, Halperin WE, Piacitelli LA. 1997/98. Review and update of the results of the NIOSH medical study of workers exposed to chemicals contaminated with 2,3,7,8-tetrachlorodibenzodioxin. *Teratogenesis, Carcinogenesis, and Mutagenesis* 17(4-5):241–247.

't Mannetje A, McLean D, Cheng S, Boffetta P, Colin D, Pearce N. 2005. Mortality in New Zealand workers exposed to phenoxy herbicides and dioxins. *Occupational and Environmental Medicine* 62(1):34–40.

Tan CE, Ma S, Wai D, Chew SK, Tai ES. 2004. Can we apply the National Cholesterol Education Program Adult Treatment Panel definition of the metabolic syndrome to Asians? *Diabetes Care* 27:1182–1186.

Tango T, Fujita T, Tanihata T, Minowa M, Doi Y, Kato N, Kunikane S, Uchiyama I, Tanaka M, Uehata T. 2004. Risk of adverse reproductive outcomes associated with proximity to municipal solid waste incinerators with high dioxin emission levels in Japan. *Journal of Epidemiology* 14(3):83–93.

Tanner CM, Kamel F, Ross GW, Hoppin JA, Goldman SM, Korell M, Marras C, Bhudhikanok GS, Kasten M, Chade AR, Comyns K, Richards MB, Meng C, Priestley B, Fernandez HH, Cambi F, Umbach DM, Blair A, Sandler DP, Langston JW. 2011. Rotenone, paraquat, and Parkinson's disease. *Environmental Health Perspectives* 119(6):866–872.

Tarone RE, Hayes HM, Hoover RN, Rosenthal JF, Brown LM, Pottern LM, Javadpour N, O'Connell KJ, Stutzman RE. 1991. Service in Vietnam and risk of testicular cancer. *Journal of the National Cancer Institute* 83:1497–1499.

Tarone RE, Alavanja MC, Zahm SH, Lubin JH, Sandler DP, McMaster SB, Rothman N, Blair A. 1997. The Agricultural Health Study: Factors affecting completion and return of self-administered questionnaires in a large prospective cohort study of pesticide applicators. *American Journal of Industrial Medicine* 31:233–242.

Tatham L, Tolbert P, Kjeldsberg C. 1997. Occupational risk factors for subgroups of non-Hodgkin's lymphoma. *Epidemiology* 8(5):551–558.

ten Tusscher GW, Stam GA, Koppe JG. 2000. Open chemical combustions resulting in a local increased incidence of orofacial clefts. *Chemosphere* 40:1263–1270.

Tenchini ML, Crimaudo C, Pacchetti G, Mottura A, Agosti S, De Carli L. 1983. A comparative cytogenetic study on cases of induced abortions in TCDD-exposed and nonexposed women. *Environmental Mutagenesis* 5:73–85.

Teschke K, Hertzman C, Fenske RA, Jin A, Ostry A, van Netten C, Leiss W. 1994. A history of process and chemical changes for fungicide application in the western Canadian lumber industry: What can we learn? *Applied Occupational and Environmental Hygiene* 9:984–993.

Thiess AM, Frentzel-Beyme R, Link R. 1982. Mortality study of persons exposed to dioxin in a trichlorophenol-process accident that occurred in the BASF AG on November 17, 1953. *American Journal of Industrial Medicine* 3:179–189.

Thomas KW, Dosemeci M, Hoppin JA, Sheldon LS, Croghan CW, Gordon SM, Jones ML, Reynolds SJ, Raymer JH, Akland GG, Lynch CF, Knott CE, Sandler DP, Blair AE, Alavanja MC. 2010. Urinary biomarker, dermal, and air measurement results for 2,4-D and chlorpyrifos farm applicators in the Agricultural Health Study. *Journal of Exposure Science and Environmental Epidemiology* 20(2):119–134.

Thomas TL. 1987. Mortality among flavour and fragrance chemical plant workers in the United States. *British Journal of Industrial Medicine* 44:733–737.

Thomas TL, Kang HK. 1990. Mortality and morbidity among Army Chemical Corps Vietnam veterans: A preliminary report. *American Journal of Industrial Medicine* 18:665–673.

Thomas TL, Kang H, Dalager N. 1991. Mortality among women Vietnam veterans, 1973–1987. *American Journal of Epidemiology* 134:973–980.

Thomaseth K, Salvan A. 1998. Estimation of occupational exposure to 2,3,7,8-tetrachlorodibenzo-*p*-dioxin using a minimal physiologic toxicokinetic model. *Environmental Health Perspectives* 106(Suppl 2):743–753.

Thörn A, Gustavsson P, Sadigh J, Westerlund-Hannestrand B, Hogstedt C. 2000. Mortality and cancer incidence among Swedish lumberjacks exposed to phenoxy herbicides. *Occupational and Environmental Medicine* 57(10):718–720.

Tonn T, Esser C, Schneider EM, Steinmann-Steiner-Haldenstatt W, Gleichmann E. 1996. Persistence of decreased T-helper cell function in industrial workers 20 years after exposure to 2,3,7,8-tetrachlorodibenzo-*p*-dioxin. *Environmental Health Perspectives* 104(4):422–426.

Torchio P, Lepore AR, Corrao G, Comba P, Settimi L, Belli S, Magnani C, di Orio F. 1994. Mortality study on a cohort of Italian licensed pesticide users. *The Science of the Total Environment* 149(3):183–191.

Townsend JC, Bodner KM, Van Peenen PFD, Olson RD, Cook RR. 1982. Survey of reproductive events of wives of employees exposed to chlorinated dioxins. *American Journal of Epidemiology* 115:695–713.

True WR, Goldberg J, Eisen SA. 1988. Stress symptomatology among Vietnam veterans. Analysis of the Veterans Administration Survey of Veterans II. *American Journal of Epidemiology* 128:85–92.

Trung CB, Chien NT. 1983. Spontaneous abortions and birth defects in area exposed to toxic chemical sprays in Giong Trom District. Summarized in: Constable JD, Hatch MC. *Reproductive Effects of Herbicide Exposure in Vietnam: Recent Studies by the Vietnamese and Others.* As cited in Constable and Hatch, 1985.

Tsukimori K, Uchi H, Mitoma C, Yasukawa F, Chiba T, Todaka T, Kajiwara J, Yoshimura T, Hirata T, Fukushima K, Wake N, Furue M. 2012. Maternal exposure to high levels of dioxins in relation to birth weight in women affected by Yusho disease. *Environment International* 38(1):79–86.

Turunen AW, Verkasalo PK, Kiviranta H, Pukkala E, Jula A, Mannisto S, Rasanen R, Marniemi J, Vartiainen T. 2008. Mortality in a cohort with high fish consumption. *International Journal of Epidemiology* 37(5):1008–1017.

Turyk M, Anderson HA, Persky VW. 2007. Relationships of thyroid hormones with polychlorinated biphenyls, dioxins, furans, and DDE in adults. *Environmental Health Perspectives* 115(8):1197–1203.

Turyk M, Anderson HA, Knobeloch L, Imm P, Persky VW. 2009. Prevalence of diabetes and body burdens of polychlorinated biphenyls, polybrominated diphenyl ethers, and p,p'-diphenyldichloroethene in Great Lakes sport fish consumers. *Chemosphere* 75(5):674–749.

Uemura H, Arisawa K, Hiyoshi M, Satoh H, Sumiyoshi Y, Morinaga K, Kodama K, Suzuki T, Nagai M, Suzuki T. 2008a. Associations of environmental exposure to dioxins with prevalent diabetes among general inhabitants in Japan. *Environmental Research* 108(1):63–68.

Uemura H, Arisawa K, Hiyoshi M, Satoh H, Sumiyoshi Y, Morinaga K, Kodama K, Suzuki T, Nagai M, Suzuki T. 2008b. PCDDs/PCDFs and dioxin-like PCBs: Recent body burden levels and their determinants among general inhabitants in Japan. *Chemosphere* 73(1):30–37.

Uemura H, Arisawa K, Hiyoshi M, Kitayama A, Takami H, Sewachika F, Dakeshita S, Nii K, Satoh H, Sumiyoshi Y, Morinaga K, Kodama K, Suzuki TI, Nagai M, Suzuki T. 2009. Prevalence of metabolic syndrome associated with body burden levels of dioxin and related compounds among Japan's general population. *Environmental Health Perspectives* 117(4):568–573.

Urban P, Pelclová D, Lukas E, Kupka K, Preiss J, Fenclová Z, Smerhovsky Z. 2007. Neurological and neurophysiological examinations on workers with chronic poisoning by 2,3,7,8-TCDD: Follow-up 35 years after exposure. *European Journal of Neurology* 14(2):213–218.

Valcin M, Henneberger PK, Kullman GJ, Umbach DM, London SJ, Alavanja MC, Sandler DP, Hoppin JA. 2007. Chronic bronchitis among nonsmoking farm women in the Agricultural Health Study. *Journal of Occupational and Environmental Medicine* 49(5):574–583.

van den Berg M, Birnbaum LS, Denison M, De Vito M, Farland W, Feeley M, Fiedler H, Hakansson H, Hanberg A, Haws L, Rose M, Safe S, Schrenk D, Tohyama C, Tritscher A, Tuomisto J, Tysklind M, Walker N, Peterson RE. 2006. The 2005 World Health Organization reevaluation of human and mammalian toxic equivalency factors for dioxins and dioxin-like compounds. *Toxicological Sciences* 93(2):223–241.

van Houdt JJ, Fransman LG, Strik JJ. 1983. Epidemiological case-control study in personnel exposed to 2,4,5-T. *Chemosphere* 12(4):575.

van Wijngaarden E, Stewart PA, Olshan AF, Savitz DA, Bunin GR. 2003. Parental occupational exposure to pesticides and childhood brain cancer. *American Journal of Epidemiology* 157(11):989–997.

Vena J, Boffetta P, Becher H, Benn T, Bueno de Mesquita HB, Coggon D, Colin D, Flesch-Janys D, Green L, Kauppinen T, Littorin M, Lynge E, Mathews JD, Neuberger M, Pearce N, Pesatori AC, Saracci R, Steenland K, Kogevinas M. 1998. Exposure to dioxin and nonneoplastic mortality in the expanded IARC international cohort study of phenoxy herbicide and chlorophenol production workers and sprayers. *Environmental Health Perspectives* 106(Suppl 2):645–653.

Viel JF, Arveux P, Baverel J, Cahn JY. 2000. Soft-tissue sarcoma and non-Hodgkin's lymphoma clusters around a municipal solid waste incinerator with high dioxin emission levels. *American Journal of Epidemiology* 152(1):13–19.

Viel JF, Clement MC, Hagi M, Grandjean S, Challier B, Danzon A. 2008a. Dioxin emissions from a municipal solid waste incinerator and risk of invasive breast cancer: A population-based case-control study with GIS-derived exposure. *International Journal of Health Geographics [Electronic Resource]* 7:4.

Viel JF, Daniau C, Goria S, Fabre P, De Crouy-Chanel P, Sauleau EA, Empereur-Bissonnet P. 2008b. Risk for non Hodgkin's lymphoma in the vicinity of French municipal solid waste incinerators. *Environmental Health* 7(51): 9 pps.

Viel JF, Floret N, Deconinck E, Focant JF, De Pauw E, Cahn JY. 2011. Increased risk of non-Hodgkin lymphoma and serum organochlorine concentrations among neighbors of a municipal solid waste incinerator. *Environment International* 37(2):449–453.

Villeneuve PJ, Steenland K. 2010. Re: "Mortality rates among trichlorophenol workers with exposure to 2,3,7,8-tetrachlorodibenzo-*p*-dioxin." *American Journal of Epidemiology* 171(1):129–130; author reply 130–121.

Vineis P, Terracini B, Ciccone G, Cignetti A, Colombo E, Donna A, Maffi L, Pisa R, Ricci P, Zanini E, Comba P. 1986. Phenoxy herbicides and soft-tissue sarcomas in female rice weeders. A population-based case-referent study. *Scandinavian Journal of Work, Environment and Health* 13:9–17.

Vineis P, Faggiano F, Tedeschi M, Ciccone G. 1991. Incidence rates of lymphomas and soft-tissue sarcomas and environmental measurements of phenoxy herbicides. *Journal of the National Cancer Institute* 83:362–363.

Visintainer PF, Barone M, McGee H, Peterson EL. 1995. Proportionate mortality study of Vietnam-era veterans of Michigan. *Journal of Occupational and Environmental Medicine* 37(4):423–428.

Waggoner JK, Kullman GJ, Henneberger PK, Umbach DM, Blair A, Alavanja MCR, Kamel F, Lynch CF, Knott C, London SJ, Hines CJ, Thomas KW, Sandler DP, Lubin JH, Beane Freeman LE, Hoppin JA. 2011. Mortality in the Agricultural Health Study, 1993–2007. *American Journal of Epidemiology* 173(1):71–83.

Wang SL, Lin CY, Guo YL, Lin LY, Chou WL, Chang LW. 2004. Infant exposure to polychlorinated dibenzo-*p*-dioxins, dibenzofurans and biphenyls (PCDD/Fs, PCBs)—correlation between prenatal and postnatal exposure. *Chemosphere* 54:1459–1473.

Wang SL, Su PH, Jong SB, Guo YL, Chou WL, Päpke O. 2005. In utero exposure to dioxins and polychlorinated biphenyls and its relations to thyroid function and growth hormone in newborns. *Environmental Health Perspectives* 113:1645–1650.

Wang SL, Chang YC, Chao HR, Li CM, Li LA, Lin LY, Päpke O. 2006. Body burdens of polychlorinated dibenzo-p-dioxins, dibenzofurans, and biphenyls and their relations to estrogen metabolism in pregnant women. *Environmental Health Perspectives* 114(5):740–745.

Warner M, Eskenazi B, Mocarelli P, Gerthoux PM, Samuels S, Needham L, Patterson D, Brambilla P. 2002. Serum dioxin concentrations and breast cancer risk in the Seveso Women's Health Study. *Environmental Health Perspectives* 110(7):625–628.

Warner M, Samuels S, Mocarelli P, Gerthoux PM, Needham L, Patterson DG Jr, Eskenazi B. 2004. Serum dioxin concentrations and age at menarche. *Environmental Health Perspectives* 112(13):1289–1292.

Warner M, Eskenazi B, Patterson DG, Clark G, Turner WE, Bonsignore L, Mocarelli P, Gerthoux PM. 2005. Dioxin-like TEQ of women from the Seveso, Italy area by ID-HRGC/HRMS and CALUX. *Journal of Exposure Analysis and Environmental Epidemiology* 15(4):310–318.

Warner M, Eskenazi B, Olive DL, Samuels S, Quick-Miles S, Vercellini P, Gerthoux PM, Needham L, Patterson DG, Mocarelli P. 2007. Serum dioxin concentrations and quality of ovarian function in women of Seveso. *Environmental Health Perspectives* 115(3):336–340.

Warner M, Mocarelli P, Samuels S, Needham L, Brambilla P, Eskenazi B. 2011. Dioxin exposure and cancer risk in the Seveso Women's Health Study. *Environmental Health Perspectives* 119(12):1700–1705.

Watanabe KK, Kang HK. 1995. Military service in Vietnam and the risk of death from trauma and selected cancers. *Annals of Epidemiology* 5(5):407–412.

Watanabe KK, Kang HK. 1996. Mortality patterns among Vietnam veterans: A 24-year retrospective analysis. *Journal of Occupational and Environmental Medicine* 38(3):272–278.

Watanabe KK, Kang HK, Thomas TL. 1991. Mortality among Vietnam veterans: With methodological considerations. *Journal of Occupational Medicine* 33:780–785.

Waterhouse D, Carman WJ, Schottenfeld D, Gridley G, McLean S. 1996. Cancer incidence in the rural community of Tecumseh, Michigan: A pattern of increased lymphopoietic neoplasms. *Cancer* 77(4):763–770.

Webb K, Evans RG, Stehr P, Ayres SM. 1987. Pilot study on health effects of environmental 2,3,7,8-TCDD in Missouri. *American Journal of Industrial Medicine* 11:685–691.

Weisglas-Kuperus N, Sas TC, Koopman-Esseboom C, van der Zwan CW, De Ridder MA, Beishuizen A, Hooijkaas H, Sauer PJ. 1995. Immunologic effects of background prenatal and postnatal exposure to dioxins and polychlorinated biphenyls in Dutch infants. *Pediatric Research* 38(3):404–410.

Weiss J, Päpke O, Bignert A, Jensen S, Greyerz E, Agostoni C, Besana R, Riva E, Giovannini M, Zetterstrom R. 2003. Concentrations of dioxins and other organochlorines (PCBs, DDTs, HCHs) in human milk from Seveso, Milan and a Lombardian rural area in Italy: A study performed 25 years after the heavy dioxin exposure in Seveso. *Acta Paediatrica* 92(4):467–472.

Wendt AS. 1985. *Iowa Agent Orange Survey of Vietnam Veterans.* Iowa State Department of Health.

Weselak M, Arbuckle TE, Wigle DT, Walker MC, Krewski D. 2008. Pre- and post-conception pesticide exposure and the risk of birth defects in an Ontario farm population. *Reproductive Toxicology* 25(4):472–480.

Wigle DT, Semenciw RB, Wilkins K, Riedel D, Ritter L, Morrison HI, Mao Y. 1990. Mortality study of Canadian male farm operators: Non-Hodgkin's lymphoma mortality and agricultural practices in Saskatchewan. *Journal of the National Cancer Institute* 82:575–582.

Wiklund K. 1983. Swedish agricultural workers: A group with a decreased risk of cancer. *Cancer* 51:566–568.

Wiklund K, Holm LE. 1986. Soft tissue sarcoma risk in Swedish agricultural and forestry workers. *Journal of the National Cancer Institute* 76:229–234.

Wiklund K, Dich J, Holm LE. 1987. Risk of malignant lymphoma in Swedish pesticide appliers. *British Journal of Cancer* 56:505–508.

Wiklund K, Lindefors BM, Holm LE. 1988a. Risk of malignant lymphoma in Swedish agricultural and forestry workers. *British Journal of Industrial Medicine* 45:19–24.

Wiklund K, Dich J, Holm LE. 1988b. Soft tissue sarcoma risk in Swedish licensed pesticide applicators. *Journal of Occupational Medicine* 30:801–804.

Wiklund K, Dich J, Holm LE, Eklund G. 1989a. Risk of cancer in pesticide applicators in Swedish agriculture. *British Journal of Industrial Medicine* 46:809–814.

Wiklund K, Dich J, Holm LE. 1989b. Risk of soft tissue sarcoma, Hodgkin's disease and non-Hodgkin lymphoma among Swedish licensed pesticide applicators. *Chemosphere* 18:395–400.

Wilmoth JM, London AS, Parker WM. 2010. Military service and men's health trajectories in later life. *Journal of Gerontology: Social Sciences* 65B(6):744–755.

Wingren G, Fredrikson M, Brage HN, Nordenskjold B, Axelson O. 1990. Soft tissue sarcoma and occupational exposures. *Cancer* 66:806–811.

Wolf N, Karmaus W. 1995. Effects of inhalative exposure to dioxins in wood preservatives on cell-mediated immunity in day-care center teachers. *Environmental Research* 68(2):96–105.

Wolfe WH, Michalek JE, Miner JC, Rahe A, Silva J, Thomas WF, Grubbs WD, Lustik MB, Karrison TG, Roegner RH, Williams DE. 1990. Health status of Air Force veterans occupationally exposed to herbicides in Vietnam. I. Physical health. *Journal of the American Medical Association* 264:1824–1831.

Wolfe WH, Michalek JE, Miner JC, Rahe AJ, Moore CA, Needham LL, Patterson DG. 1995. Paternal serum dioxin and reproductive outcomes among veterans of Operation Ranch Hand. *Epidemiology* 6(1):17–22.

Woods JS, Polissar L. 1989. Non-Hodgkin's lymphoma among phenoxy herbicide-exposed farm workers in western Washington State. *Chemosphere* 18:401–406.

Woods JS, Polissar L, Severson RK, Heuser LS, Kulander BG. 1987. Soft tissue sarcoma and non-Hodgkin's lymphoma in relation to phenoxy herbicide and chlorinated phenol exposure in western Washington. *Journal of the National Cancer Institute* 78:899–910.

Yesavage JA, Kinoshita LM, Kimball T, Zeitzer J, Friedman L, Noda A, David R, Hernandez B, Lee T, Cheng J, O'Hara R. 2012. Sleep-disordered breathing in Vietnam veterans with posttraumatic stress disorder. *American Journal of Geriatric Psychiatry* 20(3):199–204.

Yiin JH, Ruder AM, Stewart PA, Waters MA, Carrean T, Butler MA, Calvert GM, Davis-King KE, Schulte PA, Mandel JS, Morton RF, Reding DJ, Rosenman KD. 2012. The Upper Midwest Health Study: A case-control study of pesticide applicators and risk of glioma. *Environmental Health: A Global Access Science Source* 11(1):13 pps.

Yoshida J, Kumagai S, Tabuchi T, Kosaka H, Akasaka S, Kasai H, Oda H. 2006. Negative association between serum dioxin level and oxidative DNA damage markers in municipal waste incinerator workers. *International Archives of Occupational and Environmental Health* 79(2):115–122.

Zack JA, Suskind RR. 1980. The mortality experience of workers exposed to tetrachlorodibenzodioxin in a trichlorophenol process accident. *Journal of Occupational Medicine* 22:11–14.

Zack JA, Gaffey WR. 1983. A mortality study of workers employed at the Monsanto company plant in Nitro, West Virginia. *Environmental Science Research* 26:575–591.

Zahm SH, Weisenburger DD, Babbitt PA, Saal RC, Vaught JB, Cantor KP, Blair A. 1990. A case-control study of non-Hodgkin's lymphoma and the herbicide 2,4-dichlorophenoxyacetic acid (2,4-D) in eastern Nebraska. *Epidemiology* 1:349–356.

Zahm SH, Weisenburger DD, Saal RC, Vaught JB, Babbitt PA, Blair A. 1993. The role of agricultural pesticide use in the development of non-Hodgkin's lymphoma in women. *Archives of Environmental Health* 48:353–358.

Zhong Y, Rafnsson V. 1996. Cancer incidence among Icelandic pesticide users. *International Journal of Epidemiology* 25(6):1117–1124.

Zober A, Messerer P, Huber P. 1990. Thirty-four-year mortality follow-up of BASF employees exposed to 2,3,7,8-TCDD after the 1953 accident. *International Archives of Occupational and Environmental Health* 62:139–157.

Zober A, Ott MG, Messerer P. 1994. Morbidity follow-up study of BASF employees exposed to 2,3,7,8-tetrachlorodibenzo-*p*-dioxin (TCDD) after a 1953 chemical reactor incident. *Occupational and Environmental Medicine* 51:479–486.

Zober A, Messerer P, Ott MG. 1997. BASF studies: Epidemiological and clinical investigations on dioxin-exposed chemical workers. *Teratogenesis, Carcinogenesis, and Mutagenesis* 17(4-5):249–256.

7

Immune-System Disorders

As in *Veterans and Agent Orange: Update 2010* (IOM, 2012, hereafter referred to as *Update 2010*), immune-system disorders are being addressed in a separate chapter preceding those on other adverse health outcomes. In Veterans and Agent Orange (VAO) reports prior to *Update 2010—Veterans and Agent Orange: Health Effects of Herbicides Used in Vietnam*, hereafter referred to as *VAO* (IOM, 1994), *Veterans and Agent Orange: Update 1996* (IOM, 1996), *Update 1998* (IOM, 1999), *Update 2000* (IOM, 2001), *Update 2002* (IOM, 2003), *Update 2004* (IOM, 2005), *Update 2006* (IOM, 2007), and *Update 2008* (IOM, 2009)—possible adverse health outcomes arising from disruptions of the immune system were included in the "Other Health Effects" chapter. The current committee elected to revisit comprehensively the limited epidemiologic evidence concerning association of immune disease with herbicide exposure in light of the substantial volume of toxicologic evidence of 2,3,7,8-tetrachlorodibenzo-*p*-dioxin (TCDD) impairment of the immune systems of laboratory animals.

This chapter opens with an overview of the various types of health problems that can arise from malfunctioning of the human immune system. The standard VAO sections leading to the committee's assignment of a health outcome to a category of association follow, and they include a new tabulation of all the immune-related epidemiologic information that has been considered in this series and a synopsis of the information new in this update. The next section discusses factors that may lead the immune responses of animals exposed to the chemicals of interest (COIs) to be much more pronounced than any observed to date in humans. The chapter closes with the committee's thoughts regarding research on the possibility that immune perturbations in humans function as a mechanistic step in the development of disease processes in other organ systems.

The immune system plays three important roles in the body:

1. It defends the body against infection by viruses, bacteria, and other disease-producing microorganisms, known as pathogens.
2. It defends against cancer by destroying mutated cells that might otherwise develop into tumors and by providing immunity against tumors.
3. It provides resident immune cells that are specially adapted for different tissues and organs (such as microglia in the central nervous system and Kupffer cells in the liver) that help to regulate the functional activity and integrity of those tissues.

To recognize the wide array of pathogens in the environment, the immune system relies on many cell types that operate together to generate immune responses. Those cells arise from stem cells in the bone marrow; they are found in lymphoid tissues throughout the body; and they circulate in the blood as white blood cells (WBCs). The main types of WBCs are granulocytes, monocytes, and lymphocytes. Each type has many specialized cell populations that are responsible for specific functions connected to the production of specific mediators, such as immune hormones, cytokines, and other secreted factors. Imbalances in those specialized populations or in their level of functional activity can result in inadequate or improper immune responses, which may lead to pathologic outcomes. Diseases arising from immune dysfunction may be apparent immediately or observed only after an organism encounters an environmental challenge that causes immune cells to respond (such as an infection).

CATEGORIES OF IMMUNE DYSFUNCTION

Immune dysfunctions are in four major categories that need not be mutually exclusive: immune suppression, allergy, autoimmunity, and inflammatory dysfunction (inappropriate or misdirected inflammation). Although immune suppression usually is seen as an increased incidence of infections or an increased risk of cancer, allergic, autoimmune, and inflammatory disorders can be manifested as diseases that affect virtually any tissue. It is often difficult to diagnose such diseases, so they may or may not be medically categorized as immune disorders.

Immune Suppression

Suppression of immune responses can reduce resistance to infectious disease and increase the risk of cancer. Infection with the human immunodeficiency virus (HIV) is a well-recognized example of an acquired immune deficiency in which a specific type of lymphocyte (CD4+ T cell) is the target of the virus. The decline in the number of CD4+ T cells after HIV infection correlates with an increased incidence of infectious diseases, including fatal opportunistic infections, and with an increased incidence of several types of cancer. Treatment of cancer patients with toxic chemotherapeutic drugs suppresses the immune system by inhibiting the generation of new WBCs by the bone marrow and by blocking proliferation of lymphocytes during an immune response. Both those examples represent severe immune suppression in which the adverse outcome is easily detected with clinical measurements.

Immune suppression can also result from exposure to chemicals in the workplace or in the environment and be manifested as recurrent infections, opportunistic infections, a higher incidence of a specific category of infections, or a higher incidence of cancer. However, unless the immune suppression is severe, it is often difficult to obtain clinical evidence that directly links chemically induced changes in immune function to increased infectious disease or cancer because many confounding factors can influence a person's ability to combat infection. Such confounders include age, vaccination status, the virulence of the pathogen, the presence of other diseases (such as diabetes), stress, smoking, and the use of drugs or alcohol. Therefore, immunotoxicology studies are often conducted in laboratory animals to understand the scope and mechanism of chemical-induced immune suppression. Results of such studies can be used to develop biomarkers to assess effects in human populations. Infectious-disease models in animals can also be used to determine whether the pattern of disease changes with chemical exposure.

Allergic Diseases

The immune system sometimes responds to a foreign substance that is not pathogenic. Such immunogenic substances are called allergens. Like most immune-based diseases, allergic diseases have both environmental and genetic risk factors. Their prevalence has increased in many countries in recent decades (CDC, 2004; Linneberg et al., 2000; Simpson et al., 2008; Sly, 1999). Major forms of allergic diseases are asthma, allergic rhinitis, atopic dermatitis, and food allergy. In immediate hypersensitivity, the response to some allergens, such as pollen and bee venom, results in the production of immunoglobulin E (IgE) antibodies. Once produced, IgE antibodies bind to mast cells, specialized cells that occur in tissues throughout the body, including lung airways, the intestinal wall, and blood-vessel walls. When a person is exposed to the allergen again, it binds to the antibodies on the mast cells and causes them to release histamine and leukotrienes, which produce the symptoms associated with an allergic response. In delayed-type hypersensitivity (DTH) reactions, also known as cell-mediated immunity, other allergens, such as poison ivy and nickel, activate allergen-specific lymphocytes at the site of contact (usually the skin) that (memory T cells) release substances that cause inflammation and tissue damage. Some allergic responses, such as those to food allergens, may involve a combination of allergen-specific lymphocyte-driven and IgE-driven inflammation. Allergic responses may be manifested in specific tissues (such as skin, eyes, airways, and gastrointestinal tract) or may result in a system-wide response called anaphylaxis.

Autoimmune Diseases

The National Institutes of Health Autoimmune Disease Coordinating Committee recognizes 80 diseases and conditions that affect the cardiovascular, respiratory, nervous, endocrine, dermal, gastrointestinal, hepatic, and excretory systems and are classified as autoimmune diseases (NIH Autoimmune Diseases Coordinating Committee, 2005). They affect both men and women, but most affect more women than men (Fairweather et al., 2008). Genetic predisposition, age, hormone status, and such environmental factors as infectious diseases and stress are known to affect the risk of developing autoimmune diseases, and different autoimmune diseases tend to occur in the same person and to cluster in families. The existence of some autoimmune diseases is also a risk factor for the development of other immune-related diseases, such as some types of cancer (Landgren et al., 2010).

Autoimmune disease is an example of the immune system's causing rather than preventing disease: the immune system attacks the body's own cells and tissues as though they are foreign. Inappropriate immune responses that result in autoimmune disease can be promoted by different components of the immune system (such as antibodies and lymphocytes) and can be directed against a wide variety of tissues or organs. For example, the autoimmune reaction in multiple sclerosis is directed against the myelin sheath of the nervous system; in Crohn's disease, the intestine is the target of attack; in type 1 diabetes mellitus, the insulin-producing cells of the pancreas are destroyed by the immune response; and rheumatoid arthritis arises from immune attack on the joints, but can also involve the lung, heart, and additional organs.

More generalized forms of autoimmune diseases also occur. Systemic lupus erythematosus (SLE) is an autoimmune disease that has multiple target organs of immune attack. Instead, patients have a variety of symptoms that often occur in other diseases, and this makes diagnosis difficult. A characteristic rash across the cheeks and nose and sensitivity to sunlight are common symptoms; oral ulcers, arthritis, pleurisy, proteinuria, and neurologic disorders may be present. Almost all people who have SLE test positive for antinuclear antibodies in the absence of drugs known to induce them. The causes of SLE are unknown, but environmental and genetic factors have been implicated. Some of the environmental factors that may trigger it are infections, antibiotics (especially those in the sulfa and penicillin groups) and some other drugs, ultraviolet radiation, extreme stress, and hormones. Occupational exposures to such chemicals as crystalline silica, solvents, and pesticides have also been associated with SLE (Cooper and Parks, 2004; Parks and Cooper, 2005).

Inflammatory Diseases

Inflammatory diseases (also referred to as auto-inflammatory diseases) make up a more recently identified category of immune-related disorders that are characterized by exaggerated, excessively prolonged, or misdirected dysfunctional inflammatory responses (usually involving immune cells). Tissue disease can result from this inappropriate inflammation, which can affect virtually any organ. Examples of diseases and other conditions that are most often included in other disease categories but are also considered to be inflammatory diseases are coronary arterial disease, asthma, eczema, chronic sinusitis, hepatic steatosis, psoriasis, celiac disease, and prostatitis. Inflammatory diseases often occur with one another, and this has resulted in the categorizing of different but linked inflammatory diseases together as a single chronic inflammatory disorder (Borensztajn et al., 2011); among these are atherosclerosis and chronic pulmonary obstructive disease. Inappropriate inflammation also appears to play a role in promoting the growth of cancer (Bornschein et al., 2010; Hillegass et al., 2010; Landgren et al., 2010; Porta et al., 2010; Winans et al., 2010); examples can be seen in the higher prevalence of specific cancers in patients who have such inflammatory diseases as inflammatory bowel disease (Lucas et al., 2010; Viennot et al., 2009; Westbrook et al., 2010), prostatitis (Sandhu, 2008; Wang et al., 2009), and psoriasis (Ji et al., 2009).

Ordinarily, inflammation can be advantageous in fighting infectious diseases. It is one component of the normal host response to infection and is mediated by innate immune cells. Inflammatory responses have evolved to speed the trafficking of macrophages, granulocytes, and some lymphocytes to the area of infection, where they produce toxic metabolites that kill pathogens. Interactions among innate immune cells and epithelial and endothelial cells are important in regulating the magnitude of inflammation. However, improperly regulated inflammation can contribute to diseases that arise in nonlymphoid tissues, such as the lungs, skin, nervous system, endocrine system, and reproductive system.

CONCLUSIONS FROM *VAO* AND PREVIOUS UPDATES

The following comments are restricted to findings related to the immune system that occur after adult human exposure. For a discussion of potential effects on the immune system arising from early-life (such as perinatal) exposures (which would not be directly applicable to the Vietnam veterans who are the target of this report), see Chapters 4 and 9. Studies that served as the basis of prior updates of *VAO* are shown in Table 7-1.

Vietnam Veterans

A handful of the direct studies of veterans listed in Table 7-1 reported a statistically significant difference in a single immune measure (Kim et al., 2003;

TABLE 7-1 Selected Epidemiologic Studies—Immune Effects in Adult Humans (Shaded Entries Are New Information for This Update)

Study Population	**Exposure**/Results	Reference
VIETNAM VETERANS		
US Air Force Health Study—Operation Ranch Hand veterans vs SEA veterans	**All COIs**	
Participants in 1997 examination cycle, Operation Ranch Hand veterans vs comparisons (incidence)	No change in surface markers for B and T cells, no change in serum Ig, no change in autoantibodies (antinuclear antibody, smooth muscle autoantibody, parietal cell autoantibody, rheumatoid factor, and monoclonal immunoglobulins) and no dose-related change in DTH response	Michalek et al., 1999a
Participants in 1987 examination cycle, Operation Ranch Hand veterans vs comparisons (morbidity)	No change in surface markers for B and T cells	Wolfe et al., 1990
Participants in 1985 examination cycle, Operation Ranch Hand veterans vs comparisons (morbidity and mortality)	No change in surface markers for B and T cells	Wolfe et al., 1985
US CDC Vietnam Experience Study— Cross-sectional study, with medical examinations, of Army veterans: 9,324 deployed vs 8,989 nondeployed	**All COIs**	
Morbidity—Deployed vs nondeployed	No differences in infections, no changes in B and T cell-surface markers, WBC counts, or circulating serum Ig	CDC, 1988b
Mortality (1965–2000)	No increase in infectious or parasitic diseases	Boehmer et al., 2004
US VA Cohort of Monozygotic Twins	**All COIs**	
Physical health—morbidity	Increase in skin conditions of unknown etiology, no increase in blood disorders	Eisen et al., 1991
US American Legion Cohort	**All COIs**	
Physical health and reproductive outcomes	Increase in skin conditions and arthritis	Stellman et al., 1988
State Studies of US Vietnam Veterans	**All COIs**	
Michigan Vietnam Veterans (deployed vs nondeployed)	Increased mortality from infectious (including parasitic) diseases	Visintainer et al., 1995

TABLE 7-1 Immune Effects in Adult Humans, continued

Study Population	**Exposure**/Results	Reference
New Jersey Agent Orange Commission	Depressed response to tetanus in DTH tests, decrease in CD4 and SmIg+ B cells	Kahn et al., 1992
Texas Agent Orange Advisory Committee	Increase in percentage of active T rosette-forming cells	Newell, 1984
Sample of 1,000 Male Australian Vietnam Veterans–prevelance	**All COIs**	
Australian Vietnam Veterans—longitudinal cohort study of 67 conditions in randomly selected Vietnam veterans vs general population	Increase in hay fever, increases in infectious and parasitic diseases, increase in arthritis	O'Toole et al., 2009
Australian Conscripted Army National Service (18,940 deployed vs 24,642 nondeployed)	**All COIs**	
1983–1985—Australian Vietnam Veterans—longitudinal cohort study of 67 conditions in randomly selected Vietnam veterans vs general population	Increase in hay fever, increases in infectious and parasitic diseases, increase in arthritis	CDVA, 1997b
Korean Vietnam Veterans	**All COIs**	
Immunotoxicologic study	Increase in IgE and IL-4, decrease in IgG1 and IFN-gamma, no change in lymphocyte counts	Kim et al., 2003
Vietnamese Vietnam Veterans	**All COIs**	
Antinuclear and sperm autoantibodies	No change in autoantibodies to sperm, antinuclear bodies	Chinh et al., 1996
OCCUPATIONAL STUDIES		
IARC Phenoxy Herbicide Cohort— Subset of **Dutch workers** (n = 85) from 2 plants that produced and formulated chlorophenoxy herbicides (high exposure = 47, low exposure = 38); serum collected 30 yrs after exposure	**Chlorophenoxy herbicides/**General reduction in most analyte levels with the strongest effects for fractalkine, fibroblast growth factor (FGF_2), and transforming growth factor alpha (TGF-α)	Saberi Hosnijeh et al., 2012
IARC Phenoxy Herbicide Cohort— Dutch workers from 2 plants that produced and formulated chlorophenoxy herbicides (Plant A, n = 1,167; Plant B, n = 1,143).	**Chlorophenoxy herbicides/**Negative correlation between TCDD exposure and markers of humoral immunity, except perhaps for C4	Saberi Hosnijeh et al., 2012

continued

TABLE 7-1 Immune Effects in Adult Humans, continued

Study Population	**Exposure**/Results	Reference
IARC Phenoxy Herbicide Cohort—German production workers (2,479 workers at 4 plants, in IARC as of 1997)	**Dioxins, phenoxy herbicides**	
Cross-sectional study of 153 male workers in six chemical plants in Germany	**TCDD** (during production of TCP): DTH responses not correlated with dioxin concentration; slight decrease in IgM was reported with increasing dioxin exposure; overall lymphoid counts not different	Benner et al., 1994
German production workers at BASF Ludwigshafen Plant—BASF Cleanup workers from 1953 accident (n = 247); 114 with chloracne, 13 more with erythema; serum TCDD levels (not part of IARC)	**Focus on TCDD**	
138 surviving workers from a larger cohort of 254 exposed workers after an accident in a BASF TCP production facility	**TCDD**: Among 14 immune measures; regression analysis of TCDD concentration suggested marginal positive associations with IgG, IgA, C3, and C4; marginal reductions in some lymphocyte population were also reported	Ott et al., 1994
IARC Phenoxy Herbicide Cohort—German production workers at Boehringer-Ingelheim Plant in Hamburg (1,144 men working > 1 month in 1952–1984; generation of TCDD reduced after chloracne outbreak in 1954)	**Dioxins, 2,4,5-T; 2,5-DCP; 2,4,5-TCP**	
Updated and expanded evaluation of 158 workers in a German chemical plant with differing exposure studied in two trials	**TCDD** (or "TCDD toxic equivalents" from PCDD/PCDF): No differences in serum Ig or cytokine (IL1, IL6, TNF-alpha)	Neubert et al., 2000
19 highly exposed chemical workers vs 28 unexposed controls in two chemical plants in Hamburg, Germany	**TCDD** (in chemical plant): In subset of leukocytes, increase in CD8+ memory T cells and decrease in naïve T cells (CD45RA+) after TCDD exposure, as was stimulated IFN-gamma production from whole blood cultures associated with TCDD exposure	Ernst et al., 1998

TABLE 7-1 Immune Effects in Adult Humans, continued

Study Population	**Exposure**/Results	Reference
192 workers in a German pesticide plant, including 29 highly exposed and 28 controls compared for immune functional tests	**TCDD** (or TEQs from PCDD/PCDF exposure): No significant changes in TCDD and lymphocyte subsets, antibody responses to vaccination, lymphocyte proliferation, or autoantibody production; decrease in chromate resistance of PHA-stimulated lymphocytes in highest exposure group	Jung et al., 1998
Comparison of 11 2,4,5-trichlorophenol production workers 20 years after exposure vs 10 unexposed age-matched workers in the same company	**TCDD**: No differences in any lymphoid subset or in mitogen-induced proliferation; TCDD exposure was associated with decreases in MLR response and in stimulation with IL-2 in vitro	Tonn et al., 1996
Examination of eight trichlorophenol production workers who developed chloracne and were reexamined 15–25 years after initial exposure	**TCDD**: Reduced gamma globulins in the most-exposed workers; no significant effects on T4, T8 ratios.	Jansing and Korff, 1994
89 volunteers involved in decontamination work at a chemical plant in Hamburg, Germany; no control population	**TCDD** (or equivalents via PCDD/PCDF exposure): Potentially complicated by age differences among the compared groups; only subtle, clinically nonsignificant changes were seen among immune-cell surface markers in a comparison of higher exposed vs low-exposed to moderately exposed workers	Neubert et al., 1993, 1994
NIOSH Cohort (current and former workers from chemical plants in New Jersey and Missouri, 2 of the 12 plants included in the NIOSH Mortality Study)	**Dioxins, phenoxy herbicides**	
Cross-sectional study of 259 TCDD-exposed 2,4,5-trichlorophenate (and its derivatives) workers (mean serum TCDD, 223 ppt) and 243 unexposed residential controls (mean serum TCDD, 6 ppt)	**TCDD** (exposure in a chemical plant): No significant changes in serum Ig or major leukocyte categories; TCDD associated with decreased circulating CD26 cells (activated T cells)	Halperin et al., 1998
1987 cross-sectional study of 281 chemical-plant workers in NJ and MO at least 15 years after exposure vs 260 unexposed controls	**TCDD** (as a contaminant in chemical production): Increase in TCDD associated with a decrease in CD3/Ta1 (helper lymphocytes) cells	Sweeney et al., 1997/1998
Other Studies of Industrial Workers (not related to IARC or NIOSH phenoxy cohorts)		

continued

TABLE 7-1 Immune Effects in Adult Humans, continued

Study Population	**Exposure**/Results	Reference
EUROPIT Study—Prospective multicenter cohort study (Bulgaria, Finland, Italy, The Netherlands) of 238 pesticide-exposed workers vs 198 unexposed workers	**Pesticide factories** (not specifically TCDD): Reduced antibody responses to hepatitis B vaccination among exposed workers carrying a specific IL-1 allele	Baranska et al., 2008
OCCUPATIONAL—HERBICIDE-USING WORKERS (not related to IARC sprayer cohorts)		
Agricultural Health Study (AHS)—prospective study of licensed pesticide sprayers in Iowa and North Carolina: commercial (n = 4,916 men), private/farmers (n = 52,395, 97.4% men), and spouses of private sprayers (n = 32,347, 0.007% men), enrolled 1993–1997; followups with CATIs 1999–2003 and 2005–2010	**Pesticides/herbicides**	
Comparison from the AHS of 534 cases of self-reported physician-diagnosed depression vs 17,051 controls	Both high-level acute pesticide exposure (OR = 2.6, 95% CI 1.7–3.8) and cumulative pesticide exposure (OR = 1.5, 95% CI 1.2–2.0) were positively associated with increase in depression	Beseler et al., 2008
29,074 female spouses of pesticide applicators in the AHS	Depression was significantly associated with pesticide poisoning (OR = 3.3, 95% CI 1.7–6.2) but not with lower cumulative exposure	Beseler et al., 2006
Nested case-control study of rheumatoid arthritis in agricultural families (57,000 pesticide applicators and their spouses)	No strong risk factors were identified for pesticide mixing or application or for any specific class of pesticides in the AHS of rheumatoid arthritis	De Roos et al., 2005b
Other Studies of Herbicide-Using Workers		
Longitudinal study of 10 farmers during 1994 within 7 days before and 1–12 days and 50–70 days after exposure	**2,4-D and MCPA formulations**: Decreases in percentages of CD4, CD8, CTL, CD8-DR, and NK cells and in NK activity and mitogen-stimulated lymphoproliferation; CD4:CD8 ratio was unaltered; CD3 and CD8 percentages had recovered by the second assessment period; no significant correlations between immune changes and amount of pesticides applied	Faustini et al., 1996

TABLE 7-1 Immune Effects in Adult Humans, continued

Study Population	**Exposure**/Results	Reference
ENVIRONMENTAL STUDIES		
Seveso Cleanup Workers	**TCDD**	
Prospective study using analysis of samples from 36 cleanup workers (divided into three groups based on time spent in the contamination area); pre-employment samples and samples after 9 months were analyzed for comparison with samples from 31 nonexposed workers	No differences in WBC counts and platelet counts	Ghezzi et al., 1982
Seveso, Italy, Residential Cohort—Industrial accident July 10, 1976 (723 residents Zone A; 4,821 Zone B; 31,643 Zone R; 181,574 local reference group)	**TCDD**	
Study of 101 chloracne cases vs 211 controls 20 years after the accident; relatively low statistical power was available because the study examined the occurrence of individual diseases	Persistent increase in TCDD in chloracne cases; younger people seemed to be more susceptible; no major trends in disease occurrence	Baccarelli et al., 2005b
Study of 62 people from a highly exposed zone and 53 from noncontaminated areas 20 years after the accident	Plasma concentration of TCDD was determined; multivariate regression analysis showed significant decrease in plasma IgG with increasing TCDD concentration and no changes in IgM, IgA, or C3	Baccarelli et al., 2002
45 children (3–7 years of age) living in exposed areas vs 45 nonexposed children as controls	No differences in serum IG, mitogen responses of lymphocytes (PHA and pokeweed), or percentage of rosette-forming lymphocytes	Pocchiari et al., 1979
Times Beach (MO) Cohort	**TCDD**	
Regression analysis used for comparisons among 41 exposed people for adipose-tissue, TCDD vs immune measures; three exposed groups defined by tissue dioxin	No TCDD–DTH response relationships were reported; no change in mitogen responsiveness; some serum markers (A/G ratio and serum IgG) were affected	Webb et al., 1989
82 people in more highly contaminated areas vs 40 in low-risk exposure areas as controls	No differences in DTH response or T-cell subsets (T4/T8)	Webb et al., 1987
80 people in highly contaminated areas vs 40 controls in lower-risk areas	No differences in DTH induration or T-cell subset analysis (T4/T8)	Stehr et al., 1986

continued

TABLE 7-1 Immune Effects in Adult Humans, continued

Study Population	**Exposure**/Results	Reference
Pilot study of small numbers of people; for comparisons, people were assigned to two environmental-exposure groups: those in high-risk areas (27 men, 23 women, and 15 children) and those in low-risk areas (12 men, 10 women, and 8 children)	Multitest DTH evaluation to seven recall antigens was performed, no statistical differences were reported, and only trends were noted; no statistical differences were reported for T-cell markers (T3, T4, and T8) or mitogen-induced lymphocyte proliferation (PHA, Con A, and pokeweed mitogen), and . only trends were noted	Knutsen, 1984
Quail Run Mobile Home Park (MO) Cohort	**TCDD**	
A subset of the previously anergic persons in the Stehr-Green et al. (1987) study were reevaluated in the DTH test with a higher DTH test dose and highly trained, blinded readers	Retesting of DTH failed to produce the differences observed initially	Evans et al., 1988
Small (ill-defined) samples were used; comparisons of residents of the Quail Run Mobile Home Park with residents of St. Louis–area trailer parks as controls	DTH suppression in the exposed group was reported, but data from two of four readers were discarded; no differences in T-cell mitogen stimulation; decreases in percentages of T3, T4, and T11 cells in the exposed group	Knutsen et al., 1987
154 people in highly contaminated area vs 155 in three low–environmental-contamination areas as controls	Increase in anergy and decrease in induration for DTH in exposed group; data from some readers were excluded; decrease in percentages of T3, T4, and T11 cells, but no difference in cell number of T4/T8 ratio	Stehr-Green et al., 1987
80 people in a high–exposure risk group vs 40 controls	Decreases in DTH indurations, number of positive reactors, and percentages of T3, T4, and T11 cells in the exposed group	Andrews et al., 1986
154 people in the exposed area vs 155 nonexposed people in an uncontaminated area	Recall antigen multitest for DTH, increase in percentage of anergy and decrease in induration in exposed group; data from two of four readers were excluded	Hoffman et al., 1986

TABLE 7-1 Immune Effects in Adult Humans, continued

Study Population	**Exposure**/Results	Reference
Other Environmental Studies		
Belgium (Flanders)—200 people 17–18 yr of age in three areas of Flanders (Belgium); TEQ values were calculated from serum dioxin-like PCB concentrations and relationships with immune measures were examined	**Dioxins and PCBs**: Decreases in eosinophil and NK-cell counts with increasing TEQ; IgE concentrations; history of upper airway allergy, and odds of a positive RAST test correlated negatively with serum TEQ; IgA concentrations correlated positively with TEQ	Van den Heuvel et al., 2002
Germany—Cross-sectional study of 221 teachers who worked in German day-care centers treated with wood preservatives vs 189 teachers who worked in untreated facilities	**Dioxin in wood preservatives**, exposure primarily via inhalation: No effects of inhaled dioxin were seen on T4 or T8 cell numbers or on the ratio; some evidence of a dose–response relationship was seen for risk of anergy (or hypoergy) in the DTH assay	Wolf and Karmaus, 1995
US (NHANES)—1,721 adults were assessed for serum dioxin-like PCBs and self-reported arthritis	**Dioxin-like PCBs**: Association between serum dioxin-like PCBs and prevalence of arthritis particularly among women	Lee et al., 2007a
CASE-CONTROL STUDIES		
Norway—blood samples from 24 Norwegian hobby fishermen were compared with those of 10 male referents as controls	**PCDD**, exposure from food: The study generally lacks experimental details; no differences in an NK cell marker or in NK activity were seen; apparently, some effects on lymphoid markers were observed but specific details are lacking	Lovik et al., 1996
Sweden—23 high consumers of fatty fish from the Baltic Sea (containing low concentrations of PCDD) vs 20 low consumers or nonconsumers of fish as controls	**PCDD**, exposure from food: Blood PCDDs were significantly different between the groups; mercury concentrations also differed; NK cells correlated negatively with blood concentrations of persistent organic chemicals; no other	Svensson et al., 1994
South Korea (Ansan)—comparison of immune measures in 31 waste-incineration workers vs 84 controls	**TCDD** (via waste incineration): Lymphoid subsets, IFN-gamma, and Ig not statistically different; decrease in IL-4 and increase in T-cell activation (measured as combined CD3 and CD69 markers) associated with TCDD exposure	Oh et al., 2005

continued

TABLE 7-1 Immune Effects in Adult Humans, continued

Study Population	**Exposure**/Results	Reference
United Kingdom (Derbyshire)—18 chemical workers in a 2,4,5-T in the Coalite Oils and Chemical, Ltd. factory exposed as a result of an industrial accident 17 years before study vs 15 matched controls	**TCDD**: No changes in serum Ig classes, increases in antinuclear antibodies and immune complexes, and increase in circulating NK cells (Leu7+) in exposed workers	Jennings et al., 1988
United States (California)—telephone interviews concerning environmental and occupational chemical exposures were conducted with 50 AIDS patients (with Kaposi sarcoma) and 50 homosexual men as controls	**Chemical exposures, including pesticides, and Agent Orange**: No significant differences were reported in a small study that generally lacked focus	Hardell et al., 1987

NOTE: 2,4-D, 2,4-dichlorophenoxyacetic acid; 2,4,5-T, 2,4,5-trichlorophenoxyacetic acid; AHS, Agricultural Health Study; CDC, Centers for Disease Control and Prevention; CI, confidence interval; COI, chemical of interest; Con A, concanavalin A; DTH, delayed-type hypersensitivity; IFN-gamma, interferon-gamma; Ig, immunoglobulin; IL, interleukin; MCPA, methyl-4-chlorophenoxyacetic acid; MLR, mixed lymphocyte response; MO, Missouri; NHANES, National Health and Nutrition Examination Survey; NIOSH, National Institute for Occupational Safety and Health; NK, natural killer; OR, odds ratio; PCB, polychlorinated biphenyl; PCDD, polychlorinated dibenzo-*p*-dioxin (highly chlorinated, if four or more chlorines); PCDF, polychlorinated dibenzofurans; PHA, polyhydroxyalkanoates; RAST, radioallergosorbent; SEA, Southeast Asia; TCDD, 2,3,7,8-tetrachlorodibenzo-*p*-dioxin; TCP, trichlorophenol; TEQ, total toxic equivalent; TNF, tumor necrosis factor; VA, Department of Veterans Affairs; WBC, white blood cell.

Michalek et al., 1999a). But invariably the same effect was not found in other studies of Vietnam veterans, nor was support found in epidemiologic studies of other populations. Thus, there were no consistent findings indicative of immunosuppression, increased risk of autoimmunity (usually as measured with autoantibodies), or biomarkers of atopy or allergy (such as increased IgE concentrations). Much of the focus of the studies was on measuring T4:T8 ratios. The T4:T8 ratio is an effective biomarker of the progression of HIV-induced AIDS, but, on the basis of the TCDD-exposure animal data, it is not an immunologic index that is expected to be altered. The results of a survey of Australian Vietnam veterans (O'Toole et al., 2009) included purportedly significant increases in the prevalence of a number of conditions in which immune function may play a prominent role, but the study's methods were deemed unreliable.

Occupational Exposures

Occupational-exposure studies shown in Table 7-1 evaluated concentrations of lymphoid populations in circulation, such as CD4, CD8 (and the ratio of the two), and natural killer (NK) cells; cell-mediated immunity (the delayed-hypersensitivity response); serum concentrations of immunoglobulins, such as IgM, IgG, and IgA; concentrations of complement, such as C3 and C4; and concentrations of cytokines, such as IL-1, IL-2, interferon-gamma, IL-4, IL-6, and tumor necrosis factor (TNF)-alpha. A few studies also included disease or condition endpoints, such as rheumatoid arthritis, SLE, and depression. Ex vivo analyses included measures of NK activity, lymphoid mitogen-induced proliferation, and the mixed lymphocyte response (MLR) against allogeneic cells. Some studies identified one or more dioxin-related shifts in immune measures, but many reported no significant differences in the same measures. That is particularly true of the study by Neubert et al. (2000), which measured toxicity equivalents (TEQs) for dioxin but found no immunoglobulin or cytokine alterations. In general, the spectrum of occupational-exposure findings does not provide a consistent or clear picture of alterations in immune measures that could be extrapolated to an increased risk of a single disease or even a broader category of diseases. The exception may be observations of pesticide-associated autoimmunity and depression. Immune depression was rather consistently associated with very high pesticide exposures or pesticide poisonings. However, because the studies generally concerned broad categories of pesticide exposure, their relevance to herbicide exposures in Vietnam is not clear.

Environmental Exposures

Several environmental-exposure studies reported alterations, but findings were inconsistent among the studies (see Table 7-1). Some studies reported alterations in immune measures associated with TEQs for dioxin. For example, Van den Heuvel et al. (2002) reported that IgE, positive radioallergosorbent (RAST) tests in response to specific allergens, eosinophil counts, and NK-cell counts correlated negatively with dioxin TEQs but that IgA increased; these alterations, however, were not seen consistently in other studies. Baccarelli et al. (2002) found no changes in IgA but saw changes in IgG in the Seveso population. Svensson et al. (1994) found that NK-cell numbers were reduced with increasing concentrations of persistent organic chemicals, but Lovik et al. (1996) found no difference in NK numbers or activity. Similarly, the occupational-exposure studies (see Table 7-1) that examined NK concentrations reported the full spectrum of results: no alterations (Halperin et al., 1998), a decrease (Faustini et al., 1996), and even an increase in NK numbers (Jennings et al., 1988) in dioxin-exposed people.

As seen in Table 7-1, some early studies of the Quail Run Mobile Home Park population exposures reported that dioxin exposure was associated with a reduced cell-mediated immune response, the delayed-type hypersensitivity (DTH) response (Andrews et al., 1986; Hoffman et al., 1986; Knutsen et al., 1987; Stehr-Green et al., 1987). But some of those studies had technical problems in assessment and in followup analyses. Dioxin-associated changes were not confirmed (Evans et al., 1988; Webb et al., 1989). In addition, several studies of the Times

Beach population did not find any alteration of the DTH response in dioxin-exposed populations (Knutsen, 1984; Stehr et al., 1986; Webb et al., 1987).

Analysis of National Health and Nutrition Examination Survey (NHANES) data found that exposure to dioxin-like polychlorinated biphenyls was associated with an increase in self-reported arthritis (Lee et al., 2007a), but De Roos et al. (2005b) had found no such association in their study.

Prior VAO updates have concluded that human data were either insufficient or inconsistent with respect to an increased risk of immunosuppression, allergic disease, or autoimmune disease.

UPDATE OF THE EPIDEMIOLOGIC LITERATURE AND HUMAN STUDIES

Vietnam-Veteran and Case-Control Studies

No new case-control studies or studies of Vietnam veterans exposed to the COIs and adverse immunologic conditions have been published since *Update 2010*.

Occupational Studies

There were several small new studies of occupational cohorts. Endres et al. (2012) studied fungal sensitization in the Agricultural Health Study and reported that farmers had levels of fungal sensitization lower than the national levels found in the NHANES studies. It is difficult to interpret those data, although they do suggest that farmers as a group have a lower reactivity to fungal antigens.

Saberi Hosnijeh et al. (2011) studied Dutch phenoxy-herbicide workers, assessing their humoral immunity. The 45 TCDD-exposed workers had decreased concentrations of complement factor 4 but no other apparent changes in humoral immunity as measured by other complement factors or immunoglobulins. The same authors (Saberi Hosnijeh et al., 2012) reported that plasma TCDD concentrations were associated with decreases in cytokines, chemokines, and growth factors. The authors conclude that this work provided evidence of immunologic effects of TCDD.

Environmental Studies

No environmental studies of adverse immunologic conditions have been published since the 2010 review. However, a report of an investigation of the immune response of a single highly exposed person (Brembilla et al., 2011) reported some clearly TCDD-associated immune changes (such as IL-22 production by CD4+ T cells), confirming some TCDD-associated changes in immune measures. It is interesting that there was no measured effect of TCDD exposure on the person's T regulatory cells. Earlier publications cited indicate that this patient was Victor Yuchenko, whose poisoning in 2004 has provided insight into human response to and biotransformation of an extremely high dose of TCDD, exceeding by orders of magnitude the exposures experienced by Vietnam veterans.

The literature searches for the current update found two epidemiologic studies (Jusko et al., 2011; Miyashita et al., 2011) that addressed immune-related outcomes in the children of mothers potentially exposed to the COIs (the topic of Chapter 10) that are not relevant to assessing immune consequences in Vietnam veterans of their own exposure.

BIOLOGIC PLAUSIBILITY

There is an extensive body of evidence from experimental studies in animal-model systems that TCDD, other dioxins, and several dioxin-like chemicals (DLCs) are immunotoxic (Kerkvliet, 2009, 2012). Immunotoxicity is due primarily to changes in adaptive immune responses that result in suppression of both antibody-mediated and cell-mediated immunity. A new endogenous pathway, the tryptophan metabolic pathway, has recently been identified as affecting the aryl hydrocarbon receptor (AHR) and immune biology (Opitz et al., 2011). Dioxin and related chemicals with dioxin-like activity may induce a reduction in the ability to clear pathogenic infections and prevent tumor growth in a fashion that is mediated by endogenous pathways. Studies in laboratory mice have shown that the immunotoxicity of TCDD and DLCs depends on activation of the AHR. Most of the cell types involved in the immune system express the AHR, so there are many potential pathways to immunotoxicity. TCDD has also been shown to alter macrophages and neutrophils in a manner that exacerbates some forms of inflammation during infections and may contribute to the development of chronic inflammatory lung disease (Teske et al., 2005; Wong et al., 2010). Other recent work shows that the AHR is involved in hematopoiesis at multiple stages (Baba et al., 2012; Sibilano et al., 2012; Simones and Shepherd, 2011; Singh et al., 2011). Working with human B cells in vitro, Allan and Sherr (2010) demonstrated a new AHR-dependent mechanism by which exposure to environmental polycyclic aromatic hydrocarbons could suppress humoral immunity by blocking differentiation of B cells into plasma cells.

TCDD is a potent immunosuppressive chemical in laboratory animals. The relative potencies of given DLCs based on induction hepatic enzymes—their toxicity equivalence factors (TEFs)—appear to predict the degree of immunosuppression induced (Smialowicz et al., 2008). TCDD has also been shown to induce apoptosis in rabbit chondrocytes, and this supports a potential role of TCDD in contributing in a novel way to arthritis (Yang and Lee, 2010). Exposure of animals to dioxin not only suppresses some adaptive immune responses but also has been shown to increase the incidence and severity of various infectious diseases and to increase the development of cancer (Choi et al., 2003; Elizondo et al., 2011;

Fiorito et al., 2010, 2011; Head and Lawrence, 2009; Jin et al., 2010; Sanchez et al., 2010). It is consistent with its immunosuppressive effects that TCDD exposure suppresses the allergic immune response of rodents; this in turn results in decreased allergen-associated pathologic lung conditions and has recently been shown to suppress the development of experimental autoimmune disease (Quintana et al., 2008), to induce the suppression of autoimmune uveoretinitis (Zhang et al., 2010), and to affect colitis (Takamura et al., 2011), arthritis (Nakahama et al., 2011), and inflammatory lung diseases, such as silicosis (Beamer et al., 2012). A recent study of 18 people who had allergic asthma, 17 people whose asthma was controlled, and 12 controls showed that the plasma concentrations of IL-22 and the expression of the AHR in peripheral blood mononuclear cells was associated with the severity of allergic asthma; this finding strengthened the possibility that the AHR is involved in allergic asthma, thereby implying a role for dioxin exposure in this condition (Zhu et al., 2011). Thus, depending on the disease, TCDD exposure could exacerbate or ameliorate symptoms.

Recent attention has focused on the ability of the AHR to induce regulatory T cells, or Tregs (Kerkvliet, 2012; Marshall and Kerkvliet, 2010). Tregs have potent suppressive activity in the immune system, and their inappropriate induction by TCDD could account for much of the immune suppression. AHR activation in dendritic cells has also been shown to promote the development of Tregs by inducing tryptophan metabolism. AHR activation in B cells can directly disrupt the production of antibodies (Sulentic and Kaminski, 2011). The recent demonstration that AHR activation by TCDD leads to the development of Tregs helps to explain the diversity of effects seen after exposure to TCDD (Funatake et al., 2008; Kerkvliet, 2012; Marshall et al., 2008; Quintana et al., 2008; Stockinger et al., 2011; Yamamoto and Shlomchik, 2010).

Recent data indicate that the AHR pathway plays an integral role in B-cell maturation, and that TCDD and DLC exposure may alter the function of these cells and result in critical changes in the immune response. Suppression of the immune response by TCDD and similar compounds in mice has been known for over 30 years, but the effect on human cells is less clear. Some recent reports indicate that TCDD and DLC elicit similar effects in humans. Activation of non-transformed human B cells results in an increase in expression of the AHR, indicating that this pathway has a role in normal B-cell function (Allan and Sherr, 2010). Furthermore, treatment of those cells with B[a]P suppresses B-cell differentiation. Lu et al. (2010) demonstrated that although human B cells appeared less responsive to TCDD in increasing expression of AHR battery genes, the ability of TCDD to decrease IgM production was similar in both mouse and human B cells. In addition, data from human hemopoietic stem cells (HSCs) and knockout AHR mouse models show that the AHR is critical in HSC maturation and differentiation (Fracchiolla et al., 2011; Singh et al., 2011). TCDD not only alters HSC maturation but also alters proliferation and migration in vivo and in vitro (Casado et al., 2011), and this indicates that exposure may have multiple effects on immune-cell function.

SYNTHESIS

Immune Suppression

One would expect exposure to substantial doses of TCDD to result in immune suppression in Vietnam veterans. However, several studies of various measures of human immune function failed to reveal consistent correlations with TCDD exposure, probably because the exposures were inadequate to produce immune suppression or because the characteristics measured were not among those most relevant with respect to biologic plausibility. No clear pattern of an increase in infectious disease has been documented in the studies of veterans exposed to TCDD or to the herbicides used in Vietnam. However, three occupational-exposure studies provide some support for the idea that exposure to TCDD may result in an altered immune response to some exposures and an increased frequency of infections. The study of a single highly exposed person (Brembilla et al., 2011) confirmed TCDD-associated changes in immune measures that may not be applicable to people whose exposure was considerably lower. Immune alteration and the frequency and duration of specific types of infections should therefore be a focus of future studies. Suppression of the immune response by TCDD might increase the risk of some kinds of cancer in Vietnam veterans, but there is no evidence to support the connection.

Allergic and Autoimmune Diseases

Epidemiologic studies have been inconsistent with regard to TCDD's influence on IgE production in humans. No human studies have specifically addressed the influence of TCDD on autoimmune disease, but several animal studies have shown that TCDD suppresses the development of autoimmune diseases. In studying postservice mortality, Boehmer et al. (2004) found no increase in deaths of Vietnam veterans that could be attributed to immune-system disorders. There is no experimental evidence to support that finding, but increased inflammatory responses could be involved. The study of people who had allergic asthma or controlled asthma strengthened the data and suggested that the AHR (and thus dioxin exposure) is involved in the disease (Zhu et al., 2011). Future studies are needed to determine a potential mechanism of TCDD-induced allergic and autoimmune disease, including rheumatoid arthritis.

Few effects of phenoxy herbicide or cacodylic acid exposure on the immune system have been reported in animals or humans, and no clear association between such exposure and autoimmune or allergic disease has been found.

Exposure of laboratory animals to phenoxy herbicides or cacodylic acid has not been associated with immunotoxicity.

Inflammatory Diseases

There are no human data on the potential for dioxin or the herbicides of interest to induce dysregulation of inflammation that could contribute to an increased risk of inflammation-associated diseases.

Possible associations involving infectious or inflammation-related diseases should be a focus for the future. Examples of earlier studies whose results support the occurrence of such adverse outcomes are Baccarelli et al. (2002), Baranska et al. (2008), Beseler et al. (2008), Oh et al. (2005), O'Toole et al. (2009), Tonn et al. (1996), and Visintainer et al. (1995).

CONCLUSIONS

On the basis of the evidence reviewed here and in previous VAO reports, the present committee concludes that there is inadequate or insufficient evidence to determine whether there is an association between exposure to the COIs and specific infectious, allergic, or autoimmune diseases.

TRANSLATION BETWEEN ANIMAL AND HUMAN STUDIES

Animal studies and in vitro studies with human cells and cell lines are important ways of trying to understand underlying biologic mechanisms associated with immunotoxic and other responses to xenobiotics, which are "foreign" substances that do not normally occur in biologic systems. However, as discussed above, despite the vast array of data supporting the immunotoxicity of TCDD in laboratory animals, little evidence from studies of Vietnam veterans or other human populations suggests that TCDD or the herbicides of concern produce immune alterations. Many factors must be considered in examining the relevance of animal and in vitro studies to human disease and disease progression, and they are discussed in Chapter 4. Here, we present the factors that are probably most important in considering differences between the results of laboratory studies and the findings of observational epidemiologic studies.

Magnitude and Timing of Exposure

In general, the TCDD exposures used in animal studies have been orders of magnitude higher than exposures that Vietnam veterans are likely to have received during military service. It is well known that the immune system is highly susceptible to xenobiotic exposure during critical stages of development, such as gestation, and that primary immune responses are easier to alter than are secondary immune responses. In vivo studies show that exposure to antigens may be important, so the timing of antigen exposure relative to TCDD exposure may be an important variable.

Genetic Susceptibilities

Human immune diseases are likely to have complex etiologies and to be under the influence of numerous genes and gene–environment interactions (Dietert et al., 2010). Differences in AHR affinity between species may be a factor in animal-to-human extrapolation. For example, many strains of mice (AHR^b) are known to exhibit greater susceptibility of CYP1A1 induction and immune suppression than are other strains (AHR^d). In contrast, a simple single-haplotype difference in susceptibility to TCDD has not been observed in humans. Rats appear to be more similar to the resistant AHR^d phenotype of mice in their sensitivity to TCDD. Indeed, it is difficult to produce immune suppression in rats with TCDD because of that, and there probably are other genetic reasons as well.

Sex Differences

There are well-known differences in susceptibility to xenobiotic exposures between male and female animals. There are probably multiple reasons for the differences, some of which may pertain to immunomodulation by sex steroids. Similarly, evidence suggests that specific immune-based health risks in humans have important sex differences. For example, women generally are much more susceptible than are men to the development of several autoimmune diseases; such differences in humans may result from a combination of genetic factors and environmental exposures. That has ramifications for future studies. In considering the potential effects of Agent Orange on the immune system and the risk of disease, sex-based differences in chemically induced adverse immune outcomes need to be investigated. Future studies should ensure that—whether in animal models or in human studies—gene-specific or sex-specific immune effects are able to be evaluated with sufficient statistical power to support distinctions.

Stress

Stress is a well-known modifier of human immune responses. It is an ever-present variable that is difficult to assess or control for in epidemiologic studies.

REFERENCES[1]

Allan LL, Sherr DH. 2010. Disruption of human plasma cell differentiation by an environmental polycyclic aromatic hydrocarbon: A mechanistic immunotoxicological study. *Environmental Health* 9:15.

Andrews JS, Stehr-Green PA, Hoffman RE, Needham LL, Patterson DG Jr, Bagby JR Jr, Roberts DW, Webb KB, Evans RG. 1986. *Missouri dioxin studies: Some thoughts on their implications.* Proceedings of the 7th National Conference on Management of Uncontrolled Hazardous Waste Sites. December 1–3, 1986. Washington, DC. 78–83.

Baba N, Rubio M, Kenins L, Regairaz C, Woisetschlager M, Carballido JM, Sarfati M. 2012. The aryl hydrocarbon receptor (AhR) ligand VAF347 selectively acts on monocytes and naive CD4+ Th cells to promote the development of IL-22-secreting Th cells. *Human Immunology* 73(8):795–800.

Baccarelli A, Mocarelli P, Patterson DG Jr, Bonzini M, Pesatori AC, Caporaso N, Landi MT. 2002. Immunologic effects of dioxin: New results from Seveso and comparison with other studies. *Environmental Health Perspectives* 110(12):1169–1173.

Baccarelli A, Pesatori AC, Consonni D, Mocarelli P, Patterson DG Jr, Caporaso NE, Bertazzi PA, Landi MT. 2005b. Health status and plasma dioxin levels in chloracne cases 20 years after the Seveso, Italy accident. *British Journal of Dermatology* 152(3):459–465.

Baranska M, Van Amelsvoort L, Birindelli S, Fustinoni S, Corsini E, Liesivuori J, Van Loveren H. 2008. Association of pesticide exposure, vaccination response, and interleukin-1 gene polymorphisms. *Human and Experimental Toxicology* 27(9):709–713.

Beamer CA, Seaver BP, Shepherd DM. 2012. Aryl hydrocarbon receptor (AhR) regulates silica-induced inflammation but not fibrosis. *Toxicological Sciences* 126(2):554–568.

Benner A, Edler L, Mayer K, Zober A. 1994. 'Dioxin' investigation program of the chemical industry professional association. *Arbeitsmedizin Sozialmedizin Praventivmedizin* 29:11–16.

Beseler C, Stallones L, Hoppin JA, Alavanja MC, Blair A, Keefe T, Kamel F. 2006. Depression and pesticide exposures in female spouses of licensed pesticide applicators in the Agricultural Health Study cohort. *Journal of Occupational and Environmental Medicine* 48(10):1005–1013.

Beseler CL, Stallones L, Hoppin JA, Alavanja MCR, Blair A, Keefe T, Kamel F. 2008. Depression and pesticide exposures among private pesticide applicators enrolled in the Agricultural Health Study. *Environmental Health Perspectives* 116(12):1713–1719.

Boehmer TK, Flanders WD, McGeehin MA, Boyle C, Barrett DH. 2004. Postservice mortality in Vietnam veterans: 30-year follow-up. *Archives of Internal Medicine* 164(17):1908–1916.

Borensztajn KS, von der Thüsen JH, Spek CA. 2011. The role of coagulation in chronic inflammatory disorders: A jack of all trades. *Current Pharmaceutical Design* 17(1):9–16.

Bornschein J, Kandulski A, Selgrad M, Malfertheiner P. 2010. From gastric inflammation to gastric cancer. *Digestive Diseases* 28(4-5):609–614.

Brembilla NC, Ramirez JM, Chicheportiche R, Sorg O, Saurat JH, Chizzolini C. 2011. In vivo dioxin favors interleukin-22 production by human CD4+ T cells in an aryl hydrocarbon receptor (AhR)-dependent manner. *PLoS ONE* 6 (4):e18741.

Casado FL, Singh KP, Gasiewicz TA. 2011. Aryl hydrocarbon receptor activation in hematopoietic stem/progenitor cells alters cell function and pathway-specific gene modulation reflecting changes in cellular trafficking and migration. *Molecular Pharmacology* 80(4):673–682.

CDC (Centers for Disease Control). 1988b. Health status of Vietnam veterans. II. Physical health. *Journal of the American Medical Association* 259:2708–2714.

[1]Throughout this report, the same alphabetic indicator after year of publication is used consistently for a given reference when there are multiple citations by the same first author in a given year. The convention of assigning the alphabetic indicators in order of citation in a given chapter is not followed.

CDC. 2004. Fast Stats A–Z, *Advanced Data from Vital and Health Statistics, no. 346, Table 13*. http://www.cdc.gov/nchs/fastats/allergies.htm (accessed August 26, 2004).

CDVA (Commonwealth Department of Veterans' Affairs). 1997b. *Mortality of National Service Vietnam Veterans: A Report of the 1996 Retrospective Cohort Study of Australian Vietnam Veterans.* Canberra: Department of Veterans' Affairs.

Chinh TT, Phi PT, Thuy NT. 1996. Sperm auto-antibodies and anti-nuclear antigen antibodies in chronic dioxin-exposed veterans. *Chemosphere* 32(3):525–530.

Choi JY, Oughton JA, Kerkvliet NI. 2003. Functional alterations in CD11b(+)Gr-1(+) cells in mice injected with allogeneic tumor cells and treated with 2,3,7,8-tetrachlorodibenzo-*p*-dioxin. *International Journal of Immunopharmacology* 3:553–570.

Cooper GS, Parks CG. 2004. Occupational and environmental exposures as risk factors for systemic lupus erythematosus. *Current Rheumatology Reports* 6(5):367–374.

De Roos AJ, Cooper GS, Alavanja MC, Sandler DP. 2005b. Rheumatoid arthritis among women in the Agricultural Health Study: Risk associated with farming activities and exposures. *Annals of Epidemiology* 15(10):762–770.

Dietert RR, DeWitt JC, Germolec DR, Zelikoff JT. 2010. Breaking patterns of environmentally influenced disease for health risk reduction: Immune perspectives. *Environmental Health Perspectives* 118(8):1091–1099.

Eisen S, Goldberg J, True WR, Henderson WG. 1991. A co-twin control study of the effects of the Vietnam War on the self-reported physical health of veterans. *American Journal of Epidemiology* 134:49–58.

Elizondo G, Rodriguez-Sosa M, Estrada-Muniz E, Gonzalez FJ, Vega L. 2011. Deletion of the aryl hydrocarbon receptor enhances the inflammatory response to leishmania major infection. *International Journal of Biological Sciences* 7(9):1220–1229.

Endres SM, Green BJ, Henneberger PK, Germolec DR, Bledsoe TA, Beezhold DH, London SJ, Alavanja MC, Beane Freeman LE, Hoppin JA. 2012. Fungal and atopic sensitization are low among farmers in the Agricultural Health Study. *Journal of Allergy and Clinical Immunology* 130(1):267–270.

Ernst M, Flesch-Janys D, Morgenstern I, Manz A. 1998. Immunological findings in former industrial workers after high exposure to dioxins at the workplace. *Arbeitsmedizin Sozialmedizin Umweltmedizin* (Suppl 24):14–47.

Evans RG, Webb KB, Knutsen AP, Roodman ST, Roberts DW, Bagby JR, Garrett WA Jr, Andrews JS Jr. 1988. A medical follow-up of the health effects of long-term exposure to 2,3,7,8-tetrachlorodibenzo-*p*-dioxin. *Archives of Environmental Health* 43:273–278.

Fairweather D, Frisancho-Kiss S, Rose NR. 2008. Sex differences in autoimmune disease from a pathological perspective. *American Journal of Pathology* 173(3):600–609.

Faustini A, Settimi L, Pacifici R, Fano V, Zuccaro P, Forastiere F. 1996. Immunological changes among farmers exposed to phenoxy herbicides: Preliminary observations. *Occupational and Environmental Medicine* 53(9):583–585.

Fiorito F, Marfè G, Granato GE, Ciarcia R, De Blasio E, Tafani M, Florio S, De Martino L, Muzi G, Pagnini U, Giordano A. 2010. 2,3,7,8-Tetrachlorodibenzo-*p*-dioxin modifies expression and nuclear/cytosolic localization of bovine herpesvirus 1 immediate-early protein (bICP0) during infection. *Journal of Cellular Biochemistry* 111(2):333–342.

Fiorito F, Ciarcia R, Granato GE, Marfe G, Iovane V, Florio S, De Martino L, Pagnini U. 2011. 2,3,7,8-tetrachlorodibenzo-*p*-dioxin induced autophagy in a bovine kidney cell line. *Toxicology* 290(2-3):259–271.

Fracchiolla NS, Todoerti K, Bertazzi PA, Servida F, Corradini P, Carniti C, Colombi A, Cecilia Pesatori A, Neri A, Deliliers GL. 2011. Dioxin exposure of human CD34+ hemopoietic cells induces gene expression modulation that recapitulates its in vivo clinical and biological effects. *Toxicology* 283(1):18–23.

Funatake CJ, Marshall NB, Kerkvliet NI. 2008. 2,3,7,8-Tetrachlorodibenzo-*p*-dioxin alters the differentiation of alloreactive CD8+ T cells toward a regulatory T cell phenotype by a mechanism that is dependent on aryl hydrocarbon receptor in CD4+ T cells. *Journal of Immunotoxicology* 5(1):81–91.

Ghezzi I, Cannatelli P, Assennato G, Merlo F, Mocarelli P, Brambilla P, Sicurello F. 1982. Potential 2,3,7,8-tetrachlorodibenzo-*p*-dioxin exposure of Seveso decontamination workers. A controlled prospective study. *Scandinavian Journal of Work, Environment, and Health* 8:176–179.

Halperin W, Vogt R, Sweeney MH, Shopp G, Fingerhut M, Petersen M. 1998. Immunological markers among workers exposed to 2,3,7,8-tetrachlorodibenzo-*p*-dioxin. *Occupational and Environmental Medicine* 55(11):742–749.

Hardell L, Moss A, Osmond D, Volberding P. 1987. Exposure to hair dyes and polychlorinated dibenzo-*p*-dioxins in AIDS patients with Kaposi sarcoma: An epidemiological investigation. *Cancer Detection and Prevention* (Suppl 1):567–570.

Head JL, Lawrence BP. 2009. The aryl hydrocarbon receptor is a modulator of anti-viral immunity. *Biochemical Pharmacology* 77:642–653.

Hillegass JM, Shukla A, Lathrop SA, MacPherson MB, Beuschel SL, Butnor KJ, Testa JR, Pass HI, Carbone M, Steele C, Mossman BT. 2010. Inflammation precedes the development of human malignant mesotheliomas in a SCID mouse xenograft model. *Annals of the New York Academy of Sciences* 1203:7–14.

Hoffman RE, Stehr-Green PA, Webb KB, Evans RG, Knutsen AP, Schramm WF, Staake JL, Gibson BB, Steinberg KK. 1986. Health effects of long-term exposure to 2,3,7,8-tetrachlorodibenzo-*p*-dioxin. *Journal of the American Medical Association* 255:2031–2038.

IOM (Institute of Medicine). 1994. *Veterans and Agent Orange: Health Effects of Herbicides Used in Vietnam.* Washington, DC: National Academy Press.

IOM. 1996. *Veterans and Agent Orange: Update 1996.* Washington, DC: National Academy Press.

IOM. 1999. *Veterans and Agent Orange: Update 1998.* Washington, DC: National Academy Press.

IOM. 2001. *Veterans and Agent Orange: Update 2000.* Washington, DC: National Academy Press.

IOM. 2003. *Veterans and Agent Orange: Update 2002.* Washington, DC: The National Academies Press.

IOM. 2005. *Veterans and Agent Orange: Update 2004.* Washington, DC: The National Academies Press.

IOM. 2007. *Veterans and Agent Orange: Update 2006.* Washington, DC: The National Academies Press.

IOM. 2009. *Veterans and Agent Orange: Update 2008.* Washington, DC: The National Academies Press.

IOM. 2012. *Veterans and Agent Orange: Update 2010.* Washington, DC: The National Academies Press.

Jansing PJ, Korff R. 1994. Blood levels of 2,3,7,8-tetrachlorodibenzo-*p*-dioxin and gamma-globulins in a follow-up investigation of employees with chloracne. *Journal of Dermatological Science* 8:91–95.

Jennings AM, Wild G, Ward JD, Ward AM. 1988. Immunological abnormalities 17 years after accidental exposure to 2,3,7,8-tetrachlorodibenzo-*p*-dioxin. *British Journal of Industrial Medicine* 45:701–704.

Ji J, Shu X, Sundquist K, Sundquist J, Hemminki K. 2009. Cancer risk in hospitalised psoriasis patients: A follow-up study in Sweden. *British Journal of Cancer* 100(9):1499–1502.

Jin MH, Hong CH, Lee HY, Kang HJ, Han SW. 2010. Toxic effects of lactational exposure to 2,3,7,8-tetrachlorodibenzo-*p*-dioxin (TCDD) on developments of male reproductive system: Involvement of antioxidants, oxidants, and p53 protein. *Environmental Toxicology* 25(1):1–8.

Jung D, Berg PA, Edler L, Ehrenthal W, Fenner D, Flesch-Janys D, Huber C, Klein R, Koitka C, Lucier G, Manz A, Muttray A, Needham L, Päpke O, Pietsch M, Portier C, Patterson D, Prellwitz W, Rose DM, Thews A, Konietzko J. 1998. Immunologic findings in workers formerly exposed to 2,3,7,8-tetrachlorodibenzo-*p*-dioxin and its congeners. *Environmental Health Perspectives* 106(Suppl 2):689–695.

Jusko TA, De Roos AJ, Schwartz SM, Lawrence BP, Palkovicova L, Nemessanyi T, Drobna B, Fabisikova A, Kocan A, Jahnova E, Kavanagh TJ, Trnovec T, Hertz-Picciotto I. 2011. Maternal and early postnatal polychlorinated biphenyl exposure in relation to total serum immunoglobulin concentrations in 6-month-old infants. *Journal of Immunotoxicology* 8(1):95–100.

Kahn PC, Gochfeld M, Lewis WW. 1992. *Immune Status and Herbicide Exposure in the New Jersey Pointman I Project.* New Jersey Agent Orange Commission.

Kerkvliet NI. 2009. AHR-mediated immunomodulation: The role of altered gene transcription. *Biochemical Pharmacology* 77:746–760.

Kerkvliet NI. 2012. TCDD: An environmental immunotoxicant reveals a novel pathway of immunoregulation—A 30-year odyssey. *Toxicologic Pathology* 40(2):138–142.

Kim HA, Kim EM, Park YC, Yu JY, Hong SK, Jeon SH, Park KL, Hur SJ, Heo Y. 2003. Immunotoxicological effects of Agent Orange exposure to the Vietnam War Korean veterans. *Industrial Health* 41(3):158–166.

Knutsen AP. 1984. Immunologic effects of TCDD exposure in humans. *Bulletin of Environmental Contamination and Toxicology* 33:673–681.

Knutsen AP, Roodman ST, Evans RG, Mueller KR, Webb KB, Stehr-Green P, Hoffman RE, Schramm WF. 1987. Immune studies in TCDD-exposed Missouri residents: Quail Run. *Bulletin of Environmental Contamination and Toxicology* 39:481–489.

Landgren AM, Landgren O, Gridley G, Dores GM, Linet MS, Morton LM. 2010. Autoimmune disease and subsequent risk of developing alimentary tract cancers among 4.5 million US male veterans. *Cancer* 117(6):1163–1171.

Lee DH, Steffes M, Jacobs DR Jr. 2007a. Positive associations of serum concentration of polychlorinated biphenyls or organochlorine pesticides with self-reported arthritis, especially rheumatoid type, in women. *Environmental Health Perspectives* 115(6):883–888.

Linneberg A, Jørgensen T, Nielsen NH, Madsen F, Frølund L, Dirksen A. 2000. The prevalence of skin-test-positive allergic rhinitis in Danish adults: Two cross-sectional surveys 8 years apart. The Copenhagen Allergy Study. *Allergy* 55(8):767–772.

Lovik M, Johansen HR, Gaarder PI, Becher G, Aaberge IS, Gdynia W, Alexander J. 1996. Halogenated organic compounds and the human immune system: Preliminary report on a study in hobby fishermen. *Archives of Toxicology* (Suppl 18):15–20.

Lu H, Crawford RB, Suarez-Martinez JE, Kaplan BLF, Kaminski NE. 2010. Induction of the aryl hydrocarbon receptor-responsive genes and modulation of the immunoglobulin M response by 2,3,7,8-tetrachlorodibenzo-*p*-dioxin in primary human B cells. *Toxicological Sciences* 118(1):86–97.

Lucas DR, Shukla A, Thomas DG, Patel RM, Kubat AJ, McHugh JB. 2010. Dedifferentiated liposarcoma with inflammatory myofibroblastic tumor-like features. *American Journal of Surgical Pathology* 34(6):844–851.

Marshall N, Kerkvliet N. 2010. Dioxin and immune regulation: Emerging role of aryl hydrocarbon receptor in the generation of regulatory T cells. *Annals of the New York Academy of Sciences* 1183:25–37.

Marshall N, Vorachek W, Steppan L, Mourich D, Kerkvliet N. 2008. Functional characterization and gene expression analysis of CD4+ CD25+ regulatory T cells generated in mice treated with 2,3,7,8-tetrachlorodibenzo-*p*-dioxin. *Journal of Immunology* 181(4):2382–2391.

Michalek JE, Ketchum NS, Check IL. 1999a. Serum dioxin and immunologic response in veterans of Operation Ranch Hand. *American Journal of Epidemiology* 149:1038–1046.

Miyashita C, Sasaki S, Saijo Y, Washino N, Okada E, Kobayashi S, Konishi K, Kajiwara J, Todaka T, Kishi R. 2011. Effects of prenatal exposure to dioxin-like compounds on allergies and infections during infancy. *Environmental Research* 111(4):551–558.

Nakahama T, Kimura A, Trung Nguyen N, Chinen I, Hanieh H, Nohara K, Fujii-Kuriyama Y, Kishimoto T. 2011. Aryl hydrocarbon receptor deficiency in T cells suppresses the development of collagen-induced arthritis. *Proceedings of the National Academy of Sciences of the United States of America* 108(34):14222–14227.

Neubert R, Maskow L, Webb J, Jacob-Muller U, Nogueira AC, Delgado I, Helge H, Neubert D. 1993. Chlorinated dibenzo-*p*-dioxins and dibenzofurans and the human immune system. 1. Blood cell receptors in volunteers with moderately increased body burdens. *Life Sciences* 53:1995–2006.

Neubert R, Golor G, Helge H, Neubert D. 1994. Risk assessment for possible effects of 2,3,7,8-tetrachlorodibenzo-*p*-dioxin (TCDD) and related substances on components and functions of the immune system. *Experimental and Clinical Immunogenetics* 11(2-3):163–171.

Neubert R, Maskow L, Triebig G, Broding HC, Jacob-Muller U, Helge H, Neubert D. 2000. Chlorinated dibenzo-*p*-dioxins and dibenzofurans and the human immune system: 3. Plasma immunoglobulins and cytokines of workers with quantified moderately-increased body burdens. *Life Sciences* 66(22):2123–2142.

Newell GR. 1984. *Development and Preliminary Results of Pilot Clinical Studies.* Report of the Agent Orange Advisory Committee to the Texas Department of Health. University of Texas System Cancer Center.

NIH Autoimmune Diseases Coordinating Committee. 2005 (March). *Autoimmune Diseases Research Plan.*

Oh E, Lee E, Im H, Kang HS, Jung WW, Won NH, Kim EM, Sul D. 2005. Evaluation of immuno- and reproductive toxicities and association between immunotoxicological and genotoxicological parameters in waste incineration workers. *Toxicology* 210(1):65–80.

Opitz CA, Litzenburger UM, Sahm F, Ott M, Tritschler I, Trump S, Schumacher T, Jestaedt L, Schrenk D, Weller M, Jugold M, Guillemin GJ, Miller CL, Lutz C, Radlwimmer B, Lehmann I, von Deimling A, Wick W, Platten M. 2011. Anendogenous tumour-promoting ligand of the human aryl hydrocarbon receptor. *Nature* 478:197–203.

O'Toole BI, Catts SV, Outram S, Pierse KR, Cockburn J. 2009. The physical and mental health of Australian Vietnam veterans 3 decades after the war and its relation to military service, combat, and post-traumatic stress disorder. *American Journal of Epidemiology* 170(3):318–330.

Ott MG, Zober A, Germann C. 1994. Laboratory results for selected target organs in 138 individuals occupationally exposed to TCDD. *Chemosphere* 29:2423–2437.

Parks CG, Cooper GS. 2005. Occupational exposures and risk of systemic lupus erythematosus. *Autoimmunity* 38(7):497–506.

Pocchiari F, Silano V, Zampieri A. 1979. Human health effects from accidental release of tetrachlorodibenzo-*p*-dioxin (TCDD) at Seveso, Italy. *Annals of the New York Academy of Sciences* 320:311–320.

Porta C, Riboldi E, Sica A. 2010. Mechanisms linking pathogens-associated inflammation and cancer. *Cancer Letters*, Nov 17. [Epub ahead of print]

Quintana FJ, Basso AS, Iglesias AH, Korn T, Farez MF, Bettelli E, Caccamo M, Oukka M, Weiner HL. 2008. Control of T_{reg} and T_H17 cell differentiation by the aryl hydrocarbon receptor. *Nature* 453:65–72.

Saberi Hosnijeh F, Boers D, Portengen L, Bueno de Mesquita HB, Heederik D, Vermeulen R. 2011. Long-term effects on humoral immunity among workers exposed to 2,3,7,8-tetrachlorodibenzo-*p*-dioxin (TCDD). *Occupational and Environmental Medicine* 68(6):419–424.

Saberi Hosnijeh F, Boers D, Portengen L, Bueno de Mesquita HB, Heederik D, Vermeulen R. 2012. Plasma cytokine concentrations in workers exposed to 2,3,7,8-tetrachlorodibenzo-*p*-dioxin (TCDD). *Frontiers in Oncology* 2:37.

Sanchez Y, De Dios Rosado J, Vega L, Elizondo G, Estrada-Muniz E, Saavedra R, Juarez I, Rodriguez-Sosa M. 2010. The unexpected role for the aryl hydrocarbon receptor on susceptibility to experimental toxoplasmosis. *Journal of Biomedicine and Biotechnology* (article ID 303694, 15 pp).

Sandhu JS. 2008. Prostate cancer and chronic prostatitis. *Current Urology Reports* 9(4):328–332.

Sibilano R, Frossi B, Calvaruso M, Danelli L, Betto E, Dall'Agnese A, Tripodo C, Colombo MP, Pucillo CE, Gri G. 2012. The aryl hydrocarbon receptor modulates acute and late mast cell responses. *Journal of Immunology* 189(1):120–127.

Simones T, Shepherd DM. 2011. Consequences of AhR activation in steady-state dendritic cells. *Toxicological Sciences* 119 (2):293–307.

Simpson CR, Newton J, Hippisley-Cox J, Sheikh A. 2008. Incidence and prevalence of multiple allergic disorders recorded in a national primary care database. *Journal of the Royal Society of Medicine* 101:558–563.

Singh NP, Singh UP, Singh B, Price RL, Nagarkatti M, Nagarkatti PS. 2011. Activation of aryl hydrocarbon receptor (AhR) leads to reciprocal epigenetic regulation of FoxP3 and IL-17 expression and amelioration of experimental colitis. *PLoS ONE* 6 (8):e23522-e23535.

Sly RM. 1999. Changing prevalence of allergic rhinitis and asthma. *Annals of Allergy and Asthma Immunology* 82:233–248.

Smialowicz RJ, DeVito MJ, Williams WC, Birnbaum LS. 2008. Relative potency based on hepatic enzyme induction predicts immunosuppressive effects of a mixture of PCDDs/PCDFs and PCBs. *Toxicology and Applied Pharmacology* 227(3):477–484.

Stehr P, Stein G, Webb K, Schramm W, Gedney WB, Donnell HD, Ayres S, Falk H, Sampson E, Smith SJ. 1986. A pilot epidemiologic study of possible health effects associated with 2,3,7,8-tetrachlorodibenzo-*p*-dioxin contaminations in Missouri. *Archives of Environmental Health* 41:16–22.

Stehr-Green P, Hoffman R, Webb K, Evans RG, Knutsen A, Schramm W, Staake J, Gibson B, Steinberg K. 1987. Health effects of long-term exposure to 2,3,7,8-tetrachlorodibenzo-*p*-dioxin. *Chemosphere* 16:2089–2094.

Stellman SD, Stellman JM, Sommer JF Jr. 1988. Health and reproductive outcomes among American Legionnaires in relation to combat and herbicide exposure in Vietnam. *Environmental Research* 47:150–174.

Stockinger B, Hirota K, Duarte J, Veldhoen M. 2011. External influences on the immune system via activation of the aryl hydrocarbon receptor. *Seminars in Immunology* 23(2):99–105.

Sulentic CE, Kaminski NE. 2011. The long winding road toward understanding the molecular mechanisms for B-cell suppression by 2,3,7,8-tetrachlorodibenzo-*p*-dioxin. *Toxicological Science* 120(Suppl 1):S171–S191.

Svensson BG, Hallberg T, Nilsson A, Schutz A, Hagmar L. 1994. Parameters of immunological competence in subjects with high consumption of fish contaminated with persistent organochlorine compounds. *International Archives of Occupational and Environmental Health* 65:351–358.

Sweeney MH, Calvert GM, Egeland GA, Fingerhut MA, Halperin WE, Piacitelli LA. 1997/1998. Review and update of the results of the NIOSH medical study of workers exposed to chemicals contaminated with 2,3,7,8-tetrachlorodibenzodioxin. *Teratogenesis, Carcinogenesis, and Mutagenesis* 17(4-5):241–247.

Takamura T, Harama D, Fukumoto S, Nakamura Y, Shimokawa N, Ishimaru K, Ikegami S, Makino S, Kitamura M, Nakao A. 2011. *Lactobacillus bulgaricus* OLL1181 activates the aryl hydrocarbon receptor pathway and inhibits colitis. *Immunology and Cell Biology* 89(7):817–822.

Teske S, Bohn AA, Regal JF, Neumiller JJ, Lawrence BP. 2005. Activation of the aryl hydrocarbon receptor increases pulmonary neutrophilia and diminishes host resistance to influenza A virus. *American Journal of Physiology–Lung Cellular and Molecular Physiology* 289(1):L111–L124.

Tonn T, Esser C, Schneider EM, Steinmann-Steiner-Haldenstatt W, Gleichmann E. 1996. Persistence of decreased T-helper cell function in industrial workers 20 years after exposure to 2,3,7,8-tetrachlorodibenzo-*p*-dioxin. *Environmental Health Perspectives* 104(4):422–426.

Van den Heuvel RL, Koppen G, Staessen JA, Hond ED, Verheyen G, Nawrot TS, Roels HA, Vlietinck R, Schoeters GE. 2002. Immunologic biomarkers in relation to exposure markers of PCBs and dioxins in Flemish adolescents (Belgium). *Environmental Health Perspectives* 110(6):595–600.

Viennot S, Deleporte A, Moussata D, Nancey S, Flourié B, Reimund JM. 2009. Colon cancer in inflammatory bowel disease: Recent trends, questions and answers. *Gastroenterology and Clinical Biology* 33(Suppl 3):S190–S201.

Visintainer PF, Barone M, McGee H, Peterson EL. 1995. Proportionate mortality study of Vietnam-era veterans of Michigan. *Journal of Occupational and Environmental Medicine* 37(4):423–428.

Wang W, Bergh A, Damber JE. 2009. Morphological transition of proliferative inflammatory atrophy to high-grade intraepithelial neoplasia and cancer in human prostate. *Prostate* 69(13):1378–1386.

Webb K, Evans RG, Stehr P, Ayres SM. 1987. Pilot study on health effects of environmental 2,3,7,8-TCDD in Missouri. *American Journal of Industrial Medicine* 11:685–691.

Webb KZ, Evans RG, Knutsen AP, Roodman ST, Roberts DW, Schramm WF, Gibson BB, Andrews JS Jr, Needham LL, Patterson DG. 1989. Medical evaluation of subjects with known body levels of 2,3,7,8-tetrachlorodibenzo-*p*-dioxin. *Journal of Toxicology and Environmental Health* 28:183–193.

Westbrook AM, Szakmary A, Schiestl RH. 2010. Mechanisms of intestinal inflammation and development of associated cancers: Lessons learned from mouse models. *Mutation Research* 705(1):40–59.

Winans B, Humble MC, Lawrence BP. 2010. Environmental toxicants and the developing immune system: A missing link in the global battle against infectious disease? *Reproductive Toxicology* 31(3):327–336.

Wolf N, Karmaus W. 1995. Effects of inhalative exposure to dioxins in wood preservatives on cell-mediated immunity in day-care center teachers. *Environmental Research* 68(2):96–105.

Wolfe WH, Lathrop GD, Albanese RA, Moynahan PM. 1985. An epidemiologic investigation of health effects in Air Force personnel following exposure to herbicides and associated dioxins. *Chemosphere* 14:707–716.

Wolfe WH, Michalek JE, Miner JC, Rahe A, Silva J, Thomas WF, Grubbs WD, Lustik MB, Karrison TG, Roegner RH, Williams DE. 1990. Health status of Air Force veterans occupationally exposed to herbicides in Vietnam. I. Physical health. *Journal of the American Medical Association* 264(14):1824–1831.

Wong PS, Vogel CF, Kokosinski K, Matsumura F. 2010. Arylhydrocarbon receptor activation in NCI-H441 cells and C57BL/6 mice: Possible mechanisms for lung dysfunction. *American Journal of Respiratory Cell and Molecular Biology* 42(2):210–217.

Yang JH, Lee HG. 2010. 2,3,7,8-Tetrachlorodibenzo-*p*-dioxin induces apoptosis of articular chondrocytes in culture. *Chemosphere* 79(3):278–284.

Yamamoto K, Shlomchik M. 2010. Autoimmunity. *Current Opinion in Immunology* 22(6):695–697.

Zhu J, Cao Y, Li K, Wang Z, Zuo P, Xiong W, Xu Y, Xiong S. 2011. Increased expression of aryl hydrocarbon receptor and interleukin 22 in patients with allergic asthma. *Asian Pacific Journal of Allergy and Immunology* 29(3):266–272.

Zhang L, Ma J, Takeuchi M, Usui Y, Hattori T, Okunuki Y, Yamakawa N, Kezuka T, Kuroda M, Goto H. 2010. Suppression of experimental autoimmune uveoretinitis by inducing differentiation of regulatory T cells via activation of aryl hydrocarbon receptor. *Investigations in Ophthalmology and Visual Science* 51(4):2109–2117.

8

Cancer

Chapter Overview

Based on new evidence and a review of prior studies, the committee for did not find any new significant associations between the relevant exposures and particular types of cancer. Current evidence supports the findings of earlier studies that

- *There is sufficient evidence of an association with the chemicals of interest and soft tissue sarcomas and B-cell lymphomas (Hodgkin lymphoma, non-Hodgkin lymphoma, chronic lymphocytic leukemia, hairy cell leukemia).*
- *There is limited or suggestive evidence of an association between the chemicals of interest and laryngeal cancer; cancer of the lung, bronchus, or trachea; prostate cancer; multiple myeloma, and AL amyloidosis.*
- *There is inadequate or insufficient evidence to determine whether there is an association between the chemicals of interest and any other specific type of cancer.*

Cancer is the second-leading cause of death in the United States. Among men 55–69 years old, the group that includes most Vietnam veterans (see Table 8-1), however, the risk of dying from cancer exceeds the risk of dying from heart disease, the leading cause of death in the United States, and does not fall to second place until after the age of 75 years (Heron et al., 2009). About 577,000 Americans of all ages were expected to die from cancer in 2010—more than 1,500 per day. In the United States, one-fourth of all deaths are from cancer (Siegel et al., 2012).

This chapter summarizes and presents conclusions about the strength of the

TABLE 8-1 Age Distribution of Vietnam-Era and Vietnam-Theater Male Veterans, 2009–2010 (Numbers in Thousands)

Age Group (Years)	Vietnam Era n	Vietnam Era (%)	Vietnam Theater n	Vietnam Theater (%)
All ages	7,805		3,816	
≤ 54	133	(1.8)	32	(0.9)
55–59	1,109	(15.1)	369	(10.4)
60–64	3,031	(41.3)	1,676	(47.0)
65–69	2,301	(31.3)	1,090	(30.6)
70–74	675	(9.2)	280	(7.9)
75–84	511	(6.9)	322	(9.0)
≥ 85	178	(2.4)	83	(2.4)

SOURCE: IOM, 1994, Table 3-3, updated by 20 years.

evidence from epidemiologic studies regarding associations between exposure to the chemicals of interest (COIs)—2,4-dichlorophenoxyacetic acid (2,4-D), 2,4,5-trichlorophenoxyacetic acid (2,4,5-T) and its contaminant 2,3,7,8-tetrachlorodibenzo-*p*-dioxin (TCDD), picloram, and cacodylic acid—and various types of cancer. The committee also considers studies of exposure to polychlorinated biphenyls (PCBs) and other dioxin-like chemicals (DLCs) informative if their results were reported in terms of TCDD toxic equivalents (TEQs) or concentrations of specific congeners of DLCs. However, studies that report TEQs based only on mono-ortho PCBs (which are PCBs 105, 114, 118, 123, 156, 157, 167, and 189) were given very limited consideration since mono-ortho PCBs typically contribute less than 10% to total TEQs, based on the WHO revised TEFs of 2005 (La Rocca et al., 2008; Van den Berg et al., 2006). If a new study reported on only a single type of cancer and did not revisit a previously studied population, its design information is summarized here with its results; design information on all other new studies can be found in Chapter 6.

The objective of this chapter is assessment of whether the occurrence of various cancers in Vietnam veterans themselves may be associated with exposure they may have received during military service. Therefore, studies of childhood cancers in relation to parental exposure to the COIs are discussed in Chapter 10, which addresses possible adverse effects in the veterans' offspring. Studies that consider only childhood exposure are not considered relevant to the committee's charge.

In an evaluation of a possible connection between herbicide exposure and risk of cancer, the approach used to assess the exposure of study subjects is of critical importance in determining the overall relevance and usefulness of findings. As noted in Chapters 3 and 6, there is great variety in detail and accuracy of exposure assessment among studies. A few studies used biologic markers of exposure, such as the presence of a chemical in serum or tissues; some developed an index of exposure from employment or activity records; and some used other surrogate measures of exposure, such as presence in a locale when herbicides were used. As noted in Chapter 2, inaccurate assessment of exposure, a form of measurement error, can obscure the relationship between exposure and disease.

Each section on a type of cancer opens with background information, including data on its incidence in the general US population and known or suspected risk factors. Cancer-incidence data on the general US population are included in the background material to provide a context for consideration of cancer risk in Vietnam veterans; the figures presented are estimates of incidence in the entire US population, not predictions for the Vietnam-veteran cohort. The data reported are for 2004–2008 and are from the most recent dataset available (NCI, 2010). Incidence data are given for all races combined and separately for blacks and whites. The age range of 55–69 years now includes about 80% of Vietnam-era veterans, and incidences are presented for three 5-year age groups: 55–59 years, 60–64 years, and 65–69 years. The data were collected for the Surveillance, Epidemiology, and End Results (SEER) program of the National Cancer Institute and are categorized by sex, age, and race, all of which can have profound effects on risk. For example, the incidence of prostate cancer is about 2.6 times as high in men who are 65–69 years old as in men 55–59 years old and almost twice as high in blacks 55–64 years old as in whites in the same age group (NCI, 2010). Many other factors can influence cancer incidence, including screening methods, tobacco and alcohol use, diet, genetic predisposition, and medical history. Those factors can make someone more or less likely than the average to contract a given kind of cancer; they also need to be taken into account in epidemiologic studies of the possible contributions of the COIs.

Each section of this chapter pertaining to a specific type of cancer includes a summary of the findings described in the previous Agent Orange reports: *Veterans and Agent Orange: Health Effects of Herbicides Used in Vietnam*, hereafter referred to as *VAO* (IOM, 1994); *Veterans and Agent Orange: Update 1996*, referred to as *Update 1996* (IOM, 1996); *Update 1998* (IOM, 1999); *Update 2000* (IOM, 2001); *Update 2002* (IOM, 2003); *Update 2004* (IOM, 2005); *Update 2006* (IOM, 2007); *Update 2008* (IOM, 2009); and *Update 2010* (IOM, 2011). That is followed by a discussion of the most recent scientific literature, a discussion of biologic plausibility, and a synthesis of the material reviewed. When it is appropriate, the literature is discussed by exposure type (service in Vietnam, occupational exposure, or environmental exposure). Each section ends with the committee's conclusion regarding the strength of the evidence from epidemiologic studies. The categories of association and the committee's approach to categorizing the health outcomes are discussed in Chapters 1 and 2.

Biologic plausibility corresponds to the third element of the committee's congressionally mandated statement of task. In fact, the degree of biologic plausibility itself influences whether the committee perceives positive findings to be indicative of an association or the product of statistical fluctuations (chance) or bias.

Information on biologic mechanisms by which exposure to TCDD could contribute to the generic (rather than tissue-specific or organ-specific) carcinogenic potential of the COIs is summarized in Chapter 4. It distills toxicologic information concerning the mechanisms by which TCDD affects the basic process of carcinogenesis; such information, of course, applies to all the cancer sites discussed individually in this chapter. When biologic plausibility is discussed in this chapter's sections on particular cancer types, the generic information is implicit, and only experimental data peculiar to carcinogenesis at the site in question are presented. A large literature indicates that carcinogenesis is a process that involves not only genetic changes but also epigenetic changes, which modify DNA and its expression without altering its sequence of bases (Johnstone and Baylin, 2010). There is increasing evidence that TCDD and the COIs may disturb cellular processes by epigenetic mechanisms (see Chapter 4), and reference to this evidence, as it applies to cancers is included where it exists, by cancer site.

Considerable uncertainty remains about the magnitude of risk posed by exposure to the COIs. Many of the veteran, occupational, and environmental studies reviewed by the committee did not control fully for important confounders. There is not enough information about the exposure experience of individual Vietnam veterans to permit combining exposure estimates for them with any potency estimates that might be derived from scientific research studies to quantify risk. The committee therefore cannot accurately estimate the risk to Vietnam veterans that is attributable to exposure to the COIs. The (at least currently) insurmountable problems in deriving useful quantitative estimates of the risks of various health outcomes in Vietnam veterans are explained in Chapter 1 and the summary of this report, but the point is not reiterated for every health outcome addressed.

ORGANIZATION OF CANCER GROUPS

For *Update 2006*, a system for addressing cancer types was described to clarify how specific cancer diagnoses were grouped for evaluation by the committee and to ensure that the full array of cancer types would be considered. The organization of cancer groups follows major and minor categories of cause of death related to cancer sites established by the National Institute for Occupational Safety and Health (NIOSH). The NIOSH groups map the full range of *International Classification of Diseases, Ninth Revision* (ICD-9) codes for malignant neoplasms (140–208). The ICD system is used by physicians and researchers to group related diseases and procedures in a standard form for statistical evaluation. Revision 10 (ICD-10) came into use in 1999 and constitutes a marked change from the previous four revisions that evolved into ICD-9. ICD-9 was in effect from 1979 to 1998; because ICD-9 is the version most prominent in the research reviewed in this series, it is used when codes are given for a specific health outcome. Appendix C describes the correspondence between the NIOSH cause-of-death groupings and ICD-9 codes (see Table C-1); the groupings for mortality are largely congruent with those of the SEER program for cancer incidence (see Table C-2, which presents equivalences between the ICD-9 and ICD-10 systems). For the present update, the committee gave more attention to the World Health Organization's classification of lymphohematopoietic neoplasms (WHO, 2008), which stresses partitioning of the disorders first according to the lymphoid or myeloid lineage of the transformed cells rather than into lymphomas and leukemias.

The system of organization used by the committee simplifies the process for locating a particular cancer for readers and facilitated the committee's identification of ICD codes for malignancies that had not been explicitly addressed in previous updates. VAO reports' default category for any health outcome on which no epidemiologic research findings have been recovered has always been "inadequate evidence" of association with exposure to the COIs, which in principle is applicable to specific cancers. Failure to review a specific cancer or other condition separately reflects the paucity of information, so there is indeed inadequate or insufficient information to categorize an association with such a disease outcome.

BIOLOGIC PLAUSIBILITY

The studies considered with respect to the biologic plausibility of associations between exposure to the COIs and human cancers have been performed primarily in laboratory animals (rats, mice, hamsters, and monkeys) or cultured cells. Collectively, the evidence obtained from studies of TCDD indicates that a connection between human exposure to this chemical and cancers is biologically plausible, as will be discussed more fully in a generic sense below and more specifically in the biologic-plausibility sections on individual cancers. Recent reviews have affirmed the well-established mechanistic roles of the aryl hydrocarbon receptor (AHR) in cancer (Androutsopoulos et al., 2009; Barouki and Coumoul, 2010; Dietrich and Kaina, 2010; Ray and Swanson, 2009), and the data have firmly established the biologic plausibility of an association between TCDD exposure and cancer. Recently, Hernández et al. (2009) have reviewed the mechanisms of action of nongenotoxic carcinogens, including TCDD in this category.

With respect to 2,4-D, 2,4,5-T, and picloram, several studies have been performed in laboratory animals. In general, the results were negative, although some would not meet current standards of cancer bioassays; for instance, there is some question as to whether the highest doses (generally 30–50 mg/kg) in some of the studies reached a maximum tolerated dose. It is not possible to have absolute confidence that these chemicals have no carcinogenic potential. Further evidence of a lack of carcinogenic potential is provided, however, by negative findings on genotoxic effects in assays conducted primarily in vitro. The evidence indicates that 2,4-D and 2,4,5-T are genotoxic only at very high concentrations.

There is some evidence that cacodylic acid is carcinogenic. Studies performed in laboratory animals have shown that it can induce neoplasms of the kidney (Yamamoto et al., 1995) and bladder (Arnold et al., 2006; Wei et al., 2002). Treatment with cacodylic acid induced formation of neoplasms of the lung when administered to mouse strains that are genetically susceptible to them (Hayashi et al., 1998). Other studies have used the two-stage model of carcinogenesis in which animals are exposed first to a known genotoxic agent and then to a suspected tumor-promoting agent; with this model, cacodylic acid has been shown to act as a tumor-promoter with respect to lung cancer (Yamanaka et al., 1996).

Studies in laboratory animals in which only TCDD has been administered have reported that it can increase the incidence of a number of neoplasms, most notably of the liver, lungs, thyroid, and oral mucosa (Kociba et al., 1978; NTP, 2006). Some studies have used the two-stage model of carcinogenesis and shown that TCDD can act as a tumor-promoter and increase the incidence of ovarian cancer (Davis et al., 2000), liver cancer (Beebe et al., 1995), and skin cancers (Wyde et al., 2004). In exerting its carcinogenic effects, TCDD is thought to act primarily as a tumor-promoter. In many of the animal studies reviewed, treatment with TCDD has resulted in hyperplasia or metaplasia of epithelial tissues. In addition, in both laboratory animals and cultured cells, TCDD has been shown to exhibit a wide array of effects on growth regulation, hormone systems, and other factors associated with the regulation of cellular processes that involve growth, maturation, and differentiation. Thus, it may be that TCDD increases the incidence or progression of human cancers through an interplay of multiple cellular factors. Tissue-specific protective cellular mechanisms may also affect the response to TCDD and complicate our understanding of its site-specific carcinogenic effects.

As shown with long-term bioassays in both sexes of several strains of rats, mice, hamsters, and fish, there is adequate evidence that TCDD is a carcinogen in laboratory animals, increasing the incidence of tumors at sites distant from the site of treatment at doses well below the maximum tolerated. On the basis of animal studies, TCDD has been characterized as a nongenotoxic carcinogen because it does not have obvious DNA-damaging potential, but it has been known for many years that it is a potent tumor-promoter and a weak initiator in two-stage initiation–promotion models for liver, skin, and lung. Early studies demonstrated that TCDD is 2 orders of magnitude more potent than the "classic" promoter tetradecanoyl phorbol acetate and that its skin-tumor promotion depends on the AHR. Recent evidence has shown that AHR activation by TCDD in human breast and endocervical cell lines induces sustained high concentrations of the interleukin-6 cytokine, which has tumor-promoting effects in numerous tissues—including breast, prostate, ovary, and malignant cholangiocytes—and opens up the possibility that TCDD would promote carcinogenesis in these and possibly other tissues (Hollingshead et al., 2008). In rat liver, TCDD downregulates reduced folate carrier (Rfc1) mRNA and protein, whose normal levels are essential in maintaining folate homeostasis (Halwachs et al., 2010). Reduced Rfc1 activity and a functional folate deficiency may contribute to the risk of carcinogenesis posed by TCDD exposure.

Mechanisms by which TCDD induces G1 arrest in hepatic cells (Mitchell et al., 2006; Weiss et al., 2008) and decreases viability of endometrial endothelial cells (Bredhult et al., 2007), insulin-secreting beta cells (Piaggi et al., 2007), peripheral T cells (Singh et al., 2008), and neuronal cells (Bredhult et al., 2007) have been identified, and the results suggest possible carcinogenic mechanisms. TCDD may contribute to tumor progression by inhibiting p53 regulation (phosphorylation and acetylation) triggered by genotoxicants through the increased expression of the metastasis marker AGR2 (Ambolet-Camoit et al., 2010) and through a functional interaction between the AHR and FHL2—"four and a half LIM protein 2," in which the LIM domain is a highly conserved protein structure (Kollara and Brown, 2009). Borlak and Jenke (2008) demonstrated that the AHR is a major regulator of c-raf and proposed that there is cross-talk between the AHR and the mitogen-activated protein kinase signaling pathway in chemically induced hepatocarcinogenesis. TCDD inhibits ultraviolet-C radiation-induced apoptosis in primary rat hepatocytes and Huh-7 human hepatoma cells, and this supports the hypothesis that TCDD acts as a tumor-promoter by preventing initiated cells from undergoing apoptosis (Chopra et al., 2009). Additional in vitro work with mouse hepatoma cells has shown that activation of the AHR results in increased concentrations of 8-hydroxy-2′-deoxyguanosine (8-OHdG), a product of DNA-base oxidation and later excision repair and a marker of DNA damage. Induction of cytochrome P4501A1 (CYP1A1) by TCDD or indolo(3,2-b) carbazole is associated with oxidative DNA damage (Park et al., 1996). In vivo experiments in mice corroborated those findings by showing that TCDD caused a sustained oxidative stress, as determined by measurements of urinary 8-OHdG (Shertzer et al., 2002) involving AHR-dependent uncoupling of mitochondrial respiration (Senft et al., 2002). Mitochondrial reactive-oxygen production depends on the AHR. Other than the occasional observation of 8-OHdG, there is little evidence that TCDD is genotoxic, and it appears likely that some of these mechanisms of action may be induced by epigenetic modifications (events that affect gene function but do not involve a change in gene coding sequence) of the genome.

Electronics-dismantling workers who experienced complex exposures, including exposure to polychlorinated dibenzo-*p*-dioxins and dibenzofurans (PCDDs and PCDFs), had increased concentrations of urinary 8-OHdG indicative of oxidative stress and genotoxicity; this cannot, however, be ascribed directly to the DLCs (Wen et al., 2008). Clastogenic genetic disturbances arising as a consequence of confirmed exposure to Agent Orange were determined by analyzing sister-chromatid exchanges (SCEs) in lymphocytes from a group of 24 New Zealand Vietnam War veterans and 23 control volunteers (Rowland et al., 2007). The results showed a highly significant difference ($p < 0.001$) in mean SCE frequency between the experimental group and the control group. The Vietnam War veterans also had a much higher proportion of cells with SCE frequencies above the 95th percentile than did the controls (11.0% and 0.07%, respectively).

The weight of evidence that TCDD and dioxin-like PCBs make up a group of chemicals with carcinogenic potential includes unequivocal animal carcinogenesis and biologic plausibility based on mode-of-action data. Although the specific mechanisms by which dioxin causes cancer remain to be established, the intracellular factors and mechanistic pathways involved in dioxin's cancer-promoting activity all have parallels in animals and humans. No qualitative differences have been reported to indicate that humans should be considered as fundamentally different from the multiple animal species in which bioassays have demonstrated dioxin-induced neoplasia.

Thus, the toxicologic evidence indicates that a connection of TCDD and perhaps cacodylic acid with cancer in humans is, in general, biologically plausible, but (as discussed in The Committee's View of "General" Human Carcinogens below) it must be determined case by case whether such potential contributes to each individual type of cancer. Experiments with 2,4-D, 2,4,5-T, and picloram in animals and cells have not provided a strong biologic basis for either the presence or the absence of carcinogenic effects.

THE COMMITTEE'S VIEW OF "GENERAL" HUMAN CARCINOGENS

To address its charge, the committee weighed the scientific evidence linking the COIs to specific individual cancer sites. That was appropriate given the different susceptibilities of various tissues and organs to cancer and the various genetic and environmental factors that can influence the occurrence of a particular type of cancer. Before considering each site in turn, however, it is important to address the concept that cancers share some characteristics among organ sites and to clarify the committee's view regarding the implications of a chemical's being a "general" human carcinogen. All cancers share phenotypic characteristics: uncontrolled cell proliferation, increased cell survival, invasion outside normal tissue boundaries, and eventually metastasis. The current understanding of cancer development holds that a cell or group of cells must acquire a series of sufficient genetic mutations to progress and that particular epigenetic events must occur to accelerate the mutational process and provide growth advantages for the more aggressive clones of cells. Both genetic (mutational) and epigenetic (nonmutational) activities of carcinogenic agents can stimulate the process of cancer development.

In classic experiments based on the induction of cancer in mouse skin that were conducted over 40 years ago, carcinogens were categorized as initiators, those capable of causing an initial genetic insult to the target tissue, and promoters, those capable of promoting the growth of initiated tumor cells, generally through nonmutational events. Some carcinogens, such as those found in tobacco smoke, were considered "whole carcinogens"; that is, they were capable of both initiation and promotion. Today, cancer researchers recognize that the acquisition of important mutations is a continuing process in tumors and that promoters, or epigenetic processes that favor cancer growth, enhance the accumulation of genotoxic damage, which traditionally would be regarded as initiating activity.

As discussed above and in Chapter 4, 2,4-D, 2,4,5-T, and picloram have shown little evidence of genotoxicity in laboratory studies, except at very high doses, and little ability to facilitate cancer growth in laboratory animals. However, cacodylic acid and TCDD have shown the capacity to increase cancer development in animal experiments, particularly as promoters rather than as pure genotoxic agents. Extrapolating organ-specific results from animal experiments to humans is problematic because of important differences between species in overall susceptibility of various organs to cancer development and in organ-specific responses to particular putative carcinogens. Therefore, judgments about the "general" carcinogenicity of a chemical in humans are based heavily on the results of epidemiologic studies, especially on the question of whether there is evidence of excess cancer risk at multiple organ sites. As the evaluations of specific types of cancer in the remainder of this chapter indicate, the committee finds that TCDD appears to be a multisite carcinogen. That finding is in agreement with the International Agency for Research on Cancer (IARC), which has determined that TCDD is a category 1 "known human carcinogen" (Baan et al., 2009); with the US Environmental Protection Agency (EPA), which has concluded that TCDD is "likely to be carcinogenic to humans" (http://www.epa.gov/ttn/atw/hlthef/dioxin.html; updated Januarary 2000; accessed September 21, 2013); and with the National Toxicology Program (NTP), which regards TCDD as "known to be a human carcinogen" (NTP, 2011). It is important to emphasize that the goals and methods of IARC and EPA in making their determinations were different from those of the present committee: the missions of those organizations focus on evaluating risk to minimize future exposure, whereas this committee focuses on risk after exposure. Furthermore, recognition that TCDD and cacodylic acid are multisite carcinogens does not imply that they cause human cancer at every organ site.

The distinction between *general carcinogen* and *site-specific carcinogen* is more difficult to grasp in light of the common practice of beginning analyses of epidemiologic cohorts with a category of "all malignant neoplasms," which is a routine first screen for any unusual cancer activity in the study population rather than a test of a biologically based hypothesis. When the distribution of cancers among anatomic sites is lacking in the report of a cohort study, a statistical test for an increase in all cancers is not meaningless, but it is usually less scientifically supportable than are analyses based on specific sites, for which more substantial biologically based hypotheses can be developed. The size of a cohort and the length of the observation period often constrain the number of cancer cases observed and which specific types of cancer have enough observed cases to permit analysis. For instance, an analysis of cumulative results on diabetes and cancer in the prospective Air Force Health Study (Michalek and Pavuk, 2008) produced important information summarizing previous findings on the fairly common condition of diabetes, but the cancer analysis does not go beyond "all cancers." The committee does not accept the cancer findings as an indication that exposure to Agent Orange increases the risk of every variety of cancer. It acknowledges that the results of the highly stratified analyses conducted suggest that the incidence of some cancers did increase in the Operation Ranch Hand veterans, but it views the "all cancers" results as a conglomeration of information on specific cancers—most important, melanoma and prostate cancer, on which provocative results have been published (Akhtar et al., 2004; Pavuk et al., 2006)—and as meriting individual longitudinal analysis to resolve outstanding questions.

For this report, updated mortality information was available on four occupational cohorts that have been followed in VAO updates, which included risk statistics for overall cancer mortality. In three of the four (Manuwald et al., 2012; Ruder and Yiin, 2011; Waggoner et al., 2011), there was a modest increase in cancer mortality; in the fourth, the observed cancer mortality matched expectation (Boers et al., 2012).

The committee notes that current information on overall mortality in US Vietnam veterans themselves has been elusive. Considerable confusion and alarm has arisen from Internet attribution of all of the approximately 800,000 deaths among all 9.2 million US Vietnam-era veterans to the 2.7 million who served in Vietnam (Brady, 2011; Gelman, 2013). The most recent reliable information was obtained in the 30-year update of mortality through 2000 of the deployed and nondeployed veterans in the Vietnam Experience Study (Boehmer et al., 2004), which found that mortality among the deployed veterans slightly exceeded that of their nondeployed counterparts, but was only about 9%. A followup study (O'Toole et al., 2010) of a random sample of 1,000 Australian Vietnam veterans selected from Australia's comprehensive roster of 57,643 service members deployed to Vietnam may provide a somewhat newer estimate of mortality through 2004 of 11.7%, which may be fairly comparable with that of their American fellows.

The remainder of this chapter deals with the committee's review of the evidence on each individual cancer site in accordance with its charge to evaluate the statistical association between exposure and cancer occurrence, the biologic plausibility and potential causal nature of the association, and the relevance to US veterans of the Vietnam War.

A number of studies of populations that received potentially relevant exposures were identified in the literature search for this review but did not characterize exposure with sufficient specificity for their results to meet the committee's criteria for inclusion in the evidentiary database. For instance, the British Pesticide Users Health Study has followed almost 60,000 men and 4,000 women who were certified for agricultural pesticide use in Great Britain since 1987. Frost et al. (2011) reported cancer incidence and mortality in this cohort up to 2004 for the full array of anatomic sites, but exposure was defined only as being a member of this cohort. Therefore, the cancer-specific findings of Frost et al. (2011) will not be repeatedly noted in the individual sections below. That is also the case for the mortality followup of Japanese Americans in the Honolulu Heart Program reported by Charles et al. (2010). Technically, this rubric would apply to the mortality and morbidity results reported by Waggoner et al. (2011) and Koutrous et al. (2010a); because of the context provided by the extensive pesticide-specific results that have been published on individual cancers in the Agricultural Health Study (AHS) and the knowledge that 2,4-D was one of the most frequently used pesticides in this large prospective cohort, however, those results are presented below, but not given full evidentiary weight. Numerous cancer studies of the case-control design addressing particular cancers had exposure characterizations that were not more specific than job titles, farm residence, or pesticide exposure; therefore, their results are not regarded as fully relevant for the purpose of this review, and such studies are mentioned only in passing in a discussion of the cancer investigated.

ORAL, NASAL, AND PHARYNGEAL CANCER

Oral, nasal, and pharyngeal cancers are found in many anatomic sites: the structures of the mouth (inside lining of the lips, cheeks, gums, tongue, and hard and soft palate—ICD-9 codes 140–145); oropharynx (ICD-9 146); nasopharynx (ICD-9 147); hypopharynx (ICD-9 148); other buccal cavity and pharynx (ICD-9 149); and nasal cavity and paranasal sinuses (ICD-9 160). Until recently, cancers that occur in the oral cavity and pharynx have been thought to be similar in descriptive epidemiology and risk factors, and cancer of the nasopharynx is thought to have a different epidemiologic profile. However, we now recognize that human papilloma virus (HPV) is an important risk factor for squamous-cell carcinoma of the head and neck, and risk estimates are highest for the base of the tongue and tonsils (oropharynx) (Marur et al., 2010).

The American Cancer Society (ACS) estimated that about 40,250 men and women would receive diagnoses of oral, nasal, or pharyngeal cancer in the United States in 2012 and that 7,850 men and women would die from these diseases (Siegel et al., 2012). Almost 91% of those cancers originate in the oral cavity or oropharynx. Most oral, nasal, and pharyngeal cancers are squamous-cell carcinomas. Nasopharyngeal carcinoma (NPC) is the most common malignant epithelial tumor of the nasopharynx but is relatively rare in the United States. There are three types of NPC: keratinizing squamous-cell carcinoma, nonkeratinizing carcinoma, and undifferentiated carcinoma.

The average annual incidences reported in Table 8-2 show that men are at greater risk than are women for those cancers and that the incidences increase

TABLE 8-2 Average Annual Incidence (per 100,000) of Nasal, Nasopharyngeal, Oral-Cavity and Pharyngeal, and Oropharyngeal Cancers in the United States[a]

	55–59 Years Old			60–64 Years Old			65–69 Years Old		
	All Races	White	Black	All Races	White	Black	All Races	White	Black
Nose, Nasal Cavity, and Middle Ear:									
Men	1.5	1.5	2.5	2.2	1.9	3.7	2.9	2.6	3.3
Women	1.2	1.0	1.0	1.1	1.0	1.8	1.6	1.9	0.9
Nasopharynx:									
Men	2.3	1.2	2.0	2.2	1.5	0.8	2.8	1.7	2.8
Women	1.1	0.6	0.4	0.8	0.7	0.3	1.0	0.9	0.9
Oral Cavity and Pharynx:									
Men	0.8	0.7	1.8	0.8	0.6	2.3	1.4	1.2	3.9
Women	0.3	0.3	0.2	0.1	0.1	0.3	0.6	0.5	2.1
Oropharynx:									
Men	2.0	1.9	3.5	1.9	1.6	5.2	2.2	2.0	5.0
Women	0.3	0.3	0.4	0.7	0.7	0.9	0.4	0.5	0.0

[a]Surveillance, Epidemiology, and End Results program, nine standard registries, crude age-specific rates, 2005–2009 (NCI, 2013).

with age—but there are few cases, and care should be exercised in interpreting the numbers. Tobacco and alcohol use are established risk factors for oral and pharyngeal cancers. Reported risk factors for nasal cancer include occupational exposure to nickel and chromium compounds (d'Errico et al., 2009; Feron et al., 2001; Grimsrud and Peto, 2006), wood dust (d'Errico et al., 2009), leather dust (Bonneterre et al., 2007), and high doses of formaldehyde (Nielsen and Wolkoff, 2010).

Conclusions from *VAO* and Previous Updates

The committee responsible for *VAO* concluded that there was inadequate or insufficient information to determine whether there is an association between exposure to the COI and oral, nasal, and pharyngeal cancers. Additional information available to the committees responsible for *Update 1996*, *Update 1998*, *Update 2000*, *Update 2002*, *Update 2004*, *Update 2006*, *Update 2008*, and *Update 2010* did not change that conclusion.

In *Update 2006*, at the request of the Department of Veterans Affairs (VA), the committee attempted to evaluate tonsil-cancer cases separately, but it was able to identify only three cohort studies that provided the number of tonsil-cancer cases in their study populations and concluded that the studies did not provide sufficient evidence to determine whether an association existed between exposure to the COIs and tonsil cancer. No new studies have offered any important additional insight into the question. The committee responsible for *Update 2006* recommended that VA evaluate the possibility of studying health outcomes, including tonsil cancer, in Vietnam-era veterans by using existing administrative and health-services databases. Anecdotal evidence provided to that committee suggested a potential association between the exposures in Vietnam and tonsil cancer. Increasing evidence indicating that some cancers of the oropharynx and oral cavity can have a viral (HPV) etiology is consistent with the mechanistic hypothesis explaining an excess of these cancers in Vietnam veterans: immune alterations associated with Agent Orange exposure may have increased susceptibility to HPV infection in the oral cavity and tonsils of Vietnam veterans, thereby making them more prone to the development of squamous-cell carinomas in these tissues. The present committee strongly reiterates the 2006, 2008, and 2010 recommendation that VA develop a strategy that uses existing databases to evaluate tonsil cancer in Vietnam-era veterans.

The small numbers of oral, nasal, or pharyngeal cancer cases in prior studies limit interpretation of the data. Cypel and Kang (2010) updated the study of Vietnam-era Army Chemical Corps (ACC) veterans, comparing mortality through 2005 in ACC veterans by Vietnam service. They reported a nonsignificant increase in oral-cavity and pharyngeal cancers in the deployed cohort compared with cases in the nondeployed cohort—a result that is consistent with a prior report on mortality through 1991 (Dalager and Kang, 1997).

McBride et al. (2009a) reported on mortality through 2004 in the New Zealand cohort of 1,599 workers who had been employed in manufacturing phenoxy herbicides from trichlorophenol (TCP); picloram was also produced in the plant. They reported a nonsignificant excess in mortality from buccal cavity and pharyngeal cancer and no deaths from nasopharyngeal cancer in either group.

Studies evaluated previously and in the present report are summarized in Table 8-3.

Update of the Epidemiologic Literature

Vietnam-Veteran Studies

There have been no Vietnam-veteran studies of exposure to the COIs and oral, nasal, or pharyngeal cancers since *Update 2010*.

Occupational Studies

Burns et al. (2011) published an update examining the cancer incidence through 2007 in workers who were alive on January 1, 1985, and had been employed at any time from 1945 to 1994 in 2,4-D production by the Dow Chemical Company in Midland, Michigan. They found no evidence of significantly increased cancer rates overall. The incidence of lip, oral, and pharyngeal cancer

TABLE 8-3 Selected Epidemiologic Studies—Oral, Nasal, and Pharyngeal Cancer (Shaded Entries Are New Information for This Update)

Study Population[a]	Exposed Cases[b]	**Exposure of Interest**/Estimated Relative Risk (95% CI)[b]	Reference
VIETNAM VETERANS			
US Vietnam Veterans			
US Air Force Health Study—Ranch Hand veterans vs SEA veterans (unless otherwise noted)		**All COIs**	Akhtar et al., 2004
Incidence			
Ranch Hand veterans (n = 1,189)	6	0.9 (0.4–1.9)	
With tours between 1966–1970	6	1.1 (0.5–2.3)	
SEA comparison veterans (n = 1,776)	5	0.6 (0.2–1.2)	
With tours between 1966–1970	4	0.6 (0.2–1.4)	
Mortality			
Through 1999—White subjects vs national rates			
Ranch Hand veterans (n = 1,189)	0	0.0 (nr)	
SEA comparison veterans (n = 1,776)	1	0.5 (nr)	
US VA Cohort of Army Chemical Corps—Expanded as of 1997 to include all Army men with chemical MOS (2,872 deployed vs 2,737 nondeployed) serving during Vietnam era (July 1, 1965–March 28, 1973)		**All COIs**	
Mortality—Oral cavity and pharyngeal cancer			
Through 2005			Cypel and Kang, 2010
Deployed veterans (2,872) vs nondeployed (2,737)	6 vs 2	1.7 (0.3–8.7)	
Army Chemical Corps vs US men			
Vietnam cohort	6	1.5 (0.6–3.3)	
Non-Vietnam cohort	2	0.8 (0.1–2.8)	
US CDC Vietnam Experience Study—Cross-sectional study, with medical examinations, of Army veterans: 9,324 deployed vs 8,989 nondeployed		**All COIs**	
Mortality			
1965–2000 (ICD-140–149)	6	nr	Boehmer et al., 2004
US CDC Selected Cancers Study—Case-control study of incidence (Dec 1, 1984–Nov 30, 1989) among US males born 1929–1953		**All COIs**	CDC, 1990a
89 nasopharyngeal carcinomas			
Vietnam service	3	0.5 (0.2–1.8)	
62 nasal carcinomas			
Vietnam service	2	0.7 (0.2–2.9)	
State Studies of US Vietnam Veterans			
Michigan Vietnam-era veterans, PM study of deaths (1974–1989)—deployed vs nondeployed (lip, oral cavity, pharynx)	12	1.0 (0.5–1.8)	Visintainer et al., 1995

TABLE 8-3 Oral, Nasal, and Pharyngeal Cancer, continued

Study Population[a]	Exposed Cases[b]	**Exposure of Interest**/Estimated Relative Risk (95% CI)[b]	Reference
International Vietnam-Veterans Studies			
Australian Vietnam Veterans—58,077 men and 153 women served on land or in Vietnamese waters during 5/23/1962–7/1/1973 vs Australian population		**All COIs**	
Incidence			
All branches, 1982–2000 (head and neck)	247	1.5 (1.3–1.6)	ADVA, 2005a
Navy	56	1.6 (1.1–2.0)	
Army	174	1.6 (1.3–1.8)	
Air Force	17	0.9 (0.5–1.5)	
Mortality			
All branches, return–2001			ADVA, 2005b
Head and neck	101	1.4 (1.2–1.7)	
Navy	22	1.5 (0.9–2.1)	
Army	69	1.5 (1.1–1.8)	
Air Force	9	1.1 (0.5–2.0)	
Nasal	3	0.8 (0.2–2.2)	
1980–1994			CDVA, 1997a
Lip (ICD-9 140)	0	nr	
Nasopharyngeal cancer (ICD-9 147)	2	0.5 (0.1–1.7)	
Nasal cavities (ICD-9 160)	2	1.2 (0.1–4.1)	
Australian Conscripted Army National Service (18,940 deployed vs 24,642 nondeployed)		**All COIs**	
Incidence			
1982–2000			ADVA, 2005c
Head and Neck	44	2.0 (1.2–3.4)	
Mortality			
1966–2001			ADVA, 2005c
Head and neck	16	1.8 (0.8–4.3)	
Nasal	0	0.0 (0.0–48.2)	
1982–1994			CDVA, 1997b
Nasopharyngeal cancer (ICD-9 147)	1	1.3 (0.0– > 10)	
Nasal cavities (ICD-9 160)	0	0.0 (0.0– > 10)	
OCCUPATIONAL—INDUSTRIAL			
IARC Phenoxy Herbicide Cohort—Workers exposed to any phenoxy herbicide or chlorophenol (production or spraying) vs respective national mortality rates			
Mortality 1939–1992			Kogevinas et al., 1997
Oral cavity, pharynx cancer (ICD-9 140–149)	26	1.1 (0.7–1.6)	
13,831 exposed to highly chlorinated PCDDs	22	1.3 (0.8–2.0)	

continued

TABLE 8-3 Oral, Nasal, and Pharyngeal Cancer, continued

Study Population[a]	Exposed Cases[b]	**Exposure of Interest**/Estimated Relative Risk (95% CI)[b]	Reference
7,553 not exposed to highly chlorinated PCDDs	3	0.5 (0.1–1.3)	
Nasal, nasal sinus cancer (ICD-9) 160)	3	1.6 (0.3–4.7)	
13,831 exposed to highly chlorinated PCDDs	0	0.0 (0.0–3.5)	
7,553 not exposed to highly chlorinated PCDDs	3	3.8 (0.8–11.1)	
Mortality 1955–1988 of 12,492 production workers and 5,898 sprayers exposed—13,482 in exposed subcohort			Saracci et al., 1991
Bucal cavity, pharynx (ICD-8 140–149)	11	1.2 (0.6–2.1)	
Nose, nasal cavities (ICD-8 160)	3	2.9 (0.6–8.5)	
British MCPA Plant—Production 1947–1982 (n = 1,545) (included in IARC cohort) and spraying 1947–1972 (n = 2,561) (*not* included in IARC cohort)		**MCPA**	
Mortality through 1983			Coggon et al., 1986
Lip (ICD-9 140)	0	nr	
Tongue (ICD-9 141)	1	1.1 (0.0–6.2)	
Pharynx (ICD-9 146–149)	1	0.5 (0.0–3.0)	
Nose (ICD-9 160)	3	4.9 (1.0–14.4)	
Dutch production workers in Plant A (549 men exposed during production 1955–1985; 594 unexposed) (in IARC cohort)		**Dioxins, 2,4,5-T, 2,4,5-TCP**	
Mortality 1955–1991 (lip, oral cavity, pharynx)			Hooiveld et al., 1998
All working anytime in 1955–1985	1	2.3 (0.1–12.4)	
Cleaned up 1963 explosion	1	7.1 (0.2–39.6)	
German Production Workers—2,479 workers at 4 plants (in IARC cohort as of 1997)		**Dioxins, phenoxy herbicides**	
All for plants—Buccal cavity, pharynx (ICD-9 140–149)	9	3.0 (1.4–5.6)	Becher et al., 1996
Tongue	3	nr	
Floor of mouth	2	nr	
Tonsil	2	nr	
Pharynx	2	nr	
German Production Workers at Bayer Plant in Uerdingen (135 men working > 1 month in 1951–1976) (in IARC cohort as of 1997) and women—no results		**Dioxins; 2,4, 5-TCP**	
Mortality 1951–1992	0	—	Becher et al., 1996
German Production Workers at Bayer Plant in Dormagen (520 men working > 1 month in 1965–1989) (in IARC cohort as of 1997) and women—no results		**Dioxins; 2,4-D; 2,4,5-T; MCPA; MCPP; 2,4-DP**	
Mortality 1965–1989	0	—	Becher et al., 1996

TABLE 8-3 Oral, Nasal, and Pharyngeal Cancer, continued

Study Population[a]	Exposed Cases[b]	**Exposure of Interest**/Estimated Relative Risk (95% CI)[b]	Reference
German Production Workers at BASF Ludwigshafen Plant (680 men working > 1 month in 1957–1987) (in IARC cohort as of 1997) and women—no results		**Dioxins; 2,4-D; 2,4,5-T; MCPA; MCPP; 2,4-DP**	
Mortality 1956–1989	6	8.2 (3.0–17.9)	Becher et al., 1996
BASF Cleanup Workers from 1953 accident (n = 247); 114 with chloracne, 13 more with erythema; serum TCDD levels (*not* part of IARC)		**Focus on TCDD**	
Mortality			
Through 1987		*90% CI*	Zober et al., 1990
Buccal cavity, pharynx	1	4.8 (0.3–22.9)	
Squamous-cell carcinoma of tonsil	1	nr	
German Production Workers at Boehringer–Ingelheim Plant in Hamburg (1,144 men working > 1 month in 1952–1984; generation of TCDD reduced after chloracne outbreak in 1954) and women—no results (some additions to observed cancers over Manz et al., 1991) (in IARC cohort as of 1997)		**Dioxins; 2,4,5-T; 2,5-DCP; 2,4,5-TCP**	
Mortality 1952–2007 (ICD-9 140–149)	11	2.2 (1.1–3.9)	Manuwald et al., 2012
Men	9	2.0 (0.9–3.8)	
Women	2	3.4 (0.4–12.5)	
Mortality 1952–1989	3	1.8 (0.4–5.2)	Becher et al., 1996
New Zealand Phenoxy Herbicide Production Workers and Sprayers (1,599 men and women working any time in 1969–1988 at Dow plant in New Plymouth) (in IARC cohort)		**Dioxins; 2,4-D; 2,4,5-T; MCPA; MCPB; 2,4,5-TCP; Picloram**	
Mortality 1969–2004 (buccal cavity and pharynx)			McBride et al., 2009a
Ever-exposed workers	3	2.6 (0.5–7.6)	
Never-exposed workers	0	0.0 (0.0–11.5)	
Production Workers—Mortality 1969–2000			
713 men and 100 women worked > 1 month in 1969–1984	2	2.8 (0.3–9.9)	't Mannetje et al., 2005
Lip (ICD-9 140)	0	nr	
Mouth (ICD-9 141–145)	2	5.4 (0.7–20.0)	
Oropharynx (ICD-9 146)	0	nr	
Nasopharynx (ICD-9 147)	0	0.0 (0.0–41.8)	
Hypopharynx, other (ICD-9 148–149)	0	nr	
Phenoxy herbicide sprayers (> 99% men)	1	1.0 (0.0–5.7)	't Mannetje et al., 2005
Lip (ICD-9 140)	0	nr	
Mouth (ICD-9 141–145)	0	0.0 (0.0–7.5)	
Oropharynx (ICD-9 146)	0	nr	

continued

TABLE 8-3 Oral, Nasal, and Pharyngeal Cancer, continued

Study Population[a]	Exposed Cases[b]	**Exposure of Interest**/Estimated Relative Risk (95% CI)[b]	Reference
Nasopharynx (ICD-9 147)	1	8.3 (0.2–46.3)	
Hypopharynx, other (ICD-9 148–149)	0	nr	
NIOSH Mortality Cohort (12 US plants, 5,172 male production and maintenance workers 1942–1984) (included in IARC cohort as of 1997)		**Dioxins, phenoxy herbicides**	
All Dow PCP-Exposed Workers (All workers from the two plants that only made PCP (in Tacoma, Washington, and Wichita, Kansas) and workers who made PCP and TCP at two additional plants (in Midland, Michigan, and Sauget, Illinois)		**2,4,5-T; 2,4,5-TCP**	Ruder and Yiin, 2011
1940–2005 (n = 2,122) (buccal, pharynx; ICD-9 140–149)	5	0.8 (0.3–1.8)	
PCP and TCP (n = 720)	1	0.5 (0.0–2.7)	
PCP (no TCP) (n = 1,402)	4	0.9 (0.2–2.3)	
Dow 2,4-D Production Workers (1945–1982 in Midland, Michigan) (subset of all TCP-exposed workers)		**2,4-D, lower chlorinated dioxins**	
Cancer incidence through 2007 in Dow workers (n = 1,256) vs comparisons from state cancer registries (n = 23,354) (Cohort 3)	7	1.1 (0.4–2.2)	Burns et al., 2011
OCCUPATIONAL—PAPER AND PULP WORKERS		**TCDD**	
IARC cohort of pulp and paper workers—60,468 workers from 11 countries, TCDD among 27 agents assessed by JEM (oral cavity, pharynx)			McLean et al., 2006
Exposure to nonvolatile organochlorine compounds			
Never	33	0.9 (0.6–1.3)	
Ever	15	0.5 (0.3–0.9)	
Danish male, female paper workers			Rix et al., 1998
Buccal cavity (ICD-7 140–144)			
Men	24	1.0 (0.7–1.5)	
Women	4	1.5 (0.4–3.8)	
Pharynx (ICD-7 145–149)			
Men	15	2.0 (1.1–3.3)	
Women	2	2.1 (0.2–7.6)	
Tonsil cancers among pharyngeal cancers	11	nr	
Northwestern US paper and pulp workers—5 mills in Washington, Oregon, and California, 3,523 worked ≥ 1 yr 1945–1955, mortality through March 1977		*90% CI*	Robinson et al., 1986
Buccal cavity, pharynx (ICD-7 140–148)	1	0.1 (0.0–0.7)	
Nasal (ICD-7 160)	0	nr	

TABLE 8-3 Oral, Nasal, and Pharyngeal Cancer, continued

Study Population[a]	Exposed Cases[b]	**Exposure of Interest**/Estimated Relative Risk (95% CI)[b]	Reference
OCCUPATIONAL—HERBICIDE-USING WORKERS (*not* related to IARC sprayer cohorts)			
DENMARK			
Danish Farmers—incidence from linking farmers on 1970 census with national cancer registry (1970–1980)		**Herbicides**	Ronco et al., 1992
Danish self-employed farmers			
Lip	182	1.8 ($p < 0.05$)	
Tongue	9	0.6 (nr)	
Salivary glands	13	0.9 (nr)	
Mouth	14	0.5 ($p < 0.05$)	
Pharynx	13	0.3 ($p < 0.05$)	
Nasal cavities, sinuses	11	0.6 (nr)	
Danish farming employees			
Lip	43	2.1 ($p < 0.05$)	
Tongue	2	0.6 (nr)	
Salivary glands	0	0.0 (nr)	
Mouth	0	0.0 ($p < 0.05$)	
Pharynx	9	1.1 (nr)	
Nasal cavities, sinuses	5	1.3 (nr)	
Danish gardeners—incidence from 3,156 male and 859 female gardeners (buccal cavity, pharynx, ICD-7 140–148)		**Herbicides**	Hansen et al., 2007
10-yr followup (1975–1984) reported in Hansen et al. (1992)	6	1.1 (0.4–2.5)	
25-yr followup (1975–2001)			
Born before 1915 (high exposure)	3	0.7 (0.2–2.3)	
Born 1915–1934 (medium exposure)	6	0.7 (0.3–1.4)	
Born after 1934 (low exposure)	0	0.0 (0.0–1.0)	
FINNISH Phenoxy Herbicide Sprayers (1,909 men working 1955–1971 ≥ 2 wks) *not* IARC		**Phenoxy herbicides**	Asp et al., 1994
Buccal, pharynx (ICD-8 140–149)			
Incidence	5	1.0 (0.3–2.3)	
Mortality 1972–1989	0	0.0 (0.0–3.0)	
"Other Respiratory" (ICD-8 160, 161, 163)—nose, larynx, pleura			
Incidence	4	1.1 (0.3–2.7)	
Mortality 1972–1989	1	0.5 (0.0–2.9)	
ITALIAN Licensed Pesticide Users—male farmers in southern Piedmont licensed 1970–1974			
Mortality 1970–1986 (n = 23,401) (buccal cavity, pharynx)	18	0.3 (0.2–0.5)	Torchio et al., 1994

continued

TABLE 8-3 Oral, Nasal, and Pharyngeal Cancer, continued

Study Population[a]	Exposed Cases[b]	**Exposure of Interest**/Estimated Relative Risk (95% CI)[b]	Reference
Italian Farmers—mortality odds ratios from linking farmers on 1970 census with national cancer registry (1970–1980)		**Herbicides**	Ronco et al., 1992
Self-employed	13	0.9 (nr)	
Employee	4	0.5 (nr)	
NEW ZEALAND National Cancer Registry (1980–1984)—case-control study of 649 incident buccal cavity cancer cases and 49 incident nasopharynx cancer cases vs 19,904 men with any incident cancer			Reif et al., 1989
Forestry workers (n = 134)		**Herbicides**	
Buccal cavity	3	0.7 (0.2–2.2)	
Nasopharynx	2	5.6 (1.6–19.5)	
Aged 20–59	1	3.5 (0.6–22.6)	
Aged ≥ 60	1	13.4 (2.7–65.1)	
Sawmill workers (n = 139)		**Herbicides, chlorophenols**	
Nasopharynx	0	—	
NORWEGIAN farmers born 1925–1971—incidence, lip cancer		**Pesticides**	Nordby et al., 2004
Reported pesticide use	nr	0.7 (0.4–1.0)	
SWEDEN			
Swedish pesticide applicators—incidence			Wiklund et al., 1989a
Lip cancer	14	1.8 (1.0–2.9)	
Incident cancer cases 1961–1973 with agriculture as economic activity in 1960 census (male, female)		*99% CI*	Wiklund, 1983
Lip	508	1.8 (1.6–2.2)	
Tongue	32	0.4 (0.2–0.6)	
Salivary Gland	68	1.0 (0.7–1.4)	
Mouth	70	0.6 (0.5–0.8)	
Throat	84	0.5 (0.4–0.7)	
Nose, nasal sinuses	64	0.8 (0.6–1.2)	
THE NETHERLANDS			
Dutch Licensed Herbicide Sprayers—1,341 certified before 1980			
Through 2000			Swaen et al., 2004
Nose	0	—	
Pharynx	0	—	
UNITED STATES			
US farmers—usual occupation of farmer and industry of agriculture on death certificates 1984–1988 from 23 states		**Herbicides** PCMRs	Blair et al., 1993
Men			
Whites (n = 119,648)	21	2.3 (1.4–3.5)	
Nonwhites (n = 11,446)	0	—	

TABLE 8-3 Oral, Nasal, and Pharyngeal Cancer, continued

Study Population[a]	Exposed Cases[b]	**Exposure of Interest**/Estimated Relative Risk (95% CI)[b]	Reference
Women			
Whites (n = 2,400)	1	12.2 (0.2–68.0)	
Nonwhites (n = 2,066)	0	0.0 (0.0–103.6)	
US Agricultural Health Study—prospective study of licensed pesticide sprayers in Iowa and North Carolina: commercial (n = 4,916), private/farmers (n = 52,395, 97.4% men), and spouses of private sprayers (n = 32,347, 0.007% men), enrolled 1993–1997; followups with CATIs 1999–2003 and 2005–2010		**Phenoxy herbicides**	
Incidence			
Enrollment through 2006—SIRs for participants			Koutros et al., 2010a
Private applicators	93	0.6 (0.5–0.7)	
Commercial applicators	5	0.5 (0.2–1.3)	
Spouses	22	0.6 (0.4–1.0)	
Enrollment through 2002—buccal cavity			Alavanja et al., 2005
Private applicators (men and women)	66	0.7 (0.5–0.8)	
Lip	25	1.4 (0.9–2.1)	
Spouses of private applicators (> 99% women)	14	0.7 (0.4–1.2)	
Lip	2	1.4 (0.2–5.1)	
Commercial applicators	5	0.9 (0.3–2.2)	
Lip	3	2.7 (0.6–8.0)	
Mortality			
Enrollment through 2007, vs state rates (buccal cavity, pharynx)	16	0.3 (0.2–0.6)	Waggoner et al., 2011
Enrollment through 2000, vs state rates (buccal cavity, pharynx)			Blair et al., 2005a
Private applicators (men and women)	5	0.3 (0.1–0.7)	
Spouses of private applicators (> 99% women)	0	0.0 (0.0–25.4)	
White Male Residents of Iowa—Lip cancer on death certificate, usual occupation: farmers vs not		**Herbicides**	
> 20 yrs old when died 1971–1978—PMR	20	2.1 (p < 0.01)	Burmeister, 1981
ENVIRONMENTAL			
Seveso, Italy Residential Cohort—Industrial accident July 10, 1976 (723 residents Zone A; 4,821 Zone B; 31,643 Zone R; 181,574 local reference group) (ICD-9 171)		**TCDD**	

continued

TABLE 8-3 Oral, Nasal, and Pharyngeal Cancer, continued

Study Population[a]	Exposed Cases[b]	**Exposure of Interest**/Estimated Relative Risk (95% CI)[b]	Reference
Incidence			
10-yr followup to 1991—men			Bertazzi et al., 1993
Buccal cavity (ICD-9 140–149)			
Zone B	6	1.7 (0.8–3.9)	
Zone R	28	1.2 (0.8–1.7)	
Nose, nasal cavities (ICD-9 160)			
Zone R	0	nr	
10-yr followup to 1991—women			Bertazzi et al., 1993
Buccal cavity (ICD-9 140–149)			
Zone B	0	nr	
Zone R	0	nr	
Nose, nasal cavities (ICD-9 160)			
Zone R	2	2.6 (0.5–13.3)	
CASE-CONTROL STUDIES			
US Case-Control Studies			
US males born 1929–1953, all 70 nasal cancers (52 carcinomas, 11 lymphomas, 5 sarcomas) in CDC (1990a) study population		**Herbicides, pesticides**	Caplan et al., 2000
Selected landscaping, forestry occupation	26	1.8 (1.1–3.1)	
Living, working on farm	23	0.5 (0.3–0.8)	
Herbicides, pesticides	19	0.7 (0.4–1.3)	
Phenoxy herbicides	5	1.2 (0.4–3.3)	
International Case-Control Studies			
Residents of northern **Sweden** (44 nasal, 27 nasopharyngeal cancers)		**Phenoxy acids, chlorophenols**	Hardell et al., 1982
Phenoxy herbicide exposed	8	2.1 (0.9–4.7)	
Chlorophenol exposure	9	6.7 (2.8–16.2)	

NOTE: 2,4-D, 2,4-dichlorophenoxyacetic acid; 2,4-DP, 2,4-dichlorophenoxypropanoic acid; 2,4,5-T, 2,4,5-trichlorophenoxyacetic acid; 2,4,5-TCP, 2,4,5-trichlorophenol; 2,5-DCP, 2,5-dichlorophenol; AFHS, Air Force Health Study; CATI, computer-assisted telephone interviewing; CDC, Centers for Disease Control and Prevention; CI, confidence interval; COI, chemical of interest; IARC, International Agency for Research on Cancer; ICD, International Classification of Diseases; JEM, job-exposure matrix; MCPA, 2 methyl-4-chlorophenoxyacetic acid; MCPB, 4-(4-chloro-2-methylphenoxy) butanoic acid; MCPP, methylchlorophenoxypropionic acid; MOS, military occupational specialty; NIOSH, National Institute for Occupational Safety and Health; nr, not reported; PCDD, polychlorinated dibenzo-*p*-dioxins (highly chlorinated, if four or more chlorines); PCMR, proportionate cancer mortality ratios; PCP, pentachlorophenol; PM, proportionate mortality; PMR, proportionate mortality ratio; SEA, Southeast Asia; TCDD, 2,3,7,8-tetrachlorodibenzo-*p*-dioxin; TCP, trichlorophenol.

[a]Subjects are male and outcome is mortality unless otherwise noted.

[b]Given when available; results other than estimated risk explained individually.

in the most restrictively defined cohort was not increased (standardized incidence ratio [SIR] = 1.09, 95% confidence interval [CI] 0.44–2.24), as was the case for the two more inclusive but potentially more biased cohorts.

Manuwald et al. (2012) reported on mortality in 1,191 men and 398 women who had been employed for at least 3 months in 1952–1984 at a chemical plant in Hamburg (a subcohort of the IARC phenoxy herbicide cohort). During that period, the plant produced insecticides and herbicides, including 2,4,5-T, so cohort members had the possibility of exposure to TCDD. Subjects entered the cohort at the date of their first employment at the plant, and vital status was sought through 2007. Standardized mortality ratios (SMRs) calculated relative to the population of Hamburg showed that death from lip, oral-cavity, or pharyngeal cancers was not significantly increased in men (SMR = 2.00, 95% CI 0.91–3.79) or women (SMR = 3.42, 95% CI 0.39–12.45) but was significantly increased in the entire cohort (SMR = 2.17, 95% CI 1.08–3.87).

Ruder and Yiin (2011) reported mortality from 1940 to 2005 in the NIOSH pentachlorophenol (PCP) cohort of 2,122 workers in the US four plants that had been involved in PCP production. PCP production entailed exposure to PCDDs and PCDFs but not to the most toxic 2,3,7,8 dioxin congener. A subcohort of 720 workers (all men, the PCP-plus-TCDD group) had also been employed in TCP production and so had also been exposed to TCDD. In the total cohort, five deaths were attributed to buccal or pharyngeal cancer; this was consistent with the mortality experience of the US population (SMR = 0.76, 95% CI 0.25–1.77). There was only one death from this type of cancer in the PCP-plus-TCDD group, which also was not more than expected (SMR = 0.48, 95% CI 0.01–2.68). The results were effectively the same in the 1,402 workers who had not had any opportunity for occupational exposure to TCDD (SMR = 0.89, 95% CI 0.24–2.28).

The participants in the AHS are known to have had extensive exposure to the phenoxy herbicides, but the analyses of updated mortality through 2007 (Waggoner et al., 2011) and cancer incidence through 2006 (Koutros et al., 2010a) addressed only exposure to pesticides in general. The SMR was lower than expected for oral (buccal) and pharyngeal cancers in the applicators (16 deaths, SMR = 0.34, 95% CI 0.19–0.55), and only three deaths from these types of cancer were observed in their spouses. Koutros et al. (2010a) found 93 cases of oral-cavity and pharyngeal cancers in the private applicators (SIR = 0.56, 95% CI 0.45–0.69) and 22 cases in their spouses (SIR = 0.64, 95% CI 0.40–0.97). A nonsignificant increase in lip cancer was reported for the private applicators (SIR = 1.30, 95% CI 0.90–1.83), but these 33 cases may have more in common with skin cancers than with head and neck squamous-cell carcinomas. The AHS has been generating valuable information on the COIs for a number of years, but these results are not herbicide-specific and so are not regarded as being fully informative for the committee's task.

Environmental Studies

No new studies of environmental exposures to the COIs and these types of cancer have been published since *Update 2010*.

Case-Control Studies

A single case-control study of nasopharyngeal carcinoma (NPC) was identified in this publication period; it explored dietary, social, and environmental risk factors in 1,289 subjects (Aussem et al., 2012). Using a novel analytic procedure involving Baysian networks, the authors investigated whether exposure to pesticides and intake of domestic fumes from incomplete combustion of coal and wood were significantly associated with NPC risk. The characterization of exposure was insufficiently specific for the present committee to factor in the findings of the study. In any event, NPC is rare outside southern China and is known to be associated with Epstein-Barr virus infection, so it is unlikely to be a concern in American Vietnam veterans.

Biologic Plausibility

As noted above, there is increasing evidence that HPV contributes causally to cancers of the head and neck (Marur et al., 2010; Szentirmay et al., 2005) and to pharyngeal cancers in particular (Gillison and Shah, 2001; Gillison et al., 2012). It is unknown whether Agent Orange exposure contributes to a susceptibility to viral infection or action, but it warrants further exploration. The sparseness of data on the specific tumor site and a general lack of information on smoking, drinking, and viral exposure status in the few available epidemiologic studies preclude exploration of this hypothesis in the current literature.

Long-term animal studies have examined the effect of exposure to the COIs on tumor incidence (Charles et al., 1996; Stott et al., 1990; Walker et al., 2006; Wanibuchi et al., 2004). A National Toxicology Program study (Yoshizawa et al., 2005a) reported an increase in the incidence of gingival squamous-cell carcinoma in female rats treated orally (by gavage) with TCDD at 100 ng/kg 5 days/week for 104 weeks. The incidence of gingival squamous-cell hyperplasia was significantly increased in all groups treated at 3–46 ng/kg. In addition, squamous-cell carcinoma of the oral mucosa of the palate was increased. This NTP study did not, however, find any pathologic effect of TCDD on nasal tissues (Nyska et al., 2005). Increased neoplasms of the oral mucosa were previously observed and described as carcinomas of the hard palate and nasal turbinates (Kociba et al., 1978). Kociba et al. (1978) also reported a small increase in the incidence of tongue squamous-cell carcinoma.

Recently, DiNatale et al. (2011) utilized head and neck squamous-cell carcinoma cell lines to investigate mechanisms for tumor progression associated with this AHR activation. This tumor type typically produces large amounts of cytokines, and its IL6 expression levels correlate with disease aggressiveness. In this model, AHR activation by TCDD enhances IL6 production induced by another cytokine (IL 1β), so TCDD may promote head and neck squamous-cell carcinoma.

The biologic plausibility of the carcinogenicity of the COIs is discussed in general at the beginning of this chapter.

Synthesis

Most of the new studies that reported results on oral, nasal, and pharyngeal cancers noted estimated reductions or nonsignificant excesses in mortality from oral and pharyngeal cancers. With a total of 11 oral, pharyngeal, or lip cancers, however, a significantly increased risk was reported for the Hamburg cohort overall; but with nine and two cases, respectively, the increased estimates of risk for men and women did not achieve the traditional level ($p = 0.05$) of statistical significance. In the AHS, the incidence of oral and pharyngeal cancers was significantly decreased for both private applicators and their spouses. Those data are not sufficient, taken in combination with the previously reviewed literature, to suggest an association with the herbicides sprayed in Vietnam.

Conclusion

On the basis of the evidence reviewed here and in previous VAO reports, the committee concludes that there is inadequate or insufficient evidence to determine whether there is an association between exposure to the COIs and oral, nasal, or pharyngeal cancers.

CANCERS OF THE DIGESTIVE ORGANS

Until *Update 2006*, VAO committees had reviewed "gastrointestinal tract tumors" as a group consisting of stomach, colorectal, and pancreatic cancers; esophageal cancer has been formally included only since *Update 2004*. With more evidence from occupational studies available, VAO updates now address cancers of the digestive organs individually. Findings on cancers of the digestive organs as a group (ICD-9 150–159) are too broad for useful etiologic analysis and will no longer be considered.

Esophageal cancer (ICD-9 150), stomach cancer (ICD-9 151), colon cancer (ICD-9 153), rectal cancer (ICD-9 154), and pancreatic cancer (ICD-9 157) are among the most common cancers. ACS estimated that about 226,160 people would receive diagnoses of those cancers in the United States in 2012 and that 114,690 people would die from them (Siegel et al., 2012). Other digestive cancers (for example, small intestine, anal, and hepatobiliary cancers) added about 58,520 new diagnoses and 27,820 deaths to the 2012 estimates for the United States (Siegel et al., 2012). Collectively, tumors of the digestive organs were expected to account for 17% of new cancer diagnoses and 25% of cancer deaths in 2012. The average annual incidences of gastrointestinal cancers are presented in Table 8-4.

The incidences of stomach, colon, rectal, and pancreatic cancers increase with age. In general, the incidences are higher in men than in women and higher

TABLE 8-4 Average Annual Incidence (per 100,000) of Selected Gastrointestinal Cancers in the United States[a]

	55–59 Years Old			60–64 Years Old			65–69 Years Old		
	All Races	White	Black	All Races	White	Black	All Races	White	Black
Stomach:									
Men	15. 0	13.7	23.2	23.3	21.0	38.6	35.9	31.2	66.2
Women	7.0	5.3	12.4	8.8	7.1	13.9	14.6	11.3	23.0
Esophagus:									
Men	15.8	15.9	21.0	24.7	25.3	30.3	33.0	35.2	32.3
Women	3.0	2.6	6.1	4.2	3.8	9.5	7.8	7.2	13.2
Colon (excluding rectum):									
Men	52.4	48.2	83.6	80.4	76.1	127.3	123.8	120.1	170.1
Women	41.0	37.0	61.9	58.7	54.5	93.4	99.6	95.9	134.7
Rectum and rectosigmoid junction:									
Men	32.5	30.5	37.9	42.0	40.2	41.2	59.8	57.4	58.4
Women	19.9	18.1	24.6	23.2	22.4	30.7	30.7	29.3	36.7
Liver and intrahepatic bile duct:									
Men	35.9	28.5	84.6	35.5	28.2	74.5	38.0	30.2	51.7
Women	8.9	6.8	17.3	8.5	6.4	14.5	13.1	10.9	14.1
Pancreas:									
Men	22.1	21.1	33.7	36.2	35.0	55.0	54.7	53.3	80.6
Women	15.9	15.2	23.1	25.5	24.7	35.8	37.4	35.0	61.4
Small Intestine:									
Men	5.0	5.1	6.5	6.7	6.8	8.6	9.3	8.9	13.3
Women	3.6	3.5	6.5	4.5	4.0	8.6	6.7	6.6	11.9
Anus, anal canal, and anorectum:									
Men	3.4	3.6	4.2	3.4	3.8	3.0	4.2	4.7	2.8
Women	4.6	5.0	4.5	4.9	5.1	4.1	5.5	6.1	5.1
Other digestive organs:									
Men	0.8	0.7	2.0	1.7	1.2	1.9	2.3	2.5	1.1
Women	0.7	0.6	0.8	1.2	1.2	1.2	1.6	1.5	2.6
Gallbladder:									
Men	1.0	0.8	1.5	1.5	1.1	3.4	2.9	2.5	3.3
Women	1.9	1.4	4.3	2.8	2.5	4.1	4.9	4.5	6.8
Other Biliary:									
Men	2.6	2.2	5.2	5.2	4.9	5.2	7.1	6.8	5.6
Women	1.9	2.0	1.2	2.7	2.6	3.3	5.2	4.7	6.4

[a]Surveillance, Epidemiology, and End Results program, nine standard registries, crude age-specific rates, 2005–2009 (NCI, 2013).

in blacks than in whites. Risk factors for the cancers vary but always include family history of the same form of cancer, some diseases of the affected organ, and diet. Tobacco use is a risk factor for pancreatic cancer and possibly stomach cancer (Miller et al., 1996). Infection with the bacterium *Helicobacter pylori* increases the risk of stomach and pancreatic cancer. Type 2 diabetes is associated with an increased risk of colorectal and pancreatic cancers (ACS, 2013a).

It is noteworthy that there has been one report of Vietnam veterans that included all gastrointestinal cancers collectively. Cypel and Kang (2010) published an update on disease-related mortality in ACC veterans who handled or sprayed herbicides in Vietnam in comparison with their non-Vietnam veteran peers or US men. Vital status was determined through December 31, 2005. In the analyses, the site-specific rates of digestive cancers were not examined. No statistically significant excess mortality from all cancers of the digestive tract was found in ACC Vietnam veterans compared with non-Vietnam veterans (adjusted relative risk [RR] = 1.01, 95% CI 0.56–1.83).

Several studies identified for the present update did analyses that combined several digestive cancers, so the results are not particularly informative for any cancer in the group. Boers et al. (2012) reported on stomach and pancreatic cancers, leaving an additional 28 cases of other digestive cancers, which closely matched expectation. Burns et al. (2011) reported on cancers of the stomach, colon, rectum, and pancreas individually, leaving eight deaths from "other GI and digestive cancers" (SIR = 0.73, 95% CI 0.32–1.44). After reporting on cancers of the esophagus, stomach, colon, rectum, and pancreas separately, 5 of 58 digestive cancers remained unidentified in the update on mortality in the Hamburg cohort (Manuwald et al., 2012).

Esophageal Cancer

Epithelial tumors of the esophagus (squamous-cell carcinomas and adenocarcinomas) are responsible for more than 95% of all esophageal cancers (ICD-9 150); 17,460 newly diagnosed cases and 15,070 deaths were estimated for 2012 (Siegel et al., 2012). The considerable geographic variation in the incidence of esophageal tumors suggests a multifactorial etiology. Rates of esophageal cancer have been increasing in the last 2 decades. Adenocarcinoma of the esophagus has slowly replaced squamous-cell carcinoma as the most common type of esophageal malignancy in the United States and western Europe (Blot and McLaughlin, 1999). Squamous-cell esophageal carcinoma rates are higher in blacks than in whites and higher in men than in women. Smoking and alcohol ingestion are associated with the development of squamous-cell carcinoma; these risk factors have been less thoroughly studied for esophageal adenocarcinoma, but they appear to be associated. The rapid increase in obesity in the United States has been linked to increasing rates of gastroesophageal reflux disease (GERD), and the resulting rise in chronic inflammation has been hypothesized as explaining the link between GERD and esophageal adenocarcinoma. The average annual incidence of esophageal cancers is shown in Table 8-4.

Conclusions from *VAO* and Previous Updates

The committee responsible for *VAO* explicitly excluded esophageal cancer from the group of gastrointestinal tract tumors, for which it was concluded that there was limited or suggestive evidence of *no* association with exposure to the herbicides used by the US military in Vietnam. Esophageal cancer was not separately evaluated and was not categorized with this group until *Update 2004*, so by default it fell into the category of inadequate or insufficient evidence of an association. The committee responsible for *Update 2006* concluded that there was not enough evidence on each of the COIs to sustain that negative conclusion for any of the cancers in the gastrointestinal group, and that because these various types of cancer are generally regarded as separate disease entities the evidence on each should be evaluated separately. Esophageal cancer was thus formally placed into the inadequate or insufficient category. No additional studies of esophageal cancer were reviewed in *Update 2008*.

Update 2010 considered a series of papers on mortality in TCP and PCP workers employed by Dow Chemical Company in Midland, Michigan, from 1937 to 1980. Collins et al. (2009a) followed 1,615 workers who worked at least 1 day in a department that had potential TCDD exposure, among whom five esophageal-cancer deaths were observed, for an SMR of 1.0 (95% CI = 0.3–2.2); none of the five had had concurrent PCP exposure. Collins et al. (2009b) described mortality in 773 PCP workers who were exposed to chlorinated dioxins that did not include TCDD; there were two observed deaths from esophageal cancer (SMR = 0.8, 95% CI 0.1–2.9). McBride et al. (2009a) reported on a mortality followup of the workers in the Dow AgroSciences plant in New Plymouth, New Zealand, who were potentially exposed to TCDD. The SMR for esophageal-cancer deaths in exposed workers was 2.5 (95% CI 0.7–6.4) compared with an SMR of 2.1 (95% CI 0.1–12.2) in the never-exposed group. In following up cancer incidence in the men and women exposed to dioxin in the Seveso accident, Pesatori et al. (2009) observed no esophageal cancers in the high-exposure zone and no exposure-related pattern in the occurrence of esophageal cancer in the moderate- and low-exposure areas.

Table 8-5 summarizes the results of the relevant studies concerning esophageal cancer.

Update of the Epidemiologic Literature

Vietnam-Veteran and Environmental Studies No Vietnam-veterans studies or environmental studies of exposure to the COIs and esophageal cancer have been published since *Update 2010*.

TABLE 8-5 Selected Epidemiologic Studies—Esophageal Cancer (Shaded Entries Are New Information for This Update)

Study Population[a]	Exposed Cases[b]	Exposure of Interest/Estimated Relative Risk (95% CI)[b]	Reference
VIETNAM VETERANS			
US Vietnam Veterans			
US CDC Vietnam Experience Study—Cross-sectional study, with medical examinations, of Army veterans: 9,324 deployed vs 8,989 nondeployed		**All COIs**	
Mortality			
1965–2000	6	1.2 (0.4–4.0)	Boehmer et al., 2004
State Studies of US Vietnam Veterans			
Michigan Vietnam-era veterans, PM study of deaths (1974–1989)—deployed vs nondeployed	9	0.9 (0.4–1.6)	Visintainer et al., 1995
International Studies of Vietnam Veterans			
Australian Vietnam Veterans—58,077 men and 153 women served on land or in Vietnamese waters during 5/23/1962–7/1/1973 vs Australian population		**All COIs**	
Incidence			
All branches, 1982–2000	70	1.2 (0.9–1.5)	ADVA, 2005a
Navy	19	1.6 (0.9–2.4)	
Army	40	1.1 (0.7–1.4)	
Air Force	11	1.5 (0.8–2.8)	
Mortality			
All branches, return–2001	67	1.1 (0.8–1.3)	ADVA, 2005b
Navy	13	1.0 (0.5–1.7)	
Army	42	1.0 (0.7–1.3)	
Air Force	12	1.5 (0.8–2.6)	
1980–1994	23	1.2 (0.7–1.7)	CDVA, 1997a
Australian Conscripted Army National Service (18,940 deployed vs 24,642 nondeployed)		**All COIs**	
Incidence			
1982–2000	9	1.9 (0.6–6.6)	ADVA, 2005c
Mortality			
1966–2001	10	1.3 (0.5–3.6)	ADVA, 2005c
1982–1994	1	1.3 (0.0– > 10)	CDVA, 1997b
OCCUPATIONAL—INDUSTRIAL			
IARC Phenoxy Herbicide Cohort—Workers exposed to any phenoxy herbicide or chlorophenol (production or spraying) vs respective national mortality rates			

continued

TABLE 8-5 Esophageal Cancer, continued

Study Population[a]	Exposed Cases[b]	**Exposure of Interest**/Estimated Relative Risk (95% CI)[b]	Reference
Mortality 1939–1992	28	1.0 (0.7–1.4)	Kogevinas et al., 1997
13,831 exposed to highly chlorinated PCDDs	20	1.3 (0.8–1.9)	
7,553 not exposed to highly chlorinated PCDDs	6	0.5 (0.2–1.1)	
Mortality 1955–1988 of 12,492 production workers and 5,898 sprayers exposed—13,482 in exposed subcohort	8	0.6 (0.3–1.2)	Saracci et al., 1991
British MCPA Plant—Production 1947–1982 (n = 1,545) (included in IARC cohort) and spraying 1947–1972 (n = 2,561) (*not* included in IARC cohort)		**MCPA**	
Mortality through 1983	8	0.9 (0.4–1.9)	Coggon et al., 1986
German Production Workers at Boehringer–Ingelheim Plant in Hamburg (1,144 men working > 1 month in 1952–1984; generation of TCDD reduced after chloracne outbreak in 1954) and women—no results (some additions to observed cancers over Manz et al., 1991) (in IARC cohort as of 1997)		**Dioxins; 2,4,5-T; 2,5-DCP; 2,4,5-TCP**	
Mortality 1952–2007 (ICD-9 150)			Manuwald et al., 2012
Men	11	2.6 (1.3–4.6)	
Women	0	nr	
New Zealand Phenoxy Herbicide Production Workers and Sprayers (1,599 men and women working any time in 1969–1988 at Dow plant in New Plymouth) (in IARC cohort)		**Dioxins; 2,4-D; 2,4,5-T; MCPA; MCPB; 2,4,5-TCP; Picloram**	
Mortality 1969–2004			McBride et al., 2009a
Ever-exposed workers	4	2.5 (0.7–6.4)	
Never-exposed workers	1	2.1 (0.1–12.2)	
Production Workers (713 men and 100 women worked > 1 month in 1969–1984)			
Mortality 1969–2000	2	2.0 (0.2–7.0)	't Mannetje et al., 2005
Phenoxy herbicide sprayers (> 99% men)	1	0.7 (0.0–4.0)	
All Dow TCP-Exposed Workers (TCP production 1942–1979 or 2,4,5-T production 1948–1982 in Midland, Michigan) (in IARC and NIOSH cohorts)		**2,4,5-T; 2,4,5-TCP**	
1942–2003 (n = 1,615)			Collins et al., 2009a
Trichlorophenol workers	5	1.0 (0.3–2.2)	
Pentachlorophenol workers	2	0.8 (0.1–2.9)	

TABLE 8-5 Esophageal Cancer, continued

Study Population[a]	Exposed Cases[b]	**Exposure of Interest**/Estimated Relative Risk (95% CI)[b]	Reference
All Dow PCP-Exposed Workers—all workers from two plants that only made PCP (in Tacoma, Washington, and Wichita, Kansas) and workers who made PCP and TCP at two additional plants (in Midland, Michigan, and Sauget, Illinois)		**2,4,5-T; 2,4,5-TCP**	Ruder and Yiin, 2011
1940–2005 (n = 2,122)	8	1.0 (0.4–2.0)	
PCP and TCP (n = 720)	2	0.8 (0.1–3.0)	
PCP (no TCP) (n = 1,402)	6	1.1 (0.4–2.3)	
OCCUPATIONAL—PAPER AND PULP WORKERS		**TCDD**	
IARC cohort of pulp and paper workers—60,468 workers from 11 countries, TCDD among 27 agents assessed by JEM			McLean et al., 2006
Exposure to nonvolatile organochlorine compounds			
Never	27	0.7 (0.4–1.0)	
Ever	26	0.8 (0.5–1.2)	
OCCUPATIONAL—HERBICIDE-USING WORKERS (*not* related to IARC sprayer cohorts)			
DENMARK			
Danish Farmers—incidence from linking farmers on 1970 census with national cancer registry (1970–1980)		**Herbicides**	Ronco et al., 1992
Men			
Self-employed	32	0.4 ($p < 0.05$)	
Employee	13	0.9 (nr)	
Women			
Self-employed	1	1.4 (nr)	
Employee	2	0.4 (nr)	
FINNISH Phenoxy Herbicide Sprayers (1,909 men working 1955–1971 ≥ 2 wks) *not* IARC		**Phenoxy herbicides**	
Incidence	3	1.6 (0.3–4.6)	Asp et al., 1994
Mortality 1972–1989	2	1.3 (0.2–4.7)	
NEW ZEALAND National Cancer Registry (1980–1984)—case-control study of 385 incident esophageal cancer cases vs remainder of 19,904 men with any incident cancer			Reif et al., 1989
Forestry workers (n = 134)		**Herbicides**	
	4	1.8 (0.7–4.8)	
Aged 20–59	1	1.6 (0.2–11.3)	
Aged ≥ 60	3	1.9 (0.6–5.8)	

continued

TABLE 8-5 Esophageal Cancer, continued

Study Population[a]	Exposed Cases[b]	**Exposure of Interest**/Estimated Relative Risk (95% CI)[b]	Reference
Sawmill workers (n = 139)		**Herbicides, chlorophenols**	
	2	0.7 (0.2–2.9)	
SWEDEN			
Incidence cancer cases 1961–1973 with agriculture as economic activity in 1960 census (male, female)	169	*99% CI* 0.6 (0.5–0.7)	Wiklund et al., 1983
UNITED STATES			
US Agricultural Health Study—prospective study of licensed pesticide sprayers in Iowa and North Carolina: commercial (n = 4,916), private/farmers (n = 52,395, 97.4% men), and spouses of private sprayers (n = 32,347, 0.007% men), enrolled 1993–1997; followups with CATIs 1999–2003 and 2005–2010		**Phenoxy herbicides**	
Incidence			
Enrollment through 2006—SIRs for participants			Koutros et al., 2010a
Private applicators	52	0.6 (0.5–0.9)	
Commercial applicators	2	nr	
Spouses	2	nr	
Mortality			
Enrollment through 2007, vs state rates			Waggoner et al., 2011
Applicators (n = 1,641)	48	0.5 (0.4–0.7)	
Spouses (n = 676)	3	nr	
Enrollment through 2000, vs state rates			Blair et al., 2005a
Private applicators (men and women)	16	0.5 (0.3–0.9)	
Spouses of private applicators (> 99% women)	1	0.3 (0.1–1.9)	
ENVIRONMENTAL			
Seveso, Italy Residential Cohort—Industrial accident July 10, 1976 (723 residents Zone A; 4,821 Zone B; 31,643 Zone R; 181,574 local reference group)		**TCDD**	
Incidence			
20-yr followup to 1996—men and women			
Zone A	0		Pesatori et al., 2009
Zone B	1	0.3 (0.0–1.9)	
Zone R	35	1.3 (0.9–1.9)	
CASE-CONTROL STUDIES			
US Case-Control Studies			
Nebraska—agricultural pesticide use and adenocarcinoma of the esophagus	137	**Phenoxy herbicides, 2,4-D**	Lee et al., 2004a

TABLE 8-5 Esophageal Cancer, continued

Study Population[a]	Exposed Cases[b]	**Exposure of Interest**/Estimated Relative Risk (95% CI)[b]	Reference
Insecticides		0.7 (0.4–1.1)	
Herbicides		0.7 (0.4–1.2)	
International Case-Control Studies			
UK men, 18–35 yrs of age from counties with particular chemical manufacturing—mortality		**Herbicides, chlorophenols**	Magnani et al., 1987
Herbicides	nr	1.6 (0.7–3.6)	
Chlorophenols	nr	1.2 (0.7–2.2)	

NOTE: 2,4-D, 2,4-dichlorophenoxyacetic acid; 2,4-DCP, 2,4-dichlorophenol; 2,4-DP, dichlorprop; 2,4,5-T, 2,4,5-trichlorophenoxyacetic acid; 2,4,5-TCP, 2,4,5-trichlorophenol; CATI, computer-assisted telephone interviewing; CDC, Centers for Disease Control and Prevention; CI, confidence interval; COI, chemical of interest; IARC, International Agency for Research on Cancer; ICD, International Classification of Diseases; JEM, job-exposure matrix; MCPA, 2 methyl-4-chlorophenoxyacetic acid; MCPB, 4-(4-chloro-2-methylphenoxy)butanoic acid; NIOSH, National Institute for Occupational Safety and Health; nr, not reported; PM, proportionate mortality; PCDD, polychlorinated dibenzo-*p*-dioxin (highly chlorinated, if four or more chlorines); PCP, pentachlorophenol; TCDD, 2,3,7,8-tetrachlorodibenzo-*p*-dioxin; TCP, trichlorophenol.

[a]Subjects are male and outcome is mortality unless otherwise noted.

[b]Given when available; results other than estimated risk explained individually.

Occupational Studies Starting with a set of 1,316 in 2,4-D-exposed workers, Burns et al. (2011) identified cancer cases through 2007 in the Michigan's cancer registry from its start in 1985. The analysis of the third (and most stringently defined in terms of continued residence in Michigan) of the nested cohorts of workers included 1,108 men who were employed in a Dow facility in Midland during 1945–1994 and were alive on January 1, 1985. Esophageal cancers were not reported separately and so would have fallen in the category of "other GI and digestive cancers," in which there were eight cases (SIR = 1.02, 95% CI 0.44–2.02).

Manuwald et al. (2012) reported mortality in 1,191 men and 398 women who had been employed for at least 3 months during 1952–1984 in a chemical plant in Hamburg (a subcohort of the IARC phenoxy-herbicide cohort). During that period, the plant produced insecticides and herbicides, including 2,4,5-T, so cohort members had the possibility of exposure to TCDD. Subjects entered the cohort on the date of their first employment at the plant, and vital status was sought through 2007. No deaths from esophageal cancer in female workers were reported, but esophageal-cancer mortality relative to that in the population of Hamburg was increased in men (SMR = 2.56, 95% CI 1.27–4.57).

Ruder and Yiin (2011) reported mortality in 1940–2005 in the NIOSH PCP cohort of 2,122 workers in the four US plants that had been involved in PCP production. PCP production entailed exposure to PCDDs and PCDFs but not to the most toxic 2,3,7,8 dioxin congener. A subcohort of 720 workers (all men, the PCP-plus-TCDD group) had also been employed in TCP production and so had also been exposed to TCDD. In the total cohort, eight deaths were attributed to esophageal cancer; that is consistent with the mortality experience of the US population (SMR = 0.99, 95% CI 0.43–1.96). There were two deaths in the PCP-plus-TCDD group, not more than expected (SMR = 0.82, 95% CI 0.10–2.95). The results were effectively the same in the 1,402 workers who had not had any opportunity for occupational exposure to TCDD (SMR = 1.07, 95% CI 0.39–2.33).

The participants in the AHS are known to have had extensive exposure to the phenoxy herbicides, but the analyses of updated mortality (Waggoner et al., 2011) and cancer incidence (Koutros et al., 2010a) address only exposure to pesticides in general. Waggoner et al. (2011) reported lower numbers of deaths from cancer of the esophagus than expected on the basis of state rates in the applicators (SMR = 0.51, 95% CI 0.38–0.68). Only three cases of espophageal cancer were observed in the spouses. In the update of cancer incidence through 2006, Koutros et al. (2010a) found a significant decrease in the incidence of esophageal cancer in the private applicators (52 cases, SIR = 0.64, 95% CI 0.48–0.85). Only two cases of esophageal cancer were observed in the spouses. The AHS has been generating valuable information on the COIs for a number of years, but these results are not herbicide-specific and so are not regarded as being fully informative for the committee's task.

Case-Control Studies Meyer et al. (2011) conducted a case-control study of esophageal cancer in Brazilians in which occupation was obtained from death certificates. Being an agricultural worker was used as a surrogate for pesticide exposure, so exposure specificity was inadequate for the purpose of this review.

Biologic Plausibility

Long-term animal studies have examined the effect of exposure to the COIs on tumor incidence (Charles et al., 1996; Stott et al., 1990; Walker et al., 2006; Wanibuchi et al., 2004), and no increase in the incidence of esophageal cancer has been reported in laboratory animals after exposure to them. A previous biomarker study analyzed esophageal-cell samples from patients who had been exposed to indoor air pollution of different magnitudes and did or did not have high-grade squamous-cell dysplasia or a family history of upper gastrointestinal-tract (UGI) cancer (Roth et al., 2009). AHR expression was higher in patients who had a family history of UGI cancer but was not associated with indoor air pollution, esophageal squamous-cell dysplasia category, age, sex, or smoking. The results suggest that enhanced expression of the AHR in patients who had a family history of UGI cancer may contribute to UGI-cancer risk associated with AHR ligands—such as polycyclic aromatic hydrocarbons, which are found in cigarette smoke—and with TCDD.

In a small series, AHR expression was found to be higher in esophageal tumors than in corresponding normal mucosa (Zhang et al., 2012).

The biologic plausibility of the carcinogenicity of the COIs is discussed in general at the beginning of this chapter.

Synthesis

Manuwald et al. (2012) reported a significant increase in mortality from esophageal cancer in the men in the Hamburg cohort of phenoxy-herbicide workers. In combination with the studies reviewed previously, however, that single new finding did not provide adequate evidence to establish an association between exposure to the COIs and esophageal cancer. No toxicologic studies provide evidence of the biologic plausibility of an association between the COIs and tumors of the esophagus.

Conclusion

On the basis of the evidence reviewed here and in previous VAO reports, the committee concludes that there is inadequate or insufficient evidence to determine whether there is an association between exposure to the COIs and esophageal cancer.

Stomach Cancer

The incidence of stomach cancer (ICD-9 151) increases with age. ACS estimated that 13,020 men and 8,300 women would receive diagnoses of stomach cancer in the United States in 2012 and that 6,190 men and 4,350 women would die from it (Siegel et al., 2012). In general, the incidence is higher in men than in women and higher in blacks than in whites. Other risk factors include family history of this cancer, some diseases of the stomach, and diet. Infection with *Helicobacter pylori* increases the risk of stomach cancer. Tobacco use and consumption of nitrite- and salt-preserved food may also increase the risk (Brenner et al., 2009; Key et al., 2004; Miller et al., 1996). The average annual incidence of stomach cancer is shown in Table 8-4.

Conclusions from *VAO* and Previous Updates

Update 2006 considered stomach cancer independently for the first time. Prior updates developed a table of results for stomach cancer but drew conclusions about the adequacy of the evidence of its association with herbicide exposure in the context of gastrointestinal tract cancers. The committee responsible for *VAO* concluded that there was limited or suggestive evidence of *no* association between exposure to the herbicides used by the US military in Vietnam and gastrointestinal tract tumors, including stomach cancer. The committee responsible for *Update 2006* concluded that there was not enough evidence on each of the COIs to sustain that negative conclusion for any of the cancers in the gastrointestinal group and that, because these various types of cancer are generally regarded as separate disease entities, the evidence on each should be evaluated separately. Stomach cancer was thus reclassified into the default category of inadequate or insufficient evidence to determine whether there is an association.

Positive findings of an association with phenoxy-herbicide exposure from a well-conducted nested case-control study of stomach cancer in the United Farm Workers of America cohort (Mills and Yang, 2007) led the committee responsible for *Update 2008* to reconsider the results of several earlier studies. Reif et al. (1989) reported a significant relationship between stomach cancer and the nonspecific exposure of being a forestry worker. Cocco et al. (1999) had found an association with herbicide exposure but had not analyzed specific chemicals, and Ekström et al. (1999) found significant associations between the occurrence of stomach cancer and exposure to phenoxy herbicides in general and to several specific phenoxy-herbicide products. In updated mortality findings from Seveso concerning TCDD exposure, Consonni et al. (2008) found no increases in deaths from stomach cancer. In the absence of supportive findings from studies of Vietnam-veteran cohorts or IARC cohorts or from the US AHS, that committee retained stomach cancer in the inadequate or insufficient category.

Between *Update 2008* and *Update 2010*, studies of three occupational cohorts and two environmental-study populations were published. In examining mortality in workers employed by Dow Chemical Company in Midland, Michigan, during 1937–1980, Collins et al. (2009a) observed eight cases of stomach cancer in 1,615 TCP workers (SMR = 1.4, 95% CI 0.6–2.7) and four deaths from stomach cancer in 773 PCP workers (SMR = 1.2, 95% CI 0.3–3.1). McBride et al. (2009a) reported on mortality in workers in the Dow AgroSciences plant in New Plymouth, New Zealand, who were potentially exposed to TCDD; mortality from stomach cancer was somewhat higher in the never-exposed group (SMR = 2.3, 95% CI 0.3–8.4) than in exposed workers (SMR = 1.4, 95% CI 0.4–3.6). In the third followup of a retrospective cohort study of two Dutch chlorophenoxy-herbicide manufacturing factories, Boers et al. (2010) found that neither had increased mortality from stomach cancer. An update of cancer incidence in the Seveso cohort (Pesatori et al., 2009) found no evidence of an increase in stomach cancer. In a second environmental study, Turunen et al. (2008) assessed mortality in Finnish fishermen and their wives, presuming that their mortality would reflect their high consumption of contaminated fish; death from stomach cancer was not increased.

Table 8-6 summarizes the results of the relevant studies concerning stomach cancer.

TABLE 8-6 Selected Epidemiologic Studies—Stomach Cancer (Shaded Entries Are New Information for This Update)

Study Population[a]	Exposed Cases[b]	**Exposure of Interest**/Estimated Relative Risk (95% CI)[b]	Reference
VIETNAM VETERANS			
US Vietnam Veterans			
US Air Force Health Study—Ranch Hand veterans vs SEA veterans (unless otherwise noted)		**All COIs**	
Incidence			
1982–2003—White SEA comparison veterans only (n = 1,482). Serum TCDD (pg/g) based on model with exposure variable $\log_e$(TCDD)			Pavuk et al., 2005
Per unit increase of $-\log_e$(TCDD) (pg/g)	24	1.8 (0.8–3.9)	
Quartiles (pg/g):			
0.4–2.6	4	nr	
2.6–3.8	3	1.0 (0.2–4.8)	
3.8–5.2	7	2.0 (0.5–8.2)	
> 5.2	10	3.3 (0.9–12.5)	
Number of years served in SEA (per year of service)			
Quartiles (years in SEA):	24	1.2 (1.0–1.4)	
0.8–1.3	4	nr	
1.3–2.1	4	1.0 (0.2–3.8)	
2.1–3.7	5	1.1 (0.3–4.2)	
3.7–16.4	11	2.1 (0.6–7.3)	
Through 1999—White subjects vs national rates			Akhtar et al., 2004
Ranch Hand veterans (n = 1,189)	16	0.6 (0.4–1.0)	
With tours between 1966–1970	14	0.6 (0.4–1.1)	
SEA comparison veterans (n = 1,776)	31	0.9 (0.6–1.2)	
With tours between 1966–1970	24	0.9 (0.6–1.3)	
Mortality			
Through 1999—White subjects vs national rates			Akhtar et al., 2004
Ranch Hand veterans (n = 1,189)	6	0.4 (0.2–0.9)	
SEA comparison veterans (n = 1,776)	14	0.7 (0.4–1.1)	
US CDC Vietnam Experience Study—Cross-sectional study, with medical examinations, of Army veterans: 9,324 deployed vs 8,989 nondeployed		**All COIs**	
Mortality			
1965–2000	5	nr	Boehmer et al., 2004
US VA Proportionate Mortality Study—sample of deceased male Vietnam-era Army and Marine veterans who served 7/4/1965–3/1/1973		**All COIs**	

continued

TABLE 8-6 Stomach Cancer, continued

Study Population[a]	Exposed Cases[b]	**Exposure of Interest**/Estimated Relative Risk (95% CI)[b]	Reference
1965–1982			Breslin
Army, deployed (n = 19,708) vs nondeployed (n = 22,904)	88	1.1 (0.9–1.5)	et al., 1988
Marine Corps, deployed (n = 4,527) vs nondeployed (n = 3,781)	17	0.8 (0.4–1.6)	
State Studies of US Vietnam Veterans			
923 White male Vietnam veterans with **Wisconsin** death certificate (1968–1978) vs proportions for Vietnam-era veterans	1	nr	Anderson et al., 1986
International Vietnam-Veteran Studies			
Australian Vietnam Veterans—58,077 men and 153 women served on land or in Vietnamese waters during 5/23/1962–7/1/1973 vs Australian population		**All COIs**	
Incidence			
All branches, 1982–2000	104	0.9 (0.7–1.1)	ADVA,
Navy	28	1.1 (0.7–1.6)	2005a
Army	66	0.9 (0.7–1.1)	
Air Force	10	0.7 (0.3–1.3)	
Mortality			
All branches, return–2001	76	0.9 (0.7–1.2)	ADVA,
Navy	22	1.3 (0.8–1.8)	2005b
Army	50	0.9 (0.7–1.2)	
Air Force	4	0.4 (0.1–1.0)	
1980–1994	32	1.1 (0.7–1.4)	CDVA, 1997a
Australian Conscripted Army National Service (18,940 deployed vs 24,642 nondeployed)		**All COIs**	
Incidence			
1982–2000	11	0.6 (0.2–1.2)	ADVA, 2005c
Mortality			
1966–2001	7	0.7 (0.2–2.0)	ADVA, 2005c
1982–1994	4	1.7 (0.3– > 10)	CDVA, 1997b
OCCUPATIONAL—INDUSTRIAL			
IARC Phenoxy Herbicide Cohort—Workers exposed to any phenoxy herbicide or chlorophenol (production or spraying) vs respective national mortality rates		**Phenoxy herbicides, chlorophenols**	
Mortality 1939–1992	72	0.9 (0.7–1.1)	Kogevinas
13,831 exposed to highly chlorinated PCDDs	42	0.9 (0.7–1.2)	et al., 1997
7,553 not exposed to highly chlorinated PCDDs	30	0.9 (0.6–1.3)	

TABLE 8-6 Stomach Cancer, continued

Study Population[a]	Exposed Cases[b]	**Exposure of Interest**/Estimated Relative Risk (95% CI)[b]	Reference
Mortality 1955–1988 of 12,492 production workers and 5,898 sprayers exposed—13,482 in exposed subcohort			Saracci et al., 1991
Nested case-control study	40	0.9 (0.6–1.2)	
Mortality, incidence of women in production (n = 699) and spraying (n = 2) compared to national death rates and cancer incidence rates	1	**TCDD** 1.4 (nr)	Kogevinas et al, 1993
British MCPA Plant—Production 1947–1982 (n = 1,545) (included in IARC cohort) and spraying 1947–1972 (n = 2,561) (*not* included in IARC cohort)		**MCPA**	
Mortality through 1983	26	0.9 (0.6–1.3)	Coggon et al., 1986
Danish Production Workers (3,390 men and 1,069 women involved in production of phenoxy herbicides unlikely to contain TCDD at 2 plants in 1947–1987) (in IARC cohort)		**Dioxins, but TCDD unlikely; 2,4-D, 2,4-DP, MCPA, MCPP**	
Incidence 1943–1982			Lynge, 1985
Men	12	1.3 (nr)	
Women	1	0.7 (nr)	
Mortality 1955–2006	14	1.1 (0.8–1.5)	Boers et al., 2012
TCDD plasma level (hazard ratios, by tertile)			
Background (≤ 0.4)	8	—	
Low (0.4–1.9)	1	0.1 (0.0–1.0)	
Medium (1.9–9.9)	2	0.5 (0.1–2.6)	
High (≥ 9.9)	3	2.5 (0.7–9.2)	
Dutch production workers in Plant A (549 men exposed during production 1955–1985; 594 unexposed) (in IARC cohort)		**Dioxins, 2,4,5-T, 2,4,5-TCP**	
Mortality 1955–2006 (HRs for lagged TCDD plasma levels)	6	1.5 (1.1–2.2)	Boers et al., 2012
Mortality 1955–2006	5	2.2 (0.4–13.2)	Boers et al. 2010
Mortality 1955–1991	3	1.0 (0.2–2.9)	Hooiveld et al., 1998
Mortality 1955–1985	2	0.9 (0.1–3.4)	Bueno de Mesquita et al., 1993
Dutch production workers in Plant B (414 men exposed during production 1965–1986; 723 unexposed) (in IARC cohort)		**2,4-D; MCPA; MCPP; highly chlorinated dioxins unlikely**	
Mortality 1965–2006	4	1.2 (0.3–4.7)	Boers et al., 2010

continued

TABLE 8-6 Stomach Cancer, continued

Study Population[a]	Exposed Cases[b]	**Exposure of Interest**/Estimated Relative Risk (95% CI)[b]	Reference
Mortality 1965–1986	0	0.0 (0.0–6.5)	Bueno de Mesquita et al., 1993
German Production Workers at Bayer Plant in Uerdingen (135 men working > 1 month in 1951–1976) (in IARC cohort as of 1997) and women—no results		**Dioxins; 2,4,5-TCP**	
Mortality 1951–1992	0	nr	Becher et al., 1996
German Production Workers at Bayer Plant in Dormagen (520 men working > 1 month in 1965–1989) (in IARC cohort as of 1997) and women—no results		**Dioxins; 2,4-D; 2,4,5-T; MCPA; MCPP; 2,4-DP**	
Mortality 1965–1989	0	nr	Becher et al., 1996
German Production Workers at BASF Ludwigshafen Plant (680 men working > 1 month in 1957–1987) (in IARC cohort as of 1997) and women—no results		**Dioxins; 2,4-D; 2,4,5-T; MCPA; MCPP; 2,4-DP**	
Mortality 1956–1989	2	0.6 (0.1–2.3)	Becher et al., 1996
BASF Cleanup Workers from 1953 accident (n = 247); 114 with chloracne, 13 more with erythema; serum TCDD levels (*not* part of IARC)		**Focus on TCDD**	
Incidence			
1960–1992	3	1.0 (0.2–2.9)	Ott and Zober, 1996
TCDD < 0.1 μg/kg of body weight	0	0.0 (0.0–3.4)	
TCDD 0.1–0.99 μg/kg of body weight	1	1.3 (0.0–7.0)	
TCDD > 1 μg/kg of body weight	2	1.7 (0.2–6.2)	
Mortality			
Through 1987		*90% CI*	Zober et al., 1990
	3	3.0 (0.8–7.7)	
German Production Workers at Boehringer–Ingelheim Plant in Hamburg (1,144 men working > 1 month in 1952–1984; generation of TCDD reduced after chloracne outbreak in 1954) and women—no results (some additions to observed cancers over Manz et al., 1991) (in IARC cohort as of 1997)		**Dioxins; 2,4,5-T; 2,5-DCP; 2,4,5-TCP**	
Mortality 1952–2007 (ICD-9 140–149)	17	1.0 (0.6–1.6)	Manuwald et al., 2012
Men	17	1.3 (0.7–2.0)	
Women	0	nr	
Mortality 1952–1989	12	1.3 (0.7–2.2)	Becher et al., 1996

TABLE 8-6 Stomach Cancer, continued

Study Population[a]	Exposed Cases[b]	**Exposure of Interest**/Estimated Relative Risk (95% CI)[b]	Reference
Mortality 1952–1989—stats on men only, 1,184 (tables all for 1,148 men, not necessarily German nationals) vs national rates (also vs gas workers); same observation period as Becher et al., 1996	12	1.2 (0.6–2.1)	Manz et al., 1991
New Zealand Phenoxy Herbicide Production Workers and Sprayers (1,599 men and women working any time in 1969–1988 at Dow plant in New Plymouth) (in IARC cohort)		**Dioxins; 2,4-D; 2,4,5-T; MCPA; MCPB; 2,4,5-TCP; Picloram**	
Mortality 1969–2004			McBride et al., 2009a
Ever-exposed workers	4	1.4 (0.4–3.6)	
Never-exposed workers	2	2.3 (0.3–8.4)	
Production Workers (713 men and 100 women worked > 1 month in 1969–1984)			
Mortality 1969–2000	2	1.1 (0.1–4.0)	't Mannetje et al., 2005
Phenoxy herbicide sprayers (> 99% men)	3	1.4 (0.3–4.0)	
NIOSH Mortality Cohort (12 US plants, 5,172 male production and maintenance workers 1942–1984) (included in IARC cohort as of 1997)		**Dioxins, phenoxy herbicides**	
Through 1993	13	1.0 (0.6–1.8)	Steenland et al., 1999
Through 1987	10	1.0 (0.5–1.9)	Fingerhut et al., 1991
≥ 1-year exposure, ≥ 20-year latency	4	1.4 (0.4–3.5)	
Mortality—754 Monsanto workers, among most highly exposed workers from Fingerhut et al. (1991)	0	0.0 (0.0–1.1)	Collins et al., 1993
All Dow TCP-Exposed Workers (TCP production 1942–1979 or 2,4,5-T production 1948–1982 in Midland, Michigan) (in IARC and NIOSH cohorts)		**2,4,5-T; 2,4,5-TCP**	
1942–2003 (n = 1,615)	8	1.4 (0.6–2.7)	Collins et al., 2009a
1940–1994 (n = 2,187 men)	nr	1.5 (0.7–2.7)	Bodner et al., 2003
All Dow PCP-Exposed Workers—all workers from the two plants that only made PCP (in Tacoma, Washington, and Wichita, Kansas) and workers who made PCP and TCP at two additional plants (in Midland, Michigan, and Sauget, Illinois)		**2,4,5-T; 2,4,5-TCP**	Ruder and Yiin, 2011
1940–2005 (n = 2,122)	9	0.9 (0.4–1.7)	
PCP and TCP (n = 720)	3	1.0 (0.2–2.9)	
PCP (no TCP) (n = 1,402)	6	0.8 (0.3–1.8)	

continued

TABLE 8-6 Stomach Cancer, continued

Study Population[a]	Exposed Cases[b]	**Exposure of Interest**/Estimated Relative Risk (95% CI)[b]	Reference
Dow 2,4-D Production Workers (1945–1982 in Midland, Michigan) (subset of all TCP-exposed workers)		**2,4-D, lower chlorinated dioxins**	
Cancer incidence through 2007 in Dow workers (n = 1,256) vs comparisons from state cancer registries (n = 23,354) (Cohort 3)	3	0.8 (0.2–2.3)	Burns et al., 2011
Through 1994 (n = 1,517) (digestive organs, peritoneum)	16	0.7 (0.4–1.2)	Burns et al., 2001
Through 1982 (n = 878)	0	nr (0.0–3.7)	Bond et al., 1988
Dow PCP Production Workers (1937–1989 in Midland, Michigan) (*not* in IARC and NIOSH cohorts)		**Low chlorinated dioxins, 2,4-D**	
Mortality 1940–2004 (n = 577, excluding 196 also having exposure to TCP)	4	1.2 (0.3–3.1)	Collins et al., 2009b
Mortality 1940–1989 (n = 770)			Ramlow et al., 1996
0-yr latency	4	1.7 (0.5–4.3)	
15-yr latency	3	1.8 (0.4–5.2)	
Other Studies of Industrial Workers (*not* related to IARC or NIOSH phenoxy cohorts)		**Dioxins, phenoxy herbicides**	
1,412 white male US flavor and fragrance chemical plant workers (1945–1965)		**Dioxin, 2,4,5-T**	Thomas, 1987
		Expected exposed cases	
	6	4.2	
OCCUPATIONAL—PAPER AND PULP WORKERS		**TCDD**	
IARC cohort of pulp and paper workers—60,468 workers from 11 countries, TCDD among 27 agents assessed by JEM			McLean et al., 2006
Exposure to nonvolatile organochlorine compounds			
Never	146	0.9 (0.8–1.1)	
Ever	98	0.9 (0.7–1.1)	
14,362 **Danish paper workers** employed 1943–1990, followed through 1993			Rix et al., 1998
Men	48	1.1 (0.8–1.4)	
Women	7	1.0 (0.4–2.1)	
New Hampshire pulp and paper workers, 883 white men working ≥ 1 yr, mortality through July 1985	5	1.2 (0.4–2.8)	Henneberger et al., 1989
Pulp and Paper cohorts independent of IARC cohort			
United Paperworkers International, 201 white men employed ≥ 10 yrs and dying 1970–1984	1	0.5 (0.1–3.0)	Solet et al., 1989

TABLE 8-6 Stomach Cancer, continued

Study Population[a]	Exposed Cases[b]	**Exposure of Interest**/Estimated Relative Risk (95% CI)[b]	Reference
Northwestern US paper and pulp workers—5 mills in Washington, Oregon, and California, 3,523 worked ≥ 1 yr 1945–1955, mortality through March 1977	17	*90% CI* 1.2 (0.8–1.9)	Robinson et al., 1986
OCCUPATIONAL—HERBICIDE-USING WORKERS (*not* related to IARC sprayer cohorts)			
CANADA			
Canadian Farm Operator Study—156,242 men farming in Manitoba, Saskatchewan, and Alberta in 1971; mortality from stomach cancer June 1971–December 1987			
Linkage of records for ~70,000 male Saskatchewan farmers (1971–1985)	246	0.9 (0.8–1.0)	Wigle et al., 1990
DENMARK			
Danish farmers—incidence from linking farmers on 1970 census with national cancer registry (1970–1980)		**Herbicides**	Ronco et al., 1992
Men			
Self-employed	286	0.9 (nr)	
Employee	71	1.2 (nr)	
Women			
Self-employed	5	1.0 (nr)	
Employee	5	1.7 (nr)	
ITALIAN Licensed Pesticide Users—male farmers in southern Piedmont licensed 1970–1974			
Mortality 1970–1986 (n = 23,401)	126	0.7 (0.6–0.9)	Torchio et al., 1994
Italian rice growers with documented phenoxy use (n = 1,487)		**Phenoxy herbicides**	Gambini et al., 1997
	39	1.0 (0.7–1.3)	
NEW ZEALAND National Cancer Registry (1980–1984)—case-control study of incident stomach cancer cases vs remainder of 19,904 men with any incident cancer			Reif et al., 1989
Forestry workers (n = 134)		**Herbicides**	
	13	2.2 (1.3–3.9)	
Aged 20–59	3	0.7 (0.2–2.2)	
Aged ≥ 60	10	2.4 (1.2–4.5)	
Sawmill workers (n = 139)		**Herbicides, chlorophenols**	
	7	1.0 (0.4–2.1)	
SWEDEN			
348 Swedish railroad workers (1957–October, 1978)—total exposure to herbicides	3	**Phenoxy acids** 2.2 (nr)	Axelson et al., 1980

continued

TABLE 8-6 Stomach Cancer, continued

Study Population[a]	Exposed Cases[b]	**Exposure of Interest**/Estimated Relative Risk (95% CI)[b]	Reference
Incident stomach cancer cases 1961–1973 with agriculture as economic activity in 1960 census	2,599	*99% CI* 1.1 (1.0–1.2)	Wiklund, 1983
THE NETHERLANDS			
Dutch Licensed Herbicide Sprayers—1,341 certified before 1980			
Through 2000 (stomach, small intestine)	3	0.4 (0.1–1.3)	Swaen et al., 2004
Through 1987 (stomach, small intestine)	1	0.5 (0.0–2.7)	Swaen et al., 1992
UNITED STATES			
US farmers—usual occupation of farmer and industry of agriculture on death certificates 1984–1988 from 23 states		**Herbicides** PCMRs	Blair et al., 1993
Men			
Whites (n = 119,648)	657	1.0 (1.0–1.1)	
Nonwhites (n = 11,446)	115	1.1 (0.9–1.3)	
Women			
Whites (n = 2,400)	12	1.2 (0.6–2.0)	
Nonwhites (n = 2,066)	23	1.9 (1.2–2.8)	
US Agricultural Health Study—prospective study of licensed pesticide sprayers in Iowa and North Carolina: commercial (n = 4,916), private/farmers (n = 52,395, 97.4% men), and spouses of private sprayers (n = 32,347, 0.007% men), enrolled 1993–1997; followups with CATIs 1999–2003 and 2005–2010		**Phenoxy herbicides**	
Incidence			
Enrollment through 2006—SIRs for participants			Koutros et al., 2010a
Private applicators	61	0.9 (0.7–1.1)	
Commercial applicators	2	nr	
Spouses	15	0.9 (0.5–1.5)	
Enrollment through 2002			Alavanja et al., 2005
Private applicators	462	0.8 (0.8–0.9)	
Spouses of private applicators (> 99% women)	161	0.9 (0.7–1.0)	
Commercial applicators	24	1.0 (0.6–1.4)	
Mortality			
Enrollment through 2007, vs state rates			Waggoner et al., 2011
Applicators (n = 1,641)	26	0.5 (0.3–0.8)	
Spouses (n = 676)	5	0.4 (0.1–1.0)	
Enrollment through 2000, vs state rates			Blair et al., 2005a
Private applicators (men and women)	10	0.5 (0.2–1.0)	
Spouses of private applicators (> 99% women)	4	1.1 (0.3–2.8)	

TABLE 8-6 Stomach Cancer, continued

Study Population[a]	Exposed Cases[b]	**Exposure of Interest**/Estimated Relative Risk (95% CI)[b]	Reference
California United Farm Workers of America		**2,4-D**	
Nested case-control study of agricultural exposure and gastric cancer in UFW cohort			Mills and Yang, 2007
Ever worked in area where 2,4-D used	42	1.9 (1.1–3.3)	
Quartile of lifetime exposure to 2,4-D (lb)			
0	58	1.0	
1–14	17	2.2 (1.0–4.6)	
15–85	14	1.6 (0.7–3.5)	
85–1,950	11	2.1 (0.9–5.1)	
US Department of Agriculture Workers—nested case-control study of white men dying 1970–1979 of stomach cancer		**Herbicides**	
Agricultural extension agents	10	0.7 (0.4–1.4)	Alavanja et al., 1988
Forest conservationists		p-trend < over years worked	Alavanja et al., 1989
	9	0.7 (0.3–1.3)	
Soil conservationists			
Florida pesticide applicators licensed 1965–1966 (n = 3,827)—mortality through 1976		**Herbicides**	Blair et al., 1983
Any pesticide (dose-response by length of licensure)		*Expected exposed cases*	
	4	3.3	
White Male Residents of Iowa—stomach cancer on death certificate, usual occupation: farmers vs not		**Herbicides**	
> 30 yrs old when died 1964–1978—case-control	1,812	1.3 (p < 0.05)	Burmeister et al., 1983
H_0: only for "modern methods" → born after 1900			
Born before 1880	458	1.3 (p < 0.05)	
Born 1980–1900	639	1.3 (p < 0.05)	
Born after 1900	715	1.3 (p < 0.05)	
> 20 yrs old when died 1971–1978—PMR	338	1.1 (p < 0.01)	Burmeister, 1981
ENVIRONMENTAL			
Seveso, Italy Residential Cohort—Industrial accident July 10, 1976 (723 residents Zone A; 4,821 Zone B; 31,643 Zone R; 181,574 local reference group) (ICD-9 171)		**TCDD**	
Incidence			
20-yr followup to 1996—men and women			
Zone A	3	0.9 (0.3–2.7)	Pesatori et al., 2009
Zone B	19	0.9 (0.6–1.4)	

continued

TABLE 8-6 Stomach Cancer, continued

Study Population[a]	Exposed Cases[b]	**Exposure of Interest**/Estimated Relative Risk (95% CI)[b]	Reference
Zone R	131	0.8 (0.7–1.0)	
10-yr followup to 1991—men			Bertazzi et al., 1993
Zone B	7	1.0 (0.5–2.1)	
Zone R	45	0.9 (0.7–1.2)	
10-yr followup to 1991—women			Bertazzi et al., 1993
Zone B	2	0.6 (0.2–2.5)	
Zone R	25	1.0 (0.6–1.5)	
Mortality			
25-yr followup to 2001—men and women			Consonni et al., 2008
Zone A	3	0.7 (0.2–2.0)	
Zone B	24	0.8 (0.5–1.2)	
Zone R	212	1.0 (0.8–1.1)	
20-yr followup to 1996			Bertazzi et al., 2001
Zones A and B—men	16	0.9 (0.5–1.5)	
Zones A and B—women	11	1.0 (0.6–1.9)	
15-yr followup to 1991—men			Bertazzi et al., 1997, 1998
Zone B	10	0.8 (0.4–1.5)	
Zone R	76	0.9 (0.7–1.1)	
15-yr followup to 1991—women			Bertazzi et al., 1997, 1998
Zone A	1	0.9 (0.0–5.3)	
Zone B	7	1.0 (0.4–2.1)	
Zone R	58	1.0 (0.8–1.3)	
10-yr followup to 1986—men			Bertazzi et al., 1989a
Zone A, B, R	40	0.8 (0.6–1.2)	
10-yr followup to 1986—women			Bertazzi et al., 1989a
Zone A, B, R	22	1.0 (0.6–1.5)	
10-yr followup to 1986—men			Bertazzi et al., 1989b
Zone B	7	1.2 (0.6–2.6)	
Ecological Study of Residents of Chapaevsk, Russia		**Dioxin**	Revich et al., 2001
Incidence—Crude incidence rate in 1998 vs			
Men			
Regional (Samara)	nr	44.0 (nr)	
National (Russia)	nr	48.1 (nr)	
Women			
Regional (Samara)	nr	17.6 (nr)	
National (Russia)	nr	20.7 (nr)	
Mortality—1995–1998 (SMR vs regional rates)			
Men	59	1.7 (1.3–2.2)	
Women	45	0.7 (0.5–0.9)	
FINLAND			
Finnish fishermen (n = 6,410) and spouses (n = 4,260) registered between 1980 and 2002 compared to national statistics		**Serum dioxin**	Turunen et al., 2008
Fisherman	16	0.8 (0.5–1.3)	

TABLE 8-6 Stomach Cancer, continued

Study Population[a]	Exposed Cases[b]	**Exposure of Interest**/Estimated Relative Risk (95% CI)[b]	Reference
Spouses	2	0.3 (0.0–1.1)	
JAPAN			
Residents of municipalities with and without waste incineration plants (cross-sectional)		**Dioxin emissions** age-adjusted mortality (per 100,000)	Fukuda et al., 2003
Men			
With		38.2 ± 7.8 vs	
Without		39.0 ± 8.8 (p = 0.29)	
Women			
With		20.7 ± 5.0 vs	
Without		20.7 ± 5.8 (p = 0.92)	
SWEDEN			
Swedish fishermen (high consumption of fish with persistent organochlorines)		**Organochlorine compounds**	Svensson et al., 1995
Incidence			
East coast	24	1.6 (1.0–2.4)	
West coast	71	0.9 (0.7–1.2)	
Mortality			
East coast	17	1.4 (0.8–2.2)	
West coast	63	0.9 (0.7–1.2)	
CASE-CONTROL STUDIES			
US Case-Control Studies			
Eastern **Nebraska**—population-based case-control, agricultural pesticide use and adenocarcinoma of stomach	170	**Herbicides, pesticides**	Lee et al., 2004a
Insecticides		0.9 (0.6–1.4)	
Herbicides		0.9 (0.5–1.4)	
International Case-Control Studies			
Swedish—population-based case-control study of residents (40–79 yrs of age) with gastric adenocarcinoma (February 1989–January 1995)		**Phenoxy herbicides**	Ekström et al., 1999
All occupational herbicide exposures	75	1.6 (1.1–2.2)	
Phenoxyacetic acid exposure	62	1.8 (1.3–2.6)	
Hormoslyr (2,4-D, 2,4,5-T)	48	1.7 (1.2–2.6)	
2,4-D only	3	nr (vs 0 controls)	
MCPA	11	1.8 (0.8–4.1)	
Duration of Exposure			
Nonexposed to all herbicides	490	1.0	
< 1 month	11	1.6 (0.7–3.5)	
1–6 months	30	1.9 (1.1–3.2)	
7–12 months	7	1.7 (0.6–4.7)	

continued

TABLE 8-6 Stomach Cancer, continued

Study Population[a]	Exposed Cases[b]	**Exposure of Interest**/Estimated Relative Risk (95% CI)[b]	Reference
> 1 yr	13	1.4 (0.6–3.0)	
Other herbicide exposure	13	1.0 (0.5–1.9)	

NOTE: 2,4-D, 2,4-dichlorophenoxyacetic acid; 2,4-DP, dichlorprop; 2,4,5-T, 2,4,5-trichlorophenoxyacetic acid; 2,4,5-TCP, 2,4,5-trichlorophenol; 2,5-DCP, 2,5-dichlorophenol; CATI, computer-assisted telephone interviewing; CDC, Centers for Disease Control and Prevention; CI, confidence interval; COI, chemical of interest; IARC, International Agency for Research on Cancer; ICD, International Classification of Diseases; JEM, job-exposure matrix; MCPA, 2-methyl-4-chlorophenoxyacetic acid; MCPB, 4-(4-chloro-2-methylphenoxy)butanoic acid; MCPP, methylchlorophenoxypropionic acid; NIOSH, National Institute for Occupational Safety and Health; nr, not reported; PCDD, polychlorinated dibenzo-*p*-dioxin (highly chlorinated, if four or more chlorines); PCMR, proportionate cancer mortality ratios; PCP, pentachlorophenol; PMR, proportionate mortality ratio; SEA, Southeast Asia; SIR, standardized incidence ratio; SMR, standardized mortality ratio; TCDD, 2,3,7,8-tetrachlorodibenzo-*p*-dioxin; TCP, trichlorophenol; UFW, United Farm Workers of America; VA, US Department of Veterans Affairs.

[a]Subjects are male and outcome is mortality unless otherwise noted.

[b]Given when available; results other than estimated risk explained individually.

Update of the Epidemiologic Literature

Vietnam-Veteran and Environmental Studies No Vietnam-veteran studies or environmental studies of exposure to the COIs and stomach cancer have been published since *Update 2010*.

Occupational Studies Burns et al. (2011) published an update examining cancer incidence in 1985–2007 in workers employed in 2,4-D production by Dow Chemical Company in Midland, Michigan, during 1945–1994. There was no evidence of significantly increased rates of cancer overall or of stomach cancer in particular. In the cohort defined most restrictively, the SIR of stomach cancer was 0.8 (95% CI 0.16–2.34), equivalent to the findings in the two more inclusive cohorts.

Boers et al. (2012) provided a quantified, TCDD-based analysis, updated through 2006, of mortality in male workers in two Dutch phenoxy-herbicide factories, which were considered in *Update 2010* (Boers et al., 2010). The 1,020 workers in factory A had been involved in production of 2,4,5-T with its associated TCDD contamination; the 1,036 in factory B had produced only phenoxy herbicides that would not have had TCDD contamination. Contemporary TCDD concentrations measured in a subsample of 187 workers were used to derive a model incorporating job history to estimate serum TCDD concentrations of all the men at the end of their employment. Using the estimated TCDD concentrations of the workers in both factories did not indicate an increased risk of stomach cancer posed by TCDD (hazard ratio [HR] = 1.06, 95% CI 0.77–1.47). The dose–response modeling applied only to the workers in factory A, however, found a significantly increased risk of stomach cancer (HR = 1.52, 95% CI 1.05–2.20), whereas the qualitative exposure analysis in Boers et al. (2010) had not (HR = 2.23, 95% CI 0.38–13.20).

Manuwald et al. (2012) reported on mortality in 1,191 men and 398 women who had been employed for at least 3 months during 1952–1984 in a chemical plant in Hamburg (a subcohort of the IARC phenoxy-herbicide cohort). During that period, the plant produced insecticides and herbicides, including 2,4,5-T, so cohort members had the possibility of exposure to TCDD. Subjects entered the cohort on the date of their first employment in the plant, and vital status was sought through 2007. All 17 observed deaths from stomach cancer occurred in the male workers, but relative to the population of Hamburg this did not constitute an increase in stomach-cancer mortality in men (SMR = 1.27, 95% CI 0.74–2.03).

Ruder and Yiin (2011) reported mortality in 1940–2005 in the NIOSH PCP cohort of 2,122 workers in the four US plants that had been involved in PCP production. PCP production entailed exposure to PCDDs and PCDFs but not to the most toxic 2,3,7,8 dioxin congener. A subcohort of 720 workers (all men, the PCP-plus-TCDD group) had also been employed in TCP production and so had also been exposed to TCDD. In the total cohort, nine deaths were attributed to stomach cancer; this was consistent with the mortality experience of the US population (SMR = 0.89, 95% CI 0.40–1.68). There were three stomach-cancer deaths in the PCP-plus-TCDD group—also not more than expected (SMR = 0.98, 95% CI 0.20–2.88). The results were effectively the same in the 1,402 workers in the PCP-only group (SMR = 0.84, 95% CI 0.31–1.84).

The participants in the AHS are known to have had extensive exposure to the phenoxy herbicides, but the analyses of updated mortality (Waggoner et al., 2011) and cancer incidence (Koutros et al., 2010a) address only exposure to pesticides in general. Waggoner et al. (2011) updated mortality in the AHS cohort through 2007. The observed number of deaths from stomach cancer was significantly lower than expected in the applicators (26 deaths, SMR = 0.52, 95% CI 0.34–0.76), as was the case for the five deaths from this type of cancer in their spouses (SMR = 0.42, 95% CI 0.14–0.99). Reporting on cancer incidence through 2006, Koutros et al. (2010a) found 61 cases of oral-cavity and pharyngeal cancers in the private applicators (SIR = 0.86, 95% CI 0.66–1.10) and 15 cases in their spouses (SIR = 0.91, 95% CI 0.51–1.50). The AHS has been generating valuable information on the COIs for a number of years, but these results are not herbicide-specific and so are not regarded as being fully informative for the committee's task.

Case-Control Studies In a Spanish study, Santibanez et al. (2012) explored the relationship between 399 stomach cancers of varied histology and occupational exposures estimated by application of a job–exposure matrix to work histories. Of chemicals that might have been of interest, only the category of "pesticides" was used, which is not specific enough for the results to be regarded as informative for the present review.

Biologic Plausibility

Long-term animal studies have examined the effect of exposure to the COIs (2,4-D and TCDD) on tumor incidence (Charles et al., 1996; Stott et al., 1990; Walker et al., 2006; Wanibuchi et al., 2004). No increase in the incidence of gastrointestinal cancer has been reported in laboratory animals. However, studies of laboratory animals have observed dose-dependent increases in the incidence of squamous-cell hyperplasia of the forestomach or fundus of the stomach after administration of TCDD (Hebert et al., 1990; Walker et al., 2006). Similarly, in a long-term TCDD-treatment study in monkeys, hypertrophy, hyperplasia, and metaplasia were observed in the gastric epithelium (Allen et al., 1977). A transgenic mouse bearing a constitutively active form of the AHR has been shown to develop stomach tumors (Andersson et al., 2002a); the tumors are neither dysplastic nor metaplastic but are indicative of both squamous-cell and intestinal-cell metaplasia (Andersson et al., 2005). The validity of the transgenic-animal model is indicated by the similarities in the phenotype of the transgenic animal (increased relative weight of the liver and heart, decreased weight of the thymus, and increased expression of AHR target gene CYP1A1) and animals treated with TCDD (Brunnberg et al., 2006).

In a biomarker study of cancer patients, AHR expression and nuclear translocation were significantly higher in stomach-cancer tissue than in precancerous tissue (Peng et al., 2009a). The results suggest that the AHR plays an important role in stomach carcinogenesis. AHR activation in a stomach-cancer cell line (AGS) has also been shown to enhance stomach-cancer cell invasiveness potentially through a c-Jun-dependent induction of matrix metalloproteinase-9 (Peng et al., 2009b).

The biologic plausibility of the carcinogenicity of the COIs is discussed in general at the beginning of this chapter.

Synthesis

Boers et al. (2012) derived a predictive model based on job histories and current TCDD concentrations in a subset of the workers in two Dutch phenoxy-herbicide factories. Using estimates of each man's serum TCDD at the end of his employment, they found a significant increase in the risk of death from stomach cancer in the workers in the factory that had TCDD contamination, whereas an earlier categorical analysis of the same data found an increase risk with a very wide confidence interval (Boers et al., 2010); when the workers in the factory that did not have TCDD contamination were added to the continuous analysis, the risk did not remain significant (Boers et al., 2012). Several case-control studies addressing agricultural exposures reported evidence of an association of stomach cancer: both Ekström et al. (1999) and Mills and Yang (2007) found an association with herbicides, and with phenoxy herbicides in particular; Cocco et al. (1999) found a relationship with herbicide exposure, but the results were not specific as to type of herbicide. There has been no suggestion of an association between TCDD and stomach cancer in the Seveso population (Consonni et al., 2008; Pesatori et al., 2009) nor has there been any suggestion of an association between the COIs and stomach cancer in the studies of Vietnam-veteran cohorts or in the AHS.

There is some evidence of biologic plausibility in animal models, but overall the epidemiologic studies do not support an association between exposure to the COIs and stomach cancer.

Conclusion

On the basis of the evidence reviewed here and in previous VAO reports, the committee concludes that there is inadequate or insufficient evidence to determine whether there is an association between exposure to the COIs and stomach cancer.

Colorectal Cancer

Colorectal cancers include malignancies of the colon (ICD-9 153) and of the rectum and anus (ICD-9 154); less prevalent tumors of the small intestine (ICD-9 152) are often included. Findings on cancers of the retroperitoneum and other unspecified digestive organs (ICD-9 159) are considered in this category. Colorectal cancers account for about 55% of digestive tract tumors; ACS estimated that 157,760 people would receive diagnoses of colorectal cancer in the United States in 2012 and that 53,620 would die from it (Siegel et al., 2012). Excluding basal-cell and squamous-cell skin cancers, colorectal cancer is the third-most common form of cancer both in men and in women. The average annual incidence of colorectal cancers is shown in Table 8-4.

The incidence of colorectal cancer increases with age; it is higher in men than in women and higher in blacks than in whites. (Screening can affect the incidence, and it is recommended for all persons over 50 years old.) Other risk factors include family history of this form of cancer, some diseases of the intestines, and diet. Type 2 diabetes is associated with an increased risk of colorectal cancer (ACS, 2013a).

Conclusions from *VAO* and Previous Updates

Update 2006 considered colorectal cancer independently for the first time. Prior updates developed tables of results on colon and rectal cancer, but conclusions about the adequacy of the evidence of their association with herbicide exposure had been reached only in the context of gastrointestinal tract cancers. The committee responsible for *VAO* concluded that there was limited or suggestive evidence of *no* association between exposure to the herbicides used by the US military in Vietnam and gastrointestinal tract tumors, including colorectal cancer. The committee responsible for *Update 2006* concluded that there was not enough evidence on each of the COIs to sustain that negative conclusion for any of the cancers in the gastrointestinal group and that, because these various types of cancer are generally regarded as separate disease entities, the evidence on each should be evaluated separately. Colorectal cancer was thus reclassified into the default category of inadequate or insufficient evidence to determine whether there is an association. The information considered in *Update 2008* did not provide evidence to support moving colorectal cancers out of the category of inadequate or insufficient evidence.

The new information considered in *Update 2010* also did not provide evidence to suggest that colorectal cancers be moved out of the category of inadequate or insufficient evidence. Collins et al. (2009a) found no increase of deaths from colorectal cancer in PCP workers in a Dow Chemical Company plant in Midland, Michigan, compared with the general US population and the state of Michigan. In a followup study of workers in the Dow AgroSciences plant in New Plymouth, New Zealand, McBride et al. (2009a) did not find an increased SMR for colorectal-cancer deaths in the workers who were exposed to TCDD compared with the never-exposed group. In updating cancer incidence in the Seveso population (males and females combined), Pesatori et al. (2009) found no cases of rectal cancer and a lower risk of colon cancer in the high-exposure zone than in the moderate- and low-exposure zones. Turunen et al. (2008) assessed mortality in Finnish fishermen and their wives and presumed that their high consumption of fish would result in harmful exposure to dioxin-like chemicals, but found no increase in mortality from colon, rectal, or anal cancer in this cohort relative to control populations.

Table 8-7 summarizes the results of the relevant studies concerning colon and rectal cancers.

Update of the Epidemiologic Literature

Vietnam-Veteran, Environmental, and Case-Control Studies No Vietnam-veteran studies, environmental studies, or case-control studies of exposure to the COIs and colorectal cancer have been published since *Update 2010*.

Occupational Studies Burns et al. (2011) updated, through 2007, cancer incidence in workers who were alive on January 1, 1985, and had been employed at any time from 1945 to 1994 in 2,4-D production by the Dow Chemical Company in Midland, Michigan. They found no evidence of significantly increased rates of

TABLE 8-7 Selected Epidemiologic Studies—Colon and Rectal Cancer (Shaded Entries Are New Information for This Update)

Study Population[a]	Exposed Cases[b]	**Exposure of Interest**/Estimated Relative Risk (95% CI)[b]	Reference
VIETNAM VETERANS			
US Vietnam Veterans			
US CDC Vietnam Experience Study—Cross-sectional study, with medical examinations, of Army veterans: 9,324 deployed vs 8,989 nondeployed		**All COIs**	
Mortality			
1965–2000	9	1.0 (0.4–2.6)	Boehmer et al., 2004
US VA Proportionate Mortality Study—sample of deceased male Vietnam-era Army and Marine veterans who served 7/4/1965–3/1/1973		**All COIs**	
1965–1982 (Colon, other gastrointestinal, ICD-8 152–154, 158, 159)			Breslin et al., 1988
Army, deployed (n = 19,708) vs nondeployed (n = 22,904)	209	1.0 (0.7–1.3)	
Marine Corps, deployed (n = 4,527) vs nondeployed (n = 3,781)	33	1.3 (0.7–2.2)	
US VA Cohort of Female Vietnam Veterans		**All COIs**	
Mortality			
Through 2004			Cypel and Kang, 2008
US Vietnam veterans	11	0.5 (0.2–1.0)	
Vietnam-veteran nurses—colon	9	0.6 (0.2–1.4)	
Through 1991			Dalager et al., 1995
US Vietnam veterans	4	0.4 (0.1–1.2)	
Vietnam-veteran nurses—colon	4	0.5 (0.2–1.7)	
State Studies of US Vietnam Veterans			
923 White male Vietnam veterans with **Wisconsin** death certificate (1968–1978) vs proportions for Vietnam-era veterans			Anderson et al., 1986
Colon	6	1.0 (0.4–2.2)	
Rectum	1	nr	
International Studies of Vietnam-Veterans			
Australian Vietnam Veterans—58,077 men and 153 women served on land or in Vietnamese waters during 5/23/1962–7/1/1973 vs Australian population		**All COIs**	
Incidence			
Colon—All branches, 1982–2000	376	1.1 (1.0–1.2)	ADVA, 2005a
Navy	91	1.3 (1.0–1.5)	
Army	239	1.1 (0.9–1.2)	
Air Force	47	1.1 (0.8–1.5)	

continued

TABLE 8-7 Colon and Rectal Cancer, continued

Study Population[a]	Exposed Cases[b]	**Exposure of Interest**/Estimated Relative Risk (95% CI)[b]	Reference
Rectum—All branches, 1982–2000			ADVA, 2005a
Navy	54	1.1 (0.8–1.4)	
Army	152	1.0 (0.8–1.1)	
Air Force	28	1.0 (0.6–1.4)	
Validation Study		*Expected number of exposed cases*	
Men—colorectal cancer	188	221 (191–251)	AIHW, 1999
Men—self-reported colon cancer	405	117 (96–138)	CDVA, 1998a
Women—self-reported colon cancer	1	1 (0–5)	CDVA, 1998b
Mortality			
Colon—All branches, return–2001	176	1.0 (0.8–1.1)	ADVA, 2005b
Navy	49	1.3 (0.9–1.6)	
Army	107	0.9 (0.7–1.0)	
Air Force	21	0.9 (0.5–1.3)	
Rectum—All branches, return–2001			ADVA, 2005b
Navy	13	0.8 (0.4–1.4)	
Army	44	0.9 (0.6–1.1)	
Air Force	12	1.3 (0.6–2.2)	
1980–1994			CDVA, 1997a
Colon	78	1.2 (0.9–1.5)	
Rectum	16	0.6 (0.4–1.0)	
Australian Conscripted Army National Service (18,940 deployed vs 24,642 nondeployed)		**All COIs**	
Incidence			
1982–2000			ADVA, 2005c
Colon	54	0.9 (0.7–1.4)	
Rectum	46	1.4 (0.9–2.2)	
Mortality			
1966–2001			ADVA, 2005c
Colon	29	0.8 (0.5–1.3)	
Rectum	10	1.8 (0.6–5.6)	
1982–1994			CDVA, 1997b
Colon	6	0.6 (0.2–1.5)	
Rectum	3	0.7 (0.2–9.5)	
OCCUPATIONAL—INDUSTRIAL			
IARC Phenoxy Herbicide Cohort—Workers exposed to any phenoxy herbicide or chlorophenol (production or spraying) vs respective national mortality rates			

TABLE 8-7 Colon and Rectal Cancer, continued

Study Population[a]	Exposed Cases[b]	**Exposure of Interest**/Estimated Relative Risk (95% CI)[b]	Reference
Mortality 1939–1992			Kogevinas et al., 1997
13,831 exposed to highly chlorinated PCDDs			
Colon	86	1.1 (0.9–1.3)	
Rectum	44	1.1 (0.8–1.4)	
7,553 not exposed to highly chlorinated PCDDs			
Colon	52	1.0 (0.8–1.3)	
Rectum	29	1.3 (0.9–1.9)	
Mortality 1955–1988 of 12,492 production workers and 5,898 sprayers exposed—13,482 in exposed subcohort			Saracci et al., 1991
Nested case-control study			
Colon (except rectum)	41	1.1 (0.8–1.5)	
Rectum	24	1.1 (0.7–1.6)	
British MCPA Plant—Production 1947–1982 (n = 1,545) (included in IARC cohort) and spraying 1947–1972 (n = 2,561) (*not* included in IARC cohort)		**MCPA**	Coggon et al., 1986
Mortality through 1983			
Colon	19	1.0 (0.6–1.6)	
Rectum	8	0.6 (0.3–1.2)	
Danish Production Workers (3,390 men and 1,069 women involved in production of phenoxy herbicides unlikely to contain TCDD at 2 plants in 1947–1987) (in IARC cohort)		**Dioxins, but TCDD unlikely; 2,4-D, 2,4-DP, MCPA, MCPP**	
Incidence 1943–1982			Lynge, 1985
Men			
Colon	10	1.0 (nr)	
Rectum	14	1.4 (nr)	
Women			
Colon	1	0.3 (nr)	
Rectum	2	1.0 (nr)	
Dutch production workers in Plant A (549 men exposed during production 1955–1985; 594 unexposed) (in IARC cohort)		**Dioxins, 2,4,5-T, 2,4,5-TCP**	
Mortality 1955–1991			Hooiveld et al., 1998
Colon	3	1.4 (0.3–4.0)	
Rectum	1	1.0 (0.0–5.6)	
Mortality 1955–1985			Bueno de Mesquita et al., 1993
Large intestine, except colon	3	2.4 (0.5–7.0)	
Rectum	0	0.0 (0.0–5.6)	

continued

TABLE 8-7 Colon and Rectal Cancer, continued

Study Population[a]	Exposed Cases[b]	**Exposure of Interest**/Estimated Relative Risk (95% CI)[b]	Reference
Dutch production workers in Plant B (414 men exposed during production 1965–1986; 723 unexposed) (in IARC cohort)		**2,4-D; MCPA; MCPP; highly chlorinated dioxins unlikely**	
Mortality 1965–1986	3	1.8 (0.4–5.4)	Bueno de Mesquita et al., 1993
Large intestine, except rectum	0	0.0 (0.0–9.5)	
Rectum	0	0.0 (0.0–19.4)	
German Production Workers at Bayer Plant in Uerdingen (135 men working > 1 month in 1951–1976) (in IARC cohort as of 1997) and women—no results		**Dioxins; 2,4,5-TCP**	
Mortality 1951–1992			Becher et al., 1996
Colon	0	nr	
Rectum	0	nr	
German Production Workers at Bayer Plant in Dormagen (520 men working > 1 month in 1965–1989) (in IARC cohort as of 1997) and women—no results		**Dioxins; 2,4-D; 2,4,5-T; MCPA; MCPP; 2,4-DP**	
Mortality 1965–1989			Becher et al., 1996
Colon	1	2.2 (0.1–2.2)	
Rectum	0	nr	
German Production Workers at BASF Ludwigshafen Plant (680 men working > 1 month in 1957–1987) (in IARC cohort as of 1997) and women—no results		**Dioxins; 2,4-D; 2,4,5-T; MCPA; MCPP; 2,4-DP**	
Mortality 1956–1989			Becher et al., 1996
Colon	0	nr	
Rectum	1	0.9 (0.0–4.9)	
BASF Cleanup Workers from 1953 accident (n = 247); 114 with chloracne, 13 more with erythema; serum TCDD levels (*not* part of IARC)		**Focus on TCDD**	
Incidence			
1960–1992—colorectal	5	1.0 (0.3–2.3)	Ott and Zober, 1996
TCDD < 0.1 μg/kg of body weight	2	1.1 (0.1–3.9)	
TCDD 0.1–0.99 μg/kg of body weight	2	1.4 (0.2–5.1)	
TCDD > 1 μg/kg of body weight	1	0.5 (0.0–3.0)	
Mortality			
Through 1987—colon, rectum	2	*90% CI* 2.5 (0.4–7.8)	Zober et al., 1990
Through 1970—(n = 74; 70 initially exposed, 4 involved with cleaning and testing procedures)	1	0.4 (nr)	Theiss et al., 1982

TABLE 8-7 Colon and Rectal Cancer, continued

Study Population[a]	Exposed Cases[b]	**Exposure of Interest**/Estimated Relative Risk (95% CI)[b]	Reference
German Production Workers at Boehringer–Ingelheim Plant in Hamburg (1,144 men working > 1 month in 1952–1984; generation of TCDD reduced after chloracne outbreak in 1954) and women—no results (some additions to observed cancers over Manz et al., 1991) (in IARC cohort as of 1997)		**Dioxins; 2,4,5-T; 2,5-DCP; 2,4,5-TCP**	
Mortality 1952–2007 (ICD-9 140–149)			Manuwald et al., 2012
Colon (ICD-9 153)	12	0.7 (0.4–1.3)	
Men	7	0.6 (0.3–1.3)	
Women	5	0.9 (0.3–2.1)	
Rectum, rectosigmoid junction, anus (ICD-9 154)	13	1.7 (0.9–2.9)	
Men	11	2.0 (0.98–3.5)	
Women	2	1.0 (0.1–3.7)	
Mortality 1952–1989			Becher et al., 1996
Colon	2	0.4 (0.1–1.4)	
Rectum	6	1.9 (0.7–4.0)	
Mortality 1952–1989—stats on men only, 1,184 (tables for 1,148 men, not necessarily German nationals) vs national rates (also vs gas workers); same observation period as Becher et al., 1966)			Manz et al., 1991
Colon	8	0.9 (0.4–1.8)	
New Zealand Phenoxy Herbicide Production Workers and Sprayers (1,599 men and women working any time in 1969–1988 at Dow plant in New Plymouth) (in IARC cohort)		**Dioxins; 2,4-D; 2,4,5-T; MCPA; MCPB; 2,4,5-TCP; Picloram**	
Mortality 1969–2004			McBride et al., 2009a
Large intestine			
Ever-exposed workers	3	0.6 (0.1–1.7)	
Never-exposed workers	0	0.0 (0.0–2.0)	
Rectum			
Ever-exposed workers	6	2.0 (0.7–4.4)	
Never-exposed workers	2	2.1 (0.3–7.7)	
Production Workers (713 men and 100 women worked > 1 month in 1969–1984)			
Mortality 1969–2000			't Mannetje et al., 2005
Phenoxy herbicide producers (men and women)			
Colon	2	0.6 (0.0–2.3)	
Rectum, rectosigmoid junction, anus	5	2.5 (0.8–5.7)	
Phenoxy herbicide sprayers (> 99% men)			
Colon	8	1.9 (0.8–3.8)	
Rectum, rectosigmoid junction, anus	4	1.5 (0.4–3.8)	

continued

TABLE 8-7 Colon and Rectal Cancer, continued

Study Population[a]	Exposed Cases[b]	**Exposure of Interest**/Estimated Relative Risk (95% CI)[b]	Reference
NIOSH Mortality Cohort (12 US plants, 5,172 male production and maintenance workers 1942–1984) (included in IARC cohort as of 1997)		**Dioxins, phenoxy herbicides**	
Through 1993			Steenland et al., 1999
Small intestine, colon	34	1.2 (0.8–1.6)	
Rectum	6	0.9 (0.3–1.9)	
Through 1987			Fingerhut et al., 1991
Entire NIOSH cohort			
Small intestine, colon	25	1.2 (0.8–1.8)	
Rectum	5	0.9 (0.3–2.1)	
≥ 1-year exposure, ≥ 20-year latency			
Small intestine, colon	13	1.8 (1.0–3.0)	
Rectum	2	1.2 (0.1–4.2)	
Mortality, colon cancer—754 Monsanto workers, among most highly exposed workers from Fingerhut et al. (1991)	3	0.5 (0.1–1.3)	Collins et al., 1993
All Dow TCP-Exposed Workers (TCP production 1942–1979 or 2,4,5-T production 1948–1982 in Midland, Michigan) (in IARC and NIOSH cohorts)		**2,4,5-T; 2,4,5-TCP**	
1942–2003 (n = 1,615)			Collins et al., 2009a
Large intestine	18	1.2 (0.7–1.8)	
Rectum	2	0.6 (0.1–2.1)	
All Dow PCP-Exposed Workers—all workers from the two plants that only made PCP (in Tacoma, Washington, and Wichita, Kansas) and workers who made PCP and TCP at two additional plants (in Midland, Michigan, and Sauget, Illinois)		**2,4,5-T; 2,4,5-TCP**	Ruder and Yiin, 2011
Intestine (ICD-9 152–153)			
1940–2005 (n = 2,122)	26	1.1 (0.7–1.6)	
PCP and TCP (n = 720)	11	1.4 (0.7–2.6)	
PCP (no TCP) (n = 1,402)	15	0.9 (0.5–1.5)	
Rectum (ICD-9 154)			
1940–2005 (n = 2,122)	2	0.4 (0.0–1.3)	
PCP and TCP (n = 720)	1	0.5 (0.0–3.0)	
PCP (no TCP) (n = 1,402)	1	0.3 (0.0–1.5)	
Dow 2,4-D Production Workers (1945–1982 in Midland, Michigan) (subset of all TCP-exposed workers)		**2,4-D, lower chlorinated dioxins**	
Cancer incidence through 2007 in Dow workers (n = 1,256) vs comparisons from state cancer registries (n = 23,354) (Cohort 3)			Burns et al., 2011
Colon	16	1.0 (0.6–1.6)	
Rectum	6	0.8 (0.3–1.7)	

TABLE 8-7 Colon and Rectal Cancer, continued

Study Population[a]	Exposed Cases[b]	**Exposure of Interest**/Estimated Relative Risk (95% CI)[b]	Reference
Through 1982 (n = 878)			Bond et al., 1988
Colon	4	2.1 (0.6–5.4)	
Rectum	1	1.7 (0.0–9.3)	
Dow PCP Production Workers (1937–1989 in Midland, Michigan) (*not* in IARC and NIOSH cohorts)		**Low chlorinated dioxins, 2,4-D**	
Mortality 1940–2004 (n = 577, excluding 196 also having exposure to TCP)			Collins et al., 2009b
Large intestine	10	1.2 (0.6–2.3)	
Rectum	1	0.5 (0.0–2.9)	
Mortality 1940–1989 (n = 770)			Ramlow et al., 1996
0-yr latency			
Colon	4	0.8 (0.2–2.1)	
Rectum	0	nr	
15-yr latency			
Colon	4	1.0 (0.3–2.6)	
Rectum	0	nr	
Other Studies of Industrial Workers (*not* related to IARC or NIOSH phenoxy cohorts)			
1,412 white male US flavor and fragrance chemical plant workers (1945–1965)		**Dioxin, 2,4,5-T**	Thomas, 1987
Colon	4	0.6 (nr)	
Rectum	6	2.5 (nr)	
OCCUPATIONAL—PAPER AND PULP WORKERS		**TCDD**	
IARC cohort of pulp and paper workers—60,468 workers from 11 countries, TCDD among 27 agents assessed by JEM			McLean et al., 2006
Exposure to nonvolatile organochlorine compounds			
Colon	62	0.7 (0.6–1.0)	
Rectum	60	0.9 (0.7–1.1)	
Danish paper workers			Rix et al., 1998
Men			
Colon	58	1.0 (0.7–1.2)	
Rectum	43	0.9 (0.6–1.2)	
Women			
Colon	23	1.1 (0.7–1.7)	
Rectum	15	1.5 (0.8–2.4)	
New Hampshire pulp and paper workers, 883 white men working ≥ 1 yr, mortality through July 1985			Henneberger et al., 1989
Colon	9	1.0 (0.5–2.0)	
Rectum	1	0.4 (0.0–2.1)	

continued

TABLE 8-7 Colon and Rectal Cancer, continued

Study Population[a]	Exposed Cases[b]	**Exposure of Interest**/Estimated Relative Risk (95% CI)[b]	Reference
Pulp and Paper cohorts independent of IARC cohort			
United Paperworkers International, 201 white men employed ≥ 10 yrs and dying 1970–1984			Solet et al., 1989
Colon	7	1.5 (0.6–3.0)	
Northwestern US paper and pulp workers—5 mills in Washington, Oregon, and California, 3,523 worked ≥ 1 yr 1945–1955, mortality through March 1977			Robinson et al., 1986
Intestines (ICD-7 152, 153)	7	0.4 (0.2–0.7)	
OCCUPATIONAL—HERBICIDE-USING WORKERS (*not* related to IARC sprayer cohorts)			
DENMARK			
Danish Farmers—incidence from linking farmers on 1970 census with national cancer registry (1970–1980)		**Herbicides**	Ronco et al., 1992
Men			
Self-employed			
Colon	277	0.7 ($p < 0.05$)	
Rectum	309	0.8 ($p < 0.05$)	
Employee			
Colon	45	0.6 ($p < 0.05$)	
Rectum	55	0.8 (nr)	
Women			
Self-employed			
Colon	14	0.9 (nr)	
Rectum	5	0.6 (nr)	
Employee			
Colon	112	0.9 (nr)	
Rectum	55	0.8 (nr)	
ITALIAN Licensed Pesticide Users—male farmers in southern Piedmont licensed 1970–1974			
Mortality 1970–1986 (n = 23,401)			Torchio et al., 1994
Colon	84	0.6 (0.5–0.7)	
Rectum	nr	nr	
Italian rice growers with documented phenoxy use (n = 1,487)		**Phenoxy herbicides**	Gambini et al., 1997
Intestines	27	1.1 (0.7–1.6)	
NEW ZEALAND National Cancer Registry (1980–1984)—case-control study of incident cancer cases (colon, rectum, or small intestine) vs remainder of 19,904 men with any incident cancer			Reif et al., 1989
Forestry workers (n = 134)		**Herbicides**	
Colon	7	0.5 (0.2–1.1)	
Rectum	10	1.2 (0.6–2.3)	

TABLE 8-7 Colon and Rectal Cancer, continued

Study Population[a]	Exposed Cases[b]	**Exposure of Interest**/Estimated Relative Risk (95% CI)[b]	Reference
Small intestine	2	5.2 (1.4–18.9)	
Aged 20–59	2	11.2 (3.4–36.4)	
Aged ≥ 60	0	—	
Sawmill workers (n = 139)		**Herbicides, chlorophenols**	
Small intestine	0	—	
SWEDEN			
Incident cancer cases 1961–1973 with agriculture as economic activity in 1960 census			Wiklund, 1983
Colon	1,332		
Rectum		*99% CI*	
	1,083	0.8 (0.7–0.8)	
THE NETHERLANDS			
Dutch Licensed Herbicide Sprayers—1,341 certified before 1980			
Through 2000			Swaen et al., 2004
Colon	7	1.0 (0.4–2.1)	
Rectum	5	2.1 (0.7–4.8)	
Through 1987			Swaen et al., 1992
Colon	4	2.6 (0.7–6.5)	
UNITED STATES			
US farmers—usual occupation of farmer and industry of agriculture on death certificates 1984–1988 from 23 states		**Herbicides** PCMRs	Blair et al., 1993
Colon			
Men			
Whites (n = 119,648)	2,291	1.0 (0.9–1.0)	
Nonwhites (n = 11,446)	148	0.8 (0.7–0.9)	
Women			
Whites (n = 2,400)	59	1.0 (0.8–1.3)	
Nonwhites (n = 2,066)	40	1.0 (0.7–1.3)	
Rectum			
Men			
Whites (n = 119,648)	367	1.0 (0.9–1.1)	
Nonwhites (n = 11,446)	22	0.7 (0.5–1.1)	
Women			
Whites (n = 2,400)	4	0.5 (0.1–1.3)	
Nonwhites (n = 2,066)	5	1.1 (0.3–2.5)	

continued

TABLE 8-7 Colon and Rectal Cancer, continued

Study Population[a]	Exposed Cases[b]	**Exposure of Interest**/Estimated Relative Risk (95% CI)[b]	Reference
US Agricultural Health Study—prospective study of licensed pesticide sprayers in Iowa and North Carolina: commercial (n = 4,916), private/farmers (n = 52,395, 97.4% men), and spouses of private sprayers (n = 32,347, 0.007% men), enrolled 1993–1997; followups with CATIs 1999–2003 and 2005–2010		**Phenoxy herbicides**	
Incidence			
Enrollment through 2006—SIRs for participants			Koutros et al., 2010a
Colon			
Private applicators	339	0.9 (0.8–1.0)	
Commercial applicators	17	1.0 (0.6–1.6)	
Spouses	144	0.8 (0.7–1.0)	
Rectum			
Private applicators	117	0.9 (0.7–1.1)	
Commercial applicators	8	1.2 (0.5–2.3)	
Spouses	30	0.7 (0.5–1.0)	
Enrollment through 2005—Interactions between dicamba and body mass index			Andreotti et al., 2010
Trend (with dicamba use reported)	96	1.1 (1.0–1.1)	
Trend (with no dicamba use reported)	102	1.0 (1.0–1.1)	
Enrollment through 2005—colorectal cancer			Lee WJ et al., 2007
2,4-D	204	0.7 (0.5–0.9)	
2,4,5-T	65	0.9 (0.7–1.2)	
2,4,5-TP	24	0.8 (0.5–1.2)	
Dicamba	110	0.9 (0.7–1.2)	
Enrollment through 2002—colon cancer			Samanic et al., 2006
Dicamba—lifetime days exposure			
None	76	1.0	
1– < 20	9	0.4 (0.2–0.9)	
20– < 56	20	0.9 (0.5–1.5)	
56– < 116	13	0.8 (0.4–1.5)	
≥ 116	17	1.4 (0.8–2.9)	
		p-trend = 0.10	
Dicamba—intensity-weighted quartiles			
None	76	1.0	
Lowest	16	0.6 (0.4–1.1)	
Second	17	0.7 (0.4–1.2)	
Third	6	0.5 (0.2–1.2)	
Highest	20	1.8 (1.0–3.1)	
		p-trend = 0.02	
Enrollment through 2002			Alavanja et al., 2005
Colon			
Private applicators (men, women)	208	0.9 (0.8–1.0)	

TABLE 8-7 Colon and Rectal Cancer, continued

Study Population[a]	Exposed Cases[b]	**Exposure of Interest**/Estimated Relative Risk (95% CI)[b]	Reference
Spouses of private applicators (> 99% women)	87	0.9 (0.7–1.1)	
Commercial applicators (men, women)	12	0.2 (0.6–2.1)	
Rectum			
Private applicators (men, women)	94	0.8 (0.7–1.0)	
Spouses of private applicators (> 99% women)	23	0.6 (0.4–0.9)	
Commercial applicators (men, women)	7	1.3 (0.5–2.6)	
Mortality			
Enrollment through 2007, vs state rates			Waggoner et al., 2011
Intestine			
Applicators (n = 1,641)	158	0.8 (0.6–0.9)	
Spouses (n = 676)	68	0.9 (0.7–1.1)	
Rectum			
Applicators (n = 1,641)	32	0.7 (0.5–1.0)	
Spouses (n = 676)	4	nr	
Enrollment through 2000, vs state rates			Blair et al., 2005a
Colon			
Private applicators (men, women)	56	0.7 (0.6–1.0)	
Spouses of private applicators (> 99% women)	31	1.2 (0.8–1.6)	
Rectum			
Private applicators (men, women)	nr	nr	
Spouses of private applicators (> 99% women)	nr	nr	
US Department of Agriculture Workers—nested case-control study of white men dying 1970–1979 of cancer		**Herbicides**	
Agricultural extension agents			Alavanja et al., 1988
Colon	41	1.0 (0.7–1.5)	
Rectum	5	nr	
Forest conservationists		p-trend < over years worked	Alavanja et al., 1989
Colon	44	1.5 (1.1–2.0)	
Rectum	9	1.0 (0.5–1.9)	
Soil conservationists			
Florida Licensed Pesticide Applicators [common phenoxy use assumed but not documented; had been listed by Blair et al., 1983]		**Herbicides**	
Pesticide applicators in Florida licensed 1965–1966 (n = 3,827)—mortality through 1976		**Herbicides**	Blair et al., 1983
Any pesticide (dose-response by length of licensure)			
Colon	5	0.8 (nr)	

continued

TABLE 8-7 Colon and Rectal Cancer, continued

Study Population[a]	Exposed Cases[b]	**Exposure of Interest**/Estimated Relative Risk (95% CI)[b]	Reference
Rectum	2	nr	
White Male Residents of Iowa—colon cancer on death certificate, usual occupation: farmers vs not		**Herbicides**	
> 20 yrs old when died 1971–1978—PMR			Burmeister, 1981
Colon	1,064	0.9 (0.9–1.0)	
ENVIRONMENTAL			
Seveso, Italy Residential Cohort—Industrial accident July 10, 1976 (723 residents Zone A; 4,821 Zone B; 31,643 Zone R; 181,574 local reference group) (ICD-9 171)		**TCDD**	
Incidence			
20-yr followup to 1996—men and women			
Zone A			Pesatori et al., 2009
Colon	2	0.7 (0.2–2.7)	
Rectum	0		
Zone B			
Colon	19	1.0 (0.7–1.6)	
Rectum	17	1.8 (1.1–2.9)	
Zone R			
Colon	137	1.0 (0.9–1.3)	
Rectum	71	1.1 (0.8–1.4)	
10-yr followup to 1991—men			Bertazzi et al., 1993
Zone B			
Colon	2	0.5 (0.1–2.0)	
Rectum	3	1.4 (0.4–4.4)	
Zone R			
Colon	32	1.1 (0.8–1.6)	
Rectum	17	1.1 (0.7–1.9)	
10-yr followup to 1991—women			Bertazzi et al., 1993
Zone B			
Colon	2	0.6 (0.1–2.3)	
Rectum	2	1.3 (0.3–5.4)	
Zone R			
Colon	23	0.8 (0.5–1.3)	
Rectum	7	0.6 (0.3–1.3)	
Mortality			
25-yr followup to 2001—men and women			Consonni et al., 2008
Zone A			
Colon	3	1.0 (0.3–3.0)	
Rectum	1	0.9 (0.1–6.4)	
Zone B			
Colon	12	0.6 (0.3–1.1)	
Rectum	11	1.5 (0.8–2.8)	

TABLE 8-7 Colon and Rectal Cancer, continued

Study Population[a]	Exposed Cases[b]	**Exposure of Interest**/Estimated Relative Risk (95% CI)[b]	Reference
Zone R			
Colon	137	0.9 (0.7–1.3)	
Rectum	50	0.9 (0.7–1.3)	
20-yr followup to 1996			Bertazzi et al., 2001
Zones A and B—men			
Colon	10	1.0 (0.5–1.9)	
Rectum	9	2.4 (1.2–4.6)	
Zones A and B—women			
Colon	5	0.6 (0.2–1.4)	
Rectum	3	1.1 (0.4–3.5)	
15-yr followup to 1991—men			Bertazzi et al., 1997
Zone B			
Colon	5	0.8 (0.3–2.0)	
Rectum	7	2.9 (1.2–5.9)	
Zone R			
Colon	34	0.8 (0.6–1.1)	
Rectum	19	1.1 (0.7–1.8)	
15-yr followup to 1991—women			Bertazzi et al., 1997
Zone A			
Colon	2	2.6 (0.3–9.4)	
Zone B			
Colon	3	0.6 (0.1–1.8)	
Rectum	2	1.3 (0.1–4.5)	
Zone R			
Colon	33	0.8 (0.6–1.1)	
Rectum	12	0.9 (0.5–1.6)	
10-yr followup to 1986—men			Bertazzi et al., 1989a,b
Zone A, B, R—colon	20	1.0 (0.6–1.5)	
Zone A, B, R—rectum	10	1.0 (0.5–2.7)	
Zone B—rectum	2	1.7 (0.4–7.0)	
10-yr followup to 1986—women			Bertazzi et al., 1989a
Zone A, B, R—colon	12	0.7 (0.4–1.2)	
Zone A, B, R—rectum	7	1.2 (0.5–2.7)	
Ecological Study of Residents of Chapaevsk, Russia		**Dioxin**	Revich et al., 2001
Incidence—Crude incidence rate in 1998 vs			
Men			
Regional (Samara)			
Colon	nr	21.7 (nr)	
Rectum	nr	17.1 (nr)	
National (Russia)			
Colon	nr	17.9 (nr)	
Rectum	nr	16.6 (nr)	

continued

TABLE 8-7 Colon and Rectal Cancer, continued

Study Population[a]	Exposed Cases[b]	**Exposure of Interest**/Estimated Relative Risk (95% CI)[b]	Reference
Women			
Regional (Samara)			
Colon	nr	15.4 (nr)	
Rectum	nr	11.2 (nr)	
National (Russia)			
Colon	nr	14.1 (nr)	
Rectum	nr	10.3 (nr)	
Mortality—1995–1998 (SMR vs regional rates)			
Men			
Colon	17	1.3 (0.8–2.2)	
Rectum	21	1.5 (1.0–2.4)	
Women			
Colon	24	1.0 (0.7–1.5)	
Rectum	24	0.9 (0.6–1.4)	
FINLAND			
Finnish community exposed to chlorophenol contamination (men and women)		**Chlorophenol**	Lampi et al., 1992
Colon—men, women	9	1.1 (0.7–1.8)	
Finnish fishermen (n = 6,410) and spouses (n = 4,260) registered between 1980 and 2002 compared to national statistics		**Serum dioxin**	Turunen et al., 2008
Fisherman		**SMRs**	
Colon	8	0.5 (0.2–1.0)	
Rectum	8	0.8 (0.4–1.6)	
Spouses			
Colon	10	1.3 (0.6–2.4)	
Rectum	8	2.1 (0.9–4.2)	
SWEDEN			
Swedish fishermen (high consumption of fish with persistent organochlorines)		**Organochlorine compounds**	Svensson et al., 1995
Incidence			
East coast			
Colon	5	0.4 (0.1–0.9)	
Rectum	9	0.9 (0.4–1.6)	
West coast			
Colon	82	1.0 (0.8–1.2)	
Rectum	59	1.1 (0.8–1.4)	
Mortality			
East coast			
Colon	1	0.1 (0.0–0.7)	
Rectum	4	0.7 (0.2–1.9)	
West coast			
Colon	58	1.0 (0.8–1.3)	
Rectum	31	1.0 (0.7–1.5)	

TABLE 8-7 Colon and Rectal Cancer, continued

Study Population[a]	Exposed Cases[b]	**Exposure of Interest**/Estimated Relative Risk (95% CI)[b]	Reference
CASE-CONTROL STUDIES			
International Case-Control Studies			
421 **Egyptian** colorectal cancer cases and 439 hospital controls	nr	**Herbicides** 5.5 (2.4–12.3)	Lo et al., 2010
Swedish patients (1970–1977)		**Phenoxy acids, chlorophenols**	Hardell, 1981
Colon			
Exposed to phenoxy herbicides	11	1.3 (0.6–2.8)	
Exposed to chlorophenols	6	1.8 (0.6–5.3)	

NOTE: 2,4-D, 2,4-dichlorophenoxyacetic acid; 2,4-DP, dichlorprop; 2,4,5-T, 2,4,5-trichlorophenoxyacetic acid; 2,4,5-TCP, 2,4,5-trichlorophenol; 2,4,5-TP, 2-(2,4,5-trichlorophenoxy) propionic acid; 2,5-DCP, 2,5-dichlorophenol; AFHS, Air Force Health Study; CDC, Centers for Disease Control and Prevention; CI, confidence interval; COI, chemical of interest; IARC, International Agency for Research on Cancer; ICD, International Classification of Diseases; JEM, job-exposure matrix; MCPA, methyl-4-chlorophenoxyacetic acid; MCPB, 4-(4-chloro-2-methylphenoxy)butanoic acid; MCPP, methylchlorophenoxypropionic acid; NIOSH, National Institute for Occupational Safety and Health; nr, not reported; PCDD, polychlorinated dibenzo-*p*-dioxin (highly chlorinated, if four or more chlorines); PCMR, proportionate cancer mortality ratios; PCP, pentachlorophenol; PMR, proportionate mortality ratio; SIR, standardized incidence ratio; SMR, standardized mortality ratio; TCDD, 2,3,7,8-tetrachlorodibenzo-*p*-dioxin; TCP, trichlorophenol; VA, US Department of Veterans Affairs.

[a]Subjects are male and outcome is mortality unless otherwise noted.

[b]Given when available; results other than estimated risk explained individually.

cancer overall. In the most restrictively defined cohort, the SIR for colon cancer was 0.95 (95% CI 0.55–1.55), and the SIR for rectal cancer was 0.78 (95% CI 0.29–1.70). For both cancer types, the results were similar in the two more inclusive, but potentially more biased, cohorts.

Manuwald et al. (2012) reported a 23-year update of mortality in a cohort of chemical workers in Hamburg, Germany, who were exposed to dioxin. Compared to national rates, male workers had an increase in mortality from rectal cancer (SMR = 1.95, 95% CI 0.98–3.51) but not from colon cancer (SMR = 0.64, 95% CI 0.26–1.32). An increase in colorectal-cancer deaths was not seen in exposed women (SMR = 0.90, 95% C.I 0.29–2.12 for colon cancer and SMR = 1.01, 95% CI 0.11–3.65 for rectal cancer).

Ruder and Yiin (2011) reported mortality for 1940–2005 separately for intestinal cancer (ICD-9 152–153) and colon cancer in the NIOSH PCP cohort of 2,122 workers in the four US plants that had been involved in PCP production. PCP production entailed exposure to PCDDs and PCDFs but not to the most toxic 2,3,7,8 dioxin congener. A subcohort of 720 workers (all men, the PCP-plus-

TCDD group) had also been employed in TCP production and so had also been exposed to TCDD. Relative to US referent rates, deaths from intestinal cancer were not substantially changed in the entire cohort (26 deaths, SMR = 1.07, 95% CI 0.70–1.57), the PCP-only group (15 deaths, SMR = 0.90, 95% CI 0.50–1.49), or the PCP-plus-TCDD group (11 deaths, SMR = 1.44, 95% CI 0.72–2.57). Only two deaths from rectal cancer were reported in the entire cohort—one in each subcohort—which was in accord with expectations.

The participants in the AHS are known to have had extensive exposure to the phenoxy herbicides, but the analyses of updated mortality (Waggoner et al., 2011) and cancer incidence (Koutros et al., 2010a) address only exposure to pesticides in general. The updated cancer incidence in the AHS (Koutros et al., 2010a) revealed no increase in SIR of colon cancer in private applicators (339 cases, SIR = 0.87, 95% CI 0.78–0.97) or their spouses (144 cases, SIR = 0.83, 95% CI 0.70–0.98). Cancer of the rectum also was not increased in these populations of private applicators (117 cases, SIR = 0.90, 95% CI 0.74–1.08) or their spouses (30 cases, SIR = 0.69, 95% CI 0.47–0.99). In the study by Waggoner et al. (2011), mortality from both intestinal and rectal cancer in the applicators (private and commercial combined) was significantly lower than expected.

The association between obesity and cancer risk was examined (Andreotti et al., 2010) in pesticide applicators and their spouses on the basis of data from the AHS. A small increase in the risk of colon cancer in men was the only statistically significant association with increased body-mass index (BMI; trend in HR with BMI = 1.05, 95% CI 1.02–1.09, p = 0.005); no such relationship was apparent in the women. Of the many pesticides tested for an interactive role in the BMI–colon cancer relationship in men, the only one that had any bearing on the COIs and on which results were reported is dicamba (2-methoxy-3,6-dichlorobenzoic acid), which showed no evidence of interaction. The AHS has been generating valuable information on the COIs for a number of years, but these results are not herbicide-specific and so are not regarded as being fully informative for the committee's task.

Biologic Plausibility

Long-term animal studies examining the effect of exposure to the COIs on tumor incidence (Charles et al., 1996; Stott et al., 1990; Walker et al., 2006; Wanibuchi et al., 2004) have reported no increase in the incidence of colorectal cancer. Recently, Xie et al. (2012) reported that AHR activation by TCDD induces robust proliferation in two human colon-cancer cell lines through Src-mediated epidermal growth factor receptor activation. That novel finding suggests that TCDD and other AHR ligands may contribute to colon carcinogenesis, but more studies are needed to understand the potential role of AHR activation in intestinal carcinogenesis.

The biologic plausibility of the carcinogenicity of the COIs is discussed in general at the beginning of this chapter.

Synthesis

The generic findings on the applicators and their spouses in the AHS showed indications of increased mortality from both colon and intestinal cancer in agricultural workers, but earlier assessment of colorectal cancer in this study population had found no increase in risks in association with exposure to individual phenoxy herbicides (Lee WJ et al., 2007). None of the epidemiologic studies reviewed that specifically addressed the COIs, however, yielded evidence of an association between the COIs and colorectal cancer. There is no evidence of biologic plausibility of an association between exposure to any of the COIs and tumors of the colon or rectum. Overall, the available evidence does not support an association between the COIs and colorectal cancer.

Conclusion

On the basis of the evidence reviewed here and in previous VAO reports, the committee concludes that there is inadequate or insufficient evidence to determine whether there is an association between exposure to the COIs and colorectal cancer.

Hepatobiliary Cancers

Hepatobiliary cancers include cancers of the liver (ICD-9 155.0, 155.2) and the intrahepatic bile duct (ICD-9 155.1). ACS estimated that 21,370 men and 7,350 women would receive diagnoses of liver cancer or intrahepatic bile duct cancer in the United States in 2012 and that 13,980 men and 6,570 women would die from these cancers (Siegel et al., 2012). Gallbladder cancer and extrahepatic bile duct cancer (ICD-9 156) are fairly uncommon and are often grouped with liver cancers when they are addressed.

In the United States, liver cancers account for about 1.5% of new cancer cases and 3.3% of cancer deaths. Misclassification of metastatic cancers as primary liver cancer can lead to overestimation of the number of deaths attributable to liver cancer (Percy et al., 1990). In developing countries, especially those in sub-Saharan Africa and Southeast Asia, liver cancers are common and are among the leading causes of death. Known risk factors for liver cancer include chronic infection with hepatitis B or hepatitis C virus and exposure to the carcinogens aflatoxin and vinyl chloride. Alcohol cirrhosis and obesity-associated metabolic syndrome may also contribute to the risk of liver cancer. In the general population, the incidence of liver and intrahepatic bile duct cancer increases slightly with age; at the ages of 50–64 years, it is greater in men than in women and greater in blacks than in whites. The average annual incidence of hepatobiliary cancers is shown in Table 8-4.

Conclusions from *VAO* and Previous Updates

The committee responsible for *VAO* concluded that there was inadequate or insufficient information to determine whether there is an association between exposure to the COIs and hepatobiliary cancers. Additional information available to the committees responsible for *Update 1996*, *Update 1998*, *Update 2000*, *Update 2002*, *Update 2004*, *Update 2006*, and *Update 2008* did not change that conclusion.

Update 2010 considered followup reports on three previously studied populations. Collins et al. (2009a,b) examined mortality in workers employed in a Dow Chemical Company plant in Midland, Michigan, during 1937–1980. They found two cases of cancer of the hepatobiliary tract in 1,615 TCP workers (SMR = 0.5, 95% CI 0.1–1.6) but no observed deaths from that cancer in 773 PCP workers. The second occupational-mortality study was of workers in the Dow AgroSciences plant in New Plymouth, New Zealand, who were potentially exposed to TCDD; SMRs for hepatobiliary cancer calculated on the basis of national mortality figures were 1.4 (95% CI 0.2–5.1) in exposed workers and 0.0 (95% CI 0.0–8.2) in the never-exposed group (McBride et al., 2009a). The update of cancer incidence in the Seveso cohort did not find systematic evidence of hepatic or biliary cancers in any of the exposure zones (Pesatori et al., 2009).

Table 8-8 summarizes the results of the relevant studies.

Update of the Epidemiologic Literature

Vietnam-Veteran, Environmental, and Case-Control Studies No Vietnam-veteran studies, environmental studies, or case-control studies of exposure to the COIs and hepatobiliary cancer have been published since *Update 2010*.

Occupational Studies Malignant neoplasms of the hepatobiliary tract were not specifically reported in Boers et al. (2012), Burns et al. (2011), or Manuwald et al. (2012).

An update of cancer incidence in US PCP workers through 2005 reported no increase in cancers of the hepatobiliary tract (Ruder and Yiin, 2011). There were nine deaths from liver or biliary cancer for an SMR of 1.21 (95% CI 0.56–2.31) in all the workers, but they all occurred in the workers that had only PCP exposure and resulted in a somewhat higher but still nonsignificant risk estimate (SMR = 1.76, 95% CI 0.81–3.35).

Koutros et al. (2010a) published an update of cancer incidence in the AHS. In private applicators, there were 32 cases of liver cancer (SIR = 0.73, 95% CI 0.50–1.03) and eight cases of gallbladder cancer (SIR = 1.33, 95% CI 0.57–2.61).

TABLE 8-8 Selected Epidemiologic Studies—Hepatobiliary Cancers (Shaded Entries Are New Information for This Update)

Study Population[a]	Exposed Cases[b]	**Exposure of Interest**/Estimated Relative Risk (95% CI)[b]	Reference
VIETNAM VETERANS			
US CDC Vietnam Experience Study—Cross-sectional study, with medical examinations, of Army veterans: 9,324 deployed vs 8,989 nondeployed		**All COIs**	
Mortality			
1965–2000—liver, intrahepatic bile ducts (ICD-9 155)	5	nr	Boehmer et al., 2004
US CDC Selected Cancers Study—case-control study of incidence (12/1/1984–11/30/1989) among US males born 1929–1953	8	**All COIs** 1.2 (0.5–2.7)	CDC, 1990a
US VA Proportionate Mortality Study—sample of deceased male Vietnam-era Army and Marine veterans who served 7/4/1965–3/1/1973		**All COIs**	
1965–1982—liver, bile duct			Breslin et al., 1988
Army, deployed (n = 19,708) vs nondeployed (n = 22,904)	34	1.0 (0.8–1.4)	
Marine Corps, deployed (n = 4,527) vs nondeployed (n = 3,781)	6	1.2 (0.5–2.8)	
State Studies of US Vietnam Veterans			
923 White male Vietnam veterans with **Wisconsin** death certificate (1968–1978) vs proportions for Vietnam-era veterans	0	nr	Anderson et al., 1986a,b
International Vietnam-Veteran Studies			
Australian Vietnam Veterans—58,077 men and 153 women served on land or in Vietnamese waters during 5/23/1962–7/1/1973 vs Australian population		**All COIs**	
Incidence			
All branches, 1982–2000	27	0.7 (0.4–1.9)	ADVA, 2005a
Navy	8	1.0 (0.4–1.9)	
Army	18	0.7 (0.4–1.1)	
Air Force	1	0.2 (0.0–1.2)	
Mortality			
All branches, return–2001	48	0.9 (0.6–1.1)	ADVA, 2005b
Navy	11	1.0 (0.5–1.7)	
Army	33	0.9 (0.6–1.2)	
Air Force	4	0.6 (0.2–1.5)	
1980–1994			CDVA, 1997a
Liver (ICD-9 155)	8	0.6 (0.2–1.1)	
Gallbladder (ICD-9 156)	5	1.3 (0.4–2.8)	
Australian Conscripted Army National Service 18,940 deployed vs 24,642 nondeployed		**All COIs**	

continued

TABLE 8-8 Hepatobiliary Cancers, continued

Study Population[a]	Exposed Cases[b]	**Exposure of Interest**/Estimated Relative Risk (95% CI)[b]	Reference
Incidence			
1982–2000	2	2.5 (0.1–147.2)	ADVA, 2005c
Mortality			
1966–2001 (liver, gallbladder)	4	2.5 (0.4–27.1)	ADVA, 2005c
1982–1994	1	nr	CDVA, 1997b
OCCUPATIONAL—INDUSTRIAL			
IARC Phenoxy Herbicide Cohort—Workers exposed to any phenoxy herbicide or chlorophenol (production or spraying) vs respective national mortality rates			
Mortality 1939–1992	15	0.7 (0.4–1.2)	Kogevinas et al., 1997
13,831 exposed to highly chlorinated PCDDs	12	0.9 (0.5–1.5)	
7,553 not exposed to highly chlorinated PCDDs	3	0.4 (0.1–1.2)	
Mortality 1955–1988 of 12,492 production workers and 5,898 sprayers exposed—13,482 in exposed subcohort			Saracci et al., 1991
Liver, gallbladder, bileduct (ICD-8 155–156)	4	0.4 (0.1–1.1)	
Danish Production Workers (3,390 men and 1,069 women involved in production of phenoxy herbicides unlikely to contain TCDD at 2 plants in 1947–1987) (in IARC cohort)		**Dioxins, but TCDD unlikely; 2,4-D, 2,4-DP, MCPA, MCPP**	
Incidence 1943–1982			Lynge, 1985
Men	3	1.0 (nr)	
Women	0	nr	
German Production Workers at Bayer Plant in Uerdingen (135 men working > 1 month in 1951–1976) (in IARC cohort as of 1997) and women—no results		**Dioxins; 2,4,5-TCP**	
Mortality 1951–1992	0	—	Becher et al., 1996
German Production Workers at Bayer Plant in Dormagen (520 men working > 1 month in 1965–1989) (in IARC cohort as of 1997) and women—no results		**Dioxins; 2,4-D; 2,4,5-T; MCPA; MCPP; 2,4-DP**	
Mortality 1965–1989	0	—	Becher et al., 1996
German Production Workers at BASF Ludwigshafen Plant (680 men working > 1 month in 1957–1987) (in IARC cohort as of 1997) and women—no results		**Dioxins; 2,4-D; 2,4,5-T; MCPA; MCPP; 2,4-DP**	

TABLE 8-8 Hepatobiliary Cancers, continued

Study Population[a]	Exposed Cases[b]	Exposure of Interest/Estimated Relative Risk (95% CI)[b]	Reference
Mortality 1956–1989	1	1.2 (0.0–6.9)	Becher et al., 1996
BASF Cleanup Workers from 1953 accident (n = 247); 114 with chloracne, 13 more with erythema; serum TCDD levels (*not* part of IARC)		**Focus on TCDD**	
Incidence			
1960–1992—liver, gallbladder, bile duct	2	2.1 (0.3–7.5)	Ott and Zober, 1996
TCDD < 0.1 μg/kg of body weight	1	2.8 (0.1–15.5)	
TCDD 0.1–0.99 μg/kg of body weight	0	0.0 (0.0–15.4)	
TCDD > 1 μg/kg of body weight	1	2.8 (0.1–15.5)	
German Production Workers at Boehringer–Ingelheim Plant in Hamburg (1,144 men working > 1 month in 1952–1984; generation of TCDD reduced after chloracne outbreak in 1954) and women—no results (some additions to observed cancers over Manz et al., 1991) (in IARC cohort as of 1997)		**Dioxins; 2,4,5-T; 2,5-DCP; 2,4,5-TCP**	
Mortality 1952–1989	0	—	Becher et al., 1996
New Zealand Phenoxy Herbicide Production Workers and Sprayers (1,599 men and women working any time in 1969–1988 at Dow plant in New Plymouth) (in IARC cohort)		**Dioxins; 2,4-D; 2,4,5-T; MCPA; MCPB; 2,4,5-TCP; Picloram**	
Mortality 1969–2004			McBride et al., 2009a
Ever-exposed workers	2	1.4 (0.2–5.1)	
Never-exposed workers	0	0.0 (0.0–8.2)	
Production Workers (713 men and 100 women worked > 1 month in 1969–1984)			
Mortality 1969–2000—ICD-9 155			't Mannetje et al., 2005
Phenoxy herbicide producers (men and women)	1	1.6 (0.0–8.8)	
Phenoxy herbicide sprayers (> 99% men)	0	0.0 (0.0–4.2)	
NIOSH Mortality Cohort (12 US plants, 5,172 male production and maintenance workers 1942–1984) (included in IARC cohort as of 1997)		**Dioxins, phenoxy herbicides**	
Through 1993			Steenland et al., 1999
Liver, biliary tract (ICD-9 155–156)	7	0.9 (0.4–1.6)	
Through 1987 (liver, biliary tract)	6	1.2 (0.4–2.5)	Fingerhut et al., 1991
≥ 1-year exposure, ≥ 20-year latency	1	0.6 (0.0–3.3)	
Mortality—754 Monsanto workers, among most highly exposed workers from Fingerhut et al. (1991); liver, biliary tract	2	1.4 (0.2–5.2)	Collins et al., 1993

continued

TABLE 8-8 Hepatobiliary Cancers, continued

Study Population[a]	Exposed Cases[b]	**Exposure of Interest**/Estimated Relative Risk (95% CI)[b]	Reference
All Dow TCP-Exposed Workers (TCP production 1942–1979 or 2,4,5-T production 1948–1982 in Midland, Michigan) (in IARC and NIOSH cohorts)		**2,4,5-T; 2,4,5-TCP**	
1942–2003 (n = 1,615)	2	0.5 (0.1–1.6)	Collins et al., 2009a
March 1949–1978 (n = 121); 121 TCP workers with chloracne	0	nr	Zack and Suskind, 1980
Through 1982 (n = 878); liver, biliary tract (ICDA-8 155–156)	0	1.2 (nr)	Bond et al., 1988
All Dow PCP-Exposed Workers—all workers from the two plants that only made PCP (in Tacoma, Washington, and Wichita, Kansas) and workers who made PCP and TCP at two additional plants (in Midland, Michigan, and Sauget, Illinois)		**2,4,5-T; 2,4,5-TCP**	Ruder and Yiin, 2011
1940–2005 (n = 2,122) (liver and biliary; ICD–9 155–156)	9	1.2 (0.6–2.3)	
PCP and TCP (n = 720)	0	– (0.0–1.6)	
PCP (no TCP) (n = 1,402)	9	1.8 (0.8–3.4)	
Dow PCP Production Workers (1937–1989 in Midland, Michigan) (*not* in IARC and NIOSH cohorts)		**Low chlorinated dioxins, 2,4-D**	
Mortality 1940–2004 (n = 577, excluding 196 also having exposure to TCP)	0	0.0 (0.0–1.7)	Collins et al., 2009b
Mortality 1940–1989 (n = 770); liver, primary (ICDA-8 155–156)			Ramlow et al., 1996
0-yr latency	0	nr	
15-yr latency	0	nr	
OCCUPATIONAL—PAPER AND PULP WORKERS		**TCDD**	
IARC cohort of pulp and paper workers—60,468 workers from 11 countries, TCDD among 27 agents assessed by JEM			McLean et al., 2006
Exposure to nonvolatile organochlorine compounds			
Never	27	0.9 (0.6–1.3)	
Ever	16	0.7 (0.4–1.1)	
Danish paper workers			Rix et al., 1998
Men			
Liver	10	1.1 (0.5–2.0)	
Gallbladder	9	1.6 (0.7–3.0)	
Women			
Liver	1	0.6 (0.0–3.2)	
Gallbladder	4	1.4 (0.4–3.7)	

TABLE 8-8 Hepatobiliary Cancers, continued

Study Population[a]	Exposed Cases[b]	**Exposure of Interest**/Estimated Relative Risk (95% CI)[b]	Reference
Pulp and Paper cohorts independent of IARC cohort			
United Paperworkers International, 201 white men employed ≥ 10 yrs and dying 1970–1984	2	2.0 (0.2–7.3)	Solet et al., 1989
OCCUPATIONAL—HERBICIDE-USING WORKERS (*not* related to IARC sprayer cohorts)			
DENMARK			
Danish Farmers—incidence from linking farmers on 1970 census with national cancer registry (1970–1980)		**Herbicides**	Ronco et al., 1992
Men			
Liver			
Self-employed	23	0.4 ($p < 0.05$)	
Employee	9	0.8 (nr)	
Gallbladder			
Self-employed	35	0.8 (nr)	
Employee	7	0.8 (nr)	
Women			
Liver			
Family workers	5	0.5 (nr)	
Gallbladder			
Self-employed	7	2.7 ($p < 0.05$)	
Employee	1	0.7 (nr)	
Family workers	17	1.0 (nr)	
FINNISH Phenoxy Herbicide Sprayers (1,909 men working 1955–1971 ≥ 2 wks) *not* IARC (liver, biliary tract)		**Phenoxy herbicides**	
Incidence	3	0.9 (0.2–2.6)	Asp et al., 1994
Mortality 1972–1989	2	0.6 (0.1–2.2)	
ITALIAN Licensed Pesticide Users—male farmers in southern Piedmont licensed 1970–1974			
Mortality 1970–1986 (n = 23,401)	15	0.6 (0.3–0.9)	Torchio et al., 1994
Italian rice growers with documented phenoxy use (n = 1,487)	7	**Phenoxy herbicides** 1.3 (0.5–2.6)	Gambini et al., 1997
NEW ZEALAND National Cancer Registry (1980–1984)—case-control study of incident hepatobiliary cancer cases vs remainder of 19,904 men with any incident cancer			Reif et al., 1989
Forestry workers (n = 134)		**Herbicides**	
Liver	1	0.8 (0.1–5.8)	
Gallbladder	3	4.1 (1.4–12.0)	
Aged 20–59	1	6.3 (1.1–36.6)	
Aged ≥ 60	2	3.5 (0.9–13.3)	

continued

TABLE 8-8 Hepatobiliary Cancers, continued

Study Population[a]	Exposed Cases[b]	**Exposure of Interest**/Estimated Relative Risk (95% CI)[b]	Reference
Sawmill workers (n = 139)		**Herbicides, chlorophenols**	
Gallbladder	2	2.3 (0.6–9.1)	
SWEDEN			
Incident stomach cancer cases 1961–1973 with agriculture as economic activity in 1960 census		*99% CI*	Wiklund, 1983
Liver (primary)	103	0.3 (0.3–0.4)	
Biliary tract	169	0.6 (0.5–0.7)	
Liver (unspecified)	67	0.9 (0.7–1.3)	
THE NETHERLANDS			
Dutch Licensed Herbicide Sprayers—1,341 certified before 1980			
Through 2000	0	nr	Swaen et al., 2004
UNITED STATES			
US farmers—usual occupation of farmer and industry of agriculture on death certificates 1984–1988 from 23 states		**Herbicides** PCMRs	Blair et al., 1993
Men			
Whites (n = 119,648)	326	1.0 (0.9–1.1)	
Nonwhites (n = 11,446)	24	0.7 (0.5–1.1)	
Women			
Whites (n = 2,400)	6	0.7 (0.3–1.6)	
Nonwhites (n = 2,066)	2	0.4 (0.0–1.3)	
US Agricultural Health Study—prospective study of licensed pesticide sprayers in Iowa and North Carolina: commercial (n = 4,916), private/farmers (n = 52,395, 97.4% men), and spouses of private sprayers (n = 32,347, 0.007% men), enrolled 1993–1997; followups with CATIs 1999–2003 and 2005–2010		**Phenoxy herbicides**	
Incidence			
Enrollment through 2006—SIRs for participants			Koutros et al., 2010a
Liver			
Private applicators	32	0.7 (0.5–1.0)	
Commercial applicators	1	nr	
Spouses	6	0.8 (0.3–1.7)	
Gallbladder			
Private applicators	8	1.3 (0.6–2.6)	
Commercial applicators	0	nr	
Spouses			
Enrollment through 2002	7	1.1 (0.4–2.3)	Alavanja et al., 2005
Liver			
Private applicators (men, women)			

TABLE 8-8 Hepatobiliary Cancers, continued

Study Population[a]	Exposed Cases[b]	**Exposure of Interest**/Estimated Relative Risk (95% CI)[b]	Reference
Spouses of private applicators (> 99% women)	35	1.0 (0.7–1.4)	
Commercial applicators (men, women)	3	0.9 (0.2–2.5)	
Gallbladder	nr	0.0 (0.0–4.2)	
Private applicators (men, women)			
Spouses of private applicators (> 99% women)	8	2.3 (1.0–4.5)	
Commercial applicators (men, women)	3	0.9 (0.2–2.5)	
Mortality	nr	0.0 (0.0–35.8)	
Enrollment through 2007, vs state rates (liver and gallbladder)			Waggoner et al., 2011
Applicators (n = 1,641)	50	0.7 (0.5–0.9)	
Spouses (n = 676)	18	0.8 (0.5–1.3)	
Enrollment through 2000, vs state rates			Blair et al., 2005a
Liver			
Private applicators (men, women)	8	0.6 (0.2–1.1)	
Spouses of private applicators (> 99% women)	4	1.7 (0.4–4.3)	
Rectum			
Private applicators (men, women)	3	2.0 (0.4–5.7)	
Spouses of private applicators (> 99% women)	2	1.3 (0.1–4.6)	
ENVIRONMENTAL			
Seveso, Italy Residential Cohort—Industrial accident July 10, 1976 (723 residents Zone A; 4,821 Zone B; 31,643 Zone R; 181,574 local reference group) (ICD-9 171)		**TCDD**	
Incidence			
20-yr followup to 1996—men and women			Pesatori et al., 2009
Zone A			
Liver	0		
Biliary	0		
Zone B			
Liver	14	1.3 (0.8–2.2)	
Biliary	6	2.3 (1.0–5.2)	
Zone R			
Liver	56	0.7 (0.6–1.0)	
Biliary	16	0.8 (0.5–1.4)	
10-yr followup to 1991—men			Bertazzi et al., 1993
Zone B			
Liver	4	2.1 (0.8–5.8)	
Gallbladder (ICD-9 156)	1	2.3 (0.3–17.6)	

continued

TABLE 8-8 Hepatobiliary Cancers, continued

Study Population[a]	Exposed Cases[b]	**Exposure of Interest**/Estimated Relative Risk (95% CI)[b]	Reference
Zone R			
Liver	3	0.2 (0.1–0.7)	
Gallbladder (ICD-9 156)	3	1.0 (0.3–3.4)	
10-yr followup to 1991—women			Bertazzi et al., 1993
Zone B			
Gallbladder (ICD-9 156)	4	4.9 (1.8–13.6)	
Zone R			
Liver	2	0.5 (0.1–2.1)	
Gallbladder (ICD-9 156)	7	1.0 (0.5–2.3)	
Mortality			
25-yr followup to 2001—men and women			Consonni et al., 2008
Zone A			
Liver	3	1.0 (0.3–3.2)	
Biliary	0	0.0 (nr)	
Zone B			
Liver	16	0.9 (0.5–1.4)	
Biliary	2	0.6 (0.1–2.3)	
Zone R			
Liver	107	0.8 (0.7–1.0)	
Biliary	31	1.2 (0.8–1.7)	
20-yr followup to 1996			Bertazzi et al., 2001
Zones A and B—men			
Liver, gallbladder	6	0.5 (0.2–1.0)	
Liver	6	0.5 (0.2–1.1)	
Zones A and B—women			
Liver, gallbladder	7	1.0 (0.5–2.2)	
Liver	6	1.3 (0.6–2.9)	
15-yr followup to 1991—men			Bertazzi et al., 1997
Zone B			
Liver, gallbladder	4	0.6 (0.2–1.4)	
Liver	4	0.6 (0.2–1.6)	
Zone R			
Liver, gallbladder	35	0.7 (0.5–1.0)	
Liver	31	0.7 (0.5–1.0)	
15-yr followup to 1991—women			Bertazzi et al., 1997
Zone B			
Liver, gallbladder	4	1.1 (0.3–2.9)	
Liver	3	1.3 (0.3–3.8)	
Zone R			
Liver, gallbladder	25	0.8 (0.5–1.3)	
Liver	12	0.6 (0.3–1.1)	
10-yr followup to 1986—men			Bertazzi et al., 1989b
Zone B—liver	3	1.2 (0.4–3.8)	
Zone R—liver	7	0.4 (0.2–0.8)	

TABLE 8-8 Hepatobiliary Cancers, continued

Study Population[a]	Exposed Cases[b]	**Exposure of Interest**/Estimated Relative Risk (95% CI)[b]	Reference
10-yr followup to 1986—women			Bertazzi
Zone A—gallbladder (ICD-9 156)	1	12.1 (1.6–88.7)	et al., 1989b
Zone B—gallbladder (ICD-9 156)	2	3.9 (0.9–16.2)	
Zone R			
Liver	3	0.4 (0.1–1.4)	
Gallbladder (ICD-9 156)	5	1.2 (0.5–3.1)	
Quail Run Mobile Home Cohort		**TCDD**	Hoffman
154 exposed residents vs 155 unexposed area residents	0	nr	et al., 1986
SWEDEN			
Swedish fishermen (high consumption of fish with persistent organochlorines)		**Organochlorine compounds**	Svensson et al., 1995
Incidence			
East coast	1	0.5 (0.0–2.7)	
West coast	9	0.9 (0.4–1.7)	
Mortality			
East coast	6	1.3 (0.5–2.9)	
West coast	24	1.0 (0.6–1.5)	
VIETNAM			
Risk factor for hepatocellular carcinoma in Hanoi		**Herbicides**	Cordier et al., 1993
Military service in South Vietnam for ≥ 10 yrs after 1960	11	8.8 (1.9–41.0)	
CASE-CONTROL STUDIES			
International Case-Control Studies			
Swedish patients (25–80 yrs of age) diagnosed with liver cancer (ICD-7 155, 156) between 1974–June 1981 vs national rates	102	**Phenoxy acids, chlorophenols** 1.8 (0.9–4.0)	Hardell, 1984

NOTE: 2,4-D, 2,4-dichlorophenoxyacetic acid; 2,4-DP, dichlorprop; 2,4,5-T, 2,4,5-trichlorophenoxyacetic acid; 2,4,5-TCP, 2,4,5-trichlorophenol; CDC, Centers for Disease Control and Prevention; CI, confidence interval; COI, chemical of interest; IARC, International Agency for Research on Cancer; ICD, International Classification of Diseases; ICDA, International Classification of Diseases, Adapted for Use in the United States; JEM, job-exposure matrix; MCPA, methyl-4-chlorophenoxyacetic acid; MCPB, 4-(4-chloro-2-methylphenoxy)butanoic acid; MCPP, methylchlorophenoxypropionic acid; NIOSH, National Institute for Occupational Safety and Health; nr, not reported; PCDD, polychlorinated dibenzo-*p*-dioxin (highly chlorinated, if four or more chlorines); PCP, pentachlorophenol; SIR, standardized incidence ratio; TCDD, 2,3,7,8-tetrachlorodibenzo-*p*-dioxin; TCP, trichlorophenol; VA, US Department of Veterans Affairs.

[a]Subjects are male and outcome is mortality unless otherwise noted.

[b]Given when available; results other than estimated risk explained individually.

In their spouses, there were six liver-cancer cases (SIR = 0.76, 95% CI 0.28–1.66) and seven gallbladder-cancer cases (SIR = 1.09, 95% CI 0.44–2.25). Waggoner et al. (2011) compared deaths from hepataboliary from the time of enrollment (1993–1997) through 2007 to state mortality rates. Rates of hepatobiliary cancers (liver and gallbladder) in applicators was less than expected (50 deaths, SMR = 0.70, 95% CI 0.52–0.93), but not in their spouses (18 deaths, SMR = 0.81, 95% CI 0.48–1.28). The AHS has been generating valuable information on the COIs for a number of years, but these results are not herbicide-specific and so are not regarded as being fully informative for the committee's task.

Biologic Plausibility

Long-term animal studies have examined the effect of exposure to the COIs on tumor incidence (Charles et al., 1996; Stott et al., 1990; Walker et al., 2006; Wanibuchi et al., 2004). Studies performed in laboratory animals have consistently demonstrated that long-term exposure to TCDD results in the formation of liver adenomas and carcinomas (Knerr and Schrenk, 2006; Walker et al., 2006). Furthermore, TCDD increases the growth of hepatic tumors that are initiated by treatment with a complete carcinogen. Pathologic liver changes have been observed after exposure to TCDD, including nodular hyperplasia and massive inflammatory cell infiltration (Kociba et al., 1978; NTP, 2006; Walker et al., 2006; Yoshizawa et al., 2007); inflammation can be heavily involved in the development and progression of many cancers, including liver cancers (Mantovani et al., 2008). In monkeys treated with TCDD, hyperplasia and an increase in cells that stain positive for alpha-smooth muscle actin have been observed (Korenaga et al., 2007). Postive staining for alpha-smooth muscle actin is thought to be indicative of a process (epithelial–mesenchymal transition) that is associated with the progression of malignant tumors (Weinberg, 2008).

Bile duct hyperplasia (but not tumors) has been reported in rodents following chronic treatment with TCDD (Knerr and Schrenk, 2006; Walker et al., 2006; Yoshizawa et al., 2007). Similarly, monkeys treated with TCDD developed metaplasia, hyperplasia, and hypertrophy of the bile duct (Allen et al., 1977). Hollingshead et al. (2008) showed that TCDD-activated AHR in human breast and endocervical cell lines induces sustained high concentrations of the interleukin-6 cytokine, which has tumor-promoting effects in numerous tissues, including cholangiocytes; thus, TCDD might promote carcinogenesis in biliary tissue.

TCDD may contribute to tumor progression by inhibiting p53 regulation (phosphorylation and acetylation) triggered by genotoxicants through the increased expression of the metastasis marker AGR2 (Ambolet-Camoit et al., 2010) and a functional interaction between the AHR and FHL2 (Kollara and Brown, 2009). The AHR was also shown to be a regulator of c-raf and proposed cross-talk between the AHR and the mitogen-activated protein kinase signaling pathway in chemically induced hepatocarcinogenesis (Borlak and Jenke, 2008).

TCDD inhibits ultraviolet-C radiation-induced apoptosis in primary rat hepatocytes and Huh-7 human hepatoma cells, and this supports the hypothesis that TCDD acts as a tumor-promoter by preventing initiated cells from undergoing apoptosis (Chopra et al., 2009).

Elyakim et al. (2010) found that human microRNA miR-191 was upregulated in hepatocellular carcinoma and that miR-191 was upregulated after TCDD treatment and may contribute to the mechanism of the carcinogenic activity of TCDD. Ovando et al. (2010) used toxicogenomics to identify genomic responses that may be contributing to the development of hepatotoxicity in rats treated chronically with the AHR ligands, TCDD or PCB 126. They identified 24, 17, and 7 genes that were differentially expressed in the livers of rats exposed to those AHR ligands and in human cholangiocarcinoma, human hepatocellular adenoma, and rat hepatocellular adenoma, respectively. That finding may help to elucidate the mechanisms by which dioxin-like compounds induce their hepatotoxic and carcinogenic effects.

In rodents, TCDD may promote hepatocarcinogenesis through cytotoxicity, chronic inflammation, and liver regeneration and through hyperplastic and hypertrophic growth due to sustained activation of the AHR (Köhle and Bock, 2007; Köhle et al., 2008). Species differences associated with AHR activation are demonstrated by the divergence in the transcriptomic responses to TCDD in mouse, rat, and human liver (Boutros et al., 2008, 2009; Carlson et al., 2009; Kim et al., 2009), but it should be noted that the in vitro human hepatocyte studies may not reflect the in vivo response of human liver to TCDD. In vitro studies with transformed cell lines and primary hepatocytes cannot replicate the complexity of a tissue response that is important in eliciting the toxic responses observed in vivo (Dere et al., 2006).

In a recent study, gene-expression changes were compared in adult female primary human and rat hepatocytes exposed to TCDD in vitro (Black et al., 2012). Whole-genome microarrays found that TCDD produced differing gene-expression profiles in rat and human hepatocytes both on an ortholog basis (conserved genes in different species) and on a pathway basis. For commonly affected orthologs or signaling pathways, the human hepatocytes were about one-fifteenth as sensitive as rat hepatocytes. Such findings are consistent with epidemiologic studies that show humans to be less sensitive to TCDD-induced hepatotoxicity.

Chronic exposure of rats to TCDD was associated with fatty liver degeneration and necrosis (Chen X et al., 2012). Another group reported that the hepatotoxic effects of TCDD were exacerbated in mice that had glutathione deficiency (Chen YJ et al., 2012). The combined exposure to PCBs and TCDD induced significant hepatotoxicity in rats (Lu C et al., 2010). Studying the effects of environmental chemicals on nuclear hormone receptors, Shah et al. (2011) demonstrated that in vitro assays for stratifying environmental contaminants can serve as surrogates in combination with rodent toxicity evaluations.

The biologic plausibility of the carcinogenicity of the COIs is discussed in general at the beginning of this chapter.

Synthesis

The marginally significant rSMRs of hepatobiliary cancer in applicators and their spouses in the AHS (Waggoner et al., 2011) assessed exposure only to pesticides in general, so they cannot be considered fully informative for the purpose of the present review. Even in combination with the previously reported isolated finding of a barely significant increase in mortality from biliary cancer in the moderate-exposure zone at Seveso (Pesatori et al., 2009), a consistent pattern of increased risk of biliary cancer is not established. Despite the evidence of TCDD's activity as a hepatocarcinogen in animals, the evidence from epidemiologic studies remains inadequate to link the COIs with hepatobiliary cancer, which has a relatively low incidence in Western populations.

Conclusion

On the basis of the evidence reviewed here and in previous VAO reports, the committee concludes that there is inadequate or insufficient evidence to determine whether there is an association between exposure to the COIs and hepatobiliary cancer.

Pancreatic Cancer

The incidence of pancreatic cancer (ICD-9 code 157) increases with age. ACS estimated that 22,090 men and 21,830 women would receive a diagnosis of pancreatic cancer in the United States in 2012 and that 18,850 men and 18,540 women would die from it (Siegel et al., 2012). The incidence is higher in men than in women and higher in blacks than in whites. Other risk factors include family history, diet, and tobacco use. Chronic pancreatitis, obesity, and type 2 diabetes are also associated with an increased risk of pancreatic cancer (ACS, 2013a). The average annual incidence of pancreatic cancer is shown in Table 8-4.

Conclusions from *VAO* and Previous Updates

Update 2006 considered pancreatic cancer independently for the first time. Prior updates developed tables of results for pancreatic cancer but reached conclusions about the adequacy of the evidence of its association with herbicide exposure in the context of gastrointestinal tract cancers. The committee responsible for *VAO* concluded that there was limited or suggestive evidence of *no* association between exposure to the herbicides used by the US military in Vietnam and gastrointestinal tract tumors, including pancreatic cancer. The committee responsible for *Update 2006* concluded that there was not enough evidence on each of the COIs to sustain that negative conclusion for any of the cancers in the gastrointestinal group and that, because these various types of cancer are generally regarded as separate disease entities, the evidence on each should be evaluated separately. Pancreatic cancer was thus reclassified into the default category of inadequate or insufficient evidence of an association. The *Update 2006* committee reviewed the increased rates of pancreatic cancer in Australian National Service Vietnam veterans but concluded that the increased rates could be attributed to the rates of smoking in the cohort (ADVA, 2005c). The committee also noted the report of increased rates of pancreatic cancer in US female Vietnam nurse veterans (Dalager et al., 1995). That increase persisted in the followup study of the American female veterans (Cypel and Kang, 2008) considered in *Update 2008*, but the update on mortality in the Seveso population (Consonni et al., 2008) did not support an association with pancreatic cancer.

Collins et al. (2009a,b) reported on Dow Chemical Company PCP workers in Midland, Michigan, and did not find evidence of increased mortality from pancreatic cancer, whether or not they had also been engaged in TCP production, which would have provided an opportunity for exposure to TCDD and other chlorinated dioxins. McBride et al. (2009a) found no evidence of increased pancreatic-cancer deaths in either exposed workers or the never-exposed group in the Dow AgroSciences plant in New Plymouth, New Zealand. A nested case-control study of pancreatic cancer in the AHS cohort found no statistically significant associations with exposure to 2,4-D or dicamba (Andreotti et al., 2009). A followup study of two Dutch cohorts of chlorophenoxy-herbicide production workers did not find the risk of death from pancreatic cancer to be increased in either factory (Boers et al., 2010). Pesatori et al. (2009) did not find the incidence of pancreatic cancer to be increased in the Seveso cohort 20 years after the accident.

Table 8-9 summarizes the results of the relevant studies concerning pancreatic cancer.

Update of the Epidemiologic Literature

Vietnam-Veteran, Environmental, and Case-Control Studies No Vietnam-veteran studies, environmental studies, or case-control studies of exposure to the COIs and pancreatic cancer have been published since *Update 2010*.

Occupational Studies Burns et al. (2011) published an update examining cancer incidence through 2007 in workers who were alive on January 1, 1985, and had been employed at any time from 1945 to 1994 in 2,4-D production by the Dow Chemical Company in Midland, Michigan. They found no evidence of significantly increased rates of cancer overall. With two cases observed, the incidence of pancreatic cancer in the most restrictively defined cohort was not

TABLE 8-9 Selected Epidemiologic Studies—Pancreatic Cancer (Shaded Entries Are New Information for This Update)

Study Population[a]	Exposed Cases[b]	**Exposure of Interest**/Estimated Relative Risk (95% CI)[b]	Reference
VIETNAM VETERANS			
US Vietnam Veterans			
US CDC Vietnam Experience Study—Cross-sectional study, with medical examinations, of Army veterans: 9,324 deployed vs 8,989 nondeployed		**All COIs**	
Mortality			
1965–2000	5	1.0 (0.3–3.5)	Boehmer et al., 2004
US VA Proportionate Mortality Study—sample of deceased male Vietnam-era Army and Marine veterans who served 7/4/1965–3/1/1973		**All COIs**	
1965–1982			Breslin et al., 1988
Army, deployed (n = 19,708) vs nondeployed (n = 22,904)	82	0.9 (0.6–1.2)	
Marine Corps, deployed (n = 4,527) vs nondeployed (n = 3,781)	18	1.6 (0.5–5.8)	
US VA Cohort of Female Vietnam Veterans		**All COIs**	
Mortality			
Through 2004			Cypel and Kang, 2008
US Vietnam veterans	17	2.1 (1.0–4.5)	
Vietnam-veteran nurses	14	2.5 (1.0–6.0)	
Through 1991			Dalager et al., 1995
US Vietnam veterans	7	2.8 (0.8–10.2)	
Vietnam-veteran nurses	7	5.7 (1.2–27.0)	
Through 1987			Thomas et al., 1991
US Vietnam veterans	5	2.7 (0.9–6.2)	
State Studies of US Vietnam Veterans			
Michigan Vietnam-era veterans, PM study of deaths (1974–1989)—deployed vs nondeployed	14	1.0 (0.6–1.7)	Visintainer et al., 1995
Non-black	9	0.7 (0.3–1.3)	
Black	5	9.1 (2.9–21.2)	
923 White male Vietnam veterans with **Wisconsin** death certificate (1968–1978) vs proportions for Vietnam-era veterans	4	nr	Anderson et al., 1986
International Vietnam-Veteran Studies			
Australian Vietnam Veterans—58,077 men and 153 women served on land or in Vietnamese waters during 5/23/1962–7/1/1973 vs Australian population		**All COIs**	
Incidence			
All branches, 1982–2000	86	1.2 (0.9–1.4)	ADVA, 2005a
Navy	14	0.9 (0.5–1.5)	
Army	60	1.2 (0.9–1.5)	

TABLE 8-9 Pancreatic Cancer, continued

Study Population[a]	Exposed Cases[b]	**Exposure of Interest**/Estimated Relative Risk (95% CI)[b]	Reference
Air Force	12	1.3 (0.7–2.3)	
Mortality			
All branches, return–2001	101	1.2 (1.0–1.5)	ADVA, 2005b
Navy	18	1.0 (0.6–1.6)	
Army	71	1.3 (1.0–1.6)	
Air Force	11	1.1 (0.5–1.8)	
1980–1994	38	1.4 (0.9–1.8)	CDVA, 1997a
Australian Conscripted Army National Service (18,940 deployed vs 24,642 nondeployed)		**All COIs**	
Incidence			
1982–2000	17	2.5 (1.0–6.3)	ADVA, 2005c
Mortality			
1966–2001	19	3.1 (1.3–8.3)	ADVA, 2005c
1982–1994	6	1.5 (nr)	CDVA, 1997b
OCCUPATIONAL—INDUSTRIAL			
IARC Phenoxy Herbicide Cohort—Workers exposed to any phenoxy herbicide or chlorophenol (production or spraying) vs respective national mortality rates			
Mortality 1939–1992	47	0.9 (0.7–1.3)	Kogevinas et al., 1997
13,831 exposed to highly chlorinated PCDDs	30	1.0 (0.7–1.4)	
7,553 not exposed to highly chlorinated PCDDs	16	0.9 (0.5–1.4)	
Mortality 1955–1988 of 12,492 production workers and 5,898 sprayers exposed—13,482 in exposed subcohort	26	1.1 (0.7–1.6)	Saracci et al., 1991
British MCPA Plant—Production 1947–1982 (n = 1,545) (included in IARC cohort) and spraying 1947–1972 (n = 2,561) (*not* included in IARC cohort)		**MCPA**	
Mortality through 1983	9	0.7 (0.3–1.4)	Coggon et al., 1986
Danish Production Workers (3,390 men and 1,069 women involved in production of phenoxy herbicides unlikely to contain TCDD at 2 plants in 1947–1987) (in IARC cohort)		**Dioxins, but TCDD unlikely; 2,4-D, 2,4-DP, MCPA, MCPP**	
Incidence			
Incidence 1943–1982			Lynge, 1985
Men	3	0.6 (nr)	

continued

TABLE 8-9 Pancreatic Cancer, continued

Study Population[a]	Exposed Cases[b]	**Exposure of Interest**/Estimated Relative Risk (95% CI)[b]	Reference
Women	0	nr	
Mortality			
Mortality 1955–2006	7	1.2 (0.8–1.7)	Boers et al., 2012
Dutch production workers in Plant A (549 men exposed during production 1955–1985; 594 unexposed) (in IARC cohort)		**Dioxins, 2,4,5-T, 2,4,5-TCP**	
Mortality 1955–2006 (hazard ratios for lagged TCDD plasma levels)	6	0.9 (0.5–1.6)	Boers et al., 2012
Mortality 1955–2006	4	0.9 (0.2–4.2)	Boers et al. 2010
Mortality 1955–1991	4	2.5 (0.7–6.3)	Hooiveld et al., 1998
Mortality 1955–1985	3	2.9 (0.6–8.4)	Bueno de Mesquita et al., 1993
Dutch production workers in Plant B (414 men exposed during production 1965–1986; 723 unexposed) (in IARC cohort)		**2,4-D; MCPA; MCP; highly chlorinated dioxins unlikely**	
Mortality 1965–2006	1	nr	Boers et al., 2010
Mortality 1965–1986	0	0.0 (0.0–10.9)	Bueno de Mesquita et al., 1993
German Production Workers at Bayer Plant in Uerdingen (135 men working > 1 month in 1951–1976) (in IARC cohort as of 1997) and women—no results		**Dioxins; 2,4,5-TCP**	
Mortality 1951–1992	0	—	Becher et al., 1996
German Production Workers at Bayer Plant in Dormagen (520 men working > 1 month in 1965–1989) (in IARC cohort as of 1997) and women—no results		**Dioxins; 2,4-D; 2,4,5-T; MCPA; MCPP; 2,4-DP**	
Mortality 1965–1989	0	—	Becher et al., 1996
German Production Workers at BASF Ludwigshafen Plant (680 men working > 1 month in 1957–1987) (in IARC cohort as of 1997) and women—no results		**Dioxins; 2,4-D; 2,4,5-T; MCPA; MCPP; 2,4-DP**	
Mortality 1956–1989	2	1.7 (0.2–6.1)	Becher et al., 1996

TABLE 8-9 Pancreatic Cancer, continued

Study Population[a]	Exposed Cases[b]	**Exposure of Interest**/Estimated Relative Risk (95% CI)[b]	Reference
German Production Workers at Boehringer–Ingelheim Plant in Hamburg (1,144 men working > 1 month in 1952–1984; generation of TCDD reduced after chloracne outbreak in 1954) and women—no results (some additions to observed cancers over Manz et al., 1991) (in IARC cohort as of 1997)		**Dioxins; 2,4,5-T; 2,5-DCP; 2,4,5-TCP**	
Mortality 1952–2007 (ICD-9 157)	10	0.9 (0.4–1.7)	Manuwald et al., 2012
Men	7	0.9 (0.4–1.9)	
Women	3	1.0 (0.2–2.9)	
Mortality 1952–1989	2	0.6 (0.1–2.3)	Becher et al., 1996
New Zealand Phenoxy Herbicide Production Workers and Sprayers (1,599 men and women working any time in 1969–1988 at Dow plant in New Plymouth) (in IARC cohort)		**Dioxins; 2,4-D; 2,4,5-T; MCPA; MCPB; 2,4,5-TCP; Picloram**	
Mortality 1969–2004			McBride et al., 2009a
Ever-exposed workers	3	1.3 (0.3–3.9)	
Never-exposed workers	0	0.0 (0.0–4.9)	
Production Workers (713 men and 100 women worked > 1 month in 1969–1984)			
Mortality 1969–2000			't Mannetje et al., 2005
Phenoxy herbicide producers (men, women)	3	2.1 (0.4–6.1)	
Phenoxy herbicide sprayers (> 99% men)	0	0.0 (0.0–2.1)	
NIOSH Mortality Cohort (12 US plants, 5,172 male production and maintenance workers 1942–1984) (included in IARC cohort as of 1997)		**Dioxins, phenoxy herbicides**	
Through 1993	16	1.0 (0.6–1.6)	Steenland et al., 1999
Through 1987	10	0.8 (0.4–1.6)	Fingerhut et al., 1991
≥ 1-year exposure, ≥ 20-year latency	4	1.0 (0.3–2.5)	
All Dow TCP-Exposed Workers (TCP production 1942–1979 or 2,4,5-T production 1948–1982 in Midland, Michigan) (in IARC and NIOSH cohorts)		**2,4,5-T; 2,4,5-TCP**	
1942–2003 (n = 1,615)	6	0.7 (0.2–1.4)	Collins et al., 2009a

continued

TABLE 8-9 Pancreatic Cancer, continued

Study Population[a]	Exposed Cases[b]	**Exposure of Interest**/Estimated Relative Risk (95% CI)[b]	Reference
All Dow PCP-Exposed Workers—all workers from the two plants that only made PCP (in Tacoma, Washington, and Wichita, Kansas) and workers who made PCP and TCP at two additional plants (in Midland, Michigan, and Sauget, Illinois)		**2,4,5-T; 2,4,5-TCP**	Ruder and Yiin, 2011
1940–2005 (n = 2,122)	18	1.3 (0.8–2.0)	
PCP and TCP (n = 720)	6	1.4 (0.5–3.0)	
PCP (no TCP) (n = 1,402)	12	1.3 (0.7–2.2)	
Dow 2,4-D Production Workers (1945–1982 in Midland, Michigan) (subset of all TCP-exposed workers)		**2,4-D, lower chlorinated dioxins**	
Cancer incidence through 2007 in Dow workers (n = 1,256) vs comparisons from state cancer registries (n = 23,354) (Cohort 3)	2	0.4 (0.1–1.5)	Burns et al., 2011
Dow PCP Production Workers (1937–1989 in Midland, Michigan) (*not* in IARC and NIOSH cohorts)		**Low chlorinated dioxins, 2,4-D**	
Mortality 1940–2004 (n = 577, excluding 196 also having exposure to TCP)	5	1.1 (0.3–2.5)	Collins et al., 2009b
Mortality 1940–1989 (n = 770)			Ramlow et al., 1996
0-yr latency	2	0.7 (0.1–2.7)	
15-yr latency	2	0.9 (0.1–3.3)	
Other Studies of Industrial Workers (not related to IARC or NIOSH phenoxy cohorts)			
1,412 white male US flavor and fragrance chemical plant workers (1945–1965)	6	**Dioxin, 2,4,5-T** 1.4 (nr)	Thomas, 1987
OCCUPATIONAL—PAPER AND PULP WORKERS		**TCDD**	
IARC cohort of pulp and paper workers—60,468 workers from 11 countries, TCDD among 27 agents assessed by JEM			McLean et al., 2006
Exposure to nonvolatile organochlorine compounds			
Never	67	0.8 (0.7–1.1)	
Ever	69	1.1 (0.9–1.4)	
Danish paper workers			Rix et al., 1998
Men	30	1.2 (0.8–1.7)	
Women	2	0.3 (0.0–1.1)	
New Hampshire pulp and paper workers, 883 white men working ≥ 1 yr, mortality through July 1985	9	1.9 (0.9–3.6)	Henneberger et al., 1989

TABLE 8-9 Pancreatic Cancer, continued

Study Population[a]	Exposed Cases[b]	**Exposure of Interest**/Estimated Relative Risk (95% CI)[b]	Reference
United Paperworkers International, 201 white men employed ≥ 10 yrs and dying 1970–1984	1	0.4 (0.0–2.1)	Solet et al., 1989
Northwestern US paper and pulp workers—5 mills in Washington, Oregon, and California, 3,523 worked ≥ 1 yr 1945–1955, mortality through March 1977	4	*90% CI* 0.3 (0.1–0.8)	Robinson et al., 1986
OCCUPATIONAL—HERBICIDE-USING WORKERS (*not* related to IARC sprayer cohorts)			
DENMARK			
Danish Farmers—incidence from linking farmers on 1970 census with national cancer registry (1970–1980)		**Herbicides**	Ronco et al., 1992
Men			
Self-employed	137	0.6 ($p < 0.05$)	
Employee	23	0.6 ($p < 0.05$)	
Women			
Self-employed	7	1.2 (nr)	
Employee	4	1.3 (nr)	
Family workers	27	0.7 ($p < 0.05$)	
ITALIAN Licensed Pesticide Users—male farmers in southern Piedmont licensed 1970–1974			
Mortality 1970–1986 (n = 23,401)	32	0.7 (0.5–1.0)	Torchio et al., 1994
Italian rice growers with documented phenoxy use (n = 1,487)	7	**Phenoxy herbicides** 0.9 (0.4–1.9)	Gambini et al., 1997
NEW ZEALAND National Cancer Registry (1980–1984)—case-control study of incident pantreatic cancer cases vs remainder of 19,904 men with any incident cancer		**Herbicides**	Reif et al., 1989
Forestry workers (n = 134)	6	1.8 (0.8–4.1)	
Aged 20–59	0	—	
Aged ≥ 60	6	2.4 (1.1–5.4)	
Sawmill workers (n = 139)	2	**Herbicides, chlorophenols** 0.5 (0.1–1.8)	
SWEDEN			
Incident pancreatic cancer cases 1961–1973 with agriculture as economic activity in 1960 census	777	*99% CI* 0.8 (0.8–0.9)	Wiklund, 1983

continued

TABLE 8-9 Pancreatic Cancer, continued

Study Population[a]	Exposed Cases[b]	**Exposure of Interest**/Estimated Relative Risk (95% CI)[b]	Reference
THE NETHERLANDS			
Dutch Licensed Herbicide Sprayers—1,341 certified before 1980			
Through 2000	5	1.2 (0.4–2.7)	Swaen et al., 2004
Through 1987	3	2.2 (0.4–6.4)	Swaen et al., 1992
UNITED STATES			
US farmers—usual occupation of farmer and industry of agriculture on death certificates 1984–1988 from 23 states		**Herbicides** PCMRs	Blair et al., 1993
Men			
Whites (n = 119,648)	1,133	1.1 (1.1–1.2)	
Nonwhites (n = 11,446)	125	1.2 (1.0–1.4)	
Women			
Whites (n = 2,400)	23	1.0 (0.6–1.5)	
Nonwhites (n = 2,066)	16	0.7 (0.4–1.2)	
US Agricultural Health Study—prospective study of licensed pesticide sprayers in Iowa and North Carolina: commercial (n = 4,916), private/farmers (n = 52,395, 97.4% men), and spouses of private sprayers (n = 32,347, 0.007% men), enrolled 1993–1997; followups with CATIs 1999–2003 and 2005–2010		**Phenoxy herbicides**	
Incidence			
Enrollment through 2006—SIRs for participants			Koutros et al., 2010a
Private applicators	80	0.7 (0.6–0.9)	
Commercial applicators	5	1.0 (0.3–2.3)	
Spouses	32	0.7 (0.5–1.0)	
Nested case-control (applicators, spouses combined)			Andreotti et al., 2009
2,4-D	48	0.9 (0.5–1.5)	
Dicamba	23	0.9 (0.6–1.6)	
Enrollment through 2002			Alavanja et al., 2005
Private applicators	46	0.7 (0.5–1.0)	
Spouses of private applicators (> 99% women)	20	0.9 (0.6–1.4)	
Commercial applicators	3	1.1 (0.2–3.2)	
Mortality			
Enrollment through 2007, vs state rates			Waggoner et al., 2011
Applicators (n = 1,641)	171	0.8 (0.7–1.0)	
Spouses (n = 676)	1	nr	

TABLE 8-9 Pancreatic Cancer, continued

Study Population[a]	Exposed Cases[b]	**Exposure of Interest**/Estimated Relative Risk (95% CI)[b]	Reference
Enrollment through 2000, vs state rates			Blair et al., 2005a
Private applicators (men and women)	29	0.6 (0.4–0.9)	
Spouses of private applicators (> 99% women)	10	0.7 (0.3–1.2)	
US Department of Agriculture Workers—nested case-control study of white men dying 1970–1979 of pancreatic cancer		**Herbicides**	
Agricultural extension agents	21	1.3 (0.8–1.9)	Alavanja et al., 1988
Forest conservationists	22	1.5 (0.9–2.3)	Alavanja et al., 1989
Florida Licensed Pesticide Applicators (common phenoxy use assumed but not documented; had been listed by Blair et al., 1983)		**Herbicides**	
Pesticide applicators in Florida licensed 1965–1966 (n = 3,827)—mortality through 1976		**Herbicides**	Blair et al., 1983
Any pesticide (dose-response by length of licensure)		*Expected exposed cases*	
	4	4.0	
White Male Residents of Iowa—pancreatic cancer on death certificate, usual occupation: farmers vs not		**Herbicides**	
> 20 yrs old when died 1971–1978—PMR	416	1.1 (nr)	Burmeister, 1981
ENVIRONMENTAL			
Seveso, Italy Residential Cohort—Industrial accident July 10, 1976 (723 residents Zone A; 4,821 Zone B; 31,643 Zone R; 181,574 local reference group)		**TCDD**	
Incidence			
20-yr followup to 1996—men and women			
Zone A	1	1.2 (0.2–8.2)	Pesatori et al., 2009
Zone B	3	0.6 (0.2–1.7)	
Zone R	38	1.0 (0.7–1.4)	
10-yr followup to 1991—men			Pesatori et al., 1992
Zone A, B	2	1.0 (0.3–4.2)	
10-yr followup to 1991—women			Pesatori et al., 1992
Zone A, B	1	1.6 (0.2–12.0)	
Mortality			
25-yr followup to 2001—men and women			Consonni et al., 2008
Zone A	2	1.2 (0.3–4.7)	
Zone B	5	0.5 (0.2–1.1)	
Zone R	76	1.0 (0.7–1.7)	

continued

TABLE 8-9 Pancreatic Cancer, continued

Study Population[a]	Exposed Cases[b]	**Exposure of Interest**/Estimated Relative Risk (95% CI)[b]	Reference
20-yr followup to 1996			Bertazzi et al., 2001
Zones A and B—men	4	0.7 (0.3–1.9)	
Zones A and B—women	1	0.3 (0.0–2.0)	
15-yr followup to 1991—men			Bertazzi et al., 1997
Zone A	1	1.9 (0.0–10.5)	
Zone B	2	0.6 (0.1–2.0)	
Zone R	20	0.8 (0.5–1.2)	
15-yr followup to 1991—women			Bertazzi et al., 1997
Zone B	1	0.5 (0.0–3.1)	
Zone R	11	0.7 (0.4–1.3)	
10-yr followup to 1986—men			Bertazzi et al., 1989a,b
Zone A, B, R	9	0.6 (0.3–1.2)	
Zone B	2	1.1 (0.3–2.7)	
10-yr followup to 1986—women			Bertazzi et al., 1989a
Zone A, B, R	4	1.0 (0.3–2.7)	
SWEDEN			
Swedish fishermen (high consumption of fish with persistent organochlorines)		**Organochlorine compounds**	Svensson et al., 1995
Incidence			
East coast	4	0.6 (0.2–1.6)	
West coast	37	1.0 (0.7–1.4)	
Mortality			
East coast	5	0.7 (0.2–1.6)	
West coast	33	0.8 (0.6–1.2)	
CASE-CONTROL STUDIES			
International Case-Control Studies			
UK men, 18–35 yrs of age from counties with particular chemical manufacturing—mortality		**Herbicides, chlorophenols**	Magnani et al., 1987
Herbicides	nr	0.7 (0.3–1.5)	
Chlorophenols	nr	0.8 (0.5–1.4)	

NOTE: 2,4-D, 2,4-dichlorophenoxyacetic acid; 2,4-DP, dichlorprop; 2,4,5-T, 2,4,5-trichlorophenoxyacetic acid; 2,4,5-TCP, 2,4,5-trichlorophenol; 2,5-DCP, 2,5-dichlorophenol; CATI, computer-assisted telephone interviewing; CDC, Centers for Disease Control and Prevention; CI, confidence interval; COI, chemical of interest; IARC, International Agency for Research on Cancer; ICD, International Classification of Diseases; JEM, job-exposure matrix; MCPA, 2-methyl-4-chlorophenoxyacetic acid; MCPB, 4-(4-chloro-2-methylphenoxy)butanoic acid; MCPP, methylchlorophenoxypropionic acid; NIOSH, National Institute for Occupational Safety and Health; nr, not reported; PCDD, polychlorinated dibenzo-*p*-dioxin (highly chlorinated, if four or more chlorines); PCDF, polychlorinated dibenzofuran; PCMR, proportionate cancer mortality ratios; PCP, pentachlorophenol; PM, proportionate mortality; PMR, proportionate mortality ratio; SIR, standardized incidence ratio; TCDD, 2,3,7,8-tetrachlorodibenzo-*p*-dioxin; TCP, trichlorophenol; UK United Kingdom; VA, US Department of Veterans Affairs.

[a]Subjects are male and outcome is mortality unless otherwise noted.

[b]Given when available; results other than estimated risk explained individually.

increased (SIR = 0.42, 95% CI 0.05–1.52), nor was it increased in the two successively more inclusive, but potentially more biased, cohorts.

Boers et al. (2012) published the results of analyses of serum TCDD concentrations in the recently updated Dutch chlorophenoxy-herbicide cohorts, which had been published earlier. Boers et al. (2010) had published less sophisticated exposed-vs-unexposed results, which showed no increase in pancreatic-cancer deaths (HR for factory A = 0.86, 95% CI 0.18–4.19; only one pancreatic-cancer death in the factory B cohort). When the predicted serum TCDD concentrations generated by the model developed from the blood sampling were used, the risks of pancreatic cancer were not increased in the entire cohort (HR = 1.17, 95% CI 0.82–1.65) or in the factory A cohort alone (HR = 0.89, 95% CI 0.50–1.57).

Manuwald et al. (2012) reported on mortality in 1,191 men and 398 women who had been employed for at least 3 months during 1952–1984 in a chemical plant in Hamburg (a subcohort of the IARC phenoxy-herbicide cohort). During that period, the plant produced insecticides and herbicides, including 2,4,5-T, so cohort members had the possibility of exposure to TCDD. Subjects entered the cohort on the date of their first employment in the plant, and vital status was sought through 2007. The observed numbers of deaths from pancreatic cancer were near expectation in men (SMR = 0.90, 95% CI 0.36–1.85), women (SMR = 1.0, 95% CI 0.20–2.93), and the entire cohort (SMR = 0.93, 95% CI 0.44–1.70).

Ruder and Yiin (2011) reported mortality in 1940–2005 for the NIOSH PCP cohort of 2,122 workers in the US four plants that had been involved in PCP production. Relative to US referent rates, there were slightly more deaths from pancreatic cancer in each group, but results were not substantially different in the entire cohort (18 deaths, SMR = 1.29, 95% CI 0.76–2.03), the PCP-only group (12 deaths, SMR = 1.25, 95% CI 0.65–2.19), or the PCP-plus-TCDD group (six deaths, SMR = 1.36, 95% CI 0.50–2.96).

Waggoner et al. (2011) reported on mortality rates in the AHS cohort and found fewer pancreatic cancers than expected in both applicators (103 deaths, SMR = 0.75, 95% CI 0.61–0.91) and in their spouses (38 cases, SMR = 0.72, 95% CI 0.51–0.99). Koutros et al. (2010a) updated cancer incidence through 2006 in the AHS cohorts of private applicators, their spouses, and commercial applicators. There was a significant decrease in the number of pancreatic-cancer cases observed in the private applicators (80 cases, SIR = 0.72, 95% CI 0.57–0.89). A nonsignificant decrease in mortality from pancreatic cancer was observed in spouses (32 cases, SIR = 0.72, 95% CI 0.49–1.01), but the incidences did not differ from expectation in the smaller groups of commercial applicators (five cases, SIR = 0.99, 95% CI 0.32–2.31). The AHS has been generating valuable information on the COIs for a number of years, but these results are not herbicide-specific and so are not regarded as being fully informative for the committee's task.

Biologic Plausibility

Long-term animal studies have examined the effect of exposure to the COIs on tumor incidence (Charles et al., 1996; Stott et al., 1990; Walker et al., 2006; Wanibuchi et al., 2004). No increase in the incidence of pancreatic cancer in laboratory animals after the administration of cacodylic acid, 2,4-D, or picloram has been reported. A 2-year study of female rats reported increased incidences of pancreatic adenomas and carcinomas after treatment at the highest dose of TCDD (100 ng/kg per day) (Nyska et al., 2004). Other studies have observed chronic active inflammation, acinar-cell vacuolation, and an increase in proliferation of the acinar cells surrounding the vacuolated cells (Yoshizawa et al., 2005b). As previously discussed, chronic inflammation and hyperproliferation are closely linked to the formation and progression of cancers, including cancer of the pancreas (Hahn and Weinberg, 2002; Mantovani et al., 2008). Metaplastic changes in the pancreatic ducts were also observed in female monkeys treated with TCDD (Allen et al., 1977).

The biologic plausibility of the carcinogenicity of the COIs is discussed in general at the beginning of this chapter.

Synthesis

The large excess of pancreatic cancers in female Vietnam veterans vs their nondeployed counterparts observed by Thomas et al. (1991) and Dalager et al. (1995) prevailed in a study by Cypel and Kang (2008), who found a significant increase in all female Vietnam veterans and in the nurse subset. The committee responsible for *Update 2006* reported a higher incidence of and mortality from pancreatic cancer in deployed Australian National Service veterans than in nondeployed veterans (ADVA, 2005c). A limitation of all the veteran studies considered has been the lack of control for the effect of smoking. In the 31 female and 62 male cases in the AHS case-control study considered in *Update 2010* (Andreotti et al., 2009), however, the risk of pancreatic cancer was not associated with 2,4-D exposure, so the relative increase in the AHS cohort overall (Waggoner et al., 2011) would most certainly not be attributable to 2,4-D exposure. No increase in risk has been reported in US male Vietnam veterans or in IARC followup studies. The new updates on production cohorts and analyses from the AHS do not imply that exposures to the COIs are associated with the occurrence of pancreatic cancer.

Conclusion

On the basis of the evidence reviewed here and in previous VAO reports, the committee concludes that there is inadequate or insufficient evidence to determine whether there is an association between exposure to the COIs and pancreatic cancer.

LARYNGEAL CANCER

ACS estimated that 9,840 men and 2,520 women would receive diagnoses of cancer of the larynx (ICD-9 161) in the United States in 2012 and that 2,880 men and 770 women would die from it (Siegel et al., 2012). Those numbers constitute a little more than 0.9% of new cancer diagnoses and 0.7% of cancer deaths. The incidence of cancer of the larynx increases with age, and it is more common in men than in women, with a sex ratio in the United States of about 4:1 in people 50–64 years old. The average annual incidence of laryngeal cancer is shown in Table 8-10.

Established risk factors for laryngeal cancer are tobacco use and alcohol use, which are independent and act synergistically. Occupational exposures—long and intense exposures to wood dust, paint fumes, and some chemicals used in the metalworking, petroleum, plastics, and textile industries—also could increase risk (ACS, 2012a). An Institute of Medicine committee concluded that asbestos is a causal factor in laryngeal cancer (IOM, 2006); infection with human papilloma virus is also thought to raise the risk of laryngeal cancer (Baumann et al., 2009; Hobbs and Birchall, 2004).

Conclusions from *VAO* and Previous Updates

The committee responsible for *VAO* concluded that there was limited or suggestive evidence of an association between exposure to at least one of the COIs and laryngeal cancer on the basis of the evidence discussed below in the section "Synthesis." Although the small number of laryngeal cancers included in most studies generally limits their statistical power to support strong conclusions, additional information available to the committees responsible for *Update 1996*, *Update 1998*, *Update 2000*, *Update 2002*, *Update 2004*, *Update 2006*, *Update 2008*, and *Update 2010* did not change that conclusion.

Table 8-11 summarizes the results of the relevant studies.

TABLE 8-10 Average Annual Cancer Incidence (per 100,000) of Laryngeal Cancer in the United States[a]

	55–59 Years Old			60–64 Years Old			65–69 Years Old		
	All Races	White	Black	All Races	White	Black	All Races	White	Black
Men	12.0	11.3	24.5	19.2	17.8	41.2	26.5	25.9	50.6
Women	2.9	2.8	5.3	3.8	3.7	6.5	5.6	5.6	10.7

[a]Surveillance, Epidemiology, and End Results program, nine standard registries, crude age-specific rates, 2005–2009 (NCI, 2013).

TABLE 8-11 Selected Epidemiologic Studies—Laryngeal Cancer (Shaded Entries Are New Information for This Update)

Study Population[a]	Exposed Cases[b]	**Exposure of Interest**/Estimated Relative Risk (95% CI)[b]	Reference
VIETNAM VETERANS			
US Vietnam Veterans			
US CDC Vietnam Experience Study—Cross-sectional study, with medical examinations, of Army veterans: 9,324 deployed vs 8,989 nondeployed		**All COIs**	
Mortality			
1965–2000	0	0.0 (nr)	Boehmer et al., 2004
US VA Proportionate Mortality Study—sample of deceased male Vietnam-era Army and Marine veterans who served 7/4/1965–3/1/1973		**All COIs**	
1965–1988	50	1.3 (nr)	Watanabe and Kang, 1996
Army, deployed (n = 27,596) vs nondeployed (n = 31,757)	50	1.4 ($p < 0.05$)	
Marine Corps, deployed (n = 6,237) vs nondeployed (n = 5,040)	4	0.7 (nr)	
International Vietnam-Veteran Studies			
Australian Vietnam Veterans—58,077 men and 153 women served on land or in Vietnamese waters during 5/23/1962–7/1/1973 vs Australian population		**All COIs**	
Incidence			
All branches, 1982–2000	97	1.5 (1.2–1.8)	ADVA, 2005a
Navy	21	1.5 (0.9–2.1)	
Army	69	1.6 (1.2–1.9)	
Air Force	7	0.8 0.3–1.7)	
Mortality			
All branches, return–2001	28	1.1 (0.7–1.5)	ADVA, 2005b
Navy	6	1.1 (0.4–2.4)	
Army	19	1.1 (0.7–1.7)	
Air Force	3	0.9 (0.2–2.5)	
1980–1994	12	1.3 (0.7–2.2)	CDVA, 1997a
Australian Conscripted Army National Service (18,940 deployed vs 24,642 nondeployed)		**All COIs**	
Incidence			
1982–2000	8	0.7 (0.2–1.6)	ADVA, 2005c
Mortality			
1966–2001	2	0.4 (0.0–2.4)	ADVA, 2005c
1982–1994	0	0 (0– > 10)	CDVA, 1997b

TABLE 8-11 Laryngeal Cancer, continued

Study Population[a]	Exposed Cases[b]	**Exposure of Interest**/Estimated Relative Risk (95% CI)[b]	Reference
OCCUPATIONAL—INDUSTRIAL			
IARC Phenoxy Herbicide Cohort—Workers exposed to any phenoxy herbicide or chlorophenol (production or spraying) vs respective national mortality rates			
Mortality 1939–1992	21	1.6 (1.0–2.5)	Kogevinas et al., 1997
13,831 exposed to highly chlorinated PCDDs	15	1.7 (1.0–2.8)	
7,553 not exposed to highly chlorinated PCDDs	5	1.2 (0.4–2.9)	
Mortality 1955–1988 of 12,492 production workers and 5,898 sprayers exposed—13,482 in exposed subcohort	8	1.5 (0.6–2.9)	Saracci et al., 1991
British MCPA Plant—Production 1947–1982 (n = 1,545) (included in IARC cohort) and spraying 1947–1972 (n = 2,561) (*not* included in IARC cohort)		**MCPA**	
Mortality through 1983	4	1.7 (0.5–4.5)	Coggon et al., 1986
German Production Workers at Boehringer–Ingelheim Plant in Hamburg (1,144 men working > 1 month in 1952–1984; generation of TCDD reduced after chloracne outbreak in 1954) and women—no results (some additions to observed cancers over Manz et al., 1991) (in IARC cohort as of 1997)		**Dioxins; 2,4,5-T; 2,5-DCP; 2,4,5-TCP**	
Mortality 1952–2007	7	3.5 (1.4–7.2)	Manuwald et al., 2012
Men	6	3.8 (1.4–8.2)	
Women	1	2.5 (0.0–13.9)	
Mortality 1952–1989—stats on men only, 1,184 (tables all for 1,148 men, not necessarily German nationals) vs national rates (also vs gas workers); same observation period as Becher et al., 1966	2	2.0 (0.2–7.1)	Manz et al., 1991
New Zealand Phenoxy Herbicide Production Workers and Sprayers (1,599 men and women working any time in 1969–1988 at Dow plant in New Plymouth) (in IARC cohort)		**Dioxins; 2,4-D; 2,4,5-T; MCPA; MCPB; 2,4,5-TCP; Picloram**	
Mortality 1969–2004			McBride et al., 2009a
Ever-exposed workers	1	2.5 (0.1–14.0)	
Never-exposed workers	1	9.7 (0.2–54.3)	
Production Workers (713 men and 100 women worked > 1 month in 1969–1984)			
Mortality 1969–2000	0	nr	't Mannetje et al., 2005

continued

TABLE 8-11 Laryngeal Cancer, continued

Study Population[a]	Exposed Cases[b]	Exposure of Interest/Estimated Relative Risk (95% CI)[b]	Reference
NIOSH Mortality Cohort (12 US plants, 5,172 male production and maintenance workers 1942–1984) (included in IARC cohort as of 1997)		**Dioxins, phenoxy herbicides**	
Through 1987	7	2.1 (0.8–4.3)	Fingerhut et al., 1991
≥ 1-year exposure, ≥ 20-year latency	3	2.7 (0.6–7.8)	
All Dow TCP-Exposed Workers (TCP production 1942–1979 or 2,4,5-T production 1948–1982 in Midland, Michigan) (in IARC and NIOSH cohorts)		**2,4,5-T; 2,4,5-TCP**	
1942–2003 (n = 1,615)	3	1.3 (0.3–3.9)	Collins et al., 2009a
All Dow PCP-Exposed Workers—all workers from the two plants that only made PCP (in Tacoma, Washington, and Wichita, Kansas) and workers who made PCP and TCP at two additional plants (in Midland, Michigan, and Sauget, Illinois)		**2,4,5-T; 2,4,5-TCP**	Ruder and Yiin, 2011
1940–2005 (n = 2,122)	5	1.5 (0.5–3.4)	
PCP and TCP (n = 720)	1	0.9 (0.0–5.1)	
PCP (no TCP) (n = 1,402)	4	1.7 (0.5–4.3)	
Dow 2,4-D Production Workers (1945–1982 in Midland, Michigan) (subset of all TCP-exposed workers)		**2,4-D, lower chlorinated dioxins**	
Cancer incidence through 2007 in Dow workers (n = 1,256) vs comparisons from state cancer registries (n = 23,354) (Cohort 3)	4	1.1 (0.3–2.9)	Burns et al., 2011
Through 1982 (n = 878)	1	3.0 (0.0–16.8)	Bond et al., 1988
Dow PCP Production Workers (1937–1989 in Midland, Michigan) (*not* in IARC and NIOSH cohorts)		**Low chlorinated dioxins, 2,4-D**	
Mortality 1940–2004 (n = 577, excluding 196 also having exposure to TCP)	2	1.7 (0.2–6.2)	Collins et al., 2009b
Mortality 1940–1989 (n = 770)	2	2.9 (0.3–10.3)	Ramlow et al., 1996
0-yr latency	2	2.9 (0.4–10.3)	
15-yr latency	1	nr	
OCCUPATIONAL—PAPER AND PULP WORKERS		**TCDD**	
IARC cohort of pulp and paper workers—60,468 workers from 11 countries, TCDD among 27 agents assessed by JEM			McLean et al., 2006
Exposure to nonvolatile organochlorine compounds			
Never	18	0.9 (0.5–1.5)	
Ever	20	1.2 (0.8–1.9)	

TABLE 8-11 Laryngeal Cancer, continued

Study Population[a]	Exposed Cases[b]	**Exposure of Interest**/Estimated Relative Risk (95% CI)[b]	Reference
OCCUPATIONAL—HERBICIDE-USING WORKERS (*not* related to IARC sprayer cohorts)			
DENMARK			
Danish gardeners (n = 3,124) exposed to pesticides	9	0.7 (0.3–1.4)	Kenborg et al., 2012
ITALIAN Licensed Pesticide Users—male farmers in southern Piedmont licensed 1970–1974			
Mortality 1970–1986 (n = 23,401)	25	0.5 (0.3–0.7)	Torchio et al., 1994
Italian rice growers with documented phenoxy use (n = 1,487)		**Phenoxy herbicides**	Gambini et al., 1997
	7	0.9 (0.4–1.9)	
NEW ZEALAND National Cancer Registry (1980–1984)—case-control study of 303 incident laryngeal cancer cases vs remainder of 19,904 men with any incident cancer		**Herbicides**	Reif et al., 1989
Forestry workers (n = 134)	2	1.1 (0.3–4.7)	
SWEDEN			
Swedish lumberjacks—used phenoxys 1954–1967, Incidence 1958–1992			Thörn et al., 2000
Exposed (n = 154)			
Foremen (n = 15)	0	nr	
THE NETHERLANDS			
Dutch Licensed Herbicide Sprayers—1,341 certified before 1980			
Through 2000	1	1.0 (0.0–5.1)	Swaen et al., 2004
UNITED STATES			
US farmers—usual occupation of farmer and industry of agriculture on death certificates 1984–1988 from 23 states		**Herbicides** PCMRs	Blair et al., 1993
Men			
Whites (n = 119,648)	162	0.7 (0.6–0.8)	
Nonwhites (n = 11,446)	32	1.1 (0.8–1.5)	
Women			
Whites (n = 2,400)	0	nr (0.0–3.3)	
Nonwhites (n = 2,066)	0	nr (0.0–4.8)	
ENVIRONMENTAL			
Seveso, Italy Residential Cohort—Industrial accident July 10, 1976 (723 residents Zone A; 4,821 Zone B; 31,643 Zone R; 181,574 local reference group)		**TCDD**	
Mortality			
25-yr followup to 2001—men and women, all respiratory cancers (ICD-9 160–165) excluding lung cancers (ICD-9 162)			Consonni et al., 2008

continued

TABLE 8-11 Laryngeal Cancer, continued

Study Population[a]	Exposed Cases[b]	**Exposure of Interest**/Estimated Relative Risk (95% CI)[b]	Reference
Zone A	0	nr	
Zone B	≤ 8	nr	
Zone R	≤ 49	nr	
20-yr followup to 1996—men and women, all respiratory cancers (ICD-9 160–165) excluding lung cancers (ICD-9 162)			Bertazzi et al., 2001
Zone A	0	nr	
Zone B	8	nr	
15-yr followup to 1991—men			Bertazzi et al., 1997, 1998
Zone B	6	nr	
Zone R	32	nr	
15-yr followup to 1991—women			Bertazzi et al., 1997, 1998
Zone B	0	nr	
Zone R	6	nr	
Ecological Study of Residents of Chapaevsk, Russia		**Dioxin**	Revich et al., 2001
Incidence—Crude incidence rate in 1998 vs			
Men			
Regional (Samara)		0	
National (Russia)		11.3	
Women			
Regional (Samara)		0	
National (Russia)		0.4	
Mortality—1995–1998 (SMR vs regional rates)			
Men	13	2.3 (1.2–3.8)	
Women	1	0.1 (0.0–0.6)	

NOTE: 2,4-D, 2,4-dichlorophenoxyacetic acid; 2,4-DP, dichlorprop; 2,4,5-T, 2,4,5-trichlorophenoxyacetic acid; 2,4,5-TCP, 2,4,5-trichlorophenol; 2,5-DCP, 2,5-dichlorophenol; CDC, Centers for Disease Control and Prevention; CI, confidence interval; COI, chemical of interest; IARC, International Agency for Research on Cancer; ICD, International Classification of Diseases; JEM, job-exposure matrix; MCPA, 2-methyl-4-chlorophenoxyacetic acid; MCPB, 4-(4-chloro-2-methylphenoxy)butanoic acid; NIOSH, National Institute for Occupational Safety and Health; nr, not reported; PCDD, polychlorinated dibenzo-*p*-dioxin (highly chlorinated, if four or more chlorines); PCMR, proportionate cancer mortality ratios; PCP, pentachlorophenol; SMR, standardized mortality ratio; TCDD, 2,3,7,8-tetrachlorodibenzo-*p*-dioxin; TCP, trichlorophenol; VA, US Department of Veterans Affairs.

[a]Subjects are male and outcome is mortality unless otherwise noted.

[b]Given when available; results other than estimated risk explained individually.

Update of the Epidemiologic Literature

Vietnam-Veteran, Environmental, and Case-Control Studies

No Vietnam-veteran studies, environmental studies, or case-control studies of exposure to the COIs and laryngeal cancer have been published since *Update 2010*.

Occupational Studies

Burns et al. (2011) updated cancer incidence through 2007 in workers who were alive on January 1, 1985, and had been employed at any time from 1945 to 1994 in 2,4-D production by the Dow Chemical Company in Midland, Michigan. They found no evidence of significantly increased cancer rates overall. With four cases observed, the incidence of laryngeal cancer in the most restrictively defined cohort was not increased (SIR = 1.13, 95% CI 0.30–2.88), as was the case in the two successively more inclusive, but potentially more biased, cohorts.

Boers et al. (2012) did not report any deaths from laryngeal cancer in the updated Dutch chlorophenoxy-herbicide cohorts.

Manuwald et al. (2012) reported mortality in 1,191 men and 398 women who had been employed for at least 3 months during 1952–1984 in a chemical plant in Hamburg (a subcohort of the IARC phenoxy-herbicide cohort). During that period, the plant produced insecticides and herbicides, including 2,4,5-T, so cohort members had the possibility of exposure to TCDD. Subjects entered the cohort on the date of their first employment in the plant, and vital status was sought through 2007. SMRs calculated relative to the population of Hamburg showed that death from laryngeal cancer was increased in men (SMR = 3.75, 95% CI 1.37–8.16), and in the entire cohort the increase in risk was significant (SMR = 3.50, 95% CI 1.40–7.21), but a single death from laryngeal cancer did not constitute an increase in the women (SMR = 2.53, 95% CI 0.03–13.91). The prevalence of smoking was not controlled for in the study, but it has been suggested that it did not differ from that in the general population (Flesch-Janys et al., 1995).

Ruder and Yiin (2011) reported mortality in 1940–2005 in the NIOSH PCP cohort of 2,122 workers in the four US plants that had been involved in PCP production. PCP production entailed exposure to PCDDs and PCDFs but not to the most toxic 2,3,7,8 dioxin congener. A subcohort of 720 workers (all men, the PCP-plus-TCDD group) had also been employed in TCP production and so had also been exposed to TCDD. Only five deaths from laryngeal cancer were found in the entire cohort. Relative to US referent rates, that did not constitute a substantial increase (SMR = 1.45, 95% CI 0.47–3.38), nor did the four deaths in the PCP-only group (SMR = 1.69, 95% CI 0.46–4.32). There was only a single laryngeal-cancer death in the PCP-plus-TCDD group (SMR = 0.92, 95% CI 0.02–5.14).

The new publications on the AHS (Koutros et al., 2010a; Waggoner et al., 2011) did not report separate findings on laryngeal cancers.

Kenborg et al. (2012) conducted a study that focused on Parkinson disease in a Danish cohort of 3,124 male union members who worked as professional gardeners in 1975. When studying that cohort previously, Hansen et al. (1992, 2007) had reported that herbicides (including phenoxy herbicides) constituted most of their exposure. In addressing the observation that smoking has repeatedly been found to be negatively associated with the occurrence of Parkinson disease, Kenborg et al. also investigated the incidence of several cancers that are recognized as being smoking-related. The incidence of cancer of the larynx in the gardeners was similar to the age-adjusted and calendar-period–adjusted incidence in the general male Danish population (nine cases, SIR = 0.72, 95% CI 0.33–1.37).

Biologic Plausibility

Long-term animal studies have examined the effect of exposure to the COIs on tumor incidence (Charles et al., 1996; Stott et al., 1990; Walker et al., 2006; Wanibuchi et al., 2004). No increase in the incidence of laryngeal cancer in laboratory animals after the administration of any of the COIs has been reported.

The biologic plausibility of the carcinogenicity of the COIs is discussed in general at the beginning of this chapter.

Synthesis

The original *VAO* committee reviewed five studies that presented data on laryngeal cancer separately (Bond et al., 1988; Coggon et al., 1986; Fingerhut et al., 1991; Manz et al., 1991; Sarracci et al., 1991). It concluded that "although the numbers are too small to draw strong conclusions, the consistency of a mild increase in relative risk is suggestive of an association for laryngeal cancer." That committee also noted that the studies reviewed for laryngeal cancer did not control for potential confounders, such as smoking and alcohol consumption (IOM, 1994).

Since then, a combined analysis of many of the separate cohorts (the IARC Cohort of Phenoxy Herbicide Workers analyzed by Kogevinas et al., 1997) has shown significant effects in workers who were exposed to any phenoxyacetic acid herbicide or chlorophenol (21 deaths, RR = 1.6, 95% CI 1.0–2.5), especially workers who were exposed to TCDD or higher-chlorinated dioxins (15 deaths, RR = 1.7, 95% CI 1.0–2.8). Those RRs are remarkably close to the pooled estimate computed by the committee responsible for *VAO*. The study by Kogevinas et al. was a high-quality study that used an excellent method for assessing exposure, and its results were unlikely to have been affected by confounding in that the distribution of smoking in working cohorts is not likely to differ with degree of exposure (Siemiatycki et al., 1988). Another IARC cohort that was used in studying pulp and paper workers also showed an increase in risk (20 deaths, RR = 1.2, 95% CI 0.8–1.9; McLean et al., 2006).

With regard to veteran studies, a positive association was found in the study of veterans in Australia that compared mortality from laryngeal cancer with that in the general population (ADVA, 2005a) but not in the study that compared Australian veterans of the Vietnam conflict with nondeployed soldiers (ADVA, 2005c). In contrast, Watanabe and Kang (1996) found a significant 40% excess of mortality from laryngeal cancer in Army personnel deployed to the Vietnam theater. The Operation Ranch Hand study is not large enough to have sufficient power to detect an association if one exists.

An environmental study (Revich et al., 2001) of residents of Chapaevsk, Russia, which was heavily contaminated by many industrial pollutants, including dioxin, showed an association with laryngeal cancer in men (RR = 2.3, 95% CI 1.2–3.8).

The continuing updates on various occupational cohorts are largely consistent with the prior work, reporting a nonsignificant excess of laryngeal cancer. Some 10% of laryngeal cancers now being diagnosed are associated with HPV, but this small fraction is unlikely to have a substantial effect on studies over time. Most reports show an increased risk of laryngeal cancer that is not statistically significant, most likely because of the small number of cases in any individual study. In larger studies with exposure characterizations that focus on the COIs, the associations are generally strong for laryngeal cancer.

Conclusion

On the basis of the evidence reviewed here and in previous VAO reports, the committee concludes that there is limited or suggestive evidence of an association between exposure to at least one COI and laryngeal cancer.

LUNG CANCER

Lung cancer (carcinoma of the lung or bronchus, ICD-9 162.2–162.9) is the leading cause of cancer death in the United States. ACS estimated that 116,470 men and 109,690 women would receive diagnoses of lung cancer in the United States in 2012 and that about 87,750 men and 72,590 women would die from it (Siegel et al., 2012). Those numbers represent roughly 14% of new cancer diagnoses and 28% of cancer deaths in 2012. The principal types of lung neoplasms are identified collectively as bronchogenic carcinoma and carcinoma of the lung. Cancer of the trachea (ICD-9 162.0) is often grouped with cancer of the lung and bronchus under ICD-9 162. The lung is also a common site of metastatic tumors.

In men and women, the incidence of lung cancer increases greatly beginning at about the age of 40 years. The incidence in people 50–54 years old is double that in people 45–49 years old, and it doubles again in those 55–59 years old.

The incidence is consistently higher in black men than in women or white men. The average annual incidence of lung cancer in the United States is shown in Table 8-12.

ACS estimates that 87% of lung-cancer deaths are attributable to cigarette-smoking (ACS, 2011). Smoking increases the risk of all histologic types of lung cancer, but the associations with squamous-cell and small-cell carcinomas are strongest. Other risk factors include exposure to asbestos, uranium, vinyl chloride, nickel chromates, coal products, mustard gas, chloromethyl ethers, gasoline, diesel exhaust, and inorganic arsenic. The latter statement does not imply that cacodylic acid, which is a metabolite of inorganic arsenic, can be assumed to be a risk factor. Important environmental risk factors include exposure to tobacco smoke and radon (ACS, 2013a).

Conclusions from *VAO* and Previous Updates

The committee responsible for *VAO* concluded that there was limited or suggestive evidence of an association between exposure to at least one COI and lung cancer on the basis of the evidence discussed below in the section "Synthesis." Additional information available to the committees responsible for *Update 1996*, *Update 1998*, *Update 2000*, *Update 2002*, *Update 2004*, *Update 2006*, *Update 2008*, and *Update 2010* did not change that conclusion.

Table 8-13 summarizes the results of the relevant studies.

Update of the Epidemiologic Literature

Vietnam-Veteran, Environmental, and Case-Control Studies

No Vietnam-veteran studies, environmental studies, or case-control studies of exposure to the COIs and cancers of the lung, bronchus, or trachea have been published since *Update 2010*.

TABLE 8-12 Average Annual Incidence (per 100,000) of Lung and Bronchial Cancer in the United States[a]

	55–59 Years Old			60–64 Years Old			65–69 Years Old		
	All Races	White	Black	All Races	White	Black	All Races	White	Black
Men	99.7	93.6	175.7	177.3	168.5	302.9	302.2	294.6	465.8
Women	74.4	74.3	101.7	140.8	145.4	164.3	230.4	241.5	257.8

[a]Surveillance, Epidemiology, and End Results program, nine standard registries, crude age-specific rates, 2005–2009 (NCI, 2013).

TABLE 8-13 Selected Epidemiologic Studies—Lung, Bronchus, or Trachea Cancer (Shaded Entries Are New Information for This Update)

Study Population[a]	Exposed Cases[b]	**Exposure of Interest**/Estimated Relative Risk (95% CI)[b]	Reference
VIETNAM VETERANS			
US VietnamVeterans			
US Air Force Health Study—Ranch Hand veterans vs SEA veterans (unless otherwise noted)		**All COIs**	
Incidence			
1982–2003—White SEA comparison veterans only (n = 1,482). Serum TCDD (pg/g) based on model with exposure variable $\log_e$(TCDD)			Pavuk et al., 2005
Per unit increase of $-\log_e$(TCDD) (pg/g)	36	1.7 (0.9–3.2)	
Quartiles (pg/g):			
0.4–2.6	6	1.0 (nr)	
2.6–3.8	8	1.1 (0.3–3.4)	
3.8–5.2	9	1.2 (0.4–3.5)	
> 5.2	13	1.9 (0.7–5.5)	
Number of years served in SEA (per year of service)			
Quartiles (years in SEA):	36	1.1 (0.9–1.2)	
0.8–1.3	8	1.0 (nr)	
1.3–2.1	4	0.5 (0.2–1.8)	
2.1–3.7	11	0.7 (0.3–2.0)	
3.7–16.4	13	0.7 (0.3–2.0)	
Through 1999—White subjects vs national rates			Akhtar et al., 2004
Ranch Hand veterans (n = 1,189)	33	1.1 (0.8–1.6)	
With tours between 1966–1970	33	1.1 (0.8–1.6)	
SEA comparison veterans (n = 1,776)	48	1.2 (0.9–1.6)	
With tours between 1966–1970	37	1.2 (0.9–1.6)	
Mortality			
Through 1999—White subjects vs national rates			Akhtar et al., 2004
Ranch Hand veterans (n = 1,189)	21	0.9 (0.6–1.3)	
SEA comparison veterans (n = 1,776)	38	1.1 (0.8–1.5)	
US VA Cohort of Army Chemical Corps—Expanded as of 1997 to include all Army men with chemical MOS (2,872 deployed vs 2,737 nondeployed) serving during Vietnam era (7/01/1965–3/28/1973)		**All COIs**	
Mortality—Respiratory system cancers			
Through 2005			Cypel and Kang, 2010
Deployed veterans (2,872) vs nondeployed (2,737)	60 vs 26	1.3 (0.8–2.1)	
ACC deployed men in Kang et al. (2006) reported sprayed herbicide vs did not spray	19	1.4 (0.5–3.4)	

continued

TABLE 8-13 Lung, Bronchus, or Trachea Cancer, continued

Study Population[a]	Exposed Cases[b]	**Exposure of Interest**/Estimated Relative Risk (95% CI)[b]	Reference
Through 1991	11	1.4 (0.4–5.4)	Dalager and Kang, 1997
US CDC Vietnam Experience Study—Cross-sectional study, with medical examinations, of Army veterans: 9,324 deployed vs 8,989 nondeployed		**All COIs**	
Mortality—trachea, bronchus, lung			
1965–2000	41	1.0 (0.6–1.5)	Boehmer et al., 2004
Low grade pay at time of discharge	nr	1.6 (0.9–3.0)	
US VA Proportionate Mortality Study—sample of deceased male Vietnam-era Army and Marine veterans who served 7/4/1965–3/1/1973		**All COIs**	
1965–1988 (lung)			Watanabe and Kang, 1996
Army, deployed (n = 27,596) vs nondeployed (n = 31,757)	1,139	1.1 (nr) (p < 0.05)	
Marine Corps, deployed (n = 6,237) vs nondeployed (n = 5,040)	215	1.2 (1.0–1.3)	
US VA Study of Marine Post-service Mortality—sample of Marines serving 1967–1969, deployed (n = 10,716) vs nondeployed (n = 9,346)		**All COIs**	
Mortality (lung), earlier of discharge or April 1973 through 1991	42	1.3 (0.8–2.1)	Watanabe and Kang, 1995
US VA Cohort of Female Vietnam Veterans		**All COIs**	
Mortality			
Through 2004—lung	50	1.0 (0.7–1.4)	Cypel and Kang, 2008
Vietnam veteran nurses	35	0.8 (0.5–1.2)	
US VA using the Patient Treatment Files—329 Vietnam-era veterans and 269 noncancer controls and 111 colon cancer controls (1983–1990)	134	**All COIs** 1.4 (1.0–1.9)	Mahan et al., 1997
State Studies of US Vietnam Veterans			
Michigan Vietnam-era veterans, PM study of deaths (1974–1989)—deployed vs nondeployed	80	0.9 (0.7–1.1)	Visintainer et al., 1995
International Vietnam-Veteran Studies			
Australian Vietnam Veterans—58,077 men and 153 women served on land or in Vietnamese waters during 5/23/1962–7/1/1973 vs Australian population		**All COIs**	
Incidence			
All branches, 1982–2000	576	1.2 (1.1–1.3)	ADVA, 2005a
Navy	141	1.4 (1.2–1.7)	
Army	372	1.2 (1.1–1.3)	
Air Force	63	1.0 (0.7–1.2)	
Histologic type—all service branches combined			

TABLE 8-13 Lung, Bronchus, or Trachea Cancer, continued

Study Population[a]	Exposed Cases[b]	**Exposure of Interest**/Estimated Relative Risk (95% CI)[b]	Reference
Adenocarcinoma	188	1.5 (1.2–1.7)	
Squamous	152	1.2 (1.0–1.4)	
Small-cell	87	1.2 (0.97–1.5)	
Large-cell	79	1.1 (0.8–1.3)	
Other	70	1.1 (0.8–1.3)	
Validation Study		*Expected number of exposed cases*	AIHW, 1999
	46	65 (49–81)	
Men–self report	120	65 (49–89)	CDVA, 1998a
Mortality			
All branches, return–2001	544	1.2 (1.1–1.3)	ADVA, 2005b
Navy	135	1.4 (1.2–1.6)	
Army	339	1.1 (1.0–1.3)	
Air Force	71	1.1 (0.9–1.4)	
1980–1994			CDVA, 1997a
Lung (ICD-9 162)	212	1.3 (1.1–1.4)	
Respiratory systems (ICD-9 163–165)	13	1.8 (1.0–3.0)	
Australian Conscripted Army National Service (18,940 deployed vs 24,642 nondeployed)		**All COIs**	
Incidence			
1982–2000	78	1.2 (1.0–1.5)	ADVA, 2005c
Histologic type			
Adenocarcinoma	27	1.4 (0.8–1.9)	
Squamous	19	1.5 (0.9–2.3)	
Small-cell	14	1.4 (0.8–2.4)	
Large-cell	8	0.7 (0.3–1.3)	
Other	10	1.2 (0.6–2.2)	
Mortality			
1966–2001	67	1.8 (1.2–2.7)	ADVA, 2005c
1982–1994	27	2.2 (1.1–4.3)	CDVA, 1997b
OCCUPATIONAL—INDUSTRIAL			
IARC Phenoxy Herbicide Cohort—Workers exposed to any phenoxy herbicide or chlorophenol (production or spraying) vs respective national mortality rates			
Mortality 1939–1992			Kogevinas et al., 1997
Lung (ICD-9 162)	380	1.1 (1.0–1.2)	
Other respiratory organs (ICD-9 163–165)	12	2.3 (1.2–3.9)	
13,831 exposed to highly chlorinated PCDDs			
Lung (ICD-9 162)	225	1.1 (1.0–1.3)	
Other respiratory organs (ICD-9 163–165)	9	3.2 (1.5–6.1)	

continued

TABLE 8-13 Lung, Bronchus, or Trachea Cancer, continued

Study Population[a]	Exposed Cases[b]	**Exposure of Interest**/Estimated Relative Risk (95% CI)[b]	Reference
7,553 not exposed to highly chlorinated PCDDs			
Lung (ICD-9 162)	148	1.0 (0.9–1.2)	
Other respiratory organs (ICD-9 163–165)	3	1.2 (0.3–3.6)	
Mortality 1955–1988 of 12,492 production workers and 5,898 sprayers exposed—13,482 in exposed subcohort			Saracci et al., 1991
Trachea, bronchus, lung (ICD-9 162)	173	1.0 (0.9–1.2)	
Mortality, incidence of women in production (n = 699) and spraying (n = 2) compared to national death rates and cancer incidence rates (lung)	2	**TCDD** 1.4 (0.2–4.9)	Kogevinas et al, 1993
British MCPA Plant—Production 1947–1982 (n = 1,545) (included in IARC cohort) and spraying 1947–1972 (n = 2,561) (*not* included in IARC cohort)		**MCPA**	
Mortality through 1983 (lung, pleura, mediastinum, ICD-8 162–164)	117	1.2 (1.0–1.4)	Coggon et al., 1986
Background exposure	39	1.0 (0.7–1.4)	
Low-grade exposure	35	1.1 (0.8–1.6)	
High-grade exposure	43	1.3 (1.0–1.8)	
British Production Workers at 4 plants (included in IARC cohort) (lung)		**Dioxins, but TCDD unlikely; MCPA**	Coggon et al., 1991
	19	1.3 (0.8–2.1)	
Workers with exposure above background	14	1.2 (0.7–2.1)	
Danish Production Workers (3,390 men and 1,069 women involved in production of phenoxy herbicides unlikely to contain TCDD at 2 plants in 1947–1987) (in IARC cohort)		**Dioxins, but TCDD unlikely; 2,4-D, 2,4-DP, MCPA, MCPP**	
Incidence			
Incidence 1943–1987 (lung, men only)	13	1.6 (0.9–2.8)	Lynge, 1993
Incidence 1943–1982			Lynge, 1985
Men	38	1.2 (nr)	
Women	6	2.2 (nr)	
Dutch production workers in Plant A and Plant B, combined (in IARC cohort)		**Dioxins, 2,4,5-T, 2,4,5-TCP**	
Mortality 1955–2006 (Plant A, 1,020 workers; Plant B, 1,036 workers) (respiratory cancers)	54	1.0 (0.9–1.2)	Boers et al., 2012
TCDD plasma level (HRs, by tertile) (trachea, bronchus, lung)	52	1.0 (0.8–1.2)	
Background (≤ 0.4)	24	Referent	
Low (0.4–4.1)	11	0.5 (0.3–1.1)	
Medium (4.1–20.1)	12	1.2 (0.6–2.3)	
High (≥ 20.1)	5	1.2 (0.5–3.1)	

TABLE 8-13 Lung, Bronchus, or Trachea Cancer, continued

Study Population[a]	Exposed Cases[b]	**Exposure of Interest**/Estimated Relative Risk (95% CI)[b]	Reference
963 men exposed during production 1955–1985 vs 1,317 unexposed; mortality in 1986 (respiratory system cancers, ICD-8 160–163)	9 vs 3	1.7 (0.5–6.3)	Bueno de Mesquita et al., 1993
Dutch production workers in Plant A (549 men exposed during production 1955–1985; 594 unexposed) (in IARC cohort)		**Dioxins, 2,4,5-T, 2,4,5-TCP**	
Mortality 1955–2006 (hazard ratios for lagged TCDD plasma levels)			Boers et al., 2012
Respiratory cancer	30	1.1 (0.9–1.3)	
Trachea, bronchus, lung cancers	28	1.1 (0.9–1.3)	
Mortality 1955–2006			Boers et al., 2010
Respiratory cancer	21	1.1 (0.5–2.5)	
Trachea, bronchus, lung cancers	20	1.2 (0.5–2.8)	
Mortality 1955–1985			Bueno de Mesquita et al., 1993
Trachea, bronchus, lung cancers	9	1.0 (0.5–1.9)	
Dutch production workers in Plant B (414 men exposed during production 1965–1986; 723 unexposed) (in IARC cohort)		**2,4-D; MCPA; MCPP; highly chlorinated dioxins unlikely**	
Mortality 1965–2006			Boers et al., 2010
Respiratory cancer	12	1.2 (0.6–2.7)	
Trachea, bronchus, lung cancers	12	1.2 (0.6–2.7)	
Mortality 1965–1986			Bueno de Mesquita et al., 1993
Trachea, bronchus, lung cancers	0	0.0 (0.0–1.3)	
German Production Workers—2,479 workers at 4 plants (in IARC cohort as of 1997)		**Dioxins, phenoxy herbicides**	
All for plants	47	1.4 (1.1–1.9)	Becher et al., 1996
German Production Workers at Bayer Plant in Uerdingen (135 men working > 1 month in 1951–1976) (in IARC cohort as of 1997) and women—no results		**Dioxins; 2,4,5-TCP**	
Mortality 1951–1992	2	0.7 (0.0–2.5)	Becher et al., 1996
German Production Workers at Bayer Plant in Dormagen (520 men working > 1 month in 1965–1989) (in IARC cohort as of 1997) and women—no results		**Dioxins; 2,4-D; 2,4,5-T; MCPA; MCPP; 2,4-DP**	
Mortality 1965–1989	3	1.6 (0.3–4.6)	Becher et al., 1996

continued

TABLE 8-13 Lung, Bronchus, or Trachea Cancer, continued

Study Population[a]	Exposed Cases[b]	Exposure of Interest/Estimated Relative Risk (95% CI)[b]	Reference
German Production Workers at BASF Ludwigshafen Plant (680 men working > 1 month in 1957–1987) (in IARC cohort as of 1997) and women—no results		**Dioxins; 2,4-D; 2,4,5-T; MCPA; MCPP; 2,4-DP**	
Mortality 1956–1989	11	1.5 (0.7–2.6)	Becher et al., 1996
BASF Cleanup Workers from 1953 accident (n = 247); 114 with chloracne, 13 more with erythema; serum TCDD levels (*not* part of IARC)		**Focus on TCDD**	
Mortality			
1953–1992			Ott and Zober, 1996
Respiratory system	13	1.2 (0.6–2.0)	
TCDD 0.1–0.99 µg/kg of body weight	2	0.7 (0.1–2.5)	
TCDD ≥ 1 µg/kg of body weight	8	2.0 (0.9–3.9)	
Lung, bronchus	11	1.1 (0.6–2.0)	
TCDD 0.1–0.99 µg/kg of body weight	2	0.8 (0.1–2.8)	
TCDD ≥ 1 µg/kg of body weight	8	2.2 (1.0–4.3)	
Through 1987		*90% CI*	Zober et al., 1990
	4	2.0 (0.7–4.6)	
German Production Workers at Boehringer–Ingelheim Plant in Hamburg—1,144 men working > 1 month in 1952–1984 (generation of TCDD reduced after chloracne outbreak in 1954) and women—no results (some additions to observed cancers over Manz et al., 1991) (in IARC cohort as of 1997)		**Dioxins; 2,4,5-T; 2,5-DCP; 2,4,5-TCP**	
Mortality 1952–2007	73	1.4 (1.1–1.8)	Manuwald et al., 2012
Men	68	1.5 (1.2–1.9)	
Women	5	0.8 (0.3–1.9)	
Mortality 1952–1989	31	1.5 (1.0–2.1)	Becher et al., 1996
Mortality (lung) 1952–1989—stats on men only, 1,184 (tables all for 1,148 men, not necessarily German nationals) vs national rates (also vs gas workers); same observation period as Becher et al., 1966	26	1.7 (1.1–2.4)	Manz et al., 1991
New Zealand Phenoxy Herbicide Production Workers and Sprayers (1,599 men and women working any time in 1969–1988 at Dow plant in New Plymouth) (in IARC cohort)		**Dioxins; 2,4-D; 2,4,5-T; MCPA; MCPB; 2,4,5-TCP; Picloram**	
Mortality 1969–2004			McBride et al., 2009a
Ever-exposed workers			
Respiratory cancer	13	0.9 (0.5–1.6)	
Trachea, bronchus, lung	11	0.8 (0.4–1.5)	

TABLE 8-13 Lung, Bronchus, or Trachea Cancer, continued

Study Population[a]	Exposed Cases[b]	**Exposure of Interest**/Estimated Relative Risk (95% CI)[b]	Reference
Never-exposed workers			
Respiratory cancer	5	1.2 (0.4–2.7)	
Trachea, bronchus, lung	4	1.0 (0.3–2.5)	
Production Workers (713 men and 100 women worked > 1 month in 1969–1984); mortality (1969–2000)			
Trachea, bronchus, lung (ICD-9 162)	12	1.4 (0.7–2.4)	't Mannetje et al., 2005
Other respiratory system sites (ICD-9 163–165)	1	3.9 (0.1–21.5)	
Sprayers (697 men and 2 women on register of New Zealand applicators, 1973–1984); mortality 1973–2000			
Trachea, bronchus, lung (ICD-9 162)	5	0.5 (0.2–1.1)	't Mannetje et al., 2005
Other respiratory system sites (ICD-9 163–165)	1	2.5 (0.1–13.7)	
NIOSH Mortality Cohort (12 US plants, 5,172 male production and maintenance workers 1942–1984) (included in IARC cohort as of 1997)		**Dioxins, phenoxy herbicides**	
Through 1993	125	1.1 (0.9–1.3)	Steenland et al., 1999
Chloracne subcohort (n = 608)	30	1.5 (0.98–2.1)	
Through 1987 (Entire cohort)			Fingerhut et al., 1991
Trachea, bronchus, lung (ICD-9 162)	89	1.1 (0.9–1.4)	
Respiratory system (ICD-9 160–165	96	1.1 (0.9–1.4)	
≥ 1-year exposure, ≥ 20-year latency			
Trachea, bronchus, lung (ICD-9 162)	40	1.4 (1.0–1.9)	
Respiratory system (ICD-9 160–165	43	1.4 (1.0–1.9)	
All Dow TCP-Exposed Workers (TCP production 1942–1979 or 2,4,5-T production 1948–1982 in Midland, Michigan) (in IARC and NIOSH cohorts)		**2,4,5-T; 2,4,5-TCP**	
1942–2003 (n = 1,615) (bronchus, trachea, lung)	46	0.7 (0.5–0.9)	Collins et al., 2009a
1940–1994 (n = 2,187 men) (lung)	54	0.8 (0.6–1.1)	Bodner et al., 2003
All Dow PCP-Exposed Workers—all workers from the two plants that only made PCP (in Tacoma, Washington, and Wichita, Kansas) and workers who made PCP and TCP at two additional plants (in Midland, Michigan, and Sauget, Illinois)		**2,4,5-T; 2,4,5-TCP**	Ruder and Yiin, 2011
Respiratory cancer (ICD-9 160–165)			
1940–2005 (n = 2,122)	133	1.4 (1.2–1.6)[c]	
PCP and TCP (n = 720)	28	0.9 (0.6–1.3)	
PCP (no TCP) (n = 1,402)	105	1.6 (1.3–1.9)[c]	

continued

TABLE 8-13 Lung, Bronchus, or Trachea Cancer, continued

Study Population[a]	Exposed Cases[b]	**Exposure of Interest**/Estimated Relative Risk (95% CI)[b]	Reference
Trachea, bronchus, lung (ICD-9 162)			
1940–2005 (n = 2,122)	126	1.4 (1.1–1.6)[c]	
PCP and TCP (n = 720)	27	0.9 (0.6–1.3)	
PCP (no TCP) (n = 1,402)	99	1.6 (1.3–1.9)[c]	
Dow 2,4-D Production Workers (1945–1982 in Midland, Michigan) (subset of all TCP-exposed workers)		**2,4-D, lower chlorinated dioxins**	
Cancer incidence through 2007 in Dow workers (n = 1,256) vs comparisons from state cancer registries (n = 23,354) (Cohort 3) (lung, bronchus)	36	0.9 (0.6–1.3)	Burns et al., 2011
Through 1994 (n = 1,517) (respiratory system, ICD-8 160–163)	31	0.9 (0.6–1.3)	Burns et al., 2001
Through 1986 (n = 878) vs national vs 36,804 "unexposed" workers at same location			Bloemen et al., 1993
Respiratory system (ICD-8 162–163)	9	0.8 (0.4–1.5)	
Through 1982 (n = 878)			Bond et al., 1988
Lung (ICD-8 162–163)	8	1.0 (0.5–2.0)	
Respiratory (ICD-8 160–163) (exposure lagged 15 yrs)			
Low cumulative exposure	1	0.7 (nr)	
Medium cumulative exposure	2	1.0 (nr)	
High cumulative exposure	5	1.7 (nr)	
Dow PCP Production Workers (1937–1989 in Midland, Michigan) (*not* in IARC and NIOSH cohorts)		**Low chlorinated dioxins, 2,4-D**	
Mortality 1940–2004 (n = 577, excluding 196 also having exposure to TCP) (bronchus, trachea, lung)	30	1.0 (0.6–1.4)	Collins et al., 2009b
Mortality 1940–1989 (n = 770)			Ramlow et al., 1996
0-yr latency			
Respiratory system (ICD-8 160–163)	18	1.0 (0.6–1.5)	
Lung (ICD-8 162)	16	0.9 (0.5–1.5)	
15-yr latency			
Respiratory system (ICD-8 160–163)	17	1.1 (0.6–1.8)	
Lung (ICD-8 162)	16	1.1 (0.6–1.8)	
OCCUPATIONAL—PAPER AND PULP WORKERS		**TCDD**	
IARC cohort of pulp and paper workers—60,468 workers from 11 countries, TCDD among 27 agents assessed by JEM			McLean et al., 2006
Exposure to nonvolatile organochlorine compounds			

TABLE 8-13 Lung, Bronchus, or Trachea Cancer, continued

Study Population[a]	Exposed Cases[b]	**Exposure of Interest**/Estimated Relative Risk (95% CI)[b]	Reference
Lung (ICD-9 162)			
Never	356	1.0 (0.9–1.1)	
Ever	314	1.0 (0.9–1.2)	
Pleura (ICD-9 163)			
Never	17	2.8 (1.6–4.5)	
Ever	4	0.8 (0.2–2.0)	
Other respiratory (ICD-9 164–165)			
Never	8	2.1 (0.9–4.2)	
Ever	2	0.7 (0.1–2.4)	
OCCUPATIONAL—HERBICIDE-USING WORKERS (not related to IARC sprayer cohorts)			
CANADA			
Ontario Forestry Workers—1,222 men working ≥ 6 months 1950–1982		**Herbicides**	
80 deaths through 1982; 18 cancers (lung greatest with 5)	5	nr	Green, 1991
DENMARK			
Danish gardeners (n = 3,124) exposed to pesticides	139	1.0 (0.9–1.2)	Kenborg et al., 2012
Danish gardeners—incidence from 3,156 male and 859 female gardeners			Hansen et al., 2007
25-year followup (1975–2001)		**Herbicides**	
Born before 1915 (high exposure)	34	0.9 (0.6–1.3)	
Born 1915–1934 (medium exposure)	72	1.0 (0.8–1.2)	
Born after 1934 (low exposure)	8	0.8 (0.4–1.7)	
10-year followup (1975–1984) of male gardeners	41	1.0 (0.7–1.3)	Hansen et al., 1992
FINNISH Phenoxy Herbicide Sprayers (1,909 men working 1955–1971 ≥ 2 wks) *not* IARC		**Phenoxy herbicides**	
Incidence			Asp et al., 1994
Trachea, bronchus, lung (ICD-8 162)	39	0.9 (0.7–1.3)	
Other respiratory (ICD-8 160, 161, 163)	4	1.1 (0.7–1.3)	
Mortality 1972–1989			
Trachea, bronchus, lung (ICD-8 162)	37	1.0 (0.7–1.4)	
Other respiratory (ICD-8 160, 161, 163)	1	0.5 (0.0–2.9)	
ITALIAN Licensed Pesticide Users—male farmers in southern Piedmont licensed 1970–1974			
Mortality 1970–1986 (n = 23,401) (lung)	155	0.5 (0.4–0.5)	Torchio et al., 1994
Italian rice growers with documented phenoxy use (n = 1,487		**Phenoxy herbicides**	Gambini et al., 1997
Lung	45	0.8 (0.6–1.1)	
Pleura	2	2.2 (0.2–7.9)	

continued

TABLE 8-13 Lung, Bronchus, or Trachea Cancer, continued

Study Population[a]	Exposed Cases[b]	**Exposure of Interest**/Estimated Relative Risk (95% CI)[b]	Reference
NEW ZEALAND National Cancer Registry (1980–1984)—case-control study of 4,224 incident lung cancer cases vs remainder of 19,904 men with any incident cancer		**Herbicides**	Reif et al., 1989
Forestry workers (n = 134)	30	1.3 (0.8–1.9)	
SWEDEN			
Swedish pesticide applicators—incidence			Wiklund et al., 1989a
Trachea, bronchus, lung	38	0.5 (0.4–0.7)	
348 Swedish railroad workers (1957–October, 1978)—total exposure to herbicides (lung)	3	**Phenoxy acids** 1.4 (nr)	Axelson et al., 1980
Swedish lumberjacks—used phenoxys 1954–1967, Incidence 1958–1992			Thörn et al., 2000
Exposed (n = 154)			
Foremen (n = 15)	1	4.2 (0.0–23.2)	
Lumberjacks (n = 139)	0	—	
Unexposed lumberjacks (n = 241)	5	1.2 (0.4–2.7)	
THE NETHERLANDS			
Dutch Licensed Herbicide Sprayers—1,341 certified before 1980			
Through 2000 (trachea, lung)	27	0.7 (0.5–1.0)	Swaen et al., 2004
Through 1987(trachea, lung)	12	1.1 (0.6–1.9)	Swaen et al., 1992
UNITED STATES			
US farmers—usual occupation of farmer and industry of agriculture on death certificates 1984–1988 from 23 states		**Herbicides** PCMRs	Blair et al., 1993
Men			
Whites (n = 119,648)	6,473	0.9 (0.9–0.9)	
Nonwhites (n = 11,446)	664	1.0 (0.9–1.1)	
Women			
Whites (n = 2,400)	57	0.8 (0.6–1.1)	
Nonwhites (n = 2,066)	24	0.6 (0.4–0.9)	
US Agricultural Health Study—prospective study of licensed pesticide sprayers in Iowa and North Carolina: commercial (n = 4,916), private/farmers (n = 52,395, 97.4% men), and spouses of private sprayers (n = 32,347, 0.007% men), enrolled 1993–1997; followups with CATIs 1999–2003 and 2005–2010		**Phenoxy herbicides**	
Incidence			
Enrollment through 2006—SIRs for participants (lung, bronchus)			Koutros et al., 2010a
Private applicators	436	0.5 (0.4–0.5)	
Commercial applicators	26	0.8 (0.5–1.1)	
Spouses	133	0.4 (0.4–0.5)	

TABLE 8-13 Lung, Bronchus, or Trachea Cancer, continued

Study Population[a]	Exposed Cases[b]	**Exposure of Interest**/Estimated Relative Risk (95% CI)[b]	Reference
Enrollment through 2002			Samanic et al., 2006
Dicamba—lifetime days exposure			
None	95	1.0	
1– < 20	14	0.8 (0.5–1.5)	
20– < 56	11	0.6 (0.3–1.3)	
56– < 116	12	1.0 (0.5–1.9)	
≥ 116	15	1.5 (0.8–2.7	
		p-trend = 0.13	
Enrollment through 2002			Alavanja et al., 2005
Private applicators			
Lung	266	0.5 (0.4–0.5)	
Respiratory system	294	0.5 (0.4–0.5)	
Spouses of private applicators (> 99% women)			
Lung	68	0.4 (0.3–0.5)	
Respiratory system	71	0.4 (0.3–0.5)	
Commercial applicators			
Lung	12	0.6 (0.3–1.0)	
Respiratory system	14	0.6 (0.3–1.0)	
Mortality			
Enrollment through 2007, vs state rates			Waggoner et al., 2011
Respiratory			
Applicators (n = 1,641)	422	0.4 (0.4–0.5)	
Spouses (n = 676)	110	0.4 (0.3–0.5)	
Trachea, bronchus, lung			
Applicators (n = 1,641)	417	0.4 (0.4–0.5)	
Spouses (n = 676)	108	0.4 (0.3–0.5)	
Other respiratory system			
Applicators (n = 1,641)	5	0.2 (0.1–0.3)	
Spouses (n = 676)	2	nr	
Enrollment through 2000, vs state rates			Blair et al., 2005a
Private applicators (men and women)	129	0.4 (0.3–0.4)	
Years handled pesticides			
≤ 10 yrs	25	0.4 (nr) (p < 0.05)	
≥ 10 yrs	80	0.3 (nr) (p < 0.05)	
Spouses of private applicators (> 99% women)	29	0.3 (0.2–0.5)	
Florida Licensed Pesticide Applicators (common phenoxy use assumed but not documented)		**Herbicides**	
Pesticide applicators in **Florida** licensed 1965–1966 (n = 3,827)—mortality through 1976		**Herbicides**	Blair et al., 1983
Any pesticide (dose-response by length of licensure)			

continued

TABLE 8-13 Lung, Bronchus, or Trachea Cancer, continued

Study Population[a]	Exposed Cases[b]	**Exposure of Interest**/Estimated Relative Risk (95% CI)[b]	Reference
Only for lawn and ornamentals (lung, ICD-8 162–163)	7	0.9 (nr)	
Minnesota Highway Maintenance Workers (n = 4,849) who worked ≥ 1 day for the Department of Transportation and ≥ 1 day after January 1, 1945 (1984–1986)		**Herbicides**	Bender et al., 1989
Trachea, bronchus, lung (ICD-9 162.0–162.8)	54	0.7 (0.5–0.9)	
All respiratory (ICD-9 160.0–165.9)	57	0.7 (0.5–0.9)	
ENVIRONMENTAL			
Seveso, Italy Residential Cohort—Industrial accident July 10, 1976 (723 residents Zone A; 4,821 Zone B; 31,643 Zone R; 181,574 local reference group) (ICD-9 171)		**TCDD**	
Incidence			
20-yr followup to 1996—men and women (lung ICD-9 162)			Pesatori et al., 2009
Zone A	7	1.1 (0.5–2.4)	
Zone B	37	1.0 (0.7–1.3)	
Zone R	280	1.0 (0.9–1.2)	
10-yr followup to 1991—men			Bertazzi et al., 1993
Zone A	2	0.8 (0.2–3.4)	
Zone B	18	1.1 (0.7–1.8)	
Zone R	96	0.8 (0.7–1.0)	
10-yr followup to 1991—women			Bertazzi et al., 1993
Zone R	16	1.5 (0.8–2.5)	
Mortality			
25-yr followup to 2001—men and women (lung ICD-9 162)			Consonni et al., 2008
Zone A	11	1.1 (0.6–2.0)	
Zone B	62	1.1 (0.9–1.4)	
Zone R	383	1.0 (0.8–1.1)	
20-yr followup to 1996 (lung)			Bertazzi et al., 2001
Zones A, B—men	57	1.3 (1.0–1.7)	
Zones A, B—women	4	0.6 (0.2–1.7)	
15-yr followup to 1991—men (lung)			Bertazzi et al., 1998
Zone A	4	1.0 (0.4–2.6)	
Zone B	34	1.2 (0.9–1.7)	
Zone R	176	0.9 (0.8–1.1)	
15-yr followup to 1991—women (lung)			Bertazzi et al., 1998
Zone A	0	nr	
Zone B	2	0.6 (0.1–2.3)	
Zone R	29	1.0 (0.7–1.6)	
Ecological Study of Residents of Chapaevsk, Russia		**Dioxin**	Revich et al., 2001

TABLE 8-13 Lung, Bronchus, or Trachea Cancer, continued

Study Population[a]	Exposed Cases[b]	**Exposure of Interest**/Estimated Relative Risk (95% CI)[b]	Reference
Incidence—Crude incidence rate in 1998 vs			
Men			
Regional (Samara)	nr	102.4 (nr)	
National (Russia)	nr	89.4 (nr)	
Women			
Regional (Samara)	nr	11.1 (nr)	
National (Russia)	nr	9.8 (nr)	
Mortality—1995–1998 (SMR vs regional rates)			
Men	168	3.1 (2.6–3.5)	
Women	40	0.4 (0.3–0.6)	
Other International Environmental Studies			
FINLAND			
Finnish fishermen (n = 6,410) and spouses (n = 4,260) registered between 1980 and 2002 compared to national statistics (larynx, trachea, lung, combined)		**Serum dioxin**	Turunen et al., 2008
Fisherman	72	0.8 (0.6–1.0)	
Spouses	8	0.7 (0.3–1.4)	
JAPAN			
Residents of municipalities with and without waste incineration plants (cross-sectional)		**Dioxin emissions** age-adjusted mortality (per 100,000)	Fukuda et al., 2003
Men			
With Without		39.0 ± 6.7 vs 41.6 ± 9.1 (p = 0.0001)	
Women			
With Without		13.7 ± 3.8 vs 14.3 ± 4.6 (p = 0.11)	
SWEDEN			
Swedish fishermen (high consumption of fish with persistent organochlorines)		**Organochlorine compounds**	Svensson et al., 1995
Incidence			
East coast (lung)	24	1.2 (0.8–1.8)	
West coast (lung)	73	0.9 (0.7–1.1)	
Mortality			
East coast	16	0.8 (0.5–1.3)	
West coast	77	0.9 (0.7–1.1)	
CASE-CONTROL STUDIES			
International Case-Control Studies			

continued

TABLE 8-13 Lung, Bronchus, or Trachea Cancer, continued

Study Population[a]	Exposed Cases[b]	**Exposure of Interest**/Estimated Relative Risk (95% CI)[b]	Reference
Saskatchewan, Canada farmers (604 men, 223 women) diagnosed with lung cancer between November, 1983, and July, 1986		**Herbicides**	McDuffie et al., 1990
Interviews with lung cancer patients (273 men and 103 women) who sprayed herbicides	103	0.6 (nr)	

NOTE: 2,4-D, 2,4-dichlorophenoxyacetic acid; 2,4-DP, dichlorprop; 2,4,5-T, 2,4,5-trichlorophenoxyacetic acid; 2,4,5-TCP, 2,4,5-trichlorophenol; 2,5-DCP, 2,5-dichlorophenol; ACC, Army Chemical Corps; CATI, computer-assisted telephone interviewing; CDC, Centers for Disease Control and Prevention; CI, confidence interval; COI, chemical of interest; IARC, International Agency for Research on Cancer; ICD, International Classification of Diseases; JEM, job-exposure matrix; MCPA, 2-methyl-4-chlorophenoxyacetic acid; MCPB, 4-(4-chloro-2-methylphenoxy)butanoic acid; MCPP, methylchlorophenoxypropionic acid; MOS, military occupational specialty; NIOSH, National Institute for Occupational Safety and Health; nr, not reported; PCDD, polychlorinated dibenzo-*p*-dioxin (highly chlorinated, if four or more chlorines); PCMR, proportionate cancer mortality ratios; PCP, pentachlorophenol; PM, proportionate mortality; SEA, Southeast Asia; SIR, standardized incidence ratio; SMR, standardized mortality ratio; TCDD, 2,3,7,8-tetrachlorodibenzo-*p*-dioxin; TCP, trichlorophenol; VA, US Department of Veterans Affairs.

[a]Subjects are male and outcome is mortality unless otherwise noted.

[b]Given when available; results other than estimated risk explained individually.

[c]*99% CI.*

Occupational Studies

Burns et al. (2011) updated cancer incidence through 2007 in workers who were alive on January 1, 1985, and had been employed at any time from 1945 to 1994 in 2,4-D production by the Dow Chemical Company in Midland, Michigan. They found no evidence of significantly increased rates of cancer overall. With 36 cases observed, the incidence of lung or bronchial cancer in the most restrictively defined cohort was not increased (SIR = 0.92, 95% CI 0.65–1.28). The category of other respiratory cancers was significantly increased (SIR = 4.76, 95% CI 1.53–11.11), but this category consisted of only one carcinoma of the sinuses and four cases of mesothelioma, which could be attributed with some certainty to occupational asbestos exposure, although no documentation was provided.

Boers et al. (2012) updated mortality in workers in two chlorophenoxy herbicide plants in the Netherlands by using semiquantitative measures of TCDD exposure. Plasma concentrations of TCDD in a subset of 187 workers were used to develop a predictive model of TCDD exposure, and a Cox proportional-hazards model was used to investigate associations between time-varying TCDD exposure and cause-specific mortality. No relationship was found between TCDD exposure and respiratory cancers. HRs for predicted TCDD concentrations and cancers of the trachea, bronchus, and lung were not increased in the entire cohort (HR = 0.98, 95% CI 0.84–1.15 for each unit increase in TCDD exposure on a log scale) or in only the workers in factory A (HR = 1.07, 95% CI 0.86–1.33). That study was a reanalysis of the mortality data on the cohort updated through 2006; using crude exposure estimates based on job classification, Boers et al. (2010) had found that respiratory-cancer risks were not significantly increased. That finding is in contrast with the excess mortality from respiratory cancers reported in the second followup of the cohort (Hooiveld et al., 1998).

Manuwald et al. (2012) updated mortality though 2007 in a cohort of 1,589 male and female workers employed for at least 3 months during 1952–1984 in a factory in Hamburg, Germany, that produced various herbicides and insecticides, including 2,4,5-T, which was contaminated with TCDD and other higher-chlorinated dioxins and furans. SMRs were calculated by using the population of Hamburg as a reference group. Deaths due to cancer of the trachea, bronchus, and lung were significantly increased in men (68 deaths, SMR = 1.52, 95% CI 1.18–1.93) and in the total cohort (SMR = 1.43, 95% CI 1.12–1.80) but were not increased in the smaller group of women (five deaths, SMR = 0.80, 95% CI 0.26–1.88). The prevalence of smoking was not controlled for but was suggested not to differ from that in the general population (Flesch-Janys et al., 1995). Although those findings are consistent with earlier mortality reports on this cohort (Becher et al., 1996; Manz et al., 1991), an exposure–response relationship was not found ($p = 0.30$) for respiratory-cancer mortality when estimated cumulative occupational exposure to TCDD was stratified into quartiles.

Ruder and Yiin (2011) reported mortality through 2005 in a cohort of 2,122 US PCP production workers in four plants in the NIOSH Dioxin Registry relative to US referent rates. The workers in all four plants were exposed to PCP and to PCDDs and PCDFs as contaminants during the production of PCP. Two plants were also involved in TCP production, so a subcohort of 720 men was also exposed to 2,3,7,8-TCDD, a contaminant of TCP, but not of PCP. A total of 1,165 deaths occurred in 1940–2005, and overall cancer mortality was significantly increased (326 deaths, SMR = 1.17, 95% CI 1.05–1.31). There were excess deaths from tracheal, bronchial, and lung cancer (126 deaths, SMR = 1.36, 95% CI 1.13–1.62) in the entire cohort and in the PCP-only group (99 deaths, SMR = 1.56, 95% CI 1.27–1.90) but no increase in the PCP-plus-TCDD group (27 deaths, SMR = 0.91, 95% CI 0.60–1.33). The increase in the SMR for lung-cancer mortality did not increase with duration (days of work in PCP operations); it reached the concentration of statistical significance in the lowest group (up to 57 days) and in the third of the four categories (182 to < 650 days). The study has merit in that it followed all US workers employed in PCP manufacturing through 1992 for an average of 39 years from first exposure. The lack of information on smoking greatly limits conclusions regarding the contribution of the agents to the increase in mortality from tracheal, bronchial, and lung cancers. Although there was potential for occupational exposure to TEQs in the entire cohort, the smaller subcohort with potential for TCDD exposure did not have increased mortality due to tracheal, bronchial, and lung cancers. In addition, the authors noted that there was no difference in mortality between the 236 workers who had diagnoses of chloracne and other workers, as found earlier by Bodner et al. (2003).

Koutros et al. (2010a) updated cancer incidence as of 2006 in members of the large prospective AHS cohort. SIRs of lung and bronchial cancers were significantly lower in private applicators (436 cases, SIR = 0.48, 95% CI 0.43–0.53) and their spouses (133 cases, SIR = 0.42, 95% CI 0.35–0.50) and unchanged in commercial applicators (26 cases, SIR = 0.75, 95% CI 0.49–1.09) relative to the general population in Iowa and North Carolina, the states selected for the study. Lower rates of smoking and increased physical activity are factors that may contribute to the lower risk of cancer at these sites.

Waggoner et al. (2011) reported mortality in the same AHS cohort from the time of enrollment (1993–1997) through 2007 vs state-specific rates. Death from tracheal, bronchial, and lung cancer was significantly decreased in private and commercial applicators (417 deaths, SMR = 0.43, 95% CI 0.39–0.47) and their spouses (108 deaths, SMR = 0.38, 95% CI 0.31–0.45). The AHS has been generating valuable information on the COIs for a number of years, but these results are not herbicide-specific and so are not regarded as being fully informative for the committee's task.

Kenborg et al. (2012) conducted a study that focused on Parkinson disease in a Danish cohort of 3,124 male union members who worked as professional gardeners in 1975. When studying this cohort previously, Hansen et al. (1992, 2007) had reported that herbicides (including phenoxy herbicides) constituted most of their exposure. Kenborg et al. (2012) reported the incidence of several cancers recognized as being smoking-related. The incidence of lung cancer in the gardeners was similar to the age-adjusted and calendar-period–adjusted incidence in the general male Danish population (SIR = 1.02, 95% CI 0.86–1.20).

Biologic Plausibility

Long-term animal studies have examined the effects of exposure to the COIs on tumor incidence (Charles et al., 1996; Stott et al., 1990; Walker et al., 2006; Wanibuchi et al., 2004). As noted in previous VAO reports, there is evidence of an increased incidence of squamous-cell carcinoma of the lung in male and female rats exposed to TCDD at high concentrations (Kociba et al., 1978; Van Miller et al., 1977). A significant increase in neoplastic and nonneoplastic lung lesions was found in female rats exposed to TCDD for 2 years (Kociba et al., 1978; NTP, 1982a,b, 2006; Walker et al., 2006, 2007). The most common nonneoplastic lesions were bronchiolar metaplasia and squamous metaplasia of the alveolar epithelium. Cystic keratinizing epithelioma was the most commonly observed neoplasm. The lung was also identified as a target organ in an NTP tumor-promotion study after 60 weeks of exposure to TCDD in ovariectomized female Sprague Dawley rats initiated with a single dose of diethyl-*N*-nitrosamine (Beebe et al., 1995; Tritscher et al., 2000). Those studies ended with increased incidences of alveolar epithelial hyperplasia and alveolar–bronchiolar metaplasia, results that were similar to what was observed in the earlier National Toxicology Program (NTP) studies (Tritscher et al., 2000).

A 2-year study of F344 rats exposed to cacodylic acid at 0–100 ppm and B6C3F1 mice exposed at 0–500 ppm failed to detect lung neoplasms at any dose (Arnold et al., 2006); this finding is consistent with those of previous studies. However, exposure to cacodylic acid had previously been shown to increase tumor multiplicity in mouse strains that were susceptible to developing lung tumors (for example, A/J strain; Hayashi et al., 1998) or in mice pretreated with an intitiating agent (4-nitroquinoline 1-oxide; Yamanaka et al., 1996). The data indicate that cacodylic acid may act as a tumor-promoter in the lung.

The biologic plausibility of the carcinogenicity of the COIs is discussed in general at the beginning of this chapter.

Synthesis

The evidence remains limited but suggestive of an association between exposure to at least one COI and the risk of developing or dying from lung cancer. In the present update, there are new supporting data from the followup studies of mortality in the Hamburg cohort of herbicide producers (Manuwald et al., 2012) and in US PCP workers (Ruder and Yiin, 2011). In the past, the most compelling evidence has come from studies of heavily exposed occupational cohorts, including British 2-methyl-4-chlorophenoxyacetic acid (MCPA) production workers (Coggon et al., 1986), German production workers (Becher et al., 1996), a BASF cohort (Ott and Zober, 1996), a NIOSH cohort (Fingerhut et al., 1991; Steenland et al., 1999), and Danish production workers (Lynge, 1993).

In the last update, Cypel and Kang (2010) found a significantly increased lung-cancer risk in Army Chemical Corps (ACC) veterans who used herbicides in Vietnam. The most recent findings from the Operation Ranch Hand study (Pavuk et al., 2005) suggested an increase in risk with serum TCDD concentration even in subjects who made up the comparison group, whose TCDD exposure was considerably lower than that of the Ranch Hand cohort (but not zero). The American and Australian cohort studies of Vietnam veterans (ADVA, 2005a,b,c; Dalager and Kang, 1997), which presumably cover a large proportion of exposed soldiers, showed higher than expected incidence of and mortality from lung cancer. The main limitations of those studies are that there was no assessment of exposure—as there was in, for example, the Ranch Hand study—and that some potential confounding variables, notably smoking, could not be accounted for. The committee believes that it is unlikely that the distribution of smoking differed greatly between the two cohorts of veterans, so confounding by smoking is probably minimal. The studies therefore lend support to the findings of the Ranch Hand study. The methodologically sound AHS did not show any increased risk of lung cancer; however, although there was substantial 2,4-D exposure in this cohort (Blair et al., 2005b), dioxin exposure of the contemporary farmers was probably negligible.

In large part, the environmental studies have not been supportive of an association, although in the cancer-incidence update from Seveso, the highest risks occurred in the most exposed.

Also supportive of an association, however, are the numerous lines of mechanistic evidence, discussed in the section on biologic plausibility, which provide further support for the conclusion that the evidence of an association is limited or suggestive.

Conclusion

On the basis of the evidence reviewed here and in previous VAO reports, the committee concludes that there is limited or suggestive evidence of an association between exposure to at least one COI and carcinomas of the lung, bronchus, and trachea.

BONE AND JOINT CANCER

ACS estimated that about 1,600 men and 1,290 women would receive diagnoses of bone or joint cancer (ICD-9 170) in the United States in 2012 and that 790 men and 620 women would die from these cancers (Siegel et al., 2012). Primary bone cancers are among the least common malignancies, but the bones are frequent sites of tumors secondary to cancers that have metastasized. Only primary bone cancer is considered here. The average annual incidence of bone and joint cancer is shown in Table 8-14.

Bone cancer is more common in teenagers than in adults. It is rare among people in the age groups of most Vietnam veterans (50–64 years). Among the

TABLE 8-14 Average Annual Incidence (per 100,000) of Bone and Joint Cancer in the United States[a]

	55–59 Years Old			60–64 Years Old			65–69 Years Old		
	All Races	White	Black	All Races	White	Black	All Races	White	Black
Men	1.0	1.3	0.3	1.3	1.3	1.1	1.5	1.5	2.8
Women	0.8	0.9	0.4	1.5	1.5	1.5	1.2	1.4	0.4

[a]Surveillance, Epidemiology, and End Results program, nine standard registries, crude age-specific rates, 2005–2009 (NCI, 2013).

risk factors for bone and joint cancer in adults are exposure to ionizing radiation in treatment for other cancers and a history of some noncancer bone diseases, including Paget disease.

Conclusions from *VAO* and Previous Updates

The committee responsible for *VAO* concluded that there was inadequate or insufficient information to determine whether there is an association between exposure to the COIs and bone and joint cancer. Additional information available to the committees responsible for *Update 1996*, *Update 1998*, *Update 2000*, *Update 2002*, *Update 2004*, *Update 2006*, *Update 2008*, and *Update 2010* did not change that conclusion.

Table 8-15 summarizes the results of the relevant studies.

Update of the Epidemiologic Literature

Vietnam-Veteran and Case-Control Studies

No Vietnam-veteran studies or case-control studies of exposure to the COIs and bone or joint cancer have been published since *Update 2010*.

Occupational Studies

In an update of cancer incidence from 1985 through 2007 in 2,4-D production workers in the Dow Chemical Company in Midland, Michigan, Burns et al. (2011) found a single case of cancer of bone or soft tissue, with attendant nonsignificant estimates of exposure-related risk (SIR = 0.81, 95% CI 0.01–4.49 in the most restrictively defined cohort). Similarly, Waggoner et al. (2011) reported three deaths from cancer in the applicators in the AHS and two in their spouses. The numbers are too small to add significantly to the assessment of bone-cancer risk associated with exposure to the COIs.

Environmental Studies

One recent study (McNally et al., 2012) reported on the occurrence of bone cancer (Ewings sarcoma and osteosarcoma) in all of Great Britian in 1980–2005. The data on incidence from the cancer registries included 2,566 osteosarcoma cases and 1,650 Ewing sarcoma cases. There were essentially no exposure data, but the cases occurred in lower-socioeconomic areas, possibly indicating some association with agricultural exposures. This very large study has no exposure data and thus provides little information that is germane to the task of the present committee.

TABLE 8-15 Selected Epidemiologic Studies—Bone and Joint Cancer (Shaded Entries Are New Information for This Update)

Study Population[a]	Exposed Cases[b]	**Exposure of Interest**/Estimated Relative Risk (95% CI)[b]	Reference
VIETNAM VETERANS			
US Vietnam Veterans			
US VA Proportionate Mortality Study—sample of deceased male Vietnam-era Army and Marine veterans who served 7/4/1965–3/1/1973		**All COIs**	
1965–1982			Breslin et al., 1986, 1988
Army, deployed (n = 19,708) vs nondeployed (n = 22,904)	27	0.8 (0.4–1.7)	
Marine Corps, deployed (n = 4,527) vs nondeployed (n = 3,781)	11	1.4 (0.1–21.5)	
State Studies of US Vietnam Veterans			
Massachusetts Vietnam-era veterans			
Veterans aged 35–64 years in 1993—cases diagnosed 1988–1993 vs nonexposed veterans with gastrointestinal cancers	4	0.9 (0.1–11.3)	Clapp, 1997
New York			
Deployed vs nondeployed veterans	8	1.0 (0.3–3.0)	Lawrence et al., 1985
923 White male Vietnam veterans with **Wisconsin** death certificate (1968–1978) vs proportions for Vietnam-era veterans	1	nr	Anderson et al., 1986
OCCUPATIONAL—INDUSTRIAL			
IARC Phenoxy Herbicide Cohort—Workers exposed to any phenoxy herbicide or chlorophenol (production or spraying) vs respective national mortality rates			
Mortality 1939–1992	5	1.2 (0.4–2.8)	Kogevinas et al., 1997
13,831 exposed to highly chlorinated PCDDs	3	1.1 (0.2–3.1)	
7,553 not exposed to highly chlorinated PCDDs	2	1.4 (0.2–5.2)	
British MCPA Plant—Production 1947–1982 (n = 1,545) (included in IARC cohort) and spraying 1947–1972 (n = 2,561) (*not* included in IARC cohort)		**MCPA**	
Mortality through 1983	1	0.9 (0.0–5.0)	Coggon et al., 1986
BASF Cleanup Workers from 1953 accident (n = 247); 114 with chloracne, 13 more with erythema; serum TCDD levels (*not* part of IARC)		**Focus on TCDD**	
Mortality			
Through 1987		*90% CI*	Zober et al., 1990
	0	0.0 (0.0–65.5)	

TABLE 8-15 Bone and Joint Cancer, continued

Study Population[a]	Exposed Cases[b]	**Exposure of Interest**/Estimated Relative Risk (95% CI)[b]	Reference
New Zealand Phenoxy Herbicide Production Workers and Sprayers (1,599 men and women working any time in 1969–1988 at Dow plant in New Plymouth) (in IARC cohort)		**Dioxins; 2,4-D; 2,4,5-T; MCPA; MCPB; 2,4,5-TCP; Picloram**	
Mortality 1969–2004	0	0.0 (0.0–21.8)	McBride et al., 2009a
Production Workers (713 men and 100 women worked > 1 month in 1969–1984)			
Mortality 1969–2000	0	nr	't Mannetje et al., 2005
NIOSH Mortality Cohort (12 US plants, 5,172 male production and maintenance workers 1942–1984) (included in IARC cohort as of 1997)		**Dioxins, phenoxy herbicides**	
Through 1987	2	2.3 (0.3–8.2)	Fingerhut et al., 1991
≥ 1-year exposure, ≥ 20-year latency	1	5.5 (0.1–29.0)	
Mortality—754 Monsanto workers, among most highly exposed workers from Fingerhut et al. (1991)	2	5.0 (0.6–18.1)	Collins et al., 1993
Dow 2,4-D Production Workers (1945–1982 in Midland, Michigan) (subset of all TCP-exposed workers)		**2,4-D, lower chlorinated dioxins**	
Cancer incidence through 2007 in Dow workers (n = 1,256) vs comparisons from state cancer registries (n = 23,354) (Cohort 3) (bone, soft tissue)	1	0.8 (0.0–4.5)	Burns et al., 2011
Through 1982 (n = 878)	0	nr (0.0–31.1)	Bond et al., 1988
Dow PCP Production Workers (1937–1989 in Midland, Michigan) (*not* in IARC and NIOSH cohorts)		**Low chlorinated dioxins, 2,4-D**	
Mortality 1940–1989 (n = 770)	0	nr	Ramlow et al., 1996
0-yr latency	0	nr	
15-yr latency	0	nr	
OCCUPATIONAL—PAPER AND PULP WORKERS		**TCDD**	
IARC cohort of pulp and paper workers—60,468 workers from 11 countries, TCDD among 27 agents assessed by JEM			
Danish paper workers			Rix et al., 1998
Men	1	0.5 (0.0–2.7)	
Women	0	nr	

continued

TABLE 8-15 Bone and Joint Cancer, continued

Study Population[a]	Exposed Cases[b]	Exposure of Interest/Estimated Relative Risk (95% CI)[b]	Reference
OCCUPATIONAL—HERBICIDE-USING WORKERS (*not* related to IARC sprayer cohorts)			
CANADA			
Sawmill Workers in British Columbia—23,829 workers for ≥ 1 year at 11 mills using chlorophenates 1940–1985		**Chlorophenates, not TCDD**	
Incidence 1969–1989	4	1.1 (0.4–2.4)	Hertzman et al., 1997
Mortality 1950–1989	5	1.3 (0.5–2.7)	
No exposed to highly chlorinated PCDDs	2	1.4 (0.2–5.2)	
DENMARK			
Danish Farmers—incidence from linking farmers on 1970 census with national cancer registry (1970–1980)		**Herbicides**	Ronco et al., 1992
Men			
Self-employed	9	0.9 (nr)	
Employee	0	nr	
Women			
Self-employed	0	0.0	
Employee	1	6.3 ($p < 0.05$)	
ITALIAN Licensed Pesticide Users—male farmers in southern Piedmont licensed 1970–1974			
Mortality 1970–1986 (n = 23,401)	10	0.8 (0.4–1.4)	Torchio et al., 1994
Italian rice growers with documented phenoxy use (n = 1,487)		**Phenoxy herbicides**	Gambini et al., 1997
	1	0.5 (0.0–2.6)	
NEW ZEALAND National Cancer Registry (1980–1984)—case-control study of incident bone cancer cases vs remainder of 19,904 men with any incident cancer		**Herbicides**	Reif et al., 1989
Forestry workers (n = 134)	1	1.7 (0.2–13.3)	
SWEDEN			
Incident bone cancer cases 1961–1973 with agriculture as economic activity in 1960 census	44	*99% CI* 1.0 (0.6–1.4)	Wiklund, 1983
THE NETHERLANDS			
Dutch Licensed Herbicide Sprayers—1,341 certified before 1980			
Through 2000	0	nr	Swaen et al., 2004
UNITED STATES			
US farmers—usual occupation of farmer and industry of agriculture on death certificates 1984–1988 from 23 states		**Herbicides** PCMRs	Blair et al., 1993
Men			
Whites (n = 119,648)	49	1.3 (1.0–1.8)	
Nonwhites (n = 11,446)	4	1.0 (0.3–2.5)	

TABLE 8-15 Bone and Joint Cancer, continued

Study Population[a]	Exposed Cases[b]	**Exposure of Interest**/Estimated Relative Risk (95% CI)[b]	Reference
Women			
Whites (n = 2,400)	1	1.2 (0.0–6.6)	
Nonwhites (n = 2,066)	0	0.0 (0.0–6.3)	
White Male Residents of Iowa—bone cancer on death certificate, usual occupation: farmers vs not		**Herbicides**	
> 20 yrs old when died 1971–1978—PMR	56	1.1 (nr)	Burmeister, 1981
ENVIRONMENTAL			
Seveso, Italy Residential Cohort—Industrial accident July 10, 1976 (723 residents Zone A; 4,821 Zone B; 31,643 Zone R; 181,574 local reference group) (ICD-9 171)		**TCDD**	
Mortality			
15-yr followup to 1991—men			Bertazzi et al., 1998
Zone R	2	0.5 (0.1–2.0)	
15-yr followup to 1991—women			Bertazzi et al., 1998
Zone B	1	2.6 (0.3–19.4)	
Zone R	7	2.4 (1.0–5.7)	
Ecological Study of Residents of Chapaevsk, Russia		**Dioxin**	Revich et al., 2001
Mortality—1995–1998 (SMR vs regional rates)			
Men	7	2.1 (0.9–4.4)	
Women	7	1.4 (0.6–3.0)	
CASE-CONTROL STUDIES			
International Case-Control Studies			
European Multicentric study of association between occupational exposure and risk of bone sarcoma (96 cases, 35–69 yrs of age vs 2,632 hospital- and population-based controls	18	**Herbicides, pesticides** 2.6 (1.5–4.6)	Merletti et al., 2005

NOTE: 2,4-D, 2,4-dichlorophenoxyacetic acid; 2,4,5-T, 2,4,5-trichlorophenoxyacetic acid; 2,4,5-TCP, 2,4,5-trichlorophenol; CI, confidence interval; COI, chemical of interest; GI, gastrointestinal; IARC, International Agency for Research on Cancer; ICD, International Classification of Diseases; JEM, job-exposure matrix; MCPA, 2-methyl-4-chlorophenoxyacetic acid; MCPB, 4-(4-chloro-2-methylphenoxy)butanoic acid; NIOSH, National Institute for Occupational Safety and Health; nr, not reported; PCDD, polychlorinated dibenzo-*p*-dioxin (highly chlorinated, if four or more chlorines); PCMR, proportionate cancer mortality ratios; PCP, pentachlorophenol; PMR, proportionate mortality ratio; SMR, standardized mortality ratio; TCDD, 2,3,7,8-tetrachlorodibenzo-*p*-dioxin; TCP, trichlorophenol; VA, US Department of Veterans Affairs.

[a]Subjects are male and outcome is mortality unless otherwise noted.

[b]Given when available; results other than estimated risk explained individually.

No environmental studies with sufficiently specific characterization of exposure to the COIs and this health outcome have been published since *Update 2010*.

Biologic Plausibility

No animal studies have reported an increased incidence of bone and joint cancers after exposure to the COIs. The biologic plausibility of the carcinogenicity of the COIs is discussed in general at the beginning of this chapter.

Synthesis

The small amount of new data, in concert with the previous literature, summarized in Table 8-15 do not indicate an association between exposure to the COIs and bone cancer.

Conclusion

On the basis of the evidence reviewed here and in previous VAO reports, the committee concludes that there is inadequate or insufficient evidence to determine whether there is an association between exposure to the COIs and bone and joint cancers.

SOFT-TISSUE SARCOMA

Soft-tissue sarcoma (STS) (ICD-9 164.1, 171) arises in soft somatic tissues in and between organs. Three of the most common types of STS—liposarcoma, fibrosarcoma, and rhabdomyosarcoma—occur in similar numbers in men and women. Because of the diverse characteristics of STS, accurate diagnosis and classification can be difficult. ACS estimated that about 6,110 men and 5,170 women would receive diagnoses of STS in the United States in 2012 and that about 2,050 men and 1,850 women would die from it (Siegel et al., 2012). The average annual incidence of STS is shown in Table 8-16.

TABLE 8-16 Average Annual Incidence (per 100,000) of Soft-Tissue Sarcoma (Including Malignant Neoplasms of the Heart) in the United States[a]

	55–59 Years Old			60–64 Years Old			65–69 Years Old		
	All Races	White	Black	All Races	White	Black	All Races	White	Black
Men	5.4	5.4	5.2	6.8	7.2	4.5	8.6	8.7	6.7
Women	4.5	4.4	6.3	5.4	5.2	7.7	7.0	7.6	3.4

[a]Surveillance, Epidemiology, and End Results program, nine standard registries, crude age-specific rates, 2005–2009 (NCI, 2013).

Among the risk factors for STS are exposure to ionizing radiation during treatment for other cancers and some inherited conditions, including Gardner syndrome, Li-Fraumeni syndrome, and neurofibromatosis. Several chemical exposures have been identified as possible risk factors (Zahm and Fraumeni, 1997).

Conclusions from *VAO* and Previous Updates

The committee responsible for *VAO* concluded that there was sufficient epidemiologic data to support an association between exposure to the COIs and STS. Additional information available to the committees responsible for subsequent updates has not changed that finding.

As seen with Hodgkin lymphoma and non-Hodgkin lymphoma, the available epidemiologic evidence suggests that phenoxy herbicides rather than TCDD may be associated with developing STS. Some of the strongest evidence of an association between STS and exposure to phenoxy herbicides comes from a series of case-control studies conducted in Sweden (Eriksson et al., 1981, 1990; Hardell and Eriksson, 1988; Hardell and Sandstrom, 1979). The studies, involving a total of 506 cases, show an association between STS and exposure to phenoxy herbicides, chlorophenols, or both. The *VAO* committee concluded that although those studies had been criticized, there is insufficient justification to discount the consistent pattern of increased risks and the clearly described and sound methods used. In addition, a reanalysis of the data by Hardell (1981) to evaluate the potential influence of recall bias and interviewer bias confirmed the original results. Hansen et al. (2007) conducted a historical-cohort study of male gardeners who were members of the Danish Union; cancer incidence was ascertained from 1975 to 2001. Birth date served as a surrogate for potential exposure to pesticides and herbicides; older cohorts represented higher exposure potential. Men born before 1915 were much more likely to die from STS, although this finding was based on only three cases. Reif et al. (1989) performed a series of case-control analyses in a sample of specified occupations and found a significant association between STS and having recently been employed as a forestry worker.

Those findings are supported by a significantly increased risk in a NIOSH study of production workers most highly exposed to TCDD (Fingerhut et al., 1991); Steenland et al. (1999) published an update of the NIOSH cohort, but STS was not among the outcomes evaluated. A similar increased risk was seen in the IARC cohort in deaths that occurred 10–19 years after first exposure (Kogevinas et al., 1992; Saracci et al., 1991) according to a fairly crude exposure classification. An updated and expanded study of the IARC cohort by Kogevinas et al. (1997) found a nonsignificantly increased risk of STS when followup was extended to 1992. Then NIOSH and IARC cohorts are among the largest and the most highly exposed occupational cohorts. Smaller studies of workers that are included in the multinational IARC cohort—Danish herbicide manufacturers (Lynge et al., 1985, 1993) and Dow production workers in Midland, Michigan, and New Zealand

(Collins et al., 2009a; 't Mannetje et al., 2005)—showed an increased risk of STS, but the results were commonly nonsignificant, possibly because of small samples (related to the relative rarity of STS in the population).

Several studies have reported on STS in relation to living near waste incinerators that release dioxin as a contaminant. Viel et al. (2000) reported on an investigation of apparent clusters of STS and non-Hodgkin lymphoma cases in the vicinity of a municipal solid waste incinerator in Doubs, France; Comba et al. (2003) and Costani et al. (2000) examined STS in the general population living near a chemical plant in the northern Italian city of Mantua; and Zambon et al. (2007) conducted a population-based case-control study in Venice, Italy, in an area that included 26 waste incinerators and other industrial plants. Each of those studies found a statistically significant excess of STS, but none showed any direct evidence of human exposure.

No cases of STS have been reported in Zones A and B in the Seveso cohort (Consonni et al., 2008); the incidence of STS was slightly increased in Zone R but not significantly (Pesatori et al., 2009). Veteran studies have not found a significant increase in STS. No increase was seen in Operation Ranch Hand veterans (AFHS, 1996, 2000; Michalek et al., 1990) or in VA studies of US Vietnam veterans (Breslin et al., 1986, 1988; Bullman et al., 1990; Watanabe and Kang, 1995; Watanabe et al., 1991). A slight increase in the incidence of STS was seen in Australian Air Force veterans compared with the Australian population but not in Army or Navy personnel (ADVA, 2005a), and no increase in mortality was seen in Australian veterans who served in any of the military branches (ADVA, 2005b). A nonsignificant increase in mortality from STS was also seen in state studies of veterans in Massachusetts, Michigan, and New York.

Table 8-17 summarizes the relevant studies.

Update of the Epidemiologic Literature

Vietnam-Veteran and Environmental Studies

No Vietnam-veteran studies or environmental studies of exposure to the COIs and STS have been published since *Update 2010*.

Occupational Studies

In an update of cancer incidence in 1985–2007 in 2,4-D production workers of Dow Chemical Company in Midland, Michigan, Burns et al. (2011) found a single case of cancer of the bone or soft tissue in the most restrictively defined cohort of exposed workers, with attendant nonsignificant estimates of exposure-related risk (SIR = 0.8, 95% CI 0.0–4.5). The numbers were too small to add substantially to the assessment of STS risk associated with exposure to Agent Orange–associated chemicals.

TABLE 8-17 Selected Epidemiologic Studies—Soft-Tissue Sarcoma (Shaded Entries Are New Information for This Update)

Study Population[a]	Exposed Cases[b]	**Exposure of Interest**/Estimated Relative Risk (95% CI)[b]	Reference
VIETNAM VETERANS			
US Vietnam Veterans			
US Air Force Health Study—Ranch Hand veterans vs SEA veterans (unless otherwise noted)		**All COIs**	
Mortality			
Through 1987—Ranch Hand personnel (n = 1,261) vs SEA veterans (19,102)	1	nr	Michalek et al., 1990
US VA Proportionate Mortality Study—sample of deceased male Vietnam-era Army and Marine veterans who served 7/4/1965–3/1/1973		**All COIs**	
1965–1984			
Army, deployed (n = 24,145) vs nondeployed (n = 27,917)	43	1.1	Watanabe et al., 1991
Served in I Corps (n = 6,668)	10	0.9 (0.4–1.6)	Bullman et al., 1990
Marine Corps, deployed (n = 5,501) vs nondeployed (n = 4,505)	11	0.7	Watanabe et al., 1991
1965–1982			Breslin et al.,1986, 1988
Army, deployed (n = 19,708) vs nondeployed (n = 22,904)	30	1.0 (0.8–1.2)	
Marine Corps, deployed (n = 4,527) vs nondeployed (n = 3,781)	8	0.7 (0.4–1.3)	
US VA Study of Marine Post-service Mortality—sample of Marines serving 1967–1969, deployed (n = 10,716) vs nondeployed (n = 9,346)		**All COIs**	
Mortality, earlier of discharge or April 1973 through 1991	0	nr	Watanabe and Kang, 1995
US VA Case-control study			
234 Vietnam veterans vs 13,496 Vietnam-era veterans	86	0.8 (0.6–1.1)	Kang et al., 1986
State Studies of US Vietnam Veterans			
Massachusetts Vietnam-era veterans			
Veterans aged 35–65 years in 1993—cases diagnosed 1988–1993 vs gastrointestinal cancers	18	1.6 (0.5–5.4)	Clapp, 1997
Diagnosed 1972–1983	9	5.2 (2.4–11.1)	Kogan and Clapp, 1988
Michigan Vietnam-era veterans, PM study of deaths (1974–1989)—deployed vs nondeployed	8	1.1 (0.5–2.2)	Visintainer et al., 1995

continued

TABLE 8-17 Soft-Tissue Sarcoma, continued

Study Population[a]	Exposed Cases[b]	**Exposure of Interest**/Estimated Relative Risk (95% CI)[b]	Reference
New York			
—deployed vs nondeployed	2	1.1 (0.2–6.7)	Lawrence et al., 1985
281 STS cases with service in Vietnam vs live matched controls	10	0.5 (0.2–1.3)	Greenwald et al., 1984
923 White male Vietnam veterans with **Wisconsin** death certificate (1968–1978) vs proportions for Vietnam-era veterans	4	nr	Anderson et al., 1986
International Vietnam-Veteran Studies			
Australian Vietnam Veterans—58,077 men and 153 women served on land or in Vietnamese waters during 5/23/1962–7/1/1973 vs Australian population		**All COIs**	
Incidence			
All branches, 1982–2000	35	1.0 (0.7–1.3)	ADVA, 2005a
Navy	6	0.8 (0.3–1.7)	
Army	29	1.2 (0.8–1.6)	
Air Force	0	0.0 (0.0–1.1)	
Validation Study		*Expected number of exposed cases*	AIHW, 1999
	14	27 (17–37)	
Men	398	27 (17–37)	CDVA, 1998a
Women	2	0 (0–4)	CDVA, 1998b
Mortality			
All branches, return–2001	12	0.8 (0.4–1.3)	ADVA, 2005b
Navy	3	0.9 (0.2–2.4)	
Army	9	0.8 (0.4–1.5)	
Air Force	0	0.0 (0.0–2.3)	
1980–1994	9	1.0 (0.4–1.8)	CDVA, 1997a
Australian Conscripted Army National Service (18,940 deployed vs 24,642 nondeployed)		**All COIs**	
Incidence			
1982–2000	10	1.0 (0.4–2.4)	ADVA, 2005c
Mortality			
1966–2001	3	0.5 (0.1–2.0)	ADVA, 2005c
1982–1994	2	0.7 (0.6–4.5)	CDVA, 1997b
1983–1985	1	1.3 (0.1–20.0)	Fett et al., 1987

TABLE 8-17 Soft-Tissue Sarcoma, continued

Study Population[a]	Exposed Cases[b]	**Exposure of Interest**/Estimated Relative Risk (95% CI)[b]	Reference
OCCUPATIONAL—INDUSTRIAL			
IARC Phenoxy Herbicide Cohort—Workers exposed to any phenoxy herbicide or chlorophenol (production or spraying) vs respective national mortality rates			
Mortality 1939–1992			Kogevinas et al., 1997
13,831 exposed to highly chlorinated PCDDs	6	2.0 (0.8–4.4)	
7,553 not exposed to highly chlorinated PCDDs	2	1.4 (0.2–4.9)	
Mortality 1955–1988 of 12,492 production workers and 5,898 sprayers exposed—13,482 in exposed subcohort	4	2.0 (0.6–5.2)	Saracci et al., 1991
Nested case-control study			
IARC cohort (men and women)—incidence			Kogevinas et al., 1995
Exposed to 2,4,5-T	5	4.3 (0.7–26.3)	
Exposed to TCDD	5	5.2 (0.9–31.9)	
Mortality—IARC cohort (16,863 men and 1,527 women) 10–19 years since first exposure	4	6.1 (1.7–15.5)	Kogevinas et al., 1992
British MCPA Plant—Production 1947–1982 (n = 1,545) (included in IARC cohort) and spraying 1947–1972 (n = 2,561) (*not* included in IARC cohort)		**MCPA**	
Mortality through 1983	1	1.1 (0.0–5.9)	Coggon et al., 1986
Danish Production Workers (3,390 men and 1,069 women involved in production of phenoxy herbicides unlikely to contain TCDD at 2 plants in 1947–1987) (in IARC cohort)		**Dioxins, but TCDD unlikely; 2,4-D, 2,4-DP, MCPA, MCPP**	
Incidence 1943–1987 (men only)	5	2.0 (0.7–4.8)	Lynge, 1993
Incidence 1943–1982			Lynge, 1985
Men	5	2.7 (0.9–6.3)	
Women	0	nr	
Dutch production workers in Plant A (549 men exposed during production 1955–1985; 594 unexposed) (in IARC cohort)		**Dioxins, 2,4,5-T, 2,4,5-TCP**	
Mortality 1955–1991	0	nr	Hooiveld et al., 1998
Mortality 1955–1985	0	0.0 (0.0–18.4)	Bueno de Mesquita et al., 1993

continued

TABLE 8-17 Soft-Tissue Sarcoma, continued

Study Population[a]	Exposed Cases[b]	**Exposure of Interest**/Estimated Relative Risk (95% CI)[b]	Reference
Dutch production workers in Plant B (414 men exposed during production 1965–1986; 723 unexposed) (in IARC cohort)		**2,4-D; MCPA; MCPP; highly chlorinated dioxins unlikely**	
Mortality 1965–1986	0	0.0 (0.0–73.8)	Bueno de Mesquita et al., 1993
German Production Workers—2,479 workers at 4 plants (in IARC cohort as of 1997)		**Dioxins, phenoxy herbicides**	
BASF Cleanup Workers from 1953 accident (n = 247); 114 with chloracne, 13 more with erythema; serum TCDD levels (*not* part of IARC)		**Focus on TCDD**	
Incidence			
1960–1992			Ott and Zober, 1996
TCDD < 0.1 μg/kg of body weight	0	nr	
TCDD 0.1–0.99 μg/kg of body weight	0	nr	
TCDD > 1 μg/kg of body weight	0	nr	
Mortality			
Through 1987		*90% CI*	Zober et al., 1990
	0	nr	
German Production Workers at Boehringer–Ingelheim Plant in Hamburg (1,144 men working > 1 month in 1952–1984; generation of TCDD reduced after chloracne outbreak in 1954) and women—no results (some additions to observed cancers over Manz et al., 1991) (in IARC cohort as of 1997)		**Dioxins; 2,4,5-T; 2,5-DCP; 2,4,5-TCP**	
Mortality 1952–1989—stats on men only, 1,184 (tables all for 1,148 men, not necessarily German nationals) vs national rates (also vs gas workers); same observation period as Becher et al., 1966	0	nr	Manz et al., 1991
New Zealand Phenoxy Herbicide Production Workers and Sprayers (1,599 men and women working any time in 1969–1988 at Dow plant in New Plymouth) (in IARC cohort)		**Dioxins; 2,4-D; 2,4,5-T; MCPA; MCPB; 2,4,5-TCP; Picloram**	
Mortality 1969–2004			McBride et al., 2009a
Ever-exposed workers	1	3.4 (0.1–19.5)	
Never-exposed workers	0	0.0 (0.0–34.9)	
Production Workers (713 men and 100 women worked > 1 month in 1969–1984)			
Mortality 1969–2000	0	0.0 (0.0–19.3)	't Mannetje et al., 2005

TABLE 8-17 Soft-Tissue Sarcoma, continued

Study Population[a]	Exposed Cases[b]	**Exposure of Interest**/Estimated Relative Risk (95% CI)[b]	Reference
Sprayers (697 men and 2 women registered any time 1973–1984)			
Mortality 1973–2000	1	4.3 (0.1–23.8)	't Mannetje et al., 2005
NIOSH Mortality Cohort (12 US plants, 5,172 male production and maintenance workers 1942–1984) (included in IARC cohort as of 1997)		**Dioxins, phenoxy herbicides**	
Through 1993	4	2.3 (0.6–5.9)	Steenland et al., 1999
Chloracne subcohort (n = 608)	3	11.3 (2.3–33.1)	
Through 1987	4	3.4 (0.9–8.7)	Fingerhut et al., 1991
≥ 1-year exposure, ≥ 20-year latency	3	9.2 (1.9–27.0)	
All Dow TCP-Exposed Workers (TCP production 1942–1979 or 2,4,5-T production 1948–1982 in Midland, Michigan) (in IARC and NIOSH cohorts)		**2,4,5-T; 2,4,5-TCP**	
1942–2003 (n = 1,615)	4	4.1 (1.1–10.5)	Collins et al., 2009a
1940–1994 (n = 2,187 men)	2	2.4 (0.3–8.6)	Bodner et al., 2003
All Dow PCP-Exposed Workers—all workers from the two plants that only made PCP (in Tacoma, Washington, and Wichita, Kansas) and workers who made PCP and TCP at two additional plants (in Midland, Michigan, and Sauget, Illinois) (connective tissue and soft tissue)		**2,4,5-T; 2,4,5-TCP**	Ruder and Yiin, 2011
1940–2005 (n = 2,122) (connective tissue and soft tissue)	2	1.5 (0.2–5.5)	
PCP and TCP (n = 720)	1	2.3 (0.1–12.6)	
PCP (no TCP) (n = 1,402)	1	1.1 (0.0–6.4)	
Dow 2,4-D Production Workers (1945–1982 in Midland, Michigan) (subset of all TCP-exposed workers)		**2,4-D, lower chlorinated dioxins**	
Cancer incidence through 2007 in Dow workers (n = 1,256) vs comparisons from state cancer registries (n = 23,354) (Cohort 3) (bone, soft tissue)	1	0.8 (0.0–4.5)	Burns et al., 2011
Through 1982 (n = 878)	0	nr	Bond et al., 1988

continued

TABLE 8-17 Soft-Tissue Sarcoma, continued

Study Population[a]	Exposed Cases[b]	**Exposure of Interest**/Estimated Relative Risk (95% CI)[b]	Reference
Dow PCP Production Workers (1937–1989 in Midland, Michigan) (*not* in IARC and NIOSH cohorts)		**Low chlorinated dioxins, 2,4-D**	
Mortality 1940–2004 (n = 577, excluding 196 also having exposure to TCP)	1	2.2 (0.0–12.1)	Collins et al., 2009b
Mortality 1940–1989 (n = 770)	0	*Expected number of exposed cases* 0.2	Ramlow et al., 1996
OCCUPATIONAL—PAPER AND PULP WORKERS		**TCDD**	
IARC cohort of pulp and paper workers—60,468 workers from 11 countries, TCDD among 27 agents assessed by JEM			McLean et al., 2006
Exposure to nonvolatile organochlorine compounds			
Never	8	1.2 (0.5–2.4)	
Ever	4	0.8 (0.2–2.0)	
Danish paper-mill workers			Rix et al., 1998
Men employed in sorting and packing	12	1.2 (0.6–2.0)	
Women employed in sorting and packing	8	4.0 (1.7–7.8)	
OCCUPATIONAL—HERBICIDE-USING WORKERS (*not* related to IARC sprayer cohorts)			
CANADA			
Sawmill Workers in British Columbia—23,829 workers for ≥ 1 year at 11 mills using chlorophenates 1940–1985		**Chlorophenates, not TCDD**	
Incidence 1969–1989	11	1.0 (0.6–1.7)	Hertzman et al., 1997
Mortality 1950–1989	6	1.2 (0.5–2.3)	
DENMARK			
Danish gardeners—incidence from 3,156 male and 859 female gardeners			Hansen et al., 2007
25-year followup (1975–2001)		**Herbicides**	
Born before 1915 (high exposure)	3	5.9 (1.9–18.2)	
Born 1915–1934 (medium exposure)	0	0.0 (0.0–3.8)	
Born after 1934 (low exposure)	1	1.8 (0.3–12.9)	
10-year followup (1975–1984) of male gardeners	3	5.3 (1.1–15.4)	Hansen et al., 1992
ITALIAN Licensed Pesticide Users—male farmers in southern Piedmont licensed 1970–1974			
Mortality 1970–1986 (n = 23,401)	2	1.0 (0.1–3.5)	Torchio et al., 1994

TABLE 8-17 Soft-Tissue Sarcoma, continued

Study Population[a]	Exposed Cases[b]	**Exposure of Interest**/Estimated Relative Risk (95% CI)[b]	Reference
NEW ZEALAND National Cancer Registry (1980–1984)—case-control study of 142 incident STS cases vs remainder of 19,904 men with any incident cancer			
Forestry workers (n = 134)		**Herbicides**	Reif et al., 1989
Aged 20–59	4	3.2 (1.2–9.0)	
Aged ≥ 60	0	—	
SWEDEN			
Swedish pesticide applicators—incidence (n = 20,245)	7	*99% CI* 0.9 (0.8–1.1)	Wiklund et al., 1988, 1989a
354,620 Swedish agricultural and forestry workers identified from 1960 census, followed 1961–1979; compared to reference population	331	0.9 (0.8–1.0)	Wiklund and Holm, 1986
Incident STS cases 1961–1973 with agriculture as economic activity in 1960 census (connective tissue and muscle)	162	1.1 (0.9–1.3)	Wiklund, 1983
UNITED STATES			
US farmers—usual occupation of farmer and industry of agriculture on death certificates 1984–1988 from 23 states		**Herbicides** PCMRs	Blair et al., 1993
Men			
Whites (n = 119,648)	98	0.9 (0.8–1.1)	
Nonwhites (n = 11,446)	10	1.5 (0.7–2.8)	
Women			
Whites (n = 2,400)	3	1.2 (0.2–3.5)	
Nonwhites (n = 2,066)	0	0.0 (0.0–1.9)	
US Agricultural Health Study—prospective study of licensed pesticide sprayers in Iowa and North Carolina: commercial (n = 4,916), private/farmers (n = 52,395, 97.4% men), and spouses of private sprayers (n = 32,347, 0.007% men), enrolled 1993–1997; followups with CATIs 1999–2003 and 2005–2010		**Phenoxy herbicides**	
Incidence			
Enrollment through 2002			Alavanja et al., 2005
Private applicators	10	0.7 (0.3–1.2)	
Spouses of private applicators (> 99% women)	3	0.5 (0.1–1.4)	
Commercial applicators	nr	0.0 (0.0–3.8)	

continued

TABLE 8-17 Soft-Tissue Sarcoma, continued

Study Population[a]	Exposed Cases[b]	**Exposure of Interest**/Estimated Relative Risk (95% CI)[b]	Reference
Mortality			
Enrollment through 2007, vs state rates (connective tissue)			Waggoner et al., 2011
Applicators (n = 1,641)	9	0.7 (0.3–1.5)	
Spouses (n = 676)	6	1.0 (0.4–2.2)	
Enrollment through 2000, vs state rates			Blair et al., 2005a
Private applicators (men and women)	4	0.7 (0.2–1.8)	
Spouses of private applicators (> 99% women)	3	1.4 (0.3–4.1)	
US Department of Agriculture Workers—nested case-control study of white men dying 1970–1979 of STS		**Herbicides**	
USDA forest and soil	2	1.0 (0.1–3.6)	Alavanja et al., 1989
Florida Pesticide Applicators licensed 1965–1966 (n = 3,827)—mortality through 1976		**Herbicides**	Blair et al., 1983
Any pesticide (dose-response by length of licensure)	0	nr	
ENVIRONMENTAL			
Seveso, Italy Residential Cohort—Industrial accident July 10, 1976 (723 residents Zone A; 4,821 Zone B; 31,643 Zone R; 181,574 local reference group) (ICD-9 171)		**TCDD**	
Incidence			
20-yr followup to 1996—men and women			
Zone A	0	nr	Pesatori et al., 2009
Zone B	0	nr	
Zone R	9	1.3 (0.6–2.7)	
10-yr followup to 1991—men			Bertazzi et al., 1993; Pesatori et al., 1992
Zone A	0	nr	
Zone B	0	nr	
Zone R	6	2.8 (1.0–7.3)	
10-yr followup to 1991—women			Bertazzi et al., 1993; Pesatori et al., 1992
Zone A	0	nr	
Zone B	0	nr	
Zone R	2	1.6 (0.3–7.4)	
Mortality			
25-yr followup to 2001—men and women			Consonni et al., 2008
Zone A	0	nr	
Zone B	0	nr	
Zone R	4	0.8 (0.3–2.1)	

TABLE 8-17 Soft-Tissue Sarcoma, continued

Study Population[a]	Exposed Cases[b]	**Exposure of Interest**/Estimated Relative Risk (95% CI)[b]	Reference
20-yr followup to 1996			Bertazzi et al., 2001
Zone A—men and women	0	nr	
Zone B—men and women	0	nr	
Zones A and B—men	0	nr	
Zones A and B—women	0	nr	
15-yr followup to 1991—men			Bertazzi et al., 1997, 1998
Zone A	—	nr	
Zone B	0	nr	
Zone R	4	2.1 (0.7–6.5)	
15-yr followup to 1991—women			Bertazzi et al., 1997, 1998
Zone A	—	nr	
Zone B	0	nr	
Zone R	0	nr	
10-yr followup to 1986—men			Bertazzi et al., 1989a
Zone A, B, R	2	5.4 (0.8–38.6)	
Zone R	2	6.3 (0.9–45.0)	Bertazzi et al., 1989b
10-yr followup to 1986—women			Bertazzi et al., 1989a
Zone A, B, R	1	2.0 (0.2–1.9)	
Zone B	1	17.0 (1.8–163.6)	Bertazzi et al., 1989b
FINLAND			
Finnish community exposed to chlorophenol contamination (men and women)	6	**Chlorophenol** 1.6 (0.7–3.5)	Lampi et al., 1992
FRANCE			
Residents near French solid-waste incinerator—incidence		**Dioxin**	Viel et al., 2000
Spatial cluster	45	1.4 (p = 0.004)	
1994–1995	12	3.4 (p = 0.008)	
ITALY			
Italian rice growers		**Chlorophenoxy acids, chlorophenols**	Gambini et al., 1997
	1	4.0 (0.1–22.3)	
NEW ZEALAND			
Residents of New Plymouth Territorial Authority, New Zealand near plant manufacturing 2,4,5-T in 1962–1987		2,4,5-T	Read et al., 2007
Incidence	56	1.0 (0.8–1.4)[c]	
1970–1974	7	1.0 (0.4–2.1)	
1975–1979	3	0.4 (0.1–2.1)	
1980–1984	10	1.3 (0.6–2.4)	
1985–1989	11	1.2 (0.6–2.2)	
1990–1994	9	0.9 (0.4–1.7)	
1995–1999	14	1.3 (0.7–2.2)	
2000–2001	2	0.8 (0.1–3.0)	

continued

TABLE 8-17 Soft-Tissue Sarcoma, continued

Study Population[a]	Exposed Cases[b]	**Exposure of Interest**/Estimated Relative Risk (95% CI)[b]	Reference
Mortality	27	1.2 (0.8–1.8)[c]	
1970–1974	5	1.8 (0.6–4.3)	
1975–1979	1	0.4 (0.0–2.0)	
1980–1984	4	1.1 (0.3–2.9)	
1985–1989	5	1.5 (0.5–3.6)	
1990–1994	5	1.3 (0.4–3.0)	
1995–1999	5	1.3 (0.4–3.0)	
2000–2001	2	0.9 (0.1–3.1)	
SWEDEN			
Swedish fishermen (high consumption of fish with persistent organochlorines)		**Organochlorine compounds**	Svensson et al., 1995
Incidence			
East coast	0	0.0 (0.0–2.6)	
West coast	3	0.5 (0.1–1.4)	
Mortality			
East coast	0	nr	
West coast	0	nr	
CASE-CONTROL STUDIES			
US Case-Control Studies			
Kansas residents–duration and frequency of herbicide use—incidence		**Phenoxy herbicides, 2.4-D**	Hoar et al., 1986
All farmers	95	1.0 (0.7–1.6)	
Farm-use of herbicides	22	0.9 (0.5–1.6)	
Washington state residents—incidence (1983–1985)		**Phenoxy herbicides, chlorinated phenols**	Woods et al., 1987
High phenoxy exposure	nr	0.9 (0.4–1.9)	
Self-reported chloracne	nr	3.3 (0.8–14.0)	
International Case-Control Studies			
Australian residents in Victorian Cancer Registry (1982–1987)		**Phenoxy compounds**	Smith and Christophers, 1992
	30	1.0 (0.3–3.1)	
British agricultural workers		**Herbicides**	Balarajan and Acheson, 1984
Overall	42	1.7 (1.0–2.9)	
Under 75 yrs old	33	1.4 (0.8–2.6)	

TABLE 8-17 Soft-Tissue Sarcoma, continued

Study Population[a]	Exposed Cases[b]	**Exposure of Interest**/Estimated Relative Risk (95% CI)[b]	Reference
Cross-Canada Study of Pesticides and Health—Men (≥ 19 yrs of age) diagnosed September 1991–December 1994 (n = 357) vs matched population-based controls (n = 1,506); exposure to:			Pahwa et al., 2011
Phenoxy herbicides	80 vs 321	1.1 (0.8–1.5)	
2,4-D	69 vs 293	1.0 (0.7–1.4)	
Mecoprop	26 vs 81	1.3 (0.8–2.2)	
MCPA	13 vs 46	1.1 (0.6–2.2)	
Diclofop-methyl	8 vs 25	1.2 (0.4–2.9)	
Cross-Canada Study of Pesticides and Health—Men (≥ 19 yrs of age) diagnosed September 1991–December 1994 (n = 357) vs matched population-based controls (n = 1,506); exposure to:		**Phenoxy herbicides**	Pahwa et al., 2006
Any phenoxyherbicide	80 vs 321	1.1 (0.7–1.5)	
2,4-D	69 vs 293	1.0 (0.6–1.5)	
Mecoprop	26 vs 81	1.0 (0.5–1.9)	
MCPA	13 vs 46	1.1 (0.5–2.2)	
Finnish STS patients vs controls within quintiles based on TEQ in subcutaneous fat—incidence	110	**Dioxin**	Tuomisto et al., 2004
Quintile 1 (median, ~12 ng/kg TEQ)	nr	1.0	
Quintile 2 (median, ~20 ng/kg TEQ)	nr	0.4 (0.2–1.1)	
Quintile 3 (median, ~28 ng/kg TEQ)	nr	0.6 (0.2–1.7)	
Quintile 4 (median, ~40 ng/kg TEQ)	nr	0.5 (0.2–1.3)	
Quintile 5 (median, ~62 ng/kg TEQ)	nr	0.7 (0.2–2.0)	
Italy			
Population-based Veneto Tumour Registry, Italy, average exposure based on duration and distance of residence from 33 industrial sources—incidence		**Dioxin**	Zambon et al., 2007
Sarcoma (ICD-9 158, 171, 173, visceral sites)			
Men			
< 4 TCDD (fg/m^3)	31	1.0	
4–6	39	1.1 (0.6–2.0)	
≥ 6	17	1.9 (0.9–4.0)	
		p-trend = 0.15	
Women			
< 4 TCDD (fg/m^3)	24	1.0	
4–6	44	1.5 (0.8–2.7)	
≥ 6	17	2.4 (1.0–5.6)	
		p-trend = 0.04	

continued

TABLE 8-17 Soft-Tissue Sarcoma, continued

Study Population[a]	Exposed Cases[b]	**Exposure of Interest**/Estimated Relative Risk (95% CI)[b]	Reference
Men, women combined			
Connective, other soft tissue (ICD-9 171)			
< 4 TCDD (fg/m^3)	25	1.0	
4–6	39	1.4 (0.7–2.5)	
≥ 6	17	3.3 (1.4–7.9)	
		p-trend = 0.01	
Skin (ICD-9 173)			
< 4 TCDD (fg/m^3)	5	1.0	
4–6	10	0.0 (0.3–4.7)[d]	
≥ 6	2	0.3 (0.0–3.4)	
		p-trend = 0.48	
Retroperitoneum, peritoneum (ICD-9 158)			
< 4 TCDD (fg/m^3)	6	1.0	
4–6	12	1.1 (0.3–3.4)	
≥ 6	3	0.8 (0.1–4.5)	
		p-trend = 0.86	
Visceral sites			
< 4 TCDD (fg/m^3)	19	1.0	
4–6	22	1.2 (0.6–2.6)	
≥ 6	12	2.5 (1.0–6.3)	
		p-trend = 0.08	
Residents near industrial-waste incinerator in Mantua, Italy—incidence		**Dioxin**	
Residence within 2 km of incinerator	5	31.4 (5.6–176.1)	Comba et al., 2003
Residents near chemical plant in Mantua, Italy—incidence	20	**TCDD emissions** 2.3 (1.3–3.5)	Costani et al., 2000
Italian rice weeders (1981–1983)		**Phenoxy herbicides**	Vineis et al., 1986
Among all living females (n = 31)	5	2.4 (0.4–16.1)	
New Zealand Pesticide Workers		**Phenoxy herbicides** *90% CI*	
Update of New Zealand workers (1976–1982)	133	1.1 (0.7–1.8)	Smith and Pearce, 1986
Reanalysis of New Zealand workers (1976–1980)	17	1.6 (0.7–3.8)	Smith et al., 1984
New Zealand workers exposed to herbicides (1976–1980)	17	1.6 (0.8–3.2)	Smith et al., 1983
Swedish agricultural and forestry workers (1974–1979)		**Phenoxy acids, chlorophenols**	Eriksson et al., 1979, 1981
	25	(2.5–10.4) 5:1 matched	

TABLE 8-17 Soft-Tissue Sarcoma, continued

Study Population[a]	Exposed Cases[b]	**Exposure of Interest**/Estimated Relative Risk (95% CI)[b]	Reference
Swedish patients (1970–1977)		**Phenoxy acids, chlorophenols**	Hardell, 1981; Hardell and Sandström, 1979
Exposed to phenoxy herbicides	13	5.5 (2.2–13.8)	
Exposed to chlorophenols	6	5.4 (1.3–22.5)	

NOTE: 2,4-D, 2,4-dichlorophenoxyacetic acid; 2,4-DP, dichlorprop; 2,4,5-T, 2,4,5-trichlorophenoxyacetic acid; 2,4,5-TCP, 2,4,5-trichlorophenol; 2,5-DCP, 2,5-dichlorophenol; CATI, computer-assisted telephone interviewing; CI, confidence interval; COI, chemical of interest; IARC, International Agency for Research on Cancer; ICD, International Classification of Diseases; JEM, job-exposure matrix; MCPA, 2-methyl-4-chlorophenoxyacetic acid; MCPB, 4-(4-chloro-2-methylphenoxy)butanoic acid; MCPP, methylchlorophenoxypropionic acid; NIOSH, National Institute for Occupational Safety and Health; nr, not reported; PCDD, polychlorinated dibenzo-*p*-dioxin (highly chlorinated, if four or more chlorines); PCMR, proportionate cancer mortality ratios; PCP, pentachlorophenol; PM, proportionate mortality; SEA, Southeast Asia; STS, soft-tissue sarcoma; TCDD, 2,3,7,8-tetrachlorodibenzo-*p*-dioxin; TCP, trichlorophenol; TEQ, toxicity equivalent; USDA, United States Department of Agriculture; VA, US Department of Veterans Affairs.

[a]Subjects are male and outcome is mortality unless otherwise noted.

[b]Given when available; results other than estimated risk explained individually.

[c]Committee computed total SMR and SIR by dividing sum of observed values by sum of expected values over all years; 95% CIs on these total ratios were computed with exact methods.

[d]There appears to be an error in this entry because lower 95% CI (0.3) is not smaller than odds ratio (0.0).

Ruder and Yiin (2011) reported mortality in PCP production that entailed exposure to PCDDs and PCDFs but not to the most toxic 2,3,7,8 dioxin congener. A subcohort of 720 workers (all men, the PCP-plus-TCDD group) had also been employed in TCP production and so had also been exposed to TCDD. Relative to US referent rates, two deaths from STS, one in each subcohort, did not represent an important increase in the entire cohort (SMR = 1.52, 95% CI 0.18–5.48), the PCP-only group (SMR = 1.14, 95% CI 0.03–6.36), or the PCP-plus-TCDD group (SMR = 2.26, 95% CI 0.06–12.6).

In the update of mortality in the AHS cohort, Waggoner et al. (2011) reported nine deaths from cancers of connective tissue in the applicators and six in their spouses. It is unclear whether this category contained any deaths from STS, but in any case, the resulting SMRs did not differ from expectations generated from the rates of the populations of Iowa and North Carolina.

Case-Control Studies

Using information assembled in the Cross-Canada Study of Herbicides and Health, Pahwa et al. (2011) used a case-control design to examine associations between STS and specific pesticide exposures. Men who had STS (357) were compared with the study wide control group (1,506) by using conditional logistic regression stratified by age and province of residence and further adjusted for medical history (measles, rheumatoid arthritis, mononucleosis, whooping cough, or cancer in a first-degree relative). No associations were found between STS and exposure to phenoxy herbicides overall (80 exposed cases, OR = 1.09, 95% CI 0.81–1.48); to 2,4-D (69 exposed cases, OR = 0.98, 95% CI 0.71–1.35); to 2-(4-chloro-2-methylphenoxy) propionic acid (Mecoprop, MCPP; 26 exposed cases, OR = 1.34, 95% CI 0.81–2.19); to MCPA (13 exposed cases, OR = 1.11, 95% CI 0.57–2.16); to methyl 2-[4-(2,4-dichlorophenoxy) phenoxy] propanoate (diclofop-methyl; eight exposed cases, OR = 1.21, 95% CI 0.41–2.85); or to dicamba (15 exposed cases, OR = 1.31, 95% CI 0.61–2.82).

Biologic Plausibility

In a 2-year study, dermal application of TCDD to Swiss-Webster mice led to an increase in fibrosarcomas in females but not in males (NTP, 1982b). There is some concern that the increase in fibrosarcomas may be associated with the treatment protocol rather than with TCDD. The NTP gavage study (NTP, 1982a) also found an increased incidence of fibrosarcomas in male and female rats and in female mice.

The biologic plausibility of the carcinogenicity of the COIs is discussed in general at the beginning of this chapter.

Synthesis

Previous committees have concluded that the occupational, environmental, and Vietnam-veteran studies showed sufficient evidence to link herbicide exposure to STS. Although confidence intervals in the new cohort studies were broad because of the rarity of observed cases in small samples, that conclusion is consistent with the findings of Ruder and Yiin (2011). The rather extensive Canadian case-control study of pesticide exposure and STS (Pahwa et al., 2011), however, did not provide additional supportive evidence.

Conclusion

On the basis of the evidence reviewed here and in previous VAO reports, the committee concludes that there is sufficient evidence of an association between exposure to at least one of the COIs and STS.

SKIN CANCERS

Skin cancers are generally divided into two broad categories: neoplasms that develop from melanocytes (malignant melanoma, or simply melanoma) and neoplasms that do not. Nonmelanoma skin cancers (primarily basal-cell and squamous-cell carcinomas) have a far higher incidence than melanoma but are considerably less aggressive and therefore more treatable. The average annual incidence of melanoma is shown in Table 8-18.

The committee responsible for *Update 1998* first chose to address melanoma studies separately from those of nonmelanoma skin cancer. Some researchers report results by combining all types of skin cancer without specifying type. The present committee believes that combined information is not interpretable (although there is a supposition that mortality figures refer predominantly to melanoma and that high incidence figures refer to nonmelanoma skin cancer); therefore, it is interpreting data only when results specify melanoma or nonmelanoma skin cancer.

ACS estimated that about 44,250 men and 32,000 women would receive diagnoses of cutaneous melanoma (ICD-9 172) in the United States in 2012 and that about 6,060 men and 3,120 women would die from it (Siegel et al., 2012). According to one report, more than 3 million cases of nonmelanoma skin cancer (ICD-9 173), primarily basal-cell and squamous-cell carcinomas, are diagnosed in the United States each year (ACS, 2013b); it is not required to report them to registries, so the numbers of cases are not as precise as those of other cancers. ACS reports that although melanoma accounts for less than 5% of skin-cancer cases, it is responsible for about 75% of skin-cancer deaths (ACS, 2012b). It estimates that 3,010 people die each year from nonmelanoma skin cancer (ACS, 2012b).

Melanoma occurs more frequently in fair-skinned people than in dark-skinned people; the risk in whites is roughly 20 times that in dark-skinned blacks. The incidence increases with age, more strikingly in males than in females. Other risk factors include the presence of particular kinds of moles on the skin, suppression of the immune system, and excessive exposure to ultraviolet

TABLE 8-18 Average Annual Cancer Incidence (per 100,000) of Skin Cancers (Excluding Basal-Cell and Squamous-Cell Cancers) in the United States[a]

	55–59 Years Old			60–64 Years Old			65–69 Years Old		
	All Races	White	Black	All Races	White	Black	All Races	White	Black
Melanomas of the Skin:									
Men	50.7	61.1	2.5	71.1	83.9	2.6	91	108.2	5.0
Women	30.8	38.0	1.4	35.5	43.3	1.8	42.4	51.5	3.4

[a]Surveillance, Epidemiology, and End Results program, nine standard registries, crude age-specific rates, 2005–2009. SEER incidence data not available for nonmelanocytic skin cancer (NCI, 2013).

(UV) radiation, typically from the sun. A family history of the disease has been identified as a risk factor, but it is unclear whether that is attributable to genetic factors or to similarities in skin type and sun-exposure patterns. In addition to the dermal forms of melanoma, these tumors occur much more infrequently in various tissues of the eye.

Excessive exposure to UV radiation is the most important risk factor for nonmelanoma skin cancer; some skin diseases and chemical exposures have also been identified as potential risk factors. Although exposure to inorganic arsenic is recognized as a risk factor for nonmelanoma skin cancer, this does not imply that exposure to cacodylic acid, which is a metabolite of inorganic arsenic, can be assumed to be a risk factor.

Melanoma

Conclusions from *VAO* and Previous Updates

The committee responsible for *VAO* concluded that there was inadequate or insufficient information to determine whether there is an association between exposure to the COIs and skin cancer. Additional information available to the committee responsible for *Update 1996* did not change that conclusion. The committee responsible for *Update 1998* considered the literature on melanoma separately from that of nonmelanoma skin cancer and found that there was inadequate or insufficient information to determine whether there is an association between the COIs and melanoma. The committees responsible for *Update 2000*, *Update 2002*, and *Update 2004* concurred with the findings of *Update 1998*. The committee responsible for *Update 2006* was unable to reach a consensus as to whether there was limited or suggestive evidence of an association between exposure to the COIs and melanoma or inadequate or insufficient evidence to determine whether there is an association, so melanoma was left in the latter category. The committee for *Update 2008* determined that evidence of an association between exposure to the COIs and melanoma remained inadequate or insufficient to determine whether an association exists.

Cypel and Kang (2010) compared cause-specific mortality between deployed and nondeployed veterans in the Vietnam-era ACC cohort. In comparing the deployed with the nondeployed veterans, a moderate but not statistically significant increase in risk of malignant skin cancer was observed in the deployed cohort. Updates of mortality in TCP workers in New Zealand (McBride et al., 2009a) and in the Dow Chemical Company cohort in Midland, Michigan (Collins et al., 2009a) did not find evidence of an association between the COIs and melanoma. In evaluating the use of specific pesticides and melanoma in the AHS, Dennis et al. (2010) found that exposure only to arsenic-based pesticides, among the COIs, showed any increase in risk, which was weak and far from statistically significant. Updating cancer incidence in the Seveso cohort for the period 1977–1996

(Pesatori et al., 2009) continued to provide evidence that melanoma is associated with exposure to TCDD.

Table 8-19 summarizes the relevant melanoma studies.

Update of the Epidemiologic Literature

Vietnam-Veteran and Environmental Studies No Vietnam-veteran studies or environmental studies of exposure to the COIs and melanoma have been published since *Update 2010.*

Occupational Studies Burns et al. (2011) updated cancer incidence through 2007 in workers who were alive on January 1, 1985, and had been employed at any time from 1945 to 1994 in 2,4-D production by the Dow Chemical Company in Midland, Michigan. They found no evidence of significantly increased rates of cancer overall. With eight cases observed, the incidence of melanoma in the most restrictively defined cohort was not increased (SIR = 1.18, 95% CI 0.51–2.33), as was the case for the two successively more inclusive, but potentially more biased, cohorts.

Boers et al. (2012) studied an occupational cohort of 187 Dutch workers who were employed in two phenoxy-herbicide factories. Individual estimates of exposure were derived from a newly developed predictive model that used serum TCDD concentrations recently measured in a subset of the cohort. Estimates of mortality from melanoma were slightly but nonsignificantly increased (entire cohort, seven deaths, HR = 1.29, 95% CI 0.90–1.84; factory A, five deaths, HR = 1.27, 95% CI 0.76–2.23). An earlier analysis of the data (Boers et al., 2010), which categorized the subjects as exposed or not exposed on the basis of job histories, found no suggestion of a relationship between exposure to COIs and melanoma in the workers in factory A, where 2,4,5-T had been produced.

In reporting mortality in the NIOSH PCP cohort updated through 2005, Ruder and Yiin (2011) grouped an unspecified number of melanoma deaths in a classification (ICD-9 170–173, 190–199) that had 38 deaths, of which 2 were identified as STS deaths and 6 as deaths from "brain and other nervous system" cancer. The study provided no useful information on the risk of melanoma mortality in these workers.

Koutros et al. (2010a) and Waggoner et al. (2011) updated cancer incidence and overall mortality, respectively, in the AHS. Koutros et al. limited exposure characterization to job (applicators and spouses). They reported 173 incident melanomas in private applicators, for an SIR of 0.89 (95% CI 0.76–1.03), and 13 incident melanomas in commercial applicators, for an SIR of 1.09 (95% CI 0.58–1.86). They reported 92 incident cases in spouses, for an SIR of 1.17 (95% CI 0.94–1.43).

Waggoner et al. (2011) updated the vital status of the AHS cohort through 2007 and presented mortality data that differed little from the incidence data

TABLE 8-19 Selected Epidemiologic Studies—Melanoma (Shaded Entries Are New Information for This Update)

Study Population[a]	Exposed Cases[b]	**Exposure of Interest**/Estimated Relative Risk (95% CI)[b]	Reference
VIETNAM VETERANS			
US Vietnam Veterans			
US Air Force Health Study—Ranch Hand veterans vs SEA veterans (unless otherwise noted)		**All COIs**	
Incidence			
1982–2003—White SEA comparison veterans only (n = 1,482). Serum TCDD (pg/g) based on model with exposure variable $\log_e$(TCDD)			Pavuk et al., 2005
Per unit increase of $-\log_e$(TCDD) (pg/g)	25	2.7 (1.1–6.3)	
Quartiles (pg/g):			
0.4–2.6	3	1.0	
2.6–3.8	5	2.1 (0.4–11.0)	
3.8–5.2	8	3.2 (0.7–15.5)	
> 5.2	9	3.6 (0.7–17.2)	
Number of years served in SEA (per year of service)			
Quartiles (years in SEA):	25	1.1 (0.9–1.3)	
0.8–1.3	3	1.0	
1.3–2.1	4	1.9 (0.3–10.3)	
2.1–3.7	8	3.2 (0.7–15.3)	
3.7–16.4	10	4.1 (0.9–19.7)	
Through 1999—White subjects vs national rates			Akhtar et al., 2004
Ranch Hand veterans (n = 1,189)	17	2.3 (1.4–3.7)	
With tours between 1966–1970	16	2.6 (1.5–4.1)	
SEA comparison veterans (n = 1,776)	15	1.5 (0.9–2.4)	
With tours between 1966–1970	12	1.5 (0.8–2.6)	
White AFHS subjects			
Veterans who spent at most 2 yrs in SEA			
Per unit increase of $-\log_e$(TCDD) (pg/g)	14	2.2 (1.3–3.9)	
Comparison group	3	1.0	
Ranch Hand— < 10 TCDD pg/g in 1987	4	3.0 (0.5–16.8)	
Ranch Hand < 118.5 TCDD pg/g at end of service	4	7.4 (1.3–41.0)	
Ranch Hand > 118.5 TCDD pg/g at end of service	3	7.5 (1.1–50.2)	
Only Ranch Hands with 100% service in Vietnam, comparisons with no Vietnam service			
Per unit increase of $-\log_e$(TCDD) (pg/g)	14	1.7 (1.0–2.8)	
Comparison group	2	1.0	

TABLE 8-19 Melanoma, continued

Study Population[a]	Exposed Cases[b]	**Exposure of Interest**/Estimated Relative Risk (95% CI)[b]	Reference
Ranch Hand < 10 TCDD pg/g in 1987	5	3.9 (0.4–35.3)	
Ranch Hand < 118.5 TCDD pg/g at end of service	4	7.2 (0.9–58.8)	
Ranch Hand > 118.5 TCDD pg/g at end of service	3	5.5 (0.6–46.1)	
Ranch Hand veterans, comparisons through June 1997			Ketchum et al., 1999
Ranch Hand background exposure	4	1.1 (0.3–4.5)	
Ranch Hand low exposure	6	2.6 (0.7–9.1)	
Ranch Hand high exposure	2	0.9 (0.2–5.6)	
Comparisons	9	1.0	
Attended 1987 exam—Ranch Hand personnel (n = 995) vs SEA veterans (n = 1,299)	4	1.3 (0.3–5.2)	Wolfe et al., 1990
US VA Cohort of Army Chemical Corps—Expanded as of 1997 to include all Army men with chemical MOS (2,872 deployed vs 2,737 nondeployed) serving during Vietnam era (July 1, 1965–March 28, 1973)		**All COIs**	
Through 2005 (mortality)			Cypel and Kang, 2010
Deployed veterans (2,872) vs nondeployed (2,737)	5 vs 4	1.5 (0.4–6.2)	
ACC deployed men in Kang et al. (2006) reported sprayed herbicide vs did not spray			
Vietnam cohort	5	1.3 (0.4–3.1)	
Non-Vietnam cohort	4	1.3 (0.4–3.4)	
US CDC Vietnam Experience Study—Cross-sectional study, with medical examinations, of Army veterans: 9,324 deployed vs 8,989 nondeployed		**All COIs**	
1965–2000 (mortality)	6	1.4 (0.4–4.9)	Boehmer et al., 2004
US VA Proportionate Mortality Study—sample of deceased male Vietnam-era Army and Marine veterans who served 7/4/1965–3/1/1973		**All COIs**	
1965–1982			Breslin et al., 1986, 1988
Army, deployed (n = 19,708) vs nondeployed (n = 22,904)	145	1.0 (0.9–1.1)	
Marine Corps, deployed (n = 4,527) vs nondeployed (n = 3,781)	36	0.9 (0.6–1.5)	
State Studies of US Vietnam Veterans			
Massachusetts Vietnam-era veterans			
Veterans aged 35–65 years in 1993—melanoma cases diagnosed 1988–1993 vs gastrointestinal cancers	21	1.4 (0.7–2.9)	Clapp, 1997

continued

TABLE 8-19 Melanoma, continued

Study Population[a]	Exposed Cases[b]	**Exposure of Interest**/Estimated Relative Risk (95% CI)[b]	Reference
International Vietnam-Veteran Studies			
Australian Vietnam Veterans—58,077 men and 153 women served on land or in Vietnamese waters during 5/23/1962–7/1/1973 vs Australian population		**All COIs**	
Incidence			
All branches, 1982–2000	756	1.3 (1.2–1.4)	ADVA, 2005a
Navy	173	1.4 (1.2–1.6)	
Army	510	1.2 (1.2–1.4)	
Air Force	73	1.4 (1.1–1.7)	
Validation Study		*Expected number of exposed cases*	
	483	380 (342–418)	
Men	2,689	380 (342–418)	CDVA, 1998a
Women	7	3 (1–8)	CDVA, 1998b
Mortality			
All branches, return–2001	111	1.1 (0.9–1.3)	ADVA, 2005b
Navy	35	1.6 (1.0–2.1)	
Army	66	1.0 (0.7–1.2)	
Air Force	10	1.0 (0.5–1.8)	
1980–1994	51	1.3 (0.9–1.7)	CDVA, 1997a
Sample of 1,000 Male Australian Vietnam Veterans—prevalence		**All COIs**	
450 interviewed 2005–2006 vs respondents to 2004–2005 national survey	nr	4.7 (1.3–8.2)	O'Toole et al., 2009
Australian Conscripted Army National Service (18,940 deployed vs 24,642 nondeployed)		**All COIs**	
Incidence			
1982–2000	204	1.1 (0.9–1.4)	ADVA, 2005c
Mortality			
1966–2001	14	0.6 (0.3–1.1)	ADVA, 2005c
1982–1994	16	0.5 (0.2–1.3)	CDVA, 1997b

TABLE 8-19 Melanoma, continued

Study Population[a]	Exposed Cases[b]	**Exposure of Interest**/Estimated Relative Risk (95% CI)[b]	Reference
OCCUPATIONAL—INDUSTRIAL			
IARC Phenoxy Herbicide Cohort—Workers exposed to any phenoxy herbicide or chlorophenol (production or spraying) vs respective national mortality rates			
Mortality 1939–1992	9	0.6 (0.3–1.2)	Kogevinas et al., 1997
13,831 exposed to highly chlorinated PCDDs	5	0.5 (0.2–3.2)	
7,553 not exposed to highly chlorinated PCDDs	4	0.0 (0.3–2.4)	
Danish Production Workers (3,390 men and 1,069 women involved in production of phenoxy herbicides unlikely to contain TCDD at 2 plants in 1947–1987) (in IARC cohort)		**Dioxins, but TCDD unlikely; 2,4-D, 2,4-DP, MCPA, MCPP**	
Incidence			
Incidence 1943–1987 (men only)	4	4.3 (1.2–10.9)	Lynge, 1993
Mortality			
Mortality 1955–2006	7	1.3 (0.9–1.8)	Boers et al., 2012
Dutch production workers in Plant A (549 men exposed during production 1955–1985; 594 unexposed) (in IARC cohort)		**Dioxins, 2,4,5-T, 2,4,5-TCP**	
Mortality 1955–2006 (hazard ratios for lagged TCDD plasma levels)	5	1.3 (0.8–2.2)	Boers et al., 2012
Mortality 1955–1991	1	2.9 (0.1–15.9)	Hooiveld et al., 1998
New Zealand Phenoxy Herbicide Production Workers and Sprayers (1,599 men and women working any time in 1969–1988 at Dow plant in New Plymouth) (in IARC cohort)		**Dioxins; 2,4-D; 2,4,5-T; MCPA; MCPB; 2,4,5-TCP; Picloram**	
Mortality 1969–2004			McBride et al., 2009a
Ever-exposed workers	2	1.0 (0.1–3.7)	
Production Workers (713 men and 100 women worked > 1 month in 1969–1984)			
Mortality 1969–2000	0	0.0 (0.0–3.0)	't Mannetje et al., 2005
Sprayers (697 men and 2 women registered any time 1973–1984)			
Mortality 1973–2000	1	0.6 (0.0–3.4)	't Mannetje et al., 2005
NIOSH Mortality Cohort (12 US plants, 5,172 male production and maintenance workers 1942–1984) (included in IARC cohort as of 1997)		**Dioxins, phenoxy herbicides**	

continued

TABLE 8-19 Melanoma, continued

Study Population[a]	Exposed Cases[b]	**Exposure of Interest**/Estimated Relative Risk (95% CI)[b]	Reference
All Dow TCP-Exposed Workers (TCP production 1942–1979 or 2,4,5-T production 1948–1982 in Midland, Michigan) (in IARC and NIOSH cohorts)		**2,4,5-T; 2,4,5-TCP**	
1942–2003 (n = 1,615)	2	0.6 (0.1–2.3)	Collins et al., 2009a
Dow 2,4-D Production Workers (1945–1982 in Midland, Michigan) (subset of all TCP-exposed workers)		**2,4-D, lower chlorinated dioxins**	
Cancer incidence through 2007 in Dow workers (n = 1,256) vs comparisons from state cancer registries (n = 23,354) (Cohort 3)	8	1.2 (0.5–2.3)	Burns et al., 2011
Dow PCP Production Workers (1937–1989 in Midland, Michigan) (*not* in IARC and NIOSH cohorts)		**Low chlorinated dioxins, 2,4-D**	
Mortality 1940–2004 (n = 577, excluding 196 also having exposure to TCP)	1	0.7 (0.0–4.0)	Collins et al., 2009b
OCCUPATIONAL—PAPER AND PULP WORKERS		**TCDD**	
IARC cohort of pulp and paper workers—60,468 workers from 11 countries, TCDD among 27 agents assessed by JEM			McLean et al., 2006
Exposure to nonvolatile organochlorine compounds			
Never	20	0.8 (0.5–1.3)	
Ever	21	1.2 (0.7–1.8)	
OCCUPATIONAL—HERBICIDE-USING WORKERS (*not* related to IARC sprayer cohorts)			
CANADA			
Canadian Farm Operator Study—156,242 men farming in Manitoba, Saskatchewan, and Alberta in 1971; mortality from melanoma June 1971–December 1987			
Deaths among Saskatchewan farmers ≥ 35 yrs of age, 1971–1985	24	1.1 (0.7–1.6)	Wigle et al., 1990
Sawmill Workers in British Columbia—23,829 workers for ≥ 1 year at 11 mills using chlorophenates 1940–1985		**Chlorophenates, not TCDD**	
Incidence 1969–1989	38	1.0 (0.7–1.3)	Hertzman et al., 1997
Mortality 1950–1989	17	1.4 (0.9–2.0)	

TABLE 8-19 Melanoma, continued

Study Population[a]	Exposed Cases[b]	**Exposure of Interest**/Estimated Relative Risk (95% CI)[b]	Reference
DENMARK			
Danish Farmers—incidence from linking farmers on 1970 census with national cancer registry (1970–1980)		**Herbicides**	Ronco et al., 1992
Self-employed	72	0.7 ($p < 0.05$)	
Employee	17	0.6 (nr)	
Danish gardeners—incidence from 3,156 male and 859 female gardeners		**Herbicides**	Hansen et al., 2007
25-year followup (1975–2001)	31	1.3 (0.9–1.8)	
Born before 1915 (high exposure)	28	0.9 (0.6–1.4)	
Born 1915–1934 (medium exposure)	36	0.6 (0.4–0.9)	
Born after 1934 (low exposure)	5	0.3 (0.1–0.7)	
ITALIAN Licensed Pesticide Users—male farmers in southern Piedmont licensed 1970–1974			
Mortality 1970–1986 (n = 23,401)	9	1.2 (0.6–2.3)	Torchio et al., 1994
SWEDEN			
Incident melanoma cases 1961–1973 with agriculture as economic activity in 1960 census	268	0.8 (0.7–1.0)	Wiklund, 1983
Swedish lumberjacks—used phenoxys 1954–1967, Incidence 1958–1992			Thörn et al., 2000
Exposed (n = 154)	0	nr	
Foremen (n = 15)	0	nr	
Lumberjacks (n = 139)	0	nr	
Unexposed lumberjacks (n = 241)	0	nr	
THE NETHERLANDS			
Dutch Licensed Herbicide Sprayers—1,341 certified before 1980			
Through 2000	5	3.6 (1.2–8.3)	Swaen et al., 2004
UNITED STATES			
US farmers—usual occupation of farmer and industry of agriculture on death certificates 1984–1988 from 23 states		**Herbicides** PCMRs	Blair et al., 1993
Men			
Whites (n = 119,648)	244	1.0 (0.8–1.1)	
Nonwhites (n = 11,446)	5	1.2 (0.4–2.9)	
Women			
Whites (n = 2,400)	5	1.1 (0.4–2.7)	
Nonwhites (n = 2,066)	1	1.2 (0.0–6.6)	

continued

TABLE 8-19 Melanoma, continued

Study Population[a]	Exposed Cases[b]	**Exposure of Interest**/Estimated Relative Risk (95% CI)[b]	Reference
US Agricultural Health Study—prospective study of licensed pesticide sprayers in Iowa and North Carolina: commercial (n = 4,916), private/farmers (n = 52,395, 97.4% men), and spouses of private sprayers (n = 32,347, 0.007% men), enrolled 1993–1997; followups with CATIs 1999–2003 and 2005–2010		**Phenoxy herbicides**	
Incidence			
Enrollment through 2006—SIRs for participants			Koutros et al., 2010a
Private applicators	173	0.9 (0.8–1.0)	
Commercial applicators	13	1.1 (0.6–1.9)	
Spouses	92	1.2 (0.9–1.4)	
Licensed, male pesticide applicators—150 cutaneous melanomas among 24,704 pesticide applicators			Dennis et al., 2010
Ever-exposed to arsenic-based pesticides vs never-exposed	11	1.3 (0.7–2.4)	
Ever used lead arsenate insecticide	10	1.2 (0.6–2.3)	
Enrollment through 2002			Samanic et al., 2006
Dicamba—lifetime days exposure			
None	32	1.0	
1– < 20	10	1.0 (0.5–2.1)	
20– < 56	18	1.6 (0.8–3.0)	
56– < 116	6	0.7 (0.3–1.8)	
≥ 116	6	0.8 (0.3–2.1)	
		p-trend = 0.51	
Enrollment through 2002			Alavanja et al., 2005
Private applicators	100	1.0 (0.8–1.2)	
Spouses of private applicators (> 99% women)	67	1.6 (1.3–2.1)	
Commercial applicators	7	1.1 (0.4–2.2)	
Mortality			
Enrollment through 2007, vs state rates			Waggoner et al., 2011
Applicators (n = 1,641)	38	0.8 (0.5–1.1)	
Spouses (n = 676)	10	0.8 (0.4–1.4)	
Enrollment through 2000, vs state rates			Blair et al., 2005a
Private applicators (men and women)	13	0.7 (0.4–1.3)	
Spouses of private applicators (> 99% women)	2	0.4 (0.1–1.6)	

TABLE 8-19 Melanoma, continued

Study Population[a]	Exposed Cases[b]	**Exposure of Interest**/Estimated Relative Risk (95% CI)[b]	Reference
ENVIRONMENTAL			
Seveso, Italy Residential Cohort—Industrial accident July 10, 1976 (723 residents Zone A; 4,821 Zone B; 31,643 Zone R; 181,574 local reference group) (ICD-9 171)		**TCDD**	
Incidence			
20-yr followup to 1996—men and women			
Zone A	1	1.6 (0.2–11.6)	Pesatori et al., 2009
Zone B	2	0.5 (0.1–2.0)	
Zone R	19	0.7 (0.4–1.1)	
Mortality			
25-yr followup to 2001—men and women			Consonni et al., 2008
Zone A	1	3.1 (0.4–22.0)	
Zone B	2	1.0 (0.2–3.9)	
Zone R	12	0.8 (0.4–1.5)	
20-yr followup to 1996			Bertazzi et al., 2001
Zones A and B—men	1	1.5 (0.2–12.5)	
Zones A and B—women	2	1.8 (0.4–7.3)	
15-yr followup to 1991—men			Bertazzi et al., 1997
Zone A	0	0.0 (0.0–60.2)	
Zone B	0	0.0 (0.0–9.1)	
Zone R	3	1.1 (0.2–3.2)	
15-yr followup to 1991—women			Bertazzi et al., 1997
Zone A	1	9.4 (0.1–52.3)	
Zone B	0	0.0 (0.0–5.4)	
Zone R	3	0.6 (0.1–1.8)	
10-yr followup to 1986—men			Bertazzi et al., 1989a
Zone A, B, R	3	3.3 (0.8–13.9)	
10-yr followup to 1986—women			Bertazzi et al., 1989a,b
Zone A, B, R	1	0.3 (0.1–2.5)	
SWEDEN			
Swedish fishermen (high consumption of fish with persistent organochlorines)		**Organochlorine compounds**	Svensson et al., 1995
Incidence			
East coast	0	0.0 (0.0–0.7)	
West coast	20	0.8 (0.5–1.2)	
Mortality			
East coast	0	0.0 (0.0–1.7)	
West coast	6	0.7 (0.3–1.5)	

continued

TABLE 8-19 Melanoma, continued

Study Population[a]	Exposed Cases[b]	**Exposure of Interest**/Estimated Relative Risk (95% CI)[b]	Reference
CASE-CONTROL STUDIES			
International Case-Control Studies			
British Columbia—melanoma cases recruited for a study evaluating effects of ultraviolet exposure and gene variants using plasma specimens and sun-exposure data (80 cases vs 310 controls)		**PCBs**	Gallagher et al., 2011
Highest PCB-exposure quintile	29	6.0 (2.0–18.2)	
Dioxin-like PCBs	25	2.8 (1.0–8.0)	
Non-dioxin-like PCBs	30	7.0 (2.3–21.4)	
European—uveal melanoma patients (n = 323), diagnosed 1994–1997, identified from hospital records (diagnosed 1994–1995) in nine countries and matched controls (n = 3,198)		**Herbicides**	Behrens et al., 2012
Personal application of herbicides	8	0.5 (0.2–1.3)	
Personal mixing of herbicides	6	0.5 (0.2–1.5)	
UK men, 18–35 yrs of age from counties with particular chemical manufacturing—mortality		**Herbicides, chlorophenols**	Magnani et al., 1987
Herbicides	nr	1.2 (0.4–4.0)	
Chlorophenols	nr	0.9 (0.4–2.3)	

NOTE: 2,4-D, 2,4-dichlorophenoxyacetic acid; 2,4-DP, dichlorprop; 2,4,5-T, 2,4,5-trichlorophenoxyacetic acid; 2,4,5-TCP, 2,4,5-trichlorophenol; ACC, Army Chemical Corps; CATI, computer-assisted telephone interviewing; CDC, Centers for Disease Control and Prevention; CI, confidence interval; COI, chemical of interest; IARC, International Agency for Research on Cancer; ICD, International Classification of Diseases; JEM, job-exposure matrix; MCPA, 2-methyl-4-chlorophenoxyacetic acid; MCPB, 4-(4-chloro-2-methylphenoxy)butanoic acid; MCPP, methylchlorophenoxypropionic acid; MOS, military occupational specialty; NIOSH, National Institute for Occupational Safety and Health; nr, not reported; PCB, polychlorinated biphenyl; PCDD, polychlorinated dibenzo-*p*-dioxin (highly chlorinated, if four or more chlorines); PCMR, proportionate cancer mortality ratios; PCP, pentachlorophenol; SEA, Southeast Asia; SIR, standardized incidence ratio; TCDD, 2,3,7,8-tetrachlorodibenzo-*p*-dioxin; TCP, trichlorophenol; VA, US Department of Veterans Affairs.

[a]Cohorts are male and outcome mortality unless otherwise noted.

[b]Given when available; results other than estimated risk explained individually.

in Koutros et al. (2010a). Using a similar job classification as a surrogate for exposure, they reported 38 deaths compared with 50 expected for an SMR of 0.76 (95% CI 0.54–1.05). In spouses, they reported 10 deaths compared with 13 expected for an SMR of 0.75 (95% CI 0.36–1.38). The AHS has been generating valuable information on the COIs for a number of years, but these results are not herbicide-specific and so are not regarded as being fully informative for the committee's task.

Case-Control Studies Gallagher et al. (2011) studied melanoma and its association with plasma concentrations of PCBs by using an unusual case-control design. They ascertained cases by using the resources (plasma specimens and sun-exposure data) from melanoma cases originally recruited for evaluating the effects of UV exposure and gene variants on risk of melanoma in the Genes, Environment & Melanoma (GEM) study (Begg et al., 2005; Berwick et al., 2006). Controls for that study were drawn from a different study, conducted at about the same time in the same geographic region (British Columbia), that was designed to investigate the effect of solar UV exposure and plasma organochlorine compounds on risk of non-Hodgkin lymphoma (Spinelli et al., 2007). The studies were similar in design: they both recruited participants by using the population-based BC Cancer Registry, and they used the same computer-assisted telephone interview protocol to collect information on sun exposure, phenotype, and sun sensitivity. Cases from the GEM study included 153 patients, of whom 86 (56%) were able to be recontacted for drawing of additional blood for this investigation. Blood was drawn in 2002–2005 for controls and in 2008 for cases. The laboratory analyses were well controlled to ensure comparability. Plasma samples from 460 controls were assayed for 14 PCB congeners and 11 chlorine-based pesticides or their metabolites; after matching on age and area of residence, 309 were available for use in the study. A total of three cases were not included in the study because of the inability to match with controls. The exposure assessment included 14 PCB congeners (dioxin-like mono-ortho PCBs 105, 118, and 156 and non-dioxin-like PCBs 28, 52, 99, 101, 128, 138, 153, 170, 180, 183, and 187) and 11 persistent pesticides.

Many of the accepted risk factors for melanoma were found to be associated with the disease in this study. Analysis showed significant associations between PCB congeners and melanoma although they were rather imprecise. Total PCB concentrations were associated with disease, with a significant dose–response relationship. The highest risk was in the highest PCB-exposure quartile (OR = 6.02, 95% CI 2.00–18.17). The dioxin-like mono-ortho PCBs, however, showed a significant association (OR = 2.84, 95% CI 1.01–7.97), which was less pronounced than that of the non-dioxin-like PCBs (OR = 7.02, 95% CI 2.30–21.43). There was some indication of an association of pesticide exposure with melanoma but it was limited to nonachlor, Mirex, and hexachlorobenzene.

Thus, the study provided evidence of an association between chemicals that have dioxin-like activity and melanoma but with important limitations. First, the number of cases was small, and participation was low, so there is a question of unmeasured bias. In addition, although the authors attempted to control for sun exposure, this is notoriously difficult. The cases and controls arose from different studies and, although every attempt was made to match them, they may not have been comparable in some respects (such as ethnicity). The presence of disease could alter the measured exposures. The confidence limits of the point estimates are imprecise, and this lessens confidence in their generalizability. In addition, there is little exposure specificity in the association, so it is difficult to interpret in light of the biologic data. Finally, only dioxin-like mono-ortho PCBs were reported, which typically contribute only a small percentage to total TEQs, making it difficult to accurately determine whether an association exists with total TEQs, and the largest associations were found for the non-dioxin-like compounds.

Behrens et al. (2012) conducted a case-control study of uveal (ocular) melanoma and pesticide exposure, but exposure to unspecified herbicides does not reach the level of specificity that the committee has regarded as necessary for full relevance. The significant finding in the category of 1–9 years of "application of any herbicide on farm where subject worked" is intriguing but contrary to expectations of a dose–response association. The results with respect to personal application and mixing of herbicides are more pertinent for the committee's purposes, and they are firmly not positive.

Biologic Plausibility

TCDD and related herbicides have not been found to cause melanoma in animal models. In general, rodents, which are used in most toxicology studies, are not a good model for studying melanoma. TCDD does produce nonmelanoma skin cancers in animal models (Wyde et al., 2004). As discussed elsewhere in this chapter, TCDD is a known tumor-promoter and could act as a promoter for skin-cancer initiators, such as UV radiation. Ikuta et al. (2009) examined the physiologic role of the AHR in human skin and theorized that overactivation can lead to skin cancers, but they provided no evidence that melanoma incidence is increased after TCDD exposure. Recent work in this field has shown that the AHR mediates UVB-induced skin-tanning in a murine model through action on melanocytes; this is evidence that skin pigmentation and potentially the regulatory action of the target cell for melanoma may be affected by TCDD. Studies of human cells have also confirmed a role of the AHR in regulation of keratinocytes and melanocytes. Kalmes et al. (2011) have shown that AHR signaling in immortalized HaCaT cells is associated with cell-cycle progression. In human melanocytes, Luecke et al. (2010) demonstrated that TCDD exposure induced tyrosinase and tyrosinase-related protein 2 gene expression—an indication that AHR signaling after TCDD exposure modulates melanogenesis. O'Donnell et al. (2012) further showed that the activity of the AHR was associated with proliferation of melanoma cells. Finally, it was recently shown in a Han Chinese population that normal genetic variants of the AHR are associated with the occurrence of vitiligo; this strongly suggests that the AHR is associated with melanocyte distribution in humans.

The biologic plausibility of the carcinogenicity of the COIs is discussed in general at the beginning of this chapter.

Synthesis

No compelling association between the COIs and melanoma was observed in any of the three new occupational studies.

The committee responsible for *Update 2006* was unable to reach a consensus as to whether there was limited or suggestive evidence of an association between exposure to the COIs and melanoma or inadequate or insufficient evidence to determine whether there is an association. That committee considered the findings from the Air Force Health Study (AFHS) on melanoma, evaluated in terms of TCDD measurements (Akhtar et al., 2004; Pavuk et al., 2005), to be of prime interest. However, the data from the final AFHS examination cycle indicate that many more melanoma cases were diagnosed in the comparison veterans than in the Operation Ranch Hand veterans. Consequently, the committee responsible for *Update 2006* recommended that the final data on the Ranch Hand and comparison veterans be analyzed in a uniform manner to document the full melanoma experience of the AFHS subjects and to permit definitive evaluation of the possible association between the COIs and melanoma. That request remains unaddressed.

This is the first update in which any information on ocular melanoma has been identified. The case-control study of Behrens et al. (2012) found some increases in the incidence of uveal melanoma in association with unspecified herbicides; this is not the degree of herbicide specificity required for results to be considered fully relevant. A Vietnam veteran submitted information (Data from Rutz [2012] available in the National Academies Public Access Records Office [http://www8.nationalacademies.org/cp/ManageRequest.aspx?key=49448]) received in response to a Freedom of Information Act request to VA about the frequency with which choroidal melanoma (a specific type of uveal melanoma) was diagnosed in VA facilities; the document indicated that a large number of such cases had been seen, but the lack of documentation explaining how the VA had gathered the data and exactly what they represented prevented the committee from being able to assess their import. Because literature searches did not identify any epidemiology studies of ocular melanoma in association with the COIs, the committee submitted an inquiry to Carol and Mark Shields, who responded (Data from Shields [2012] available in the National Academies Public Access Records Office [http://www8.nationalacademies.org/cp/ManageRequest.aspx?key=49448]) that their analyses of more than 2,000 cases of uveal melanoma had not revealed any association with the COIs.

Conclusion

On the basis of the evidence reviewed here and in previous VAO reports, the committee concludes that there is inadequate or insufficient evidence to determine whether there is an association between exposure to the COIs and melanoma (dermal or ocular).

Basal-Cell Cancer and Squamous-Cell Cancer (Nonmelanoma Skin Cancer)

Conclusions from *VAO* and Previous Updates

The committee responsible for *VAO* concluded that there was inadequate or insufficient information to determine whether there is an association between exposure to the COIs and skin cancer, and additional information available to the committee responsible for *Update 1996* did not change that conclusion. The committee responsible for *Update 1998* considered the literature on nonmelanoma skin cancer separately from that on melanoma and concluded that there was inadequate or insufficient information to determine whether there is an association between exposure to the COIs and basal-cell or squamous-cell cancer. The committees responsible for *Update 2000*, *Update 2002*, *Update 2004*, *Update 2006*, *Update 2008*, and *Update 2010* did not change that conclusion.

Table 8-20 summarizes the relevant studies.

Update of the Epidemiologic Literature

No epidemiology studies of exposure to the COIs and basal-cell or squamous-cell cancer have been published since *Update 2010*.

Biologic Plausibility

There are no new studies on animal models of skin cancer that are relevant to this update. TCDD has been shown to produce nonmelanoma skin cancer in animal models (Wyde et al., 2004). As discussed elsewhere in this chapter, TCDD is a known tumor-promoter and could act as a promoter for skin-cancer initiators, such as UV radiation, but no experiments have been conducted specifically to support this potential mechanism.

The biologic plausibility of the carcinogenicity of the COIs is discussed in general at the beginning of this chapter.

Synthesis

In accord with the results of reports previously assessed, the committee concludes that there is inadequate or insufficient evidence to determine whether there is an association between exposure to the COIs and basal-cell or squamous-cell cancer.

TABLE 8-20 Selected Epidemiologic Studies—Other Nonmelanoma (Basal-Cell and Squamous-Cell) Skin Cancer (Shaded Entries Are New Information for This Update)

Study Population[a]	Exposed Cases[b]	**Exposure of Interest**/Estimated Relative Risk (95% CI)[b]	Reference
VIETNAM VETERANS			
US Vietnam Veterans			
US Air Force Health Study—Ranch Hand veterans vs SEA veterans (unless otherwise noted)		**All COIs**	
Incidence—basal cell, squamous cell			
1982–2003—White SEA comparison veterans only (n = 1,482). Serum TCDD (pg/g) based on model with exposure variable $\log_e$(TCDD)	253	1.2 (0.9–1.4)	Pavuk et al., 2005
Per unit increase of $-\log_e$(TCDD) (pg/g)			
Quartiles (pg/g):			
0.4–2.6	50	nr	
2.6–3.8	59	1.2 (0.8–1.8)	
3.8–5.2	71	1.5 (1.1–2.3)	
> 5.2	73	1.4 (0.9–2.0)	
Number of years served in SEA (per year of service)	253	1.0 (0.9–1.1)	
Quartiles (years in SEA):			
0.8–1.3	55	nr	
1.3–2.1	50	0.9 (0.6–1.4)	
2.1–3.7	73	1.1 (0.8–1.6)	
3.7–16.4	75	1.2 (0.8–1.7)	
Attended 1987 exam—Ranch Hand personnel (n = 995) vs SEA veterans (n = 1,299)			Wolfe et al., 1990
Basal-cell carcinoma	78	1.5 (1.0–2.1)	
Squamous-cell carcinoma	6	1.6 (0.5–5.1)	
International Vietnam-Veteran Study			
Australian Vietnam Veterans—58,077 men and 153 women served on land or in Vietnamese waters during 5/23/1962–7/1/1973 vs Australian population		**All COIs**	
Incidence			
Validation Study (expected number of exposed cases)			
Men	6,936	nr	CDVA, 1998a
Women	37	nr	CDVA, 1998b
OCCUPATIONAL—INDUSTRIAL			
IARC Phenoxy Herbicide Cohort—Workers exposed to any phenoxy herbicide or chlorophenol (production or spraying) vs respective national mortality rates	4	0.9 (0.3–2.4)	

continued

TABLE 8-20 Other Nonmelanoma (Basal-Cell and Squamous-Cell) Skin Cancer, continued

Study Population[a]	Exposed Cases[b]	**Exposure of Interest**/Estimated Relative Risk (95% CI)[b]	Reference
Mortality 1939–1992			Kogevinas et al., 1997
13,831 exposed to highly chlorinated PCDDs	4	1.3 (0.3–3.2)	
7,553 not exposed to highly chlorinated PCDDs	0	0.0 (0.0–3.4)	
British MCPA Plant—Production 1947–1982 (n = 1,545) (included in IARC cohort) and spraying 1947–1972 (n = 2,561) (*not* included in IARC cohort)		**MCPA**	
Mortality through 1983	3	3.1 (0.6–9.0)	Coggon et al., 1986
NIOSH Mortality Cohort (12 US plants, 5,172 male production and maintenance workers 1942–1984) (included in IARC cohort as of 1997)		**Dioxins, phenoxy herbicides**	
Dow 2,4-D Production Workers (1945–1982 in Midland, Michigan) (subset of all TCP-exposed workers)		**2,4-D, lower chlorinated dioxins**	
Through 1994 (n = 1,517)	0	nr	Burns et al., 2001
OCCUPATIONAL—HERBICIDE-USING WORKERS (*not* related to IARC sprayer cohorts)			
DENMARK			
Danish Farmers—incidence from linking farmers on 1970 census with national cancer registry (1970–1980)		**Herbicides**	Ronco et al., 1992
Men			
Self-employed	493	0.7 (p < 0.05)	
Employee	98	0.7 (p < 0.05)	
Women			
Self-employed	5	0.3 (p < 0.05)	
Employee	10	0.9 (nr)	
Family worker	90	0.6 (p < 0.05)	
Danish gardeners—incidence from 3,156 male and 859 female gardeners (skin, ICD-7 190–191)	31	**Herbicides** 1.3 (0.9–1.8)	Hansen et al., 2007
25-year followup (1975–2001)			
Born before 1915 (high exposure)	28	0.9 (0.6–1.4)	
Born 1915–1934 (medium exposure)	36	0.6 (0.4–0.9)	
Born after 1934 (low exposure)	5	0.3 (0.1–0.7)	
ICELANDIC pesticide users (n = 2,449, 1,860 men and 589 women), 2,4-D used most often, little 2,4,5-T			Zhong and Rafnsson, 1996
Men	5	2.8 (0.9–6.6)	
Men, women combined	5	2.6 (0.8–6.1)	

TABLE 8-20 Other Nonmelanoma (Basal-Cell and Squamous-Cell) Skin Cancer, continued

Study Population[a]	Exposed Cases[b]	**Exposure of Interest**/Estimated Relative Risk (95% CI)[b]	Reference
ITALIAN Licensed Pesticide Users—male farmers in southern Piedmont licensed 1970–1974			
Mortality 1970–1986 (n = 23,401)	3	0.6 (0.1–1.8)	Torchio et al., 1994
SWEDEN			
Incident melanoma cases 1961–1973 with agriculture as economic activity in 1960 census	708	*99% CI* 1.1 (1.0–1.2)	Wiklund, 1983
Swedish lumberjacks—used phenoxys 1954–1967, Incidence 1958–1992			Thörn et al., 2000
Exposed (n = 154)			
Foremen (n = 15)	1	16.7 (0.2–92.7)	
Lumberjacks (n = 139)	0	—	
Unexposed lumberjacks (n = 241)	3	2.0 (0.4–5.8)	
THE NETHERLANDS			
Dutch Licensed Herbicide Sprayers—1,341 certified before 1980			
Through 2000—melanoma, squamous-cell carcinoma, unknown skin cancer (mortality presumably attributable to melanoma)	5	3.6 (1.2–8.3)	Swaen et al., 2004
UNITED STATES			
US farmers—usual occupation of farmer and industry of agriculture on death certificates 1984–1988 from 23 states (skin, including melanoma)		**Herbicides** PCMRs	Blair et al., 1993
Men			
Whites (n = 119,648)	425	1.1 (1.0–1.2)	
Nonwhites (n = 11,446)	13	1.0 (0.5–1.7)	
Women			
Whites (n = 2,400)	6	1.0 (0.4–2.1)	
Nonwhites (n = 2,066)	3	1.8 (0.4–5.4)	
ENVIRONMENTAL			
Seveso, Italy Residential Cohort—Industrial accident July 10, 1976 (723 residents Zone A; 4,821 Zone B; 31,643 Zone R; 181,574 local reference group)		**TCDD**	
Incidence			
20-yr followup to 1996—men and women			Pesatori et al., 2009
Zone A	3	1.4 (0.5–4.3)	
Zone B	5	0.4 (0.2–0.9)	
Zone R	88	0.9 (0.8–1.2)	
10-yr followup to 1991—men			Bertazzi et al., 1993
Zone A	1	2.4 (0.3–17.2)	
Zone B	2	0.7 (0.2–2.9)	
Zone R	20	1.0 (0.6–1.6)	

continued

TABLE 8-20 Other Nonmelanoma (Basal-Cell and Squamous-Cell) Skin Cancer, continued

Study Population[a]	Exposed Cases[b]	**Exposure of Interest**/Estimated Relative Risk (95% CI)[b]	Reference
10-yr followup to 1991—women			Bertazzi et al., 1993
Zone A	1	3.9 (0.5–28.1)	
Zone B	2	1.3 (0.3–5.1)	
Zone R	13	1.0 (0.6–1.9)	
Other International Environmental Study			
Swedish fishermen (high consumption of fish with persistent organochlorines)		**Organochlorine compounds**	Svensson et al., 1995
Incidence			
East coast	22	2.3 (1.5–3.5)	
West coast	69	1.1 (0.9–1.4)	
Mortality			
East coast	0	0.0 (0.0–15.4)	
West coast	5	3.1 (1.0–7.1)	
CASE-CONTROL STUDIES			
International Case-Control Studies			
Alberta, **Canada** residents—squamous-cell carcinoma—incidence		**Herbicides**	Gallagher et al., 1996
All herbicide exposure	79	1.5 (1.0–2.3)	
Low herbicide exposure	33	1.9 (1.0–3.6)	
High herbicide exposure	46	3.9 (2.2–6.9)	
Alberta, **Canada** residents—basal-cell carcinoma		**Herbicides**	Gallagher et al., 1996
All herbicide exposure	70	1.1 (0.8–1.7)	

NOTE: 2,4-D, 2,4-dichlorophenoxyacetic acid; 2,4,5-T, 2,4,5-trichlorophenoxyacetic acid; CI, confidence interval; COI, chemical of interest; IARC, International Agency for Research on Cancer; ICD, International Classification of Diseases; MCPA, 2-methyl-4-chlorophenoxyacetic acid; NIOSH, National Institute for Occupational Safety and Health; nr, not reported; PCDD, polychlorinated dibenzo-*p*-dioxin (highly chlorinated, if four or more chlorines); PCMR, proportionate cancer mortality ratios; SEA, Southeast Asia; TCDD, 2,3,7,8-tetrachlorodibenzo-*p*-dioxin; TCP, trichlorophenol.

[a]Subjects are male and outcome is mortality unless otherwise noted.

[b]Given when available; results other than estimated risk explained individually.

Conclusion

On the basis of the evidence reviewed here and in previous VAO reports, the committee concludes that there is inadequate or insufficient evidence to determine whether there is an association between exposure to the COIs and basal-cell or squamous-cell cancer.

BREAST CANCER

Breast cancer (ICD-9 174 for females, ICD-9 175 for males) is the second-most common type of cancer (after nonmelanoma skin cancer) in women in the United States. ACS estimated that 226,870 women would receive diagnoses of breast cancer in the United States in 2012 and that 39,510 would die from it (Siegel et al., 2012). Overall, those numbers represent about 29% of the new cancers and 14% of cancer deaths in women. Incidence data on breast cancer are presented in Table 8-21.

Breast-cancer incidence generally increases with age. In the age groups of most Vietnam veterans, the incidence is higher in whites than in blacks. Established risk factors other than age include personal or family history of breast cancer and some characteristics of reproductive history—specifically, early menarche, late onset of menopause, and either no pregnancies or first full-term pregnancy after the age of 30 years. A pooled analysis of six large-scale prospective studies of invasive breast cancer showed that alcohol consumption up to a daily average of 60 g (2.1 oz), which spanned the consumption reported by more than 99% of the women, was associated with a small linear increase in incidence in comparison with nondrinkers (Smith-Warner et al., 1998). It is generally accepted that breast-cancer risk is increased by prolonged use of hormone-replacement therapy, particularly preparations that combine estrogen and progestins (Chlebowski et al., 2003). The potential of other personal behavioral and environmental factors (including use of exogenous hormones) to affect breast-cancer incidence is being studied extensively.

Most of the roughly 10,000 female Vietnam veterans who were potentially exposed to herbicides in Vietnam are approaching or have reached menopause. Given the high incidence of breast cancer in older and postmenopausal women in general, it is expected on the basis of demographics alone that the breast-cancer burden in female Vietnam veterans will increase in the near future.

The vast majority of breast-cancer epidemiologic studies involve women, but the disease also occurs rarely in men, with 2,190 new cases expected in 2012

TABLE 8-21 Average Annual Incidence (per 100,000) of Breast Cancer in the United States[a]

	55–59 Years Old			60–64 Years Old			65–69 Years Old		
	All Races	White	Black	All Races	White	Black	All Races	White	Black
Men	2.0	2.0	2.8	3.4	3.3	4.9	5.0	5.3	3.3
Women	279.6	284.3	273.8	359.9	373.0	348.0	420.8	438.5	389.5

[a]Surveillance, Epidemiology, and End Results program, nine standard registries, crude age-specific rates, 2005–2009 (NCI, 2013).

(Siegel et al., 2012). Reported instances of male breast cancer are noted below, but the committee's conclusions are based on the studies in women.

Conclusions from *VAO* and Previous Updates

The committee responsible for *VAO* concluded that there was inadequate or insufficient information to determine whether there is an association between exposure to the COIs and breast cancer. Additional information available to the committees responsible for *Update 1996*, *Update 1998*, *Update 2000*, *Update 2002*, and *Update 2004* did not change that conclusion. After consideration of a new study with positive findings on an association between 2,4-D exposure and breast cancer in female farmworkers in California (Mills and Yang, 2005)—in conjunction with the earlier findings of Kang et al. (2000), Kogevinas et al. (1997), Revich et al. (2001), and Warner et al. (2002)—the committee responsible for *Update 2006* was unable to reach consensus as to whether there might be limited or suggestive evidence of an association between the COIs and breast cancer. An increase in the incidence of breast cancer in the residents of Zone A in Seveso may be emerging with greater latency (Pesatori et al., 2009), but in light of null findings on mortality from breast cancer in the important cohorts of female Vietnam-era veterans (Cypel and Kang, 2008) and Seveso residents (Consonni et al., 2008), all members of the committees for *Update 2008* and *Update 2010* concurred that breast cancer should remain in the category of inadequate or insufficient evidence to determine whether there is an association.

Table 8-22 summarizes the relevant research.

Update of the Epidemiologic Literature

Vietnam-Veteran Studies

No Vietnam-veteran studies of exposure to the COIs and breast cancer have been published since *Update 2010*.

Occupational Studies

Burns et al. (2011) updated the incidence of cancer through 2007 in workers who were alive on January 1, 1985, and had been employed at any time from 1945 to 1994 in 2,4-D production by the Dow Chemical Company in Midland, Michigan. They found no evidence of significantly increased rates of cancer overall. One case of male breast cancer was observed in Cohorts 1 and 2, but the residience requirements excluded it from Cohort 3.

There were 398 women in the Hamburg cohort (a subcohort of the IARC phenoxy-herbicide cohort). They had been employed for at least 3 months during 1952–1984 in a chemical plant that produced insecticides and herbicides,

TABLE 8-22 Selected Epidemiologic Studies—Breast Cancer (Shaded Entries Are New Information for This Update)

Study Population[a]	Exposed Cases[b]	**Exposure of Interest**/Estimated Relative Risk (95% CI)[b]	Reference
VIETNAM VETERANS			
US Vietnam Veterans			
US CDC Vietnam Experience Study—Cross-sectional study, with medical examinations, of Army veterans: 9,324 deployed vs 8,989 nondeployed		**All COIs**	
Mortality			
1965–2000	0	nr	Boehmer et al., 2004
US VA Cohort of Female Vietnam Veterans		**All COIs**	
Incidence			
Breast cancer	170	1.2 (0.9–1.5)	Kang et al., 2000
Mortality			
Through 2004	57	1.0 (0.7–1.4)	Cypel and
Vietnam-veteran nurses	44	0.9 (0.6–1.4)	Kang, 2008
Through 1991	26	1.0 (0.6–1.8)	Dalager et al., 1995
Through 1987	17	1.2 (0.6–2.5)	Thomas et al., 1991
International Vietnam-Veteran Studies			
Australian Vietnam Veterans—58,077 men and 153 women served on land or in Vietnamese waters during 5/23/1962–7/1/1973 vs Australian population		**All COIs**	
Incidence			
All branches, 1982–2000	7	0.9 (0.4–1.9)	ADVA,
Navy	1	0.6 (0.0–3.3)	2005a
Army	5	1.0 (0.3–2.2)	
Air Force	1	1.1 (0.0–6.3)	
Validation Study		*Expected number of exposed cases*	
Women	17	5 (2–11)	CDVA, 1998b
Mortality			
All branches, return–2001	4	2.2 (0.6–5.4)	ADVA,
Navy	1	2.5 (0.0–13.5)	2005b
Army	3	2.5 (0.5–7.2)	
Air Force	0	0.0 (0.0–14.6)	
1980–1994 (men)	3	5.5 (1.0– > 10.0)	CDVA, 1997a
Australian Conscripted Army National Service (18,940 deployed vs 24,642 nondeployed)		**All COIs**	

continued

TABLE 8-22 Breast Cancer, continued

Study Population[a]	Exposed Cases[b]	**Exposure of Interest**/Estimated Relative Risk (95% CI)[b]	Reference
Incidence			
1982–2000	0	0.0 (0.0–2.4)	ADVA, 2005c
Mortality			
1966–2001	nr		ADVA, 2005c
OCCUPATIONAL—INDUSTRIAL			
IARC Phenoxy Herbicide Cohort—Workers exposed to any phenoxy herbicide or chlorophenol (production or spraying) vs respective national mortality rates			
Mortality 1939–1992 (13,831 exposed to highly chlorinated PCDDs vs 7,553 unexposed)		**Phenoxy herbicides**	Kogevinas et al., 1997
Men	2	1.6 (0.2–2.1)	
Exposed to highly chlorinated PCDDs	2	2.6 (0.3–9.3)	
Not exposed to highly chlorinated PCDDs	0	nr	
Women	12	1.2 (0.6–2.1)	
Exposed to highly chlorinated PCDDs	9	2.2 (1.0–4.1)	
Not exposed to highly chlorinated PCDDs	3	0.5 (0.1–1.6)	
Mortality 1955–1988 of 12,492 production workers and 5,898 sprayers exposed—13,482 in exposed subcohort			Saracci et al., 1991
Men	2	3.5 (0.4–12.5)	
Women	1	0.3 (0.0–1.7)	
Mortality, incidence of women in production (n = 699) and spraying (n = 2) compared to national death rates and cancer incidence rates	7	**TCDD** 0.9 (0.4–1.9)	Kogevinas et al, 1993
Danish Production Workers (3,390 men and 1,069 women involved in production of phenoxy herbicides unlikely to contain TCDD at 2 plants in 1947–1987) (in IARC cohort)		**Dioxins, but TCDD unlikely; 2,4-D, 2,4-DP, MCPA, MCPP**	
Incidence 1943–1982 (women)	13	0.9 (nr)	Lynge, 1985
German Production Workers at Boehringer–Ingelheim Plant in Hamburg (1,144 men working > 1 month in 1952–1984; generation of TCDD reduced after chloracne outbreak in 1954) and women—no results (some additions to observed cancers over Manz et al., 1991) (in IARC cohort as of 1997)		**Dioxins; 2,4,5-T; 2,5-DCP; 2,4,5-TCP**	
Mortality 1952–2007			Manuwald et al., 2012
Women	19	1.9 (1.1–2.9)	
Mortality 1952–1989—stats on men only, 1,184 (tables all for 1,148 men, not necessarily German nationals) vs national rates (also vs gas workers); same observation period as Becher et al., 1966	9	2.2 (1.0–4.1)	Manz et al., 1991

TABLE 8-22 Breast Cancer, continued

Study Population[a]	Exposed Cases[b]	Exposure of Interest/Estimated Relative Risk (95% CI)[b]	Reference
New Zealand Phenoxy Herbicide Production Workers and Sprayers (1,599 men and women working any time in 1969–1988 at Dow plant in New Plymouth) (in IARC cohort)		**Dioxins; 2,4-D; 2,4,5-T; MCPA; MCPB; 2,4,5-TCP; Picloram**	
Mortality 1969–2004			McBride et al., 2009a
Ever-exposed workers	2	1.4 (0.2–5.0)	
Production Workers (713 men and 100 women worked > 1 month in 1969–1984)			
Mortality 1969–2000			't Mannetje et al., 2005
Phenoxy herbicide producers			
Men	1	32 (0.8–175)	
Women	1	1.3 (0.0–7.2)	
Phenoxy herbicide sprayers (> 99% men)			
Men	0	0.0 (0.0–214)	
Women	0	0.0 (0.0–86.0)	
NIOSH Mortality Cohort (12 US plants, 5,172 male production and maintenance workers 1942–1984) (included in IARC cohort as of 1997)		**Dioxins, phenoxy herbicides**	
All Dow PCP-Exposed Workers—all workers from the two plants that only made PCP (in Tacoma, Washington, and Wichita, Kansas) and workers who made PCP and TCP at two additional plants (in Midland, Michigan, and Sauget, Illinois)		**2,4,5-T; 2,4,5-TCP**	Ruder and Yiin, 2011
1940–2005 (n = 2,122)	1	0.5 (0.0–2.9)	
PCP and TCP (n = 720)	0	nr	
PCP (no TCP) (n = 1,402)	1	0.6 (0.0–3.1)	
Dow 2,4-D Production Workers (1945–1982 in Midland, Michigan) (subset of all TCP-exposed workers)		**2,4-D, lower chlorinated dioxins**	
Cancer incidence through 2007 in Dow workers (n = 1,256) vs comparisons from state cancer registries (n = 23,354) (Cohort 3)	0	nr	Burns et al., 2011
OCCUPATIONAL—PAPER AND PULP WORKERS		**TCDD**	
IARC cohort of pulp and paper workers—60,468 workers from 11 countries, TCDD among 27 agents assessed by JEM			McLean et al., 2006
Exposure to nonvolatile organochlorine compounds			
Never	21	0.9 (0.6–1.4)	
Ever	32	0.9 (0.6–1.3)	

continued

TABLE 8-22 Breast Cancer, continued

Study Population[a]	Exposed Cases[b]	**Exposure of Interest**/Estimated Relative Risk (95% CI)[b]	Reference
OCCUPATIONAL—HERBICIDE-USING WORKERS (*not* related to IARC sprayer cohorts)			
DENMARK			
Danish Farmers—incidence from linking farmers on 1970 census with national cancer registry (1970–1980)		**Herbicides**	Ronco et al., 1992
Men			
Self-employed	5	0.5 (nr)	
Employee	3	1.4 (nr)	
Women			
Self-employed	41	0.9 (nr)	
Employee	25	0.6 ($p < 0.05$)	
Family worker	429	0.8 ($p < 0.05$)	
SWEDEN			
Incident breast cancer cases 1961–1973 with agriculture as economic activity in 1960 census			Wiklund, 1983
Men, women		*99% CI*	
	444	0.8 (0.7–0.9)	
Men	nr	1.0 (nr)	
UNITED STATES			
US farmers—usual occupation of farmer and industry of agriculture on death certificates 1984–1988 from 23 states		**Herbicides** PCMRs	Blair et al., 1993
Men			
Whites (n = 119,648)	18	0.7 (0.4–1.2)	
Nonwhites (n = 11,446)	4	1.7 (0.5–4.4)	
Women			
Whites (n = 2,400)	71	1.0 (0.8–1.3)	
Nonwhites (n = 2,066)	30	0.7 (0.5–1.0)	
US Agricultural Health Study—prospective study of licensed pesticide sprayers in Iowa and North Carolina: commercial (n = 4,916), private/farmers (n = 52,395, 97.4% men), and spouses of private sprayers (n = 32,347, 0.007% men), enrolled 1993–1997; followups with CATIs 1999–2003 and 2005–2010		**Phenoxy herbicides**	
Incidence			
Enrollment through 2006—SIRs for participants			Koutros et al., 2010a
Private applicators	33	1.0 (0.7–1.3)	
Commercial applicators	0	nr	
Spouses	770	1.0 (0.9–1.1)	
Enrollment through 2002			Alavanja et al., 2005
Private applicators	27	1.1 (0.7–1.6)	

TABLE 8-22 Breast Cancer, continued

Study Population[a]	Exposed Cases[b]	**Exposure of Interest**/Estimated Relative Risk (95% CI)[b]	Reference
Spouses of private applicators (> 99% women)	474	1.0 (0.9–1.1)	
Commercial applicators	1	0.6 (0.1–3.5)	
Enrollment through 2001			Engel et al., 2005
Wives' own use of phenoxy herbicides	41	0.8 (0.6–1.1)	
2,4-D	41	0.8 (0.6–1.1)	
Husbands' own use of phenoxy herbicides	110	1.1 (0.7–1.8)	
2,4-D	107	0.9 (0.6–1.4)	
2,4,5-T	44	1.3 (0.9–1.9)	
2,4,5-TP	19	2.0 (1.2–3.2)	
Mortality			
Enrollment through 2007, vs state rates			Waggoner et al., 2011
Applicators (n = 1,641)	11	0.9 (0.5–1.7)	
Spouses (n = 676)	136	0.8 (0.7–0.9)	
Enrollment through 2000, vs state rates			Blair et al., 2005a
Private applicators (men and women)	3	0.9 (0.2–2.7)	
Spouses of private applicators (> 99% women)	54	0.9 (0.7–1.1)	
ENVIRONMENTAL			
Seveso, Italy Residential Cohort—Industrial accident July 10, 1976 (723 residents Zone A; 4,821 Zone B; 31,643 Zone R; 181,574 local reference group)		**TCDD**	
Incidence			
20-yr followup to 1996—men and women			
Zone A	8	1.4 (0.7–2.9)	Pesatori et al., 2009
Zone B	30	0.9 (0.6–1.2)	
Zone R	249	1.0 (0.9–1.2)	
Zone A only (15+ yrs after accident)	5	2.6 (1.1–6.2)	
Zone A only (10–14 yrs after accident)	2	1.4 (0.4–5.7)	
Zone A only (5–9 yrs after accident)	1	0.8 (0.1–5.7)	
10-yr followup to 1991—men			Bertazzi et al., 1993
Zone R	1	1.2 (0.1–10.2)	
10-yr followup to 1991—women			Bertazzi et al., 1993
Zone A	1	0.5 (0.1–3.3)	
Zone B	10	0.7 (0.4–1.4)	
Zone R	106	1.1 (0.9–1.3)	
Mortality			
25-yr followup to 2001—men and women			Consonni et al., 2008
Zone A	2	0.6 (0.2–2.4)	
Zone B	13	0.6 (0.3–1.2)	
Zone R	133	0.9 (0.7–1.1)	

continued

TABLE 8-22 Breast Cancer, continued

Study Population[a]	Exposed Cases[b]	**Exposure of Interest**/Estimated Relative Risk (95% CI)[b]	Reference
20-yr followup to 1996			Bertazzi et al., 2001
Zones A and B—women	14	0.7 (0.4–1.3)	
15-yr followup to 1991—women			Bertazzi et al., 1997
Zone A	1	0.6 (0.0–3.1)	
Zone B	9	0.8 (0.4–1.5)	
Zone R	67	0.8 (0.6–1.0)	
10-yr followup to 1986—women			Bertazzi et al., 1989a,b
Zone A	1	1.1 (0.1–7.5)	
Zone B	5	0.9 (0.4–2.1)	
Zone R	28	0.6 (0.4–0.9)	
Seveso (Italy) Women's Health Study—981 women who were infants to 10–40 yrs of age when exposed—incidence		**TCDD**	
Cancer incidence (1976–2009)			Warner et al., 2011
Hazard ratios from lipid-adjusted serum TCDD levels and breast cancer; TCDD (ppt):			
Log10 TCDD (ppt)	33	1.4 (0.9–2.3)	
11–20 yrs followup (1987–1996)	10	2.2 (1.1–4.6)	
21–32 yrs followup (1997–2009)	20	1.1 (0.6–1.9)	
With 10-fold increase in TCDD	15	2.1 (1.0–4.6)	Warner et al., 2002
Ecological Study of Residents of Chapaevsk, Russia		**Dioxin**	Revich et al., 2001
Women			
Regional (Samara)	nr	50.7 (nr)	
National (Russia)	nr	46.2 (nr)	
Mortality—1995–1998 (SMR vs regional rates)			
Women	58	2.1 (1.6–2.7)	
FINLAND			
Finnish fishermen (n = 6,410) and spouses (n = 4,260) registered between 1980 and 2002 compared to national statistics		**Serum dioxin**	Turunen et al., 2008
Fisherman's wives	18	0.8 (0.5–1.3)	
CASE-CONTROL STUDIES			
US Case-Control Studies			
California—Women undergoing breast biopsies in San Francisco area hospitals—79 breast-cancer cases vs 52 controls with benign breasts conditions—incidence		**PCDDs, PCDFs**	Reynolds et al., 2005
Total TEQs (pg/g) in adipose breast tissue			
≤ 14.0	24	1.0	
14.1–20.9	22	0.7 (0.3–1.9)	
≤ 21.0	33	0.3 (0.3–2.0) p-trend = 0.99	

TABLE 8-22 Breast Cancer, continued

Study Population[a]	Exposed Cases[b]	**Exposure of Interest**/Estimated Relative Risk (95% CI)[b]	Reference
California—Registry-based study of 128 Hispanic agricultural farmworkers (women) diagnosed 1988–2001 and 640 cancer-free controls.		**Herbicides**	Mills and Yang, 2005
Cancer diagnosis 1987–1994			
Low 2,4-D use	12	0.6 (0.2–1.9)	
High 2,4-D use	8	0.6 (0.2–1.7)	
Cancer diagnosis 1995–2001			
Low 2,4-D use	19	2.2 (1.0–4.9)	
High 2,4-D use	21	2.1 (1.1–4.3)	
California Teachers Study Cohort—residential proximity to use of "endocrine disruptors" (including 2,4-D, cacodylic acid)		**2,4-D, cacodylic acid**	Reynolds et al., 2004
Quartiles of use (lb/mi^2)			
< 1	1,027	1.0	
1–21	274	1.0 (0.8–1.1)	
22–323	114	0.9 (0.7–1.1)	
≥ 324	137	1.0 (0.9–1.3)	
California women (n = 146) receiving medical care in Woodland Hills (1995–1996), 73 breast-cancer cases vs 73 controls undergoing mammoplasty	73	**Organochlorines** nr	Bagga et al., 2000
New York—Population-based study of lifetime residential pesticide use in Long Island; 1,508 newly diagnosed cases and 1,556 matched controls (1996–1997)		**Pesticides**	Teitelbaum et al., 2007
Used lawn and garden pesticides			
Never	240	1.0	
Ever	1,254	1.3 (1.1–1.6)	
Product for weeds	1,109	1.4 (1.2–1.8)	
North Carolina—862 female farmworkers, residents diagnosed 1993–1996 and 790 controls.		**Herbicides**	Duell et al., 2000
Used pesticides in garden	228	2.3 (0.7–3.1)	
Laundered clothes for pesticide user	119	4.1 (2.8–5.9)	
Connecticut patient at Yale–New Haven hospital with breast related surgery; dl-congener 156	nr	**dl-PCBs** 0.9 (0.8–1.0)	Holford et al., 2000
International Case-Control Studies			
Canadian women in Quebec City—315 newly diagnosed breast-cancer cases (and plasma concentrations) vs hospital- and population-based controls	314	**Organochlorines**, nr	Demers et al., 2000

continued

TABLE 8-22 Breast Cancer, continued

Study Population[a]	Exposed Cases[b]	**Exposure of Interest**/Estimated Relative Risk (95% CI)[b]	Reference
Denmark females with breast cancer in Copenhagen City Heart Study (n = 195), 2 blood samples taken (1987–1978, 1981–1983)		**Organochlorines** *Overall survival* *RR*	Høyer et al., 2000
	195	2.8 (1.4–5.6)	
France—Besançon residents in zones of dioxin exposure around solid-waste incinerator (434 incident breast-cancer cases; 2,170 randomly selected controls) (1996–2002)		**Dioxin**	Viel et al., 2008
Women, 20–59 yrs of age			
Very low	41	1.0	
Low	81	1.1 (0.7–1.6)	
Intermediate	64	1.3 (0.8–1.9)	
High	11	0.9 (0.4–1.8)	
Women, 20–59 yrs of age			
Very low	50	1.0	
Low	111	0.9 (0.6–1.3)	
Intermediate	72	1.0 (0.7–1.4)	
High	4	0.3 (0.1–0.9)	
Greenland Inuit women with breast cancer (n = 31) vs 115 matched controls, 2000–2003		**POPs, dl PCBs**	Bonefeld-Jorgensen et al., 2011
Dl-PCbs in serum (median: cases vs controls)		56.8 vs 65.4 pg/g lipid p = 0.0009	

NOTE: 2,4-D, 2,4-dichlorophenoxyacetic acid; 2,4-DP, dichlorprop; 2,4,5-T, 2,4,5-trichlorophenoxyacetic acid; 2,4,5-TCP, 2,4,5-trichlorophenol; 2,4,5-TP, 2 (2,4,5-trichlorophenoxy) propionic acid; 2,5-DCP, 2,5-dichlorophenol; CATI, computer-assisted telephone interviewing; CDC, Centers for Disease Control and Prevention; CI, confidence interval; COI, chemical of interest; dl, dioxin-like; IARC, International Agency for Research on Cancer; JEM, job-exposure matrix; MCPA, 2-methyl-4-chlorophenoxyacetic acid; MCPB, 4-(4-chloro-2-methylphenoxy)butanoic acid; MCPP, methylchlorophenoxypropionic acid; NIOSH, National Institute for Occupational Safety and Health; nr, not reported; PCDD, polychlorinated dibenzo-*p*-dioxin (highly chlorinated, if four or more chlorines); PCDF, polychlorinated dibenzofurans; PCMR, proportionate cancer mortality ratios; PCP, pentachlorophenol; PM, proportionate mortality; ppt, parts per trillion; RR, relative risk; SIR, standardized incidence ratio; SMR, standardized mortality rate; TCDD, 2,3,7,8-tetrachlorodibenzo-*p*-dioxin; TCP, trichlorophenol; TEQ, toxicity equivalent; VA, US Department of Veterans Affairs.

[a]Subjects are female and outcome is mortality unless otherwise noted.

[b]Given when available; results other than estimated risk explained individually.

including 2,4,5-T, so they had the possibility of exposure to TCDD. Manuwald et al. (2012) reported on their mortality through 2007. Relative to the population of Hamburg, 19 breast-cancer deaths represented a significantly increased risk in the women (SMR = 1.86, 95% CI 1.12–2.91). A Cochran–Armitage trend test on deaths from breast cancer according to quartiles of cumulative exposure did not find evidence of a dose–response relationship; the second and fourth quartiles had significantly increased risks, but the third quartile matched the lowest quartile, with only two breast-cancer deaths. That constitutes a somewhat stronger finding than had previously been reported by Manz et al. (1991).

Ruder and Yiin (2011) reported mortality in 1940–2005 in the NIOSH PCP cohort of 2,122 workers in the four US plants that had been involved in PCP production. An SMR for breast cancer in the 1,402 PCP production workers (including 67 women) who had not been exposed to TCDD was derived on a sex- and race-specific basis using 5-year intervals of age and calendar time. With only a single death, the resulting finding (SMR = 0.55, 95% CI 0.01–3.07) was not informative.

In that the members of the applicator cohort in the AHS are largely men and those in the spouse cohort predominantly women, for this cancer it is the spouses who are more informative. Koutros et al. (2010a) did not find an increase in the incidence of female breast cancer through 2006 (770 cases, SIR = 1.00, 95% CI 0.93–1.08); Waggoner et al. (2011) found that mortality from breast cancer through 2007 was significantly below expectation (136 deaths, SMR = 0.80, 95% CI 0.67–0.94). The AHS has been generating valuable information on the COIs for a number of years, but these results are not herbicide-specific and so are not regarded as being fully informative for the committee's task.

Environmental Studies

Warner et al. (2011) added more than 10 years of observation of cancer incidence in the women in the Seveso Women's Health Study, updating the borderline significant results on breast cancer published earlier (Warner et al., 2002) to cover the period from the 1976 explosion through 2009. Of the 981 women participating in the earlier study, 833 were reinterviewed. A total of 66 cases were reported, which represented a distinct increase in the risk of any cancer (HR = 1.86, 95% CI 1.29–2.52) in association with lipid-adjusted, log-transformed serum TCDD concentrations at the time of the accident; 33 of the cases were breast cancers. After adjustment for age at the time of the explosion, marital status, parity, and family history of breast cancer, the occurrence of breast cancer was not as clearly associated with serum TCDD concentrations (HR = 1.46, 95% CI 0.89–2.33) as Warner et al. (2002) had found it to be up to 1998 (HR = 2.1, 95% CI 1.0–4.6). With stratification by decade since the industrial accident in 1976, the breast-cancer risk appeared to have peaked in the interval 11–20 years after (HR = 2.23, 95% CI 1.09–4.56) and to have subsided in the period 21–32 years after (HR = 1.06,

95% CI 0.58–1.93). The small size of the cohort curtails the analyses that can be conducted, but the availability of serum TCDD concentrations measured from blood samples gathered fairly soon after the single-substance accident (which minimizes uncertainty about what exposure had been experienced and reduces the need for back-extrapolation) contributes substantially to the value of the results.

Case-Control Studies

The incidence of breast cancer in Inuits has traditionally been much lower that that in other Western populations, but there has been a notable increase in the frequency in this population over the last several decades. Bonefeld-Jorgensen et al. (2011) conducted a case-control study of breast cancer in Greenland Inuits. The registry of breast-cancer cases in Greenland during 2000–2003 was screened for Inuits (defined as women who had at least two grandparents born in Greenland), and 31 (80%) were entered into the study. They were matched by age and district to 115 controls assembled in a previous study of serum concentrations of persistant organic pollutants. The focus of this study was on perfluorinated compounds, but there also was reporting of serum concentrations of 12 PCB congeners—including dioxin-like, mono-ortho PCBs 105, 118, and 156—and overall AHR-mediated transcriptional activity. The median concentrations of dioxin-like, mono-ortho PCBs did not differ between cases and controls (149 and 198 pg/g lipid, respectively; $p = 0.36$). Further, AHR TEQs were significantly lower in cases than in controls (median, 56.8 and 65.4 pg/g lipid, respectively; $p = 0.009$). Therefore, the study results did not provide evidence of an association between dioxin-like activity and the occurrence of breast cancer in this population. However, since these values are based solely on mono-ortho PCBs, which typically contribute only a small percentage to total TEQs, no conclusions can be drawn.

Biologic Plausibility

The experimental evidence indicates that 2,4-D, 2,4,5-T, and TCDD are weakly genotoxic at most. However, TCDD is a demonstrated carcinogen in animals and is recognized as having carcinogenic potential in humans because of the mechanisms discussed in Chapter 4.

With respect to breast cancer, experimental data have shown a role of TCDD in carcinogenesis and promotion and evidence of a protective effect, particularly with regard to metastasis. Studies performed in laboratory animals (Sprague-Dawley rats) indicate that the effect of TCDD may depend on the age of the animal. For example, TCDD exposure was found to inhibit mammary-tumor growth in the adult rat (Holcombe and Safe, 1994) but to increase tumor growth in the neonatal rat (21 days old) (Desaulniers et al., 2001). Other studies have failed to demonstrate an effect of TCDD on mammary-tumor incidence or growth (Desaulniers et al., 2004).

Fenton (2009) recently reviewed the literature on TCDD and breast cancer and suggested that a mechanism may be related to endocrine disruption, which might indicate a close association between the development of mammary cancers and mammary gland differentiation. Agents capable of disrupting the ability of the normal mammary epithelial cell to enter or maintain its appropriate status (a proliferative, differentiated, apoptotic state), to maintain its appropriate architecture, or to conduct normal hormone (estrogen) signaling are likely to act as carcinogens (Fenton, 2006; McGee et al., 2006). In that light, it is interesting that postnatal exposure of pregnant rats to TCDD has been found to alter proliferation and differentiation of cells in the mammary gland (Birnbaum and Fenton, 2003; Vorderstrasse et al., 2004). A recent study has shown that TCDD directly targets mammary epithelial cells and the surrounding stromal fat cells during pregnancy-induced mammary gland differentiation; this indicates interference with stromal–epithelial cross-talk as one of several underlying pathways (Lew et al., 2011). Jenkins et al. (2007) used a rat carcinogen-induced mammary-cancer model to show that prenatal exposure to TCDD alters mammary gland differentiation and increases susceptibility to mammary cancer by altering the expression of estrogen-receptor (ER) genes and of genes involved in oxidative-stress defense. Thus, the effect of TCDD may depend on the timing of the exposure and on the magnitude of gene expression at the time of exposure; TCDD may influence mammary-tumor development only if exposure to it occurs during a specific window during breast development (Rudel et al., 2011). The breast is the only human organ that does not fully differentiate until it becomes ready for use; nulliparous women have less-differentiated breast lobules, which are presumably more susceptible to carcinogenesis.

Paradoxically, activation of the AHR by dioxin or by the nondioxin ligand indole-3-carbinol has also been shown to protect against breast cancer by mechanisms that disrupt migration and metastasis (Bradlow, 2008; Hsu et al., 2007). Administration of TCDD to mice that harbor highly metastatic breast-cancer cells in the mammary fat pad reduced the metastasis by 50% without suppressing primary tumor size—indication that TCDD's protective effects are selective to the metastatic process (Wang et al., 2011). It is possible that some protective effects may be mediated through the known cross-talk between the AHR and ERα, which has been studied extensively at the molecular level for potential therapeutic benefit. Recent data show that AHR controls ERα-mediated gene stimulation through recruitment of receptor interacting protein 140 (RIP140), which can both activate and repress ER actions (Madak-Erdogan and Katzenellenbogen, 2012). In the presence of dioxin, the AHR can repress specific estrogen-dependent genes in MCF-7 breast-cancer cells (Labrecque et al., 2012). TCDD can also activate AHR-mediated G_1cell-cycle arrest (Barhoover et al., 2010); however, in the presence of a progesterone receptor, TCDD enriches the G2/M phase and stimulates proliferation of MCF-7 cells (Chen YJ et al., 2012). Together, those results demonstrate a complicated interplay between the AHR and other nuclear transcription factors that can either stimulate or inhibit breast-cancer growth in a manner that depends on cell-context.

TCDD has been shown to modulate the induction of DNA-chain breaks in human breast-cancer cells by regulating the activity of the enzymes responsible for estradiol catabolism and generating more reactive intermediates, which might contribute to TCDD-induced carcinogenesis by altering the ratio of 4-OH-estradiol to 2-OH-estradiol, a marker of breast-cancer risk (Lin et al., 2007, 2008). A similar imbalance in metabolite ratios has been observed in pregnant Taiwanese women, in whom the ratio of 4-OH-estradiol to 2-OH-estradiol decreased with increasing exposure to TCDD (Wang et al., 2006). Expression of CYP1B1—the cytochrome P450 enzyme responsible for 2-OH-estradiol formation—but not CYP1A1—the one responsible for 4-OH-estradiol formation—was found to be highly increased in premalignant and malignant rat mammary tissues in which the AHR was constitutively active in the absence of ligand (Yang et al., 2008). On the basis of recent mechanistic data, it has been proposed that the AHR contributes to mammary-tumor cell growth by inhibiting apoptosis while promoting transition to an invasive, metastatic phenotype (Marlowe et al., 2008; Schlezinger et al, 2006; Vogel et al., 2011).

Recent evidence has shown that AHR activation by TCDD in human breast and endocervical cell lines induces sustained high concentrations of the interleukin-6 (IL-6) cytokine, which has tumor-promoting effects in numerous tissues, including breast tissue, so TCDD might promote carcinogenesis in these tissues (DiNatale et al., 2010; Hollingshead et al., 2008). Similarly, TCDD induced IL-8 expression in an AHR-dependent manner and may contribute to the inflammatory type of breast cancer (Vogel et al., 2011). Degner et al. (2009) have shown that AHR ligands can upregulate the expression of COX-2, and this may lead to a proinflammatory environment that can support tumor development.

The biologic plausibility of the carcinogenicity of the COIs is discussed in general at the beginning of this chapter.

Synthesis

In the early 1990s, it was suggested that exposure to some environmental chemicals, such as organochlorine compounds, might play a role in the etiology of breast cancer through estrogen-related pathways. The relationship between organochlorines and breast-cancer risk has been studied extensively, especially in the last decade; TCDD and dioxin-like compounds have been among the organochlorines so investigated. Today, there is no clear evidence of a causal role of most organochlorines in human breast cancer (Salehi et al., 2008).

Because of concerns raised by a combination of a new study that had good exposure assessment and positive findings (Mills and Yang, 2005) and several earlier studies (Kang et al., 2000; Kogevinas et al., 1997; Revich et al., 2001; Warner et al., 2002), some members of the committee responsible for *Update*

2006 believed that there was suggestive evidence of an association, but that committee was unable to reach a consensus. After reviewing new studies that had null findings on mortality from breast cancer in the important cohorts of female Vietnam-era veterans (Cypel and Kang, 2008) and Seveso residents (Consonni et al., 2008), the committee for *Update 2008* readily reached a consensus that breast cancer should remain in the category of inadequate or insufficient evidence of an association. The committee for *Update 2010* concurred, although the 20-year followup of cancer incidence in Seveso (Pesatori et al., 2009) had reported a significantly increasing relationship between breast-cancer incidence and time from the accident until diagnosis in the women in Zone A: 15 or more years (RR = 2.57, 95% CI 1.07–6.20), 10–14 years (RR = 1.42, 95% CI 0.35–5.68), and 5–9 years (RR = 0.81, 95% CI 0.11–5.74); that is, accounting for latency led to stronger associations.

In the present update, the followup of the Seveso Women's Health Study through 2009 by Warner et al. (2011) showed an abating of the risk of breast cancer (HR = 1.46, 95% CI 0.89–2.33) from what Warner et al. (2002) had reported through 1998 (HR = 2.1, 95% CI 1.0–4.6) and in contrast with the findings in the entire cohort through 1996 reported by Pesatori et al. (2009). The marginal increase in the Hamburg cohort (Manuwald et al., 2012) was counterbalanced by null results in the Dow Chemical Company 2,4-D production workers (Burns et al., 2011). The case-control study of Greenland Inuits provided no evidence of an association with dioxin-like activity.

Conclusion

Having considered the new evidence and the results of studies reviewed in previous updates, the present committee concludes that there is inadequate or insufficient evidence to determine whether there is an association (either positive or negative) between exposure to the COIs and breast cancer.

CANCERS OF THE FEMALE REPRODUCTIVE SYSTEM

This section addresses cancers of the cervix (ICD-9 180), endometrium (also referred to as the corpus uteri; ICD-9 182.0–182.1, 182.8), and ovary (ICD-9 183.0). Additional cancers of the female reproductive system that are infrequently reported separately are cancers of the uterus (ICD-9 179), placenta (ICD-9 181), fallopian tube and other uterine adnexa (ICD-9 183.2–183.9), and other female genital organs (ICD-9 184); findings on these cancers are included in this section. ACS estimates of the numbers of new female reproductive-system cancers in the United States in 2012 are presented in Table 8-23; they represent roughly 11% of new cancer cases and 11% of cancer deaths in women (Siegel et al., 2012).

Cervical cancer occurs more often in blacks than in whites, but endometrial and ovarian cancers occur more often in whites. The incidence of endometrial and

TABLE 8-23 Estimates of New Cases of Deaths from Selected Cancers of the Female Reproductive System in the United States in 2012

Site	New Cases	Deaths
Cervix	12,170	4,220
Endometrium	47,130	8,010
Ovary	22,280	15,500
Other female genital [organs]	2,680	840

SOURCE: Siegel et al., 2012.

ovarian cancers is higher in older women and in those who have family histories of these cancers. Use of unopposed (without progestogen) estrogen-hormone therapy and obesity, which increases endogenous concentrations of estrogen, both increase the risk of endometrial cancer. HPV infection, particularly infection with HPV types 16 and 18, is the most important risk factor for cervical cancer. Use of oral contraceptives is associated with a substantial reduction in the risk of ovarian cancer.

Conclusions from *VAO* and Previous Updates

The committee responsible for *VAO* concluded that there was inadequate or insufficient information to determine whether there is an association between exposure to the COIs and female reproductive cancers. Additional information available to the committees responsible for *Update 1996*, *Update 1998*, *Update 2000*, *Update 2002*, *Update 2004*, *Update 2006*, *Update 2008*, and *Update 2010* has been sparse and has not changed that conclusion.

Tables 8-24, 8-25, and 8-26 summarize the results of the relevant studies on cancers of the cervix, uterus, and ovary, respectively.

Update of the Epidemiologic Literature

Vietnam-Veteran, Environmental, and Case-Control Studies

No Vietnam-veteran studies, environmental studies, or case-control studies of exposure to the COIs and female reproductive cancers have been published since *Update 2010*.

TABLE 8-24 Selected Epidemiologic Studies—Cervical Cancer (Shaded Entries Are New Information for This Update)

Study Population[a]	Exposed Cases[b]	**Exposure of Interest**/Estimated Relative Risk (95% CI)[b]	Reference
VIETNAM VETERANS			
US Vietnam Veterans			
US VA Cohort of Female Vietnam Veterans			
Incidence		**All COIs**	
Female Vietnam veterans	57	1.1 (0.7–1.7)	Kang et al., 2000
International Vietnam-Veterans Studies			
Australian Vietnam Veterans—58,077 men and 153 women served on land or in Vietnamese waters during 5/23/1962–7/1/1973 vs Australian population		**All COIs**	
Incidence		*Expected number of exposed cases*	CDVA, 1998b
Validation Study			
Self-reported cervical cancer	8	1 (0–5)	
OCCUPATIONAL—INDUSTRIAL			
IARC Phenoxy Herbicide Cohort—Workers exposed to any phenoxy herbicide or chlorophenol (production or spraying) vs respective national mortality rates		**Dioxin, phenoxy herbicides**	
Mortality 1939–1992	3	1.1 (0.2–3.3)	Kogevinas et al., 1997
13,831 exposed to highly chlorinated PCDDs	0	0.0 (0.0–3.8)	
7,553 not exposed to highly chlorinated PCDDs	3	1.8 (0.4–5.2)	
Danish Production Workers (3,390 men and 1,069 women involved in production of phenoxy herbicides unlikely to contain TCDD at 2 plants in 1947–1987) (in IARC cohort)		**Dioxins, but TCDD unlikely; 2,4-D, 2,4-DP, MCPA, MCPP**	
Incidence 1943–1987	7	3.2 (1.3–6.6)	Lynge, 1993
New Zealand Phenoxy Herbicide Production Workers and Sprayers (1,599 men and women working any time in 1969–1988 at Dow plant in New Plymouth) (in IARC cohort)		**Dioxins; 2,4-D; 2,4,5-T; MCPA; MCPB; 2,4,5-TCP; Picloram**	
Mortality 1969–2004			McBride et al., 2009a
Cervix uteri (ICD-10 C53)	0	0.0 (0.0–14.6)	
OCCUPATIONAL—HERBICIDE-USING WORKERS (*not* related to IARC sprayer cohorts)			
DENMARK			
Danish Farmers—incidence from linking farmers on 1970 census with national cancer registry (1970–1980)		**Herbicides**	Ronco et al., 19922
Self-employed	7	0.5 ($p < 0.05$)	

continued

TABLE 8-24 Cervical Cancer, continued

Study Population[a]	Exposed Cases[b]	**Exposure of Interest**/Estimated Relative Risk (95% CI)[b]	Reference
Employees	12	0.8 (nr)	
Family workers	100	0.5 ($p < 0.05$)	
ITALIAN Licensed Pesticide Users—male farmers in southern Piedmont licensed 1970–1974			
Incident cervical cancer cases 1961–1973 with agriculture as economic activity in 1960 census	82	*99% CI* 0.6 (0.4–0.8)	Wiklund, 1983
UNITED STATES			
US farmers—usual occupation of farmer and industry of agriculture on death certificates 1984–1988 from 23 states		**Herbicides** PCMRs	Blair et al., 1993
Women			
Whites (n = 2,400)	6	0.9 (0.3–2.0)	
Nonwhites (n = 2,066)	21	2.0 (1.3–3.1)	
ENVIRONMENTAL			
Seveso, Italy Residential Cohort—Industrial accident July 10, 1976 (723 residents Zone A; 4,821 Zone B; 31,643 Zone R; 181,574 local reference group) (ICD-9 171)		**TCDD**	
Incidence			
20-yr followup to 1996—men and women			
Zone A	2	2.7 (0.7–10.8)	Pesatori et al., 2009
Zone B	7	1.5 (0.7–3.1)	
Zone R	28	0.8 (0.6–1.3)	
Ecological Study of Residents of Chapaevsk, Russia		**Dioxin**	Revich et al., 2001
Incidence—Crude incidence rate in 1998 vs			
Regional (Samara)	nr	11.7 (nr)	
National (Russia)	nr	13.2 (nr)	
Mortality—1995–1998 (SMR vs regional rates)	13	1.8 (1.0–3.1)	

NOTE: 2,4-D, 2,4-dichlorophenoxyacetic acid; 2,4-DP, dichlorprop; 2,4,5-T, 2,4,5-trichlorophenoxyacetic acid; 2,4,5-TCP, 2,4,5-trichlorophenol; CI, confidence interval; COI, chemical of interest; IARC, International Agency for Research on Cancer; ICD, International Classification of Diseases; MCPA, 2-methyl-4-chlorophenoxyacetic acid; MCPB, 4-(4-chloro-2-methylphenoxy)butanoic acid; MCPP, methylchlorophenoxypropionic acid; nr, not reported; PCDD, polychlorinated dibenzo-*p*-dioxin (highly chlorinated, if four or more chlorines); PCMR, proportionate cancer mortality ratios; SMR, standardized mortality rate; TCDD, 2,3,7,8-tetrachlorodibenzo-*p*-dioxin; VA, US Department of Veterans Affairs.

[a]Subjects are female and outcome is mortality unless otherwise noted.

[b]Given when available; results other than estimated risk explained individually.

TABLE 8-25 Selected Epidemiologic Studies—Uterine Cancer (Shaded Entries Are New Information for This Update)

Study Population[a]	Exposed Cases[b]	**Exposure of Interest**/Estimated Relative Risk (95% CI)[b]	Reference
VIETNAM VETERANS			
US Vietnam Veterans			
US VA Cohort of Female Vietnam Veterans			
Incidence		**All COIs**	
Female Vietnam veterans	41	1.0 (0.6–1.6)	Kang et al., 2000
Mortality			
Through 2004—US non-Vietnam veterans	5	0.8 (0.2–2.8)	Cypel and Kang, 2008
vs non-Vietnam nurses	5	1.3 (0.3–5.0)	
Through 1991—US Vietnam veterans	4	2.1 (0.6–5.4)	Dalager et al., 1995
International Vietnam-Veterans Studies			
Australian Vietnam Veterans—58,077 men and 153 women served on land or in Vietnamese waters during 5/23/1962–7/1/1973 vs Australian population		**All COIs**	
Incidence		*Expected number of exposed cases*	
Validation Study			
Self-reported uterine cancer	4	1 (0–5)	CDVA, 1998b
OCCUPATIONAL—INDUSTRIAL			
IARC Phenoxy Herbicide Cohort—Workers exposed to any phenoxy herbicide or chlorophenol (production or spraying) vs respective national mortality rates		**Dioxin, phenoxy herbicides**	
Mortality 1939–1992	3	3.4 (0.7–10.0)	Kogevinas et al., 1997
13,831 exposed to highly chlorinated PCDDs	1	1.2 (0.0–6.5)	
7,553 not exposed to highly chlorinated PCDDs	4	2.3 (0.6–5.9)	
New Zealand Phenoxy Herbicide Production Workers and Sprayers (1,599 men and women working any time in 1969–1988 at Dow plant in New Plymouth) (in IARC cohort)		**Dioxins; 2,4-D; 2,4,5-T; MCPA; MCPB; 2,4,5-TCP; Picloram**	
Mortality 1969–2004			McBride et al., 2009a
Corpus uteri (ICD-10 C54–C55)	0	0.0 (0.0–30.6)	
OCCUPATIONAL—HERBICIDE-USING WORKERS (*not* related to IARC sprayer cohorts)			
DENMARK			
Danish Farmers—incidence from linking farmers on 1970 census with national cancer registry (1970–1980)		**Herbicides**	Ronco et al., 1992
Self-employed	8	0.6 (nr)	

continued

TABLE 8-25 Uterine Cancer, continued

Study Population[a]	Exposed Cases[b]	**Exposure of Interest**/Estimated Relative Risk (95% CI)[b]	Reference
Employees	9	0.9 (nr)	
Family workers	103	0.8 ($p < 0.05$)	
ITALIAN Licensed Pesticide Users—male farmers in southern Piedmont licensed 1970–1974			
Incident NHL cases 1961–1973 with agriculture as economic activity in 1960 census	135	*99% CI* 0.9 (0.7–1.1)	Wiklund, 1983
UNITED STATES			
US farmers—usual occupation of farmer and industry of agriculture on death certificates 1984–1988 from 23 states		**Herbicides** PCMRs	Blair et al., 1993
Women			
Whites (n = 2,400)	15	1.2 (0.7–2.1)	
Nonwhites (n = 2,066)	17	1.4 (0.8–2.2)	
US Agricultural Health Study—prospective study of licensed pesticide sprayers in Iowa and North Carolina: commercial (n = 4,916), private/farmers (n = 52,395, 97.4% men), and spouses of private sprayers (n = 32,347, 0.007% men), enrolled 1993–1997; followups with CATIs 1999–2003 and 2005–2010		**Phenoxy herbicides**	
Enrollment through 2006—SIRs for participants			Koutros et al., 2010a
Private applicators	4	nr	
Commercial applicators	1	nr	
Spouses	148	0.9 (0.8–1.1)	
ENVIRONMENTAL			
Seveso, Italy Residential Cohort—Industrial accident July 10, 1976 (723 residents Zone A; 4,821 Zone B; 31,643 Zone R; 181,574 local reference group)		**TCDD**	
Incidence			
20-yr followup to 1996 (Uterus, ICD-9 179–182)			
Zone A	4	2.3 (0.9–6.3)	Pesatori et al., 2009
Zone B	10	0.9 (0.5–1.7)	
Zone R	61	0.8 (0.6–1.0)	
20-yr followup to 1996 (Endometrium, ICD-9 182)			
Zone A	1	1.2 (0.2–8.8)	
Zone B	3	0.6 (0.2–1.9)	
Zone R	27	0.7 (0.5–1.1)	

TABLE 8-25 Uterine Cancer, continued

Study Population[a]	Exposed Cases[b]	**Exposure of Interest**/Estimated Relative Risk (95% CI)[b]	Reference
Mortality			
25-yr followup to 2001			
Zone A	0	0	Consonni et al., 2008
Zone B	2	0.5 (0.1–1.9)	
Zone R	41	1.3 (0.9–1.8)	
20-yr followup to 1996			
Zone A, B	2	0.5 (0.1–1.9)	Bertazzi et al., 2001
15-yr followup to 1991			
Zone B	1	0.3 (0.0–2.4)	Bertazzi et al., 1997, 1998
Zone R	27	1.1 (0.8–1.7)	
CASE-CONTROL STUDIES			
International Case-Control studies			
Swedish women—endometrial cancer and serum concentrations of chlorinated pesticides and PCB congeners	154	**Pesticides, PCB congeners** 1.0 (0.6–2.0)	Weiderpass et al., 2000

NOTE: 2,4-D, 2,4-dichlorophenoxyacetic acid; 2,4,5-T, 2,4,5-trichlorophenoxyacetic acid; 2,4,5-TCP, 2,4,5-trichlorophenol; CATI, computer-assisted telephone interviewing; CI, confidence interval; COI, chemical of interest; IARC, International Agency for Research on Cancer; ICD, International Classification of Diseases; MCPA, 2-methyl-4-chlorophenoxyacetic acid; MCPB, 4-(4-chloro-2-methylphenoxy)butanoic acid; NHL, non-Hodgkin lymphoma; nr, not reported; PCB, polychlorinated biphenyl; PCDD, polychlorinated dibenzo-*p*-dioxin (highly chlorinated, if four or more chlorines); PCMR, proportionate cancer mortality ratios; SIR, standardized incidence ratio; TCDD, 2,3,7,8-tetrachlorodibenzo-*p*-dioxin; VA, US Department of Veterans Affairs.

[a]Subjects are female and outcome is mortality unless otherwise noted.

[b]Given when available; results other than estimated risk explained individually.

Occupational Studies

Ruder and Yiin (2011) reported mortality in 1940–2005 in the NIOSH PCP cohort of 2,122 workers in the four US plants that had been involved in PCP production. They reported a single death, specified only as female genital cancer (ICD-9 179–184) in the 1,402 PCP production workers (including 67 women) who had not been exposed to TCDD (SMR = 0.90, 95% CI 0.02–5.03). That finding is not informative

Updated information from the AHS on incidence of and mortality from both uterine and ovarian cancers were presented by Koutros et al. (2010a) and Waggoner et al. (2011). Five incident cases of uterine cancer were reported in the applicators, most of whom were male, whereas the incidence in the predomi-

TABLE 8-26 Selected Epidemiologic Studies—Ovarian Cancer (Shaded Entries Are New Information for This Update)

Study Population[a]	Exposed Cases[b]	**Exposure of Interest**/Estimated Relative Risk (95% CI)[b]	Reference
VIETNAM VETERANS			
US Vietnam Veterans			
US VA Cohort of Female Vietnam Veterans			
Incidence		**All COIs**	
Female Vietnam veterans	16	1.8 (0.7–4.6)	Kang et al., 2000
International Vietnam-Veteran Studies			
Australian Vietnam Veterans—58,077 men and 153 women served on land or in Vietnamese waters during 5/23/1962–7/1/1973 vs Australian population		**All COIs**	
Incidence		*Expected number of exposed cases*	
Validation Study			
Self-reported uterine cancer	1	0 (0–4)	CDVA, 1998b
OCCUPATIONAL—INDUSTRIAL			
IARC Phenoxy Herbicide Cohort—Workers exposed to any phenoxy herbicide or chlorophenol (production or spraying) vs respective national mortality rates		**Dioxin, phenoxy herbicides**	
Mortality 1939–1992	1	0.3 (0.0–1.5)	Kogevinas et al., 1997
13,831 exposed to highly chlorinated PCDDs	0	0.0 (0.0–2.6)	
7,553 not exposed to highly chlorinated PCDDs	1	0.5 (0.0–2.5)	
Mortality, incidence of women in production (n = 699) and spraying (n = 2) compared to national death rates and cancer incidence rates	1	**TCDD** 0.7 (nr)	Kogevinas et al, 1993
New Zealand Phenoxy Herbicide Production Workers and Sprayers (1,599 men and women working any time in 1969–1988 at Dow plant in New Plymouth) (in IARC cohort)		**Dioxins; 2,4-D; 2,4,5-T; MCPA; MCPB; 2,4,5-TCP; Picloram**	McBride et al., 2009a
Mortality 1969–2004			
Ovarian cancer (ICD-10 C56)	0	0.0 (0.0–9.5)	
OCCUPATIONAL—HERBICIDE-USING WORKERS (not related to IARC sprayer cohorts)			
DENMARK			
Danish Farmers—incidence from linking farmers on 1970 census with national cancer registry (1970–1980)		**Herbicides**	Ronco et al., 1992
Self-employed	12	0.9 (nr)	
Employees	5	0.5 (nr)	
Family workers	104	0.8 ($p < 0.05$)	

TABLE 8-26 Ovarian Cancer, continued

Study Population[a]	Exposed Cases[b]	**Exposure of Interest**/Estimated Relative Risk (95% CI)[b]	Reference
UNITED STATES			
US Agricultural Health Study—prospective study of licensed pesticide sprayers in Iowa and North Carolina: commercial (n = 4,916), private/farmers (n = 52,395, 97.4% men), and spouses of private sprayers (n = 32,347, 0.007% men), enrolled 1993–1997; followups with CATIs 1999–2003 and 2005–2010			
Incidence			
Enrollment through 2006—SIRs for participants			Koutros et al., 2010a
Private applicators	9	2.5 (1.1–4.7)	
Commercial applicators	0	nr	
Spouses	58	0.7 (0.6–0.9)	
Enrollment through 2002			Alavanja et al., 2005
Private applicators (men, women)	8	3.0 (1.3–5.9)	
Spouses of private applicators (> 99% women)	32	0.6 (0.4–0.8)	
Commercial applicators (men, women)	0	0.0 (0.0–16.0)	
Mortality			
Enrollment through 2007, vs state rates			Waggoner et al., 2011
Applicators (n = 1,641)	5	1.6 (0.5–3.8)	
Spouses (n = 676)	45	0.7 (0.5–0.9)	
Enrollment through 2000, vs state rates			Blair et al., 2005a
Private applicators (men, women)	4	3.9 (1.1–10.1)	
Spouses of private applicators (> 99% women)	13	0.7 (0.4–1.2)	
ENVIRONMENTAL			
Seveso, Italy Residential Cohort—Industrial accident July 10, 1976 (723 residents Zone A; 4,821 Zone B; 31,643 Zone R; 181,574 local reference group) (ICD-9 171)		**TCDD**	
Incidence			
20-yr followup to 1996 (Uterus, ICD-9 179–182)			
Zone A	1	1.1 (0.2–7.9)	Pesatori et al., 2009
Zone B	1	0.2 (0.0–1.3)	
Zone R	45	1.1 (0.8–1.5)	
Mortality			
25-yr followup to 2001			
Zone A	1	1.2 (0.2–8.5)	Consonni et al., 2008
Zone B	2	0.4 (0.1–1.6)	
Zone R	37	1.0 (0.7–1.4)	

continued

TABLE 8-26 Ovarian Cancer, continued

Study Population[a]	Exposed Cases[b]	**Exposure of Interest**/Estimated Relative Risk (95% CI)[b]	Reference
20-yr followup to 1996			
Zone A, B	3	0.7 (0.2–2.0)	Bertazzi et al., 2001
15-yr followup to 1991			
Zone B	1	2.3 (0.3–16.5)	Bertazzi et al., 1997, 1998
Zone R	21	1.0 (0.6–1.6)	
CASE-CONTROL STUDIES			
International Case-Control studies			
Italian women—hospital-based study of women with primary mesothelial ovarian tumors (n = 60) and 127 subjects with non-ovarian malignancies	18	**Herbicides** 4.4 (1.9–16.1)	Donna et al., 1984

NOTE: 2,4-D, 2,4-dichlorophenoxyacetic acid; 2,4,5-T, 2,4,5-trichlorophenoxyacetic acid; CATI, computer-assisted telephone interviewing; CI, confidence interval; COI, chemical of interest; IARC, International Agency for Research on Cancer; ICD, International Classification of Diseases; MCPA, 2-methyl-4-chlorophenoxyacetic acid; MCPB, 4-(4-chloro-2-methylphenoxy)butanoic acid; nr, not reported; PCDD, polychlorinated dibenzo-*p*-dioxin (highly chlorinated, if four or more chlorines; SIR, standardized incidence ratio; TCDD, 2,3,7,8-tetrachlorodibenzo-*p*-dioxin; VA, US Department of Veterans Affairs.

[a]Subjects are female and outcome is mortality unless otherwise noted.

[b]Given when available; results other than estimated risk explained individually.

nantly female spouses did not differ from expectation (148 cases, SIR = 0.94, 95% CI 0.79–1.10) (Koutros et al., 2010a). Waggoner et al. (2011) did not find any change in mortality in the spouses from uterine cancer through 2007 (19 deaths, SMR = 0.70, 95% CI 0.42–1.09). Nine incident cases of ovarian cancer in the private applicators in the study by Koutros et al. (2010a) constituted a significant increase (SIR = 2.45, 95% CI 1.12–4.65), whereas 58 cases in spouses resulted in a decreased estimate of risk (SIR = 0.72, 95% CI 0.55–0.93). In the study by Waggoner et al. (2011), five deaths from ovarian cancer in the applicators did not suggest any difference from the general state populations (SMR = 1.61, 95% CI 0.54–3.76), and a deficit in observed ovarian cancer deaths in the spouses was reported (45 deaths, SMR = 0.70, 95% CI 0.51–0.94). The AHS has been generating valuable information on the COIs for a number of years, but these results are not herbicide-specific and so are not regarded as being fully informative for the committee's task.

Biologic Plausibility

Yoshizawa et al. (2009) have shown that chronic administration of TCDD and other AHR ligands to adult female Harlan Sprague-Dawley rats results in chronic inflammation and increases in reproductive-tissue tumors, including cystic endometrial hyperplasia and uterine squamous-cell carcinoma. The mechanism of action might be related to endocrine disruption and chronic inflammation. Hollingshead et al. (2008) showed that TCDD activation of the AHR in human breast and endocervical cell lines induces sustained high concentrations of the IL-6 cytokine. It is noteworthy that effects of TCDD treatment differed between MCF-7 breast-cancer cells and ECC-1 endometrial carcinoma cells with respect to activation and repression of genes; this shows the role of cell context and organ specificity in responses to TCDD with regard to cancer promotion (Labrecque et al., 2012).

The biologic plausibility of the carcinogenicity of the COIs is discussed in general at the beginning of this chapter.

Synthesis

New information on specific female reproductive cancers since *Update 2010* was limited to findings from the AHS, which were inconsistent and not specific for any of the COIs.

Conclusion

On the basis of the evidence reviewed here and in previous VAO reports, the committee concludes that there is inadequate or insufficient evidence to determine whether there is an association between exposure to the COIs and uterine, ovarian, or cervical cancer.

PROSTATE CANCER

ACS estimated that 241,740 new cases of prostate cancer (ICD-9 185) would be diagnosed in the United States in 2012 and that 28,170 men would die from it (Siegel et al., 2012). That makes prostate cancer the second-most common cancer in men (after nonmelanoma skin cancers); it is expected to account for about 29% of new cancer diagnoses and 9% of cancer deaths in men in 2012. The average annual incidence of prostate cancer is shown in Table 8-27.

The incidence of prostate cancer varies widely with age and race. The risk more than doubles from the ages of 50–54 years to the ages of 55–59 years, and it nearly doubles again from the ages of 55–59 years to the ages of 60–64 years. As a group, American black men have the highest recorded incidence of prostate cancer in the world (Miller et al., 1996); their risk is roughly twice that in whites

TABLE 8-27 Average Annual Incidence (per 100,000) of Prostate Cancer in the United States[a]

55–59 Years Old			60–64 Years Old			65–69 Years Old		
All Races	White	Black	All Races	White	Black	All Races	White	Black
347.6	329.6	611.7	609.1	585.6	1,026.5	892.0	865.22	1,416.7

[a]Surveillance, Epidemiology, and End Results program, nine standard registries, crude age-specific rates, 2005–2009 (NCI, 2013).

in the United States, 5 times that in Alaska natives, and nearly 8.5 times that in Korean Americans. Little is known about the causes of prostate cancer. Other than race and age, risk factors include a family history of the disease and possibly some elements of the Western diet, such as high consumption of animal fats. The drug finasteride, which has been widely used to treat benign enlargement of the prostate, was found to decrease the prevalence of prostate cancer substantially in a major randomized trial (Thompson et al., 2003). Finasteride acts by decreasing the formation of potent androgen hormones in the prostate.

The study of the incidence of and mortality from prostate cancer is complicated by trends in screening for the disease. The widespread adoption of serum prostate-specific antigen (PSA) screening in the 1990s led to very large increases in prostate-cancer incidence in the United States, which have recently subsided as exposure to screening has become saturated. The long-term influence of better screening on incidence and mortality in any country or population is difficult to predict and will depend on the rapidity with which the screening tool is adopted, its differential use in men of various ages, and the aggressiveness of tumors detected early with this test (Gann, 1997). Because exposure to PSA testing is such a strong determinant of prostate-cancer incidence, epidemiologic studies must be careful to exclude differential PSA testing as an explanation of a difference in risk observed between two populations.

Prostate cancer tends not to be fatal, so mortality studies might miss an increase in incidence of the disease. Findings that show an association between an exposure and prostate-cancer mortality should be examined closely to determine whether the exposed group might have had poorer access to treatment that would have increased the likelihood of survival.

Conclusions from *VAO* and Previous Updates

The committee responsible for *VAO* concluded that there was limited or suggestive evidence of an association between exposure to the COIs and prostate cancer. Additional information available to the committees responsible for

Update 1996, *Update 1998*, *Update 2000*, *Update 2002*, *Update 2004*, *Update 2006*, and *Update 2008* did not change that conclusion.

Eight studies that addressed whether exposure to the COIs is associated with prostate cancer were considered in *Update 2010*, and they were all effectively neutral, small sample size being the primary limitation. The only strong result that was in any way related to prostate cancer was the finding by Shah et al. (2009) that of 1,495 veterans who had undergone radical prostatectomy and were followed for 5 years, those who were exposed to Agent Orange had an increased risk of biochemical progression of 1.47 (95% CI 1.08–2.00). Accordingly, the committee for *Update 2010* agreed with the conclusion of its predecessors.

Table 8-28 summarizes results of the relevant studies, including both morbidity and mortality studies.

Update of the Epidemiologic Literature

Vietnam-Veteran and Environmental Studies

No Vietnam-veteran studies or environmental studies of exposure to the COIs and prostate cancer have been published since *Update 2010*.

Occupational Studies

Burns et al. (2011) updated cancer incidence through 2007 in workers who were alive on January 1, 1985, and had been employed at any time from 1945 to 1994 in 2,4-D production by the Dow Chemical Company in Midland, Michigan. They found no evidence of significantly increased rates of cancer overall. With 51 cases observed, the incidence of prostate cancer in the most restrictively defined cohort was not increased (SIR = 0.76, 95% CI 0.57–1.00), as was the case in the two successively more inclusive, but potentially more biased, cohorts.

Boers et al. (2012) provided a quantified, TCDD-based analysis of the mortality, updated through 2006, in male workers in two Dutch phenoxy-herbicide factories, which were considered in *Update 2010* (Boers et al., 2010). The 1,020 workers in factory A had been involved in production of 2,4,5-T with its associated TCDD contamination, whereas the 1,036 working in factory B had produced only phenoxy herbicides that would not have had TCDD contamination. Contemporary TCDD concentrations measured in a subsample of 187 workers were used to derive a model incorporating job history to estimate serum TCDD concentrations of all the men at the end of their employment. Using the estimated TCDD concentrations of the workers in both factories did not provide evidence of an increased risk of prostate-cancer death associated with TCDD (HR = 1.08, 95% CI 0.79–1.49). The dose–response modeling applied only to the workers in factory A also did not find a significantly increased risk of prostate-cancer death (HR

TABLE 8-28 Selected Epidemiologic Studies—Prostate Cancer (Shaded Entries Are New Information for This Update)

Study Population[a]	Exposed Cases[b]	**Exposure of Interest**/Estimated Relative Risk (95% CI)[b]	Reference
VIETNAM VETERANS			
US Vietnam Veterans			
US Air Force Health Study—Ranch Hand veterans vs SEA veterans (unless otherwise noted)		**All COIs**	
Incidence			
2,516 veterans (1,019 Ranch Hand, 1,497 SEA veterans) who participated in ≥ 1 physical examination and had recorded serum TCDD measurements			Pavuk et al., 2006
20-yr cumulative TCDD (ppt-yr)			
Comparison group	81	1.0	
Ranch Hand low (≤ 434 ppt-yr)	31	1.0 (0.7–1.6)	
Ranch Hand high (> 434 ppt-yr)	28	1.2 (0.8–1.9)	
		p-trend = 0.42	
Last tour in SEA before 1969 (heavy spraying)			
Yes			
Comparison group	17	1.0	
Ranch Hand low (≤ 434 ppt-yr)	9	1.0 (0.4–2.3)	
Ranch Hand high (> 434 ppt-yr)	15	2.3 (1.1–4.7)	
		p-trend = 0.04	
No			
Comparison group	64	1.0	
Ranch Hand low (≤ 434 ppt-yr)	22	1.1 (0.7–1.8)	
Ranch Hand high (> 434 ppt-yr)	13	0.9 (0.5–1.6)	
		p-trend = 0.75	
Less than 2 yrs served in SEA			
Yes			
Comparison group	16	1.0	
Ranch Hand low (≤ 434 ppt-yr)	20	1.9 (1.0–3.7)	
Ranch Hand high (> 434 ppt-yr)	14	2.2 (1.0–4.5)	
		p-trend = 0.03	
No			
Comparison group	65	1.0	
Ranch Hand low (≤ 434 ppt-yr)	11	0.8 (0.4–1.5)	
Ranch Hand high (> 434 ppt-yr)	14	1.1 (0.6–1.9)	
		p-trend = 0.89	
1982–2003—White SEA comparison veterans only (n = 1,482). Serum TCDD (pg/g) based on model with exposure variable $\log_e$(TCDD)			Pavuk et al., 2005
Per unit increase of $-\log_e$(TCDD) (pg/g)	83	1.1 (0.7–1.5)	
Quartiles (pg/g):			
0.4–2.6	13	1.0	
2.6–3.8	24	1.7 (0.8–3.3)	

TABLE 8-28 Prostate Cancer, continued

Study Population[a]	Exposed Cases[b]	**Exposure of Interest**/Estimated Relative Risk (95% CI)[b]	Reference
3.8–5.2	24	1.5 (0.7–2.9)	
> 5.2	22	1.2 (0.6–2.4)	
Number of years served in SEA (per year of service)	83	1.1 (1.0–1.2)	
Quartiles (years in SEA):			
0.8–1.3	8	1.0	
1.3–2.1	11	1.3 (0.5–3.2)	
2.1–3.7	28	2.2 (1.0–4.9)	
3.7–16.4	36	2.4 (1.1–5.2)	
Through 1999—White subjects vs national rates			Akhtar et al., 2004
Ranch Hand veterans (n = 1,189)	36	1.5 (1.0–2.0)	
With tours between 1966–1970	34	1.7 (1.2–2.3)	
SEA comparison veterans (n = 1,776)	54	1.6 (1.2–2.1)	
With tours between 1966–1970	42	1.6 (1.2–2.2)	
White AFHS subjects who spent at most 2 yrs in SEA			
Per unit increase of $-\log_e$(TCDD)	28	1.5 (0.9–2.4)	
Comparison group	7	1.0	
Ranch Hand— < 10 TCDD pg/g in 1987	10	1.5 (0.5–4.4)	
Ranch Hand— < 118.5 TCDD pg/g at end of service	6	2.2 (0.7–6.9)	
Ranch Hand— > 118.5 TCDD pg/g at end of service	5	6.0 (0.4–24.6)	
Only Ranch Hands with 100% service in Vietnam and comparisons with no service in Vietnam			
Per unit increase of $-\log_e$(TCDD)	20	1.1 (0.6–1.8)	
Comparison group	3	1.0	
Ranch Hand— < 10 TCDD pg/g in 1987	9	2.5 (0.4–16.1)	
Ranch Hand— < 118.5 TCDD pg/g at end of service	4	2.4 (0.4–16.0)	
Ranch Hand— > 118.5 TCDD pg/g at end of service	4	4.7 (0.8–29.1)	
Mortality			
Through 1999—White subjects vs national rates			Akhtar et al., 2004
Ranch Hand veterans (n = 1,189)	2	0.7 (0.1–2.3)	
SEA comparison veterans (n = 1,776)	3	0.8 (0.2–2.1)	
US VA Cohort of Army Chemical Corps—Expanded as of 1997 to include all Army men with chemical MOS (2,872 deployed vs 2,737 nondeployed) serving during Vietnam era (July 1, 1965–March 28, 1973)		**All COIs**	

continued

TABLE 8-28 Prostate Cancer, continued

Study Population[a]	Exposed Cases[b]	**Exposure of Interest**/Estimated Relative Risk (95% CI)[b]	Reference
Mortality—Prostate cancers			
Through 2005			Cypel and Kang, 2010
Deployed veterans (2,872) vs nondeployed (2,737)	5 vs 2	1.0 (0.2–5.6)	
ACC veterans vs US men			
Vietnam cohort	5	1.1 (0.3–2.5)	
Non-Vietnam cohort	2	1.0 (0.1–3.4)	
US CDC Vietnam Experience Study—Cross-sectional study, with medical examinations, of Army veterans: 9,324 deployed vs 8,989 nondeployed		**All COIs**	
Mortality			
1965–2000	1	0.4 (nr)	Boehmer et al., 2004
US VA Proportionate Mortality Study—sample of deceased male Vietnam-era Army and Marine veterans who served 7/4/1965–3/1/1973		**All COIs**	
1965–1988			Watanabe and Kang, 1996
Army, deployed (n = 27,596) vs nondeployed (n = 31,757)	58	0.9 (nr)	
Marine Corps, deployed (n = 6,237) vs nondeployed (n = 5,040)	9	0.8 (nr)	
1965–1982			Breslin et al.,1986, 1988
Army, deployed (n = 19,708) vs nondeployed (n = 22,904)	30	0.9 (0.6–1.2)	
Marine Corps, deployed (n = 4,527) vs nondeployed (n = 3,781)	5	1.3 (0.2–10.3)	
State Studies of US Vietnam Veterans			
Veterans with radical prostatectomies examined in VA Healthcare facilities (California, Georgia, North Carolina)			Shah et al., 2009
AO-exposed veterans with biochemical progression	nr	1.5 (1.1–2.0)	
Northern California—prostate cancer (self-reported [before diagnosis] of AO expo vs not)	239	2.9 (2.3–3.6)	Chamie et al., 2008
Massachusetts veterans aged 35–65 years in 1993—prostate cases diagnosed 1988–1993 vs gastrointestinal cancers	15	0.8 (0.4–1.6)	Clapp, 1997
Michigan Vietnam veterans using the VA Medical Center in Ann Arbor, Michigan (n = 47); 142 frequency-matched controls			Giri et al., 2004
Cases reporting AO exposure	11	OR 2.1 (0.8–5.2)	
Cases in white veterans reporting AO exposure	nr	OR 2.7 (0.9–8.2)	

TABLE 8-28 Prostate Cancer, continued

Study Population[a]	Exposed Cases[b]	**Exposure of Interest**/Estimated Relative Risk (95% CI)[b]	Reference
Michigan Vietnam-era veterans, PM study of deaths (1974–1989)—deployed vs nondeployed			Visintainer et al., 1995
Male genital system	19	1.1 (0.6–1.7)	Clapp, 1997
923 White male Vietnam veterans with **Wisconsin** death certificate (1968–1978) vs proportions for Vietnam-era veterans	0	nr	Anderson et al., 1986a,b
International Vietnam-Veteran Studies			
Australian Vietnam Veterans—58,077 men and 153 women served on land or in Vietnamese waters during 5/23/1962–7/1/1973 vs Australian population		**All COIs**	
Incidence			
All branches, 1982–2000	692	1.3 (1.2–1.3)	ADVA, 2005a
Navy	137	1.2 (1.0–1.4)	
Army	451	1.8 (1.2–1.4)	
Air Force	104	1.3 (1.0–1.5)	
Validation Study		*Expected number of exposed cases*	AIHW, 1999
	212	147 (123–171)	
Men	428	147 (123–171)	CDVA, 1998a
Mortality			
All branches, return–2001	107	1.2 (1.0–1.5)	ADVA, 2005b
Navy	22	1.3 (0.8–1.8)	
Army	65	1.2 (0.9–1.5)	
Air Force	19	1.4 (0.8–2.1)	
Sample of 1,000 Male Australian Vietnam Veterans—prevalence		**All COIs**	
450 interviewed 2005–2006 vs respondents to 2004–2005 national survey	nr	1.3 (0.3–6.7)	O'Toole et al., 2009
Australian Conscripted Army National Service (18,940 deployed vs 24,642 nondeployed)		**All COIs**	
Incidence			
1982–2000	65	1.2 (0.9–1.5)	ADVA, 2005c
Mortality			
1966–2001	0	0.0 (0.0–0.7)	ADVA, 2005c
1982–1994	36	1.5 (1.0–2.0)	CDVA, 1997b
Other Australian Vietnam veterans		**All COIs**	
606 prostate cancer cases in Western Australia			Leavy et al., 2006
Vietnam service	25	2.1 (0.9–5.1)	

continued

TABLE 8-28 Prostate Cancer, continued

Study Population[a]	Exposed Cases[b]	**Exposure of Interest**/Estimated Relative Risk (95% CI)[b]	Reference
OCCUPATIONAL—INDUSTRIAL			
IARC Phenoxy Herbicide Cohort—Workers exposed to any phenoxy herbicide or chlorophenol (production or spraying) vs respective national mortality rates			
Mortality 1939–1992	68	1.1 (0.9–1.4)	Kogevinas et al., 1997
13,831 exposed to highly chlorinated PCDDs	43	1.1 (0.8–1.5)	
7,553 not exposed to highly chlorinated PCDDs	25	1.1 (0.7–1.6)	
Mortality 1955–1988 of 12,492 production workers and 5,898 sprayers exposed—13,482 in exposed subcohort	30	1.1 (0.8–1.6)	Saracci et al., 1991
British MCPA Plant—production 1947–1982 (n = 1,545) (included in IARC cohort) and spraying 1947–1972 (n = 2,561) (*not* included in IARC cohort)		**MCPA**	
Mortality through 1983	18	1.3 (0.8–2.1)	Coggon et al., 1986
Danish Production Workers (3,390 men and 1,069 women involved in production of phenoxy herbicides unlikely to contain TCDD at 2 plants in 1947–1987) (in IARC cohort)		**Dioxins, but TCDD unlikely; 2,4-D, 2,4-DP, MCPA, MCPP**	
Mortality 1955–2006	14	1.1 (0.8–1.5)	Boers et al., 2012
Incidence 1943–1982	9	0.8 (nr)	Lynge, 1985
Dutch production workers in Plant A (549 men exposed during production 1955–1985; 594 unexposed) (in IARC cohort)		**Dioxins, 2,4,5-T, 2,4,5-TCP**	
Mortality 1955–2006 (hazard ratios for lagged TCDD plasma levels)	8	1.3 (0.9–1.9)	Boers et al., 2012
Mortality 1955–2006	6 vs 2	2.9 (0.6–14.2)	Boers et al., 2010
Mortality 1955–1985	2	2.2 (0.3–7.8)	Bueno de Mesquita et al., 1993
Dutch production workers in Plant B (414 men exposed during production 1965–1986; 723 unexposed) (in IARC cohort)		**2,4-D; MCPA; MCPP; highly chlorinated dioxins unlikely**	
Mortality 1965–2006	4 vs 2	2.7 (0.5–14.9)	Boers et al., 2010
Mortality 1965–1986	1	4.8 (0.1–26.5)	Bueno de Mesquita et al., 1993

TABLE 8-28 Prostate Cancer, continued

Study Population[a]	Exposed Cases[b]	**Exposure of Interest**/Estimated Relative Risk (95% CI)[b]	Reference
German Production Workers at Bayer Plant in Uerdingen (135 men working > 1 month in 1951–1976) (in IARC cohort as of 1997) and women—no results		**Dioxins; 2,4,5-TCP**	
Mortality 1951–1992	1	1.5 (0.0–8.5)	Becher et al., 1996
German Production Workers at Bayer Plant in Dormagen (520 men working > 1 month in 1965–1989) (in IARC cohort as of 1997) and women—no results		**Dioxins; 2,4-D; 2,4,5-T; MCPA; MCPP; 2,4-DP**	
Mortality 1965–1989	0	—	Becher et al., 1996
German Production Workers at BASF Ludwigshafen Plant (680 men working > 1 month in 1957–1987) (in IARC cohort as of 1997) and women—no results		**Dioxins; 2,4-D; 2,4,5-T; MCPA; MCPP; 2,4-DP**	
Mortality 1956–1989	1	0.7 (0.0–3.7)	Becher et al., 1996
BASF Cleanup Workers from 1953 accident (n = 247); 114 with chloracne, 13 more with erythema; serum TCDD levels (*not* part of IARC)		**Focus on TCDD**	
Incidence			
1960–1992			Ott and Zober, 1996
TCDD < 0.1 μg/kg of body weight	3	2.5 (0.5–7.4)	
TCDD 0.1–0.99 μg/kg of body weight	1	1.1 (0.0–5.9)	
TCDD > 1 μg/kg of body weight	0	0.0 (0.0–2.5)	
Mortality			
1953–1992			Ott and Zober, 1996
TCDD < 0.1 μg/kg of body weight	0	0.0 (0.0–5.7)	
TCDD 0.1–0.99 μg/kg of body weight	0	0.0 (0.0–7.5)	
TCDD > 1 μg/kg of body weight	0	0.0 (0.0–4.6))	
Through 1987		*90% CI*	Zober et al., 1990
	0	0.0 (0.0–6.1)	
German Production Workers at Boehringer–Ingelheim Plant in Hamburg (1,144 men working > 1 month in 1952–1984; generation of TCDD reduced after chloracne outbreak in 1954) and women—no results (some additions to observed cancers over Manz et al., 1991) (in IARC cohort as of 1997)		**Dioxins; 2,4,5-T; 2,5-DCP; 2,4,5-TCP**	
Mortality 1952–2007	19	1.4 (0.8–2.1)	Manuwald et al., 2012

continued

TABLE 8-28 Prostate Cancer, continued

Study Population[a]	Exposed Cases[b]	**Exposure of Interest**/Estimated Relative Risk (95% CI)[b]	Reference
Mortality 1952–1989	7	1.5 (0.6–3.0)	Becher et al., 1996
Mortality 1952–1989—stats on men only, 1,184 (tables all for 1,148 men, not necessarily German nationals) vs national rates (also vs gas workers); same observation period as Becher et al., 1966	7	1.4 (0.6–2.9)	Manz et al., 1991
New Zealand Phenoxy Herbicide Production Workers and Sprayers (1,599 men and women working any time in 1969–1988 at Dow plant in New Plymouth) (in IARC cohort)		**Dioxins; 2,4-D; 2,4,5-T; MCPA; MCPB; 2,4,5-TCP; Picloram**	
Mortality 1969–2004			McBride et al., 2009a
Ever-exposed workers	1	0.2 (0.0–1.2)	
Never-exposed workers	2	1.9 (0.2–6.7)	
Production Workers (713 men and 100 women worked > 1 month in 1969–1984)			
Mortality 1969–2000	1	0.4 (0.0–2.1)	't Mannetje et al., 2005
Sprayers (697 men and 2 women on register of New Zealand applicators, 1973–1984)			
Mortality 1973–2000	2	0.6 (0.1–2.2)	't Mannetje et al., 2005
NIOSH Mortality Cohort (12 US plants, 5,172 male production and maintenance workers 1942–1984) (included in IARC cohort as of 1997)		**Dioxins, phenoxy herbicides**	
Through 1993	28	1.2 (0.8–1.7)	Steenland et al., 1999
Through 1987	17	1.2 (0.7–2.0)	Fingerhut et al., 1991
≥ 1-year exposure, ≥ 20-year latency	9	1.5 (0.7–2.9)	
Mortality—754 Monsanto workers, among most highly exposed workers from Fingerhut et al. (1991)	9	1.6 (0.7–3.0)	Collins et al., 1993
All Dow TCP-Exposed Workers (TCP production 1942–1979 or 2,4,5-T production 1948–1982 in Midland, Michigan) (in IARC and NIOSH cohorts)		**2,4,5-T; 2,4,5-TCP**	
1942–2003 (n = 1,615)	21	1.4 (0.9–2.2)	Collins et al., 2009a
1940–1994 (n = 2,187 men)	nr	1.7 (1.0–2.6)	Bodner et al., 2003

TABLE 8-28 Prostate Cancer, continued

Study Population[a]	Exposed Cases[b]	**Exposure of Interest**/Estimated Relative Risk (95% CI)[b]	Reference
All Dow PCP-Exposed Workers—all workers from the two plants that only made PCP (in Tacoma, Washington, and Wichita, Kansas) and workers who made PCP and TCP at two additional plants (in Midland, Michigan, and Sauget, Illinois)		**2,4,5-T; 2,4,5-TCP**	Ruder and Yiin, 2011
1940–2005 (n = 2,122)	26	1.0 (0.7–1.5)	
PCP and TCP (n = 720)	8	1.1 (0.5–2.1)	
PCP (no TCP) (n = 1,402)	18	1.0 (0.6–1.6)	
Dow 2,4-D Production Workers (1945–1982 in Midland, Michigan) (subset of all TCP-exposed workers)		**2,4-D, lower chlorinated dioxins**	
Cancer incidence through 2007 in Dow workers (n = 1,256) vs comparisons from state cancer registries (n = 23,354) (Cohort 3)	51	0.8 (0.6–1.0)	Burns et al., 2011
Through 1994 (n = 1,517)	7	1.3 (0.5–2.8)	Burns et al., 2001
Through 1982 (n = 878)	1	1.0 (0.0–5.8)	Bond et al., 1988
Dow PCP Production Workers (1937–1989 in Midland, Michigan) (*not* in IARC and NIOSH cohorts)		**Low chlorinated dioxins, 2,4-D**	
Mortality 1940–2004 (n = 577, excluding 196 also having exposure to TCP)	8	1.0 (0.4–1.9)	Collins et al., 2009b
OCCUPATIONAL—PAPER AND PULP WORKERS		**TCDD**	
IARC cohort of pulp and paper workers—60,468 workers from 11 countries, TCDD among 27 agents assessed by JEM			McLean et al., 2006
Exposure to nonvolatile organochlorine compounds			
Never	117	0.9 (0.7–1.0)	
Ever	84	0.9 (0.7–1.2)	
New Hampshire pulp and paper workers, 883 white men working ≥ 1 yr, mortality through July 1985	9	1.0 (0.5–1.9)	Henneberger et al., 1989
United Paperworkers International, 201 white men employed ≥ 10 yrs and dying 1970–1984	4	1.1 (0.3–2.9)	Solet et al., 1989
Northwestern US paper and pulp workers—5 mills in Washington, Oregon, and California, 3,523 worked ≥ 1 yr 1945–1955, mortality through March 1977	17	*90% CI* 1.2 (0.7–1.7)	Robinson et al., 1986

continued

TABLE 8-28 Prostate Cancer, continued

Study Population[a]	Exposed Cases[b]	**Exposure of Interest**/Estimated Relative Risk (95% CI)[b]	Reference
OCCUPATIONAL—HERBICIDE-USING WORKERS (not related to IARC sprayer cohorts)			
CANADA			
Canadian Farm Operator Study—156,242 men farming in Manitoba, Saskatchewan, and Alberta in 1971; mortality from prostate cancer June 1971–December 1987		**Herbicides**	Morrison et al., 1993
Herbicides sprayed on ≥ 250 acres vs 0 acres	20	2.2 (1.3–3.8)	
Sawmill Workers in British Columbia—23,829 workers for ≥ 1 year at 11 mills using chlorophenates 1940–1985		**Chlorophenates, not TCDD**	
Incidence 1969–1989	282	1.0 (0.9–1.1)	Hertzman
Mortality 1950–1989	116	1.2 (1.0–1.4)	et al., 1997
DENMARK			
Danish Farmers—incidence from linking farmers on 1970 census with national cancer registry (1970–1980)		**Herbicides**	Ronco et al., 1992
Men			
Self-employed	399	0.9 ($p < 0.05$)	
Employee	63	0.8 ($p < 0.05$)	
Danish gardeners—incidence from 3,156 male and 859 female gardeners			Hansen et al., 2007
25-year followup (1975–2001)		**Herbicides**	
Born before 1915 (high exposure)	39	1.3 (1.0–1.8)	
Born 1915–1934 (medium exposure)	35	0.9 (0.6–1.2)	
Born after 1934 (low exposure)	3	0.4 (0.1–1.3)	
10-year followup (1975–1984) of male gardeners	20	1.2 (0.7–1.8)	Hansen et al., 1992
FINNISH Phenoxy Herbicide Sprayers (1,909 men working 1955–1971 ≥ 2 wks) *not* IARC		**Phenoxy herbicides**	
Incidence	6	0.4 (0.1–0.8)	Asp et al.,
Mortality 1972–1989	5	0.8 (0.3–1.8)	1994
ICELAND			
Icelandic men (1,860), women (859) exposed to agricultural pesticides, primarily 2,4-D (other endocrine organs, ICD-9 194)—incidence	10	**2,4-D** 0.7 (0.3–1.3)	Zhong and Rafnsson, 1996
ITALIAN Licensed Pesticide Users—male farmers in southern Piedmont licensed 1970–1974			
Mortality 1970–1986 (n = 23,401)	66	1.0 (0.7–1.2)	Torchio et al., 1994
Italian rice growers with documented phenoxy use (n = 1,487)		**Phenoxy herbicides**	Gambini et al., 1997
	19	1.0 (0.6–1.5)	

TABLE 8-28 Prostate Cancer, continued

Study Population[a]	Exposed Cases[b]	**Exposure of Interest**/Estimated Relative Risk (95% CI)[b]	Reference
NEW ZEALAND National Cancer Registry (1980–1984)—case-control study of incident prostate cancer cases vs remainder of 19,904 men with any incident cancer		**Herbicides**	Reif et al., 1989
Forestry workers (n = 134)	12	0.7 (0.4–1.3)	
SWEDEN			
Swedish Cancer-Environment Registry—National cancer registry linked to census		**Herbicides**	Sharma-Wagner et al., 2000
36,269 incident prostate cancer cases 1961–1979 with 1960 census occupation of:			
Agriculture, stock raising	6,080	1.1 (1.0–1.1) ($p < 0.01$)	
Farmers, foresters, gardeners	5,219	1.1 (1.0–1.1) ($p < 0.01$)	
Paper-mill workers	304	0.9 (0.8–1.0)	
Pulp grinding	39	1.4 (1.0–1.9) ($p < 0.05$)	
Incident prostate cancer cases 1961–1973 with agriculture as economic activity in 1960 census	3,890	*99% CI* 1.0 (0.9–1.0)	Wiklund, 1983
Licensed Swedish Pesticide Sprayers—Incidence of prostate cancer		**Phenoxy herbicides**	Dich and Wiklund, 1998
	401	1.1 (1.0–1.2)	
Born 1935 or later	7	2.0 (0.8–4.2)	
Born before 1935	394	1.1 (1.0–1.2)	
Swedish lumberjacks—used phenoxys 1954–1967, Incidence 1958–1992			Thörn et al., 2000
Exposed (n = 154)			
Foremen (n = 15)	2	4.7 (nr)	
Lumberjacks (n = 139)	3	0.9 (nr)	
THE NETHERLANDS			
Dutch Licensed Herbicide Sprayers—1,341 certified before 1980			
Through 2000	6	1.0 (0.4–2.2)	Swaen et al., 2004
Through 1987	1	1.3 (0.0–7.3)	Swaen et al., 1992
UNITED STATES			
US farmers—usual occupation of farmer and industry of agriculture on death certificates 1984–1988 from 23 states		**Herbicides** PCMRs	Blair et al., 1993
Men			
Whites (n = 119,648)	3,765	1.2 (1.1–1.2)	
Nonwhites (n = 11,446)	564	1.1 (1.1–1.2)	

continued

TABLE 8-28 Prostate Cancer, continued

Study Population[a]	Exposed Cases[b]	**Exposure of Interest**/Estimated Relative Risk (95% CI)[b]	Reference
US Agricultural Health Study—prospective study of licensed pesticide sprayers in Iowa and North Carolina: commercial (n = 4,916), private/farmers (n = 52,395, 97.4% men), and spouses of private sprayers (n = 32,347, 0.007% men), enrolled 1993–1997; followups with CATIs 1999–2003 and 2005–2010		**Phenoxy herbicides**	
Incidence			
Enrollment through 2006—SIRs for participants			Koutros et al., 2010a
Private applicators	1,719	1.2 (1.1–1.3)	
Commercial applicators	73	1.3 (1.0–1.6)	
Spouses	7	1.1 (0.4–2.2)	
Enrollment through 2002			Samanic et al., 2006
Dicamba—lifetime days exposure			
None	343	1.0	
1– < 20	106	1.0 (0.8–1.3)	
20– < 56	102	0.9 (0.7–1.2)	
56– < 116	76	1.0 (0.7–1.3)	
≥ 116	67	1.1 (0.8–1.5)	
		p-trend 0.45	
Enrollment through 2002			Alavanja et al., 2005
Private applicators	1,046	1.3 (1.2–1.3)	
Spouses of private applicators (> 99% women)	5	1.2 (0.4–2.8)	
Commercial applicators	41	1.4 (1.0–1.9)	
Enrollment through 1999 (n = 55,332)	566	1.1 (1.1–1.2)	Alavanja et al., 2003
Mortality			
Enrollment through 2007, vs state rates			Waggoner et al., 2011
Applicators (n = 1,641)	171	0.8 (0.7–1.0)	
Enrollment through 2000, vs state rates			Blair et al., 2005a
Private applicators (men and women)	48	0.7 (0.5–0.8)	
Spouses of private applicators (> 99% women)	0	0.0 (0.0–1.6)	
US Department of Agriculture Workers—nested case-control study of white men dying 1970–1979 of prostate cancer		**Herbicides**	
Agricultural extension agents	nr	1.0 (0.7–1.5)	Alavanja et al., 1988
Forest conservationists		p-trend < over years worked	Alavanja et al., 1989
	nr	p < 0.05	
Soil conservationists	nr	P < 0.26	

TABLE 8-28 Prostate Cancer, continued

Study Population[a]	Exposed Cases[b]	**Exposure of Interest**/Estimated Relative Risk (95% CI)[b]	Reference
Florida Licensed Pesticide Applicators (common phenoxy use assumed but not documented; had been listed by Blair et al., 1983)		**Herbicides**	
30,155 white men licensed 1975–1993			
Incidence 1975–1993	353	1.9 (1.7–2.1)	Fleming et al., 1999a
Mortality 1975–1993	64	2.4 (1.8–3.0)	Fleming et al., 1999b
Pesticide applicators in Florida licensed 1965–1966 (n = 3,827)—mortality through 1976		**Herbicides**	Blair et al., 1983
Any pesticide (dose-response by length of licensure)		*Expected number of exposed cases*	
	2	3.8 (nr)	
> 30 yrs old when died 1964–1978—case-control	4,827	1.2 ($p < 0.05$)	Burmeister et al., 1983
H_0: only for "modern methods" → born after 1900			
Born before 1880	1,539	1.5 (nr)	
Born 1980–1900	2,081	1.3 (nr)	
Born after 1900	1,207	0.8 (nr)	
> 20 yrs old when died 1971–1978—PMR	1,138	1.1 ($p < 0.01$)	Burmeister, 1981
ENVIRONMENTAL			
Seveso, Italy Residential Cohort—Industrial accident July 10, 1976 (723 residents Zone A; 4,821 Zone B; 31,643 Zone R; 181,574 local reference group) (ICD-9 171)		**TCDD**	
Incidence			
20-yr followup to 1996—men and women			
Zone A	0		Pesatori et al., 2009
Zone B	7	0.9 (0.5–2.0)	
Zone R	39	0.8 (0.5–1.1)	
10-yr followup to 1991—men			Bertazzi et al., 1993
Zone R	16	0.9 (0.5–1.5)	
Mortality			
25-yr followup to 2001—men and women			Consonni et al., 2008
Zone A	1	0.9 (0.1–6.2)	
Zone B	8	0.9 (0.4–1.8)	
Zone R	65	1.1 (0.8–1.4)	
20-yr followup to 1996			Bertazzi et al., 2001
Zones A, B—men	8	1.1 (0.5–2.2)	
15-yr followup to 1991—men			Bertazzi et al., 1997
Zone B	6	1.2 (0.5–2.7)	
Zone R	39	1.2 (0.8–1.6)	

continued

TABLE 8-28 Prostate Cancer, continued

Study Population[a]	Exposed Cases[b]	**Exposure of Interest**/Estimated Relative Risk (95% CI)[b]	Reference
10-yr followup to 1986—men			Bertazzi et al., 1989b
Zone B	3	2.2 (0.7–6.9)	
Zone R	16	1.6 (0.9–2.7)	
Other International Environmental Studies			
FINLAND			
Finnish fishermen (n = 6,410) and spouses (n = 4,260) registered between 1980 and 2002 compared to national statistics		**Serum dioxin**	Turunen et al., 2008
Fishermen	36	1.0 (0.7–1.4)	
Spouses	—	—	
SWEDEN			
Swedish fishermen (high consumption of fish with persistent organochlorines)		**Organochlorine compounds**	Svensson et al., 1995
Incidence			
East coast	38	1.1 (0.8–1.5)	
West coast	224	1.0 (0.9–1.1)	
Mortality			
East coast	12	1.0 (0.5–1.8)	
West coast	123	1.1 (0.9–1.3)	
CASE-CONTROL STUDIES			
CANADA—1,516 prostate cancer patients identified in the British Columbia Cancer Registry vs 4,994 matched controls; estimated lifetime exposure to:		**Pesticides**	Band et al., 2011
2,4-D	11	2.7 (1.1–6.6)	
2,4-DB	24	1.8 (1.0–3.0)	
MCPA	14	1.8 (1.0–3.2)	
Dicamba	22	2.0 (1.0–4.2)	

NOTE: 2,4-D, 2,4-dichlorophenoxyacetic acid; 2,4-DB, 4-(2,4-dichlorophenoxy)butyric acid; 2,4-DP, dichlorprop; 2,4,5-T, 2,4,5-trichlorophenoxyacetic acid; 2,4,5-TCP, 2,4,5-trichlorophenol; 2,5-DCP, 2,5-dichlorophenol; ACC, Army Chemical Corps; AFHS, Air Force Health Study; AO, Agent Orange; CATI, computer-assisted telephone interviewing; CDC, Centers for Disease Control and Prevention; CI, confidence interval; COI, chemical of interest; IARC, International Agency for Research on Cancer; ICD, International Classification of Diseases; JEM, job-exposure matrix; MCPA, 2-methyl-4-chlorophenoxyacetic acid; MCPB, 4-(4-chloro-2-methylphenoxy)butanoic acid; MCPP, methyl-chlorophenoxypropionic acid; MOS, military occupation specialty; NIOSH, National Institute for Occupational Safety and Health; nr, not reported; PCDD, polychlorinated dibenzo-*p*-dioxin (highly chlorinated, if four or more chlorines); PCMR, proportionate cancer mortality ratios; PCP, pentachlorophenol; PM, proportionate mortality; PMR, proportionate mortality ratio; SEA, Southeast Asia; SIR, standardized incidence ratio; TCDD, 2,3,7,8-tetrachlorodibenzo-*p*-dioxin; TCP, trichlorophenol; VA, US Department of Veterans Affairs.

[a]Subjects are male and outcome is mortality unless otherwise noted.

[b]Given when available; results other than estimated risk explained individually.

[c]Statistically significant with the 95% CI not including 1.0.

= 1.29, 95% CI 0.85–1.94), and the estimate of risk from the qualitative exposure analysis in Boers et al. (2010) was imprecise (HR = 1.93, 95% CI 0.61–14.15).

Manuwald et al. (2012) reported on mortality through 2007 in 1,191 men in the Hamburg cohort (a subcohort of the IARC phenoxy-herbicide cohort). They had been employed for at least 3 months during 1952–1984 in a chemical plant producing insecticides and herbicides, including 2,4,5-T, so they had the possibility of exposure to TCDD. SMRs showed that mortality from prostate cancer was not higher than that in the population of Hamburg (SMR = 1.37, 95% CI 0.82–2.13).

Ruder and Yinn (2011) reported mortality from 1940–2005 for the NIOSH PCP cohort of 2,053 male workers from the four US plants that had been involved in PCP production. PCP production entailed exposure to PCDDs and PCDFs but not to the most toxic 2,3,7,8 dioxin congener. A subcohort of 720 workers (all men, the PCP-plus-TCDD group) had also been employed in TCP production and so had also been exposed to TCDD. In the total cohort, 26 deaths were attributed to prostate cancer; this was consistent with mortality in the US population (SMR = 1.03, 95% CI 0.67–1.51). There were eight deaths from this type of cancer in the PCP-plus-TCDD group, which also was as expected (SMR = 1.08, 95% CI 0.47–2.12). The results were comparable in the 1,333 men in the PCP-only group (SMR = 1.01, 95% CI 0.60–1.60).

In the update of cancer incidence in the AHS through 2006, Koutros et al. (2010a) found significant increases in the incidence of prostate cancer in both the private (1,719 cases, SIR = 1.19, 95% CI 1.14–1.25) and the commercial applicators (73 cases, SIR = 1.28, 95% CI 1.00–1.61); the seven cases of prostate cancer reported in the spouses (most of whom were female) did not represent any deviation from expectation (7 cases, SIR = 1.05, 95% CI 0.42–2.15). Waggoner et al. (2011) found that mortality from prostate cancer in the applicators was lower than predicted on the basis of the state rates (171 deaths, SMR = 0.81, 95% CI 0.70–0.95). The AHS has been generating valuable information on the COIs for a number of years, but these results are not herbicide-specific and so are not regarded as being fully informative for the committee's task.

Case-Control Studies

Band et al. (2011) identified all cases of cancer entered into the British Columbia Cancer Registry in 1983–1990. In a case-control study, the 1,516 cases of prostate cancer identified and enrolled in the study (% participation rate) were matched by age to 4,944 men who had other cancers (excluding those of the lung and unknown primary site). All cases were histologically confirmed. Participants completed a questionnaire that requested a complete job history, alcohol and smoking behaviors, and other demographic information. A job–exposure matrix derived for the province's agricultural industry in eight regions for the period 1950–1998 was used to estimate cumulative exposures to 290 chemicals—including 180 pesticides, of which 53 were herbicides—from the work histories of every farmer in the sample. The herbicides reported on included 2,4-D, 4-(2,4-dichlorophenoxy)butyric acid (2,4-DB), MCPA, and dicamba. Because the job–exposure matrix was specific for British Columbia, subjects who had worked as farmers but only outside British Columbia were excluded, leaving a working sample of 1,153 cases and 3,999 controls, who included 113 and 316 farmers, respectively. Conditional logistic regressions were adjusted for the nonagricultural potentially confounding variables marital status, education, smoking, alcohol consumption, ethnicity, and whether the questionnaire had been completed by a proxy using an exposure of ever or never for each agent; analysis for trend was conducted over the categories none, low, or high when there were at least 15 exposed cases.

Correlations between the occurrence of prostate cancer and exposure to the various pesticides were calculated and were fairly substantial among the COIs, but not with particular fungicides or insecticides. Associations with prostate cancer were significant for 19 (13.7%) of the 139 pesticide active ingredients to which any of the subjects had been exposed, including 2,4-D (11 exposed cases, OR = 2.72, 95% CI 1.12–6.57), 2,4-DB (24 exposed cases, OR = 1.77, 95% CI 1.04–3.03), and MCPA (22 exposed cases, OR = 1.83, 95% CI 1.04–3.23); associations were marginally significant for dicamba (14 exposed cases, OR = 2.02, 95% CI 0.98–4.15). 2,4-D did not have enough exposed cases for the trend analysis, but for both 2,4-DB and MCPA there were significant trends with degree of exposure ($p = 0.02$ for both). The assumption that none of the non-farmers had any occupational exposure to those agricultural chemicals is probably valid, but some misclassification may have arisen from personal use.

Several recent publications (Andreotti and Silverman, 2012; Barry et al., 2011, 2012; Koutros et al., 2010b, 2011) reported on a nested case-control substudy within the AHS on relationships among prostate cancer, pesticide exposure (including exposure to the COIs, such as 2,4-D and 2,4,5-T), and genetic markers. All men eligible for inclusion in the study were white applicators who had not had any cancer other than nonmelanoma skin cancer before enrollment in the AHS and had provided a buccal cell sample. Two controls, matched on age and alive at the time of the case's diagnosis, were sought for each case. The final study sample consisted of 776 prostate-cancer cases diagnosed in 1993–2004 and 1,444 controls. The focus of the substudy was on the interaction between pesticide exposure and genetic markers; how pesticide exposure modified the association between genetic markers and prostate cancer. Some useful information about the effect of exposure to the COIs and prostate cancer can be gleaned as a byproduct of the interaction analyses, but it came primarily from the perspective of biologic plausibility. Koutros et al. (2011) did report main effects adjusted for age, state, and family history of prostate cancer and trend for low and for high exposure vs no exposure to the various pesticides and prostate cancer. The results did not support significantly increased risks associated with 2,4-D, 2,4,5-T, and 2,4,5-TP; for the high-exposure group for 2,4,5-T there was a significant decrease in risk (OR = 0.60, 95% CI 0.42–0.84). The AHS has been generating valuable information on the COIs for a number of years, but these results are not herbicide-specific and so are not regarded as being fully informative for the committee's task.

Biologic Plausibility

Prostate cells and prostate-cancer cell lines are responsive to TCDD in induction of various genes, including those involved in drug metabolism. Simanainen et al. (2004) used different rat lines (TCDD-resistant Hans/Wistar and TCDD-sensitive Long Evans) and showed that TCDD treatment resulted in a significant decrease in the weight of prostate lobes; the effect did not appear to be line-specific. Different responses to TCDD in human prostate-cancer cell lines LNCaP and PC3 have been reported, including increased proliferation or no growth and stimulation or repression of AHR activity, which may be a function of coactivator–corepressor concentrations in the cells (Kollara and Brown, 2009, 2010). TCDD suppressed expression of genes associated with cell-cycle progression in LNCaP cells but also suppressed DNA-repair genes and increased Wnt5a concentrations; these effects could lead to divergent responses with regard to prostate-cancer progression (Hruba et al., 2011). In utero and lactational exposure to TCDD increases aging-associated cribiform hyperplasia in the murine prostate, which may be a precancerous lesion (Fritz et al., 2005). In a followup, progeny of a genetic cross between AHR-null mice and the transgenic adenocarcinoma of the mouse-prostate (TRAMP) strain that models prostate cancer showed that the presence of the AHR inhibited the formation of prostate tumors that have a neuroendocrine phenotype (Fritz et al., 2008). In agreement with a possible protective role, negative associations were found in the AFHS between the risk of benign prostate hyperplasia and both TCDD exposure and serum testosterone concentration (Gupta et al., 2006). As in breast cancer, this suggests that timing of exposure may be critical in adult-onset prostate disease, with early-life exposures increasing prostate-cancer susceptibility and adult AHR activation reducing it. Inasmuch as male Vietnam veterans were exposed to Agent Orange during adulthood, the early-life exposure findings are not relevant to this population.

The biologic plausibility of the carcinogenicity of the COIs is discussed in general at the beginning of this chapter.

Synthesis

The occupational studies reviewed in this update did not contain much evidence of an association between the COIs and prostate cancer. However, the increased risks reported from the non-pesticide-specific analysis of the AHS cohort were consistent with earlier positive findings concerning prostate cancer, and the case-control study of specific agricultural exposures in British Columbia

(Band et al., 2011) was fully supportive of there being an association between phenoxy herbicides and prostate cancer. The existing body of epidemiologic evidence supporting an association between exposure to the COIs and prostate cancer is robust enough that this committee finds no justification for reversing the conclusion of prior VAO committees that there is limited or suggestive evidence of an association.

Conclusion

On the basis of the evidence reviewed here and in previous VAO reports, the committee concludes that there remains limited or suggestive evidence of an association between exposure to at least one of the COIs and prostate cancer.

TESTICULAR CANCER

ACS estimated that 8,590 men would receive diagnoses of testicular cancer (ICD-9 186.0–186.9) in the United States in 2012 and that 360 men would die from it (Siegel et al., 2012). Other cancers of the male reproductive system that are infrequently reported separately are cancers of the penis and other male genital organs (ICD-9 187). The average annual incidence of testicular cancer is shown in Table 8-29.

Testicular cancer occurs more often in men under 40 years old than in older men. On a lifetime basis, the risk in white men is about four times that in black men. Cryptorchidism (undescended testes) is a major risk factor for testicular cancer. Family history of the disease also appears to be a risk factor. Several other hereditary, medical, and environmental risk factors have been suggested, but the results of research are inconsistent (Bosl and Motzer, 1997).

Conclusions from *VAO* and Previous Updates

The committee responsible for *VAO* concluded that there was inadequate or insufficient information to determine whether there is an association between

TABLE 8-29 Average Annual Incidence (per 100,000) of Testicular Cancer in the United States[a]

55–59 Years Old			60–64 Years Old			65–69 Years Old		
All Races	White	Black	All Races	White	Black	All Races	White	Black
2.9	3.4	0.5	1.7	1.8	0.8	1.2	1.3	0.0

[a]Surveillance, Epidemiology, and End Results program, nine standard registries, crude age-specific rates, 2005–2009 (NCI, 2013).

exposure to the COIs and testicular cancer. Additional information available to the committees responsible for *Update 1996*, *Update 1998*, *Update 2000*, *Update 2002*, *Update 2004*, *Update 2006*, *Update 2008*, and *Update 2010* did not change that conclusion.

Table 8-30 summarizes the results of the relevant studies.

Update of the Epidemiologic Literature

Vietnam-Veteran, Environmental, and Case-Control Studies

No Vietnam veteran studies, environmental studies, or case-control studies of exposure to the COIs and testicular cancer have been published since *Update 2010*.

Occupational Studies

Ruder and Yiin (2011) did not report any deaths from testicular cancer in the 2,053 men in the updated NIOSH PCP cohort.

In an update of cancer incidence in the AHS by Koutros et al. (2010a), no increases in the incidence of testicular cancer were found in private applicators (32 cases, SIR = 0.97, 95% CI 0.67–1.37) or in commercial applicators (six cases, SIR = 1.21, 95% CI 0.45–2.64). Waggoner et al. (2011) did not report on mortality from this type of cancer. The AHS has been generating valuable information on the COIs for a number of years, but these results are not herbicide-specific and so are not regarded as being fully informative for the committee's task.

Biologic Plausibility

No animal studies of the incidence of testicular cancer after exposure to any of the COIs have been published since *Update 2010*. That is undoubtedly due to the lack of a valid animal model of testicular cancer. The biologic plausibility of the carcinogenicity of the COIs is discussed in general at the beginning of this chapter.

Synthesis

The evidence from epidemiologic studies is inadequate to link herbicide exposure and testicular cancer. The relative rarity of this cancer makes it difficult to develop risk estimates with any precision. Most cases occur in men 25–35 years old, and men who have received such a diagnosis could be excluded from military service; this could explain the slight reduction in risk observed in some veteran studies.

TABLE 8-30 Selected Epidemiologic Studies—Testicular Cancer (Shaded Entries Are New Information for This Update)

Study Population[a]	Exposed Cases[b]	**Exposure of Interest**/Estimated Relative Risk (95% CI)[b]	Reference
VIETNAM VETERANS			
US Vietnam Veterans			
US VA Cohort of Army Chemical Corps—Expanded as of 1997 to include all Army men with chemical MOS (2,872 deployed vs 2,737 nondeployed) serving during Vietnam era (July 1, 1965–March 28, 1973)		**All COIs**	
Mortality			
Through 2005			Cypel and Kang, 2010
Deployed veterans (2,872) vs nondeployed (2,737)	2	—	
Through 1991	2	4.0 (0.5–14.5)	Dalager and Kang, 1997
US VA Proportionate Mortality Study—sample of deceased male Vietnam-era Army and Marine veterans who served 7/4/1965–3/1/1973		**All COIs**	
1965–1988			Watanabe and Kang, 1996
Army, deployed (n = 27,596) vs nondeployed (n = 31,757)	114	1.1 (nr)	
Marine Corps, deployed (n = 6,237) vs nondeployed (n = 5,040)	28	1.0 (nr)	
1965–1984			Watanabe et al., 1991
Army, deployed (n = 24,145) vs nondeployed (n = 27,917)	109	1.2 (ns)	
Served in I Corps (n = 6,668)	12	2.6 (1.1–6.2)	Bullman et al., 1990
Marine Corps, deployed (n = 5,501) vs nondeployed (n = 4,505)	28	0.8 (ns)	Watanabe et al., 1991
1965–1982			Breslin et al., 1988
Army, deployed (n = 19,708) vs nondeployed (n = 22,904)	90	1.1 (0.8–1.5)	
Marine Corps, deployed (n = 4,527) vs nondeployed (n = 3,781)	26	1.3 (0.5–3.6)	
State Studies of US Vietnam Veterans			
District of Columbia patients (18–42 yrs of age) in 3 hospitals, diagnosed with testicular cancer (1976–June 30, 1981)	31	2.3 (1.0–5.5)	Tarone et al., 1991
Massachusetts Vietnam-era veterans			
Veterans aged 35–65 years in 1993—cases diagnosed 1988–1993 vs gastrointestinal cancers	30	1.2 (0.4–3.3)	Clapp, 1997

TABLE 8-30 Testicular Cancer, continued

Study Population[a]	Exposed Cases[b]	**Exposure of Interest**/Estimated Relative Risk (95% CI)[b]	Reference
923 White male Vietnam veterans with **Wisconsin** death certificate (1968–1978) vs proportions for Vietnam-era veterans	9	1.0 (0.5–1.9)	Anderson et al., 1986
International Vietnam-Veterans Studies			
Australian Vietnam Veterans—58,077 men and 153 women served on land or in Vietnamese waters during 5/23/1962–7/1/1973 vs Australian population		**All COIs**	
Incidence			
All branches, 1982–2000	54	0.9 (0.6–1.1)	ADVA, 2005a
Navy	17	1.2 (0.7–1.8)	
Army	34	0.8 (0.5–1.0)	
Air Force	3	0.8 (0.2–2.3)	
Validation Study		*Expected number of exposed cases*	AIHW, 1999
	59	110 (89–139)	
Men	151	110 (89–131)	
Mortality			
All branches, return–2001	14	0.9 (0.4–1.4)	ADVA, 2005b
Navy	3	0.8 (0.2–2.4)	
Army	10	0.9 (0.4–1.7)	
Air Force	0	0.0 (0.0–3.3)	
1980–1994	4	ns	CDVA, 1997a
Australian Conscripted Army National Service (18,940 deployed vs 24,642 nondeployed)		**All COIs**	
Incidence			
1982–2000	17	0.7 (0.4–1.2)	ADVA, 2005c
Mortality			
1966–2001	4	0.8 (0.2–2.0)	ADVA, 2005c
1982–1994	1	1.3 (nr)	CDVA, 1997b
OCCUPATIONAL—INDUSTRIAL			
IARC Phenoxy Herbicide Cohort—Workers exposed to any phenoxy herbicide or chlorophenol (production or spraying) vs respective national mortality rates			
Mortality 1939–1992	68	1.1 (0.9–1.4)	Kogevinas et al., 1997
13,831 exposed to highly chlorinated PCDDs	43	1.1 (0.8–1.5)	
7,553 not exposed to highly chlorinated PCDDs	25	1.1 (0.3–1.6)	

continued

TABLE 8-30 Testicular Cancer, continued

Study Population[a]	Exposed Cases[b]	**Exposure of Interest**/Estimated Relative Risk (95% CI)[b]	Reference
Mortality 1955–1988 of 12,492 production workers and 5,898 sprayers exposed—13,482 in exposed subcohort	7	2.3 (0.9–4.6)	Saracci et al., 1991
British MCPA Plant—Production 1947–1982 (n = 1,545) (included in IARC cohort) and spraying 1947–1972 (n = 2,561) (*not* included in IARC cohort)		**MCPA**	
Mortality through 1983	4	2.2 (0.6–5.7)	Coggon et al., 1986
New Zealand Phenoxy Herbicide Production Workers and Sprayers (1,599 men and women working any time in 1969–1988 at Dow plant in New Plymouth) (in IARC cohort)		**Dioxins; 2,4-D; 2,4,5-T; MCPA; MCPB; 2,4,5-TCP; Picloram**	
Mortality 1969–2004			McBride et al., 2009a
Ever-exposed workers	0	0.0 (0.0–15.6)	
Never-exposed workers			
All Dow TCP-Exposed Workers (TCP production 1942–1979 or 2,4,5-T production 1948–1982 in Midland, Michigan) (in IARC and NIOSH cohorts)		**2,4,5-T; 2,4,5-TCP**	
1942–2003; testes and other male genital (n = 1,615)	1	1.6 (0.0–8.9)	Collins et al., 2009a
Dow 2,4-D Production Workers (1945–1982 in Midland, Michigan) (subset of all TCP-exposed workers)		**2,4-D, lower chlorinated dioxins**	
Through 1994 (n = 1,517)	1	2.2 (0.0–12.5)	Burns et al., 2001
Through 1982 (n = 878)	1	4.6 (0.0–25.7)	Bond et al., 1988
Dow PCP Production Workers (1937–1989 in Midland, Michigan) (*not* in IARC and NIOSH cohorts)		**Low chlorinated dioxins, 2,4-D**	
Mortality 1940–2004 (n = 577, excluding 196 also having exposure to TCP); testes and other male genital	0	0.0 (0.0–12.5)	Collins et al., 2009b
Mortality 1940–1989 (n = 770)	0	nr	Ramlow et al., 1996
OCCUPATIONAL—PAPER AND PULP WORKERS		**TCDD**	
IARC cohort of pulp and paper workers—60,468 workers from 11 countries, TCDD among 27 agents assessed by JEM			McLean et al., 2006
Exposure to nonvolatile organochlorine compounds			
Never	2	1.1 (0.1–4.1)	
Ever	5	3.6 (1.2–8.4)	

TABLE 8-30 Testicular Cancer, continued

Study Population[a]	Exposed Cases[b]	**Exposure of Interest**/Estimated Relative Risk (95% CI)[b]	Reference
OCCUPATIONAL—HERBICIDE-USING WORKERS (*not* related to IARC sprayer cohorts)			
CANADA			
Sawmill Workers in British Columbia—23,829 workers for ≥ 1 year at 11 mills using chlorophenates 1940–1985		**Chlorophenates, not TCDD**	
Incidence 1969–1989	18	1.0 (0.6–1.4)	Hertzman et al., 1997
Mortality 1950–1989 (male genital cancers)	116	1.0 (0.8–1.1)	
DENMARK			
Danish Farmers—incidence from linking farmers on 1970 census with national cancer registry (1970–1980)		**Herbicides**	Ronco et al., 1992
Men			
Self-employed	74	0.9 (nr)	
Employee	23	0.6 ($p < 0.05$)	
ICELANDIC men (1,860), women (859) exposed to agricultural pesticides, primarily 2,4-D—incidence	2	**2,4-D** 1.2 (0.1–4.3)	Zhong and Rafnsson, 1996
NEW ZEALAND National Cancer Registry (1980–1984)—case-control study of 339 incident testicular cancer cases vs remainder of 19,904 men with any incident cancer		**Herbicides**	Reif et al., 1989
Forestry workers (n = 134)	6	1.0 (0.4–2.6)	
SWEDEN			
Incident testicular cancer cases 1961–1973 with agriculture as economic activity in 1960 census	101	*99% CI* 1.0 (0.7–1.2)	Wiklund, 1983
UNITED STATES			
US farmers—usual occupation of farmer and industry of agriculture on death certificates 1984–1988 from 23 states		**Herbicides** PCMRs	Blair et al., 1993
Men			
Whites (n = 119,648)	32	0.8 (0.6–1.2)	
Nonwhites (n = 11,446)	6	1.3 (0.5–2.9)	
US Agricultural Health Study—prospective study of licensed pesticide sprayers in Iowa and North Carolina: commercial (n = 4,916), private/farmers (n = 52,395, 97.4% men), and spouses of private sprayers (n = 32,347, 0.007% men), enrolled 1993–1997; followups with CATIs 1999–2003 and 2005–2010		**Phenoxy herbicides**	

continued

TABLE 8-30 Testicular Cancer, continued

Study Population[a]	Exposed Cases[b]	**Exposure of Interest**/Estimated Relative Risk (95% CI)[b]	Reference
Incidence			
Enrollment through 2006—SIRs for participants			Koutros et al., 2010a
Private applicators	32	1.0 (0.7–1.4)	
Commercial applicators	6	1.2 (0.5–2.6)	
Spouses	0	nr	
Enrollment through 2002			Alavanja et al., 2005
Private applicators	23	1.1 (0.7–1.6)	
Spouses of private applicators (> 99% women)	nr	0.0 (0.0–50.2)	
Commercial applicators	4	1.2 (0.3–3.2)	
Mortality			
Enrollment through 2000, vs state rates			Blair et al., 2005a
Private applicators (men and women)	0	nr	
Spouses of private applicators (> 99% women)	0	nr	
Florida Licensed Pesticide Applicators (common phenoxy use assumed but not documented; had been listed by Blair et al., 1983)		**Herbicides**	
Mortality 1975–1993	23	2.5 (1.6–3.7)	Fleming et al., 1999b
ENVIRONMENTAL			
Seveso, Italy Residential Cohort—Industrial accident July 10, 1976 (723 residents Zone A; 4,821 Zone B; 31,643 Zone R; 181,574 local reference group) (ICD-9 171)		**TCDD**	
Incidence			
20-yr followup to 1996—men and women			
Zone A	0		Pesatori et al., 2009
Zone B	2	0.8 (0.2–3.3)	
Zone R	22	1.4 (0.9–2.3)	
10-yr followup to 1991—men			Bertazzi et al., 1993
Zone B	1	1.0 (0.1–7.5)	
Zone R	9	1.4 (0.7–3.0)	
Mortality			
20-yr followup to 1996			Bertazzi et al., 2001
Zones A, B—men	17	1.0 (0.6–1.7)	
15-yr followup to 1991—men			Bertazzi et al., 1998
Zone B	10	1.0 (0.5–1.8)	
Zone R	73	1.0 (0.8–1.3)	

TABLE 8-30 Testicular Cancer, continued

Study Population[a]	Exposed Cases[b]	**Exposure of Interest**/Estimated Relative Risk (95% CI)[b]	Reference
CASE-CONTROL STUDIES			
International Case-Control Studies			
Swedish Cancer Registry (1989–1992)—testicular cancer patients (20–75 yrs old) (n = 148)		**Herbicides**	Hardell et al., 1998
Exposed to herbicides	4	0.3 (0.1–1.0)	

NOTE: 2,4-D, 2,4-dichlorophenoxyacetic acid; 2,4,5-T, 2,4,5-trichlorophenoxyacetic acid; 2,4,5-TCP, 2,4,5-trichlorophenol; CATI, computer-assisted telephone interviewing; CI, confidence interval; COI, chemical of interest; IARC, International Agency for Research on Cancer; ICD, International Classification of Diseases; JEM, job-exposure matrix; MCPA, 2-methyl-4-chlorophenoxyacetic acid; MCPB, 4-(4-chloro-2-methylphenoxy)butanoic acid; MOS, military occupation specialty; NIOSH, National Institute for Occupational Safety and Health; nr, not reported; PCDD, polychlorinated dibenzo-*p*-dioxin (highly chlorinated, if four or more chlorines); PCMR, proportionate cancer mortality ratios; PCP, pentachlorophenol; SIR, standardized incidence ratio; TCDD, 2,3,7,8-tetrachlorodibenzo-*p*-dioxin; TCP, trichlorophenol; VA, US Department of Veterans Affairs.

[a]Subjects are male and outcome is mortality unless otherwise noted.

[b]Given when available; results other than estimated risk explained individually.

Conclusion

On the basis of the evidence reviewed here and in previous VAO reports, the committee concludes that there is inadequate or insufficient evidence to determine whether there is an association between exposure to the COIs and testicular cancer.

BLADDER CANCER

Urinary bladder cancer (ICD-9 188) is the most common urinary tract cancer. Cancers of the urethra and paraurethral glands and other and unspecified urinary cancers (ICD-9 189.3–189.9) are infrequently reported separately; any findings on these cancers would be reported in this section. ACS estimated that 55,600 men and 17,910 women would receive a diagnosis of bladder cancer in the United States in 2012 and that 10,510 men and 4,370 women would die from it (Siegel et al., 2012). In males, in whom this cancer is about twice as common as it is in females, those numbers represent about 7% of new cancer diagnoses and 3% of cancer deaths. Overall, bladder cancer is fourth in incidence in men in the United States.

Bladder-cancer risk rises rapidly with age. In men in the age groups that characterize most Vietnam veterans, bladder-cancer incidence is about twice as high in whites as in blacks. The average annual incidence of urinary bladder cancer is shown in Table 8-31.

The most important known risk factor for bladder cancer is tobacco use, which accounts for about half the bladder cancers in men and one-third of them in women (Miller et al., 1996). Occupational exposure to aromatic amines (also called arylamines), polycyclic aromatic hydrocarbons, and some other organic chemicals used in the rubber, leather, textile, paint-products, and printing industries is associated with higher incidence. In some parts of Africa and Asia, infection with the parasite *Schistosoma haematobium* contributes to the high incidence.

Exposure to inorganic arsenic is also a risk factor for bladder cancer. Although cacodylic acid is a metabolite of inorganic arsenic, as discussed in Chapter 4, the data are insufficient to conclude that studies of inorganic-arsenic exposure are directly relevant to exposure to cacodylic acid, so the literature on inorganic arsenic is not considered in this section.

Conclusions from *VAO* and Previous Updates

The committees responsible for *VAO* and *Update 1996* concluded that there was limited or suggestive evidence of *no* association between exposure to the COIs and urinary bladder cancer. Additional information available to the committee responsible for *Update 1998* led it to change that conclusion to one of inadequate or insufficient information to determine whether there is an association. The committees responsible for *Update 2000*, *Update 2002*, *Update 2004*, *Update 2006*, *Update 2008*, and *Update 2010* did not change that conclusion.

Table 8-32 summarizes the results of the relevant studies.

TABLE 8-31 Average Annual Incidence (per 100,000) of Bladder Cancer in the United States[a]

	55–59 Years Old			60–64 Years Old			65–69 Years Old		
	All Races	White	Black	All Races	White	Black	All Races	White	Black
Men	43.4	46.9	26.2	77.3	84.6	48.7	130.6	141.4	95.1
Women	12.2	13.5	7.7	21.4	23.2	14.5	33.6	36.5	27.7

[a]Surveillance, Epidemiology, and End Results program, nine standard registries, crude age-specific rates, 2005–2009 (NCI, 2013).

TABLE 8-32 Selected Epidemiologic Studies—Urinary Bladder Cancer (Shaded Entries Are New Information for This Update)

Study Population[a]	Exposed Cases[b]	**Exposure of Interest**/Estimated Relative Risk (95% CI)[b]	Reference
VIETNAM VETERANS			
US Vietnam Veterans			
US Air Force Health Study—Ranch Hand veterans vs SEA veterans (unless otherwise noted)		**All COIs**	
Incidence			
Through 1999—White subjects vs national rates			Akhtar et al., 2004
Ranch Hand veterans (n = 1,189)	14	1.1 (0.6–1.7)	
With tours between 1966–1970	14	1.3 (0.7–2.1)	
SEA comparison veterans (n = 1,776)	8	0.4 (0.2–0.8)	
With tours between 1966–1970	4	0.3 (0.1–0.7)	
Mortality			
Through 1999—White subjects vs national rates			
Ranch Hand veterans	1	0.9 (nr)	
SEA comparison veterans	1	0.6 (nr)	
US CDC Vietnam Experience Study—Cross-sectional study, with medical examinations, of Army veterans: 9,324 deployed vs 8,989 nondeployed		**All COIs**	
Mortality			
1965–2000	1	nr	Boehmer et al., 2004
US VA Proportionate Mortality Study—sample of deceased male Vietnam-era Army and Marine veterans who served 7/4/1965–3/1/1973		**All COIs**	
1965–1982			Breslin et al., 1988
Army, deployed (n = 19,708) vs nondeployed (n = 22,904)	9	0.6 (0.3–1.2)	
Marine Corps, deployed (n = 4,527) vs nondeployed (n = 3,781)	4	2.4 (0.1–66.4)	
State Studies of US Vietnam Veterans			
Massachusetts Vietnam-era veterans			
Veterans served 1958–1973—cases diagnosed 1988–1993 (served in Vietnam) (updates Clapp et al., 1991)	80	0.6 (0.2–1.3)	Clapp et al., 1997
923 White male Vietnam veterans with **Wisconsin** death certificate (1968–1978) vs proportions for Vietnam-era veterans (includes lymphosarcoma, reticulosarcoma)	1	nr	Anderson et al., 1986
International Vietnam-Veteran Studies			
Australian Vietnam Veterans—58,077 men and 153 women served on land or in Vietnamese waters during 5/23/1962–7/1/1973 vs Australian population		**All COIs**	

continued

TABLE 8-32 Urinary Bladder Cancer, continued

Study Population[a]	Exposed Cases[b]	**Exposure of Interest**/Estimated Relative Risk (95% CI)[b]	Reference
Incidence			
All branches, 1982–2000	164	1.0 (0.9–1.2)	ADVA, 2005a
Navy	34	1.0 (0.7–1.4)	
Army	104	1.0 (0.8–1.2)	
Air Force	26	1.3 (0.8–1.8)	
Mortality			
All branches, return–2001	22	0.7 (0.4–1.0)	ADVA, 2005b
Navy	4	0.6 (0.2–1.6)	
Army	13	0.7 (0.3–1.1)	
Air Force	5	1.1 (0.4–2.5)	
1980–1994	11	1.1 (0.6–1.9)	CDVA, 1997a
Australian Conscripted Army National Service (18,940 deployed vs 24,642 nondeployed)		**All COIs**	
Incidence—1982–2000	19	0.7 (0.4–1.1)	ADVA, 2005c
Mortality			
1966–2001	1	0.3 (0.0–1.7)	
1982–1994	1	0.6 (nr)	CDVA, 1997b
OCCUPATIONAL—INDUSTRIAL			
IARC Phenoxy Herbicide Cohort—Workers exposed to any phenoxy herbicide or chlorophenol (production or spraying) vs respective national mortality rates			
Mortality 1939–1992	34	1.0 (0.7–1.5)	Kogevinas et al., 1997
13,831 exposed to highly chlorinated PCDDs	24	1.4 (0.9–2.1)	
7,553 not exposed to highly chlorinated PCDDs	10	0.7 (0.3–1.2)	
Mortality 1955–1988 of 12,492 production workers and 5,898 sprayers exposed—13,482 in exposed subcohort	13	0.8 (0.4–1.4)	Saracci et al., 1991
British MCPA Plant—Production 1947–1982 (n = 1,545) (included in IARC cohort) and spraying 1947–1972 (n = 2,561) (*not* included in IARC cohort)		**MCPA**	
Mortality through 1983	8	0.9 (0.4–1.7)	Coggon et al., 1986
Danish Production Workers (3,390 men and 1,069 women involved in production of phenoxy herbicides unlikely to contain TCDD at 2 plants in 1947–1987) (in IARC cohort)		**Dioxins, but TCDD unlikely; 2,4-D, 2,4-DP, MCPA, MCPP**	
Incidence 1943–1982 (men only)	11	0.8 (nr)	Lynge, 1985

TABLE 8-32 Urinary Bladder Cancer, continued

Study Population[a]	Exposed Cases[b]	**Exposure of Interest**/Estimated Relative Risk (95% CI)[b]	Reference
Mortality 1955–2006	15	1.1 (0.8–1.4)	Boers et al., 2012
TCDD plasma level (hazard ratios, by tertile)			
Background (≤ 0.4)	4	nr	
Low (0.4–4.1)	10	2.4 (0.8–8.3)	
Medium (4.1–20.1)	7	4.0 (1.1–14.3)	
High (≥ 20.1)	2	3.1 (0.6–17.0)	
Dutch production workers in Plant A (549 men exposed during production 1955–1985; 594 unexposed) (in IARC cohort)		**Dioxins, 2,4,5-T, 2,4,5-TCP**	
Mortality 1955–2006 (hazard ratios for lagged TCDD plasma levels)	11	1.0 (0.7–1.5)	Boers et al., 2012
Mortality 1955–2006	9 vs 2	2.3 (0.5–10.3)	Boers et al., 2010
Mortality 1955–1991	4	3.7 (1.0–9.5)	Hooiveld et al., 1998
Accidentally exposed subcohort	1	2.8 (0.1–15.5)	
Mortality 1955–1985	1	1.5 (0.0–8.8)	Bueno de Mesquita et al., 1993
Dutch production workers in Plant B (414 men exposed during production 1965–1986; 723 unexposed) (in IARC cohort)		**2,4-D; MCPA; MCPP; highly chlorinated dioxins unlikely**	
Mortality 1965–2006	2 vs 2	1.1 (0.2–7.2)	Boers et al., 2010
Mortality 1965–1986	0	0.0 (0.0–20.5)	Bueno de Mesquita et al., 1993
German Production Workers at BASF Ludwigshafen Plant (680 men working > 1 month in 1957–1987) (in IARC cohort as of 1997) and women—no results		**Dioxins; 2,4-D; 2,4,5-T; MCPA; MCPP; 2,4-DP**	
BASF Cleanup Workers from 1953 accident (n = 247); 114 with chloracne, 13 more with erythema; serum TCDD levels (*not* part of IARC)		**Focus on TCDD**	
Incidence			
1960–1992			Ott and Zober, 1996
TCDD < 0.1 µg/kg of body weight	1	0.7 (0.0–4.0)	
TCDD 0.1–0.99 µg/kg of body weight	3	3.0 (0.6–8.9)	
TCDD > 1 µg/kg of body weight	1	0.8 (0.0–4.4)	
Mortality			
1960–1992			
TCDD < 0.1 µg/kg of body weight	0	0.0 (0.0–5.7)	
TCDD 0.1–0.99 µg/kg of body weight	2	4.1 (0.5–14.7)	
TCDD > 1 µg/kg of body weight	0	0.0 (0.0–5.4)	

continued

TABLE 8-32 Urinary Bladder Cancer, continued

Study Population[a]	Exposed Cases[b]	**Exposure of Interest**/Estimated Relative Risk (95% CI)[b]	Reference
Through 1987	0	*90% CI* nr (0.0–15.0)	Zober et al., 1990
German Production Workers at Boehringer–Ingelheim Plant in Hamburg (1,144 men working > 1 month in 1952–1984; generation of TCDD reduced after chloracne outbreak in 1954) and women—no results (some additions to observed cancers over Manz et al., 1991) (in IARC cohort as of 1997)		**Dioxins; 2,4,5-T; 2,5-DCP; 2,4,5-TCP**	
Mortality 1952–2007	13	1.8 (1.0–3.1)	Manuwald et al., 2012
Men	11	1.8 (0.9–3.3)	
Women	2	1.8 (0.2–6.6)	
New Zealand Phenoxy Herbicide Production Workers and Sprayers (1,599 men and women working any time in 1969–1988 at Dow plant in New Plymouth) (in IARC cohort)		**Dioxins; 2,4-D; 2,4,5-T; MCPA; MCPB; 2,4,5-TCP; Picloram**	
Mortality 1969–2004			McBride et al., 2009a
Ever-exposed workers	0	0.0 (0.0–2.9)	
Production Workers (713 men and 100 women worked > 1 month in 1969–1984)			
Mortality 1969–2000	0	nr	't Mannetje et al., 2005
Sprayers (697 men and 2 women registered any time 1973–1984)			
Mortality 1973–2000	0	nr	't Mannetje et al., 2005
NIOSH Mortality Cohort (12 US plants, 5,172 male production and maintenance workers 1942–1984) (included in IARC cohort as of 1997)		**Dioxins, phenoxy herbicides**	
Through 1993	16	2.0 (1.1–3.2)	Steenland et al., 1999
Chloracne subcohort (n = 608)	6	3.0 (1.4–8.5)	
Through 1987 (bladder, other)	9	1.6 (0.7–3.0)	Fingerhut et al., 1991
≥ 1-year exposure, ≥ 20-year latency	4	1.9 (0.5–4.8)	
Mortality—754 Monsanto workers, among most highly exposed workers from Fingerhut et al. (1991)	16	6.8 (3.9–11.1)	Collins et al., 1993
All Dow TCP-Exposed Workers (TCP production 1942–1979 or 2,4,5-T production 1948–1982 in Midland, Michigan) (in IARC and NIOSH cohorts)		**2,4,5-T; 2,4,5-TCP**	
1942–2003 (n = 1,615)	6	1.2 (0.5–2.7)	Collins et al., 2009a
1940–1994 (n = 2,187 men)	nr	0.7 (0.1–2.0)	Bodner et al., 2003

TABLE 8-32 Urinary Bladder Cancer, continued

Study Population[a]	Exposed Cases[b]	**Exposure of Interest**/Estimated Relative Risk (95% CI)[b]	Reference
All Dow PCP-Exposed Workers—all workers from the two plants that only made PCP (in Tacoma, Washington, and Wichita, Kansas) and workers who made PCP and TCP at two additional plants (in Midland, Michigan, and Sauget, Illinois)		**2,4,5-T; 2,4,5-TCP**	Ruder and Yiin, 2011
1940–2005 (n = 2,122) (bladder and other urinary organs, ICD-9 188, 189.3, 189.9)	8	1.1 (0.5–2.1)	
PCP and TCP (n = 720)	1	0.4 (0.0–2.3)	
PCP (no TCP) (n = 1,402)	7	1.4 (0.6–2.9)	
Dow 2,4-D Production Workers (1945–1982 in Midland, Michigan) (subset of all TCP-exposed workers)		**2,4-D, lower chlorinated dioxins**	
Cancer incidence through 2007 in Dow workers (n = 1,256) vs comparisons from state cancer registries (n = 23,354) (Cohort 3)	19	1.2 (0.7–1.9)	Burns et al., 2011
Through 1994 (n = 1,517)	1	0.5 (0.1–2.8)	Burns et al., 2001
Through 1982 (n = 878)	0	nr (0.0–7.2)	Bond et al., 1988
Dow PCP Production Workers (1937–1989 in Midland, Michigan) (*not* in IARC and NIOSH cohorts)		**Low chlorinated dioxins, 2,4-D**	
Mortality 1940–2004 (n = 577, excluding 196 also having exposure to TCP)	2	0.7 (0.1–2.7)	Collins et al., 2009b
OCCUPATIONAL—PAPER AND PULP WORKERS		**TCDD**	
IARC cohort of pulp and paper workers—60,468 workers from 11 countries, TCDD among 27 agents assessed by JEM			McLean et al., 2006
Exposure to nonvolatile organochlorine compounds			
Never	50	1.0 (0.7–1.3)	
Ever	43	1.1 (0.8–1.5)	
New Hampshire pulp and paper workers, 883 white men working ≥ 1 yr, mortality through July 1985	4	1.2 (0.3–3.2)	Henneberger et al., 1989
Pulp and Paper cohorts independent of IARC cohort			
Northwestern US paper and pulp workers—5 mills in Washington, Oregon, and California, 3,523 worked ≥ 1 yr 1945–1955, mortality through March 1977	8	*90% CI* 1.2 (0.6–2.6)	Robinson et al., 1986

continued

TABLE 8-32 Urinary Bladder Cancer, continued

Study Population[a]	Exposed Cases[b]	**Exposure of Interest**/Estimated Relative Risk (95% CI)[b]	Reference
OCCUPATIONAL—HERBICIDE-USING WORKERS (*not* related to IARC sprayer cohorts)			
CANADA			
Sawmill Workers in British Columbia—23,829 workers for ≥ 1 year at 11 mills using chlorophenates 1940–1985		**Chlorophenates, not TCDD**	
Incidence 1969–1989	33	0.9 (0.7–1.2)	Hertzman et al., 1997
Mortality 1950–1989	94	1.0 (0.8–1.2)	
Herbicide sprayers routinely exposed to herbicides for 6 months or more (1950–1982)		**Phenoxy herbicides**	Green, 1991
Diseases of genitourinary system	1	1.0 (0.0–5.6)	
DENMARK			
Danish gardeners (n = 3,124) exposed to pesticides	59	0.8 (0.6–1.1)	Kenborg et al., 2012
Danish farmers—incidence from linking farmers on 1970 census with national cancer registry (1970–1980)		**Herbicides**	Ronco et al., 1992
Men			
Self-employed	300	0.6 ($p < 0.05$)	
Employee	70	0.7 ($p < 0.05$)	
Women			
Self-employed	1	0.2 (nr)	
Employee	2	0.6 (nr)	
Family worker	25	0.6 ($p < 0.05$)	
Danish gardeners—incidence from 3,156 male and 859 female gardeners (urinary system, ICD-7 180–181)			Hansen et al., 2007
25-year followup (1975–2001)		**Herbicides**	
Born before 1915 (high exposure)	25	1.1 (0.7–1.6)	
Born 1915–1934 (medium exposure)	23	0.5 (0.4–0.8)	
Born after 1934 (low exposure)	1	0.2 (0.0–1.1)	
10-year followup (1975–1984) of male gardeners	18	0.9 (0.5–1.4)	Hansen et al., 1992
FINNISH Phenoxy Herbicide Sprayers (1,909 men working 1955–1971 ≥ 2 wks) *not* IARC		**Phenoxy herbicides**	
Incidence			Asp et al., 1994
No latency	12	1.6 (0.8–2.8)	
10-yr latency	11	1.7 (0.8–3.0)	
Mortality			
No latency	1	0.5 (0.0–2.6)	
10-yr latency	1	0.5 (0.0–3.0)	
ITALIAN Licensed Pesticide Users—male farmers in southern Piedmont licensed 1970–1974			
Mortality 1970–1986 (n = 23,401)	31	0.5 (0.4–0.8)	Torchio et al., 1994

TABLE 8-32 Urinary Bladder Cancer, continued

Study Population[a]	Exposed Cases[b]	**Exposure of Interest**/Estimated Relative Risk (95% CI)[b]	Reference
Italian rice growers with documented phenoxy use (n = 1,487)		**Phenoxy herbicides**	Gambini et al., 1997
	12	1.0 (0.5–1.8)	
NEW ZEALAND National Cancer Registry (1980–1984)—case-control study of incident stomach cancer cases vs remainder of 19,904 men with any incident cancer			Reif et al., 1989
Forestry workers (n = 134)		**Herbicides**	
	4	0.7 (0.3–1.8)	
THE NETHERLANDS			
Dutch Licensed Herbicide Sprayers—1,341 certified before 1980			
Through 2000	2	0.7 (0.1–2.4)	Swaen et al., 2004
UNITED STATES			
US Agricultural Health Study—prospective study of licensed pesticide sprayers in Iowa and North Carolina: commercial (n = 4,916), private/farmers (n = 52,395, 97.4% men), and spouses of private sprayers (n = 32,347, 0.007% men), enrolled 1993–1997; followups with CATIs 1999–2003 and 2005–2010		**Phenoxy herbicides**	
Incidence			
Enrollment through 2006—SIRs for participants			Koutros et al., 2010a
Private applicators	191	0.6 (0.5–0.7)	
Commercial applicators	16	0.2 (0.7–1.9)	
Spouses	29	0.6 (0.4–0.9)	
Enrollment through 2002			Samanic et al., 2006
Dicamba—lifetime days exposure			
None	43	1.0	
1– < 20	6	0.5 (0.2–1.3)	
20– < 56	9	0.7 (0.3–1.4)	
56– < 116	6	0.6 (0.3–1.5)	
≥ 116	8	0.8 (0.4–1.9)	
		p-trend = 0.66	
Enrollment through 2002			Alavanja et al., 2005
Private applicators	184	0.7 (0.6–0.8)	
Spouses of private applicators (> 99% women)	17	0.7 (0.4–1.1)	
Commercial applicators	13	1.1 (0.6–1.8)	

continued

TABLE 8-32 Urinary Bladder Cancer, continued

Study Population[a]	Exposed Cases[b]	**Exposure of Interest**/Estimated Relative Risk (95% CI)[b]	Reference
Mortality			
Enrollment through 2007, vs state rates			Waggoner et al., 2011
Applicators (n = 1,641)	35	0.6 (0.4–0.8)	
Spouses (n = 676)	9	0.8 (0.4–1.6)	
Enrollment through 2000, vs state rates			Blair et al., 2005a
Private applicators (men and women)	7	0.4 (0.1–0.7)	
Spouses of private applicators (> 99% women)	2	0.8 (0.1–2.7)	
US Department of Agriculture Workers—nested case-control study of white men dying 1970–1979 of NHL		**Herbicides**	
Agricultural extension agents	8	0.7 (0.4–1.4)	Alavanja et al., 1988
Forest conservationists		p- trend < over years worked	Alavanja et al., 1989
	8	0.8 (0.3–1.6)	
Florida Licensed Pesticide Applicators (common phenoxy use assumed but not documented; had been listed by Blair et al., 1983)		**Herbicides**	
Pesticide applicators in Florida licensed 1965–1966 (n = 3,827)—mortality through 1976		**Herbicides**	Blair et al., 1983
Any pesticide (dose-response by length of licensure)		*Expected exposed cases*	
	3	1.6 (nr)	
White Male Residents of Iowa—NHL cancer on death certificate, usual occupation: farmers vs not		**Herbicides**	
> 20 yrs old when died 1971–1978—PMR	274	0.9 (nr)	Burmeister, 1981
ENVIRONMENTAL			
Seveso, Italy Residential Cohort—Industrial accident July 10, 1976 (723 residents Zone A; 4,821 Zone B; 31,643 Zone R; 181,574 local reference group) (ICD-9 171)		**TCDD**	
Incidence			
20-yr followup to 1996—men and women			
Zone A	3	1.4 (0.5–4.5)	Pesatori et al., 2009
Zone B	17	1.3 (0.8–2.2)	
Zone R	84	0.9 (0.8–1.2)	
10-yr followup to 1991—men			Pesatori et al., 1992
Zone A, B	10	1.6 (0.9–3.1)	
Zone R	39	1.0 (0.7–1.4)	
10-yr followup to 1991—women			
Zone A, B	1	0.9 (0.1–6.8)	
Zone R	4	0.6 (0.2–1.5)	

TABLE 8-32 Urinary Bladder Cancer, continued

Study Population[a]	Exposed Cases[b]	**Exposure of Interest**/Estimated Relative Risk (95% CI)[b]	Reference
Mortality			
25-yr followup to 2001—men and women			Consonni et al., 2008
Zone A	1	1.0 (0.2–7.4)	
Zone B	6	0.9 (0.4–2.0)	
Zone R	42	0.9 (0.6–1.2)	
20-yr followup to 1996			Bertazzi et al., 2001
Zones A and B—men	6	1.2 (0.5–2.7)	
15-yr followup to 1991—men			Bertazzi et al., 1998
Zone B	1	2.4 (0.3–16.8)	
Zone R	21	0.9 (0.6–1.5)	
15-yr followup to 1991—women			Bertazzi et al., 1998
Zone B	3	0.9 (0.3–3.0)	
Zone R	4	0.6 (0.2–1.8)	
Ecological Study of Residents of Chapaevsk, Russia		**Dioxin**	Revich et al., 2001
Mortality—1995–1998 (SMR vs regional rates)			
Men	31	2.6 (1.7–3.6)	
Women	17	0.8 (0.5–1.3)	
Other International Environmental Studies			
FINLAND			
Finnish community exposed to chlorophenol contamination (men and women)—incidence	14	**Chlorophenol** 1.0 (0.6–1.9)	Lampi et al., 1992
SWEDEN			
Swedish fishermen (high consumption of fish with persistent organochlorines)		**Organochlorine compounds**	Svensson et al., 1995
Incidence			
East coast	10	0.7 (0.4–1.3)	
West coast	55	0.9 (0.7–1.1)	
Mortality			
East coast	5	1.3 (0.4–3.1)	
West coast	20	1.0 (0..6–1.6)	

NOTE: 2,4-D, 2,4-dichlorophenoxyacetic acid; 2,4-DP, dichlorprop; 2,4,5-T, 2,4,5-trichlorophenoxyacetic acid; 2,4,5-TCP, 2,4,5-trichlorophenol; 2,5-DCP, 2,5-dichlorophenol; CATI, computer-assisted telephone interviewing; CDC, Centers for Disease Control and Prevention; CI, confidence interval; COI, chemical of interest; IARC, International Agency for Research on Cancer; ICD, International Classification of Diseases; JEM, job-exposure matrix; MCPA, 2-methyl-4-chlorophenoxyacetic acid; MCPB, 4-(4-chloro-2-methylphenoxy)butanoic acid; MCPP, methylchlorophenoxypropionic acid; NHL, non-Hodgkin lymphoma; NIOSH, National Institute for Occupational Safety and Health; nr, not reported; PCDD, polychlorinated dibenzo-*p*-dioxin (highly chlorinated, if four or more chlorines); PCMR, proportionate cancer mortality ratios; PCP, pentachlorophenol; PMR, proportional mortality ratio; SEA, Southeast Asia; SIR, standardized incidence ratio; SMR, standardized mortality rate; TCDD, 2,3,7,8-tetrachlorodibenzo-*p*-dioxin; TCP, trichlorophenol; VA, US Department of Veterans Affairs.

[a]Subjects are male and outcome is mortality unless otherwise noted.

[b]Given when available; results other than estimated risk explained individually.

Update of the Epidemiologic Literature

Vietnam-Veteran, Environmental, and Case-Control Studies

No Vietnam-veteran studies, environmental studies, or case-control studies of exposure to the COIs and bladder cancer have been published since *Update 2010*.

Occupational Studies

Burns et al. (2011) updated cancer incidence through 2007 in workers who were alive on January 1, 1985, and had been employed at any time from 1945 to 1994 in 2,4-D production by the Dow Chemical Company in Midland, Michigan. They found no evidence of significantly increased rates of cancer overall. With 19 cases observed, the incidence of bladder cancer in the most restrictively defined cohort was not increased (SIR = 1.22, 95% CI 0.73–1.90), as was the case in the two successively more inclusive, but potentially more biased, cohorts.

Boers et al. (2012) provided a quantified, TCDD-based analysis of mortality updated through 2006 in male workers in two Dutch phenoxy-herbicide factories, which were considered in *Update 2010* (Boers et al., 2010). The 1,020 workers in factory A had been involved in production of 2,4,5-T with its associated TCDD contamination, whereas the 1,036 working in factory B had produced only phenoxy herbicides that would not have had TCDD contamination. Contemporary TCDD concentrations measured in a subsample of 187 workers were used to derive a model incorporating job history to estimate serum TCDD concentrations of all the men at the end of their employment. Using the estimated TCDD concentrations of the workers in both factories did not indicate an increased risk of bladder-cancer mortality associated with TCDD (HR = 1.07, 95% CI 0.83–1.38). The dose–response modeling applied only to the workers in factory A did not find an increased risk of death from bladder cancer (HR = 0.98, 95% CI 0.66–1.45), whereas the estimated risk from the qualitative exposure analysis in Boers et al. (2010) was imprecise (HR = 2.27, 95% CI 0.50–10.28).

Manuwald et al. (2012) reported mortality in 1,191 men and 398 women who had been employed for at least 3 months during 1952–1984 in a chemical plant in Hamburg (a subcohort of the IARC phenoxy-herbicide cohort). During that period, the plant produced insecticides and herbicides, including 2,4,5-T, so cohort members had the possibility of exposure to TCDD. Subjects entered the cohort on the date of their first employment in the plant, and vital status was sought through 2007. SMRs calculated relative to the population of Hamburg showed that death from bladder cancer was not increased in men (SMR = 1.83, 95% CI 0.91–3.28) or in women (SMR = 1.82, 95% CI 0.20–6.56), but in the entire cohort the increase in risk was marginally significant (SMR = 1.83, 95% CI 0.97–3.13).

Ruder and Yiin (2011) reported mortality in 1940–2005 in the NIOSH PCP cohort of 2,122 workers in the four US plants that had been involved in PCP production. PCP production entailed exposure to PCDDs and PCDFs but not to the most toxic 2,3,7,8 dioxin congener. A subcohort of 720 workers (all men, the PCP-plus-TCDD group) had also been employed in TCP production and so had also been exposed to TCDD. Relative to US referent rates, deaths from cancers of the bladder or other urinary organs were not substantially increased in the entire cohort (eight deaths, SMR = 1.08, 95% CI 0.47–2.13) or in the PCP-only group (seven deaths, SMR = 1.41, 95% CI 0.57–2.90). Only a single death from cancer of the urinary organs was observed in the PCP-plus-TCDD group (SMR = 0.41, 95% CI 0.01–2.90).

In the update of cancer incidence through 2006, Koutros et al. (2010a) found decreased incidences of bladder cancer in private applicators (191 cases, SIR = 0.59, 95% CI 0.51–0.68) and in their spouses (29 cases, SIR = 0.60, 95% CI 0.40–0.86). Waggoner et al. (2011) found mortality due to bladder cancer to be lower than expected in the applicators (35 deaths, SMR = 0.55, 95% CI 0.38–0.76) but not significantly so in their spouses (nine deaths, SMR = 0.83, 95% CI 0.38–1.58). The AHS has been generating valuable information on the COIs for a number of years, but these results are not herbicide-specific and so are not regarded as being fully informative for the committee's task.

Kenborg et al. (2012) conducted a study focused on Parkinson disease in a Danish cohort of 3,124 male union members who worked as professional gardeners in 1975. When previously studying this cohort, Hansen et al. (1992, 2007) had reported that herbicides (including phenoxy herbicides) constituted most of their exposure. In conjunction with addressing the observation that smoking has been repeatedly found to be negatively associated with the occurrence of Parkinson disease, Kenborg et al. (2012) also investigated the incidence of several cancers that are recognized as being smoking-related. The incidence of bladder cancer in the gardeners was similar to the age-specific and calendar-period–specific incidence in the general male Danish population (59 cases, SIR = 0.82, 95% CI 0.62–1.05).

Biologic Plausibility

In laboratory animals, cacodylic acid has been shown to induce primarily bladder tumors (Cohen et al., 2006; Wang et al., 2009). In a study of male F344 rats, cacodylic acid administered in drinking water resulted in formation of bladder tumors at the highest concentrations (50 and 200 ppm) (Wei et al., 2002). In another report (Arnold et al., 2006), administration of cacodylic acid in the diet resulted in formation of papillomas and carcinomas in the bladders of female and male F344 rats but not B6C3F1 mice. In a study that used a rat-cancer initiation–promotion model, cacodylic acid was found to be a weak cancer-initiator but a tumor-promoter at high doses (Fukushima et al., 2005). Direct intravesical administration of cacodylic acid (DMA^V) in female adult rats resulted in increased bromodeoxyuridine labeling in urothelial cells indicating DNA damage, weak neutrophil infiltration, and modest increases in oxidative-stress indexes (Takahashi et al., 2011). Other recent studies have shown cacodylic acid concentrations to be lower in bladder-cancer patients than in matched controls (Pu et al., 2007) and to be negatively associated with the incidence of urinary cancer (Huang et al., 2008). In contrast, greater oxidative DNA damage has been found in association with higher cacodylic acid concentrations in urothelial-cancer patients (Chung et al., 2008), although this was not the case in primary human hepatocytes (Dopp et al., 2008).

No studies have reported an increased incidence of urinary bladder cancer in TCDD-treated animals. Working with tissues from urothelial-cancer patients, Ishida et al. (2010) found that activation of the AHR pathway by TCDD enhances cancer-cell invasion by upregulating matrix metalloproteinase-1 and -9 expression and is associated with poor prognosis in upper urinary tract urothelial cancer. In contrast, transgenic mice that have deletion of the AHR exhibit immune-cell infiltration in bladder submucosa and loss of e-cadherin in some epithelial cells with local invasion in aged mice (Butler et al., 2012); although direct studies with TCDD were not undertaken, these findings suggest a protective effect of AHR signaling in bladder cancer.

The biologic plausibility of the carcinogenicity of the COIs is discussed in general at the beginning of this chapter.

Synthesis

Available analyses of an association between exposure to the COIs and bladder-cancer risk are characterized by low precision because of the small numbers, low exposure specificity, and lack of ability to control for confounding. Over the last several updates, laboratory data have emerged suggesting that cacodylic acid may be a bladder-tumor–promoter, but there have also been observations that cacodylic acid concentrations are lower in patients who have urinary cancer than in controls without any cancer diagnosis. The evidence in either direction remains too preliminary to alter the conclusion that the cumulative evidence of such an association is inadequate or insufficient.

Conclusion

On the basis of the evidence reviewed here and in previous VAO reports, the committee concludes that there is inadequate or insufficient evidence to determine whether there is an association between exposure to the COIs and bladder cancer.

RENAL CANCER

Cancers of the kidney other than the renal pelvis (ICD-9 189.0) and cancer of the renal pelvis (ICD-9 189.1) are often grouped in epidemiologic studies; cancer of the ureter (ICD-9 189.2) is sometimes also included. Although diseases of those organs have different characteristics and could have different risk factors, there is some logic to grouping them: the structures are all exposed to filterable chemicals, such as polycyclic aromatic hydrocarbons, that appear in urine. ACS estimated that 40,250 men and 24,520 women would receive diagnoses of renal cancer (ICD-9 189.0, 189.1) in the United States in 2012 and that 8,650 men and 4,920 women would die from it (Siegel et al., 2012). Those figures represent 2–4% of all new cancer diagnoses and cancer deaths. The average annual incidence of renal cancer is shown in Table 8-33.

Renal cancer is twice as common in men as in women. In the age groups that include most Vietnam veterans, black men have a higher incidence than do white men. With the exception of Wilms tumor, which is more likely to occur in children, renal cancer is more common in people over 50 years old.

Tobacco use is a well-established risk factor for renal cancer. People who have some rare syndromes—notably, von Hippel–Lindau syndrome and tuberous sclerosis—are at higher risk. Other potential risk factors include obesity, heavy acetaminophen use, kidney stones, and occupational exposure to asbestos, cadmium, and organic solvents. Firefighters, who are routinely exposed to numerous pyrolysis products, are in a known higher-risk group.

Conclusions from *VAO* and Previous Updates

The committee responsible for *VAO* concluded that there was inadequate or insufficient information to determine whether there is an association between exposure to the COIs and renal cancer. Additional information available to the committees responsible for *Update 1996*, *Update 1998*, *Update 2000*, *Update 2002*, *Update 2004*, *Update 2006*, *Update 2008*, and *Update 2010* did not change that conclusion.

Table 8-34 summarizes the results of the relevant studies.

TABLE 8-33 Average Annual Incidence (per 100,000) of Kidney and Renal Pelvis Cancer in the United States[a]

	55–59 Years Old			60–64 Years Old			65–69 Years Old		
	All Races	White	Black	All Races	White	Black	All Races	White	Black
Men	42.1	40.5	62.9	61.1	60.2	85.4	80.7	80.6	102.3
Women	20.5	20.5	24.6	28.5	29.3	33.1	36.3	35.9	48.2

[a]Surveillance, Epidemiology, and End Results program, nine standard registries, crude age-specific rates, 2005–2009 (NCI, 2013).

TABLE 8-34 Selected Epidemiologic Studies—Renal Cancer (Shaded Entries Are New Information for This Update)

Study Population[a]	Exposed Cases[b]	**Exposure of Interest**/Estimated Relative Risk (95% CI)[b]	Reference
VIETNAM VETERANS			
US Vietnam Veteran			
US CDC Vietnam Experience Study—Cross-sectional study, with medical examinations, of Army veterans: 9,324 deployed vs 8,989 nondeployed		**All COIs**	
Mortality			
1965–2000	1	nr	Boehmer et al., 2004
US VA Proportionate Mortality Study—sample of deceased male Vietnam-era Army and Marine veterans who served 7/4/1965–3/1/1973		**All COIs**	
1965–1982			Breslin et al., 1988
Army, deployed (n = 19,708) vs nondeployed (n = 22,904)	55	0.9 (0.5–1.5)	
Marine Corps, deployed (n = 4,527) vs nondeployed (n = 3,781)	13	0.9 (0.5–1.5)	
State Studies of US Vietnam Veterans			
Massachusetts Vietnam veterans diagnosed 1972–1983	9	1.8 (1.0–3.5)	Kogan and Clapp, 1988
Michigan Vietnam-era veterans, PM study of deaths (1974–1989)—deployed vs nondeployed	21	1.4 (0.9–2.2)	Visintainer et al., 1995
923 White male Vietnam veterans with **Wisconsin** death certificate (1968–1978) vs proportions for Vietnam-era veterans (includes lymphosarcoma, reticulosarcoma)	2	nr	Anderson et al., 1986
International Vietnam-Veteran Studies			
Australian Vietnam Veterans—58,077 men and 153 women served on land or in Vietnamese waters during 5/23/1962–7/1/1973 vs Australian population		**All COIs**	
Incidence			
All branches, 1982–2000	125	1.0 (0.8–1.2)	ADVA, 2005a
Navy	34	1.3 (0.9–1.7)	
Army	77	0.9 (0.7–1.1)	
Air Force	14	1.1 (0.6–1.8)	
Mortality			
All branches, return–2001	50	1.0 (0.7–1.2)	ADVA, 2005b
Navy	12	1.1 (0.6–1.9)	
Army	33	0.9 (0.6–1.3)	
Air Force	5	0.8 (0.3–1.8)	
1980–1994	22	1.2 (0.7–1.8)	

TABLE 8-34 Renal Cancer, continued

Study Population[a]	Exposed Cases[b]	**Exposure of Interest**/Estimated Relative Risk (95% CI)[b]	Reference
Australian Conscripted Army National Service (18,940 deployed vs 24,642 nondeployed)		**All COIs**	
Incidence—1982–2000	19	0.7 (0.4–1.0)	ADVA, 2005c
Mortality			
1966–2001	4	0.4 (0.1–1.1)	
1982–1994	3	3.9 (nr)	CDVA, 1997b
OCCUPATIONAL—INDUSTRIAL			
IARC Phenoxy Herbicide Cohort—Workers exposed to any phenoxy herbicide or chlorophenol (production or spraying) vs respective national mortality rates		**Dioxin, phenoxy herbicides**	
Mortality 1939–1992	29	1.1 (0.7–1.6)	Kogevinas et al., 1997
13,831 exposed to highly chlorinated PCDDs	26	1.6 (1.1–2.4)	
7,553 not exposed to highly chlorinated PCDDs	3	0.3 (0.1–0.9)	
Mortality 1955–1988 of 12,492 production workers and 5,898 sprayers exposed—13,482 in exposed subcohort	11	1.0 (0.5–1.7)	Saracci et al., 1991
British MCPA Plant—Production 1947–1982 (n = 1,545) (included in IARC cohort) and spraying 1947–1972 (n = 2,561) (*not* included in IARC cohort)		**MCPA**	
Mortality through 1983	5	1.0 (0.3–2.3)	Coggon et al., 1986
Danish Production Workers (3,390 men and 1,069 women involved in production of phenoxy herbicides unlikely to contain TCDD at 2 plants in 1947–1987) (in IARC cohort)		**Dioxins, but TCDD unlikely; 2,4-D, 2,4-DP, MCPA, MCPP**	
Incidence 1943–1982 (men only)	3	0.6 (nr)	Lynge, 1985
Mortality 1955–2006	8	1.2 (0.8–1.6)	Boers et al., 2012
Dutch production workers in Plant A (549 men exposed during production 1955–1985; 594 unexposed) (in IARC cohort)		**Dioxins, 2,4,5-T, 2,4,5-TCP**	
Mortality 1955–2006 (HRs for lagged TCDD plasma levels)	8	0.8 (0.5–1.5)	Boers et al., 2012
Mortality 1955–2006	8	HR = "infinitively large"	Boers et al., 2010
Mortality 1955–1991	4	3.7 (1.0–9.5)	Hooiveld et al., 1998

continued

TABLE 8-34 Renal Cancer, continued

Study Population[a]	Exposed Cases[b]	**Exposure of Interest**/Estimated Relative Risk (95% CI)[b]	Reference
Total cohort—kidney cancer	4	4.1 (1.1–10.4)	
Total cohort—"urinary organs"	8	3.9 (0.7–7.6)	
German Production Workers at Boehringer–Ingelheim Plant in Hamburg (1,144 men working > 1 month in 1952–1984; generation of TCDD reduced after chloracne outbreak in 1954) and women—no results (some additions to observed cancers over Manz et al., 1991) (in IARC cohort as of 1997)		**Dioxins; 2,4,5-T; 2,4,5-TCP; 2,5-DCP**	
Mortality 1952–2007 (kidney and other and unspecified urinary organs)	9	2.1 (0.9–3.9)	Manuwald et al., 2012
Men	7	2.0 (0.8–4.1)	
Women	2	2.3 (0.3–8.1)	
Mortality 1952–1989—stats on men only, 1,184 (tables all for 1,148 men, not necessarily German nationals) vs national rates (also vs gas workers); same observation period as Becher et al., 1966	3	1.6 (0.3–4.6)	Manz et al., 1991
New Zealand Phenoxy Herbicide Production Workers and Sprayers (1,599 men and women working any time in 1969–1988 at Dow plant in New Plymouth) (in IARC cohort)		**Dioxins; 2,4-D; 2,4,5-T; MCPA; MCPB; 2,4,5-TCP; Picloram**	
Mortality 1969–2004			McBride et al., 2009a
Ever-exposed workers	3	2.3 (0.5–6.7)	
Production Workers (713 men and 100 women worked > 1 month in 1969–1984)			
Mortality 1969–2000	1	1.2 (0.0–6.6)	't Mannetje et al., 2005
Sprayers (697 men and 2 women registered any time 1973–1984)			
Mortality 1973–2000	3	2.7 (0.6–8.0)	't Mannetje et al., 2005
NIOSH Mortality Cohort (12 US plants, 5,172 male production and maintenance workers 1942–1984) (included in IARC cohort as of 1997)		**Dioxins, phenoxy herbicides**	
Through 1993	13	1.6 (0.8–2.7)	Steenland et al., 1999
Through 1987 (bladder, other)	8	1.4 (0.6–2.8)	Fingerhut et al., 1991
≥ 1-year exposure, ≥ 20-year latency	2	1.1 (0.1–3.8)	
All Dow TCP-Exposed Workers (TCP production 1942–1979 or 2,4,5-T production 1948–1982 in Midland, Michigan) (in IARC and NIOSH cohorts)		**2,4,5-T; 2,4,5-TCP**	
1942–2003 (n = 1,615)	2	0.4 (0.1–1.5)	Collins et al., 2009a

TABLE 8-34 Renal Cancer, continued

Study Population[a]	Exposed Cases[b]	**Exposure of Interest**/Estimated Relative Risk (95% CI)[b]	Reference
All Dow PCP-Exposed Workers—all workers from the two plants that only made PCP (in Tacoma, Washington, and Wichita, Kansas) and workers who made PCP and TCP at two additional plants (in Midland, Michigan, and Sauget, Illinois)		**2,4,5-T; 2,4,5-TCP**	Ruder and Yiin, 2011
1940–2005 (n = 2,122) (kidney, ICD-9 189.0–189.2)	8	1.2 (0.5–2.4)	
PCP and TCP (n = 720)	4	1.8 (0.5–4.6)	
PCP (no TCP) (n = 1,402)	4	0.9 (0.3–2.3)	
Dow 2,4-D Production Workers (1945–1982 in Midland, Michigan) (subset of all TCP-exposed workers)		**2,4-D, lower chlorinated dioxins**	
Cancer incidence through 2007 in Dow workers (n = 1,256) vs comparisons from state cancer registries (n = 23,354) (Cohort 3) (kidney, renal pelvis)	5	0.8 (0.3–1.8)	Burns et al., 2011
Through 1994 (n = 1,517)	2	0.9 (0.1–3.3)	Burns et al., 2001
Through 1982 (n = 878)	0	nr (0.0–6.2)	Bond et al., 1988
Dow PCP Production Workers (1937–1989 in Midland, Michigan) (not in IARC and NIOSH cohorts)		**Low chlorinated dioxins, 2,4-D**	
Mortality 1940–2004 (n = 577, excluding 196 also having exposure to TCP)	4	1.7 (0.5–4.4)	Collins et al., 2009b
OCCUPATIONAL—PAPER AND PULP WORKERS		**TCDD**	
IARC cohort of pulp and paper workers—60,468 workers from 11 countries, TCDD among 27 agents assessed by JEM			McLean et al., 2006
Exposure to nonvolatile organochlorine compounds			
Never	41	0.9 (0.7–1.3)	
Ever	18	0.5 (0.3–0.8)	
New Hampshire pulp and paper workers, 883 white men working ≥ 1 yr, mortality through July 1985	3	1.5 (0.3–4.4)	Henneberger et al., 1989
Pulp and Paper cohorts independent of IARC cohort			
Northwestern US paper and pulp workers—5 mills in Washington, Oregon, and California, 3,523 worked ≥ 1 yr 1945–1955, mortality through March 1977	6	*90% CI* 1.2 (0.5–3.0)	Robinson et al., 1986

continued

TABLE 8-34 Renal Cancer, continued

Study Population[a]	Exposed Cases[b]	**Exposure of Interest**/Estimated Relative Risk (95% CI)[b]	Reference
OCCUPATIONAL—HERBICIDE-USING WORKERS (*not* related to IARC sprayer cohorts)			
DENMARK			
Danish farmers—incidence from linking farmers on 1970 census with national cancer registry (1970–1980)		**Herbicides**	Ronco et al., 1992
Men			
Self-employed	141	0.6 ($p < 0.05$)	
Employee	18	0.4 ($p < 0.05$)	
Women			
Self-employed	4	0.9 (nr)	
Employee	3	1.0 (nr)	
Family Worker	30	0.8 (nr)	
Danish gardeners—incidence from 3,156 male and 859 female gardeners (urinary system, ICD-7 180–181)			Hansen et al., 2007
25-year followup (1975–2001)		**Herbicides**	
Born before 1915 (high exposure)	25	1.1 (0.7–1.6)	
Born 1915–1934 (medium exposure)	23	0.5 (0.4–0.8)	
Born after 1934 (low exposure)	1	0.2 (0.0–1.1)	
10-year followup (1975–1984) of male gardeners (lymphohematopoietic, ICD-7 200–2005)	18	0.9 (0.7–1.8)	Hansen et al., 1992
ITALIAN Licensed Pesticide Users—male farmers in southern Piedmont licensed 1970–1974			
Mortality 1970–1986 (n = 23,401)	16	0.6 (0.4–1.0)	Torchio et al., 1994
NEW ZEALAND National Cancer Registry (1980–1984)—case-control study of incident stomach cancer cases vs remainder of 19,904 men with any incident cancer			Reif et al., 1989
Forestry workers (n = 134)		**Herbicides**	
	2	0.6 (0.2–2.3)	
SWEDEN			
Incident cancer cases 1961–1973 with agriculture as economic activity in 1960 census (male, female)	775	*99% CI* 0.8 (0.7–0.9)	Wiklund, 1983
THE NETHERLANDS			
Dutch Licensed Herbicide Sprayers—1,341 certified before 1980			
Through 2000	4	1.3 (0.4–3.4)	Swaen et al., 2004

TABLE 8-34 Renal Cancer, continued

Study Population[a]	Exposed Cases[b]	**Exposure of Interest**/Estimated Relative Risk (95% CI)[b]	Reference
UNITED STATES			
US farmers—usual occupation of farmer and industry of agriculture on death certificates 1984–1988 from 23 states		**Herbicides** PCMRs	Blair et al., 1993
Men			
Whites (n = 119,648)	522	1.1 (1.0–1.2)	
Nonwhites (n = 11,446)	30	0.8 (0.5–1.1)	
Women			
Whites (n = 2,400)	6	0.8 (0.3–1.7)	
Nonwhites (n = 2,066)	6	1.4 (0.5–3.1)	
US Agricultural Health Study—prospective study of licensed pesticide sprayers in Iowa and North Carolina: commercial (n = 4,916), private/farmers (n = 52,395, 97.4% men), and spouses of private sprayers (n = 32,347, 0.007% men), enrolled 1993–1997; followups with CATIs 1999–2003 and 2005–2010		**Phenoxy herbicides**	
Incidence			
Enrollment through 2006—SIRs for participants			Koutros et al., 2010a
Private applicators	148	0.8 (0.7–1.0)	
Commercial applicators	2	nr	
Spouses	39	0.7 (0.5–1.0)	
Mortality			
Enrollment through 2007, vs state rates			Waggoner et al., 2011
Applicators (n = 1,641)	71	0.9 (0.7–1.1)	
Spouses (n = 676)	12	0.6 (0.3–1.1)	
US Department of Agriculture Workers—nested case-control study of white men dying 1970–1979 of NHL		**Herbicides**	
Agricultural extension agents	nr	1.7 (0.9–3.3)	Alavanja et al., 1988
Forest conservationists		p- trend < over years worked	Alavanja et al., 1989
	2.3	0.1	
Soil conservationists	2.1	0.6	
Florida Licensed Pesticide Applicators (common phenoxy use assumed but not documented; had been listed by Blair et al., 1983)		**Herbicides**	
Pesticide applicators in Florida licensed 1965–1966 (n = 3,827)—mortality through 1976	1	0.5 (nr)	Blair et al., 1983

continued

TABLE 8-34 Renal Cancer, continued

Study Population[a]	Exposed Cases[b]	**Exposure of Interest**/Estimated Relative Risk (95% CI)[b]	Reference
White Male Residents of Iowa—NHL cancer on death certificate, usual occupation: farmers vs not		**Herbicides**	
> 20 yrs old when died 1971–1978—PMR	178	1.1 (ns)	Burmeister, 1981
ENVIRONMENTAL			
Seveso, Italy Residential Cohort—Industrial accident July 10, 1976 (723 residents Zone A; 4,821 Zone B; 31,643 Zone R; 181,574 local reference group) (ICD-9 171)		**TCDD**	
Incidence			
20-yr followup to 1996—men and women			Pesatori et al., 2009
Zone B	6	0.9 (0.4–2.0)	
Zone R	43	0.9 (0.7–1.2)	
10-yr followup to 1991 (kidney, other urinary organs)			Bertazzi et al., 1993
Zone R—men	10	0.9 (0.4–1.7)	
Zone R—women	7	1.2 (0.5–2.7)	
10-yr followup to 1991—men			Pesatori et al., 1992
Zone A, B	0	nr	
Zone R	11	0.9 (0.5–1.7)	
10-yr followup to 1991—women			
Zone A, B	1	1.1 (0.2–8.1)	
Zone R	7	1.2 (0.5–2.6)	
Mortality			
25-yr followup to 2001—men and women			Consonni et al., 2008
Zone A	0	nr	
Zone B	3	0.6 (0.2–2.0)	
Zone R	39	1.2 (0.8–1.6)	
20-yr followup to 1996			Bertazzi et al., 2001
Zones A and B—men	3	0.8 (0.3–2.6)	
Zones A and B—women	3	1.8 (0.6–5.8)	
CASE-CONTROL STUDIES			
International Case-Control Studies			
Danish Cancer Registry patients (n = 365) and 396 referents, occupational herbicide exposure		**Herbicides**	Mellemgaard et al., 1994
Men	13	1.7 (0.7–4.3)	
Women	3	5.7 (0.6–58.0)	

TABLE 8-34 Renal Cancer, continued

Study Population[a]	Exposed Cases[b]	**Exposure of Interest**/Estimated Relative Risk (95% CI)[b]	Reference
UK men, 18–35 yrs of age from counties with particular chemical manufacturing—mortality		**Herbicides, chlorophenols**	Magnani et al., 1987
Herbicides	nr	1.3 (0.6–3.1)	
Chlorophenols	nr	0.9 (0.4–1.9)	

NOTE: 2,4-D, 2,4-dichlorophenoxyacetic acid; 2,4-DP, dichlorprop; 2,4,5-T, 2,4,5-trichlorophenoxyacetic acid; 2,4,5-TCP, 2,4,5-trichlorophenol; 2,5-DCP, 2,5-dichlorophenol; CATI, computer-assisted telephone interviewing; CDC, Centers for Disease Control and Prevention; CI, confidence interval; COI, chemical of interest; HR, hazard ratio; IARC, International Agency for Research on Cancer; ICD, International Classification of Diseases; JEM, job-exposure matrix; MCPA, 2-methyl-4-chlorophenoxyacetic acid; MCPB, 4-(4-chloro-2-methylphenoxy)butanoic acid; MCPP, methylchlorophenoxypropionic acid; NHL, non-Hodgkin lymphoma; NIOSH, National Institute for Occupational Safety and Health; nr, not reported; PCDD, polychlorinated dibenzo-*p*-dioxin (highly chlorinated, if four or more chlorines); PCMR, proportionate cancer mortality ratios; PCP, pentachlorophenol; PMR, proportional mortality ratio; SIR, standardized incidence ratio; TCDD, 2,3,7,8-tetrachlorodibenzo-*p*-dioxin; TCP, trichlorophenol; VA, US Department of Veterans Affairs.

[a]Subjects are male, and outcome is mortality unless otherwise noted.

[b]Given when available; results other than estimated risk explained individually.

Update of the Epidemiologic Literature

Vietnam-Veteran, Environmental, and Case-Control Studies

No Vietnam-veteran studies, environmental studies, or case-control studies of exposure to the COIs and renal cancer have been published since *Update 2010*.

Occupational Studies

Burns et al. (2011) updated cancer incidence through 2007 in workers who were alive on January 1, 1985, and had been employed at any time from 1945 to 1994 in 2,4-D production by the Dow Chemical Company in Midland, Michigan. They found no evidence of significantly increased rates of cancer overall. With five cases observed, the incidence of cancer of the kidney or renal pelvis in the most restrictively defined cohort was not increased (SIR = 0.76, 95% CI 0.25–1.78), as was the case in the two successively more inclusive, but potentially more biased, cohorts.

Boers et al. (2012) provided a quantified, TCDD-based analysis of mortality updated through 2006 in male workers in two Dutch phenoxy-herbicide factories, which were considered in *Update 2010* (Boers et al., 2010). The 1,020 workers in factory A had been involved in production of 2,4,5-T with its associated TCDD contamination, whereas the 1,036 working in factory B had produced only phenoxy herbicides that would not have had TCDD contamination. Contemporary TCDD concentrations measured in a subsample of 187 workers were used to derive a model incorporating job history to estimate serum TCDD concentrations of all the men at the end of their employment. Using the estimated TCDD concentrations of the workers in both factories did not indicate increased mortality from renal cancer associated with TCDD (HR = 1.16, 95% CI 0.82–1.63). The dose–response modeling applied only to the workers in factory A did not find an increased renal-cancer mortality (HR = 0.83, 95% CI 0.46–1.49), whereas Boers et al. (2010) had been unable to calculate a risk of renal cancer because none of the eight deaths from renal cancer occurred in the workers in the nonexposed category.

Manuwald et al. (2012) reported mortality through 2007 in 1,191 men and 398 women who had been employed for at least 3 months during 1952–1984 in a chemical plant in Hamburg (a subcohort of the IARC phenoxy-herbicide cohort). During that period, the plant produced insecticides and herbicides, including 2,4,5-T, so cohort members had the possibility of exposure to TCDD. SMRs calculated relative to the population of Hamburg showed that mortality from cancer of the "kidney or other and unspecified urinary organs" was not increased in men (seven deaths, SMR = 2.00, 95% CI 0.80–4.12) or in women (two deaths, SMR = 2.25, 95% CI 0.25–8.11), but in the entire cohort the increase neared significance (SMR = 2.05, 95% CI 0.94–3.89).

Ruder and Yiin (2011) reported mortality in 1940–2005 in the NIOSH PCP cohort of 2,122 workers in the four US plants that had been involved in PCP production. PCP production entailed exposure to PCDDs and PCDFs but not to the most toxic 2,3,7,8 dioxin congener. A subcohort of 720 workers (all men, the PCP-plus-TCDD group) had also been employed in TCP production and so had also been exposed to TCDD. Relative to US referent rates, mortality from renal cancer was not substantially increased in the entire cohort (eight deaths, SMR = 1.20, 95% CI 0.52–2.37) or in the PCP-plus-TCDD group (four deaths, SMR = 1.80, 95% CI 0.49–4.61). In the larger PCP-only group, four deaths from renal cancer were reported (SMR = 0.90, 95% CI 0.25–2.31).

In the update of cancer incidence through 2006 in the AHS, Koutros et al. (2010a) reported decreased rates of renal cancer in both the private applicators (148 cases, SIR = 0.82, 95% CI 0.69–0.96) and their spouses (39 cases, SIR = 0.71, 95% CI 0.50–0.97). Similar findings were reported in Waggoner et al. (2011) in both applicators (71 cases, SIR = 0.87, 95% CI 0.68–1.09) and their spouses (12 cases, SIR = 0.61, 95% CI 0.32–1.07). The AHS has been generating valuable information on the COIs for a number of years, but these results are not herbicide-specific and so are not regarded as being fully informative for the committee's task.

Biologic Plausibility

No animal studies have reported an increased incidence of renal cancer after exposure to the COIs. Working with tissues from urothelial-cancer patients, Ishida et al. (2010) found that activation of the AHR pathway by TCDD enhances cancer-cell invasion by upregulating matrix metalloproteinase-1 and -9 expression and is associated with poor prognosis in upper urinary tract urothelial cancer. The biologic plausibility of the carcinogenicity of the COIs is discussed in general at the beginning of this chapter.

Synthesis

Available analyses of an association between exposure to the COIs and renal-cancer risk are limited by the small number of cases and lack of exposure specificity. No data have emerged since *Update 2010* to alter the committee's conclusion that the evidence is inadequate or insufficient to determine whether there is an association.

Conclusion

On the basis of the evidence reviewed here and in previous VAO reports, the committee concludes that there is inadequate or insufficient evidence to determine whether there is an association between exposure to the COIs and renal cancer.

BRAIN CANCER

Nervous-system cancers (ICD-9 191–192) involve the central nervous system (CNS) and include tumors of the brain and spinal cord, the cranial nerves, and the meninges (the outer coverings of the brain and spinal cord). Any of the cell types in the CNS can develop into cancer. Tumors of the peripheral nervous system and autonomic nervous system are considered soft-tissue tumors (ICD-9 171). Most cancers in the CNS are not primary tumors arising from nervous system tissues, but originated in other parts of the body, such as the lung or breast, and have metastasized to the brain or spinal cord. This section focuses on cancers that originate in the CNS.

Cancer of the eye (ICD-9 190) was considered in *Update 2006*, but the present committee decided that findings concerning cancer of the eye would be tracked with results on brain cancer because when it is reported it is often grouped with brain cancer.

The average annual incidence of primary CNS cancer is shown in Table 8-35. About 95% of cases originate in the brain, cranial nerves, and cranial meninges. In people over 45 years old, about 90% of tumors that originate in the brain are

TABLE 8-35 Average Annual Incidence (per 100,000) of Brain and Other Nervous System Cancers in the United States[a]

	55–59 Years Old			60–64 Years Old			65–69 Years Old		
	All Races	White	Black	All Races	White	Black	All Races	White	Black
Men	13.6	15.0	9.2	16.4	18.5	9.0	19.6	22.3	12.2
Women	7.9	8.7	5.7	11.0	12.2	7.0	13.1	14.5	9.4

[a]Surveillance, Epidemiology, and End Results program, nine standard registries, crude age-specific rates, 2005–2009 (NCI, 2013).

gliomas—astrocytoma, ependymoma, oligodendroglioma, or glioblastoma multiforme. Astrocytoma is the most common; glioblastoma multiforme has the worst prognosis. Meningiomas make up 20–40% of CNS cancers; they tend to occur in middle age and are more common in women than in men. Most meningiomas are benign and can be removed surgically.

ACS estimated that about 12,630 men and 10,280 women would receive diagnoses of brain and other nervous-system cancers in the United States in 2012 and that 7,720 men and 5,980 women would die from them (Siegel et al., 2012). Those numbers represent about 1.5% of new cancer diagnoses and 2.3% of cancer deaths. ACS estimated that 1,310 men and 1,300 women would receive diagnoses of cancers of the eye and orbit in the United States in 2012 and that 120 men and 150 women would die from them (Siegel et al., 2012).

In reviewing the descriptive epidemiology of these cancers, it is important to recognize the variation with which specific cancers are included in published reports, many of which distinguish between benign and malignant tumors. Another variation is whether cancers derived from related tissues (such as the pituitary or the eye) are included with CNS cancers. Various types of cancer are usually grouped; although this may bias results in unpredictable ways, the most likely consequence is dilution of risk estimates toward the null.

The only well-established environmental risk factor for brain tumors is exposure to high doses of ionizing radiation (ACS, 2012c; Wrensch et al., 2002). Other environmental exposures—such as to vinyl chloride, petroleum products, electromagnetic fields, and cell-phone use—are unproved as risk factors. The causes of most cancers of the brain and other portions of the nervous system are not known.

Conclusions from *VAO* and Previous Updates

The committee responsible for *VAO* concluded that there was limited or suggestive evidence of *no* association between exposure to the COIs and brain cancer. The committees responsible for *Update 1996*, *Update 1998*, *Update 2000*, *Update 2002*, and *Update 2004* did not change that conclusion.

The committee responsible for *Update 2006* changed the classification for brain cancer (formally expanding it to include cancers of the eye and orbit) to inadequate or insufficient evidence to determine whether there is an association between exposure to the COIs and brain cancer. That committee considered one study that suggested a relationship between phenoxy acid herbicides and adult gliomas (Lee et al., 2005); studies that reported slightly but not statistically significantly higher risks of brain cancer in deployed than in nondeployed Australian Vietnam-era veterans (ADVA, 2005a,b) and in pesticide applicators in the AHS (Alavanja et al., 2005); and several studies that had essentially neutral findings (Carreon et al., 2005; Magnani et al., 1987; McLean et al., 2006; Ruder et al., 2004; Torchio et al., 1994). Overall, the studies discussed in *Update 2006* suggested that a conclusion of *no* association between exposure to the COIs and brain cancer had been too definitive.

The committee for *Update 2008* agreed that brain cancers should remain in the inadequate or insufficient category after review of two new studies. The relevance of the largely null findings on association with occupational exposure to herbicides from a case-control study of gliomas and meningiomas (Samanic et al., 2008) was limited in that no specific compounds were addressed. In evaluating mortality through 2001 in the Seveso cohort, Consonni et al. (2008) found no increase in mortality from brain cancer in any of the three exposure zones with increasing exposure and no indication of a dose–response relationship.

Update 2010 considered several new studies. A study of Vietnam-era Army Chemical Corps veterans found no difference in brain cancer rates between deployed and nondeployed veterans (Cypel and Kang, 2010), and studies of TCP and 2,4,5-T production workers in two settings also found no difference in brain-cancer incidence (Collins et al., 2009a) or brain-cancer mortality (Collins et al., 2009b; McBride et al, 2009a) compared with general population rates. A 20-year followup of brain cancer after the Seveso exposure incident found a nonstatistically significantly increased rate of brain cancer in those in the closest zone (RR = 2.43, 95% CI 0.60–9.79), but not in Zones B and R (Pesatori et al., 2009).

Table 8-36 summarizes the results of the relevant studies.

Update of the Epidemiologic Literature

Vietnam-Veteran and Environmental Studies

No Vietnam-veteran studies or environmental studies of exposure to the COIs and brain cancer have been published since *Update 2010*.

Occupational Studies

Burns et al. (2011) updated cancer incidence through 2007 in workers who were alive on January 1, 1985, and had been employed at any time from 1945 to 1994 in 2,4-D production by the Dow Chemical Company in Midland, Michigan. They found no evidence of significantly increased rates of cancer overall. Three brain-cancer cases were identified; this was not significantly different from popu-

TABLE 8-36 Selected Epidemiologic Studies—Brain Tumors (Shaded Entries Are New Information for This Update)

Study Population[a]	Exposed Cases[b]	**Exposure of Interest**/Estimated Relative Risk (95% CI)[b]	Reference
VIETNAM VETERANS			
US Vietnam Veterans			
US Air Force Health Study—Ranch Hand veterans vs SEA veterans (unless otherwise noted)		**All COIs**	
Incidence			
Through 1999—White subjects vs national rates (brain and nervous system)			Akhtar et al., 2004
Ranch Hand veterans (n = 1,189)	5	1.8 (0.7–4.1)	
With tours between 1966–1970	5	2.2 (0.8–4.8)	
SEA comparison veterans (n = 1,776)	2	0.5 (0.1–1.8)	
With tours between 1966–1970	2	0.7 (0.1–2.3)	
Mortality			
Through 1999—White subjects vs national rates			Akhtar et al., 2004
Ranch Hand veterans (n = 1,189)	3	1.3 (0.3–3.6)	
SEA comparison veterans (n = 1,776)	1	0.3 (nr)	
US VA Cohort of Army Chemical Corps—Expanded as of 1997 to include all Army men with chemical MOS (2,872 deployed vs 2,737 nondeployed) serving during Vietnam era (7/1/1965–3/28/1973)		**All COIs**	
Mortality—brain tumors			
Through 2005			Cypel and Kang, 2010
Deployed veterans (2,872) vs nondeployed (2,737)	4 vs 2	1.7 (0.3–10.2)	
ACC veterans vs US men			
Vietnam cohort	4	0.9 (0.2–2.2)	
Non-Vietnam cohort	2	0.5 (0.1–2.0)	
Through 1991	2	1.9 (nr)	Dalager and Kang, 1997
894 ACC members assigned to Vietnam in 1966–1971—Through 1987	2	nr	Thomas and Kang, 1990
US CDC Vietnam Experience Study—Cross-sectional study, with medical examinations, of Army veterans: 9,324 deployed vs 8,989 nondeployed		**All COIs**	
Mortality			
1965–2000 (meninges, brain, other CNS)	9	1.2 (0.4–3.2)	Boehmer et al., 2004
Post-service–1983	3	nr	Boyle et al., 1987

TABLE 8-36 Brain Tumors, continued

Study Population[a]	Exposed Cases[b]	**Exposure of Interest**/Estimated Relative Risk (95% CI)[b]	Reference
US VA Proportionate Mortality Study—sample of deceased male Vietnam-era Army and Marine veterans who served 7/4/1965–3/1/1973		**All COIs**	
1965–1982			Breslin et al., 1988
Army, deployed (n = 19,708) vs nondeployed (n = 22,904)	116	1.0 (0.3–3.2)	
Marine Corps, deployed (n = 4,527) vs nondeployed (n = 3,781)	25	1.1 (0.2–7.1)	
US VA Cohort of Female Vietnam Veterans		**All COIs**	
Mortality—brain, CNS			
Through 2004 (all female Vietnam veterans)	8	2.0 (0.7–5.9)	Cypel and Kang, 2008
Vietnam veteran nurses only	8	3.6 (0.9–14.5)	
Through 1991	4	1.4 (0.4–3.7)	Dalager et al., 1995
State Studies of US Vietnam Veterans			
Michigan Vietnam-era veterans, PM study of deaths (1974–1989)—deployed vs nondeployed	36	1.1 (0.8–1.5)	Visintainer et al., 1995
New York			
—deployed vs nondeployed (brain, CNS)	4	0.5 (0.2–1.5)	Lawrence et al., 1985
923 White male Vietnam veterans with **Wisconsin** death certificate (1968–1978) vs proportions for Vietnam-era veterans	8	0.8 (0.3–1.5)	Anderson et al., 1986a,b
International Vietnam-Veteran Studies			
Australian Vietnam Veterans—58,077 men and 153 women served on land or in Vietnamese waters during 5/23/1962–7/1/1973 vs Australian population		**All COIs**	
Incidence			
All branches, 1982–2000 (brain)	97	1.1 (0.9–1.2)	ADVA, 2005a
Navy	24	1.2 (0.7–1.7)	
Army	63	1.0 (0.8–1.3)	
Air Force	10	1.1 (0.6–2.1)	
Mortality			
All branches, return–2001 (brain, CNS)	99	1.0 (0.8–1.1)	ADVA, 2005b
Navy	23	1.0 (0.6–1.4)	
Army	66	0.9 (0.7–1.2)	
Air Force	9	0.9 (0.4–1.6)	
1980–1994	39	1.1 (0.7–1.4)	CDVA, 1997a
Australian Conscripted Army National Service (18,940 deployed vs 24,642 nondeployed)		**All COIs**	
Incidence (brain, CNS)			

continued

TABLE 8-36 Brain Tumors, continued

Study Population[a]	Exposed Cases[b]	**Exposure of Interest**/Estimated Relative Risk (95% CI)[b]	Reference
1982–2000	23	1.4 (0.7–2.6)	ADVA, 2005c
Mortality (brain, CNS)			
1966–2001	27	1.6 (0.9–3.1)	ADVA, 2005c
1982–1994	13	1.4 (nr)	CDVA, 1997b
OCCUPATIONAL—INDUSTRIAL			
IARC Phenoxy Herbicide Cohort—Workers exposed to any phenoxy herbicide or chlorophenol (production or spraying) vs respective national mortality rates			
Mortality 1939–1992	22	0.7 (0.4–1.0)	Kogevinas et al., 1997
13,831 exposed to highly chlorinated PCDDs	12	0.6 (0.3–1.1)	
7,553 not exposed to highly chlorinated PCDDs	10	0.8 (0.4–1.5)	
Mortality 1955–1988 of 12,492 production workers and 5,898 sprayers exposed—13,482 in exposed subcohort	6	0.4 (0.1–0.8)	Saracci et al., 1991
British MCPA Plant—Production 1947–1982 (n = 1,545) (included in IARC cohort) and spraying 1947–1972 (n = 2,561) (*not* included in IARC cohort)		**MCPA**	
Mortality through 1983 (brain, CNS)	11	1.2 (0.6–2.2)	Coggon et al., 1986
Danish Production Workers (3,390 men and 1,069 women involved in production of phenoxy herbicides unlikely to contain TCDD at 2 plants in 1947–1987) (in IARC cohort)		**Dioxins, but TCDD unlikely; 2,4-D, 2,4-DP, MCPA, MCPP**	
Incidence 1943–1982	4	0.7 (nr)	Lynge, 1985
German Production Workers at Bayer Plant in Uerdingen (135 men working > 1 month in 1951–1976) (in IARC cohort as of 1997) and women—no results		**Dioxins; 2,4,5-TCP**	
Mortality 1951–1992	0	—	Becher et al., 1996
German Production Workers at Bayer Plant in Dormagen (520 men working > 1 month in 1965–1989) (in IARC cohort as of 1997) and women—no results		**Dioxins; 2,4-D; 2,4,5-T; MCPA; MCPP; 2,4-DP**	
Mortality 1965–1989	0	—	Becher et al., 1996

TABLE 8-36 Brain Tumors, continued

Study Population[a]	Exposed Cases[b]	**Exposure of Interest**/Estimated Relative Risk (95% CI)[b]	Reference
German Production Workers at BASF Ludwigshafen Plant (680 men working > 1 month in 1957–1987) (in IARC cohort as of 1997) and women—no results		**Dioxins; 2,4-D; 2,4,5-T; MCPA; MCPP; 2,4-DP**	
Mortality 1956–1989	0	—	Becher et al., 1996
German Production Workers at Boehringer–Ingelheim Plant in Hamburg (1,144 men working > 1 month in 1952–1984; generation of TCDD reduced after chloracne outbreak in 1954) and women—no results (some additions to observed cancers over Manz et al., 1991) (in IARC cohort as of 1997)		**Dioxins; 2,4,5-T; 2,5-DCP; 2,4,5-TCP**	
Mortality 1952–1989	3	2.3 (0.5–6.8)	Becher et al., 1996
New Zealand Phenoxy Herbicide Production Workers and Sprayers (1,599 men and women working any time in 1969–1988 at Dow plant in New Plymouth) (in IARC cohort)		**Dioxins; 2,4-D; 2,4,5-T; MCPA; MCPB; 2,4,5-TCP; Picloram**	
Mortality 1969–2004			McBride et al., 2009a
Ever-exposed workers	4	2.0 (0.6–5.2)	
Never-exposed workers	0	0.0 (0.0–5.5)	
Production Workers (713 men and 100 women worked > 1 month in 1969–1984)			
Mortality 1969–2000	1	0.8 (0.0–4.6)	't Mannetje et al., 2005
Sprayers (697 men and 2 women on register of New Zealand applicators, 1973–1984)			
Mortality 1973–2000	1	0.6 (0.0–3.4)	't Mannetje et al., 2005
NIOSH Mortality Cohort (12 US plants, 5,172 male production and maintenance workers 1942–1984) (included in IARC cohort as of 1997)		**Dioxins, phenoxy herbicides**	
Through 1993 (brain, CNS)	8	0.8 (0.4–1.6)	Steenland et al., 1999
Through 1987 (brain, CNS)			Fingerhut et al., 1991
≥ 1-year exposure, ≥ 20-year latency	2	1.1 (0.1–3.8)	
All Dow TCP-Exposed Workers (TCP production 1942–1979 or 2,4,5-T production 1948–1982 in Midland, Michigan) (in IARC and NIOSH cohorts)		**2,4,5-T; 2,4,5-TCP**	
1942–2003 (n = 1,615)	3	0.6 (0.1–1.7)	Collins et al., 2009a

continued

TABLE 8-36 Brain Tumors, continued

Study Population[a]	Exposed Cases[b]	**Exposure of Interest**/Estimated Relative Risk (95% CI)[b]	Reference
1940–1994 (n = 2,187 men)	nr	0.6 (0.1–1.8)	Bodner et al., 2003
All Dow PCP-Exposed Workers—all workers from the two plants that only made PCP (in Tacoma, Washington, and Wichita, Kansas) and workers who made PCP and TCP at two additional plants (in Midland, Michigan, and Sauget, Illinois)		**2,4,5-T; 2,4,5-TCP**	Ruder and Yiin, 2011
1940–2005 (n = 2,122) (brain, other nervous system)	6	0.9 (0.3–1.9)	
PCP and TCP (n = 720)	1	0.4 (0.0–2.4)	
PCP (no TCP) (n = 1,402)	5	1.1 (0.4–2.6)	
Dow 2,4-D Production Workers (1945–1982 in Midland, Michigan) (subset of all TCP-exposed workers)		**2,4-D, lower chlorinated dioxins**	
Cancer incidence through 2007 in Dow workers (n = 1,256) vs comparisons from state cancer registries (n = 23,354) (Cohort 3) (brain, other CNS)	3	1.1 (0.2–3.2)	Burns et al., 2011
Through 1994 (n = 1,517)	3	1.1 (0.1–3.2)	Burns et al., 2001
Through 1982 (n = 878) (brain, other system tissues)	0	nr (0.0–4.1)	Bond et al., 1988
Dow PCP Production Workers (1937–1989 in Midland, Michigan) (*not* in IARC and NIOSH cohorts)		**Low chlorinated dioxins, 2,4-D**	
Mortality 1940–2004 (n = 577, excluding 196 also having exposure to TCP)	1	0.4 (0.0–2.3)	Collins et al., 2009b
Mortality 1940–1989 (n = 770)			Ramlow et al., 1996
0-yr latency	1	nr	
15-yr latency	1	nr	
OCCUPATIONAL—PAPER AND PULP WORKERS		**TCDD**	
IARC cohort of pulp and paper workers—60,468 workers from 11 countries, TCDD among 27 agents assessed by JEM			McLean et al., 2006
Exposure to nonvolatile organochlorine compounds			
Never	44	1.0 (0.7–1.4)	
Ever	28	0.8 (0.5–1.2)	
New Hampshire pulp and paper workers, 883 white men working ≥ 1 yr, mortality through July 1985	2	1.2 (0.1–4.2)	Henneberger et al., 1989

TABLE 8-36 Brain Tumors, continued

Study Population[a]	Exposed Cases[b]	**Exposure of Interest**/Estimated Relative Risk (95% CI)[b]	Reference
Northwestern US paper and pulp workers—5 mills in Washington, Oregon, and California, 3,523 worked ≥ 1 yr 1945–1955, mortality through March 1977	4	0.6 (0.2–2.1)	Robinson et al., 1986
OCCUPATIONAL—HERBICIDE-USING WORKERS (*not* related to IARC sprayer cohorts)			
CANADA			
Canadian Farm Operator Study—156,242 men farming in Manitoba, Saskatchewan, and Alberta in 1971; mortality from brain cancer June 1971–December 1987			
210 histologically confirmed deaths attributed to brain cancer in farmers ≥ 35 yrs of age			Morrison et al., 1992
Herbicides sprayed on ≥ 250 acres vs 0 acres	24	0.8 (0.5–1.2)	
70,000 male Saskatchewan farmers identified in 1971 census data linked to mortality records (brain)	96	1.0 (0.8–1.3)	Wigle et al., 1990
DENMARK			
Danish Farmers—incidence from linking farmers on 1970 census with national cancer registry (1970–1980)		**Herbicides**	Ronco et al., 1992
Men			
Self-employed	194	1.1 (nr)	
Employee	39	0.9 (nr)	
Women			
Self-employed	5	1.0 (nr)	
Employee	2	0.5 (nr)	
FINNISH Phenoxy Herbicide Sprayers (1,909 men working 1955–1971 ≥ 2 wks) *not* IARC (eye, brain)		**Phenoxy Herbicides**	
Incidence	3	0.7 (0.1–2.0)	Asp et al., 1994
Mortality 1972–1989	3	1.2 (0.3–3.6)	
ITALIAN Licensed Pesticide Users—male farmers in southern Piedmont licensed 1970–1974			
Mortality 1970–1986 (n = 23,401)			Torchio et al., 1994
Brain, nervous system	15	0.5 (0.3–0.9)	
Eye	4	2.4 (0.7–6.1)	
Italian rice growers with documented phenoxy use (n = 1,487) (brain, CNS)		**Phenoxy herbicides**	Gambini et al., 1997
	4	0.9 (0.2–2.3)	

continued

TABLE 8-36 Brain Tumors, continued

Study Population[a]	Exposed Cases[b]	**Exposure of Interest**/Estimated Relative Risk (95% CI)[b]	Reference
NEW ZEALAND National Cancer Registry (1980–1984)—case-control study of incident brain cancer cases vs remainder of 19,904 men with any incident cancer		**Herbicides**	Reif et al., 1989
Forestry workers (n = 134) (brain, CNS)	4	1.2 (0.4–3.3)	
SWEDEN			
Swedish lumberjacks—used phenoxys 1954–1967, Incidence 1958–1992			Thörn et al., 2000
Exposed (n = 154)	0	—	
Foremen (n = 15)	0	—	
Lumberjacks (n = 139)	0	—	
Unexposed lumberjacks (n = 241)	1	0.9 (0.0–5.1)	
THE NETHERLANDS			
Dutch Licensed Herbicide Sprayers—1,341 certified before 1980			
Through 2000	4	1.6 (0.4–4.1)	Swaen et al., 2004
Through 1987	3	3.2 (0.6–9.3)	Swaen et al., 1992
UNITED STATES			
US farmers—usual occupation of farmer and industry of agriculture on death certificates 1984–1988 from 23 states		**Herbicides** PCMRs	Blair et al., 1993
Men			
Whites (n = 119,648)			
Brain	447	1.2 (1.1–1.3)	
Eye	17	1.6 (0.9–2.5)	
Nonwhites (n = 11,446) (brain)	16	1.0 (0.6–1.6)	
Women			
Whites (n = 2,400) (brain)	9	1.1 (0.5–2.1)	
Nonwhites (n = 2,066) (brain)	1	0.4 (0.0–2.1)	
US Agricultural Health Study—prospective study of licensed pesticide sprayers in Iowa and North Carolina: commercial (n = 4,916), private/farmers (n = 52,395, 97.4% men), and spouses of private sprayers (n = 32,347, 0.007% men), enrolled 1993–1997; followups with CATIs 1999–2003 and 2005–2010		**Phenoxy herbicides**	
Incidence			
Enrollment through 2006—SIRs for participants			Koutros et al., 2010a
Private applicators	51	0.8 (0.6–1.0)	
Commercial applicators	5	1.2 (0.4–2.8)	
Spouses	26	0.9 (0.6–1.4)	

TABLE 8-36 Brain Tumors, continued

Study Population[a]	Exposed Cases[b]	**Exposure of Interest**/Estimated Relative Risk (95% CI)[b]	Reference
Enrollment through 2002			Alavanja et al., 2005
Private applicators	33	0.8 (0.6–0.8)	
Spouses of private applicators (> 99% women)	15	0.9 (0.5–1.4)	
Commercial applicators	5	1.9 (0.6–4.3)	
Mortality			
Enrollment through 2007, vs state rates			Waggoner et al., 2011
Applicators (n = 1,641) (brain, other nervous system)	59	0.8 (0.6–1.0)	
Spouses (n = 676)	25	0.8 (0.5–1.2)	
Enrollment through 2000, vs state rates			Blair et al., 2005a
Private applicators (men and women)	19	0.7 (0.4–1.1)	
Years handled pesticides			
≤ 10 yrs	5	0.9 (ns)	
> 10 yrs	12	0.6 (ns)	
Spouses of private applicators (> 99% women)	11	1.1 (0.5–1.8)	
US Department of Agriculture Workers—nested case-control study of white men dying 1970–1979 of brain cancer		**Herbicides**	
Agricultural extension agents	nr	1.0 (0.4–2.4)	Alavanja et al., 1988
Forest conservationists	6	1.7 (0.6–3.7)	Alavanja et al., 1989
Soil conservationists			
Pesticide applicators in Florida licensed 1965–1966 (n = 3,827)—mortality through 1976	5	**Herbicides** 2.0 (nr)	Blair et al., 1983
White Male Residents of Iowa—brain cancer on death certificate, usual occupation: farmers vs not		**Herbicides**	
> 20 yrs old when died 1971–1978—PMR	111	1.1 (ns)	Burmeister, 1981
ENVIRONMENTAL			
Seveso, Italy Residential Cohort—Industrial accident July 10, 1976 (723 residents Zone A; 4,821 Zone B; 31,643 Zone R; 181,574 local reference group) (ICD-9 171)		**TCDD**	
Incidence			
20-yr followup to 1996—men and women			
Zone A	2	2.4 (0.6–9.8)	Pesatori et al., 2009
Zone B	4	0.8 (0.3–2.1)	
Zone R	37	1.0 (0.7–1.5)	
10-yr followup to 1991—men			Bertazzi et al., 1993
Zone R	6	0.6 (0.3–1.4)	
10-yr followup to 1991—women			Bertazzi et al., 1993
Zone R	6	1.4 (0.6–3.4)	

continued

TABLE 8-36 Brain Tumors, continued

Study Population[a]	Exposed Cases[b]	**Exposure of Interest**/Estimated Relative Risk (95% CI)[b]	Reference
Mortality			
25-yr followup to 2001—men and women			Consonni et al., 2008
Zone A	0	nr	
Zone B	3	0.7 (0.2–2.1)	
Zone R	34	1.1 (0.8–1.6)	
20-yr followup to 1996			Bertazzi et al., 2001
Zones A, B—men	1	0.4 (0.1–3.0)	
Zones A, B—women	3	1.9 (0.6–6.0)	
15-yr followup to 1991—men			Bertazzi et al., 1998
Zone B	1	0.8 (0.1–5.5)	
Zone R	12	1.3 (0.7–2.5)	
15-yr followup to 1991—women			Bertazzi et al., 1998
Zone B	3	3.2 (1.0–10.3)	
Zone R	8	1.1 (0.5–2.4)	
10-yr followup to 1986—men			Bertazzi et al., 1989a
Zone A, B, R	5	1.2 (0.4–3.1)	
10-yr followup to 1986—women			Bertazzi et al., 1989a
Zone A, B, R	5	2.1 (0.8–5.9)	
Other International Environmental Studies			
SWEDEN			
Swedish fishermen (high consumption of fish with persistent organochlorines)		**Organochlorine compounds**	Svensson et al., 1995
Incidence			
East coast	3	0.5 (0.1–1.5)	
West coast	24	0.9 (0.6–1.4)	
Mortality			
East coast	2	0.6 (0.1–2.1)	
West coast	15	1.1 (0.6–1.7)	
CASE-CONTROL STUDIES			
US Case-Control Studies			
NIOSH UMHS—farm pesticide exposure and glioma risk in adults (18–80 yrs of age) living in Iowa, Michigan, Minnesota, Wisconsin (glioma cases diagnosed 1995–January 1997)		**Arsenicals, phenoxy herbicides, 2.4-D**	
798 glioma cases vs 1,175 population-based controls (excluding proxy, 438 vs 1,141)			Yiin et al., 2012
Herbicide use—including proxy (160 vs 265)		0.8 (0.6–1.0)	
Herbicide use—excluding proxy (90 vs 260)		0.8 (0.6–1.1)	
341 female glioma cases vs 528 population-based controls			Carreon et al., 2005
Arsenicals	13	1.0 (0.5–1.9)	
Phenoxy herbicides	25	0.9 (0.5–1.5)	
2,4-D	24	0.9 (0.5–1.6)	

TABLE 8-36 Brain Tumors, continued

Study Population[a]	Exposed Cases[b]	**Exposure of Interest**/Estimated Relative Risk (95% CI)[b]	Reference
457 male glioma cases vs 648 population-based controls			Ruder et al., 2004
Arsenicals	15	0.7 (0.4–1.4)	
Phenoxy herbicides	67	0.9 (0.6–1.2)	
2,4-D	nr	nr	
US hospital-based study of 462 glioma and 195 meningioma patients vs 765 patient controls; cumulative lifetime occupational exposure to herbicides vs unexposed		**Herbicides**	Samanic et al., 2008
Gliomas			
Men	65	0.9 (0.6–1.3)	
Low quartile	20	1.0 (0.5–1.9)	
Second quartile	16	1.0 (0.5–2.1)	
Third quartile	12	0.6 (0.3–1.3)	
Fourth quartile	17	0.8 (0.4–1.6)	
		p-trend = 0.50	
Women	35	1.3 (0.8–2.0)	
Below median	23	1.5 (0.8–2.7)	
Above median	12	1.0 (0.5–2.1)	
		p-trend = 0.91	
Meningiomas (women only)	33	2.4 (1.4–4.3)	
Below median	16	2.1 (1.0–4.4)	
Above median	17	2.9 (1.3–6.2)	
		p-trend = 0.01	
Nebraska men and women diagnosed with gliomas between 1988 and 1993; association between farming and pesticide use (251 cases vs 498 controls)			Lee et al., 2005
Phenoxy herbicides—combined reports (identical with results for 2,4-D specifically)	32	1.8 (1.0–3.3)	
By self	7	0.6 (0.2–1.6)	
By proxy	25	3.3 (1.5–7.2)	
2,4,5-T—combined reports	7	1.3 (0.5–3.6)	
By self	2	0.4 (0.1–2.3)	
By proxy	5	2.7 (0.7–9.8)	
International Case-Control Studies			
Irish farmers and farmworkers		**Herbicides**	Dean, 1994
Men	195	nr	
Women	72	nr	
Italian hospital-based study of 240 brain glioma patients vs 742 controls		**Herbicides**	Musicco et al., 1988
Male, female farmers	61	1.6 (1.1–2.4)	
French hospital-based study of 125 brain glioma patients vs 238 controls		**Herbicides**	Cordier et al., 1988
Woodworkers		OR = 1.6 ($p > 0.05$)	

continued

TABLE 8-36 Brain Tumors, continued

Study Population[a]	Exposed Cases[b]	**Exposure of Interest**/Estimated Relative Risk (95% CI)[b]	Reference
UK men, 18–35 yrs of age from counties with particular chemical manufacturing—mortality		**Herbicides, chlorophenols**	Magnani et al., 1987
Herbicides	nr	1.2 (0.7–2.1)	
Chlorophenols	nr	1.1 (0.7–1.8)	

NOTE: 2,4-D, 2,4-dichlorophenoxyacetic acid; 2,4-DP, dichlorprop; 2,4,5-T, 2,4,5-trichlorophenoxyacetic acid; 2,4,5-TCP, 2,4,5-trichlorophenol; ACC, Army Chemical Corps; CATI, computer-assisted telephone interviewing; CDC, Centers for Disease Control and Prevention; CI, confidence interval; CNS, central nervous system; COI, chemical of interest; IARC, International Agency for Research on Cancer; ICD, International Classification of Diseases; JEM, job-exposure matrix; MCPA, 2-methyl-4-chlorophenoxyacetic acid; MCPB, 4-(4-chloro-2-methylphenoxy)butanoic acid; MCPP, methylchlorophenoxypropionic acid; MOS, military occupation specialty; NIOSH, National Institute for Occupational Safety and Health; nr, not reported; ns, not statistically significant; OR, odds ratio; PCDD, polychlorinated dibenzo-*p*-dioxin (highly chlorinated, if four or more chlorines); PCMR, proportionate cancer mortality ratios; PCP, pentachlorophenol; PMR, proportional mortality ratio; SEA, Southeast Asia; SIR, standardized incidence ratio; TCDD, 2,3,7,8-tetrachlorodibenzo-*p*-dioxin; TCP, trichlorophenol; VA, US Department of Veterans Affairs.

[a]Subjects are male and outcome is mortality unless otherwise noted.

[b]Given when available; results other than estimated risk explained individually.

lation rates in any of three approaches used by Burns et al. for handling possible movement of workers outside of Michigan. In the cohort defined with the most stringency the SIR was 1.09 (95% CI 0.22–3.19).

Mortality in a cohort of 2,122 PCP production workers in four plants in the NIOSH Dioxin Registry was compared with US population rates (Ruder and Yiin, 2011). Causes of death were determined by nosologist review of death certificates or linkage with the National Death Index. In the total cohort, six deaths were attributed to cancers of the brain and other parts of the CNS; this was consistent with mortality in the US population (SMR = 0.89, 95% CI 0.33–1.94). There was only one death from this type of cancer in the PCP-plus-TCDD group, and this also was not more than expected (SMR = 0.43, 95% CI 0.01–2.41). The results in the 1,402 workers in the PCP-only group were similar and again generally uninformative (SMR = 1.13, 95% CI 0.37–2.64).

In the AHS, no difference in the incidence of brain cancer through 2006 was observed in private applicators (SIR = 0.78, 95% CI 0.58–1.03), in commercial applicators (SIR = 1.19, 95% CI 0.39–2.78), or in spouses (SIR = 0.94, 95% CI 0.61–1.37) (Koutros et al., 2010a). Similar results were reported when Waggoner et al. (2011) compared the AHS cohort's mortality through 2007 with the mortality in the general populations in Iowa and North Carolina. Mortality from brain and other nervous system cancers was not increased in pesticide applicators (SMR = 0.76, 95% CI 0.58–0.98) or in their spouses (SMR = 0.83, 95% CI 0.54–1.23). The AHS has been generating valuable information on the COIs for a number of years, but these results are not herbicide-specific and so are not regarded as being fully informative for the committee's task.

Case-Control Studies

In the NIOSH Upper Midwest Health Study, Yiin et al. (2012) analyzed risk factors for 798 glioma cases identified in Iowa, Michigan, Minnesota, and Wisconsin from medical facilities and screening of state cancer registries. Controls (1,175) were randomly selected from state driver's license and nondriver ID records and Health Care Financing Administration Medicare data and were frequency-matched by state and age group. Over 90% of eligible cases and over 70% of eligible controls participated. Histories of use of specific pesticides and job histories were collected by questionnaire, which was administered to a proxy if a person was unable to complete the questionnaire. No increased risk of glioma was seen in association with use of herbicides in general, phenoxy herbicides, or most specifically 2,4-D, whether self-reported exposure or exposure based on industrial-hygienist assessment of job history was used. In some cases, significant reductions in risk were seen, although these did not remain significant in analyses that excluded data from proxy respondents.

In an older study that was not previously reviewed, Cordier et al. (1988) analyzed 125 glioma cases and 238 controls (65% and 71% participation, respectively) recruited from a hospital in France. Occupations and work descriptions were obtained by questionnaire. A nonsignificantly increased risk of glioma with adjustment for age and residence was seen in woodworkers (OR = 1.6, 95% CI not provided, but $p > 0.05$), a group potentially exposed to organochlorine-based preservatives that include chlorophenols and dioxins. In a post hoc exploratory analysis of the 20 woodworkers (nine cases, 11 controls), there was a trend ($p < 0.10$) toward greater odds of glioma with exposure to the chemicals as determined by blinded review of the work descriptions, but these findings need to be interpreted with caution given the small numbers of woodworkers and the post hoc nature of the analysis.

Several other case-control studies explored the association between pesticide exposure and brain cancer, but the unclear methods and the lack of exposure specificity beyond "pesticides" limited the informativeness of these studies with reference to the COIs (Bhat et al., 2010; Prochazka et al., 2010; Rashid et al., 2010).

Biologic Plausibility

No animal studies have reported an association between exposure to the COIs and brain cancer. The biologic plausibility of the carcinogenicity of the COIs is discussed in general at the beginning of this chapter.

Synthesis

Since *Update 2010*, several studies relevant to the possibility of an association between the COIs and brain cancer have been identified, including cohort and case-control studies. Most recent studies do not identify a relationship between exposure to the COIs and the development of brain cancers. A few studies are somewhat suggestive of an association, but these studies have limited exposure specificity or limited precision because of small sample size.

Conclusion

On the basis of the epidemiologic evidence from new and previously reported studies of populations that had potential exposure to the COIs, the committee concludes that there is inadequate or insufficient evidence to determine whether there is an association between exposure to the COIs and brain cancer or other nervous system cancers.

ENDOCRINE CANCERS

Cancers of the endocrine system as grouped by the Surveillance, Epidemiology, and End Results program (see Table B-2 in Appendix B) have a disparate group of ICD codes: thymus cancer (ICD-9 164.0), thyroid cancer (ICD-9 193), and other endocrine cancer (ICD-9 194).

ACS estimated that 13,250 men and 43,210 women would receive diagnoses of thyroid cancer in the United States in 2012 and that 780 men and 1,000 women would die from it, and it estimated that 1,350 men and 1,170 women would receive diagnoses of other endocrine cancers in 2012 and that 460 men and 460 women would die from them (Siegel et al., 2012). Incidence data on cancers of the endocrine system are presented in Table 8-37.

Thyroid cancer is the most prevalent endocrine cancer. Many types of tumors can develop in the thyroid, most of them benign. The thyroid contains two

TABLE 8-37 Average Annual Incidence (per 100,000) of Endocrine System Cancer in the United States[a]

	55–59 Years Old			60–64 Years Old			65–69 Years Old		
	All Races	White	Black	All Races	White	Black	All Races	White	Black
Men	14.7	15.3	10.0	16.1	16.7	11.2	18.5	19.5	11.1
Women	31.8	32.2	21.3	31.9	32.9	24.2	34.0	34.0	26.0

[a]Surveillance, Epidemiology, and End Results program, nine standard registries, crude age-specific rates, 2005–2009 (NCI, 2013).

main types of cells: follicular cells make and store thyroid hormones and make thyroglobulin; C cells make the hormone calcitonin, which helps to regulate calcium metabolism. Different cancers of varied severity can develop from each kind of cell, and the classification of thyroid cancer is still evolving (Liu et al., 2006; Nikiforov, 2011). Papillary carcinoma is the most common and usually affects women of childbearing age; it metastasizes slowly and is the least malignant type of thyroid cancer. Follicular carcinoma accounts for about 15% of all cases and has greater rates of recurrence and metastasis. Medullary carcinoma is a cancer of parafollicular cells in the thyroid and tends to occur in families; it requires treatment different from other types of thyroid cancer. Anaplastic carcinoma (also called giant-cell cancer and spindle-cell cancer) is rare but is the most aggressive form of thyroid cancer; it does not respond to radioiodine therapy and metastasizes quickly, invading such nearby structures as the trachea and causing compression and breathing difficulties.

Thyroid cancer can occur in all age groups. Radiation exposure is recognized as a risk factor for thyroid cancer, so increased incidence is observed in people who received radiation therapy directed at the neck (a common treatment in the 1950s for enlarged thymus, adenoids, and tonsils and for skin disorders) or who were exposed to iodine-125 from the Chernobyl nuclear power plant accident. If radiation exposure occurred in childhood, the risk of thyroid cancer is further increased. Other risk factors are a family history of thyroid cancer and chronic goiter.

Conclusions from *VAO* and Previous Updates

The committees responsible for *VAO*, *Update 1996*, *Update 1998*, *Update 2000*, *Update 2002*, and *Update 2004* did not consider endocrine cancers separately and therefore reached no conclusion as to whether there was an association between exposure to the COIs and endocrine cancers. The committees responsible for *Update 2006*, *Update 2008*, and *Update 2010* did consider endocrine cancers separately and concluded that there was inadequate or insufficient evidence to determine whether there is an association between the COIs and endocrine cancers.

Table 8-38 summarizes the pertinent results of the relevant studies.

Update of the Epidemiologic Literature

Vietnam-Veteran, Environmental, and Case-Control Studies

No Vietnam-veteran studies, environmental studies, or case-control studies of exposure to the COIs and thyroid or other endocrine cancers have been published since *Update 2010*.

TABLE 8-38 Selected Epidemiologic Studies—Endocrine Cancers (Thyroid, Thymus, and Other) (Shaded Entries Are New Information for This Update)

Study Population[a]	Exposed Cases[b]	**Exposure of Interest**/Estimated Relative Risk (95% CI)[b]	Reference
VIETNAM VETERANS			
US Vietnam Veterans			
US VA Proportionate Mortality Study—sample of deceased male Vietnam-era Army and Marine veterans who served 7/4/1965–3/1/1973			**All COIs**
1965–1982 (thyroid and other endocrine, ICD-9 193–194)			Breslin et al.,1986, 1988
Army, deployed (n = 19,708) vs nondeployed (n = 22,904)	15	0.6 (0.3–1.2)	
Marine Corps, deployed (n = 4,527) vs nondeployed (n = 3,781)	4	0.6 (0.1–3.4)	
State Studies of US Vietnam Veterans			
Massachusetts Vietnam-era veterans			
Veterans aged 35–65 years in 1993—cases diagnosed 1988–1993 vs thyroid cancer	4	1.2 (0.3–4.5)	Clapp, 1997
International Vietnam-Veterans Studies			
Australian Vietnam Veterans—58,077 men and 153 women served on land or in Vietnamese waters during 5/23/1962–7/1/1973 vs Australian population		**All COIs**	
Incidence—thyroid			
All branches, 1982–2000	17	0.6 (0.3–0.9)	ADVA, 2005a
Navy	3	0.5 (0.1–1.3)	
Army	11	0.5 (0.3–1.0)	
Air Force	3	1.2 (0.2–3.5)	
Mortality—thyroid			
All branches, return–2001	2	0.5 (0.0–1.8)	ADVA, 2005b
Navy	1	1.2 (0.0–6.5)	
Army	1	0.4 (0.0–2.0)	
Air Force	0	0.0 (0.0–7.8)	
Australian Conscripted Army National Service (18,940 deployed vs 24,642 nondeployed)		**All COIs**	
Incidence—thyroid			
1982–2000	4	0.6 (0.1–2.2)	ADVA, 2005c
Mortality—thyroid			
1966–2001	1	1.2 (0.0–91.7)	ADVA, 2005c
OCCUPATIONAL—INDUSTRIAL			
IARC Phenoxy Herbicide Cohort—Workers exposed to any phenoxy herbicide or chlorophenol (production or spraying) vs respective national mortality rates			

TABLE 8-38 Endocrine Cancers (Thyroid, Thymus, and Other), continued

Study Population[a]	Exposed Cases[b]	**Exposure of Interest**/Estimated Relative Risk (95% CI)[b]	Reference
Mortality 1939–1992			Kogevinas et al., 1997
Thyroid (ICD-9 193)	4	1.7 (0.5–4.3)	
13,831 exposed to highly chlorinated PCDDs	2	1.4 (0.2–4.9)	
7,553 not exposed to highly chlorinated PCDDs	2	2.2 (0.3–7.9)	
Other endocrine organs (ICD-9 194)	5	3.6 (1.2–8.4)	
13,831 exposed to highly chlorinated PCDDs	2	2.3 (0.3–8.1)	
7,553 not exposed to highly chlorinated PCDDs	3	6.4 (1.3–18.7)	
British MCPA Plant—Production 1947–1982 (n = 1,545) (included in IARC cohort) and spraying 1947–1972 (n = 2,561) (*not* included in IARC cohort)		**MCPA**	
Mortality through 1983 (thyroid)	1	1.8 (0.4–9.8)	Coggon et al., 1986
New Zealand Phenoxy Herbicide Production Workers and Sprayers (1,599 men and women working any time in 1969–1988 at Dow plant in New Plymouth) (in IARC cohort)		**Dioxins; 2,4-D; 2,4,5-T; MCPA; MCPB; 2,4,5-TCP; Picloram**	
Mortality 1969–2004 (thyroid, other endocrine)			McBride et al., 2009a
Ever-exposed workers	0	0.0 (0.0–19.8)	
Production Workers (713 men and 100 women worked > 1 month in 1969–1984)			
Mortality 1969–2000	0	nr	't Mannetje et al., 2005
Sprayers (697 men and 2 women registered any time 1973–1984)			
Mortality 1973–2000	0	nr	't Mannetje et al., 2005
NIOSH Mortality Cohort (12 US plants, 5,172 male production and maintenance workers 1942–1984) (included in IARC cohort as of 1997)		**Dioxins, phenoxy herbicides**	
Dow 2,4-D Production Workers (1945–1982 in Midland, Michigan) (subset of all TCP-exposed workers)		**2,4-D, lower chlorinated dioxins**	
Through 1982 (n = 878)	0	nr	Bond et al., 1988
Dow PCP Production Workers (1937–1989 in Midland, Michigan) (*not* in IARC and NIOSH cohorts)		**Low chlorinated dioxins, 2,4-D**	
Mortality 1940–1989 (n = 770)	0	nr	Ramlow et al., 1996

continued

TABLE 8-38 Endocrine Cancers (Thyroid, Thymus, and Other), continued

Study Population[a]	Exposed Cases[b]	**Exposure of Interest**/Estimated Relative Risk (95% CI)[b]	Reference
OCCUPATIONAL—HERBICIDE-USING WORKERS (*not* related to IARC sprayer cohorts)			
CANADA			
Herbicide sprayers routinely exposed to herbicides for 6 months or more (1950–1982)	1	**Phenoxy herbicides** nr	Green, 1991
DENMARK			
Danish Farmers—incidence from linking farmers on 1970 census with national cancer registry (1970–1980)		**Herbicides**	Ronco et al., 1992
Men			
Self-employed	13	0.7 (nr)	
Employee	5	1.1 (nr)	
Women			
Self-employed	1	1.3 (nr)	
Employee	1	1.4 (nr)	
Family worker	15	1.7 ($p < 0.05$)	
FINNISH Phenoxy Herbicide Sprayers (1,909 men working 1955–1971 ≥ 2 wks), *not* IARC		**Phenoxy herbicides**	
Incidence (thyroid, other endocrine)			Asp et al., 1994
No latency	2	1.9 (0.3–7.0)	
10-yr latency	2	2.4 (0.3–8.6)	
15-yr latency	2	3.4 (0.4–12.2)	
Mortality (thyroid)			
No latency	1	3.8 (0.1–21.3)	
10-yr latency	1	4.7 (0.1–26.4)	
15-yr latency	1	6.5 (0.2–36.2)	
ICELANDIC men (1,860), women (859) exposed to agricultural pesticides, primarily 2,4-D (other endocrine organs, ICD-9 194)—incidence	2	**2,4-D** 1.3 (0.1–4.7)	Zhong and Rafnsson, 1996
SWEDEN			
Swedish pesticide applicators—incidence	6	1.1 (0.4–2.4)	Wiklund et al., 1989a
Incident NHL cases 1961–1973 with agriculture as economic activity in 1960 census		*99% CI*	Wiklund, 1983
Thyroid	126	0.9 (0.7–1.1)	
Other endocrine gland	117	0.7 (0.5–0.9)	
UNITED STATES			
US farmers—usual occupation of farmer and industry of agriculture on death certificates 1984–1988 from 23 states		**Herbicides** PCMRs	Blair et al., 1993
Men			
Whites (n = 119,648)	39	1.3 (1.0–1.8)	
Nonwhites (n = 11,446)	1	0.6 (0.0–3.0)	
Women			

TABLE 8-38 Endocrine Cancers (Thyroid, Thymus, and Other), continued

Study Population[a]	Exposed Cases[b]	**Exposure of Interest**/Estimated Relative Risk (95% CI)[b]	Reference
Whites (n = 2,400)	1	0.8 (0.0–4.4)	
Nonwhites (n = 2,066)	1	1.1 (0.0–6.4)	
US Agricultural Health Study—prospective study of licensed pesticide sprayers in Iowa and North Carolina: commercial (n = 4,916), private/farmers (n = 52,395, 97.4% men), and spouses of private sprayers (n = 32,347, 0.007% men), enrolled 1993–1997; followups with CATIs 1999–2003 and 2005–2010		**Phenoxy herbicides**	
Incidence			
Enrollment through 2006—SIRs for participants			Koutros et al., 2010a
Private applicators	39	1.0 (0.7–1.3)	
Commercial applicators	5	1.4 (0.5–3.3)	
Spouses	49	0.9 (0.7–1.2)	
Enrollment through 2002 (thyroid, other endocrine)			Alavanja et al., 2005
Private applicators	29	1.3 (0.8–1.8)	
Spouses of private applicators (> 99% women)	24	0.9 (0.5–1.4)	
Commercial applicators	3	1.6 (0.3–5.0)	
Mortality			
Enrollment through 2007, vs state rates			Waggoner et al., 2011
Applicators (n = 1,641)	8	1.5 (0.7–3.0)	
Spouses (n = 676)	1	nr	
Enrollment through 2000, vs state rates (thyroid)			Blair et al., 2005a
Private applicators (men and women)	3	1.8 (0.4–5.3)	
Spouses of private applicators (> 99% women)	0	0.0 (0.0–2.2)	
ENVIRONMENTAL			
Seveso, Italy Residential Cohort—Industrial accident July 10, 1976 (723 residents Zone A; 4,821 Zone B; 31,643 Zone R; 181,574 local reference group) (ICD-9 171)		**TCDD**	
Incidence			
20-yr followup to 1996—men and women			
Zone A	1	2.6 (0.4–18.9)	Pesatori et al., 2009
Zone B	4	1.6 (0.6–4.4)	
Zone R	19	1.2 (0.7–1.9)	
Seveso population (1976–1996); incidence cases identified by hospital discharge records			

continued

TABLE 8-38 Endocrine Cancers (Thyroid, Thymus, and Other), continued

Study Population[a]	Exposed Cases[b]	**Exposure of Interest**/Estimated Relative Risk (95% CI)[b]	Reference
Zone A (prolactinoma)	1	6.2 (0.9–45.5)	Pesatori et al., 2008
Zone B (nonfunctioning pituitary tumors)	2	1.9 (0.5–7.7)	
Zone R (2 nonfunctioning pituitary adenomas and 3 prolactinomas)	5	0.7 (0.3–1.8)	
Mortality			
15-yr followup to 1991—men			Bertazzi et al., 1997, 1998
Zone B	1	4.9 (0.6–39.0)	
Zone R	0	nr	
15-yr followup to 1991—women			Bertazzi et al., 1997, 1998
Zone B	1	3.2 (0.4–24.5)	
Zone R	2	0.8 (0.2–3.6)	
CASE-CONTROL STUDIES			
International Case-Control Studies			
Sweden—male, female thyroid cancers from Swedish Cancer Registry, 1980–1989		**Phenoxy herbicides, chlorophenols**	Hallquist et al., 1993
Phenoxy herbicide exposure	3	0.5 (0.0–2.0)	
Chlorophenols	4	2.8 (0.5–18.0)	

NOTE: 2,4-D, 2,4-dichlorophenoxyacetic acid; 2,4,5-T, 2,4,5-trichlorophenoxyacetic acid; 2,4,5-TCP, 2,4,5-trichlorophenol; CATI, computer-assisted telephone interviewing; CDC, Centers for Disease Control and Prevention; CI, confidence interval; COI, chemical of interest; IARC, International Agency for Research on Cancer; ICD, International Classification of Diseases; MCPA, 2-methyl-4-chlorophenoxyacetic acid; MCPB, 4-(4-chloro-2-methylphenoxy)butanoic acid; NHL, non-Hodgkin lymphoma; NIOSH, National Institute for Occupational Safety and Health; nr, not reported; PCDD, polychlorinated dibenzo-*p*-dioxin (highly chlorinated, if four or more chlorines); PCMR, proportionate cancer mortality ratios; PCP, pentachlorophenol; SIR, standardized incidence ratio; TCDD, 2,3,7,8-tetrachlorodibenzo-*p*-dioxin; TCP, trichlorophenol; VA, US Department of Veterans Affairs.

[a]Subjects are male and outcome is mortality unless otherwise noted.

[b]Given when available; results other than estimated risk explained individually.

Occupational Studies

In the update of cancer incidence in the AHS through 2006, Koutros et al. (2010a) found that the incidence of thyroid cancer was not significantly increased in private applicators (39 cases, SIR = 0.98, 95% CI 0.69–1.33), in commercial applicators (five cases, SIR = 1.40, 95% CI 0.45–3.26), or in their spouses (49 cases, SIR = 0.90, 95% CI 0.67–1.19). Updated mortality in the AHS cohort through 2007 (Waggoner et al., 2011) included only one death from thyroid cancer in spouses, but eight deaths in applicators (SMR = 1.53, 95% CI 0.66–3.02). The AHS has been generating valuable information on the COIs for a number of years, but these results are not herbicide-specific and so are not regarded as being fully informative for the committee's task.

Biologic Plausibility

The NTP conducted carcinogenesis bioassays in Osborne-Mendel rats and B6C3F1 mice that were exposed to TCDD by gavage (NTP, 1982a). The incidence of follicular-cell adenoma, but not of carcinoma, increased with increasing TCDD dose in male and female rats; the increase was significant in male but not in female rats. There was a significant increase in follicular-cell adenoma in female but not in male mice. The NTP carried out a similar study in female Sprague-Dawley rats more recently (NTP, 2006), and Walker et al. (2006) compared the data from that study and the results of the Dow Chemical Company assessment of TCDD carcinogenicity (Kociba et al, 1978). In the NTP and Dow studies, the incidence of thyroid cancer (C-cell adenoma and carcinoma) decreased with increasing dose of TCDD. However, an increased incidence of slight thyroid follicular-cell hypertrophy was noted in rats that were given TCDD at 22 ng/kg of body weight or more. A more recent 2-year NTP study (Yoshizawa et al., 2010) treated female Sprague-Dawley rats with either TCDD, 2,3,4,7,8-pentachlorodibenzofuran, dioxin-like PCB congeners (PCB 126 or 118), a non-dioxin-like PCB (PCB 153), or mixtures of these chemicals; it failed to find any increases in either thyroid adenoma or carcinoma. Thus, although studies show that dioxin and dioxin-like compounds alter thyroid hormones and increase follicular-cell hyperplasia, there is little evidence of an increase in thyroid cancer.

As indicated in Chapter 4, 2,4-D and 2,4,5-T are at most weakly mutagenic or carcinogenic. No studies that addressed a possible association between exposure to those herbicides and thyroid cancer in animal models have been identified.

The biologic plausibility of the carcinogenicity of the COIs is discussed in general at the beginning of this chapter.

Synthesis

The studies reviewed previously did not provide sufficient evidence to determine whether there is an association between exposure to the COIs and thyroid or other endocrine cancers. The participants in the AHS are known to have had extensive exposure to the phenoxy herbicides, but the analyses of updated mortality (Waggoner et al., 2011) and cancer incidence (Koutros et al., 2010a) address only exposure to pesticides in general, so they cannot be considered fully informative for the purpose of this review. Consequently, the present committee retained the categorization for endocrine cancers assigned by previous VAO committees.

Conclusion

On the basis of the epidemiologic evidence reviewed here, the committee concludes that there is insufficient evidence to determine whether there is an association between exposure to the COIs and thyroid or other endocrine cancers.

LYMPHOHEMATOPOIETIC CANCERS

Lymphohematopoietic cancers (LHCs) constitute a heterogeneous group of clonal hematopoietic and lymphoid-cell disorders, including leukemias, lymphomas, and multiple myeloma. They are among the most common types of cancer induced by environmental and therapeutic agents. As in the case of other cancers that are subject to idiosyncratic grouping in reports of results of epidemiologic studies (notably, head and neck cancers and gastrointestinal cancers), the conclusions that the VAO committees have drawn about associations between herbicide exposure to the COIs and specific LHCs have been complicated and curtailed by the lack of specificity and by inconsistencies in groupings in the available evidence. For LHCs, that has been a function not only of epidemiologists' seeking to combine related cancers to produce categories that have enough cases to permit statistical analysis but also of alterations in the prevailing system used by the medical community to classify these malignancies. Categorization of cancers of the lymphatic and hematopoietic systems has continued to evolve, guided by growing information about gene expression and lineage of the clonal cancer cells that characterize each of a broad spectrum of neoplasms arising in these tissues (Jaffe, 2009). The World Health Organization (WHO) categorization presented in the *WHO Classification of Tumours of Haematopoietic and Lymphoid Tissue* (WHO, 2008) bases its primary partition on whether the cancer cells are of myeloid or lymphoid origin (see Figure 8-1).

Stem cells arising in the bone marrow generate two major lineages of leukocytes: myeloid and lymphoid. Myeloid cells include monocytes and three types of granulocytes (neutrophils, eosinophils, and basophils). Lymphoid cells include T and B lymphocytes and a smaller set of cells called natural killer (NK) cells. All those cells circulate in the blood and are collectively referred to as white blood cells or leukocytes. Monocytes move out of the bloodstream into inflamed tissues, where they differentiate into macrophages or dendritic cells. Stem cells that are destined to become T lymphocytes migrate from the bone marrow to the thymus, where they acquire antigen-specific receptors. Antigen stimulation induces the T cells to differentiate into the several types involved in cell-mediated immunity. Progenitor or pre-B cells mature in the bone marrow into antigen-specific B cells. On encountering their cognate antigens, B cells differentiate into antibody-secreting plasma cells involved in humoral immunity; these result in multiple myeloma when they undergo malignant transformation.

LHCs originate in specific pluripotent or lineage-restricted cells at different

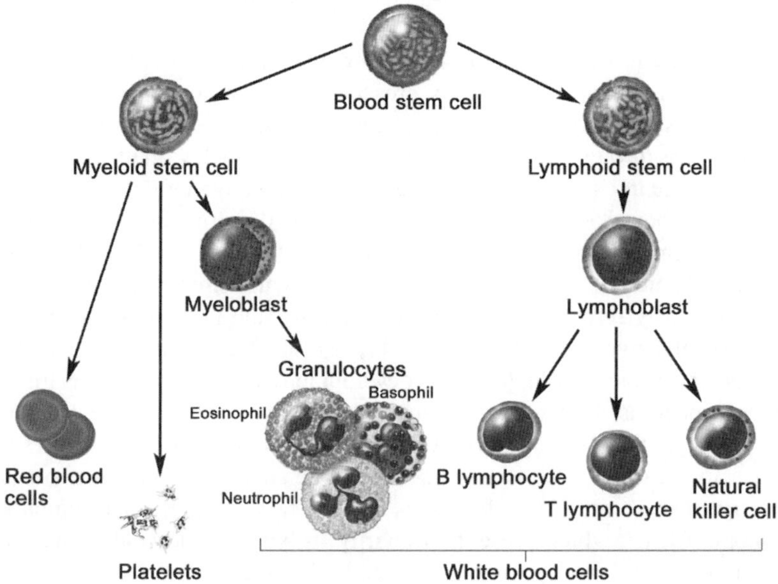

FIGURE 8-1 Hematopoiesis of stem cell differentiation.
SOURCE: © Terese Winslow, 2007; US government has certain rights.

stages in hematopoiesis and immune-cell development. The normal cells are transformed into a malignant tumor through multistep processes that involve genetic and epigenetic alterations. Traditionally, LHCs have been divided into leukemias, lymphomas, myelomas, and so on, according to their cell and site of origin (see Figure 8-1). That information and morphologic, cytochemical, and immunophenotypic data are used to characterize LHCs further by their distinct subtypes.

Leukemias occur when a cell residing in the bone marrow becomes cancerous and its daughter cells crowd normal cells in the bone marrow or are released from the bone marrow and circulate in the blood. Leukemias have generally been classified as myeloid or lymphoid, depending on the lineage of the original mutated cell. If the original mutated cell of a cancer of the blood arises in a lymphocytic cell line, the cancer is called lymphocytic leukemia; lymphocytic leukemias have been partitioned into acute lymphocytic leukemia (ALL) forms if they are derived from precursor B or T lymphoid cells, and indolent lymphoproliferative disorders (ILDs) derived from more mature lymphoid cells, which tend to replicate less rapidly. Although "chronic lymphocytic leukemia" is commonly used to refer to this group of ILDs, CLL is actually a specific form of ILD. Similarly, myeloid leukemias arise from a myeloid cell line and are classified into acute (AML) and chronic (CML) forms.

Lymphoma is a general term for cancers that arise from lymphocytes (B, T, or NK cells). Lymphomas generally present as solid tumors at lymphoid proliferative sites, such as lymph nodes and spleen. As stem cells mature into B or T cells, they pass through several developmental stages, each with unique functions. The developmental stage at which a cell becomes malignant defines the kind of lymphoma. About 85% of lymphomas are of B-cell origin, and 15% of NK-cell or T-cell origin, referred to as NKTCL by WHO (Jaffe et al., 2001) and Liao et al. (2012). There are two major types of B-cell lymphoma: Hodgkin lymphoma (HL), previously referred to as Hodgkin disease, and non-Hodgkin lymphoma (NHL). B cells give rise to a number of types of neoplasms that are given names based on the stage at which B-cell development was arrested when the cells became cancerous. Follicular, large-cell, and immunoblastic lymphomas result when a malignancy develops *after* a B cell has been exposed to antigens (such as bacteria and viruses). CLL is now believed to be a tumor of antigen-experienced (memory) B cells, not naïve B cells (Chiorazzi et al., 2005); small lymphocytic lymphoma (SLL), which presents primarily in lymph nodes rather than in the bone marrow and blood, is now considered to be the same disease as CLL at a different stage (Jaffe et al., 2008).

Myeloma is another type of lymphohematopoietic malignancy derived from antibody-secreting plasma cells, which also have a B-cell lineage, that accumulate in the marrow of various bones. In most cases (90%), tumors are formed at multiple sites, and the disease is called *multiple myeloma* (MM). The related premalignant condition AL amyloidosis also arises from B-cell–derived plasma cells. It occurs in 5–15% of patients who have MM and causes abnormal deposition of antibody fragments. Monoclonal gammopathy of undetermined significance (MGUS) is also recognized as a clonal condition that may progress to MM.

ICD partitions these malignancies into leukemias and lymphomas primarily on the basis of whether cancer cells circulated in the blood (disseminated) or appeared in the lymphatic system (solid tissue), respectively, before subdividing according to cell type. The emerging WHO classification of lymphohematopoietic malignancies (Campo et al., 2008; Jaffe, 2009) stratifies cancers of the blood and lymph nodes into disease categories according to their cell lineages—lymphoid or myeloid—as shown in Figure 8-1. It represents a substantial advance in understanding the biologic paths by which these cancers develop. The present committee decided, however, that it would not be productive to reformulate this entire section to correspond to the WHO categories. In practice, LHCs have routinely been reported in a variety of groupings, so it is a continuing challenge to parse out results, noting when results for broader groupings are presented in the results tables for several more specific diagnoses while recognizing that the specific results will be muted by being "misclassified" with other entities. Most epidemiologic studies already in the evidentiary database that did specify diseases precisely used ICD-9 or earlier versions, but some recent studies have applied ICD-10. Furthermore, the existing records that will serve as the basis of many current and even future studies will use earlier and evolving classifications, so this is likely to remain the case even in new literature for a considerable period. The nomenclature has become more uniform in recent studies, but the possibility of ambiguity remains if earlier researchers did not use a unique code in accordance with some established system.

Because it has been the objective of VAO committees to address disease entities in as great specificity as possible with the available data, overall results on the coarser grouping of LHCs are of little consequence for the conclusions of association that have been drawn for the more specific entities. The committee for *Update 2010* noted, however, that the common biologic origin of LHCs that have been judged to have a substantial amount of evidence supporting association with the COIs (HL, NHL, CLL, hairy cell leukemia [HCL], MM, and AL amyloidosis) means that the WHO approach is supportive of and consistent with these decisions on the part of VAO committees.

VA has asked previous VAO committees to address CLL, AML, and HCL individually. Scrutiny of the entire body of epidemiologic results on leukemia for findings on particular types (as had been the most common manner of grouping) revealed several studies that showed increased risks specifically of CLL (or ILDs more generally), but did not provide support for an association of AML with exposure to the COIs. The committee for *Update 2002* advised VA that CLL is recognized as a form of the already recognized-as-service-related condition NHL, whereas the committee for *Update 2006* did not recognize an association between the COIs and AML. Later, the committee responsible for *Update 2008* advised VA that HCL should be grouped with ILDs. In light of the history and in accord with the current WHO classification, the present committee has incorporated data specifically on CLL and HCL into the section on NHL. After a brief synopsis of biologic plausibility of the LHCs overall, the more common cancers of the lymphatic system are described in the sections below on HL, NHL, and MM (with a section on the related condition, AL amyloidosis), and then evidence on leukemias in general is discussed with a focus on information regarding those of myeloid origin.

Biologic Plausibility

Recent data indicate that the AHR pathway plays an integral role in B-cell maturation and that TCDD and dioxin-like chemical (DLC) exposure may alter the function of these cells and lead to critical changes in the immune response. Suppression of the immune response by TCDD and similar chemicals in rodents and primates has been known for over 30 years, but the effect on human cells is less clear. Some recent reports indicate that TCDD and DLCs elicit similar effects in humans. Activation of nontransformed human B cells results in an increase in expression of the AHR, and additional data indicate that this pathway has a role in normal B-cell function (Allan and Sherr, 2010). Furthermore, treatment of these cells with benzo[a]pyrene suppresses B-cell differentiation. Lu H et al. (2010) demonstrated that although human B cells appeared less responsive to TCDD in terms of increasing expression of AHR battery genes the ability of TCDD to decrease immunoglobulin M production was similar in both mouse and human B cells. Data on human hematopoietic stem cells (HSCs) and from the use of knockout AHR mouse models show that the AHR is critical in HSC maturation and differentiation (Fracchiolla et al., 2011; Singh et al., 2011). TCDD not only alters HSC maturation but also alters proliferation and migration in vivo and in vitro (Casado et al., 2011); this indicates that exposure may have multiple effects on how these immune cells function.

On occasion, the observed number of cases is so small that researchers cannot perform useful analyses for each type of LHC and will provide summary statistics for the entire group of them. In updating mortality in the Hamburg cohort in 1952–2007, Manuwald et al. (2012) found nonsignificant increases in mortality from LHC in both men (SMR = 1.53, 95% CI 0.89–2.45) and women (SMR = 1.84, 95% CI 0.74–3.80), which combined to give a significant association between TCDD and all LHC deaths in the whole cohort (SMR = 1.61, 95% CI 1.03–2.40). In a Dutch cohort of workers in two phenoxy-herbicide plants, Boers et al. (2012) assessed plasma TCDD concentrations at the time of the assumed last exposure and reported a modest but nearly significant increase in the hazard ratio for LHC in the total cohort (HR = 1.12, 95% CI 0.94–1.35) but no increase in plant A, where workers were occupationally exposed to TCDD (HR = 0.96, 95% CI 0.71–1.30).

Hodgkin Lymphoma

HL (ICD-9 201), also known as Hodgkin disease, is distinguished from NHL primarily on the basis of its neoplastic cells, mononucleated Hodgkin cells, and multinucleated Reed–Sternberg cells originating in germinal-center B cells (Küppers et al., 2002). HL's demographics and genetics are also characteristic. ACS estimated that 4,960 men and 4,100 women would receive diagnoses of HL in the United States in 2012 and that 670 men and 520 women would die from it (Siegel et al., 2012). The average annual incidence is shown in Table 8-39.

The possibility that HL has an infectious etiology has been a topic of discussion since its earliest description. A higher incidence in people who have a history of infectious mononucleosis has been observed in some studies, and a link with Epstein–Barr virus has been proposed. In addition to the occupational associations discussed below, higher rates of the disease have been observed in people who have suppressed or compromised immune systems.

TABLE 8-39 Average Annual Incidence (per 100,000) of Hodgkin Disease in the United States[a]

	55–59 Years Old			60–64 Years Old			65–69 Years Old		
	All Races	White	Black	All Races	White	Black	All Races	White	Black
Men	3.7	4.1	2.8	3.8	4.0	4.5	5.0	5.3	5.0
Women	1.9	1.7	3.9	2.1	2.2	2.4	3.7	4.1	4.3

[a]Surveillance, Epidemiology, and End Results program, nine standard registries, crude age-specific rates, 2005–2009 (NCI, 2013).

Conclusions from *VAO* and Previous Updates

The committee responsible for *VAO* determined that there were sufficient epidemiologic data to support an association between exposure to the COIs and HL. Additional studies available to the committees responsible for later updates have not changed that conclusion.

Of the 32 studies reviewed by the committee responsible for *VAO*, two well-conducted Swedish studies with good exposure characterization provide the most comprehensive information on the association between exposure to phenoxy herbicides (2,4-D and 2,4,5-T), picloram, or chlorophenols and HL. Hardell et al. (1981) considered NHL and HL together, and Hardell and Bengtsson (1983) considered HL separately; they found statistically significant associations with exposure to phenoxy acids (after excluding people who were exposed to chlorophenols) and with exposure to chlorophenols. In a study of 54 HL cases, Persson et al. (1989) found a large but not statistically significant risk associated with exposure to phenoxy acids. Several of the other case-control and occupational-cohort studies reviewed in *VAO* showed increased risk of HL, but only a few of the results were statistically significant. As with NHL, even the largest studies of production workers who were exposed to TCDD did not indicate an increased risk. The few studies of HL in Vietnam veterans tended to show increased risks, but only one (Holmes et al., 1986) was statistically significant.

Update 1996 reviewed studies that showed no excess of HL in the IARC phenoxy-herbicide cohort (Kogevinas et al., 1993) or in US farmers in 23 states (Blair et al., 1993). A smaller study of Finnish herbicide appliers (Asp et al., 1994) showed a nonsignificant increase, whereas Persson et al. (1993) reported a significant increase in Swedish farmers who were exposed to phenoxy acid herbicides. Studies of the Seveso cohort (Bertazzi et al., 1993) and of Vietnam-era veterans in Michigan (Visintainer et al., 1995) did not provide data that strengthened the association.

In *Update 1998*, a proportionate mortality ratio analysis that compared the experience of 33,833 US Army and Marine Corps Vietnam veterans who died during 1965–1988 with that of 36,797 deceased non-Vietnam veterans found a significant increase in Marine Corps veterans, but not Army veterans, who had served in Vietnam (Watanabe and Kang, 1996). Two studies of manufacturing workers found no association between TCDD and HL (Becher et al., 1996) or between PCP and HL (Ramlow et al., 1996). An update of the large IARC phenoxy herbicide cohort (Kogevinas et al., 1997) showed no association between phenoxy herbicides or chlorophenols and HL but did show a nonsignificant increase in HL in workers who were exposed to TCDD or higher-chlorinated hydrocarbons. Waterhouse et al. (1996) demonstrated a significant increase in the combined incidence of lymphopoietic neoplasms in a prospective study of a Michigan farming community. A 15-year followup study of the Seveso cohort (Bertazzi et al., 1997) found no deaths from HL in Zone A and a nonsignificant increase in deaths from HL in men and women in Zone B.

The committee responsible for *Update 2000* reviewed the 15-year update of the Operation Ranch Hand study (AFHS, 2000), but the findings on HL were nonsignificant. In a retrospective cohort study of Dutch production and contract workers who were exposed to phenoxy herbicides, chlorophenols, and contaminants during 1950–1976, Hooiveld et al. (1998) reported increased but nonsignificant findings. Rix et al. (1998) compared mortality in a cohort of Danish paper-mill workers with that in the general Danish population and found a statistically significant increase in men but not women. In an update and expansion of cohorts involved in the NIOSH study, Steenland et al. (1999) found that the three deaths attributed to HL were consistent with the number expected. The 20-year mortality update after the Seveso accident reported no additional HL deaths in Zone A or B (Bertazzi et al., 2001).

The only new study reviewed in *Update 2002* followed mortality to 1994 in a cohort of Dow Chemical Company workers (Burns et al., 2001); the single death attributed to HL resulted in a slight but nonsignificant increase.

Update 2004 reviewed a study by Akhtar et al. (2004) that found no excess of lymphopoietic cancers when comparing incidence and mortality between Ranch Hand veterans and veterans who had not served in Southeast Asia. Swaen et al. (2004) extended followup of mortality by 13 years in a cohort of Dutch herbicide appliers; with no additional deaths observed, the earlier increase in HL remained nonsignificant (Swaen et al., 1992).

Update 2006 reviewed reports on the cancer experience of Australian Vietnam veterans. In comparison with the general population, the incidence of HL was significantly higher when veterans from the different armed forces were combined (ADVA, 2005a); there was a significant association between HL and service in the Army, but Navy and Air Force veterans showed nonsignificant increases. Mortality from HL was nonsignificantly higher in the Army veterans but not in all veterans combined or in the other branches (ADVA, 2005b). A comparison of deployed and nondeployed Vietnam-era Australian conscripted

Army National Service veterans (ADVA, 2005c) found no association between deployment and the incidence of or mortality from HL. In a multinational IARC cohort of 60,468 pulp and paper industry workers, McLean et al. (2006) found that death from HL was significantly higher in those who had ever been exposed to nonvolatile organochlorine compounds (which would include TCDD) but not in those who had never been exposed. Two reports from the US AHS (Alavanja et al., 2005; Blair et al., 2005a) found no excess risk of HL in pesticide applicators, commercial applicators, and their spouses. In the Cross-Canada Study of Pesticides and Health, Pahwa et al. (2006) found no association of any exposure to phenoxy herbicides, 2,4-D, Mecoprop, or MCPA and HL.

The committee responsible for *Update 2008* reviewed a study by Cypel and Kang (2008) that compared mortality from lymphopoietic cancers in female Vietnam veterans with that of female era veterans and the US population; deaths from lymphopoietic cancers were not higher in those who served in Vietnam. Consonni et al. (2008) reported no statistically significant increase in deaths from HL in the Seveso cohort 25 years after the accident.

The committee for *Update 2010* reviewed several occupational cohorts, a case-control study, and an update of cancer incidence in the Seveso cohort. No deaths from HL were identified in Dow PCP workers in Midland, Michigan (Collins et al., 2009b), but the TCP workers (Collins et al., 2009a) had an increased SMR of HL with a wide confidence interval. McBride et al. (2009a) examined mortality in TCP manufacturing workers in the Dow AgroSciences plant in New Plymouth, New Zealand, but a single observed HL death yielded inconclusive results. A French hospital-based case-control study of lymphoid neoplasms (Orsi et al., 2009) found a modest increase in the risk of HL after occupational exposure to herbicides in general and a greater increase after occupational exposure to phenoxy herbicides in particular, but neither was statistically significant; no association was observed with domestic use of herbicides. In the 20-year followup of cancer incidence in the Seveso cohort (Pesatori et al., 2009), there were still no cases of HL in Zone A, whereas a modest nonsignificant increase in HL risk was found in Zone R and a less clear increase in Zone B.

Table 8-40 summarizes the results of the relevant studies.

Update of the Epidemiologic Literature

Vietnam-Veteran and Environmental Studies No Vietnam-veteran studies or environmental studies of exposure to the COIs and HL specifically have been published since *Update 2010*.

Occupational Studies Only a single case of HL was diagnosed in the period January 1987–December 2007 in 1,316 men who had worked at any time during 1945–1994 at Dow Chemical Company's 2,4-D production plant in Midland,

TABLE 8-40 Selected Epidemiologic Studies—Hodgkin Lymphoma (Shaded Entries Are New Information for This Update)

Study Population[a]	Exposed Cases[b]	Exposure of Interest/Estimated Relative Risk (95% CI)[b]	Reference
VIETNAM VETERANS			
US Vietnam Veterans			
US Air Force Health Study—Ranch Hand veterans vs SEA veterans (unless otherwise noted)		**All COIs**	
Incidence			
Through 1999—white subjects vs national rates (lymphopoietic cancer[c])			Akhtar et al., 2004
Ranch Hand veterans (n = 1,189)	10	0.9 (0.4–1.5)	
With tours between 1966–1970	7	0.7 (0.3–1.4)	
SEA comparison veterans (n = 1,776)	9	0.6 (0.3–1.0)	
With tours between 1966–1970	4	0.3 (0.1–0.8)	
Attended 1987 exam—Ranch Hand personnel (n = 995) vs SEA veterans (n = 1,299)	0	nr	Wolfe et al., 1990
Mortality			
Through 1987—Ranch Hand personnel (n = 1,261) vs SEA veterans (19,102)	0	nr	Michalek et al., 1990
US CDC Vietnam Experience Study—Cross-sectional study, with medical examinations, of Army veterans: 9,324 deployed vs 8,989 nondeployed		**All COIs**	
Mortality			
1965–2000	2	0.9 (nr)	Boehmer et al., 2004
Post-service–1983	0	nr	Boyle et al., 1987
US CDC Selected Cancers Study—case-control study of incidence (Dec 1, 1984–Nov 30, 1989) among US males born 1929–1953 (CDC, 1990a)		**All COIs**	CDC, 1990a
Vietnam veterans	28	1.2 (0.7–2.4)	
Army	12	1.0 (0.5–2.0)	
Marine Corps	4	1.7 (0.5–5.9)	
Air Force	5	1.7 (0.6–4.9)	
Navy	7	1.1 (0.4–2.6)	
US VA Proportionate Mortality Study—sample of deceased male Vietnam-era Army and Marine veterans who served 7/4/1965–3/1/1973		**All COIs**	
1965–1988			Watanabe and Kang, 1996
Army, deployed (n = 27,596) vs nondeployed (n = 31,757)	125	1.0 (nr)	
Marine Corps, deployed (n = 6,237) vs nondeployed (n = 5,040)	25	1.9 (1.2–2.7)	

TABLE 8-40 Hodgkin Lymphoma, continued

Study Population[a]	Exposed Cases[b]	**Exposure of Interest**/Estimated Relative Risk (95% CI)[b]	Reference
1965–1984			Watanabe et al., 1991
Army, deployed (n = 24,145) vs nondeployed (n = 27,917)			
Vs Army non-Vietnam veterans	116	1.0 (nr)	
Vs all non-Vietnam veterans	116	1.1 (nr)	
Marine Corps, deployed (n = 5,501) vs nondeployed (n = 4,505)			
Vs Marine non-Vietnam veterans	25	1.9 (nr)	
Vs all non-Vietnam veterans	25	1.0 (nr)	
1965–1982			Breslin et al., 1988
Army, deployed (n = 19,708) vs nondeployed (n = 22,904)	92	1.2 (0.7–1.9)	
Marine Corps, deployed (n = 4,527) vs nondeployed (n = 3,781)	22	1.3 (0.7–2.6)	
US VA Cohort of Female Vietnam Veterans		**All COIs**	
Mortality			
Through 2004	18	0.7 (0.4–1.3)	Cypel and Kang, 2008
Vietnam-veteran nurses	14	0.7 (0.3–1.3)	
State Studies of US Vietnam Veterans			
Michigan Vietnam-era veterans, PM study of deaths (1974–1989)—deployed vs nondeployed	20	1.1 (0.7–1.8)	Visintainer et al., 1995
New York—deployed vs nondeployed (lymphoma, HD)	10	*99% CI* 1.0 (0.4–2.2)	Lawrence et al., 1985
West Virginia—deployed vs nondeployed	5	8.3 (2.7–19.5)	Holmes et al., 1986
923 White male Vietnam veterans with **Wisconsin** death certificate (1968–1978) vs proportions for Vietnam-era veterans	4	nr	Anderson et al., 1986
International Vietnam-Veteran Studies			
Australian Vietnam Veterans—58,077 men and 153 women served on land or in Vietnamese waters during 5/23/1962–7/1/1973 vs Australian population		**All COIs**	
Incidence			
All branches, 1982–2000	51	2.1 (1.5–2.6)	ADVA, 2005a
Navy	7	1.3 (0.5–2.6)	
Army	40	2.3 (1.6–3.0)	
Air Force	4	2.1 (0.6–5.3)	
Mortality			
All branches, return–2001	13	0.9 (0.5–1.5)	ADVA, 2005b
Navy	2	0.6 (0.1–2.1)	
Army	11	1.1 (0.5–1.9)	
Air Force	0	0.0 (0.0–2.9)	

continued

TABLE 8-40 Hodgkin Lymphoma, continued

Study Population[a]	Exposed Cases[b]	**Exposure of Interest**/Estimated Relative Risk (95% CI)[b]	Reference
Australian Conscripted Army National Service (18,940 deployed vs 24,642 nondeployed)		**All COIs**	
Incidence			
1982–2000	12	0.9 (0.4–2.0)	ADVA, 2005c
Mortality			
1982–2000	12	0.9 (0.4–2.0)	ADVA, 2005c
1966–2001	4	1.7 (0.3–11.8)	ADVA, 2005c
1983–1985	0	nr	Fett et al., 1987
OCCUPATIONAL—INDUSTRIAL			
IARC Phenoxy Herbicide Cohort—Workers exposed to any phenoxy herbicide or chlorophenol (production or spraying) vs respective national mortality rates			
Mortality 1939–1992	10	1.0 (0.5–1.8)	Kogevinas et al., 1997
13,831 exposed to highly chlorinated PCDDs	8	1.3 (0.6–2.5)	
7,553 not exposed to highly chlorinated PCDDs	1	0.3 (0.0–1.5)	
Mortality 1955–1988 of 12,492 production workers and 5,898 sprayers exposed—13,482 in exposed subcohort	2	0.4 (0.1–1.4)	Saracci et al., 1991
Mortality, incidence of women in production (n = 699) and spraying (n = 2) compared to national death rates and cancer incidence rates	1	**TCDD** nr	Kogevinas et al, 1993
Mortality—IARC cohort (16,863 men and 1,527 women) 10–19 years since first exposure	3	0.6 (0.1–1.7)	Kogevinas et al, 1992
Danish Production Workers (3,390 men and 1,069 women involved in production of phenoxy herbicides unlikely to contain TCDD at 2 plants in 1947–1987) (in IARC cohort)		**Dioxins, but TCDD unlikely; 2,4-D, 2,4-DP, MCPA, MCPP**	
Dutch production workers in Plant A (549 men exposed during production 1955–1985; 594 unexposed) (in IARC cohort)		**Dioxins, 2,4,5-T, 2,4,5-TCP**	
Mortality 1955–1991	1	3.2 (0.1–17.6)	Hooiveld et al., 1998
German Production Workers at Bayer Plant in Uerdingen (135 men working > 1 month in 1951-1976) (in IARC cohort as of 1997) and women—no results		**Dioxins; 2,4,5-TCP**	
Mortality 1951–1992	0	nr	Becher et al., 1996

TABLE 8-40 Hodgkin Lymphoma, continued

Study Population[a]	Exposed Cases[b]	**Exposure of Interest**/Estimated Relative Risk (95% CI)[b]	Reference
German Production Workers at Bayer Plant in Dormagen (520 men working > 1 month in 1965–1989) (in IARC cohort as of 1997) and women—no results		**Dioxins; 2,4-D; 2,4-DP; 2,4,5-T; MCPA; MCPP**	
Mortality 1965–1989	0	nr	Becher et al., 1996
German Production Workers at BASF Ludwigshafen Plant (680 men working > 1 month in 1957–1987) (in IARC cohort as of 1997) and women—no results		**Dioxins; 2,4-D; 2,4-DP; 2,4,5-T; MCPA; MCPP**	
Mortality 1956–1989	0	nr	Becher et al., 1996
BASF Cleanup Workers from 1953 accident (n = 247); 114 with chloracne, 13 more with erythema; serum TCDD levels (*not* part of IARC)		**Focus on TCDD**	
Mortality			
Through 1987 [Table 2]	0	nr	Zober et al., 1990
German Production Workers at Boehringer–Ingelheim Plant in Hamburg (1,144 men working > 1 month in 1952–1984; generation of TCDD reduced after chloracne outbreak in 1954) and women—no results (some additions to observed cancers over Manz et al., 1991) (in IARC cohort as of 1997)		**Dioxins; 2,4,5-T; 2,5-DCP; 2,4,5-TCP**	
Mortality 1952–1989	0	nr	Becher et al., 1996
New Zealand Phenoxy Herbicide Production Workers and Sprayers (1,599 men and women working any time in 1969–1988 at Dow plant in New Plymouth) (in IARC cohort)		**Dioxins; 2,4-D; 2,4,5-T; 2,4,5-TCP; MCPA; MCPB; Picloram**	
Mortality 1969–2004			McBride et al., 2009a
Ever-exposed workers	1	4.2 (0.1–23.3)	
Never-exposed workers	0	0.0 (0.0–47.1)	
Production Workers (713 men and 100 women worked > 1 month in 1969–1984)			
Mortality 1969–2000	1	5.6 (0.1–31.0)	't Mannetje et al., 2005
Sprayers (697 men and 2 women on register of New Zealand applicators, 1973–1984)			
Mortality 1973–2000	0	0.0 (0.0–16.1)	't Mannetje et al., 2005

continued

TABLE 8-40 Hodgkin Lymphoma, continued

Study Population[a]	Exposed Cases[b]	Exposure of Interest/Estimated Relative Risk (95% CI)[b]	Reference
NIOSH Mortality Cohort (12 US plants, 5,172 male production and maintenance workers 1942–1984) (included in IARC cohort as of 1997)		**Dioxins, phenoxy herbicides**	
Through 1993	3	1.1 (0.2–3.2)	Steenland et al., 1999
Chloracne subcohort (n = 608) (lymphatic, hematopoietic; ICD-9 200–208)	6	1.1 (0.4–2.5)	
Through 1987	3	1.2 (0.3–3.5)	Fingerhut et al., 1991
≥ 1-year exposure, ≥ 20-year latency	1	2.8 (0.1–15.3)	
All Dow TCP-Exposed Workers (TCP production 1942–1979 or 2,4,5-T production 1948–1982 in Midland, Michigan) (in IARC and NIOSH cohorts)		**2,4,5-T; 2,4,5-TCP**	
1942–2003 (n = 1,615)	0	0.0 (0.0–6.4)	Collins et al., 2009a
All Dow PCP-Exposed Workers—all workers from the two plants that only made PCP (in Tacoma, Washington, and Wichita, Kansas) and workers who made PCP and TCP at two additional plants (in Midland, Michigan, and Sauget, Illinois)		**2,4,5-T; 2,4,5-TCP**	Ruder and Yiin, 2011
1940–2005 (n = 2,122)	1	0.6 (0.0–3.6)	
PCP and TCP (n = 720)	0	nr (0.0–6.9)	
PCP (no TCP) (n = 1,402)	1	1.0 (0.0–5.4)	
Dow 2,4-D Production Workers (1945–1982 in Midland, Michigan) (subset of all TCP-exposed workers)		**2,4-D, lower chlorinated dioxins**	
Cancer incidence through 2007 in Dow workers (n = 1,256) vs comparisons from state cancer registries (n = 23,354) (Cohort 3)	1	1.3 (0.0–7.2)	Burns et al., 2011
Through 1994 (n = 1,517)	1	1.5 (0.0–8.6)	Burns et al., 2001
Through 1982 (n = 878)	1	2.7 (0.0–14.7)	Bond et al., 1988
Dow PCP Production Workers (1937–1989 in Midland, Michigan) (*not* in IARC and NIOSH cohorts)		**Low chlorinated dioxins, 2,4-D**	
Mortality 1940–2004 (n = 577, excluding 196 also having exposure to TCP)	2	1.8 (0.2–6.4)	Collins et al., 2009b
Mortality 1940–1989 (n = 770)			Ramlow et al., 1996
0-yr latency	0	nr	
15-yr latency	0	nr	

TABLE 8-40 Hodgkin Lymphoma, continued

Study Population[a]	Exposed Cases[b]	**Exposure of Interest**/Estimated Relative Risk (95% CI)[b]	Reference
OCCUPATIONAL—PAPER AND PULP WORKERS		**TCDD**	
IARC cohort of pulp and paper workers—60,468 workers from 11 countries, TCDD among 27 agents assessed by JEM			McLean et al., 2006
Exposure to nonvolatile organochlorine compounds			
Never	7	0.6 (0.2–1.2)	
Ever	17	1.8 (1.0–2.8)	
Danish paper workers			Rix et al., 1998
Men	18	2.0 (1.2–3.2)	
Women	2	1.1 (0.1–3.8)	
OCCUPATIONAL—HERBICIDE-USING WORKERS (*not* related to IARC sprayer cohorts)			
CANADA			
Ontario Forestry Workers—1,222 men working ≥ 6 months 1950–1982			
80 deaths through 1982; 18 cancers (lung greatest with 5)	0	nr	Green, 1991
DENMARK			
Danish Farmers—incidence from linking farmers on 1970 census with national cancer registry (1970–1980)		**Herbicides**	Ronco et al., 1992
Men			
Self-employed	27	0.6 ($p < 0.05$)	
Employee	13	1.0 (nr)	
Women			
Self-employed	1	1.1 (nr)	
Employee	1	1.2 (nr)	
FINNISH Phenoxy Herbicide Sprayers (1,909 men working 1955–1971 ≥ 2 wks) *not* IARC		**Phenoxy herbicides**	
Incidence	2	1.7 (0.2–6.0)	Asp et al., 1994
Mortality 1972–1989	0	0.0 (0.0–5.0)	
Except for lung cancer, numbers too small for reporting mortality 1972–1980	0	nr	Riihimaki et al., 1982
ITALIAN Licensed Pesticide Users—male farmers in southern Piedmont licensed 1970–1974			
Mortality 1970–1986 (n = 23,401)	11	1.0 (0.5–1.7)	Torchio et al., 1994
Italian rice growers with documented phenoxy use (n = 1,487)		**Phenoxy herbicides**	Gambini et al., 1997
	1	0.7 (0.0–3.6)	

continued

TABLE 8-40 Hodgkin Lymphoma, continued

Study Population[a]	Exposed Cases[b]	**Exposure of Interest**/Estimated Relative Risk (95% CI)[b]	Reference
SWEDEN			
Swedish Cancer-Environment Registry—National Cancer Registry linked to census		**Herbicides**	
Incidence data from Swedish Cancer Environment Register (1971–1984) linked to 1970 census			Eriksson et al., 1992
Male sawmill workers	10	2.1 (1.0–4.0)	
Male farmers	97	1.2 (nr)	
Male forestry workers	35	1.2 (nr)	
Male horticulture workers	11	1.2 (nr)	
20,245 Swedish pesticide applicators with license issued between 1965 and 1976	15	1.5 (0.8–2.4)	Wiklund et al., 1989a
354,620 Swedish agriculture, forestry workers			Wiklund et al., 1988a
Workers in land or in animal husbandry	242	1.0 (0.9–1.2)	
Workers in silviculture	15	2.3 (1.3–3.7)	
Incident HD cases 1961–1973 with agriculture as economic activity in 1960 census	226	*99% CI* 1.0 (0.9–1.2)	Wiklund, 1983
THE NETHERLANDS			
Dutch Licensed Herbicide Sprayers—1,341 certified before 1980			
Through 2000	0	nr	Swaen et al., 2004
Through 1987	1	3.3 (0.0–18.6)	Swaen et al., 1992
UNITED STATES			
US farmers—usual occupation of farmer and industry of agriculture on death certificates 1984–1988 from 23 states		**Herbicides** PCMRs	Blair et al., 1993
Men			
Whites (n = 119,648)	56	1.0 (0.8–1.3)	
Nonwhites (n = 11,446)	2	0.7 (0.1–2.6)	
Women			
Whites (n = 2,400)	0	0.0 (0.0–3.4)	
Nonwhites (n = 2,066)	0	0.0 (0.0–7.2)	
US Agricultural Health Study—prospective study of licensed pesticide sprayers in Iowa and North Carolina: commercial (n = 4,916), private/farmers (n = 52,395, 97.4% men), and spouses of private sprayers (n = 32,347, 0.007% men), enrolled 1993–1997; followups with CATIs 1999–2003 and 2005–2010		**Phenoxy herbicides**	
Incidence			
Enrollment through 2006—SIRs for participants			Koutros et al., 2010a

TABLE 8-40 Hodgkin Lymphoma, continued

Study Population[a]	Exposed Cases[b]	**Exposure of Interest**/Estimated Relative Risk (95% CI)[b]	Reference
Private applicators	18	1.0 (0.6–1.5)	
Commercial applicators	1	nr	
Spouses	7	0.9 (0.3–1.7)	
Enrollment through 2002			Alavanja et al., 2005
Private applicators	11	0.9 (0.4–1.6)	
Spouses of private applicators (> 99% women)	4	0.7 (0.2–1.9)	
Commercial applicators	1	0.8 (0.1–4.2)	
Mortality			
Enrollment through 2007, vs state rates			Waggoner et al., 2011
Applicators (n = 1,641)	5	1.0 (0.3–2.4)	
Spouses (n = 676)			
Enrollment through 2000, vs state rates	3	1.1 (0.2–3.3)	Blair et al., 2005a
Private applicators (men and women)	3	1.7 (0.3–4.8)	
Spouses of private applicators (> 99% women)	0	0.0 (0.0–2.5)	
US Department of Agriculture Workers—nested case-control study of white men dying 1970–1979 of HD		**Herbicides**	
Agricultural extension agents			Alavanja et al., 1988
PM analysis	6	2.7 (1.2–6.3)	
Case-control analysis	6	1.1 (0.3–3.5)	
USDA forest, soil conservationists	4	2.2 (0.6–5.6)	Alavanja et al., 1989
White Male Residents of Iowa—HD on death certificate, usual occupation: farmers vs not		**Herbicides**	
> 20 yrs old when died 1971–1978—PMR	47	1.2 (ns)	Burmeister, 1981
ENVIRONMENTAL			
Seveso, Italy, Residential Cohort—Industrial accident July 10, 1976 (723 residents Zone A; 4,821 Zone B; 31,643 Zone R; 181,574 local reference group) (ICD-9 171)		**TCDD**	
Incidence			
20-yr followup to 1996—men and women			
Zone A	0	nr	Pesatori et al., 2009
Zone B	3	1.2 (0.4–3.8)	
Zone R	23	1.5 (0.9–2.3)	
10-yr followup to 1991—men			Bertazzi et al., 1993
Zone B	1	1.7 (0.2–12.8)	
Zone R	4	1.1 (0.4–3.1)	

continued

TABLE 8-40 Hodgkin Lymphoma, continued

Study Population[a]	Exposed Cases[b]	**Exposure of Interest**/Estimated Relative Risk (95% CI)[b]	Reference
10-yr followup to 1991—women			Bertazzi et al., 1993
Zone B	1	2.1 (0.3–15.7)	
Zone R	3	1.0 (0.3–3.2)	
Mortality			
25-yr followup to 2001—men and women			Consonni et al., 2008
Zone A	0	nr	
Zone B	3	2.2 (0.7–6.9)	
Zone R	9	0.9 (0.5–1.9)	
20-yr followup to 1996			Bertazzi et al., 2001
Zones A, B—men	2	2.6 (0.6–10.9)	
Zones A, B—women	2	3.7 (0.9–16.0)	
15-yr followup to 1991—men			Bertazzi et al., 1997
Zone B	2	3.3 (0.4–11.9)	
15-yr followup to 1991—women			Bertazzi et al., 1997
Zone B	2	6.5 (0.7–23.5)	
Zone R	4	1.9 (0.5–4.9)	
Other International Environmental Studies			
FRANCE			
Residents near French solid-waste incinerator—incidence		**Dioxin**	Viel et al., 2000
1980–1995	9	1.5 (nr) ($p = 0.89$)	
NEW ZEALAND			
Residents of New Plymouth Territorial Authority, New Zealand, near plant manufacturing 2,4,5-T in 1962–1987		2,4,5-T	Read et al., 2007
Incidence	49	1.1 (0.8–1.5)[d]	
1970–1974	9	1.2 (0.6–2.3)	
1975–1979	9	1.1 (0.5–2.2)	
1980–1984	8	1.1 (0.5–2.1)	
1985–1989	9	1.3 (0.6–2.5)	
1990–1994	7	1.3 (0.5–2.7)	
1995–1999	4	0.7 (0.2–1.7)	
2000–2001	3	1.0 (0.2–3.1)	
Mortality	22	1.3 (0.8–2.0)[d]	
1970–1974	7	1.6 (0.7–3.3)	
1975–1979	4	1.2 (0.3–3.0)	
1980–1984	6	2.1 (0.8–4.5)	
1985–1989	3	1.2 (0.2–3.5)	
1990–1994	1	0.6 (0.0–3.5)	
1995–1999	1	0.6 (0.0–3.6)	
2000–2001	0	nr	
CASE-CONTROL STUDIES			
US Case-Control Studies			
Kansas residents–duration and frequency of herbicide use—incidence		**Phenoxy herbicides, 2.4-D**	Hoar et al., 1986
All farmers	71	0.8 (0.5–1.2)	

TABLE 8-40 Hodgkin Lymphoma, continued

Study Population[a]	Exposed Cases[b]	**Exposure of Interest**/Estimated Relative Risk (95% CI)[b]	Reference
Farm-use of herbicides (phenoxy acids, others)	28	0.9 (0.5–1.5)	
Farmers using herbicides > 20 days/yr	3	1.0 (0.2–4.1)	
Farmers using herbicides > 15 days/yr	10	1.2 (0.5–2.6)	
Tecumseh, Michigan, residents participating in longitudinal study (1959–1987)	13	**Herbicides** 2.0 (1.1–3.4)	Waterhouse et al., 1996
Hancock County, **Ohio,** residents—farmers	3	2.7 (nr)	Dubrow et al., 1988
International Case-Control Studies			
Canadian residents (≥ 19 yrs of age) in any of 6 provinces		**Phenoxy herbicides**	Karunanayake et al., 2012
Any phenoxy herbicide	65	0.9 (0.7–1.3)	
2,4-D	57	0.9 (0.6–1.3)	
Mecoprop	20	1.4 (0.8–2.4)	
MCPA	11	1.0 (0.4–2.2)	
Diclofopmethyl	10	1.8 (0.7–4.5)	
Canadian residents (≥ 19 yrs of age) in any of 6 provinces		**Phenoxy herbicides**	Pahwa et al., 2006
Any phenoxy herbicide	65	1.0 (0.7–1.4)	
2,4-D	57	1.0 (0.7–1.4)	
Mecoprop	20	1.3 (0.7–2.2)	
MCPA	11	1.2 (0.6–2.6)	
France hospital-based case-control study		**Herbicides**	Orsi et al., 2009
Occupational use of herbicides	7	1.5 (0.6–4.1)	
Phenoxy herbicides	6	2.5 (0.8–7.7)	
Domestic use of herbicides	19	0.8 (0.4–1.6)	
Italian incident cases of malignancies of hematolymphopoietic system (HD = 258) in men and women (20–74 yrs of age) from agricultural and mixed use areas		**Herbicides**	Miligi et al., 2006
Men	5	0.4 (0.1–1.3)	
Women	1	0.5 (0.1–4.0)	
Italy—Residents of Milan area (men and women)—incidence		**Herbicides**	LaVecchia et al., 1989
Agricultural occupations	nr	2.1 (1.0–3.8)	
Chemical-industry occupations	nr	4.3 (1.4–10.2)	
New Zealand National Cancer Registry (1977–1981) (≥ 20 yrs of age) with agricultural occupations—incidence (ICD-9 200, 202)	107	**Herbicides** 1.1 (0.6–2.0)	Pearce et al., 1985
Swedish Regional Cancer Registry—HD patients		**Phenoxy herbicides**	Persson et al., 1993
Exposed to phenoxy herbicides		*90% CI*	
	5	7.4 (1.4–40.0)	

continued

TABLE 8-40 Hodgkin Lymphoma, continued

Study Population[a]	Exposed Cases[b]	**Exposure of Interest**/Estimated Relative Risk (95% CI)[b]	Reference
Örebro (**Sweden**) Hospital (men and women)—incidence		**Phenoxy herbicides, chlorophenols** *90% CI*	Persson et al., 1989
Farming	6	1.2 (0.4–3.5)	
Exposed to phenoxy acids	4	3.8 (0.7–21.0)	
Sweden—Umea Hospital patients (men and women, 25–85 yrs of age) (1974–1978)		**Phenoxys, chlorophenols**	Hardell and Bengtsson, 1983
Exposed to phenoxy acids	14	5.0 (2.4–10.2)	
Exposed to high-grade chlorophenols	6	6.5 (2.2–19.0)	
Exposed to low-grade chlorophenols	5	2.4 (0.9–6.5)	
Swedish patients (1970–1977)		**Phenoxy acids, chlorophenols**	Hardell, 1981
Exposed to phenoxy herbicides	41	4.8 (2.9–8.1)	
Exposed to chlorophenols	50	4.3 (2.7–6.9)	

NOTE: 2,4-D, 2,4-dichlorophenoxyacetic acid; 2,4-DP, dichlorprop; 2,4,5-T, 2,4,5-trichlorophenoxyacetic acid; 2,4,5-TCP, 2,4,5-trichlorophenol; CATI, computer-assisted telephone interviewing; CDC, Centers for Disease Control and Prevention; CI, confidence interval; COI, chemical of interest; HD, Hodgkin disease; IARC, International Agency for Research on Cancer; ICD, International Classification of Diseases; JEM, job-exposure matrix; MCPA, 2-methyl-4-chlorophenoxyacetic acid; MCPB, 4-(4-chloro-2-methylphenoxy)butanoic acid; MCPP, methylchlorophenoxypropionic acid; NHL, non-Hodgkin lymphoma; NIOSH, National Institute for Occupational Safety and Health; nr, not reported; PCDD, polychlorinated dibenzo-*p*-dioxin (highly chlorinated, if four or more chlorines); PCMR, proportionate cancer mortality ratios; PCP, pentachlorophenol; PM, proportionate mortality; PMR, proportional mortality ratio; SEA, Southeast Asia; SIR, standardized incidence ratio; TCDD, 2,3,7,8-tetrachlorodibenzo-*p*-dioxin; TCP, trichlorophenol; USDA, United States Department of Agriculture; VA, US Department of Veterans Affairs.

[a]Subjects are male and outcome is mortality unless otherwise noted.

[b]Given when available; results other than estimated risk explained individually.

[c]Lymphopoietic cancers comprise all forms of lymphoma (including Hodgkin disease and non-Hodgkin lymphoma) and leukemia (ALL, AML, CLL, CML).

[d]Committee computed total SMR and SIR by dividing sum of observed values by sum of expected values over all years; 95% CIs on these total ratios were computed with exact methods.

Michigan (Burns et al., 2011). That provides little information about whether HL is associated with 2,4-D exposure (SIR = 1.30, 95% CI 0.02–7.23) in the most restrictively defined cohort.

In the NIOSH cohort of 2,122 PCP workers, Ruder and Yiin (2011) reported a single death from HL (ICD-9 201), which occurred in the 1,402 people in the PCP-only group (SMR = 0.97, 95% CI 0.02–5.41); there were none in the 720 men in the PCP-plus-TCDD group.

In the update of cancer incidence through December 31, 2006, in participants in the AHS, Koutros et al. (2010a) did not find increases in the incidence of HL in the private applicators (SIR = 0.96, 95% CI 0.57–1.52) or in their spouses (SIR = 0.85, 95% CI 0.34–1.74). The preponderance of the HL cases occurred in the subsample drawn from Iowa (15 of 18 cases in applicators [SIR = 1.27, 95% CI 0.71–2.09] and 6 of 7 cases in their spouses [SIR = 1.02, 95% CI 0.37–2.21]). In the update of mortality in the AHS cohort through 2007, Waggoner et al. (2011) observed only five deaths from HL in the applicators (SMR = 1.03, 95% CI 0.34–2.41) and a single death from HL in their spouses. The AHS has been generating valuable information on the COIs for a number of years, but these results are not herbicide-specific and so are not regarded as being fully informative for the committee's task.

Case-Control Studies In an early report of the Cross-Canada Study of Pesticides and Health, Pahwa et al. (2003) had not found an increased risk of HL in those exposed to any type of herbicide for at least 10 hours/year. Karunanayake et al. (2012) presented results on exposure of any duration to individual pesticides. The 316 HL cases had been diagnosed during September 1, 1991–December 31, 1994, and age-matched to 1,506 controls randomly selected from provincial insurance, voter, or telephone lists. With adjustment for age, province, and several aspects of medical history, herbicides of interest in this review showed no statistically significant associations with the incidence of HL; for all phenoxy herbicides, 65 exposed cases, OR = 0.94 , 95% CI 0.66–1.34; for 2,4-D, 57 exposed cases, OR = 0.88, 95% CI 0.61–1.34; for Mecoprop, 20 exposed cases, OR = 1.35, 95% CI 0.76–2.40; for MCPA, 11 exposed cases, OR = 0.97, 95% CI 0.42–2.22; for diclofop-methyl, 10 exposed cases, OR = 1.77, 95% CI 0.70–4.47; and for dicamba, 32 exposed cases, OR = 1.16, 95% CI 0.71–1.90.

Zakerinia et al. (2012) conducted an Iranian hospital-based case-control study of 200 cases of lymphoma (54 HL, 100 NHL, and 46 MM admitted from January 2007 through April 2008) and 200 controls admitted through the emergency room and matched on age, sex, and state of residence. A detailed job history gathered by interview was the source of information on exposure to pesticides (herbicides, insecticides, and fungicides). The analyses for the subtypes of pesticides were conducted only on the full set of lymphomas, so this study does not provide fully relevant information for the purpose of this review.

Biologic Plausibility

HL arises from the malignant transformation of a germinal-center B cell and is characterized by malignant cells that have a distinctive structure and phenotype; these binucleate cells are known as Reed–Sternberg cells (Jaffe et al., 2008). No animal studies have shown an increase in HL after exposure to the COIs. Reed–Sternberg cells have not been demonstrated in mice or rats, so there is no good animal model of HL. Thus, there are no specific animal data to support the biologic plausibility of an association between the COIs and HL.

The biologic plausibility of the carcinogenicity of the COIs is discussed in general at the beginning of this chapter.

Synthesis

The relative rarity of HL complicates the evaluation of epidemiologic studies because their statistical power is generally low. Earlier studies (Eriksson et al., 1992; Hardell et al., 1981; Holmes et al., 1986; LaVecchia et al., 1989; Persson et al., 1993; Rix et al., 1998; Waterhouse et al., 1996; Wiklund et al., 1988) were generally well conducted and included excellent characterization of exposure, and they formed the basis of previous VAO committees' conclusions. Later findings have not contradicted those conclusions, especially given that most studies have had low statistical power. Although it has not been demonstrated as clearly as for NHL, a positive association between the COIs and the development of HL is biologically plausible because of the common lymphoreticular origin of HL and NHL and their common risk factors.

Conclusion

On the basis of the evidence reviewed here and in previous VAO reports, the committee concludes that there is sufficient evidence of an association between exposure to at least one of the COIs and HL.

Non-Hodgkin Lymphoma

NHL (ICD-9 200.0–200.8, 202.0–202.2, 202.8–202.9) is a general name for cancers of the lymphatic system other than HL or MM. NHL consists of a large group of lymphomas that can be partitioned into acute and aggressive (fast-growing) or chronic and indolent (slow-growing) types of either B-cell or T-cell origin. B-cell NHL includes Burkitt lymphoma, diffuse large B-cell lymphoma, follicular lymphoma, large-cell lymphoma, precursor B-lymphoblastic lymphoma, and mantle-cell lymphoma. T-cell NHL includes mycosis fungoides and anaplastic large-cell lymphoma. Precursor T-lymphoblastic lymphoma is not considered a type of NHL; it is considered part of T-lymphoblastic lymphoma/leukemia, a precursor lymphoid neoplasm included with the broad group of "acute lymphoid leukemias," which can be of either T-cell or B-cell origin.

As noted in earlier VAO updates, in response to requests from VA, CLL and HCL have been recognized as sharing many traits with NHL (including B-cell origin and immunohistochemical properties). The proposed WHO classification of NHL notes that CLL (ICD-9 204.1) and its lymphomatous form, SLL, are both derived from mature B cells (Chiorazzi et al., 2005; IARC, 2001). The present

VAO committee has determined that it is more appropriate to consider those lymphatic malignancies with other forms of NHL. Therefore, discussion of CLL and HCL will no longer follow the general section on leukemia but has been moved into the NHL grouping.

ACS estimated that 38,160 men and 31,970 women would receive diagnoses of NHL in the United States in 2012 and that 10,320 men and 8,620 women would die from it (Siegel et al., 2012). The incidence of NHL is uniformly higher in men than in women and typically higher in whites than in blacks. In the groups that characterize most Vietnam veterans, incidence increases with age. In addition, ACS estimated that about 9,490 men and 6,570 women would receive diagnoses of CLL in the United States in 2012 and that 2,730 men and 1,850 women would die from it (Siegel et al., 2012). Nearly all cases occur after the age of 50 years. Average annual incidences of NHL are shown in Table 8-41 with the additional incidences of CLL.

The causes of NHL are poorly understood. People who have suppressed or compromised immune systems are known to be at higher risk, and some studies show an increased incidence in people who have HIV, human T-cell leukemia virus type I, Epstein–Barr virus, or gastric *Helicobacter pylori* infections. The human retrovirus HTLV-1 causes adult T-cell lymphoma, but early reports that HTLV-2 might play a role in the etiology of HCL have not been substantiated. A broad spectrum of behavioral, occupational, and environmental risk factors have been proposed as contributors to the occurrence of NHL, but given the diversity of malignancies included under this name, it is not too surprising that—aside from infectious agents, immune problems, and particular chemotherapies—specific risk factors have not been definitively established (Morton et al., 2008; Wang and Nieters, 2010).

Conclusions from *VAO* and Previous Updates

The committee responsible for *VAO* concluded that there was sufficient evidence to support an association between exposure to at least one of the COIs and

TABLE 8-41 Average Annual Incidence (per 100,000) of Non-Hodgkin Lymphoma in the United States[a]

	55–59 Years Old			60–64 Years Old			65–69 Years Old		
	All Races	White	Black	All Races	White	Black	All Races	White	Black
Men	38.1	39.1	36.7	55.4	57.8	42.7	78.4	82.7	51.7
Women	27.0	28.3	21.9	39.3	41.1	33.4	52.3	55.8	35.8

[a]Surveillance, Epidemiology, and End Results program, nine standard registries, crude age-specific rates, 2005–2009 (NCI, 2013).

NHL. Additional information available to the committees responsible for later updates has not changed that conclusion.

As with HL, epidemiologic data reviewed by previous VAO committees suggest that the phenoxy herbicides (including 2,4-D) rather than TCDD may be associated with NHL. The original VAO committee concluded that a positive association existed between exposure to herbicides and the development of NHL, and studies reviewed by later committees have continued to support that finding. A large, well-conducted case-control study in Sweden by Hardell (1981) examined NHL and HL together and found a significantly increased risk associated with exposure to phenoxy acids or chlorophenols on the basis of 105 cases. Those results were replicated in further investigations of the validity of the exposure assessment and potential biases (Hardell, 1981). Another Swedish case-control study by Hardell et al. (1994) showed a statistically significant risk in a comparison of the occupational histories of 105 people who were exposed to phenoxy herbicides and chlorophenols and received diagnoses of NHL in 1974–1978 with 335 control subjects. Similar data by Persson et al. (1989) showed an increased risk of NHL in those exposed to phenoxy acids on the basis of a logistic regression analysis of 106 cases.

Studies of production workers have shown some association between TCDD exposure and NHL. A larger study of 21,863 workers in the IARC phenoxy-herbicide cohort by Kogevinas et al. (1997) found a nonsignificant increase in NHL risk. Subjects in that expanded multinational study were followed from 1939 to 1992. Other studies of Danish and Dutch phenoxy-herbicide workers who were part of the IARC cohort have shown a nonsignificant increased risk of NHL (Boers et al., 2010; Bueno de Mesquita et al., 1993; Hooiveld et al., 1998; Lynge, 1993). A cohort of 2,479 workers in four plants in Germany with exposure to phenoxy herbicide and contaminants (dioxins and furans) had significantly increased risk of NHL on the basis of five cases (Becher et al., 1996). A variety of herbicides were produced in the plants, including those known to have been contaminated with TCDD. Increases in risk—but nonsignificant ones—have also been found in the NIOSH mortality study (Steenland et al., 1999). Risks were not significantly increased in the Dow Chemical Company Midland, Michigan, or Plymouth, New Zealand, chemical production workers, phenoxy-herbicide sprayers, or 2,4-D production workers (Bloemen et al., 1993; Bodner et al., 2003; Burns et al., 2001; Collins et al., 2009a,b; McBride et al., 2009a,b; Ramlow et al., 1996; 't Mannetje et al., 2005). A multinational IARC cohort study of paper and pulp workers found a statistically significant increase in workers who were exposed to chlorophenols (McLean et al., 2006).

Studies of farmers and agricultural workers have been generally positive for an association between herbicides or TCDD and NHL; however, only a few were statistically significant. A meta-analysis of several studies of the association between employment as a farmer in the central United States and NHL showed a statistically significant risk (Keller-Bryne et al., 1997). All the studies of US agricultural workers reviewed showed increased RRs, and two NCI studies of farmers in Kansas and Nebraska (Hoar et al., 1986; Zahm et al., 1990) showed patterns of increased risk linked to use of 2,4-D. A study of a subcohort of Hispanic workers in a larger cohort of 139,000 California members of the United Farm Workers of America (Mills et al., 2005) and a population-based case-control study in Italy of NHL and CLL cases (combined) identified during 1991–1993 (Miligi et al., 2006) both showed statistically significant associations with 2,4-D.

A large, well-conducted, population-based, Cross-Canada Study of Pesticides and Health reported on pesticide use and NHL incidence in men identified from cancer registries of six Canadian provinces in 1991–1994. Statistically significant associations were found between exposure to phenoxy herbicides, 2,4-D, or Mecocrop and NHL. A reanalysis of the data from that study confirmed the findings on phenoxy herbicides but found that the association with 2,4-D, although still increased, was no longer significantly so (McDuffie et al., 2001). A population-based case-control study in 2000–2001 in men and women 20–74 years old living in New South Wales, Australia, found an increased risk of NHL associated with "substantial" exposure to phenoxy herbicides (Fritschi et al., 2005). Spinelli et al. (2007) reported on a population-based case-control study in Vancouver and Victoria, British Columbia, and found strong monotonic increases in serum concentrations of two dioxin-like PCBs (PCB 118 and 156). Chiu et al. (2004) and Lee et al. (2004b) conducted a pooled (combined) analysis of two case-control studies that were carried out in three Midwestern US states—Iowa and Minnesota (Cantor et al., 1992) and Nebraska (Zahm et al., 1990)—and found that risks were increased in farmers by use of herbicides, including 2,4-D and 2,4,5-T. In a study of NHL incidence in people who lived in the vicinity of 13 French municipal waste incinerators, Viel et al. (2008) found a small but statistically significant increase in the risk of NHL and evidence of a dose–response relationship with increased exposure to dioxin. A case-control study of NHL rates in people who lived near a municipal solid-waste incinerator in Bensaçon, France, found that incidence of NHL was significantly increased in the area determined to have the highest dioxin contamination, but no increases were found in the low and intermediate categories (Floret et al., 2003). A French hospital-based case-control study of lymphoid neoplasms (Orsi et al., 2009) did not find the occurrence of NHL to be associated with occupational or domestic use of pesticides or phenoxy herbicides in particular.

Evidence of an association between the COIs and NHL in Vietnam veterans, the primary population of interest in the VAO updates, has been lacking. The Centers for Disease Control and Prevention (CDC) Selected Cancers Study (CDC, 1990a) showed a significantly increased risk of NHL in all Vietnam veterans; however, in analysis according to branch of service, Army and Air Force personnel were not at increased risk. Marine Corps veterans had higher mortality in the CDC Selected Cancers Study and significantly increased risks in several other studies (Breslin et al., 1988; Burt et al., 1987; Watanabe and Kang, 1996;

Watanabe et al., 1991), but the implications of these findings are unclear. No increased risk has been seen in Operation Ranch Hand veterans (AFHS, 2000; Akhtar et al., 2004; Michalek et al., 1990; Wolfe et al., 1990) or in members of the Army Chemical Corps (Boehmer et al., 2004).

With 25 years of followup of the Seveso population and a relatively small number of observed cases, evidence of an increased incidence of NHL is emerging in the subgroup in the most highly exposed zones (Bertazzi et al., 1989b, 1993, 1997, 2001; Consonni et al., 2008; Pesatori et al., 1992, 2009).

The findings of several PCB-focused studies (Bertrand et al., 2010; Engel et al., 2007; Laden et al., 2010) are consistent with the associations with NHL repeatedly observed in connection with the COIs in the VAO series, but the extent of intercorrelation of these persistent organic pollutants greatly curtails the degree to which any effect can be specifically attributed to dioxin-like activity.

Table 8-42 summarizes the results of the relevant studies of all forms of NHL.

Update 2002 was the first to discuss CLL separately from other leukemias. The epidemiologic studies indicated that farming, especially with exposure to 2,4-D and 2,4,5-T, is associated with significant mortality from CLL. Many more studies support the hypothesis that herbicide exposure can contribute to NHL risk. Most cases of CLL and NHL reflect malignant transformation of germinal-center B cells, so these diseases could have a common etiology.

Studies concerning CLL reviewed in *Update 2002*, *Update 2004*, *Update 2006*, *Update 2008*, and *Update 2010* are summarized in Table 8-43.

Update of the Epidemiologic Literature

Vietnam-Veteran and Environmental Studies No Vietnam-veteran studies or environmental studies of exposure to the COIs and NHL have been published since *Update 2010*.

Occupational Studies Burns et al. (2011) published an update of cancer incidence through 2007 in workers who were alive on January 1, 1985, and had been employed at any time from 1945 to 1994 in 2,4-D production by the Dow Chemical Company in Midland, Michigan. They found no evidence of significantly increased rates of cancer overall. With 14 cases observed, the increase in risk of NHL in the most restrictively defined cohort did not reach statistical significance (SIR = 1.71, 95% CI 0.93–2.87), as was the case in the two successively more inclusive, but potentially more biased, cohorts.

Boers et al. (2012) provided a quantified, TCDD-based analysis of the mortality data updated through 2006 in male workers in two Dutch phenoxy-herbicide factories, which were considered in *Update 2010* (Boers et al., 2010). The 1,020 workers in factory A had been involved in production of 2,4,5-T with its associated TCDD contamination, whereas the 1,036 working in factory B had

TABLE 8-42 Selected Epidemiologic Studies—Non-Hodgkin Lymphoma (Shaded Entries Are New Information for This Update)

Study Population[a]	Exposed Cases[b]	**Exposure of Interest**/Estimated Relative Risk (95% CI)[b]	Reference
VIETNAM VETERANS			
US Air Force Health Study—Ranch Hand veterans vs SEA veterans (unless otherwise noted)		**All COIs**	
Incidence			
Through 1999—White subjects vs national rates (lymphopoietic cancer[c])			Akhtar et al., 2004
Ranch Hand veterans (n = 1,189)	10	0.9 (0.4–1.5)	
With tours between 1966–1970	7	0.7 (0.3–1.4)	
SEA comparison veterans (n = 1,776)	9	0.6 (0.3–1.0)	
With tours between 1966–1970	4	0.3 (0.1–0.8)	
Attended 1987 exam—Ranch Hand personnel (n = 995) vs SEA veterans (n = 1,299)	1	nr	Wolfe et al., 1990
Mortality			
Through 1987—Ranch Hand personnel (n = 1,261) vs SEA veterans (19,102)	0	nr	Michalek et al., 1990
US CDC Vietnam Experience Study—Cross-sectional study, with medical examinations, of Army veterans: 9,324 deployed vs 8,989 nondeployed		**All COIs**	
Army enlisted Vietnam veterans (all lymphomas) (1965–1983)	7	1.8 (nr)	O'Brien et al., 1991
Mortality			
1965–2000	6	0.9 (0.3–2.9)	Boehmer et al., 2004
US CDC Selected Cancers Study—case-control study of incidence (12/1/1984–11/30/1989) among US males born 1929–1953 (CDC, 1990a)	99	**All COIs** 1.5 (1.1–2.0)	CDC, 1990b
Army Vietnam veterans	45	1.2 (0.8–1.8)	
Marine Vietnam veterans	10	1.8 (0.8–4.3)	
Air Force Vietnam veterans	12	1.0 (0.5–2.2)	
Navy Vietnam veterans	32	1.9 (1.1–3.2)	
Blue Water Navy Vietnam veterans	28	2.2 (1.2–3.9)	
US VA Proportionate Mortality Study—sample of deceased male Vietnam-era Army and Marine veterans who served 7/4/1965–3/1/1973		**All COIs**	
1965–1988			Watanabe and Kang, 1996
Army, deployed (n = 27,596) vs nondeployed (n = 31,757)	171	—	
Marine Corps, deployed (n = 6,237) vs nondeployed (n = 5,040)	46	1.7 (1.2–2.2)	

continued

TABLE 8-42 Non-Hodgkin Lymphoma, continued

Study Population[a]	Exposed Cases[b]	**Exposure of Interest**/Estimated Relative Risk (95% CI)[b]	Reference
1965–1984—Army, deployed (n = 24,145) vs nondeployed (n = 27,917) (ICD-8 200, 202)	140	1.7 (1.2–2.2)	Watanabe et al., 1991
Army Vietnam veterans vs combined Army and Marine Vietnam-era veterans	140	0.9 (nr)	
Marine Vietnam veterans vs non-Vietnam veterans	42	1.8 (1.3–2.4)	
Marine Vietnam veterans vs combined Army and Marine Vietnam-era veterans	42	1.2 (nr)	
1965–1982 (ICDA-8 200, 202)			Breslin et al., 1986, 1988
Army, deployed (n = 19,708) vs nondeployed (n = 22,904)	108	0.8 (0.6–1.0)	
Marine Corps, deployed (n = 4,527) vs nondeployed (n = 3,781)	35	2.1 (1.2–3.8)	
Nested case-control study of NHL	39	1.1 (0.7–1.5)	Burt et al., 1987
Army combat Vietnam veterans	17	3.2 (1.4–7.4)	
Marine combat Vietnam veterans	64	0.9 (0.7–1.3)	
Army Vietnam veterans (service 1967–1969)	17	2.5 (1.1–5.8)	
Marine Vietnam veterans (service 1967–1969)	4	1.8 (0.4–8.0)	
US VA Cohort of Female Vietnam Veterans		**All COIs**	
Mortality			
Through 2004 (lymphopoietic cancers[c])	18	0.7 (0.4–1.3)	Cypel and Kang, 2008
Vietnam–veteran nurses	14	0.7 (0.3–1.3)	
Through 1987 (ICD-8 200, 200–203, 208)	3	1.3 (0.3–1.8)	Thomas et al., 1991
US Navy Enlisted Personnel (1974–1983)			
Active duty	68	0.7 (0.5–0.9)	Garland et al., 1988
VA Case-Control Studies			
US Vietnam veterans—incidence	100	1.0 (0.7–1.5)	Dalager et al., 1991
State Studies of US Vietnam Veterans			
Massachusetts Vietnam-era veterans who served 1958–1973—cases diagnosed 1982–1988 (served in Vietnam)	—	1.2 (0.6–2.4)	Clapp et al., 1991
Michigan Vietnam-era veterans, PM study of deaths (1974–1989)—deployed vs nondeployed	32	1.5 (1.0–2.1)	Visintainer et al., 1995
New York—deployed vs nondeployed	10	1.0 (0.4–2.2)	Lawrence et al., 1985
West Virginia—deployed vs nondeployed	2	1.1 (nr)	Holmes et al., 1986

TABLE 8-42 Non-Hodgkin Lymphoma, continued

Study Population[a]	Exposed Cases[b]	**Exposure of Interest**/Estimated Relative Risk (95% CI)[b]	Reference
923 White male Vietnam veterans with **Wisconsin** death certificate (1968–1978) vs proportions for Vietnam-era veterans (includes lymphosarcoma, reticulosarcoma)	4	nr	Anderson et al., 1986a,b
International Vietnam-Veteran Studies			
Australian Vietnam Veterans—58,077 men and 153 women served on land or in Vietnamese waters during 5/23/1962–7/1/1973 vs Australian population		**All COIs**	
Incidence			
All branches, 1982–2000	126	0.7 (0.6–0.8)	ADVA, 2005a
Navy	31	0.8 (0.5–1.0)	
Army	86	0.7 (0.5–0.8)	
Air Force	9	0.5 (0.2–0.9)	
Validation Study		*Expected number of exposed cases*	AIHW, 1999
	62	48 (34–62)	
Men	137	48 (34–62)	CDVA, 1998a
Women	2	0 (0–4)	CDVA, 1998b
Mortality			
All branches, return–2001	70	0.8 (0.6–1.0)	ADVA, 2005b
Navy	10	0.5 (0.3–0.9)	
Army	52	0.9 (0.6–1.1)	
Air Force	8	0.9 (0.4–1.6)	
1980–1994	33	0.9 (0.6–1.2)	CDVA, 1997a
Australian Conscripted Army National Service (18,940 deployed vs 24,642 nondeployed)		**All COIs**	
Incidence			
1982–2000	35	1.1 (0.7–1.9)	ADVA, 2005c
Mortality			
1966–2001	21	1.4 (0.7–2.8)	ADVA, 2005c
1983–1985 (ICD-8 200, 202)	4	1.8 (0.4–8.0)	Fett et al., 1987

continued

TABLE 8-42 Non-Hodgkin Lymphoma, continued

Study Population[a]	Exposed Cases[b]	**Exposure of Interest**/Estimated Relative Risk (95% CI)[b]	Reference
OCCUPATIONAL—INDUSTRIAL			
IARC Phenoxy Herbicide Cohort—Workers exposed to any phenoxy herbicide or chlorophenol (production or spraying) vs respective national mortality rates			
Mortality 1939–1992	34	1.3 (0.9–1.8)	Kogevinas et al., 1997
13,831 exposed to highly chlorinated PCDDs	24	1.4 (0.9–2.1)	
7,553 not exposed to highly chlorinated PCDDs	9	1.0 (0.5–1.9)	
Mortality 1955–1988 of 12,492 production workers and 5,898 sprayers exposed—13,482 in exposed subcohort			Saracci et al., 1991
Nested case-control study			
IARC cohort (men and women)—incidence			Kogevinas et al, 1995
Exposed to 2,4,5-T	10	1.9 (0.7–4.8)	
Exposed to TCDD	11	1.9 (0.7–5.1)	
Mortality—IARC cohort (16,863 men and 1,527 women) 10–19 years since first exposure	11	1.0 (0.5–1.7)	Kogevinas et al, 1992
Danish Production Workers (3,390 men and 1,069 women involved in production of phenoxy herbicides unlikely to contain TCDD at 2 plants in 1947–1987) (in IARC cohort)		**Dioxins, but TCDD unlikely; 2,4-D, 2,4-DP, MCPA, MCPP**	
Mortality 1955–2006	7	1.4 (1.1–1.7)	Boers et al., 2012
TCDD plasma level (HRs, by tertile)			
Background (≤ 0.4)	1	nr	
Low (0.4–4.1)	3	3.8 (0.4–34.3)	
Medium (4.1–20.1)	2	7.8 (0.7–89.3)	
High (≥ 20.1)	1	8.1 (0.4–149.1)	
Incidence 1943–1987 (men only)	10	1.7 (0.5–4.5)	Lynge, 1993
Dutch production workers in Plant A (549 men exposed during production 1955–1985; 594 unexposed) (in IARC cohort)		**Dioxins, 2,4,5-T, 2,4,5-TCP**	
Mortality 1955–2006 (HRs for lagged TCDD plasma levels)	6	1.3 (1.0–1.7)	Boers et al., 2012
Mortality 1955–2006	4 vs 3	0.9 (0.2–4.5)	Boers et al., 2010
Mortality 1955–1991	3	3.8 (0.8–11.0)	Hooiveld et al., 1998
Mortality 1955–1985	1	2.0 (0.1–11.4)	Bueno de Mesquita et al., 1993

TABLE 8-42 Non-Hodgkin Lymphoma, continued

Study Population[a]	Exposed Cases[b]	**Exposure of Interest**/Estimated Relative Risk (95% CI)[b]	Reference
Dutch production workers in Plant B (414 men exposed during production 1965–1986; 723 unexposed) (in IARC cohort)		**2,4-D; MCPA; MCPP; highly chlorinated dioxins unlikely**	
Mortality 1965–2006	1 vs 0	nr	Boers et al., 2010
Mortality 1965–1986	1	5.6 (0.1–31.0)	Bueno de Mesquita et al., 1993
German Production Workers—2,479 workers at 4 plants (in IARC cohort as of 1997)		**Dioxins, phenoxy herbicides**	
All for plants	6	3.3 (1.2–7.1)	Becher et al., 1996
German Production Workers at Bayer Plant in Uerdingen (135 men working > 1 month in 1951–1976) (in IARC cohort as of 1997) and women—no results		**Dioxins; 2,4,5-TCP**	
Mortality 1951–1992	2	12.0 (1.5–43.5)	Becher et al., 1996
German Production Workers at Bayer Plant in Dormagen (520 men working > 1 month in 1965–1989) (in IARC cohort as of 1997) and women—no results		**Dioxins; 2,4-D; 2,4-DP; 2,4,5-T; MCPA; MCPP**	
Mortality 1965–1989	0	—	Becher et al., 1996
German Production Workers at BASF Ludwigshafen Plant (680 men working > 1 month in 1957–1987) (in IARC cohort as of 1997) and women—no results		**Dioxins; 2,4-D; 2,4-DP; 2,4,5-T; MCPA; MCPP**	
Mortality 1956–1989	0	—	Becher et al., 1996
German Production Workers at Boehringer–Ingelheim Plant in Hamburg (1,144 men working > 1 month in 1952–1984; generation of TCDD reduced after chloracne outbreak in 1954) and women—no results (some additions to observed cancers over Manz et al., 1991) (in IARC cohort as of 1997)		**Dioxins; 2,5-DCP; 2,4,5-T; 2,4,5-TCP**	
Mortality 1952–2007	7	1.6 (0.6–3.3)	Manuwald et al., 2012
Men	5	1.6 (0.5–3.7)	
Women	2	1.7 (0.2–6.0)	
Mortality 1952–1989	4	3.8 (1.0–9.6)	Becher et al., 1996

continued

TABLE 8-42 Non-Hodgkin Lymphoma, continued

Study Population[a]	Exposed Cases[b]	Exposure of **Interest**/Estimated Relative Risk (95% CI)[b]	Reference
New Zealand Phenoxy Herbicide Production Workers and Sprayers (1,599 men and women working any time in 1969–1988 at Dow plant in New Plymouth) (in IARC cohort)		**Dioxins; 2,4-D; 2,4,5-T; MCPA; MCPB; 2,4,5-TCP; Picloram**	
Mortality 1969–2004			McBride et al., 2009a
Ever-exposed workers	3	1.6 (0.3–4.7)	
Never-exposed workers	1	1.6 (0.0–8.7)	
Production Workers (713 men and 100 women worked > 1 month in 1969–1984)			
Mortality 1969–2000	1	0.9 (0.0–4.9)	't Mannetje et al., 2005
Sprayers (697 men and 2 women registered any time 1973–1984)			
Mortality 1973–2000	1	0.7 (0.0–3.8)	't Mannetje et al., 2005
NIOSH Mortality Cohort (12 US plants, 5,172 male production and maintenance workers 1942–1984) (included in IARC cohort as of 1997)		**Dioxins, phenoxy herbicides**	
Through 1993	12	1.1 (0.6–1.9)	Steenland et al., 1999
Chloracne subcohort (n = 608) (Lymphatic and hematopoietic, ICD-9 200–208)	6	1.1 (0.4–2.5)	
All Dow TCP-Exposed Workers (TCP production 1942–1979 or 2,4,5-T production 1948–1982 in Midland, Michigan) (in IARC and NIOSH cohorts)		**2,4,5-T; 2,4,5-TCP**	
1942–2003 (n = 1,615)	9	1.3 (0.6–2.5)	Collins et al., 2009a
1940–1994 (n = 2,187 men)	nr	1.4 (0.6–2.7)	Bodner et al., 2003
All Dow PCP-Exposed Workers—all workers from the two plants that only made PCP (in Tacoma, Washington, and Wichita, Kansas) and workers who made PCP and TCP at two additional plants (in Midland, Michigan, and Sauget, Illinois)		**2,4,5-T; 2,4,5-TCP**	Ruder and Yiin, 2011
1940–2005 (n = 2,122) (ICD-9 200, 202, 273.3)	17	1.8 (1.0–2.8)	
PCP and TCP (n = 720)	8	2.5 (1.1–4.9)	
PCP (no TCP) (n = 1,402)	9	1.4 (0.6–2.7)	
Dow 2,4-D Production Workers (1945–1982 in Midland, Michigan) (subset of all TCP-exposed workers)		**2,4-D, lower chlorinated dioxins**	

TABLE 8-42 Non-Hodgkin Lymphoma, continued

Study Population[a]	Exposed Cases[b]	**Exposure of Interest**/Estimated Relative Risk (95% CI)[b]	Reference
Cancer incidence through 2007 in Dow workers (n = 1,256) vs comparisons from state cancer registries (n = 23,354) (Cohort 3)	14	1.7 (0.9–2.9)	Burns et al., 2011
Through 1994 (n = 1,517)	3	1.0 (0.2–2.9)	Burns et al., 2001
Through 1986 (n = 878) vs national vs 36,804 "unexposed" workers at same location	2	2.0 (0.2–7.1)	Bloemen et al., 1993
Dow PCP Production Workers (1937–1989 in Midland, Michigan) (*not* in IARC and NIOSH cohorts)		**Low chlorinated dioxins, 2,4-D**	
Mortality 1940–2004 (n = 577, excluding 196 also having exposure to TCP)	8	2.4 (1.0–4.7)	Collins et al., 2009b
Mortality 1940–1989 (n = 770)			Ramlow et al., 1996
All lymphopoietic cancer (ICDA-8 200–209)			
0-yr latency	7	1.4 (0.6–2.9)	
15-yr latency	5	1.3 (0.4–3.1)	
Other, unspecified lymphopoietic cancer (ICDA-8 200, 202–203, 209)			
0-yr latency	5	2.0 (0.7–4.7)	
15-yr latency	4	2.0 (0.5–5.1)	
OCCUPATIONAL—PAPER AND PULP WORKERS		**TCDD**	
IARC cohort of pulp and paper workers—60,468 workers from 11 countries, TCDD among 27 agents assessed by JEM			McLean et al., 2006
Exposure to nonvolatile organochlorine compounds			
Never	35	0.9 (0.7–1.3)	
Ever	25	0.9 (0.6–1.3)	
Exposure to chlorophenols	50	4.3 (2.7–6.9)	
OCCUPATIONAL—HERBICIDE-USING WORKERS (*not* related to IARC sprayer cohorts)			
CANADA			
Canadian Farm Operator Study—156,242 men farming in Manitoba, Saskatchewan, and Alberta in 1971; mortality from NHL June 1971–December 1987			

continued

TABLE 8-42 Non-Hodgkin Lymphoma, continued

Study Population[a]	Exposed Cases[b]	**Exposure of Interest**/Estimated Relative Risk (95% CI)[b]	Reference
Farm operators ≥ 35 yrs of age (June 1971–December 1987)			Morrison et al., 1994
All farm operators	nr	0.8 (0.7–0.9)	
Highest quartile of herbicides sprayed	19	2.1 (1.1–3.9)	
Highest quartile of herbicide sprayed relative to no spraying	6	3.0 (1.1–8.1)	
Farm operators ≥ 35 yrs of age during study period (June 1971–December 1985)			Wigle et al., 1990
All farmers	103	0.9 (0.8–1.1)	
Spraying herbicides on 250+ acres	10	2.2 (1.0–4.6)	
DENMARK			
Danish gardeners—incidence from 3,156 male and 859 female gardeners			Hansen et al., 2007
25-year followup (1975–2001)		**Herbicides**	
Born before 1915 (high exposure)	16	1.4 (0.9–2.3)	
Born 1915–1934 (medium exposure)	25	1.2 (0.8–1.8)	
Born after 1934 (low exposure)	1	0.2 (0.0–1.0)	
10-year followup (1975–1984) of male gardeners (lymphohematopoietic, ICD-7 200–2005)	15	1.4 (0.8–2.4)	Hansen et al., 1992
NHL (ICD-7 200, 202, 205)	6	1.7 (0.6–3.8)	
FINNISH Phenoxy Herbicide Sprayers (1,909 men working 1955–1971 ≥ 2 wk) *not* IARC		**Phenoxy herbicides**	
Incidence			Asp et al., 1994
No latency	1	0.4 (0.0–2.0)	
10-yr latency	1	0.4 (0.0–2.4)	
Except for lung cancer, numbers too small for reporting mortality 1972–1980	0	nr	Riihimaki et al., 1982
ITALIAN Licensed Pesticide Users—male farmers in southern Piedmont licensed 1970–1974			
Mortality 1970–1986 (n = 23,401) (ICD-8 202.0–202.9)	15	0.9 (0.5–1.5)	Torchio et al., 1994
Incidence 1976–1983 (n = 25,945)			Corrao et al., 1989
Licensed pesticide users and nonusers	45	1.4 (1.0–1.9)	
Farmers in arable land areas	31	1.8 (1.2–2.5)	
Italian rice growers with documented phenoxy use (n = 1,487)	4	**Phenoxy herbicides** 1.3 (0.3–3.3)	Gambini et al., 1997
SWEDEN			
20,245 Swedish pesticide applicators with license issued between 1965 and 1976	27	1.1 (0.7–1.6)	Wiklund et al., 1989b

TABLE 8-42 Non-Hodgkin Lymphoma, continued

Study Population[a]	Exposed Cases[b]	**Exposure of Interest**/Estimated Relative Risk (95% CI)[b]	Reference
354,620 Swedish agriculture, forestry workers			Wiklund et al., 1988
Workers in land, animal husbandry	670	1.0 (0.9–1.1)	
Timber cutters	111	0.9 (0.7–1.1)	
Incident NHL cases 1961–1973 with agriculture as economic activity in 1960 census	476	*99% CI* 1.1 (0.9–1.2)	Wiklund, 1983
Swedish lumberjacks—used phenoxys 1954–1967, Incidence 1958–1992			Thörn et al., 2000
Exposed (n = 154)			
Foremen (n = 15)	0	—	
Lumberjacks (n = 139)	1	1.9 (0.0–10.7)	
Unexposed lumberjacks (n = 241)	1	0.8 (0.0–4.5)	
THE NETHERLANDS			
Dutch Licensed Herbicide Sprayers—1,341 certified before 1980			
Through 1987	0	nr	Swaen et al., 1992
UNITED STATES			
US farmers—usual occupation of farmer and industry of agriculture on death certificates 1984–1988 from 23 states		**Herbicides** PCMRs	Blair et al., 1993
Men			
Whites (n = 119,648)	843	1.2 (1.1–1.3)	
Nonwhites (n = 11,446)	24	0.7 (0.5–1.1)	
Women			
Whites (n = 2,400)	18	1.1 (0.6–1.7)	
Nonwhites (n = 2,066)	6	1.1 (0.4–2.3)	
US Agricultural Health Study—prospective study of licensed pesticide sprayers in Iowa and North Carolina: commercial (n = 4,916), private/farmers (n = 52,395, 97.4% men), and spouses of private sprayers (n = 32,347, 0.007% men), enrolled 1993–1997; followups with CATIs 1999–2003 and 2005–2010		**Phenoxy herbicides**	
Incidence			
Enrollment through 2006—SIRs for participants			Koutros et al., 2010a
NHL			
Private applicators	195	1.0 (0.9–1.1)	
Commercial applicators	9	0.8 (0.4–1.6)	
Spouses	86	1.0 (0.8–1.2)	

continued

TABLE 8-42 Non-Hodgkin Lymphoma, continued

Study Population[a]	Exposed Cases[b]	**Exposure of Interest**/Estimated Relative Risk (95% CI)[b]	Reference
B-cell			
Private applicators	167	1.0 (0.9–1.2)	
Commercial applicators	8	0.9 (0.4–1.7)	
Spouses	78	1.1 (0.8–1.3)	
Enrollment through 2002			Samanic et al., 2006
Dicamba—lifetime days exposure			
None	39	1.0	
1– < 20	18	1.8 (1.0–3.2)	
20– < 56	14	1.3 (0.7–2.5)	
56– < 116	7	0.9 (0.4–2.2)	
≥ 116	7	1.2 (0.5–2.9)	
		p-trend = 0.92	
Enrollment through 2002			Alavanja et al., 2005
Private applicators	114	1.0 (0.8–1.2)	
Spouses of private applicators (> 99% women)	42	0.9 (0.6–1.2)	
Commercial applicators	6	1.0 (0.4–2.1)	
Mortality			
Enrollment through 2007, vs state rates			Waggoner et al., 2011
Applicators (n = 1,641)	90	0.8 (0.7–1.0)	
Spouses (n = 676)	42	1.1 (0.8–1.5)	
Enrollment through 2000, vs state rates			Blair et al., 2005a
Private applicators (men and women)	33	0.9 (0.6–1.2)	
Spouses of private applicators (> 99% women)	16	1.2 (0.7–2.0)	
California United Farm Workers of America			
Nested case-control analysis of Hispanic workers in cohort of 139,000 CA United Farm Workers			Mills et al., 2005
Ever used 2,4-D	nr	3.8 (1.9–7.8)	
US Department of Agriculture Workers—nested case-control study of white men dying 1970–1979 of NHL		**Herbicides**	
Agricultural extension agents (from Table 3)	nr	1.2 (0.7–2.3)	Alavanja et al., 1988
White Male Residents of Iowa—NHL cancer on death certificate, usual occupation: farmers vs not		**Herbicides**	
> 30 yrs old when died 1964–1978—case-control	1,101	1.3 (nr)	Burmeister et al., 1983
H_0: only for "modern methods" → born after 1900			

TABLE 8-42 Non-Hodgkin Lymphoma, continued

Study Population[a]	Exposed Cases[b]	**Exposure of Interest**/Estimated Relative Risk (95% CI)[b]	Reference
Born before 1880	154	2.9 (nr)	
Born 1980–1900	336	1.6 (nr)	
Born after 1900	611	0.9 (nr)	
ENVIRONMENTAL			
Seveso, Italy Residential Cohort—Industrial accident July 10, 1976 (723 residents Zone A; 4,821 Zone B; 31,643 Zone R; 181,574 local reference group) (ICD-9 171)		**TCDD**	
Incidence			
20-yr followup to 1996—men and women			
Zone A	1	0.8 (0.1–5.7)	Pesatori et al., 2009
Zone B	12	1.5 (0.9–2.7)	
Zone R	49	0.9 (0.7–1.2)	
10-yr followup to 1991—men			Bertazzi et al., 1993
Zone A	0	nr	
Zone B	3	2.3 (0.7–7.4)	
Zone R	12	1.3 (0.7–2.5)	
10-yr followup to 1991—women			Bertazzi et al., 1993
Zone A	0	nr	
Zone B	1	0.9 (0.1–6.4)	
Zone R	10	1.2 (0.6–2.3)	
Mortality			
25-yr followup to 2001—men and women			Consonni et al., 2008
Zone A	3	3.4 (1.1–10.5)	
Zone B	7	1.2 (0.6–2.6)	
Zone R	40	1.0 (0.7–1.4)	
20-yr followup to 1996			Bertazzi et al., 2001
Zone A—men and women	2	3.3 (0.8–13.1)	
Zone B—men and women	5	1.2 (0.5–3.0)	
Zones A and B—men	3	1.2 (0.4–3.9)	
Zones A and B—women	4	1.8 (0.7–4.9)	
15-yr followup to 1991—men			Bertazzi et al., 1997, 1998
Zone A	0	0.0 (0.0–18.1)	
Zone B	2	1.5 (0.2–5.3)	
Zone R	10	1.1 (0.5–2.0)	
15-yr followup to 1991—women			Bertazzi et al., 1997, 1998
Zone A	0	0.0 (0.0–19.6)	
Zone B	0	0.0 (0.0–3.0)	
Zone R	8	0.9 (0.4–1.7)	
10-yr followup to 1986—men			Bertazzi et al., 1989a,b
Zone B	nr	nr	
Zone R	3	1.0 (0.3–3.4)	
10-yr followup to 1986—women			
Zone B	2	1.0 (0.3–4.2)	
Zone R	4	1.6 (0.5–4.7)	

continued

TABLE 8-42 Non-Hodgkin Lymphoma, continued

Study Population[a]	Exposed Cases[b]	**Exposure of Interest**/Estimated Relative Risk (95% CI)[b]	Reference
Other International Environmental Studies			
FINLAND			
Finnish community exposed to chlorophenol contamination (men and women)—incidence	16	**Chlorophenol** 2.8 (1.4–5.6)	Lampi et al., 1992
FRANCE			
Residents near French solid-waste incinerator in Besançon. NHL cases diagnosed 2003–2005—incidence		**Dioxin, furans, PCBs**	Viel et al., 2011
pg WHO_{1998}-TEQ/g lipid:			
Σ PCDD	13.4	1.1 (1.0–1.3) (p-trend < 0.01)	
Σ PCDF	9.4	1.2 (1.0–1.4) (p-trend = 0.01)	
Σ dl-PCBs	33.1	1.0 (1.0–1.1) (p-trend = 0.01)	
Residents near French solid-waste incinerator—incidence		**Dioxin**	Viel et al., 2008
Highly exposed census group vs slightly exposed	nr	1.1 (1.0–1.3)	
Residents near municipal solid-waste incinerator—incidence		**Dioxin**	Floret et al., 2003
High-exposure category	31	2.3 (1.4–3.8)	
Residents near municipal solid-waste incinerator—incidence		**Dioxin**	Viel et al., 2000
Spatial cluster	286	1.3 (p = 0.00003)	
1994–1995	109	1.8 (p = 0.00003)	
NEW ZEALAND			
Residents of New Plymouth Territorial Authority, New Zealand, near plant manufacturing 2,4,5-T in 1962–1987		2,4,5-T	Read et al., 2007
Incidence	223	1.0 (0.9–1.1)[d]	
1970–1974	33	1.8 (1.2–2.5)	
1975–1979	29	1.3 (0.9–1.9)	
1980–1984	22	0.8 (0.5–1.3)	
1985–1989	24	0.7 (0.5–1.1)	
1990–1994	35	0.8 (0.6–1.1)	
1995–1999	61	1.1 (0.8–1.4)	
2000–2001	19	0.8 (0.5–1.3)	
Mortality	138	1.1 (0.9–1.3)[d]	
1970–1974	19	1.6 (0.9–2.4)	
1975–1979	24	1.6 (1.0–2.4)	
1980–1984	14	1.0 (0.5–1.6)	
1985–1989	25	1.3 (0.9–2.0)	
1990–1994	23	0.9 (0.6–1.4)	

TABLE 8-42 Non-Hodgkin Lymphoma, continued

Study Population[a]	Exposed Cases[b]	**Exposure of Interest**/Estimated Relative Risk (95% CI)[b]	Reference
1995–1999	21	0.7 (0.4–1.1)	
2000–2001	12	1.0 (0.5–1.8)	
CASE-CONTROL STUDIES			
US Case-Control Studies			
Cental US—meta-analysis of NHL and farmers	nr	**Pesticides** 1.3 (1.2–1.6)	Keller-Byrne et al., 1997
Pooled incidence data on herbicide use from 3 case-control studies in **Iowa/Minnesota**, **Kansas**, and **Nebraska** (n = 973)		**Herbicides**	Chiu et al., 2004
Farmers (no herbicide use)	294	1.2 (1.0–1.5)	
Farmers (herbicide use)	273	1.0 (0.8–1.2)	
Pooled data from case-control studies in **Iowa**, **Minnesota**, and **Nebraska**—effect of asthma on NHL and pesticide use (n = 872)		**Pesticides**	Lee et al., 2004b
Asthmatics—incidence			
Herbicide exposure—phenoxy acid	17	1.3 (0.7–2.4)	
Exposure among farmers			
2,4-D	17	1.3 (0.7–2.5)	
2,4,5-T	7	2.2 (0.8–6.1)	
Nonasthmatics—incidence			
Herbicide exposure—phenoxy acid	176	1.0 (0.8–1.3)	
Exposure among farmers			
2,4-D	172	1.0 (0.8–1.3)	
2,4,5-T	36	1.1 (0.7–1.8)	
Kansas residents–duration and frequency of herbicide use—incidence		**Phenoxy herbicides, 2.4-D**	Hoar et al., 1986
All farmers	133	1.4 (0.9–2.1)	
Farm-use of herbicides	7	6.0 (1.9–19.5)	
NCI SEER study (Iowa, Los Angeles County, Detroit, Seattle), 1998–2000; 1,321 NHL patients and 1,057 controls—residential exposures		**2,4-D**	Hartge et al., 2005
2,4-D exposure in carpet dust (ng/g)			
Under detection limit	147	1.0	
< 500	257	1.1 (0.8–1.6)	
500–999	86	0.9 (0.6–1.5)	
1,000–9,999	165	0.7 (0.5–1.0)	
> 10,000	24	0.8 (0.4–1.7)	
Nebraska residents (men and women), NHL reclassified according to specific chromosomal translocation (t[14;18] [q32;q21])—incidence		**Herbicides**	Chiu et al., 2006
Translocation present in cases			
Herbicides	25	2.9 (1.1–7.9)	

continued

TABLE 8-42 Non-Hodgkin Lymphoma, continued

Study Population[a]	Exposed Cases[b]	**Exposure of Interest**/Estimated Relative Risk (95% CI)[b]	Reference
Translocation present in cases			
Herbicides	22	0.7 (0.3–1.2)	
Females on Eastern **Nebraska** farms		**Herbicides**	Zahm et al., 1993
	119	1.0 (0.7–1.4)	
Eastern **Nebraska** residents—incidence		**2,4-D**	Zahm et al., 1990
Ever done farm work	147	0.9 (0.6–1.4)	
Ever mixed or applied 2,4-D	43	1.5 (0.9–2.5)	
Upstate New York—population-based study, women (20–79 yrs old), 1995–1998 (376 cases vs 463 controls)		**Herbicides, pesticides**	Kato et al., 2004
Home use only of herbicides, pesticides (times)			
0	231	1.0	
1–4	33	0.9 (0.5–1.5)	
5–17	30	0.7 (0.4–1.3)	
18–39	27	1.0 (0.6–1.7)	
≥ 40	40	0.9 (0.5–1.5)	
Hancock County, **Ohio**, residents—farmers	15	1.6 (0.8–3.4)	Dubrow et al., 1988
Washington state residents—incidence (1983–1985)		**Phenoxy herbicides, chlorinated phenols**	Woods et al., 1987
Phenoxy herbicide use	nr	1.1 (0.8–1.4)	
Chlorophenol use	nr	1.0 (0.8–1.2)	
Farming occupations	nr	1.3 (1.0–1.7)	
Forestry herbicide appliers	nr	4.8 (1.2–19.4)	
Self-reported chloracne	nr	2.1 (0.6–7.0)	
Wisconsin residents—farmers (ICD-8 200.0, 200.1, 202.2)		**Herbicides**	Cantor, 1982
	175	1.2 (1.0–1.5)	
International Case-Control Studies			
Asian patients (≥ 20 yrs old) from China, Korea, and Japan diagnosed with NKTCL between March 2000 and March 2005–occupational exposures		**Herbicides, pesticides**	Xu et al., 2006
Pesticide use	23	4.0 (2.0–8.1)	
Herbicide	13	3.2 (1.4–7.4)	
Insecticide	20	3.5 (1.7–7.1)	
Fungicide	10	6.1 (2.0–18.5)	
Australian population-based study in New Wales (2000–2001)		**Phenoxy compounds**	Fritschi et al., 2005
Phenoxy herbicides			
Nonsubstantial exposures	10	0.7 0.3–1.7)	

TABLE 8-42 Non-Hodgkin Lymphoma, continued

Study Population[a]	Exposed Cases[b]	**Exposure of Interest**/Estimated Relative Risk (95% CI)[b]	Reference
Australian residents in Victorian Cancer Registry (1982–1987)		**Phenoxy compounds**	Smith and Christophers, 1992
Exposure > 1 day	15	1.5 (0.6–3.7)	
Exposure > 30 days	7	2.7 (0.7–9.6)	
Canadian population based study (March 2000–February 2004), men and women subjects and matched controls (20–79 yrs of age)—organochlorines and NHL		**dl-PCBs**	Spinelli et al., 2007
Total dl–PCBs			
Lowest quartile	82	1.0	
Second quartile	96	1.4 (0.9–2.2)	
Third quartile	82	1.6 (1.0–2.5)	
Highest quartile	143	2.4 (1.5–3.7)	
		p-trend < 0.001	
Canadian multicenter population-based study (September 1991–December 1994), male NHL patients (n = 517) and controls (n = 1,506) and impact of exposure to multiple pesticides		**Phenoxy herbicides, 2,4-D**	Hohenadel et al., 2011
Exposure to multiple herbicides			
0	369	1.0 (nr)	
1	45	1.2 (0.9–1.8)	
2–4	73	1.6 (1.2–2.2)	
5+	26	1.6 (1.0–2.6)	
Exposure to phenoxy herbicides			
0	384	1.0 (nr)	
1	66	1.3 (1.0–1.8)	
2+	63	1.8 (1.3–2.5)	
Exposure to Mecoprop	23	2.1 (1.2–5.4)	
Exposure to 2,4-D	49	0.9 (0.7–1.3)	
Canadian multicenter population-based study (September 1991–December 1994), male NHL patients (n = 517) and controls (n = 1,506) and pesticide exposure of ≥ 10 h/yr		**Phenoxy herbicides, 2,4-D**	McDuffie et al., 2001
Exposed to phenoxy herbicides	131	1.4 (1.1–1.8)	
2,4-D	111	1.3 (1.0–1.7)	
Mecoprop	53	2.3 (1.6–3.4)	
Danish residents (Copenhagen and Aarhus) in the Diet, Cancer and Health prospective study diagnosed with NHL from enrollment (1994–5/1977) through 2008		**Organochlorines**	Bräuner et al., 2012
Organochlorines in adipose tissue (ug/kg lipids)			
dl-PCB 118			

continued

TABLE 8-42 Non-Hodgkin Lymphoma, continued

Study Population[a]	Exposed Cases[b]	**Exposure of Interest**/Estimated Relative Risk (95% CI)[b]	Reference
10–25	53	1.0 (nr)	
25–34	63	0.9 (0.5–1.6)	
34–48	58	1.0 (0.6–1.7)	
48–62	34	0.7 (0.3–1.3)	
62–150	25	0.7 (0.4–1.4)	
dl-PCB 156			
13–28	62	1.0 (nr)	
28–34	51	0.6 (0.3–1.0)	
34–41	54	0.7(0.4–1.2)	
41–50	45	0.9 (0.5–1.8)	
50–88	23	0.7 (0.3–1.4)	
Denmark—Danish farmworkers—incidence	147	**Phenoxy herbicides** 1.0 (nr)	Ronco et al., 1992
Italian farmworkers—mortality	14	1.3 (nr)	
France hospital-based case-control study		**Herbicides**	Orsi et al., 2009
Occupational use of herbicides	25	1.3 (0.7–2.2)	
Phenoxy herbicides	11	0.9 (0.4–1.9)	
Domestic use of herbicides	86	1.0 (0.7–1.5)	
German population-based study (1986–1998), men and women, 15–75 yrs of age—occupational factors associated with NHL		**TCDD, herbicides**	Richardson et al., 2008
Chlorophenols			
NHL—high-grade malignancy	61	2.0 (1.3–2.9)	
NHL—low-grade malignancy	77	1.3 (1.0–1.8)	
CLL	44	0.9 (0.6–1.3)	
Herbicides			
NHL—high-grade malignancy	56	2.2 (1.4–3.3)	
NHL—low-grade malignancy	79	1.4 (1.0–1.9)	
CLL	43	1.2 (0.8–1.7)	
Irish farmers and farmworkers		**Herbicides**	Dean, 1994
Other malignant neoplasms of lymphoid and histiocytic tissue (including some types of NHL) (ICD-9 202)	164	1.8 (1.2–2.6)	
Italian incident cases of malignancies of the hematolymphopoietic system in men and women (20–74 yrs of age) from agricultural and mixed use areas (HD cases = 258)		**Herbicides**	Miligi et al., 2006
Men, women	73	1.0 (0.7–1.4)	
Men	49	0.8 (0.5–1.3)	
Women	24	1.3 (0.7–2.5)	
NHL (men, women)			
Phenoxy herbicides—ever	32	1.1 (0.6–1.8)	
Probability of use more than "low," lack of protective equipment	13	2.4 (0.9–7.6)	

TABLE 8-42 Non-Hodgkin Lymphoma, continued

Study Population[a]	Exposed Cases[b]	**Exposure of Interest**/Estimated Relative Risk (95% CI)[b]	Reference
2,4-D—ever	17	0.9 (0.5–1.8)	
Probability of use more than "low," lack of protective equipment	9	4.4 (1.1–29.1)	
MCPA—ever	18	0.9 (0.4–1.8)	
Probability of use more than "low," lack of protective equipment	7	3.4 (0.8–23.2)	
Italian residents of 11 areas (NHL other than lymphosarcoma and reticulosarcoma)—incidence		**Herbicides**	Miligi et al., 2003
Phenoxy acid herbicides exposure			
Men	18	1.0 (0.5–2.0)	
Women	11	1.3 (0.5–3.7)	
2,4-D exposure			
Men	6	0.7 (0.3–1.9)	
Women	7	1.5 (0.4–5.7)	
Italian farming and animal-breeding workers (men and women) (NHL other than lymphosarcoma and reticulosarcoma)—incidence		**Herbicides**	Nanni et al., 1996
Exposure to herbicides	3	1.4 (0.4–5.7)	
Italian farming and animal-breeding workers (men and women)—incidence		**Herbicides**	Amadori et al., 1995
NHL, CLL combined	164	1.8 (1.2–2.6)	
Residents of selected **Italian** provinces		**Herbicides**	Vineis et al., 1991
Male residents of contaminated areas	nr	2.2 (1.4–3.5)	
Residents of Milan, **Italy**, area (men and women)—incidence		**Herbicides**	LaVecchia et al., 1989
Agricultural occupations	nr	2.1 (1.3–3.4)	
New Zealand National Cancer Registry (1980–1984)—case-control study of 652 incident NHL cases vs remainder of 19,904 men with any incident cancer		**Herbicides**	Reif et al., 1989
Forestry workers (n = 134)			
Aged 20–59	4	2.0 (0.7–5.6)	
Aged ≥ 60	3	1.7 (0.5–5.4)	
Sawmill workers (n = 139)		**Herbicides, chlorophenols**	
	4	1.2 (0.4–3.2)	
New Zealand National Cancer Registry (1977–1981) (< 70 yrs of age)—incidence (1977–1981) (ICD-9 200 and 202)		**Herbicides**	Pearce et al., 1987
Farming occupations	33	1.0 (0.7–1.5)	
Fencing work	68	1.4 (1.0–2.0)	

continued

TABLE 8-42 Non-Hodgkin Lymphoma, continued

Study Population[a]	Exposed Cases[b]	**Exposure of Interest**/Estimated Relative Risk (95% CI)[b]	Reference
New Zealand National Cancer Registry (1977–1981) (< 70 yrs of age)—incidence (1977–1981) (ICD-9 202 only)		**Phenoxy herbicides**	Pearce et al., 1986
Agricultural sprayers	19	1.5 (0.7–3.3)	
New Zealand National Cancer Registry (1977–1981) (≥ 20 yrs of age) with agricultural occupations—incidence (ICD-9 200 and 202)	nr	**Herbicides** 1.4 (0.9–2.0)	Pearce et al., 1985
Sweden—male, female subjects (18–74 yrs of age) with NHL living in Sweden between December 1, 1999 and April 30, 2002 vs controls from national population registry		**Pesticides, herbicides**	Eriksson et al., 2008
Herbicides, total	74	1.7 (1.2–2.5)	
≤ 20 days	36	1.6 (1.0–2.7)	
> 20 days	38	1.9 (1.1–3.2)	
Phenoxyacetic acids	47	2.0 (1.2–3.4)	
≤ 45 days	32	2.8 (1.5–5.5)	
> 45 days	15	1.3 (0.6–2.7)	
MCPA	21	2.8 (1.3–6.2)	
≤ 32 days	15	3.8 (1.4–10.5)	
> 32 days	6	1.7 (0.5–6.0)	
2,4,5-T, 2,4-D	33	1.6 (0.9–3.0)	
≤ 29 days	21	2.1 (1.0–4.4)	
> 29 days	12	1.3 (0.6–3.1)	
Sweden—male and female patients (18–74 yrs of age) diagnosed December 1999–April 2002		**Pesticides, herbicides**	Hardell et al., 2002
Chlorophenols			
NHL—high grade malignancy	61	2.0 (1.3–2.9)	
Sweden—pooled analysis of case-control NHL, hairy cell leukemia studies		**Herbicides**	Hardell et al., 2002
Herbicide exposure	77	1.8 (1.3–2.4)	
Phenoxyacetic acids	64	1.7 (1.2–2.3)	
MCPA	21	2.6 (1.4–4.9)	
2,4-D, 2,4,5-T	48	1.5 (1.0–2.2)	
Other	15	2.9 (1.3–6.4)	
Substantial exposure	5	1.8 (0.4–7.4)	
Sweden—adipose tissue from 33 NHL patients and 39 surgical controls from Örebro-Uppsala medical region (1994–1997)		**Dioxin, dibenzofurans**	Hardell et al., 2001
TEQ > 27.8, EA > 80	8	2.8 (0.5–18.0)	
Umea (**Sweden**) Hospital patients—incidence		**Phenoxy herbicides, chlorophenols**	Hardell et al., 1994
Exposed to phenoxy herbicides	25	5.5 (2.7–11.0)	

TABLE 8-42 Non-Hodgkin Lymphoma, continued

Study Population[a]	Exposed Cases[b]	**Exposure of Interest**/Estimated Relative Risk (95% CI)[b]	Reference
Exposed to chlorophenols	35	4.8 (2.7–8.8)	
Swedish Regional Cancer Registry—NHL patients		**Phenoxy herbicides**	Persson et al., 1993
Exposed to phenoxy herbicides	10	2.3 (0.7–7.2)	
Exposed to chlorophenols	9	6.0 (1.1–31.0)	
Örebro (**Sweden**) Hospital (men and women)—incidence		**Phenoxy herbicides, chlorophenols**	Persson et al., 1989
Exposed to phenoxy acids	6	4.9 (1.0–27.0)	
Lund (**Sweden**) Hospital patients—incidence		**Herbicides**	Olsson and Brandt, 1988
Exposed to herbicides	nr	1.3 (0.8–2.1)	
Exposed to chlorophenols	nr	1.2 (0.7–2.0)	
Swedish patients (1970–1977)		**Phenoxy acids, chlorophenols**	Hardell, 1981
Exposed to phenoxy herbicides	41	4.8 (2.9–8.1)	
Exposed to chlorophenols	50	4.3 (2.7–6.9)	

NOTE: 2,4-D, 2,4-dichlorophenoxyacetic acid; 2,4-DP, dichlorprop; 2,4,5-T, 2,4,5-trichlorophenoxyacetic acid; 2,4,5-TCP, 2,4,5-trichlorophenol; 2,5-DCP, 2,5-dichlorophenol; ACC, Army Chemical Corps; CA, California; CATI, computer-assisted telephone interviewing; CDC, Centers for Disease Control and Prevention; CI, confidence interval; CLL, chronic lymphocytic leukemia; COI, chemical of interest; dl, dioxin-like; HD, Hodgkin disease; HR, hazard ratio; IARC, International Agency for Research on Cancer; ICD, International Classification of Diseases; ICDA, International Classification of Diseases, Adapted for Use in the United States; JEM, job-exposure matrix; MCPA, 2-methyl-4-chlorophenoxyacetic acid; MCPB, 4-(4-chloro-2-methylphenoxy)butanoic acid; MCPP, methylchlorophenoxypropionic acid; MOS, military occupation specialty; NCI, National Cancer Institute; NHL, non-Hodgkin lymphoma; NIOSH, National Institute for Occupational Safety and Health; NKTCL, NK/T-cell lymphoma; nr, not reported; PCDD, polychlorinated dibenzo-*p*-dioxin (highly chlorinated, if four or more chlorines); PCMR, proportionate cancer mortality ratios; PCP, pentachlorophenol; PM, proportionate mortality; SEA, Southeast Asia; SEER, Surveillance, Epidemiology, and End Results; SIR, standardized incidence ratio; SMR, standardized mortality rate; TCDD, 2,3,7,8-tetrachlorodibenzo-*p*-dioxin; TCP, trichlorophenol; TEQ, toxicity equivalent; USDA, United States Department of Agriculture; VA, US Department of Veterans Affairs.

[a]Subjects are male and outcome is mortality unless otherwise noted.

[b]Given when available; results other than estimated risk explained individually.

[c]Lymphopoietic cancers comprise all of forms of lymphoma (including Hodgkin disease and non-Hodgkin lymphoma) and leukemia (ALL, AML, CLL, CML).

[d]Committee computed total SMR and SIR by dividing sum of observed values by sum of expected values over all years; 95% CIs on these total ratios were computed with exact methods.

TABLE 8-43 Selected Epidemiologic Studies—Chronic Lymphocytic Leukemia (Shaded Entries Are New Information for This Update)

Study Population[a]	Exposed Cases[b]	**Exposure of Interest**/Estimated Relative Risk (95% CI)[b]	Reference
VIETNAM VETERANS			
International Vietnam-Veteran Study			
Australian Vietnam Veterans—58,077 men and 153 women served on land or in Vietnamese waters during 5/23/1962–7/1/1973 vs Australian population		**All COIs**	
Incidence			
All branches, 1982–2000	58	1.2 (0.7–1.7)	ADVA, 2005a
Navy	12	1.5 (0.8–2.6)	
Army	42	1.7 (1.2–2.2)	
Air Force	4	0.9 (0.2–2.2)	
OCCUPATIONAL—HERBICIDE-USING WORKERS (*not* related to IARC sprayer cohorts)			
CANADA			
Sawmill Workers in British Columbia—23,829 workers for ≥ 1 year at 11 mills using chlorophenates 1940–1985		**Chlorophenates, not TCDD**	
Incidence—all leukemias (1969–1989)	47	1.2 (0.9–1.5)	Hertzman et al., 1997
ALL	2	1.0 (0.2–3.1)	
CLL	24	1.7 (1.2–2.4)	
AML	5	0.8 (0.3–1.7)	
CML	7	1.1 (0.5–2.0)	
Other, unspecified	5	0.5 (0.2–1.0)	
DENMARK			
Danish gardeners—incidence from 3,156 male and 859 female gardeners		**Herbicides**	Hansen et al., 2007
10-year followup (1975–1984) of Danish gardeners			Hansen et al., 1992
All gardeners	6	2.5 (0.9–5.5)	
Male gardeners	6	2.8 (1.0–6.0)	
UNITED STATES			
White Male Residents of Iowa—chronic lymphocytic leukemia on death certificate, usual occupation: farmers vs not		**Herbicides**	
> 30 yrs old when died 1964–1978—case-control (1,675 leukemia deaths, 1968–1978)			Burmeister et al., 1982
Farmer usual occupation on death certificate		1.2 ($p < 0.05$))	
CLL	132	1.7 (1.2–2.4)	
Lived in counties with highest herbicide use	nr	1.9 (1.2–3.1)	
White Male Residents of Iowa and Minnesota— > 30 yrs old diagnosed 1981–1983 in Iowa or 1980–1982 in Minnesota—case-control		**Herbicides**	

TABLE 8-43 Chronic Lymphocytic Leukemia, continued

Study Population[a]	Exposed Cases[b]	**Exposure of Interest**/Estimated Relative Risk (95% CI)[b]	Reference
> 30 yrs old diagnosed 1981–1983 in Iowa or 1980–1982 in Minnesota—case-control (ever farmer)			Brown et al., 1990
Ever farmed	156	1.4 (1.1–1.9)	
Any herbicide used	74	1.4 (1.0–2.0)	
Ever used 2,4,5-T	10	1.6 (0.7–3.4)	
Use at least 20 yrs before interview	7	3.3 (1.2–8.7)	
ENVIRONMENTAL			
Seveso, Italy Residential Cohort—Industrial accident July 10, 1976 (723 residents Zone A; 4,821 Zone B; 31,643 Zone R; 181,574 local reference group) (ICD-9 171)		**TCDD**	
Incidence			
20-yr followup to 1996—men and women (lymphatic leukemia, ICD-9 204)			
Zone A	1	2.8 (0.4–19.9)	Pesatori et al., 2009
Zone B	0	nr	
Zone R	13	0.8 (0.5–1.5)	
Mortality			
25-yr followup to 2001—men and women (lymphatic leukemia, ICD-9 204)			Consonni et al., 2008
Zone A	0	nr	
Zone B	3	1.3 (0.4–4.1)	
Zone R	23	1.4 (0.9–2.2)	
20-yr followup to 1996 (lymphatic leukemia)			Bertazzi et al., 2001
Zones A, B—men	2	1.6 (0.4–6.8)	
Zones A, B—women	0	nr	
Other International Environmental Studies			
NEW ZEALAND			
Residents of New Plymouth Territorial Authority, New Zealand, near plant manufacturing 2,4,5-T in 1962–1987		2,4,5-T	Read et al., 2007
Incidence	104	1.3 (1.1–1.6)[c]	
1970–1974	16	2.5 (1.4–4.1)	
1975–1979	7	0.9 (0.4–1.8)	
1980–1984	21	2.6 (1.6–3.9)	
1985–1989	16	1.4 (0.8–2.3)	
1990–1994	13	0.9 (0.5–1.6)	
1995–1999	19	0.9 (0.5–1.4)	
2000–2001	12	1.1 (0.6–1.9)	
Mortality	40	1.3 (0.9–1.8)[c]	
1970–1974	7	1.7 (0.7–3.5)	
1975–1979	7	1.8 (0.7–3.6)	
1980–1984	6	1.4 (0.5–3.0)	
1985–1989	4	0.8 (0.2–2.2)	

continued

TABLE 8-43 Chronic Lymphocytic Leukemia, continued

Study Population[a]	Exposed Cases[b]	**Exposure of Interest**/Estimated Relative Risk (95% CI)[b]	Reference
1990–1994	6	1.1 (0.4–2.5)	
1995–1999	8	1.3 (0.6–2.6)	
2000–2001	2	0.8 (0.1–2.8)	
CASE-CONTROL STUDIES			
US Case-Control Studies			
Tecumseh, Michigan, residents participating in longitudinal study (1959–1987)	10	**Herbicides** 1.8 (0.8–3.2)	Waterhouse et al., 1996
Nebraska—1,084 leukemia deaths in 1957–1974; farmers–usual occupation on death certificate	nr	**Herbicides, pesticides** 1.3 ($p < 0.05$)	Blair and White, 1985
248 CLL cases	nr	1.7 ($p < 0.05$)	
International Case-Control Studies			
France hospital-based case-control study		**Herbicides**	Orsi et al., 2009
Occupational use of herbicides	5	0.5 (0.2–1.3)	
Phenoxy herbicides	3	0.4 (0.1–1.7)	
German population-based study (1986–1998), men and women, 15–75 yrs of age—occupational factors associated with CLL		**TCDD, herbicides**	Richardson et al., 2008
Chlorophenols	44	0.9 (0.6–1.3)	
Lowest tertile cumulative exposure	12	0.9 (0.4–1.8)	
Middle tertile	15	0.9 (0.5–1.8)	
Highest tertile	17	0.9 (0.5–1.6)	
		p-trend = 0.770	
Herbicides	43	1.2 (0.8–1.7)	
Lowest tertile cumulative exposure	13	1.3 (0.7–2.7)	
Middle tertile	15	1.3 (0.7–2.5)	
Highest tertile	15	1.0 (0.5–1.9)	
		p-trend = 0.755	
Italian farming and animal-breeding workers (men and women)—incidence	15	**Herbicides** 2.3 (0.9–5.8)	Amadori et al., 1995
Farming workers only	5	1.6 (0.5–5.2)	
Breeding workers only	10	3.1 (1.1–8.3)	

NOTE: 2,4,5-T, 2,4,5-trichlorophenoxyacetic acid; ALL, acute lymphocytic leukemia; AML, acute myelogenous leukemia; CI, confidence interval; CLL, chronic lymphocytic leukemia; CML, chronic myelogenous leukemia; COI, chemical of interest; ICD, International Classification of Diseases; nr, not reported; TCDD, 2,3,7,8-tetrachlorodibenzo-*p*-dioxin.

[a]Subjects are male and outcome is mortality unless otherwise noted.

[b]Given when available; results other than estimated risk explained individually.

[c]The total SMR/SIR were computed by dividing sum of observed values by sum of expected values over all years; 95% CIs on these total ratios were computed with exact methods.

produced only phenoxy herbicides that would not have had TCDD contamination. Contemporary TCDD concentrations measured in a subsample of 187 workers were used to derive a model incorporating job history to estimate serum TCDD concentrations of all the men at the end of their employment. Use of the estimated TCDD concentrations of the workers in both factories showed a significant increase in death due to NHL in association with TCDD exposure (HR = 1.36, 95% CI 1.06–1.74). Dose–response modeling applied only to the workers in factory A estimated an increased risk of NHL mortality that neared significance (HR = 1.27, 95% CI 0.95–1.71), whereas an increase in risk had not been evident (HR = 0.98, 95% CI 0.19–4.47) in the qualitative exposure analysis by Boers et al. (2010).

Manuwald et al. (2012) reported mortality in 1,191 men and 398 women who had been employed for at least 3 months during 1952–1984 in a chemical plant in Hamburg (a subcohort of the IARC phenoxy-herbicide cohort). During that period, the plant produced insecticides and herbicides, including 2,4,5-T, so cohort members had the possibility of exposure to TCDD. Subjects entered the cohort on the date of their first employment in the plant, and vital status was sought through 2007. SMRs that were calculated relative to the population of Hamburg showed that mortality from NHL was not increased in men (five deaths, SMR = 1.56, 95% CI 0.50–3.65) or in women (two deaths, SMR = 1.67, 95% CI 0.19–6.02), but for the entire cohort the increase in risk was significant (SMR = 1.59, 95% CI 0.64–3.28).

Ruder and Yiin (2011) reported mortality in 1940–2005 in the NIOSH PCP cohort of 2,122 workers in the four US plants that had been involved in PCP production. PCP production entailed exposure to PCDDs and PCDFs but not to the most toxic 2,3,7,8 dioxin congener. A subcohort of 720 workers (all men, the PCP-plus-TCDD group) had also been employed in TCP production and so had also been exposed to TCDD. Relative to US referent rates, deaths from NHL were significantly increased in the entire cohort (17 deaths, SMR = 1.77, 95% CI 1.03–2.84) and in the PCP-plus-TCDD group (eight deaths, SMR = 2.50, 95% CI 1.08–4.93) but not in the PCP-only group (nine deaths, SMR = 1.41, 95% CI 0.64–2.67).

Koutros et al. (2010a) and Waggoner et al. (2011) assessed cancer incidence and mortality, respectively, in private applicators, commercial applicators, and their spouses in the AHS cohort vs the general population of Iowa and North Carolina. Koutros et al. (2010a) updated their previously reported incidence study through December 31, 2006, and found no association between pesticide exposure and NHL incidence in private applicators (195 cases, SIR = 0.99, 95% CI 0.86–1.14), commercial applicators (9 cases, SIR = 0.82, 95% CI 0.38–1.56) and their spouses (86 cases, SIR = 0.99, 95% CI 0.79–1.22). Waggoner et al. (2011) reported similar findings in applicators (90 cases, SMR = 0.84, 95% CI 0.67–1.03) and in their spouses (42 cases, SMR = 1.11, 95% CI 0.80–1.50). The AHS has been generating valuable information on the COIs for a number of years, but these results are not herbicide-specific and so are not regarded as being fully informative for the committee's task.

Case-Control Studies Using information assembled in the Cross-Canada Study of Pesticides and Health, Hohenadel et al. (2011) tested for interaction effects on the risk of NHL when exposures involved various combinations of pesticides. Men who had NHL (513) were compared with the studywide control group (1,506) to assess NHL risk associated with exposure to multiple pesticides. When exposure to multiple herbicides (144 cases exposed to any herbicide) was considered, there was a trend ($p = 0.02$) in those who had been exposed to more herbicides to have a higher risk of NHL. When the analysis was limited to phenoxy-herbicide exposures (129 cases exposed to any phenoxy herbicide), the trend was a bit stronger ($p = 0.01$). When 36 combinations of differing types of pesticides were assessed, five pairs (all including the insecticide malathion) showed higher risk when exposure was to both, but none of the interaction terms was statistically significant; two of the combinations with malathion involved the phenoxy herbicides 2,4-D and Mecoprop. That is consistent with results on associations between NHL and individual pesticides published previously (McDuffie et al., 2001), in which exposure to the two phenoxy herbicides individually increased the risk of NHL significantly, whereas this was not the case for the two other phenoxy herbicides considered (MCP and diclofop-methyl). For the subsets of those exposed to the particular phenoxy herbicide, but not to malathion, the risk remained significant for Mecoprop (23 cases exposed only to phenoxy herbicide, OR = 2.09, 95% CI 1.23–3.54) but not for 2,4-D (49 cases exposed only to phenoxy herbicide, OR = 0.94, 95% CI 0.67–1.3).

Bräuner et al. (2012) measured the concentrations of 10 PCBs and eight organochlorine pesticides in adipose tissues and examined their relationship with NHL risk. There were no associations between PCBs and other organochlorine pesticides tested except DDT, which was associated with an increased NHL risk.

Viel et al. (2011) found a strong and consistent association between serum concentrations of PCDDs, PCDFs, and dioxin-like PCBs and NHL risk in people who lived in the vicinity of a municipal solid-waste incinerator that had high dioxin emission concentrations (Viel et al., 2011).

The literature search for the present update identified two additional case-control studies in which the exposures considered were not sufficiently specific for this review's COIs. In an Iranian hospital-based case-control study of exposure to pesticides, Zakerinia et al. (2012) found a significant increase in NHL incidence in people who were exposed (OR = 3.9, 95% CI 2.2–6.8). Similarly, a case-control study in the Shanghai Health Watch project reported statistically significant increases in NHL risks in agriculture and farmworkers and in workers who were exposed to general herbicides (OR = 1.77, 95% CI 1.02–3.05) (Wong et al., 2010).

Biologic Plausibility

The diagnosis of NHL encompasses a wide variety of lymphoma subtypes. In humans, about 85% are of B-cell origin and 15% of T-cell origin. In commonly used laboratory mice, the lifetime incidence of spontaneous B-cell lymphomas is about 30% in females and about 10% in males. Although researchers seldom note the subtypes of B-cell lymphomas observed, lymphoblastic, lymphocytic, follicular, and plasma-cell lymphomas are seen in mice and are similar to types of NHL seen in humans. Laboratory rats, however, are less prone to develop lymphomas, but Fisher 344 rats do have an increased incidence of spontaneous mononuclear-cell leukemia of nonspecific origin. The lifetime incidence of leukemia is about 50% in male rats and about 20% in female rats. Neither mice nor rats develop T-cell lymphomas spontaneously at a predictable incidence, but T-cell–derived tumors can be induced by exposure to some carcinogens.

Several long-term feeding studies of various strains of mice and rats have been conducted over the last 30 years to determine the effects of TCDD on cancer incidence. Few of them have shown effects of TCDD on lymphoma or leukemia incidence. The NTP (1982a) reported no increase in overall incidence of lymphoma in female B6C3F1 mice exposed to TCDD at 0.04, 0.2, or 2.0 μg/kg per week for 104 weeks but found that histiocytic lymphomas (now considered to be equivalent to large B-cell lymphomas) were more common in the high-dose group. No effects on lymphoma incidence were seen in Osborne–Mendel rats treated with TCDD at 0.01, 0.05, or 0.5 μg/kg per week. Sprague–Dawley rats treated with TCDD at 0.003, 0.010, 0.022, 0.046, or 0.100 μg/kg per day showed no change in incidence of malignant lymphomas. Long-term exposure to phenoxy herbicides or cacodylic acid also has not resulted in an increased incidence of lymphomas in laboratory animals. Thus, few laboratory animal data support the biologic plausibility of promotion of NHL by TCDD or other COIs, but it should be noted that standard rodent models are not particularly sensitive for detection of chemicals that cause lymphohematopoietic cancers.

In contrast, more recent studies at the cellular level indicate that activation of the AHR by TCDD inhibits apoptosis, a mechanism of cell death that controls the growth of cancer cells. Vogel et al. (2007) studied human cancer cells in tissue culture and showed that addition of TCDD inhibited apoptosis in histiocytic-lymphoma cells, Burkitt-lymphoma cells, and NHL cell lines. The reduction in apoptosis was associated with an increase in the expression of *Cox-2*, *C/EBP* β, and *Bcl-xL* mRNA in the cells. Those genes code for proteins that protect cells from apoptosis. The effects of TCDD on apoptosis were blocked when an AHR antagonist or a Cox-2 inhibitor was added to the culture; this demonstrated the underlying AHR-dependent mechanism of the effects. More important, when C57Bl/10J mice were given multiple doses of TCDD over a period of 140 days, premalignant lymphoproliferation of B cells was induced before the appearance of any spontaneous lymphomas in the control mice. When the B cells were examined, they were found to manifest changes in gene expression similar to those induced by TCDD in the human cell lines, which provided support for this mechanism of lymphoma promotion by TCDD.

Recent evidence has shown that AHR activation by TCDD in human breast and endocervical cell lines induces sustained high concentrations of the interleukin-6 (IL-6) cytokine, which has tumor-promoting effects in numerous tissues (Hollingshead et al., 2008). IL-6 plays a roll in B-cell maturation and induces a transcriptional inflammatory response. It is known to be increased in B-cell neoplasms, including MM and various lymphomas, especially diffuse large B-cell lymphomas (Hussein et al., 2002; Kato et al., 1998; Kovacs, 2006).

An alternative link that could help to explain the association between TCDD and NHL has been explored in human studies. Chromosomal rearrangements, with consequent dysregulation of expression of various genes, are prevalent in B-cell lymphomas, and the t(14;18) reciprocal translocation, which juxtaposes the BCL2 with the locus of the immunoglobin heavy chain, is found in tumor cells in most cases of follicular lymphoma. Roulland et al. (2004) investigated the prevalence of the t(14;18) translocation that is characteristic of most cases of follicular lymphoma in 53 never-smoking and pesticide-using men in a cohort of French farmers whose pesticide exposures and confounding information had previously been well characterized; blood samples had been gathered from 21 during periods of high pesticide use and samples from the other 32 during a period of low pesticide use. The authors found a higher prevalence of cells carrying the translocation in the farmers whose blood had been drawn during a period of high pesticide use than in those whose blood had been drawn during a low-use period. Baccarelli et al. (2006) reported an increase in t(14;18) chromosomal translocation in lymphocytes from humans who were exposed to TCDD in the Seveso accident. In most cases of follicular lymphoma, tumor cells carry the t(14;18) chromosomal translocation, and there is evidence that an increased frequency of lymphocytes from the peripheral blood carrying this tumor marker may be a necessary but not sufficient step toward development of follicular lymphoma (Roulland et al., 2006).

Synthesis

The first VAO committee found the evidence to be sufficient to support an association between exposure to at least one of the COIs and NHL. The evidence was drawn from occupational and other studies in which subjects were exposed to a variety of herbicides and herbicide components. As has generally been the case in previous updates, the new studies were largely concordant with the conclusion that there is an association with the COIs. Of the seven studies newly evaluated for this update that investigated the association between NHL and adequately specified exposures to the COIs, three found statistically significant positive associations (Boers et al., 2012; Ruder and Yiin, 2011; Viel et al., 2011).

Individual findings on CLL are fairly few compared with the considerable number of studies supporting an association between exposure to the COIs and NHL. Results of some high-quality studies show that exposure to 2,4-D and 2,4,5-T appears to be associated with CLL, including the incidence study of Australian veterans (ADVA, 2005a); the case-control study by Hertzman et al. (1997) of British Columbia sawmill workers who were exposed to chlorophenates; the Danish-gardener study (Hansen et al., 1992); and the population-based case-control study in two US states by Brown et al. (1990) that showed increased risks associated with any herbicide use and specifically use of 2,4,5-T for at least 20 years before the subjects were interviewed. Other studies that showed positive associations but do not contribute greatly to the overall conclusion include the population-based case-control study by Amadori et al. (1995) that used occupational titles but did not include specific assessments of exposure to the chemicals; the cancer-incidence study in Tecumseh County, Michigan, in which no exposure assessments were available (Waterhouse et al., 1996); and proportionate-mortality studies by Blair and White (1985) and Burmeister et al. (1982).

Conclusion

On the basis of the evidence reviewed here and in previous VAO reports, the committee concludes that there is sufficient evidence of an association between exposure to at least one of the COIs and NHL.

Multiple Myeloma

MM (ICD-9 203.0) is characterized by proliferation of bone-marrow stem cells that results in an excess of neoplastic plasma cells and in the production of excess abnormal proteins, usually fragments of immunoglobulins. MM is sometimes grouped with other immunoproliferative neoplasms (ICD-9 203.8). ACS estimated that 12,190 men and 9,510 women would receive diagnoses of MM in the United States in 2012 and that 6,020 men and 4,690 women would die from it (Siegel et al., 2012). The average annual incidence of MM is shown in Table 8-44.

TABLE 8-44 Average Annual Incidence (per 100,000) of Multiple Myeloma in the United States[a]

	55–59 Years Old			60–64 Years Old			65–69 Years Old		
	All Races	White	Black	All Races	White	Black	All Races	White	Black
Men	11.6	10.5	25.0	18.8	16.6	47.2	28.7	27.0	61.7
Women	8.6	7.7	17.1	13.1	11.5	30.7	18.5	15.7	46.9

[a]Surveillance, Epidemiology, and End Results program, nine standard registries, crude age-specific rates, 2005–2009 (NCI, 2013).

The incidence of MM is highly age-dependent and is relatively low in people under 40 years old. The incidence is slightly higher in men than in women, and the difference becomes more pronounced with age.

An increased incidence of MM has been observed in several occupational groups, including farmers and other agricultural workers and those with workplace exposure to rubber, leather, paint, and petroleum (Riedel et al., 1991). People who have high exposure to ionizing radiation and those who suffer from other plasma-cell diseases, such as monoclonal gammopathy of unknown significance or solitary plasmacytoma, are also at greater risk.

Conclusions from *VAO* and Previous Updates

The committee responsible for *VAO* concluded that there was limited or suggestive evidence of an association between exposure to the COIs and MM. Additional information available to the committees responsible for *Update 1996*, *Update 1998*, *Update 2000*, *Update 2002*, *Update 2004*, *Update 2006*, *Update 2008*, and *Update 2010* did not change that conclusion.

Table 8-45 summarizes the results of the relevant studies.

Update of the Epidemiologic Literature

Vietnam-Veteran and Environmental Studies No Vietnam-veteran studies or environmental studies of exposure to the COIs and MM have been published since *Update 2010*.

Occupational Studies Burns et al. (2011) updated cancer incidence through 2007 in workers who were alive on January 1, 1985, and had been employed at any time from 1945 to 1994 in 2,4-D production by the Dow Chemical Company in Midland, Michigan. They found no evidence of significantly increased rates of cancer overall. With two cases observed, the incidence of MM in the most restrictively defined cohort was not increased (SIR = 0.79, 95% CI 0.09–2.87), as was the case for the two successively more inclusive, but potentially more biased, cohorts.

Ruder and Yiin (2011) reported mortality in 1940–2005 in the NIOSH PCP cohort of 2,122 workers in the four US plants that had been involved in PCP production. PCP production entailed exposure to PCDDs and PCDFs but not to the most toxic 2,3,7,8 dioxin congener. A subcohort of 720 workers (all men, the PCP-plus-TCDD group) had also been employed in TCP production and so had also been exposed to TCDD. In the total cohort, seven deaths attributed to MM were identified, which was consistent with the mortality experience of the US population (SMR = 1.50, 95% CI 0.60–3.10). The results were similar for the 1,402 workers in the PCP-only group (six deaths, SMR = 1.84, 95% CI

TABLE 8-45 Selected Epidemiologic Studies—Multiple Myeloma

Study Population[a]	Exposed Cases[b]	**Exposure of Interest**/Estimated Relative Risk (95% CI)[b]	Reference
VIETNAM VETERANS			
US Vietnam Veterans			
US Air Force Health Study—Ranch Hand veterans vs SEA veterans (unless otherwise noted)		**All COIs**	
Incidence			
Through 1999—White subjects vs national rates			Akhtar et al., 2004
Ranch Hand veterans (n = 1,189)	10	0.9 (0.4–1.5)	
With tours between 1966–1970	7	0.7 (0.3–1.4)	
SEA comparison veterans (n = 1,776)	9	0.6 (0.3–1.0)	
With tours between 1966–1970	4	0.3 (0.1–0.8)	
US CDC Vietnam Experience Study—Cross-sectional study, with medical examinations, of Army veterans: 9,324 deployed vs 8,989 nondeployed		**All COIs**	
Mortality			Boehmer et al., 2004
1965–2000	1	0.4 (nr)	
US VA Proportionate Mortality Study—sample of deceased male Vietnam-era Army and Marine veterans who served 7/4/1965–3/1/1973		**All COIs**	
1965–1988			Watanabe and Kang, 1996
Army, deployed (n = 27,596) vs nondeployed (n = 31,757)	36	0.9 (nr)	
Marine Corps, deployed (n = 6,237) vs nondeployed (n = 5,040)	4	0.6 (nr)	
1965–1982			Breslin et al., 1988
Army, deployed (n = 19,708) vs nondeployed (n = 22,904)	18	0.8 (0.2–2.5)	
Marine Corps, deployed (n = 4,527) vs nondeployed (n = 3,781)	2	0.5 (0.0–17.1)	
US VA Cohort of Female Vietnam Veterans		**All COIs**	
Mortality, through 2004	18	0.7 (0.4–1.3)	Cypel and Kang, 2008
Vietnam-veteran nurses only	14	0.7 (0.3–1.3)	
International Vietnam-Veteran Studies			
Australian Vietnam Veterans—58,077 men and 153 women served on land or in Vietnamese waters during 5/23/1962–7/1/1973 vs Australian population		**All COIs**	
Incidence			
All branches, 1982–2000	31	0.7 (0.4–0.9)	ADVA, 2005a
Navy	4	0.4 (0.1–1.0)	
Army	21	0.7 (0.4–1.0)	
Air Force	6	1.1 (0.4–2.4)	

continued

TABLE 8-45 Multiple Myeloma, continued

Study Population[a]	Exposed Cases[b]	**Exposure of Interest**/Estimated Relative Risk (95% CI)[b]	Reference
Mortality			
All branches, return–2001	24	0.9 (0.5–1.2)	ADVA, 2005b
Navy	3	0.5 (0.1–1.5)	
Army	15	0.8 (0.4–1.3)	
Air Force	6	1.7 (0.6–3.6)	
1980–1994	6	0.6 (0.2–1.3)	CDVA, 1997a
Australian Conscripted Army National Service (18,940 deployed vs 24,642 nondeployed)		**All COIs**	
Incidence			
1982–2000	8	2.1 (0.7–6.0)	ADVA, 2005c
Mortality			
1966–2001	5	0.9 (0.2–3.4)	ADVA, 2005c
1982–1994	0	nr	CDVA, 1997b
OCCUPATIONAL—INDUSTRIAL			
IARC Phenoxy Herbicide Cohort—Workers exposed to any phenoxy herbicide or chlorophenol (production or spraying) vs respective national mortality rates			
Mortality 1939–1992	17	1.3 (0.8–2.1)	Kogevinas et al., 1997
13,831 exposed to highly chlorinated PCDDs	9	1.2 (0.6–2.3)	
7,553 not exposed to highly chlorinated PCDDs	8	1.6 (0.7–3.1)	
Mortality 1955–1988 of 12,492 production workers and 5,898 sprayers exposed—13,482 in exposed subcohort	4	0.7 (0.2–1.8)	Saracci et al., 1991
Danish Production Workers (3,390 men and 1,069 women involved in production of phenoxy herbicides unlikely to contain TCDD at 2 plants in 1947–1987) (in IARC cohort)		**Dioxins, but TCDD unlikely; 2,4-D, 2,4-DP, MCPA, MCPP**	
Incidence 1943–1987 (men only)	0	nr	Lynge, 1993
Dutch production workers in Plant A (549 men exposed during production 1955–1985; 594 unexposed) (in IARC cohort)		**Dioxins, 2,4,5-T, 2,4,5-TCP**	
Mortality 1955–1991	0	0.0 (nr)	Hooiveld et al., 1998
German Production Workers at Bayer Plant in Uerdingen (135 men working > 1 month in 1951–1976) (in IARC cohort as of 1997) and women—no results		**Dioxins; 2,4,5-TCP**	
Mortality 1951–1992	0	nr	Becher et al., 1996

TABLE 8-45 Multiple Myeloma, continued

Study Population[a]	Exposed Cases[b]	**Exposure of Interest**/Estimated Relative Risk (95% CI)[b]	Reference
German Production Workers at Bayer Plant in Dormagen (520 men working > 1 month in 1965–1989) (in IARC cohort as of 1997) and women—no results		**Dioxins; 2,4-D; 2,4-DP; 2,4,5-T; MCPA; MCPP**	
Mortality 1965–1989	0	nr	Becher et al., 1996
German Production Workers at BASF Ludwigshafen Plant (680 men working > 1 month in 1957–1987) (in IARC cohort as of 1997) and women—no results		**Dioxins; 2,4-D; 2,4-DP; 2,4,5-T; MCPA; MCPP**	
Mortality 1956–1989	0	nr	Becher et al., 1996
German Production Workers at Boehringer–Ingelheim Plant in Hamburg (1,144 men working > 1 month in 1952–1984; generation of TCDD reduced after chloracne outbreak in 1954) and women—no results (some additions to observed cancers over Manz et al., 1991) (in IARC cohort as of 1997)		**Dioxins; 2,5-DCP; 2,4,5-T; 2,4,5-TCP**	
Mortality 1952–1989	3	5.4 (1.1–15.9)	Becher et al., 1996
New Zealand Phenoxy Herbicide Production Workers and Sprayers (1,599 men and women working any time in 1969–1988 at Dow plant in New Plymouth) (in IARC cohort)		**Dioxins; 2,4-D; 2,4,5-T; MCPA; MCPB; 2,4,5-TCP; Picloram**	
Mortality 1969–2004			McBride et al., 2009a
Ever-exposed workers	2	2.2 (0.2–8.1)	
Never-exposed workers	0	0.0 (0.0–12.2)	
Production Workers (713 men and 100 women worked > 1 month in 1969–1984)			't Mannetje et al., 2005
Mortality 1969–2000	3	5.5 (1.1–16.1)	
Sprayers (697 men and 2 women on register of New Zealand applicators, 1973–1984)			
Mortality 1973–2000	0	0.0 (0.0–5.3)	
NIOSH Mortality Cohort (12 US plants, 5,172 male production and maintenance workers 1942–1984) (included in IARC cohort as of 1997)		**Dioxins, phenoxy herbicides**	
Through 1993	10	2.1 (1.0–3.8)	Steenland et al., 1999
Through 1987	5	1.6 (0.5–3.9)	Fingerhut et al., 1991
≥ 1-year exposure, ≥ 20-year latency	3	2.6 (0.5–7.7)	

continued

TABLE 8-45 Multiple Myeloma, continued

Study Population[a]	Exposed Cases[b]	**Exposure of Interest**/Estimated Relative Risk (95% CI)[b]	Reference
All Dow PCP-Exposed Workers—all workers from the two plants that only made PCP (in Tacoma, Washington, and Wichita, Kansas) and workers who made PCP and TCP at two additional plants (in Midland, Michigan, and Sauget, Illinois)		**2,4,5-T; 2,4,5-TCP**	Ruder and Yiin, 2011
1940–2005 (n = 2,122)	7	1.5 (0.6–3.1)	
PCP and TCP (n = 720)	1	0.7 (0.0–4.0)	
PCP (no TCP) (n = 1,402)	6	1.8 (0.7–4.0)	
Dow 2,4-D Production Workers (1945–1982 in Midland, Michigan) (subset of all TCP-exposed workers)		**2,4-D, lower chlorinated dioxins**	
Cancer incidence through 2007 in Dow workers (n = 1,256) vs comparisons from state cancer registries (n = 23,354) Cohort 3)	2	0.8 (0.1–2.9)	Burns et al., 2011
Through 1994 (n = 1,517)	1	0.8 (0.0–4.5)	Burns et al., 2001
OCCUPATIONAL—PAPER AND PULP WORKERS		**TCDD**	
IARC cohort of pulp and paper workers—60,468 workers from 11 countries, TCDD among 27 agents assessed by JEM			McLean et al., 2006
Exposure to nonvolatile organochlorine compounds			
Never	21	0.8 (0.5–1.3)	
Ever	20	1.1 (0.7–1.7)	
OCCUPATIONAL—HERBICIDE-USING WORKERS (*not* related to IARC sprayer cohorts)			
CANADA			
Canadian Farm Operator Study—156,242 men farming in Manitoba, Saskatchewan, and Alberta in 1971; mortality from MM June 1971–December 1987			
Farmers from Canadian prairie provinces	160	0.8 (0.7–1.0)	Semenciw et al., 1994
FINNISH Phenoxy Herbicide Sprayers (1,909 men working 1955–1971 ≥ 2 wks) *not* IARC		**Phenoxy herbicides**	
Incidence	2	1.5 (0.2–5.2)	Asp et al., 1994
Mortality 1972–1989	3	2.6 (0.5–7.7)	
Except for lung cancer, numbers too small for reporting mortality 1972–1980		*Expected number of exposed cases*	Riihimaki et al., 1982
	1	0.2 (nr)	
ITALIAN Licensed Pesticide Users—male farmers in southern Piedmont licensed 1970–1974			
Mortality 1970–1986 (n = 23,401)	5	0.4 (0.1–1.0)	Torchio et al., 1994

TABLE 8-45 Multiple Myeloma, continued

Study Population[a]	Exposed Cases[b]	**Exposure of Interest**/Estimated Relative Risk (95% CI)[b]	Reference
Italian rice growers with documented phenoxy use (n = 1,487)		**Phenoxy herbicides**	Gambini et al., 1997
	0	nr	
NEW ZEALAND National Cancer Registry (1980–1984)—case-control study of incident multiple myeloma cancer cases vs remainder of 19,904 men with any incident cancer		**Herbicides**	Reif et al., 1989
Forestry workers (n = 134)	1	0.5 (0.1–3.7)	
SWEDISH lumberjacks—used phenoxys 1954–1967, incidence (1958–1992)			Thörn et al., 2000
Exposed (n = 154)			
Foremen (n = 15)	0		
Lumberjacks (n = 139)	0		
Unexposed lumberjacks (n = 241)	1	1.5 (0.0–8.6)	
THE NETHERLANDS			
Dutch Licensed Herbicide Sprayers—1,341 certified before 1980			
Through 2000	3	2.1 (0.4–6.1)	Swaen et al., 2004
Through 1987	3	8.2 (1.6–23.8)	Swaen et al., 1992
UNITED STATES			
US farmers—usual occupation of farmer and industry of agriculture on death certificates 1984–1988 from 23 states		**Herbicides** PCMRs	Blair et al., 1993
Men			
Whites (n = 119,648)	413	1.2 (1.0–1.3)	
Nonwhites (n = 11,446)	51	0.9 (0.7–1.2)	
Women			
Whites (n = 2,400)	14	1.8 (0.97–3.0)	
Nonwhites (n = 2,066)	11	1.1 (0.6–2.0)	
US Agricultural Health Study—prospective study of licensed pesticide sprayers in Iowa and North Carolina: commercial (n = 4,916), private/farmers (n = 52,395, 97.4% men), and spouses of private sprayers (n = 32,347, 0.007% men), enrolled 1993–1997; followups with CATIs 1999–2003 and 2005–2010		**Phenoxy herbicides**	
Incidence			
Enrollment through 2006—SIRs for participants			Koutros et al., 2010a
Private applicators	71	1.2 (0.9–1.5)	
Commercial applicators	1	nr	
Spouses	21	0.9 (0.6–1.4)	
Nested case-control study of MGUS among male private and commercial applicators			Landgren et al., 2009

continued

TABLE 8-45 Multiple Myeloma, continued

Study Population[a]	Exposed Cases[b]	**Exposure of Interest**/Estimated Relative Risk (95% CI)[b]	Reference
2,4-D	33	1.8 (0.7–4.8)	
Dicamba	17	0.9 (0.5–1.8)	
Enrollment through 2002			Alavanja et al., 2005
Private applicators	43	1.3 (1.0–1.8)	
Spouses of private applicators (> 99% women)	13	1.1 (0.6–1.9)	
Commercial applicators	0	0.0 (0.0–2.7)	
Mortality			
Enrollment through 2007, vs state rates			Waggoner et al., 2011
Applicators (n = 1,641)	52	1.0 (0.8–1.3)	
Spouses (n = 676)	10	0.6 (0.3–1.0)	
Enrollment through 2000, vs state rates			Blair et al., 2005a
Private applicators (men and women)	11	0.6 (0.3–1.2)	
Spouses of private applicators (> 99% women)	5	0.9 (0.3–2.1)	
US Department of Agriculture Workers—nested case-control study of white men dying 1970–1979 of MM		**Herbicides**	
Forest conservationists	1.3	nr (p-trend = 0.35)	Alavanja et al., 1989
Soil conservationists	1.3	nr (p-trend = 0.32)	
White Male Residents of Iowa—MM on death certificate, usual occupation: farmers vs not		**Herbicides**	
> 30 yrs old diagnosed 1981–1984—case-control (ever farmer)	111	1.2 (0.8–1.7)	Brown et al., 1993
> 30 yrs old when died 1964–1978—case-control			Burmeister et al., 1983
H_0: only for "modern methods" → born after 1900			
Born 1980–1900	nr	2.7 ($p < 0.05$)	
Born after 1900	nr	2.4 ($p < 0.05$)	
ENVIRONMENTAL			
Seveso, Italy Residential Cohort—Industrial accident July 10, 1976 (723 residents Zone A; 4,821 Zone B; 31,643 Zone R; 181,574 local reference group) (ICD-9 171)		**TCDD**	
Incidence			
20-yr followup to 1996—men and women			
Zone A	1	2.9 (0.4–20.7)	Pesatori et al., 2009
Zone B	6	2.8 (1.2–6.3)	
Zone R	18	1.2 (0.7–1.9)	
10-yr followup to 1991—men			Bertazzi et al., 1993
Zone B	2	3.2 (0.8–13.3)	
Zone R	1	0.2 (0.0–1.6)	

TABLE 8-45 Multiple Myeloma, continued

Study Population[a]	Exposed Cases[b]	**Exposure of Interest**/Estimated Relative Risk (95% CI)[b]	Reference
10-yr followup to 1991—women			Bertazzi et al., 1993
Zone B	2	5.3 (1.2–22.6)	
Zone R	2	0.6 (0.2–2.8)	
Mortality			
25-yr followup to 2001—men and women			Consonni et al., 2008
Zone A	2	4.3 (1.1–17.5)	
Zone B	5	1.7 (0.7–4.1)	
Zone R	24	1.1 (0.7–1.7)	
20-yr followup to 1996			Bertazzi et al., 2001
Zones A, B—men	1	0.6 (0.1–4.3)	
Zones A, B—women	4	3.2 (1.2–8.8)	
15-yr followup to 1991—men			Bertazzi et al., 1997
Zone B	1	1.1 (0.0–6.2)	
Zone R	5	0.8 (0.3–1.9)	
15-yr followup to 1991—women			Bertazzi et al., 1997
Zone B	4	6.6 (1.8–16.8)	
Zone R	5	1.0 (0.3–2.3)	
CASE-CONTROL STUDIES			
US Case-Control Studies			
ACS Prevention Study II subjects, MM on death certificate (128 MM cases vs 154 controls)	12	**Herbicides, pesticides** 2.1 (1.0–4.2)	Boffetta et al., 1989
Farmers using herbicides, pesticides	8	4.3 (1.7–10.9)	
Residents of four SEER program areas, 698 cases (< 80 yrs of age) vs 1,683 controls (July 1977–June 1981)	nr	**Pesticides** 2.9 (1.5–5.5)	Morris et al., 1986
Nebraska herbicide and pesticide use by Nebraska residents		**Herbicides**	Zahm et al., 1992
Eastern Nebraska users of herbicides			
Men	8	0.6 (0.2–1.7)	
Women	10	2.3 (0.8–7.0)	
Eastern Nebraska users of insecticides			
Men	11	0.6 (0.2–1.4)	
Women	21	2.8 (1.1–7.3)	
Wisconsin mortality listings (1968–1976)—farmers (30–39 yrs of age) in counties with highest herbicide use	nr	**Herbicides** 1.4 (0.8–2.3)	Cantor and Blair, 1984
International Case-Control Studies			
Canadian multicenter population-based study (September 1991–December 1994), male MM patients (n = 342) and controls (n = 1,506) and non-trivial exposure to pesticides		**Phenoxy herbicides**	Pahwa et al., 2012
Expose to any phenoxy herbicide	87	1.3 (1.0–1.8)	
2,4-D	80	1.3 (0.9–1.8)	
Mecoprop	27	0.9 (1.2–3.1)	
MCPA	8	0.7 (0.3–1.5)	

continued

TABLE 8-45 Multiple Myeloma, continued

Study Population[a]	Exposed Cases[b]	**Exposure of Interest**/Estimated Relative Risk (95% CI)[b]	Reference
Canadian residents		**Phenoxy herbicides**	Pahwa et al., 2006
Any phenoxy herbicide	62	1.2 (0.8–1.8)	
2,4-D	59	1.3 (0.9–1.9)	
Mecoprop	16	1.2 (0.7–2.8)	
MCPA	7	0.5 (0.2–1.2)	
France hospital-based case-control study		**Herbicides**	Orsi et al., 2009
Occupational use of herbicides	12	2.9 (1.3–6.5)	
Phenoxy herbicides	7	2.6 (0.9–7.0)	
Domestic use of herbicides	22	1.0 (0.6–2.0)	
Irish farmers and farm workers		**Herbicides**	Dean, 1994
Other malignant neoplasms of lymphoid and histiocytic tissue (including some types of NHL) (ICD-9 202)	171	1.0 (nr)	
Italian residents of 11 areas (NHL other than lymphosarcoma and reticulosarcoma)—incidence		**Herbicides**	Miligi et al., 2003
Herbicide exposure	11	1.6 (0.8–3.5)	
Men	8	1.4 (0.6–3.5)	
Women	3	3.2 (0.7–14.7)	
Residents of Milan, **Italy**, area (men and women)—incidence		**Herbicides**	LaVecchia et al., 1989
Agricultural occupations	nr	2.0 (1.1–3.5)	
New Zealand National Cancer Registry (1977–1981)—agricultural workers (< 70 yrs of age) (76 MM cases vs 315 controls)—incidence		**Phenoxy herbicides, chlorophenols**	Pearce et al., 1986
Use of agricultural spray	16	1.3 (0.7–2.5)	
Likely sprayed 2,4,5-T	14	1.6 (0.8–3.1)	
Swedish residents from 4 counties diagnosed with MM (n = 275) vs 275 controls from population registry (July 1982–June 1986)		**Phenoxy herbicides** *90% CI*	Eriksson and Karlsson, 1992
Exposed to phenoxy herbicides	20	2.2 (1.2–4.7)	

NOTE: 2,4-D, 2,4-dichlorophenoxyacetic acid; 2,4-DP, dichlorprop; 2,4,5-T, 2,4,5-trichlorophenoxyacetic acid; 2,4,5-TCP, 2,4,5-trichlorophenol; 2,5-DCP, 2,5-dichlorophenol; CATI, computer-assisted telephone interviewing; CDC, Centers for Disease Control and Prevention; CI, confidence interval; COI, chemical of interest; IARC, International Agency for Research on Cancer; ICD, International Classification of Diseases; JEM, job-exposure matrix; MCPA, 2-methyl-4-chlorophenoxyacetic acid; MCPB, 4-(4-chloro-2-methylphenoxy)butanoic acid; MCPP, methylchlorophenoxypropionic acid; MGUS, monoclonal gammopathy of undetermined significance; MM, multiple myeloma; NHL, non-Hodgkin lymphoma; NIOSH, National Institute for Occupational Safety and Health; nr, not reported; PCDD, polychlorinated dibenzo-*p*-dioxin (highly chlorinated, if four or more chlorines); PCMR, proportionate cancer mortality ratios; PCP, pentachlorophenol; SEA, Southeast Asia; SEER, Surveillance, Epidemiology, and End Results; TCDD, 2,3,7,8-tetrachlorodibenzo-*p*-dioxin; TCP, trichlorophenol; TEQ, toxicity equivalent; VA, US Department of Veterans Affairs.

[a]Subjects are male and outcome is mortality unless otherwise noted.

[b]Given when available; results other than estimated risk explained individually.

0.68–4.00). Only one of the deaths occurred in the PCP-plus-TCDD group (SMR = 0.72, 95% CI 0.02–3.99).

Koutros et al. (2010a) and Waggoner et al. (2011) assessed cancer incidence and mortality, respectively, in private and commercial pesticide applicators and their spouses in the AHS cohort vs the general population of Iowa and North Carolina. Koutros et al. (2010a) updated their previously reported incidence study through December 31, 2006, and found nonsignificant associations for MM in private pesticide applicators (71 cases, SIR = 1.2, 95% CI 0.93–1.51) and their spouses (21 cases, SIR = 0.94, 95% CI 0.58–1.44). Similarly, in an analysis of MM mortality in agricultural applicators and their spouses in 1993–2007 in this AHS cohort, Waggoner et al. (2011) reported a nonsignificant SMR in applicators (52 cases, SMR = 1.01, 95% CI 0.76–1.33) and their spouses (10 cases, SMR = 0.56, 95% CI 0.27–1.04). The AHS has been generating valuable information on the COIs for a number of years, but these results are not herbicide-specific and so are not regarded as being fully informative for the committee's task.

Case-Control Studies The Cross-Canada Study of Pesticides and Health is a population-based case-control study of several rare cancers conducted in men who lived in six Canadian provinces. Pahwa et al. (2012) assessed the effect of exposure to several specific phenoxy herbicides on 342 MM cases in comparison with the study's standard set of 1,506 controls with adjustment for age, province of residence, and several aspects of personal and family history. Mecoprop was found to be positively associated with the risk of MM (OR = 1.89, 95% CI 1.15–3.12), whereas this was not the case for 2,4-D (OR = 1.23, 95% CI 0.93–1.76) or for the less frequently used phenoxy herbicides MCPA (OR = 0.68, 95% CI 0.30–1.53) and diclofop-methyl (OR = 1.49, 95% CI 0.60–3.72).

Additional studies identified in the literature search for the present update presented results on MM in association with exposures that were not sufficiently specific with respect to the COIs in the VAO reviews. Perrotta et al. (2012) published findings from the EPILYMPH study, which applied a detailed occupational exposure-assessment approach to a large multicenter case-control study conducted in six European countries. The study included 227 MM cases and four age-matched controls per case, and ORs and 95% CIs were calculated for MM risk associated with level of education, individual occupations, and specific exposures. An increased risk was observed in general farmers (OR = 1.77, 95% CI 1.05–2.99) after adjustment for level of education. Pesticide exposure over a period of 10 years or more increased MM risk (OR = 1.62, 95% CI 1.01–2.58). In an Iranian hospital-based case-control study of exposure to pesticides, Zakerinia et al. (2012) found a significant increase in MM incidence (OR = 2.48, 95% CI 1.16–5.20).

Biologic Plausibility

No animal studies have reported an association between exposure to the COIs and MM. Thus, there are no specific animal data to support the biologic plausibility of such an association between the COIs and MM.

Recent evidence has shown that AHR activation by TCDD in human breast and endocervical cell lines induces sustained high concentrations of the IL-6 cytokine, which has tumor-promoting effects in numerous tissues (Hollingshead et al., 2008). IL-6 plays a roll in B-cell maturation and induces a transcriptional inflammatory response. It is known to be increased in B-cell neoplasms, including MM and various lymphomas (Hussein et al., 2002; Kovacs, 2006).

In comparing the frequency of specific variants of several metabolic genes between MM cases and controls, Gold et al. (2009) found some indication of differences, particularly in *CYP1B1* and *AHR* alleles, that might reflect increased suspectibility to MM after exposure to particular chemicals. A biochemical link to the COIs, however, is far from being established.

The biologic plausibility of the carcinogenicity of the COIs is discussed in general at the beginning of this chapter.

Synthesis

Previous VAO reports found limited or suggestive evidence of an association between exposure to at least one of the COIs and MM. MM is a type of lymphohematopoietic malignancy that is derived from antibody-secreting plasma cells from the B-cell lineage. The evidence of an association between the COIs and lymphomas (NHL, HL, and CLL/HCL) has been classified as sufficient. Most of these cancers also arise from B cells, so the committee hypothesized that it would be etiologically plausible for the association with MM to belong with the lymphomas in the sufficient category. Although many studies of exposure to pesticides in general and MM found strong or at least positive associations, review of studies that addressed an association between the specific COIs and MM found that the results were considerably weaker than those for the other B-cell neoplasms and did not justify advancing MM out of the limited or suggestive category.

Conclusion

On the basis of the evidence reviewed here and in previous VAO reports, the committee concludes that there is limited or suggestive evidence of an association between exposure to at least one of the COIs and MM.

AL Amyloidosis

The committee responsible for *Update 2006* moved the discussion of AL amyloidosis from the chapter on miscellaneous nonneoplastic health conditions to the cancer chapter to put it closer to related neoplastic conditions, such as MM and some types of B-cell lymphoma. The conditions share several biologic features, notably clonal hyperproliferation of B-cell–derived plasma cells and production of abnormal amounts of immunoglobulins.

The primary feature of amyloidosis (ICD-9 277.3) is the accumulation and deposition in various tissues of insoluble proteins that were historically denoted by the generic term *amyloid*. Amyloid protein accumulates in the extracellular spaces of various tissues. The pattern of organ involvement depends on the nature of the protein; some amyloid proteins are more fibrillogenic than are others. Amyloidosis is classified according to the biochemical properties of the fibril-forming protein. Excessive amyloid protein can have modest clinical consequences or can produce severe, rapidly progressive multiple–organ-system dysfunction. The annual incidence is estimated at 1/100,000; there are about 2,000 new cases each year in the United States (http://www.cancer.net/cancer-types/amyloidosis/statistics, as of June 13, 2013). Amyloidosis occurs mainly in people 50–70 years old and occurs more often in males than in females.

AL amyloidosis is the most common form of systemic amyloidosis; the *A* stands for *amyloid*, and the *L* indicates that the amyloid protein is derived from immunoglobin *light* chains. That links AL amyloidosis with other B-cell disorders that involve overproduction of immunoglobin, such as MM and some types of B-cell lymphomas. AL amyloidosis results from the overproduction of immunoglobulin light-chain protein from a monoclonal population of plasma cells. Clinical findings can include excessive AL protein or immunoglobulin fragments in the urine or serum, renal failure with nephrotic syndrome, liver failure with hepatomegaly, heart failure with cardiomegaly, marcroglossia, carpal tunnel syndrome, and peripheral neuropathy. Bone marrow biopsies commonly show an increased density of plasma cells, which suggests a premalignant state. Historically, that test emphasized routine histochemical analysis, but modern immunocytochemistry and flow cytometry now commonly identify monoclonal populations of plasma cells with molecular techniques. AL amyloidosis can progress rapidly and is often far advanced by the time it is diagnosed (Buxbaum, 2004).

Conclusions from *VAO* and Previous Updates

VA identified AL amyloidoisis as of concern after the publication of *Update 1998*. The committees responsible for *Update 2000*, *Update 2002*, and *Update 2004* concluded that there was inadequate or insufficient evidence to determine whether there is an association between exposure to the COIs and AL amyloidosis. Although there are few epidemiologic data specifically on AL amyloidosis, the committee responsible for *Update 2006* changed the categorization to limited or suggestive evidence of an association on the basis of commonalities in its cellular lineage with MM and B-cell lymphomas. Later committees have not changed that categorization.

Update of the Epidemiologic Literature

No studies of exposure to the COIs and amyloidosis of any sort have been published since *Update 2010.*

Biologic Plausibility

A 1979 study reported the dose-dependent development of a "generalized lethal amyloidosis" in Swiss mice that were treated with TCDD for 1 year (Toth et al., 1979). That finding has not been validated in 2-year carcinogenicity studies of TCDD in mice or rats. Thus, few animal data support an association between TCDD exposure and AL amyloidosis in humans, and no animal data support an association between the other COIs and AL amyloidosis.

It is known, however, that AL amyloidosis is associated with B-cell diseases, and 15–20% of cases of AL amyloidosis occur with MM. Other diagnoses associated with AL amyloidosis include B-cell lymphoma (Cohen et al., 2004), monoclonal gammopathy, and agammaglobulinemia (Rajkumar et al., 2006).

Synthesis

AL amyloidosis is very rare, and it is not likely that population-based epidemiology will ever provide substantial direct evidence regarding its causation. However, the biologic and pathophysiologic features linking AL amyloidosis, MM, and some types of B-cell lymphoma—especially clonal hyperproliferation of plasma cells and abnormal immunoglobulin production—indicate that AL amyloidosis is pathophysiologically related to these conditions.

Conclusion

On the basis of the evidence reviewed here and in previous VAO reports, the committee concludes that there is limited or suggestive evidence of an association between exposure to the COIs and AL amyloidosis.

Leukemia

Leukemias (ICD-9 202.4, 203.1, 204.0–204.9, 205.0–205.9, 206.0–206.9, 207.0–207.2, 207.8, 208.0–208.9) have traditionally been divided into four primary types: acute and chronic lymphocytic leukemia and acute and chronic myeloid leukemia. There are numerous subtypes of AML (ICD-9 205), which is also called acute myelogenous leukemia, granulocytic leukemia, or acute non-lymphocytic leukemia.

ACS estimated that 26,380 men and 20,320 women would receive diagnoses of some form of leukemia in the United States in 2012 and that 13,500 men and

10,040 women would die from it (Siegel et al., 2012). Collectively, leukemia was expected to account for 2.9% of all new diagnoses of cancer and 4.1% of deaths from cancer in 2012. The different forms of leukemia have different patterns of incidence and in some cases different risk factors. The incidences of the various forms of leukemia are presented in Table 8-46.

Myeloid Leukemias

In adults, acute leukemia is nearly always in the form of AML (ICD-9 205.0, 207.0, 207.2). ACS estimated that about 7,350 men and 6,430 women would receive new diagnoses of AML in the United States in 2012 and that 5,790 men and 4,410 women would die from it (Siegel et al., 2012). In the age groups that include most Vietnam veterans, AML makes up roughly one-fourth of cases of leukemia in men and one-third in women. Overall, AML is slightly more common in men than in women. Risk factors associated with AML include high doses of ionizing radiation, occupational exposure to benzene, and exposure to some medications used in cancer chemotherapy (such as melphalan). Fanconi anemia

TABLE 8-46 Average Annual Incidence (per 100,000) of Leukemias in the United States[a]

	55–59 Years Old			60–64 Years Old			65–69 Years Old		
	All Races	White	Black	All Races	White	Black	All Races	White	Black
All leukemias:									
Men	20.9	22.2	14.5	31.8	33.6	31.1	47.2	50.8	31.7
Women	12.8	13.5	10.4	18.9	20.0	14.8	27.4	28.9	23.4
Acute lymphocytic leukemia:									
Men	1.0	1.1	0.3	1.2	1.2	1.1	1.4	1.4	1.1
Women	0.7	0.8	0.6	1.1	1.1	0.6	1.3	1.1	2.6
Acute myeloid leukemia:									
Men	4.9	5.1	3.7	6.8	6.8	8.2	10.5	11.0	7.8
Women	4.3	4.5	3.9	5.0	5.1	3.6	8.1	8.5	5.5
Chronic lymphocytic leukemia:									
Men	10.1	11.0	5.5	16.1	17.7	13.5	25.5	28.2	15.0
Women	4.9	5.3	2.8	9.1	10.2	5.3	12.3	13.5	8.5
Chronic myeloid leukemia:									
Men	2.6	2.6	3.2	3.8	3.8	4.5	5.3	5.5	3.3
Women	1.6	1.7	1.2	2.1	2.0	3.6	2.8	3.1	2.1
All other leukemia[b]									
Men	0.6	0.6	0.8	1.4	1.2	2.6	1.7	1.8	1.7
Women	0.5	0.4	1.0	0.7	0.5	1.5	1.2	1.2	2.6

[a]Surveillance, Epidemiology, and End Results program, nine standard registries, crude age-specific rates, 2005–2009 (NCI, 2013).

[b]Includes leukemic reticuloendotheliosis (hairy cell leukemia), plasma-cell leukemia, monocytic leukemia, and acute and chronic erythremia and erythroleukemia.

and Down syndrome are associated with an increased risk of AML, and tobacco use is thought to account for about 20% of AML cases.

Vietnam veterans have expressed concern about whether myelodysplastic syndromes, most often precursors to AML, are associated with Agent Orange exposure. However, no results on those conditions in conjunction with the COIs have been found in VAO literature searches. Epidemiologic research on those hematologic disorders has been undertaken fairly recently; for instance, the LATIN case-control study (Maluf et al., 2009) has undertaken investigation of aplastic anemia in South America, but the reported exposures have been only as specific as "herbicides" and "agricultural pesticides."

The incidence of CML increases steadily with age in people over 30 years old. Its lifetime incidence is roughly equal in whites and blacks and is slightly higher in men than in women. CML accounts for about one-fifth of cases of leukemia in people in the age groups that include most Vietnam veterans. It is associated with an acquired chromosomal abnormality known as the Philadelphia chromosome, for which exposure to high doses of ionizing radiation is a known risk factor.

Lymphoid Leukemias

ALL is a disease of young children (peak incidence at the age of 2–5 years) and of people over 70 years old. It is relatively uncommon in the age groups that include most Vietnam veterans. The lifetime incidence of ALL is slightly higher in whites than in blacks and higher in men than in women. Exposure to high doses of ionizing radiation is a known risk factor for ALL, but there is little consistent evidence on other factors.

CLL shares many traits with lymphomas (such as immunohistochemistry, B-cell origin, and progression to an acute, aggressive form of NHL), so the committee now considers it in the section above on NHL, as classified in the WHO system.

Conclusions from *VAO* and Previous Updates

The committee responsible for *VAO* concluded that there was inadequate or insufficient information to determine whether there is an association between exposure to the COIs and all types of leukemia. Additional information available to the committees responsible for *Update 1996*, *Update 1998*, *Update 2000*, *Update 2002*, *Update 2004*, *Update 2006*, *Update 2008*, and *Update 2010* did not change that conclusion.

The committee responsible for *Update 2002*, however, considered CLL separately and judged that there was sufficient evidence of an association with the herbicides used in Vietnam and CLL alone, and *Update 2008* noted that HCL is closely related to CLL.

The committee responsible for *Update 2006* considered AML individually but did not find evidence to suggest that its occurrence is associated with exposure to the COIs, and there is still not sufficient evidence to support such an association, so AML has been retained with other non-CLL leukemias in the category of inadequate and insufficient evidence.

Table 8-47 summarizes the results of the relevant studies.

Update of the Epidemiologic Literature

Vietnam-Veteran, Environmental, and Case-Control Studies No Vietnam-veteran studies, environmental studies, or case-control studies of exposure to the COIs and leukemia have been published since *Update 2010*.

Occupational Studies Burns et al. (2011) updated cancer incidence through 2007 in workers who were alive on January 1, 1985, and had been employed at any time from 1945 to 1994 in 2,4-D production by the Dow Chemical Company in Midland, Michigan. They found no evidence of significantly increased rates of cancer overall. With five cases observed, the incidence of leukemia in the most restrictively defined cohort was not increased (SIR = 0.86, 95% CI 0.28–2.02), as was the case for the two successively more inclusive, but potentially more biased, cohorts.

Boers et al. (2012) provided a quantified, TCDD-based analysis of mortality updated through 2006 in male workers in two Dutch phenoxy-herbicide factories, which were considered in *Update 2010* (Boers et al., 2010). The 1,020 workers in factory A had been involved in production of 2,4,5-T with its associated TCDD contamination, whereas the 1,036 working in factory B had produced only phenoxy herbicides that would not have had TCDD contamination. Contemporary TCDD concentrations measured in a subsample of 187 workers were used to derive a model incorporating job history to estimate serum TCDD concentrations of all the men at the end of their employment. The estimated TCDD concentrations in the workers in both factories did not indicate an increased risk of leukemia mortality in association with TCDD (HR = 0.90, 95% CI 0.59–1.37). The dose–response modeling, applied only to the workers in factory A, also did not find an increased risk of death from leukemia (HR = 0.74, 95% CI 0.38–1.42), whereas the qualitative exposure analysis in Boers et al. (2010) had found an HR of 0.28 (95% CI 0.03–2.61).

Ruder and Yiin (2011) reported mortality in 1940–2005 in the NIOSH PCP cohort of 2,122 workers in the four US plants that had been involved in PCP production. PCP production entailed exposure to PCDDs and PCDFs but not to the most toxic 2,3,7,8 dioxin congener. A subcohort of 720 workers (all men, the PCP-plus-TCDD group) had also been employed in TCP production and so had also been exposed to TCDD. Relative to US referent rates, deaths from leukemia were not substantially altered in the entire cohort (nine deaths, SMR =

TABLE 8-47 Selected Epidemiologic Studies—Leukemia (Shaded Entries Are New Information for This Update)

Study Population[a]	Exposed Cases[b]	Exposure of Interest/Estimated Relative Risk (95% CI)[b]	Reference
VIETNAM VETERANS			
US Vietnam Veterans			
US Air Force Health Study—Ranch Hand veterans vs SEA veterans (unless otherwise noted)		**All COIs**	
Incidence			
Through 1999—White subjects vs national rates (lymphopoietic cancer[c])			Akhtar et al., 2004
Ranch Hand veterans (n = 1,189)	10	0.9 (0.4–1.5)	
With tours between 1966–1970	7	0.7 (0.3–1.4)	
SEA comparison veterans (n = 1,776)	9	0.6 (0.3–1.0)	
With tours between 1966–1970	4	0.3 (0.1–0.8)	
Mortality			
Through 1999—White subjects vs national rates (lymphopoietic cancer[c])		Akhtar et al., 2004	
Ranch Hand veterans (n = 1,189)	6	1.0 (0.4–2.0)	
SEA comparison veterans (n = 1,776)	5	0.6 (0.2–1.2)	
US VA Cohort of Army Chemical Corps—Expanded as of 1997 to include all Army men with chemical MOS (2,872 deployed vs 2,737 nondeployed) serving during Vietnam era (7/1/1965–3/28/1973)		**All COIs**	
Mortality—Through 2005			Cypel and Kang, 2010
All lymphopoietic			
Deployed vs nondeployed	6 vs 6	1.1 (0.4–2.5)	
ACC veterans vs US men			
Vietnam cohort	6	0.5 (0.2–1.0)	
Non-Vietnam cohort	6	0.6 (0.2–1.4)	
Leukemia			
Deployed vs nondeployed	2 vs 4	0.6 (0.1–3.2)	
ACC veterans vs US men			
Vietnam cohort	2	0.4 (0.1–1.5)	
Non-Vietnam cohort	4	1.2 (0.3–3.0)	
Mortality—Through 2001		1.0 (0.1–3.8)	Dalager and Kang, 1997
US CDC Vietnam Experience Study—Cross-sectional study, with medical examinations, of Army veterans: 9,324 deployed vs 8,989 nondeployed		**All COIs**	
Mortality			
1965–2000	8	1.0 (0.4–2.5)	Boehmer et al., 2004
US VA Cohort of Female Vietnam Veterans		**All COIs**	
Mortality			

TABLE 8-47 Leukemia, continued

Study Population[a]	Exposed Cases[b]	**Exposure of Interest**/Estimated Relative Risk (95% CI)[b]	Reference
Through 2004 (lymphopoietic cancers[c])	18	0.7 (0.4–1.3)	Cypel and Kang, 2008
Vietnam–veteran nurses	14	0.7 (0.3–1.3)	
State Studies of US Vietnam Veterans			
Michigan Vietnam-era veterans, PM study of deaths (1974–1989)—deployed vs nondeployed	30	1.0 (0.7–1.5)	Visintainer et al., 1995
International Vietnam-Veteran Studies			
Australian Vietnam Veterans—58,077 men and 153 women served on land or in Vietnamese waters during 5/23/1962–7/1/1973 vs Australian population		**All COIs**	
Incidence			
All branches, 1982–2000	130	1.1 (1.0–1.4)	ADVA, 2005a
Lymphocytic leukemia	72	1.4 (1.1–1.7)	
Myeloid leukemia	54	1.0 (0.8–1.3)	
Navy	35	1.5 (1.0–2.0)	
Lymphocytic leukemia	14	1.3 (0.7–2.1)	
Myeloid leukemia	19	1.7 (1.0–2.6)	
Army	80	1.1 (0.8–1.3)	
Lymphocytic leukemia	50	1.4 (1.0–1.8)	
Myeloid leukemia	28	0.8 (0.5–1.1)	
Air Force	15	1.2 (0.7–2.0)	
Lymphocytic leukemia	8	1.4 (0.6–2.7)	
Myeloid leukemia	7	1.3 (0.5–2.6)	
Validation Study		*Expected number of exposed cases*	AIHW, 1999
	27	26 (16–36)	
Men	64	26 (16–36	CDVA, 1998a
Women	1	0 (0–4)	CDVA, 1998b
Mortality			
All branches, return–2001	84	1.0 (0.8–1.3)	ADVA, 2005b
Lymphocytic leukemia	24	1.2 (0.7–1.7)	
Myeloid leukemia	55	1.1 (0.8–1.3)	
Army	48	0.1 (0.7–1.2)	
Lymphocytic leukemia	17	1.3 (0.7–2.0)	
Myeloid leukemia	30	0.8 (0.5–1.1)	
Air Force	14	1.6 (0.8–2.6)	
Lymphocytic leukemia	6	2.7 (1.0–5.8)	
Myeloid leukemia	8	1.3 (0.5–2.5)	
1980–1994	33	1.3 (0.8–1.7)	CDVA, 1997a
Australian Conscripted Army National Service (18,940 deployed vs 24,642 nondeployed)		**All COIs**	

continued

TABLE 8-47 Leukemia, continued

Study Population[a]	Exposed Cases[b]	**Exposure of Interest**/Estimated Relative Risk (95% CI)[b]	Reference
Incidence—1982–2000	16	0.6 (0.3–1.1)	ADVA, 2005c
Lymphocytic leukemia	9	0.8 (0.3–2.0)	
Myeloid leukemia	7	0.5 (0.2–1.3)	
Mortality—1966–2001	11	0.6 (0.3–1.3)	ADVA, 2005c
Lymphocytic leukemia	2	0.4 (0.0–2.4)	
Myeloid leukemia	8	0.7 (0.3–1.7)	
OCCUPATIONAL—INDUSTRIAL			
IARC Phenoxy Herbicide Cohort—Workers exposed to any phenoxy herbicide or chlorophenol (production or spraying) vs respective national mortality rates			
Mortality 1939–1992	34	1.0 (0.7–1.4)	Kogevinas et al., 1997
13,831 exposed to highly chlorinated PCDDs	16	0.7 (0.4–1.2)	
7,553 not exposed to highly chlorinated PCDDs	17	1.4 (0.8–2.3)	
Mortality 1955–1988 of 12,492 production workers and 5,898 sprayers exposed—13,482 in exposed subcohort	18	1.2 (0.7–1.9)	Saracci et al., 1991
Mortality, incidence of women in production (n = 699) and spraying (n = 2) compared to national death rates and cancer incidence rates (myeloid leukemia)	1	**TCDD** 2.0 (0.2–7.1)	Kogevinas et al., 1993
Danish Production Workers (3,390 men and 1,069 women involved in production of phenoxy herbicides unlikely to contain TCDD at 2 plants in 1947–1987) (in IARC cohort)		**Dioxins, but TCDD unlikely; 2,4-D, 2,4-DP, MCPA, MCPP**	
Mortality 1955–2006	9	0.9 (0.6–1.4)	Boers et al., 2012
Dutch production workers in Plant A (549 men exposed during production 1955–1985; 594 unexposed) (in IARC cohort)		**Dioxins, 2,4,5-T, 2,4,5-TCP**	
Mortality 1955–2006 (hazard ratios for lagged TCDD plasma levels)	5	0.7 (0.4–1.4)	Boers et al., 2012
Mortality 1955–2006			Boers et al., 2010
LHC	11 vs 7	0.9 (0.3–2.6)	
Leukemia	2 vs 3	0.3 (0.0–2.6)	
Mortality 1955–1991	1	1.0 (0.0–5.7)	Hooiveld et al., 1998
Mortality 1955–1985			Bueno de Mesquita et al., 1993
Leukemia, aleukemia (ICD-9 204–207)	1	1.5 (0.0–8.2)	
Myeloid leukemia (ICD-8 205)	1	2.9 (0.0–15.9)	

TABLE 8-47 Leukemia, continued

Study Population[a]	Exposed Cases[b]	Exposure of Interest/Estimated Relative Risk (95% CI)[b]	Reference
Dutch production workers in Plant B (414 men exposed during production 1965–1986; 723 unexposed) (in IARC cohort)		**2,4-D; MCPA; MCPP; highly chlorinated dioxins unlikely**	
Mortality 1965–2006			Boers et al., 2010
LHC	3 vs 3	1.5 (0.3–7.5)	
Leukemia	2 vs 2	1.5 (0.2–10.8)	
Mortality 1965–1986			Bueno de Mesquita et al., 1993
Leukemia, aleukemia (ICD-9 204–207)	1	4.4 (0.1–24.2)	
Myeloid leukemia (ICD-8 205)	1	7.7 (0.2–42.9)	
German Production Workers—2,479 workers at 4 plants (in IARC cohort as of 1997)		**Dioxins, phenoxy herbicides**	
BASF Cleanup Workers from 1953 accident (n = 247); 114 with chloracne, 13 more with erythema; serum TCDD levels (*not* part of IARC)		**Focus on TCDD**	
Mortality			
Through 1987		*90% CI*	Zober et al., 1990
All cohorts (n = 247)	1	1.7 (nr)	
Cohort 3	1	5.2 (0.4–63.1)	
German Production Workers at Bayer Plant in Uerdingen (135 men working > 1 month in 1951–1976) (in IARC cohort as of 1997) and women—no results		**Dioxins; 2,4,5-TCP**	
Mortality 1951–1992	0	—	Becher et al., 1996
German Production Workers at Bayer Plant in Dormagen (520 men working > 1 month in 1965–1989) (in IARC cohort as of 1997) and women—no results		**Dioxins; 2,4-D; 2,4,5-T; MCPA; MCPP; 2,4-DP**	
Mortality 1965–1989	0	—	Becher et al., 1996
German Production Workers at BASF Ludwigshafen Plant (680 men working > 1 month in 1957–1987) (in IARC cohort as of 1997) and women—no results		**Dioxins; 2,4-D; 2,4,5-T; MCPA; MCPP; 2,4-DP**	
Mortality 1956–1989	0	—	Becher et al., 1996

continued

TABLE 8-47 Leukemia, continued

Study Population[a]	Exposed Cases[b]	**Exposure of Interest**/Estimated Relative Risk (95% CI)[b]	Reference
German Production Workers at Boehringer–Ingelheim Plant in Hamburg (1,144 men working > 1 month in 1952–1984; generation of TCDD reduced after chloracne outbreak in 1954) and women—no results (some additions to observed cancers over Manz et al., 1991) (in IARC cohort as of 1997)		**Dioxins; 2,4,5-T; 2,5-DCP; 2,4,5-TCP**	
Mortality 1952–1989	4	1.8 (0.5–4.7)	Becher et al., 1996
New Zealand Phenoxy Herbicide Production Workers and Sprayers (1,599 men and women working any time in 1969–1988 at Dow plant in New Plymouth) (in IARC cohort)		**Dioxins; 2,4-D; 2,4,5-T; MCPA; MCPB; 2,4,5-TCP; Picloram**	
Mortality 1969–2004 (leukemia, aleukemia)			McBride et al., 2009a
Ever-exposed workers	1	0.6 (0.0–3.1)	
Never-exposed workers	0	0.0 (0.0–6.0)	
Production Workers (713 men and 100 women worked > 1 month in 1969–1984)			
Mortality 1969–2000	0	0.0 (0.0–5.3)	't Mannetje et al., 2005
Sprayers (697 men and 2 women registered any time 1973–1984)			
Mortality 1973–2000	1	1.2 (0.0–6.4)	't Mannetje et al., 2005
NIOSH Mortality Cohort (12 US plants, 5,172 male production and maintenance workers 1942–1984) (included in IARC cohort as of 1997)		**Dioxins, phenoxy herbicides**	
Through 1993	10	0.8 (0.4–1.5)	Steenland et al., 1999
Through 1987	6	0.7 (0.2–1.5)	Fingerhut et al., 1991
All Dow TCP-Exposed Workers (TCP production 1942–1979 or 2,4,5-T production 1948–1982 in Midland, Michigan) (in IARC and NIOSH cohorts)		**2,4,5-T; 2,4,5-TCP**	
1942–2003 (n = 1,615) (leukemia, aleukemia)	13	1.9 (1.0–3.2)	Collins et al., 2009a
Excluding subset with PCP exposure	2	1.9 (1.0–3.4)	
1942–2003 (n = 1,615) (other lymphopoietic)	2	0.6 (0.1–2.3)	
Excluding subset with PCP exposure	2	0.7 (0.1–2.6)	

TABLE 8-47 Leukemia, continued

Study Population[a]	Exposed Cases[b]	Exposure of Interest/Estimated Relative Risk (95% CI)[b]	Reference
All Dow PCP-Exposed Workers—all workers from the two plants that only made PCP (in Tacoma, Washington, and Wichita, Kansas) and workers who made PCP and TCP at two additional plants (in Midland, Michigan, and Sauget, Illinois)		**2,4,5-T; 2,4,5-TCP**	Ruder and Yiin, 2011
1940–2005 (n = 2,122)	9	0.9 (0.4–1.7)	
PCP and TCP (n = 720)	2	0.6 (0.1–2.2)	
PCP (no TCP) (n = 1,402)	7	1.0 (0.4–2.1)	
Dow PCP Production Workers (1937–1989 in Midland, Michigan) (*not* in IARC and NIOSH cohorts)		**Low chlorinated dioxins, 2,4-D**	
Mortality 1940–2004 (n = 577, excluding 196 also having exposure to TCP)			Collins et al., 2009b
1942–2003 (n = 773) (leukemia, aleukemia)	2	0.6 (0.1–2.0)	
Excluding subset with TCP exposure	1	0.4 (0.0–2.0)	
1942–2003 (n = 773) (other lymphopoietic)	2	1.3 (0.2–4.6)	
Excluding subset with TCP exposure	2	1.7 (0.2–6.0)	
Mortality 1940–1989 (n = 770)			Ramlow et al., 1996
0-yr latency	2	1.0 (0.1–3.6)	
15-yr latency	1	nr	
Dow 2,4-D Production Workers (1945–1982 in Midland, Michigan)		**2,4-D, lower chlorinated dioxins**	
Cancer incidence through 2007 in Dow workers (n = 1,256) vs comparisons from state cancer registries (n = 23,354) (Cohort 3)	5	0.9 (0.3–2.0)	Burns et al., 2011
Through 1994 (n = 1,517)—lymphopoietic mortality in workers with high 2,4-D exposure	4	1.3 (0.4–3.3)	Burns et al., 2001
Through 1982 (n = 878)	2	3.6 (0.4–13.2)	Bond et al., 1988
OCCUPATIONAL—PAPER AND PULP WORKERS		**TCDD**	
IARC cohort of pulp and paper workers—60,468 workers from 11 countries, TCDD among 27 agents assessed by JEM			McLean et al., 2006
Exposure to nonvolatile organochlorine compounds			
Never	49	1.0 (0.7–1.3)	
Ever	35	0.9 (0.6–1.2)	

continued

TABLE 8-47 Leukemia, continued

Study Population[a]	Exposed Cases[b]	**Exposure of Interest**/Estimated Relative Risk (95% CI)[b]	Reference
Danish paper workers			Rix et al., 1998
Men	20	0.8 (0.5–1.2)	
Women	7	1.3 (0.5–2.7)	
OCCUPATIONAL—HERBICIDE-USING WORKERS (*not* related to IARC sprayer cohorts)			
CANADA			
Canadian Farm Operator Study—156,242 men farming in Manitoba, Saskatchewan, and Alberta in 1971; mortality from leukemia June 1971–December 1987		**Herbicides**	
Farm operators ≥ 35 yrs of age (June 1971–December 1987)	357	0.9 (0.8–1.0)	Semenciw et al., 1994
Lymphatic	132	0.9 (0.8–1.1)	
Myeloid	127	0.8 (0.7–0.9)	
Farm operators ≥ 35 yrs of age during study period (June 1971–December 1985)	138	0.9 (0.7–1.0)	Wigle et al., 1990
Sawmill workers in British Columbia—23,829 workers for ≥ 1 yr at 11 mills using chlorophenates 1940–1985		**Chlorophenates, not TCDD**	Hertzman et al., 1997
All leukemias—incidence	47	1.2 (0.9–1.5)	
ALL	2	1.0 (0.2–3.1)	
CLL	24	1.7 (1.2–2.4)	
AML	5	0.8 (0.3–1.7)	
CML	7	1.1 (0.5–2.0)	
Other, unspecified	5	0.5 (0.2–1.0)	
DENMARK			
Danish gardeners—incidence from 3,156 male and 859 female gardeners		**Herbicides**	Hansen et al., 2007
25-year followup (1975–2001)	42	1.1 (0.8–1.4)	
Leukemia (ICD-7 204)	22	1.4 (0.9–2.1)	
Born before 1915 (high exposure)	16	1.4 (0.9–2.3)	
Leukemia (ICD-7 204)	12	2.3 (1.3–4.1)	
Born 1915–1934 (medium exposure)	25	1.2 (0.8–1.8)	
Leukemia (ICD-7 204)	9	1.0 (0.5–2.0)	
Born after 1934 (low exposure)	1	0.2 (0.0–1.0)	
Leukemia (ICD-7 204)	1	0.5 (0.0–3.4)	
10-year followup (1975–1984) reported in Hansen et al. (1992)	15	1.4 (0.8–2.4)	
NHL (ICD-7 200, 202, 205)	6	1.7 (0.6–3.8)	
HD (ICD-7 201)	0	nr	
Multiple myeloma (ICD-7 203)	0	nr	
CLL (ICD-7 204.0)	6	2.8 (1.0–6.0)	
Other leukemia (ICD-7 204.1–204.4)	3	1.4 (0.3–4.2)	
10-year followup (1975–1984) of male gardeners			Hansen et al., 1992
All gardeners—CLL	6	2.5 (0.9–5.5)	
Men	6	2.8 (1.0–6.0)	

TABLE 8-47 Leukemia, continued

Study Population[a]	Exposed Cases[b]	**Exposure of Interest**/Estimated Relative Risk (95% CI)[b]	Reference
All gardeners—all other types of leukemia	3	1.2 (0.3–3.6)	
Men	3	1.4 (0.3–4.2)	
Danish Farmers—incidence from linking farmers on 1970 census with national cancer registry (1970–1980)		**Herbicides**	Ronco et al., 1992
Men			
Self-employed	145	0.9 (nr)	
Employee	33	1.0 (nr)	
Women			
Self-employed	8	2.2 ($p < 0.05$)	
Employee	3	1.3 (nr)	
Family worker	27	0.9 (nr)	
FINNISH Phenoxy Herbicide Sprayers (1,909 men working 1955–1971 ≥ 2 wks) *not* IARC		**Phenoxy herbicides**	
Incidence			Asp et al., 1994
Lymphatic	3	1.0 (0.2–3.0)	
Mortality	2	nr	
Lymphatic	1	0.9 (0.0–5.1)	
Myeloid	1	0.7 (0.0–3.7)	
ITALIAN Licensed Pesticide Users—male farmers in southern Piedmont licensed 1970–1974			
Mortality 1970–1986 (n = 23,401) (ICD-8 202.0–202.9)	27	0.8 (0.5–1.1)	Torchio et al., 1994
Italian rice growers with documented phenoxy use (n = 1,487)	4	**Phenoxy herbicides** 0.6 (0.2–1.6)	Gambini et al., 1997
NEW ZEALAND National Cancer Registry (1980–1984)—case-control study of 571 incident pancreatic cancer cases vs remainder of 19,904 men with any incident cancer		**Herbicides**	Reif et al., 1989
Forestry workers (n = 134) (leukemia)	4	1.0 (0.4–2.6)	
Aged 20–59 (AML)	2	2.8 (0.7–11.0)	
Aged ≥ 60 (AML)	1	1.6 (0.2–11.5)	
Sawmill workers (n = 139)		**Herbicides, chlorophenols**	
Leukemia (ICD-7 204–248)	2	0.5 (0.1–2.1)	
AML (ICD-7 205.0)	1	0.9 (0.1–6.4)	
SWEDEN			
Swedish lumberjacks—used phenoxys 1954–1967, Incidence 1958–1992	0	nr	Thörn et al., 2000
THE NETHERLANDS			
Dutch Licensed Herbicide Sprayers—1,341 certified before 1980			
Through 2000	3	1.3 (0.3–3.7)	Swaen et al., 2004

continued

TABLE 8-47 Leukemia, continued

Study Population[a]	Exposed Cases[b]	**Exposure of Interest**/Estimated Relative Risk (95% CI)[b]	Reference
UNITED STATES			
US farmers—usual occupation of farmer and industry of agriculture on death certificates 1984–1988 from 23 states		**Herbicides** PCMRs	Blair et al., 1993
Men			
Whites (n = 119,648)	1,072	1.3 (1.2–1.4)	
Nonwhites (n = 11,446)	55	0.9 (0.7–1.3)	
Women			
Whites (n = 2,400)	24	1.5 (0.9–2.2)	
Nonwhites (n = 2,066)	8	0.9 (0.4–1.9)	
US Agricultural Health Study—prospective study of licensed pesticide sprayers in Iowa and North Carolina: commercial (n = 4,916), private/farmers (n = 52,395, 97.4% men), and spouses of private sprayers (n = 32,347, 0.007% men), enrolled 1993–1997; followups with CATIs 1999–2003 and 2005–2010		**Phenoxy herbicides**	
Incidence			
Enrollment through 2006—SIRs for participants			Koutros et al., 2010a
Private applicators	133	1.0 (0.8–1.1)	
Commercial applicators	7	0.9 (0.4–1.9)	
Spouses	37	0.8 (0.6–1.1)	
Enrollment through 2002			Alavanja et al., 2005
Private applicators	70	0.9 (0.7–1.2)	
Spouses of private applicators (> 99% women)	17	0.7 (0.4–1.2)	
Commercial applicators	4	0.9 (0.3–2.4)	
Mortality			
Enrollment through 2007, vs state rates			Waggoner et al., 2011
Applicators (n = 1,641)	91	0.9 (0.7–1.0)	
Spouses (n = 676)	33	1.1 (0.8–1.5)	
Enrollment through 2000, vs state rates			Blair et al., 2005a
Private applicators (men and women)	27	0.8 (0.5–1.1)	
Spouses of private applicators (> 99% women)	14	1.4 (0.8–2.4)	
California United Farm Workers of America			
Nested case-control analysis of Hispanic workers in cohort of 139,000 CA United Farm Workers			Mills et al., 2005
Ever used 2,4-D—total leukemia	nr	1.0 (0.4–2.6)	
Lymphocytic leukemia	nr	1.5 (0.3–6.6)	
Granulocytic (myeloid) leukemia	nr	1.3 (0.3–5.4)	

TABLE 8-47 Leukemia, continued

Study Population[a]	Exposed Cases[b]	Exposure of Interest/Estimated Relative Risk (95% CI)[b]	Reference
US Department of Agriculture Workers—nested case-control study of white men dying 1970–1979 of NHL		**Herbicides**	
Agricultural extension agents	23	1.9 (1.0–3.5)	Alavanja et al., 1988
Lymphatic	nr	2.1 (0.7–6.4)	
Trend over years worked		($p < 0.01$)	
Myeloid	nr	2.8 (1.1–7.2)	
Trend over years worked		($p < 0.01$)	
White Male Residents of Iowa—leukemia cancer on death certificate, usual occupation: farmers vs not		**Herbicides**	
> 30 yrs old when died 1964–1978—case-control		1.2 ($p < 0.05$)	Burmeister et al., 1983
ALL	28	0.7 (0.4–1.2)	
CLL	132	1.7 (1.2–2.4)	
Lived in one of 33 counties with highest herbicide use	nr	1.9 (1.2–3.1)	
Unspecified lymphatic	64	1.7 (1.0–2.7)	
AML	86	1.0 (0.8–1.5)	
CML	46	1.0 (0.7–1.7)	
Unspecified myeloid	36	0.8 (0.5–1.4)	
Acute monocytic	10	1.1 (0.4–2.6)	
Unspecified leukemia	31	1.1 (0.6–2.0)	
White Male Residents of Iowa and Minnesota— > 30 yrs old diagnosed 1981–1983 in Iowa or 1980–1982 in Minnesota (ever farmer, used herbicides)	578	**Herbicides**	Brown et al., 1990
Ever farmed	335	1.2 (1.0–1.5)	
AML	81	1.2 (0.8–1.8)	
CML	27	1.1 (0.6–2.0)	
CLL	156	1.4 (1.1–1.9)	
ALL	7	0.9 (0.3–2.5)	
Myelodysplasias	32	0.8 (0.5–1.4)	
Any herbicide use	157	1.2 (0.9–1.6)	
AML	39	1.3 (0.8–2.0)	
CML	16	1.3 (0.7–2.6)	
CLL	74	1.4 (1.0–2.0)	
ALL	2	0.5 (0.1–2.2)	
Myelodysplasias	10	0.7 (0.3–1.5)	
Phenoxy acid use	120	1.2 (0.9–1.6)	
2,4-D use	98	1.2 (0.9–1.6)	
2,4,5-T use	22	1.3 (0.7–2.2)	
First use > 20 yrs before	11	1.8 (0.8–4.0)	
MCPA	11	1.9 (0.8–4.3)	
First use > 20 yrs before	5	2.4 (0.7–8.2)	

continued

TABLE 8-47 Leukemia, continued

Study Population[a]	Exposed Cases[b]	**Exposure of Interest**/Estimated Relative Risk (95% CI)[b]	Reference
ENVIRONMENTAL			
Seveso, Italy Residential Cohort—Industrial accident July 10, 1976 (723 residents Zone A; 4,821 Zone B; 31,643 Zone R; 181,574 local reference group) (ICD-9 171)		**TCDD**	
Incidence—20-yr followup to 1996—men and women			
Leukemia (ICD-9 204–208)			Pesatori et al., 2009
Zone A	2	2.2 (0.5–8.8)	
Zone B	8	1.4 (0.7–2.7)	
Zone R	31	0.8 (0.5–2.1)	
Lymphatic leukemia (ICD-9 204)			
Zone A	1	2.8 (0.4–19.9)	
Zone B	0	nr	
Zone R	13	0.8 (0.5–1.5)	
Myeloid leukemia (ICD-9 205)			
Zone A	1	2.2 (0.3–16.0)	
Zone B	7	2.4 (1.1–5.2)	
Zone R	15	0.8 (0.4–1.3)	
Leukemia, unspecified (ICD-9 208)			
Zone A	0	nr	
Zone B	1	2.2 (0.3–16.1)	
Zone R	2	0.6 (0.1–2.6)	
10-yr followup to 1991—men			Bertazzi et al., 1993
Zone B	2	1.6 (0.4–6.5)	
Myeloid leukemia (ICD-9 205)	1	2.0 (0.3–14.6)	
Zone R	8	0.9 (0.4–1.9)	
Myeloid leukemia (ICD-9 205)	5	1.4 (0.5–3.8)	
10-yr followup to 1991—women			Bertazzi et al., 1993
Zone B	2	1.8 (0.4–7.3)	
Myeloid leukemia (ICD-9 205)	2	3.7 (0.9–15.7)	
Zone R	3	0.4 (0.1–1.2)	
Myeloid leukemia (ICD-9 205)	2	0.5 (0.1–2.1)	
Mortality—25-yr followup to 2001 (men and women)			
Leukemia (ICD-9 204–208)			Consonni et al., 2008
Zone A	1	0.9 (0.1–6.3)	
Zone B	13	1.7 (1.0–3.0)	
Zone R	51	1.0 (0.7–1.3)	
Lymphatic leukemia (ICD-9 204)			
Zone A	0	nr	
Zone B	3	1.3 (0.4–4.1)	
Zone R	23	1.4 (0.9–2.2)	
Myeloid leukemia (ICD-9 205)			
Zone A	1	2.1 (0.3–15.2)	
Zone B	6	2.0 (0.9–4.5)	

TABLE 8-47 Leukemia, continued

Study Population[a]	Exposed Cases[b]	**Exposure of Interest**/Estimated Relative Risk (95% CI)[b]	Reference
Zone R	16	0.7 (0.4–1.2)	
Monocytic leukemia (ICD-9 206)	0	nr	
Leukemia, unspecified (ICD-9 208)			
Zone A	0	nr	
Zone B	4	2.4 (0.9–6.5)	
Zone R	10	0.8 (0.4–1.6)	
20-yr followup to 1996			Bertazzi et al., 2001
Zones A, B—men	9	2.1 (1.1–4.1)	
Zones A, B—women	3	1.0 (0.3–3.0)	
15-yr followup to 1991—men			Bertazzi et al., 1998
Zone B	7	3.1 (1.4–6.7)	
Zone R	12	0.8 (0.4–1.5)	
15-yr followup to 1991—women			Bertazzi et al., 1998
Zone B	1	0.6 (0.1–4.0)	
Zone R	12	0.9 (0.5–1.6)	
Chapaevsk, Russia Residential Cohort		**Dioxin**	Revich et al., 2001
Incidence—Crude incidence rate in 1998 vs			
Men			
Regional (Samara)	nr	14.6 (nr)	
National (Russia)	nr	15.2 (nr)	
Women			
Regional (Samara)	nr	13.9 (nr)	
National (Russia)	nr	10.7 (nr)	
Mortality—1995–1998 (SMR vs regional rates)			
Men	11	1.5 (0.8–2.7)	
Women	15	1.5 (0.8–2.4)	
Other International Environmental Studies			
SWEDEN			
Swedish fishermen (high consumption of fish with persistent organochlorines)		**Organochlorine compounds**	Svensson et al., 1995
Incidence			
Lymphocytic			
East coast (higher serum TEQs)	4	1.2 (0.3–3.3)	
West coast (lower serum TEQs)	16	1.3 (0.8–2.2)	
Myeloid			
East coast (higher serum TEQs)	2	0.9 (0.1–3.1)	
West coast (lower serum TEQs)	6	0.5 (0.2–1.1)	
Mortality—all leukemias			
East coast (higher serum TEQs)	5	1.4 (0.5–3.2)	
West coast (lower serum TEQs)	24	1.0 (0.6–1.5)	
CASE-CONTROL STUDIES			
US Case-Control Studies			
1,084 leukemia deaths in Nebraska in 1957–1974; farmers–usual occupation on death certificate		**Herbicides, pesticides** 1.3 ($p < 0.05$)	Blair and White, 1985
99 ALL cases	nr	1.3 (nr)	

continued

TABLE 8-47 Leukemia, continued

Study Population[a]	Exposed Cases[b]	**Exposure of Interest**/Estimated Relative Risk (95% CI)[b]	Reference
248 CLL cases	nr	1.7 ($p < 0.05$)	
105 unspecified lymphatic cases	nr	0.9 (nr)	
235 AML cases	nr	1.2 (nr)	
96 CML cases	nr	1.1 (nr)	
39 unspecified myeloid cases	nr	1.0 (nr)	
39 acute monocytic cases	nr	1.9 (nr)	
52 acute unspecified leukemia cases	nr	2.4 (nr)	
65 unspecified leukemia cases	nr	1.2 (nr)	
Tecumseh, Michigan, residents participating in longitudinal study (1959–1987)		**Herbicides**	Waterhouse et al., 1996
All leukemias			
Men	42	1.4 (1.0–1.9)	
Women	32	1.2 (0.9–1.8)	
CLL	10	1.4 (1.0–1.9)	
International Case-Control Studies			
Italian residents of 11 areas (incidence of leukemia excluding CLL)		**Herbicides**	Miligi et al., 2003
Exposure to phenoxy herbicides	6	2.1 (0.7–6.2)	
Italian farming and animal-breeding workers (men and women)—incidence (CLL)	15	**Herbicides** 2.3 (0.9–5.8)	Amadori et al., 1995
Farmers	5	1.6 (0.5–5.2)	
Breeders	10	3.1 (1.1–8.3)	

NOTE: 2,4-D, 2,4-dichlorophenoxyacetic acid; 2,4-DP, dichlorprop; 2,4,5-T, 2,4,5-trichlorophenoxyacetic acid; 2,4,5-TCP, 2,4,5-trichlorophenol; 2,5-DCP, 2,5-dichlorophenol; ACC, Army Chemical Corps; ALL, acute lymphocytic leukemia; AML, acute myeloid leukemia; CA, California; CATI, computer-assisted telephone interviewing; CDC, Centers for Disease Control and Prevention; CI, confidence interval; CLL, chronic lymphocytic leukemia; CML, chronic myeloid leukemia; COI, chemical of interest; HD, Hodgkin disease; IARC, International Agency for Research on Cancer; ICD, International Classification of Diseases; JEM, job-exposure matrix; LHC, lymphohematopoietic cancers; MCPA, 2-methyl-4-chlorophenoxyacetic acid; MCPB, 4-(4-chloro-2-methylphenoxy) butanoic acid; MCPP, methylchlorophenoxypropionic acid; MOS, military occupation specialty; NHL, non-Hodgkin lymphoma; NIOSH, National Institute for Occupational Safety and Health; nr, not reported; PCDD, polychlorinated dibenzo-*p*-dioxin (highly chlorinated, if four or more chlorines); PCMR, proportionate cancer mortality ratios; PCP, pentachlorophenol; PM, proportionate mortality; SEA, Southeast Asia; SIR, standardized incidence ratio; SMR, standardized mortality rate; TCDD, 2,3,7,8-tetrachlorodibenzo-*p*-dioxin; TCP, trichlorophenol; TEQ, toxicity equivalent; VA, US Department of Veterans Affairs.

[a]Subjects are male and outcome is mortality unless otherwise noted.

[b]Given when available; results other than estimated risk explained individually.

[c]Lymphopoietic cancers comprise all forms of lymphoma (including Hodgkin lymphoma and non-Hodgkin lymphoma) and leukemia (ALL, AML, CLL, CML).

0.89, 95% CI 0.41–1.68), the PCP-only group (seven deaths, SMR = 1.03, 95% CI 0.41–2.12), or the PCP-plus-TCDD group (two deaths, SMR = 0.60, 95% CI 0.07–2.16). Of the nine leukemia deaths, four occurred in the small group of 277 nonwhite males and resulted in a significant increase in SMR (4.57, 95% CI 1.25–11.7).

Koutros et al. (2010a) updated cancer incidence data in the AHS through 2006 and found nonsignificant associations with leukemia in the private pesticide applicators (133 cases, SIR = 0.96, 95% CI 0.81–1.14) and their spouses (37 cases, SIR = 0.83, 95% CI 0.58–1.14). Similarly, in an analysis of leukemia mortality in agricultural pesticide applicators and their spouses (1993–2007), Waggoner et al. (2011) reported no increased risk of leukemia in applicators (91 deaths, SMR = 0.85, 95% CI 0.68–1.04) or in their spouses (33 deaths, SMR = 1.09, 95% CI 0.75–1.53). The AHS has been generating valuable information on the COIs for a number of years, but these results are not herbicide-specific and so are not regarded as being fully informative for the committee's task.

In the British PUHS cohort of 62,960 subjects, neither leukemia incidence nor leukemia mortality was significantly increased by pesticide exposure in men or women (Frost et al., 2011).

Biologic Plausibility

Leukemia is a relatively rare spontaneous neoplasm in mice, but it is less rare in some strains of rats. A small study reported that five of 10 male rats fed TCDD at 1 ng/kg per week for 78 weeks showed an increased incidence of various cancers, one of which was lymphocytic leukemia (Van Miller et al., 1977). Later studies of TCDD's carcinogenicity have not shown an increased incidence of lymphocytic leukemia in mice or rats.

Two studies that used cells in tissue culture suggested that TCDD exposure does not promote leukemia. Proliferation of cultured human bone marrow stem cells (the source of leukemic cells) was not influenced by addition of TCDD to the culture medium (van Grevenynghe et al., 2005). Likewise, Mulero-Navarro et al. (2006) reported that the AHR promoter is silenced in ALL—an effect that could lead to reduced expression of the receptor, which binds TCDD and mediates its toxicity. No reports of animal studies have noted an increased incidence of leukemia after exposure to the phenoxy herbicides or other COIs.

The biologic plausibility of the carcinogenicity of the COIs is discussed in general at the beginning of this chapter.

Synthesis

The new findings from three cohorts of production workers (Boers et al., 2012; Burns et al., 2011; Ruder and Yiin, 2011) provide no evidence to support an association between exposure to the COIs and the occurrence of leukemia. The committee has some concern about misclassification of leukemia types and finds the correspondence between intensity of exposure and magnitude of risk for leukemias (other than CLL) to be erratic.

Conclusion

On the basis of the evidence reviewed here and in previous VAO reports, the committee concludes that there is inadequate or insufficient evidence to determine whether there is an association between exposure to the COIs and leukemias in general. An exception is the specific leukemia subtypes of chronic B-cell hematoproliferative diseases, including CLL and HCL, which are more appropriately grouped with lymphomas.

Nonmalignant Myeloid Diseases

The myelodysplastic syndromes (MDSs) are a collection of proliferative diseases (ICD-9 238.7, ICD-10 D46) that involve myeloid dysplasia. Patients often develop anemia and cytopenia caused by progressive bone marrow failure. MDSs are not malignancies, nor are they necessarily fatal, but aggressive cases of MDS frequently progress to AML. On the basis of Surveillance, Epidemiology, and End Results program data collected from 2001 to 2003, the age-adjusted incidence of MDS in the United States was estimated to be 3.4 per 100,000 people per year, which means about 10,000 new cases per year (Sekeres, 2011). Various factors determine prognosis, and several scoring systems are used. Most involve the number of cytopenias, dependence on transfusion, cytogenetic abnormalities, and the number of blasts in the marrow. For low-risk disease, the median survival is about 7 years; for high risk, it is less than 1 year. MDS does not always progress to AML, and the incidence of progression varies with risk category. Of cases with high-risk MDS, around 25–35% progress to AML. More people die from complications of infection or bleeding than through transformation to AML. Myeloproliferative neoplasms (ICD-9 205.1, 238.4, 289.89, 289.9; ICD-10 D47.1) are generally less serious clonal diseases of the myeloid lineage, but they may progress into MDS or AML.

Aplastic anemia (AA) (ICD-9 284, ICD-10 D60-D61) is another disease of the bone marrow in which stem cells are damaged in such a way that there are simultaneous decreases in red blood cells (anemia), white blood cells (leukopenia), and platelets (thrombocytopenia)—pancytopenia. Exposures to radiation, a number of drugs, and some industrial chemicals (such as benzene) are recognized as risk factors for this condition, but it may also arise from an autoimmune disease.

Update of the Epidemiologic Literature

No Vietnam-veteran, occupational, or environmental studies of MDS with adequate specification of exposure to the COIs have been published since *Update 2010*, but two hospital-based case-control studies have investigated possible association between herbicides and MDS, and another has addressed pesticides and AA.

Case-Control Studies In a study comprising 403 newly diagnosed MDS patients and 806 sex- and age-matched patient controls in 27 major hospitals in Shanghai, China, Lv et al. (2011) examined the relation of lifestyle, environmental, and occupational factors to risk of MDS. Exposure to herbicides was associated with an increased risk of MDS (OR = 5.33, 95% CI 1.41–20.10) and with the MDS subtype refractory cytopenia with multilineage dysplasia (OR = 12, 95% CI 1.44–99.67).

Shorter constitutive telomeres in proliferative mononuclear cells has been associated with MDS and is thus a plausible mechanism by which associated exposures could induce MDS. Rollison et al. (2011) measured telomere length (TL) in peripheral blood leukocytes of MDS cases identified in a hospital-based case-control study in Florida, with (n = 8) and without (n = 47) self-reported herbicide exposure (Rollison et al., 2011). Telomere length was significantly reduced ($p = 0.05$) in the exposed people, with a mean ± SD of 2.52 ± 0.95 compared with that in unexposed people (4.23 ± 2.44).

AA is a severe disease of bone marrow failure involving stem cells from different lineages. It has a fatality rate of 34% 1 year after diagnosis. Its causes are unknown, but may be associated with pesticide exposure. Risk of AA from occupational exposures to pesticides in the preceding 6 months was assessed in a hospital-based case-control study in Thailand with 541 cases and 2,261 controls (Prihartono et al., 2011). The time frame of AA does not correspond to the situation of concern in the present review. An increased risk of AA was found to be associated with exposure to several classes of pesticides measured by either self-report or expert assessment (organophosphates, carbamates, organochlorines, and paraquat), but there was no indication that exposures to phenoxy herbicides, picloram, or cacodylic acid were assessed.

Synthesis

There are no data with which to assess the role that specific COIs may play in the occurrence of the various nonmalignant bone-marrow–derived diseases.

Conclusion

On the basis of the available tangential information, the committee concludes that there is inadequate or insufficient evidence to determine whether there is an association between exposure to the COIs and nonmalignant myeloid diseases.

REFERENCES[1]

ACS (American Cancer Society). 2011. Skin cancer: Basal and squamous cell. Atlanta, GA. American Cancer Society.

ACS. 2012a. Laryngeal and hypopharyngeal cancer. Atlanta, GA: American Cancer Society. http://www.cancer.org/acs/groups/cid/documents/webcontent/003108-pdf.pdf (accessed May 15, 2013).

ACS. 2012b. *Cancer Facts and Figures 2012*. Atlanta, GA: American Cancer Society.

ACS.2012c. Brain and spinal cord tumors in adults. Atlanta, GA: American Cancer Society. http://www.cancer.org/acs/groups/cid/documents/webcontent/003088-pdf.pdf (accessed May 15, 2013).

ACS. 2013a. *Cancer Facts and Figures 2013*. Atlanta, GA: American Cancer Society. http://www.cancer.org/research/cancerfactsstatistics/cancerfactsfigures2013/index (accessed May 15, 2013).

ACS. 2013b. Skin cancer: Basal and squamous cell overview. Atlanta, GA: American Cancer Society. http://www.cancer.org/acs/groups/cid/documents/webcontent/003075-pdf.pdf (accessed May 15, 2013).

ADVA (Australia Department of Veterans' Affairs). 2005a. *Cancer Incidence in Australian Vietnam Veteran Study 2005.* Canberra, Australia: Department of Veterans' Affairs.

ADVA. 2005b. *The Third Australian Vietnam Veterans Mortality Study 2005.* Canberra, Australia: Department of Veterans' Affairs.

ADVA. 2005c. *Australian National Service Vietnam Veterans: Mortality and Cancer Incidence 2005.* Canberra, Australia: Department of Veterans' Affairs.

AFHS (Air Force Health Study). 1996. *An Epidemiologic Investigation of Health Effects in Air Force Personnel Following Exposure to Herbicides. Mortality Update 1996.* Brooks AFB, TX: Epidemiologic Research Division. Armstrong Laboratory. AL/AO-TR-1996-0068. 31 pps.

AFHS. 2000. *An Epidemiologic Investigation of Health Effects in Air Force Personnel Following Exposure to Herbicides. 1997 Follow-up Examination Results.* Brooks AFB, TX: Epidemiologic Research Division, Armstrong Laboratory. AFRL-HE-BR-TR-2000-02.

AIHW (Australian Institute of Health and Welfare). 1999. *Morbidity of Vietnam Veterans: A Study of the Health of Australia's Vietnam Veteran Community, Volume 3: Validation Study.* Canberra, Australia.

Akhtar FZ, Garabrant DH, Ketchum NS, Michalek JE. 2004. Cancer in US Air Force veterans of the Vietnam War. *Journal of Occupational and Environmental Medicine* 46(2):123–136.

Alavanja MC, Blair A, Merkle S, Teske J, Eaton B. 1988. Mortality among agricultural extension agents. *American Journal of Industrial Medicine* 14(2):167–176.

Alavanja MC, Blair A, Merkle S, Teske J, Eaton B, Reed B. 1989. Mortality among forest and soil conservationists. *Archives of Environmental Health* 44:94–101.

[1]Throughout this report, the same alphabetic indicator after year of publication is used consistently for a given reference when there are multiple citations by the same first author in a given year. The convention of assigning the alphabetic indicators in order of citation in a given chapter is not followed.

Alavanja MC, Samanic C, Dosemeci M, Lubin J, Tarone R, Lynch CF, Knott C, Thomas K, Hoppin JA, Barker J, Coble J, Sandler DP, Blair A. 2003. Use of agricultural pesticides and prostate cancer risk in the Agricultural Health Study cohort. *American Journal of Epidemiology* 157(9):800–814.

Alavanja MCR, Sandler DP, Lynch CF, Knott C, Lubin JH, Tarone R, Thomas K, Dosemeci M, Barker J, Hoppin JA, Blair A. 2005. Cancer incidence in the Agricultural Health Study. *Scandinavian Journal of Work, Environment and Health* 31(Suppl 1):39–45.

Allan LL, Sherr DH. 2010. Disruption of human plasma cell differentiation by an environmental polycyclic aromatic hydrocarbon: A mechanistic immunotoxicological study. *Environmental Health* 9:15.

Allen JR, Barsotti DA, Van Miller JP, Abrahamson LJ, Lalich JJ. 1977. Morphological changes in monkeys consuming a diet containing low levels of 2,3,7,8-tetrachlorodibenzo-*p*-dioxin. *Food and Cosmetics Toxicology* 15:401–410.

Amadori D, Nanni O, Falcini F, Saragoni A, Tison V, Callea A, Scarpi E, Ricci M, Riva N, Buiatti E. 1995. Chronic lymphocytic leukaemias and non-Hodgkin's lymphomas by histological type in farming-animal breeding workers: A population case-control study based on job titles. *Occupational and Environmental Medicine* 52(6):374–379.

Ambolet-Camoit A, Bui L, Pierre S, Chevallier A, Marchand A, Coumoul X, Garlatti M, Andreau K, Barouki R, Aggerbeck M. 2010. 2,3,7,8-tetrachlorodibenzo-*p*-dioxin counteracts the p53 response to a genotoxicant by upregulating expression of the metastasis marker AGR2 in the hepatocarcinoma cell line HepG2. *Toxicological Sciences* 115(2):501–512.

Anderson HA, Hanrahan LP, Jensen M, Laurin D, Yick WY, Wiegman P. 1986. *Wisconsin Vietnam Veteran Mortality Study: Final Report.* Madison: Wisconsin Division of Health.

Andersson P, McGuire J, Rubioi C, Gradin K, Whitelaw ML, Pettersson S, Hanberg A, Poellinger L. 2002a. A constitutively active dioxin/aryl hydrocarbon receptor induces stomach tumors. *Proceedings of the National Academy of Sciences of the United States* 99(15):9990–9995.

Andersson P, Rubio C, Poellinger L, Hanberg A. 2005. Gastric hamartomatous tumours in a transgenic mouse model expressing an activated dioxin/Ah receptor. *Anticancer Research* 25(2A):903–911.

Andreotti G, Freeman LE, Hou L, Coble J, Rusiecki J, Hoppin JA, Silverman DT, Alavanja MC. 2009. Agricultural pesticide use and pancreatic cancer risk in the Agricultural Health Study cohort. *International Journal of Cancer* 124(10):2495–2500.

Andreotti G, Hou L, Beane Freeman LE, Mahajan R, Koutros S, Coble J, Lubin J, Blair A, Hoppin JA, Alavanja M. 2010. Body mass index, agricultural pesticide use, and cancer incidence in the Agricultural Health Study cohort. *Cancer Causes and Control* 21(11):1759–1775.

Andreotti G, Silverman DT. 2012. Occupational risk factors and pancreatic cancer: A review of recent findings. *Molecular Carcinogenesis* 51(1):98–108.

Androutsopoulos VP, Tsatsakis AM, Spandidos DA. 2009. Cytochrome P450 CYP1A1: Wider roles in cancer progression and prevention. *BMC Cancer* 9:187.

Arnold LL, Eldan M, Nyska A, van Gemert M, Cohen SM. 2006. Dimethylarsinic acid: Results of chronic toxicity/oncogenicity studies in F344 rats and in B6C3F1 mice. *Toxicology* 223(1-2):82–100.

Asp S, Riihimaki V, Hernberg S, Pukkala E. 1994. Mortality and cancer morbidity of Finnish chlorophenoxy herbicide applicators: An 18-year prospective follow-up. *American Journal of Industrial Medicine* 26(2):243–253.

Aussem A, de Morais SR, Corbex M. 2012. Analysis of nasopharyngeal carcinoma risk factors with Bayesian networks. *Artificial Intelligence in Medicine* 54(1):53–62.

Axelson O, Sundell L, Andersson K, Edling C, Hogstedt C, Kling H. 1980. Herbicide exposure and tumor mortality. An updated epidemiologic investigation on Swedish railroad workers. *Scandinavian Journal of Work, Environment, and Health* 6(1):73–79.

Baan R, Grosse Y, Straif K, Secretan B, El Ghissassi F, Bouvard V, Benbrahim-Tallaa L, Guha N, Freeman C, Galichet L, Cogliano V; WHO International Agency for Research on Cancer Monograph Working Group. 2009. A review of human carcinogens—Part F: Chemical agents and related occupations. *Lancet Oncology* 10(12):1143–1144.

Baccarelli A, Hirt C, Pesatori AC, Consonni D, Patterson DG Jr, Bertazzi PA, Dolken G, Landi MT. 2006. t(14;18) translocations in lymphocytes of healthy dioxin-exposed individuals from Seveso, Italy. *Carcinogenesis* 27(10):2001–2007.

Bagga D, Anders KH, Wang HJ, Roberts E, Glaspy JA. 2000. Organochlorine pesticide content of breast adipose tissue from women with breast cancer and control subjects. *Journal of the National Cancer Institute* 92(9):750–753.

Balarajan R, Acheson ED. 1984. Soft tissue sarcomas in agriculture and forestry workers. *Journal of Epidemiology and Community Health* 38(2):113–116.

Band PR, Abanto Z, Bert J, Lang B, Fang R, Gallagher RP, Le ND. 2011. Prostate cancer risk and exposure to pesticides in British Columbia farmers. *The Prostate* 71:168–183.

Barhoover MA, Hall JM, Greenlee WF, Thomas RS. 2010. Aryl hydrocarbon receptor regulates cell cycle progression in human breast cancer cells via a functional interaction with cyclin-dependent kinase 4. *Molecular Pharmacology* 77(2):195–201.

Barouki R, Coumoul X. 2010. Cell migration and metastasis markers as targets of environmental pollutants and the aryl hydrocarbon receptor. *Cell Adhesion and Migration* 4(1):72–76.

Barry KH, Koutros S, Berndt SI, Andreotti G, Hoppin JA, Sandler DP, Burdette LA, Yeager M, Freeman LE, Lubin JH, Ma X, Zheng T, Alavanja MC. 2011. Genetic variation in base excision repair pathway genes, pesticide exposure, and prostate cancer risk. *Environmental Health Perspectives* 119(12):1726–1732.

Barry KH, Koutros S, Andreotti G, Sandler DP, Burdette LA, Yeager M, Beane Freeman LE, Lubin JH, Ma X, Zheng T, Alavanja MC, Berndt SI. 2012. Genetic variation in nucleotide excision repair pathway genes, pesticide exposure and prostate cancer risk. *Carcinogenesis* 33(2):331–337.

Baumann JL, Cohen S, Evjen AN, Law JH, Vadivelu S, Attia A, Schindler JS, Chung CH, Wirth PS, Meijer CJ, Yarbrough WG, Slebos RJ. 2009. Human papillomavirus in early laryngeal carcinoma. *Laryngoscope* 119:1531–1537.

Becher H, Flesch-Janys D, Kauppinen T, Kogevinas M, Steindorf K, Manz A, Wahrendorf J. 1996. Cancer mortality in German male workers exposed to phenoxy herbicides and dioxins. *Cancer Causes and Control* 7(3):312–321.

Beebe LE, Fornwald LW, Diwan BA, Anver MR, Anderson LM. 1995. Promotion of N-nitrosodiethylamine-initiated hepatocellular tumors and hepatoblastomas by 2,3,7,8-tetrachlorodibenzo-*p*-dioxin or Aroclor 1254 in C57BL/6, DBA/2, and B6D2F1 mice. *Cancer Research* 55(21):4875–4880.

Begg CB, Orlow I, Hummer AJ, Armstrong BK, Kricker A, Marrett LD, Millikan R, Gruber S, Anton-Culver H, Zanetti R, Gallagher RP, Dwyer T, Rebbeck TR, Mitra N, Busam K, From L, Berwick M; the Genes Environment and Melanoma (GEM) Study Group. 2005. Lifetime risk of melanoma in CDKN2A mutation carriers in a population-based sample. *Journal of the National Cancer Institute* 97:1507–1515.

Behrens T, Lynge E, Cree I, Lutz JM, Eriksson M, Guenel P, Merletti F, Morales-Suarez-Varela M, Afonso N, Stengrevics A, Fevotte J, Sabroe S, Llopis-Gonzalez A, Gorini G, Hardell L, Stang A, Ahrens W. 2012. Pesticide exposure in farming and forestry and the risk of uveal melanoma. *Cancer Causes and Control* 23(1):141–151.

Bender AP, Parker DL, Johnson RA, Scharber WK, Williams AN, Marbury MC, Mandel JS. 1989. Minnesota highway maintenance worker study: Cancer mortality. *American Journal of Industrial Medicine* 15(5):545–556.

Bertazzi PA, Zocchetti C, Pesatori AC, Guercilena S, Sanarico M, Radice L. 1989a. Mortality in an area contaminated by TCDD following an industrial incident. *Medicina Del Lavoro* 80(4):316–329.

Bertazzi PA, Zocchetti C, Pesatori AC, Guercilena S, Sanarico M, Radice L. 1989b. Ten-year mortality study of the population involved in the Seveso incident in 1976. *American Journal of Epidemiology* 129(6):1187–1200.

Bertazzi A, Pesatori AC, Consonni D, Tironi A, Landi MT, Zocchetti C. 1993. Cancer incidence in a population accidentally exposed to 2,3,7,8-tetrachlorodibenzo-*para*-dioxin. *Epidemiology* 4(5):398–406.

Bertazzi PA, Zochetti C, Guercilena S, Consonni D, Tironi A, Landi MT, Pesatori AC. 1997. Dioxin exposure and cancer risk: A 15-year mortality study after the "Seveso accident." *Epidemiology* 8(6):646–652.

Bertazzi PA, Bernucci I, Brambilla G, Consonni D, Pesatori AC. 1998. The Seveso studies on early and long-term effects of dioxin exposure: A review. *Environmental Health Perspectives* 106(Suppl 2):625–633.

Bertazzi PA, Consonni D, Bachetti S, Rubagotti M, Baccarelli A, Zocchetti C, Pesatori AC. 2001. Health effects of dioxin exposure: A 20-year mortality study. *American Journal of Epidemiology* 153(11):1031–1044.

Bertrand KA, Spiegelman D, Aster JC, Altshul LM, Korrick SA, Rodig SJ, Zhang SM, Kurth T, Laden F. 2010. Plasma organochlorine levels and risk of non-Hodgkin lymphoma in a cohort of men. *Epidemiology* 21(2):172–180.

Berwick M, Orlow I, Hummer AJ, Armstrong BK, Kricker A, Marrett LD, Millikan RC, Gruber S, Anton-Culver H, Zanetti R, Gallagher RP, Dwyer T, Rebbeck TR, Kanetsky PA, Busan K, From L, Mujumdar U, Wilcox H, Begg CB; the GEM Study Group. 2006. The prevalence of CDKN2A germ-line mutations and relative risk for cutaneous malignant melanoma: An international population-based study. *Cancer Epidemiology, Biomarkers and Prevention* 15:1520–1525.

Birnbaum LS, Fenton SE. 2003. Cancer and developmental exposure to endocrine disruptors. *Environmental Health Perspectives* 111(4):389–394.

Bhat AR, Wani MA, Kirmani AR, Raina TH. 2010. Pesticides and brain cancer linked in orchard farmers of Kashmir. *Indian Journal of Medical and Paediatric Oncology* 31(4):110–120.

Black MB, Budinsky RA, Dombkowski A, Cukovic D, LeCluyse EL, Ferguson SS, Thomas RS, Rowlands JC. 2012. Cross-species comparisons of transcriptomic alterations in human and rat primary hepatocytes exposed to 2,3,7,8-tetrachlorodibenzo-*p*-dioxin. *Toxicological Sciences* 127(1):199–215.

Blair A, White DW. 1985. Leukemia cell types and agricultural practices in Nebraska. *Archives of Environmental Health* 40(4):211–214.

Blair A, Grauman DJ, Lubin JH, Fraumeni JF Jr. 1983. Lung cancer and other causes of death among licensed pesticide applicators. *Journal of the National Cancer Institute* 71(1):31–37.

Blair A, Dosemeci M, Heineman EF. 1993. Cancer and other causes of death among male and female farmers from twenty-three states. *American Journal of Industrial Medicine* 23(5):729–742.

Blair A, Sandler DP, Tarone R, Lubin J, Thomas K, Hoppin JA, Samanic C, Coble J, Kamel F, Knott C, Dosemeci M, Zahm SH, Lynch CF, Rothman N, Alavanja MC. 2005a. Mortality among participants in the Agricultural Health Study. *Annals of Epidemiology* 15(4):279–285.

Blair A, Sandler D, Thomas K, Hoppin JA, Kamel F, Coble J, Lee WJ, Rusiecki J, Knott C, Dosemeci M, Lynch CF, Lubin J, Alavanja M. 2005b. Disease and injury among participants in the Agricultural Health Study. *Journal of Agricultural Safety and Health* 11(2):141–150.

Bloemen LJ, Mandel JS, Bond GG, Pollock AF, Vitek RP, Cook RR. 1993. An update of mortality among chemical workers potentially exposed to the herbicide 2,4-dichlorophenoxyacetic acid and its derivatives. *Journal of Occupational Medicine* 35(12):1208–1212.

Blot WJ, McLaughlin JK. 1999. The changing epidemiology of esophageal cancer. *Seminars in Oncology* 26(5 Suppl 15):2–8.

Bodner KM, Collins JJ, Bloemen LJ, Carson ML. 2003. Cancer risk for chemical workers exposed to 2,3,7,8-tetrachlorodibenzo-*p*-dioxin. *Occupational and Environmental Medicine* 60(9):672–675.

Boehmer TK, Flanders WD, McGeehin MA, Boyle C, Barrett DH. 2004. Postservice mortality in Vietnam veterans: 30-year follow-up. *Archives of Internal Medicine* 164(17):1908–1916.

Boers D, Portengen L, Bueno de Mesquita HB, Heederik D, Vermeulen R. 2010. Cause-specific mortality of Dutch chlorophenoxy herbicide manufacturing workers. *Occupational and Environmental Medicine* 67(1):24–31.

Boers D, Portengen L, Turner WE, Bueno de Mesquita HB, Heederik D, Vermeulen R. 2012. Plasma dioxin levels and cause-specific mortality in an occupational cohort of workers exposed to chlorophenoxy herbicides, chlorophenols and contaminants. *Occupational and Environmental Medicine* 69(2):113–118.

Boffetta P, Stellman SD, Garfinkel L. 1989. A case-control study of multiple myeloma nested in the American Cancer Society prospective study. *International Journal of Cancer* 43(4):554–559.

Bond GG, Wetterstroem NH, Roush GJ, McLaren EA, Lipps TE, Cook RR. 1988. Cause specific mortality among employees engaged in the manufacture, formulation, or packaging of 2,4-dichlorophenoxyacetic acid and related salts. *British Journal of Industrial Medicine* 45(2):98–105.

Bonefeld-Jorgensen EC, Long M, Bossi R, Ayotte P, Asmund G, Kruger T, Ghisari M, Mulvad G, Kern P, Nzulumiki P, Dewailly E. 2011. Perfluorinated compounds are related to breast cancer risk in Greenlandic Inuit: A case control study. *Environmental Health: A Global Access Science Source* 10(1):88.

Bonneterre V, Deschamps E, Persoons R, Bernardet C, Liaudy S, Maitre A, de Gaudemaris R. 2007. Sino-nasal cancer and exposure to leather dust. *Occupational Medicine* 57(6):438–443.

Borlak J, Jenke HS. 2008. Cross-talk between aryl hydrocarbon receptor and mitogen-activated protein kinase signaling pathway in liver cancer through c-raf transcriptional regulation. *Molecular Cancer Research* 6(8):1326–1336.

Bosl GJ, Motzer RJ. 1997. Testicular germ-cell cancer. *New England Journal of Medicine* 337(4):242–253.

Boutros PC, Yan R, Moffat ID, Pohjanvirta R, Okey AB. 2008. Transcriptomic responses to 2,3,7,8-tetrachlorodibenzo-*p*-dioxin (TCDD) in liver: Comparison of rat and mouse. *BMC Genomics* 9:419.

Boutros PC, Bielefeld KA, Pohjanvirta R, Harper PA. 2009. Dioxin-dependent and dioxin-independent gene batteries: Comparison of liver and kidney in AHR-null mice. *Toxicological Sciences* 112(1):245–256.

Boyle C, Decoufle P, Delaney RJ, DeStefano F, Flock ML, Hunter MI, Joesoef MR, Karon JM, Kirk ML, Layde PM, McGee DL, Moyer LA, Pollock DA, Rhodes P, Scally MJ, Worth RM. 1987. *Postservice Mortality Among Vietnam Veterans.* Atlanta, GA: Centers for Disease Control. CEH 86-0076. 143 pps.

Bradlow H. 2008. Review: Indole-3-carbinol as a chemoprotective agent in breast and prostate cancer. *In Vivo* 22(4):441–445.

Brady PS. 2011. Not dead yet. *The VVA Veteran* (March/April). http://digitaledition.qwinc.com/display_article.php?id=675095 (accessed October 29, 2013).

Bräuner EV, Sørensen M, Gaudreau E, LeBlanc A, Eriksen KT, Tjønneland A, Overvad K, Raaschou-Nielsen O. 2012. A prospective study of organochlorines in adipose tissue and risk of non-Hodgkin lymphoma. *Environmental Health Perspectives* 120(1):105–111.

Bredhult C, Backlin BM, Olovsson M. 2007. Effects of some endocrine disruptors on the proliferation and viability of human endometrial endothelial cells in vitro. *Reproductive Toxicology* 23(4):550–559.

Brenner J, Rothenbacher D, Arndt V. 2009. Epidemiology of stomach cancer. *Methods in Molecular Biology* 472:467–477.

Breslin P, Lee Y, Kang H, Burt V, Shepard BM. 1986. *A Preliminary Report: The Vietnam Veterans Mortality Study.* Washington, DC: Veterans Administration, Office of Environmental Epidemiology.

Breslin P, Kang H, Lee Y, Burt V, Shepard BM. 1988. Proportionate mortality study of US Army and US Marine Corps veterans of the Vietnam War. *Journal of Occupational Medicine* 30(5):412–419.

Brown LM, Blair A, Gibson R, Everett GD, Cantor KP, Schuman LM, Burmeister LF, Van Lier SF, Dick F. 1990. Pesticide exposures and other agricultural risk factors for leukemia among men in Iowa and Minnesota. *Cancer Research* 50(20):6585–6591.

Brown LM, Burmeister LF, Everett GD, Blair A. 1993. Pesticide exposures and multiple myeloma in Iowa men. *Cancer Causes and Control* 4(2):153–156.

Brunnberg S, Andersson P, Lindstam M, Paulson I, Poellinger L, Hanberg A. 2006. The constitutively active Ah receptor (CA-Ahr) mouse as a potential model for dioxin exposure—Effects in vital organs. *Toxicology* 224(3):191–201.

Bueno de Mesquita HB, Doornbos G, Van der Kuip DA, Kogevinas M, Winkelmann R. 1993. Occupational exposure to phenoxy herbicides and chlorophenols and cancer mortality in the Netherlands. *American Journal of Industrial Medicine* 23(2):289–300.

Bullman TA, Kang HK, Watanabe KK. 1990. Proportionate mortality among US Army Vietnam veterans who served in Military Region I. *American Journal of Epidemiology* 132(4):670–674.

Burmeister LF. 1981. Cancer mortality in Iowa farmers, 1971–1978. *Journal of the National Cancer Institute* 66(3):461–464.

Burmeister LF, Van Lier SF, Isacson P. 1982. Leukemia and farm practices in Iowa. *American Journal of Epidemiology* 115(5):720–728.

Burmeister LF, Everett GD, Van Lier SF, Isacson P. 1983. Selected cancer mortality and farm practices in Iowa. *American Journal of Epidemiology* 118(1):72–77.

Burns CJ, Beard KK, Cartmill JB. 2001. Mortality in chemical workers potentially exposed to 2,4-dichlorophenoxyacetic acid (2,4-D) 1945–1994: An update. *Occupational and Environmental Medicine* 58(1):24–30.

Burns C, Bodner K, Swaen G, Collins J, Beard K, Lee M. 2011. Cancer incidence of 2,4-D production workers. *International Journal of Environmental Research and Public Health* 8(9):3579–3590.

Burt VL, Breslin PP, Kang HK, Lee Y. 1987. *Non-Hodgkin's Lymphoma in Vietnam Veterans.* Washington, DC, Department of Medicine and Surgery, Veterans Administration. 33 pps.

Butler R, Inzunza J, Suzuki H, Fujii-Kuriyama Y, Warner M, Gustafsson JA. 2012. Uric acid stones in the urinary bladder of aryl hydrocarbon receptor (AhR) knockout mice. *Proceedings of the National Academy of Sciences of the United States of America* 109(4):1122–1126.

Buxbaum JN. 2004. The systemic amyloidoses. *Current Opinion in Rheumatology* 16(1):67–75.

Campo E, Swerdlow SH, Harris NL, Pileri S, Stein H, Jaffe ES. 2008. The 2008 WHO classification of lymphoid neoplasms and beyond: Evolving concepts and practical applications. *Blood* 117(19):5019–5032.

Cantor KP. 1982. Farming and mortality from non-Hodgkin's lymphoma: A case-control study. *International Journal of Cancer* 29(3):239–247.

Cantor KP, Blair A. 1984. Farming and mortality from multiple myeloma: A case control study with the use of death certificates. *Journal of the National Cancer Institute* 72(2):251–255.

Cantor KP, Blair A, Everett G, Gibson R, Burmeister LF, Brown LM, Schuman L, Dick FR. 1992. Pesticides and other agricultural risk factors for non-Hodgkin's lymphoma among men in Iowa and Minnesota. *Cancer Research* 52:2447–2455.

Caplan LS, Hall HI, Levine RS, Zhu K. 2000. Preventable risk factors for nasal cancer. *Annals of Epidemiology* 10(3):186–191.

Carlson E, McCulloch C, Koganti A, Goodwin S, Sutter T, Silkworth J. 2009. Divergent transcriptomic responses to aryl hydrocarbon receptor agonists between rat and human primary hepatocytes. *Toxicological Sciences* 112(1):257–272.

Carreon T, Butler MA, Ruder AM, Waters MA, Davis-King KE, Calvert GM, Schulte PA, Connally B, Ward EM, Sanderson WT, Heineman EF, Mandel JS, Morton RF, Reding DJ, Rosenman KD, Talaska G; Brain Cancer Collaborative Group. 2005. Gliomas and farm pesticide exposure in women: The Upper Midwest Health Study. *Environmental Health Perspectives* 113(5):546–551.

Casado FL, Singh KP, Gasiewicz TA. 2011. Aryl hydrocarbon receptor activation in hematopoietic stem/progenitor cells alters cell function and pathway-specific gene modulation reflecting changes in cellular trafficking and migration. *Molecular Pharmacology* 80(4):673–682.

CDC (Centers for Disease Control and Prevention). 1990a. The association of selected cancers with service in the US military in Vietnam. III. Hodgkin's disease, nasal cancer, nasopharyngeal cancer, and primary liver cancer. The Selected Cancers Cooperative Study Group. *Archives of Internal Medicine* 150(12):2495–2505.

CDC. 1990b. The association of selected cancers with service in the US military in Vietnam. I. Non-Hodgkin's lymphoma. *Archives of Internal Medicine* 150:2473–2483.

CDVA (Commonwealth Department of Veterans' Affairs). 1997a. *Mortality of Vietnam Veterans: The Veteran Cohort Study. A Report of the 1996 Retrospective Cohort Study of Australian Vietnam Veterans.* Canberra, Australia: Department of Veterans' Affairs.

CDVA. 1997b. *Mortality of National Service Vietnam Veterans: A Report of the 1996 Retrospective Cohort Study of Australian Vietnam Veterans.* Canberra, Australia: Department of Veterans' Affairs.

CDVA. 1998a. *Morbidity of Vietnam Veterans: A Study of the Health of Australia's Vietnam Veteran Community. Volume 1: Male Vietnam Veterans Survey and Community Comparison Outcomes.* Canberra, Australia: Department of Veterans' Affairs.

CDVA. 1998b. *Morbidity of Vietnam Veterans: A Study of the Health of Australia's Vietnam Veteran Community. Volume 2: Female Vietnam Veterans Survey and Community Comparison Outcomes.* Canberra, Australia: Department of Veterans' Affairs.

Chamie K, deVere White R, Volpp B, Lee D, Ok J, Ellison L. 2008. Agent Orange exposure, Vietnam War veterans, and the risk of prostate cancer. *Cancer* 113(9):2464–2470.

Charles JM, Bond DM, Jeffries TK, Yano BL, Stott WT, Johnson KA, Cunny HC, Wilson RD, Bus JS. 1996. Chronic dietary toxicity/oncogenicity studies on 2,4-dichlorophenoxyacetic acid in rodents. *Fundamental and Applied Toxicology* 33:166–172.

Charles LE, Burchfiel CM, Fekedulegn D, Gu JK, Petrovich H, Sanderson WT, Masaki K, Rodriguez BL, Ross GW. 2010. Occupational exposure to pesticides, metals, and solvents: The impact on mortality in the Honolulu Heart Program. *Work* 37:205–215.

Chen X, Ma SW, Ma XM, Xu YJ, Tang NJ. 2012. Changes in fibrinopeptide A peptides in the sera of rats chronically exposed to low doses of 2,3,7,8-tetrachlorodibenzo-*p*-dioxin (TCDD). *Environmental Toxicology and Pharmacology* 33:191–196.

Chen YJ, Hung CM, Kay N, Chen CC, Kao YH, Yuan SS. 2012. Progesterone receptor is involved in 2,3,7,8-tetrachlorodibenzo-*p*-dioxin-stimulated breast cancer cells proliferation. *Cancer Letters* 319(2):223–231.

Chiorazzi N, Rai KR, Ferrarini M. 2005. Mechanisms of disease: Chronic lymphocytic leukemia. *The New England Journal of Medicine* 352(8):804–815.

Chiu BC, Weisenburger DD, Zahm SH, Cantor KP, Gapstur SM, Holmes F, Burmeister LF, Blair A. 2004. Agricultural pesticide use, familial cancer, and risk of non-Hodgkin lymphoma. *Cancer Epidemiology, Biomarkers and Prevention* 13(4):525–531.

Chiu BC, Dave BJ, Blair A, Gapstur SM, Zahm SH, Weisenburger DD. 2006. Agricultural pesticide use and risk of t(14;18)-defined subtypes of non-Hodgkin lymphoma. *Blood* 108(4):1363–1369.

Chlebowski RT, Hendrix SL, Langer RD, Stefanick ML, Gass M, Lane D, Rodabough RJ, Gilligan MA, Cyr MG, Thomson CA, Khandekar J, Petrovitch H, McTiernan A; WHI Investigators. 2003. Influence of estrogen plus progestin on breast cancer and mammography in healthy postmenopausal women: The Women's Health Initiative Randomized Trial. *Journal of the American Medical Association* 289(24):3243–3253.

Chopra M, Dharmarajan AM, Meiss G, Schrenk D. 2009. Inhibition of UV-C light-induced apoptosis in liver cells by 2,3,7,8-tetrachlorodibenzo-*p*-dioxin. *Toxicological Sciences* 111(1):49–63.

Chung CJ, Huang CJ, Pu YS, Su CT, Huang YK, Chen YT, Hsueh YM. 2008. Urinary 8-hydroxydeoxyguanosine and urothelial carcinoma risk in low arsenic exposure area. *Toxicology and Applied Pharmacology* 226(1):14–21.

Clapp RW. 1997. Update of cancer surveillance of veterans in Massachusetts, USA. *International Journal of Epidemiology* 26(3):679–681.

Clapp RW, Cupples LA, Colton T, Ozonoff DM. 1991. Cancer surveillance of veterans in Massachusetts, 1982–1988. *International Journal of Epidemiology* 20(1):7–12.

Cocco P, Heineman EF, Dosemeci M. 1999. Occupational risk factors for cancer of the central nervous system (CNS) among US women. *American Journal of Industrial Medicine* 36(1):70–74.

Coggon D, Pannett B, Winter PD, Acheson ED, Bonsall J. 1986. Mortality of workers exposed to 2-methyl-4-chlorophenoxyacetic acid. *Scandinavian Journal of Work, Environment, and Health* 12(5):448–454.

Coggon D, Pannett B, Winter P. 1991. Mortality and incidence of cancer at four factories making phenoxy herbicides. *British Journal of Industrial Medicine* 48(3):173–178.

Cohen AD, Zhou P, Xiao Q, Fleisher M, Kalakonda N, Akhurst T, Chitale DA, Moscowitz MV, Dhodapkar J, Teruya-Feldstein D, Filippa D, Comenzo RL. 2004. Systemic AL amyloidosis due to non-Hodgkin's lymphoma: An unusual clinicopathologic association. *British Journal of Haematology* 124:309–314.

Cohen SM, Arnold LL, Eldan M, Lewis AS, Beck BD. 2006. Methylated arsenicals: The implications of metabolism and carcinogenicity studies in rodents to human risk assessment. *Critical Reviews in Toxicology* 36(2):99–133.

Collins JJ, Strauss ME, Levinskas GJ, Conner PR. 1993. The mortality experience of workers exposed to 2,3,7,8-tetrachlorodibenzo-*p*-dioxin in a trichlorophenol process accident. *Epidemiology* 4(1):7–13.

Collins JJ, Bodner K, Aylward LL, Wilken M, Bodner CM. 2009a. Mortality rates among trichlorophenol workers with exposure to 2,3,7,8-tetrachlorodibenzo-*p*-dioxin. *American Journal of Epidemiology* 170(4):501–506.

Collins JJ, Bodner K, Aylward LL, Wilken M, Swaen G, Budinsky R, Rowlands C, Bodnar CM. 2009b. Mortality rates among workers exposed to dioxins in the manufacture of pentachlorophenol. *Journal of Occupational and Environmental Medicine* 51(10):1212–1219.

Comba P, Ascoli V, Belli S, Benedetti M, Gatti L, Ricci P, Tieghi A. 2003. Risk of soft tissue sarcomas and residence in the neighbourhood of an incinerator of industrial wastes. *Occupational and Environmental Medicine* 60(9):680–683.

Consonni D, Pesatori AC, Zocchetti C, Sindaco R, D'Oro LC, Rubagotti M, Bertazzi PA. 2008. Mortality in a population exposed to dioxin after the Seveso, Italy, accident in 1976: 25 Years of follow-up. *American Journal of Epidemiology* 167(7):847–858.

Cordier S, Poisson M, Gerin M, Varin J, Conso F, Hemon D. 1988. Gliomas and exposure to wood preservatives. *British Journal of Industrial Medicine* 45:705–709.

Cordier S, Le TB, Verger P, Bard D, Le CD, Larouze B, Dazza MC, Hoang TQ, Abenhaim L. 1993. Viral infections and chemical exposures as risk factors for hepatocellular carcinoma in Vietnam. *International Journal of Cancer* 55(2):196–201.

Corrao G, Caller M, Carle F, Russo R, Bosia S, Piccioni P. 1989. Cancer risk in a cohort of licensed pesticide users. *Scandinavian Journal of Work, Environment, and Health* 15(3):203–209.

Costani G, Rabitti P, Mambrini A, Bai E, Berrino F. 2000. Soft tissue sarcomas in the general population living near a chemical plant in northern Italy. *Tumori* 86(5):381–383.

Cypel Y, Kang H. 2008. Mortality patterns among women Vietnam-era veterans: Results of a retrospective cohort study. *Annals of Epidemiology* 18(3):244–252.

Cypel Y, Kang H. 2010. Mortality patterns of Army Chemical Corps veterans who were occupationally exposed to herbicides in Vietnam. *Annals of Epidemiology* 20(5):339–346.

Dalager NA, Kang HK. 1997. Mortality among Army Chemical Corps Vietnam veterans. *American Journal of Industrial Medicine* 31(6):719–726.

Dalager NA, Kang HK, Burt VL, Weatherbee L. 1991. Non-Hodgkin's lymphoma among Vietnam veterans. *Journal of Occupational Medicine* 33(7):774–779.

Dalager NA, Kang HK, Thomas TL. 1995. Cancer mortality patterns among women who served in the military: The Vietnam experience. *Journal of Occupational and Environmental Medicine* 37(3):298–305.

Davis BJ, McCurdy EA, Miller BD, Lucier GW, Tritscher AM. 2000. Ovarian tumors in rats induced by chronic 2,3,7,8-tetrachlorodibenzo-*p*-dioxin treatment. *Cancer Research* 60(19):5414–5419.

Dean G. 1994. Deaths from primary brain cancers, lymphatic and haematopoietic cancers in agricultural workers in the Republic of Ireland. *Journal of Epidemiology and Community Health* 48(4):364–368.

Degner SC, Papoutsis AJ, Selmin O, Romagnolo DF. 2009. Targeting of aryl hydrocarbon receptor-mediated activation of cyclooxygenase-2 expression by the indole-3-carbinol metabolite 3,3′-diindolylmethane in breast cancer cells. *Journal of Nutrition* 139(1):26–32.

Demers A, Ayotte P, Brisson J, Dodin S, Robert J, Dewailly E. 2000. Risk and aggressiveness of breast cancer in relation to plasma organochlorine concentrations. *Cancer Epidemiology, Biomarkers and Prevention* 9(2):161–166.

Dennis LK, Lynch CF, Sandler DP, Alavanja M. 2010. Pesticide use and cutaneous melanoma in pesticide applicators in the Agricultural Health Study. *Environmental Health Perspectives* 118(6):812–817.

Dere E, Boverhof DR, Burgoon LD, Zacharewski TR. 2006. In vivo-in vitro toxicogenomic comparison of TCDD-elicited gene expression in Hepa1c1c7 mouse hepatoma cells and C57BL/6 hepatic tissue. *BMC Genomics* 7:80.

d'Errico A, Pasian S, Baratti A, Zanelli R, Alfonzo S, Gilardi L, Beatrice F, Bena A, Costa G. 2009. A case-control study on occupational risk factors for sino-nasal cancer. *Occupational and Environmental Medicine* 66(7):448–455.

Desaulniers D, Leingartner K, Russo J, Perkins G, Chittim BG, Archer MC, Wade M, Yang J. 2001. Modulatory effects of neonatal exposure to TCDD or a mixture of PCBs, p,p′-DDT, and p-p′-DDE on methylnitrosourea-induced mammary tumor development in the rat. *Environmental Health Perspectives* 109:739–747.

Desaulniers D, Leingartner K, Musicki B, Cole J, Li M, Charboneau M, Tsang BK. 2004. Lack of effects of postnatal exposure to a mixture of aryl hydrocarbon-receptor agonists on the development of methylnitrosourea-induced mammary tumors in Sprague-Dawley rats. *Journal of Toxicology and Environmental Health, Part A* 67(18):1457–1475.

Dich J, Wiklund K. 1998. Prostate cancer in pesticide applicators in Swedish agriculture. *Prostate* 34(2):100–112.

Dietrich C, Kaina B. 2010. The aryl hydrocarbon receptor (AHR) in the regulation of cell-cell contact and tumor growth. *Carcinogenesis* 31(8):1319–1328.

DiNatale BC, Schroeder JC, Francey LJ, Kusnadi A, Perdew GH. 2010. Mechanistic insights into the events that lead to synergistic induction of interleukin 6 transcription upon activation of the aryl hydrocarbon receptor and inflammatory signaling. *Journal of Biological Chemistry* 285(32):24388–24397.

DiNatale BC, Schroeder JC, Perdew GH. 2011. Ah receptor antagonism inhibits constitutive and cytokine inducible IL6 production in head and neck tumor cell lines. *Molecular Carcinogenesis* 50(3):173–183.

Donna A, Betta PG, Robutti F, Crosignani P, Berrino F, Bellingeri D. 1984. Ovarian mesothelial tumors and herbicides: A case-control study. *Carcinogenesis* 5(7):941–942.

Dopp E, Von Recklinghausen U, Hartmann LM, Stueckradt I, Pollok I, Rabieh S, Hao L, Nussler A, Katier C, Hirner AV, Rettenmeier AW. 2008. Subcellular distribution of inorganic and methylated arsenic compounds in human urothelial cells and human hepatocytes. *Drug Metabolism and Disposition* 36(5):971–979.

Dubrow R, Paulson JO, Indian RW. 1988. Farming and malignant lymphoma in Hancock County, Ohio. *British Journal of Industrial Medicine* 45(1):25–28.

Duell EJ, Millikan RC, Savitz DA, Newman B, Smith JC, Schell MJ, Sandler DP. 2000. A population-based case-control study of farming and breast cancer in North Carolina. *Epidemiology* 11(5):523–531.

Ekström AM, Eriksson M, Hansson LE, Lindgren A, Signorello LB, Nyrén O, Hardell L. 1999. Occupational exposures and risk of gastric cancer in a population-based case-control study. *Cancer Research* 59:5932–5937.

Elyakim E, Sitbon E, Faerman A, Tabak S, Montia E, Belanis L, Dov A, Marcusson EG, Bennett CF, Chajut A, Cohen D, Yerushalmi N. 2010. Hsa-miR-191 is a candidate oncogene target for hepatocellular carcinoma therapy. *Cancer Research* 70(20):8077–8087.

Engel LS, Hill DA, Hoppin JA, Lubin JH, Lynch CF, Pierce J, Samanic C, Sandler DP, Blair A, Alavanja MC. 2005. Pesticide use and breast cancer risk among farmers' wives in the Agricultural Health Study. *American Journal of Epidemiology* 161(2):121–135.

Engel LS, Laden F, Andersen A, Strickland PT, Blair A, Needham LL, Barr DB, Wolff MS, Helzlsouer K, Hunter DJ, Lan Q, Cantor KP, Comstock GW, Brock, JW, Bush D, Hoover RN, Rothman N. 2007. Polychlorinated biphenyl levels in peripheral blood and non-Hodgkin's lymphoma: A report from three cohorts. *Cancer Research* 67(11):5545–5552.

Eriksson M, Karlsson M. 1992. Occupational and other environmental factors and multiple myeloma: A population based case-control study. *British Journal of Industrial Medicine* 49(2):95–103.

Eriksson M, Hardell L, Berg NO, Moller T, Axelson O. 1979. Case-control study on malignant mesenchymal tumor of the soft tissue and exposure to chemical substances. *Lakartidningen* 76(44):3872–3875.

Eriksson M, Hardell L, Berg NO, Moller T, Axelson O. 1981. Soft-tissue sarcomas and exposure to chemical substances: A case-referent study. *British Journal of Industrial Medicine* 38(1):27–33.

Eriksson M, Hardell L, Adami HO. 1990. Exposure to dioxins as a risk factor for soft tissue sarcoma: A population-based case-control study. *Journal of the National Cancer Institute* 82:486–490.

Eriksson M, Hardell L, Malker H, Weiner J. 1992. Malignant lymphoproliferative diseases in occupations with potential exposure to phenoxyacetic acids or dioxins: A register-based study. *American Journal of Industrial Medicine* 22:305–312.

Eriksson M, Hardell L, Carlberg M, Akerman M. 2008. Pesticide exposure as risk factor for non-Hodgkin lymphoma including histopathological subgroup analysis. *International Journal of Cancer* 123(7):1657–1663.

Fenton SE. 2006. Endocrine-disrupting compounds and mammary gland development: Early exposure and later life consequences. *Endocrinology* 147(6):S18–S24.

Fenton SE. 2009. The mammary gland: A tissue sensitive to environmental exposures. *Reviews on Environmental Health* 24(4):319–325.

Feron VJ, Arts JH, Kuper CF, Slootweg PJ, Woutersen RA. 2001. Health risks associated with inhaled nasal toxicants. *Critical Reviews in Toxicology* 31(3):313–347.

Fett MJ, Nairn JR, Cobbin DM, Adena MA. 1987. Mortality among Australian conscripts of the Vietnam conflict era. II. Causes of death. *American Journal of Epidemiology* 125(15):878–884.

Fingerhut MA, Halperin WE, Marlow DA, Piacitelli LA, Honchar PA, Sweeney MH, Greife AL, Dill PA, Steenland K, Suruda AJ. 1991. Cancer mortality in workers exposed to 2,3,7,8-tetrachlorodibenzo-*p*-dioxin. *New England Journal of Medicine* 324(4):212–218.

Fleming LE, Bean JA, Rudolph M, Hamilton K. 1999a. Mortality in a cohort of licensed pesticide applicators in Florida. *Journal of Occupational and Environmental Medicine* 56(1):14–21.

Fleming LE, Bean JA, Rudolph M, Hamilton K. 1999b. Cancer incidence in a cohort of licensed pesticide applicators in Florida. *Journal of Occupational and Environmental Medicine* 41(4):279–288.

Flesch-Janys D, Berger J, Gurn P, Manz A, Nagel S, Waltsgott H, Dwyer JH. 1995. Exposure to polychlorinated dioxins and furans (PCDD/F) and mortality in a cohort of workers from a herbicide-producing plant in Hamburg, Federal Republic of Germany. *American Journal of Epidemiology* 142(11):1165–1175.

Floret N, Mauny F, Challier B, Arveux P, Cahn JY, Viel JF. 2003. Dioxin emissions from a solid waste incinerator and risk of non-Hodgkin lymphoma. *Epidemiology* 14(4):392–398.

Fracchiolla NS, Todoerti K, Bertazzi PA, Servida F, Corradini P, Carniti C, Colombi A, Pesatori AC, Neri A, Deliliers GL. 2011. Dioxin exposure of human CD34+ hemopoietic cells induces gene expression modulation that recapitulates its in vivo clinical and biological effects. *Toxicology* 283:18–23.

Fritschi L, Benke G, Hughes AM, Kricker A, Turner J, Vajdic CM, Grulich A, Milliken S, Kaldor J, Armstrong BK. 2005. Occupational exposure to pesticides and risk of non-Hodgkin's lymphoma. *American Journal of Epidemiology* 162(9):849–857.

Fritz WA, Lin TM, Moore RW, Cooke PS, Peterson RE. 2005. In utero and lactational 2,3,7,8-tetrachlorodibenzo-*p*-dioxin exposure: Effects on the prostate and its response to castration in senescent C57BL/6J mice. *Toxicological Sciences* 86(2):387–395.

Fritz WA, Lin TM, Peterson RE. 2008. The aryl hydrocarbon receptor (AhR) inhibits vanadate-induced vascular endothelial growth factor (VEGF) production in TRAMP prostates. *Carcinogenesis* 29(5):1077–1082.

Frost G, Brown T, Harding AH. 2011. Mortality and cancer incidence among British agricultural pesticide users. *Occupational Medicine* 61(5):303–310.

Fukuda Y, Nakamura K, Takano T. 2003. Dioxins released from incineration plants and mortality from major diseases: An analysis of statistical data by municipalities. *Journal of Medical and Dental Sciences* 50(4):249–255.

Fukushima S, Morimura K, Wanibuchi H, Kinoshita A, Salim EI. 2005. Current and emerging challenges in toxicopathology: Carcinogenic threshold of phenobarbital and proof of arsenic carcinogenicity using rat medium-term bioassays for carcinogens. *Toxicology and Applied Pharmacology* 207(Suppl 2):225–229.

Gallagher RP, Bajdik CD, Fincham S, Hill GB, Keefe AR, Coldman A, McLean DI. 1996. Chemical exposures, medical history, and risk of squamous and basal cell carcinoma of the skin. *Cancer Epidemiology, Biomarkers and Prevention* 5(6):419–424.

Gallagher RP, MacArthur AC, Lee TK, Weber JP, Leblanc A, Mark Elwood J, Borugian M, Abanto Z, Spinelli JJ. 2011. Plasma levels of polychlorinated biphenyls and risk of cutaneous malignant melanoma: A preliminary study. *International Journal of Cancer* 128(8):1872–1880.

Gambini GF, Mantovani C, Pira E, Piolatto PG, Negri E. 1997. Cancer mortality among rice growers in Novara Province, northern Italy. *American Journal of Industrial Medicine* 31(4):435–441.

Gann PH. 1997. Interpreting recent trends in prostate cancer incidence and mortality. *Epidemiology* 8(2):117–120.

Garland FC, Gorham ED, Garland CF, Ferns JA. 1988. Non-Hodgkin's lymphoma in US Navy personnel. *Archives of Environmental Health* 43(6):425–429.

Gelman A. 2013. How many Vietnam veterans are still alive? *New York Times* (March 25, 2013). http://www.nytimes.com/2013/03/26/science/how-many-vietnam-veterans-are-still-alive.html (accessed October 29, 2013).

Gillison ML, Shah KV. 2001. Human papillomavirus-associated head and neck squamous cell carcinoma: A mounting evidence for an etiologic role for human papillomavirus in a subset of head and neck cancers. *Current Opinions in Oncology* 13:183–188.

Gillison, ML, Alemany L, Snijders PJ, Chaturvedi A, Steinberg BM, Schwartz S, Castellsaque X. 2012. Human papillomavirus and diseases of the upper airway: Head and neck cancer and respiratory papillomatosis. *Vaccine* 30(Suppl 5):F34–F54.

Giri VN, Cassidy AE, Beebe-Dimmer J, Smith DC, Bock CH, Cooney KA. 2004. Association between Agent Orange and prostate cancer: A pilot case-control study. *Urology* 63(4):757–760; discussion 760–761.

Gold LS, De Roos AJ, Brown EE, Lan Q, Milliken K, Davis S, Chanock SJ, Zhang Y, Severson R, Zahm SH, Zheng T, Rothman N, Baris D. 2009. Association of common varients in genes involved in metabolism and response to exogenous chemicals with risk of multiple myeloma. *Cancer Epidemiology* 33:276–280.

Green LM. 1991. A cohort mortality study of forestry workers exposed to phenoxy acid herbicides. *British Journal of Industrial Medicine* 48(4):234–238.

Greenwald P, Kovasznay B, Collins DN, Therriault G. 1984. Sarcomas of soft tissues after Vietnam service. *Journal of the National Cancer Institute* 73(5):1107–1109.

Grimsrud TK, Peto J. 2006. Persisting risk of nickel related lung cancer and nasal cancer among Clydach refiners. *Occupational and Environmental Medicine* 63(5):365–366.

Gupta A, Ketchum N, Roehrborn CG, Schecter A, Aragaki CC, Michalek JE. 2006. Serum dioxin, testosterone, and subsequent risk of benign prostatic hyperplasia: A prospective cohort study of Air Force veterans. *Environmental Health Perspectives* 114(11):1649–1654.

Hahn WC, Weinberg RA. 2002. Rules for making human tumor cells. *New England Journal of Medicine* 347(20):1593–1603.

Hallquist A, Hardell L, Degerman A, Boquist L. 1993. Occupational exposures and thyroid cancer: Results of a case-control study. *European Journal of Cancer Prevention* 2(4):345–349.

Halwachs S, Lakoma C, Gebhardt R, Schafer I, Seibel P, Honscha W. 2010. Dioxin mediates down-regulation of the reduced folate carrier transport activity via the arylhydrocarbon receptor signalling pathway. *Toxicology and Applied Pharmacology* 246(1-2):100–106.

Hansen ES, Hasle H, Lander F. 1992. A cohort study on cancer incidence among Danish gardeners. *American Journal of Industrial Medicine* 21(5):651–660.

Hansen ES, Lander F, Lauritsen JM. 2007. Time trends in cancer risk and pesticide exposure, a long-term follow-up of Danish gardeners. *Scandinavian Journal of Work, Environment, and Health* 33(6):465–469.

Hardell L. 1981. Relation of soft-tissue sarcoma, malignant lymphoma and colon cancer to phenoxy acids, chlorophenols and other agents. *Scandinavian Journal of Work, Environment, and Health* 7(2):119–130.

Hardell L, Sandström A. 1979. Case-control study: Soft-tissue sarcomas and exposure to phenoxy-acetic acids or chlorophenols. *British Journal of Cancer* 39:711–717.

Hardell L, Bengtsson NO. 1983. Epidemiological study of socioeconomic factors and clinical findings in Hodgkin's disease, and reanalysis of previous data regarding chemical exposure. *British Journal of Cancer* 48(2):217–225.

Hardell L, Eriksson M. 1988. The association between soft tissue sarcomas and exposure to phenoxyacetic acids: A new case-referent study. *Cancer* 62:652–656.

Hardell L, Eriksson M, Lenner P, Lundgren E. 1981. Malignant lymphoma and exposure to chemicals, especially organic solvents, chlorophenols and phenoxy acids: A case-control study. *British Journal of Cancer* 43:169–176.

Hardell L, Johansson B, Axelson O. 1982. Epidemiological study of nasal and nasopharyngeal cancer and their relation to phenoxy acid or chlorophenol exposure. *American Journal of Industrial Medicine* 3(3):247–257.

Hardell L, Bengtsson NO, Jonsson U, Eriksson S, Larsson LG. 1984. Aetiological aspects on primary liver cancer with special regard to alcohol, organic solvents and acute intermittent porphyria: An epidemiological investigation. *British Journal of Cancer* 50(3):389–397.

Hardell L, Eriksson M, Degerman A. 1994. Exposure to phenoxyacetic acids, chlorophenols, or organic solvents in relation to histopathology, stage, and anatomical localization of non-Hodgkin's lymphoma. *Cancer Research* 54(9):2386–2389.

Hardell L, Nasman A, Ohlson CG, Fredrikson M. 1998. Case-control study on risk factors for testicular cancer. *International Journal of Oncology* 13(6):1299–1303.

Hardell L, Lindström G, van Bavel B, Hardell K, Linde A, Carlberg M, Liljegren G. 2001. Adipose tissue concentrations of dioxins and dibenzofurans, titers of antibodies to Epstein-Barr virus early antigen and the risk for non-Hodgkin's lymphoma. *Environmental Research* 87(2):99–107.

Hardell L, Eriksson M, Nordstrom M. 2002. Exposure to pesticides as risk factor for non-Hodgkin's lymphoma and hairy cell leukemia: Pooled analysis of two Swedish case-control studies. *Leukemia and Lymphoma* 43(5):1043–1049.

Hartge P, Colt JS, Severson RK, Cerhan JR, Cozen W, Camann D, Zahm SH, Davis S. 2005. Residential herbicide use and risk of non-Hodgkin lymphoma. *Cancer Epidemiology, Biomarkers and Prevention* 14(4):934–937.

Hayashi H, Kanisawa M, Yamanaka K, Ito T, Udaka N, Ohji H, Okudela K, Okada S, Kitamura H. 1998. Dimethylarsinic acid, a main metabolite of inorganic arsenics, has tumorigenicity and progression effects in the pulmonary tumors of A/J mice. *Cancer Letters* 125(1-2):83–88.

Hebert CD, Harris MW, Elwell MR, Birnbaum LS. 1990. Relative toxicity and tumor-promoting ability of 2,3,7,8-tetrachlorodibenzo-*p*-dioxin (TCDD), 2,3,4,7,8-pentachlorodibenzofuran (PCDF), and 1,2,3,4,7,8-hexachlorodibenzofuran (HCDF) in hairless mice. *Toxicology and Applied Pharmacology* 102(2):362–377.

Henneberger PK, Ferris BG Jr, Monson RR. 1989. Mortality among pulp and paper workers in Berlin, New Hampshire. *British Journal of Industrial Medicine* 46(9):658–664.

Hernández LG, van Steeg H, Luijten M, van Benthem J. 2009. Review: Mechanisms of non-genotoxic carcinogens and importance of a weight of evidence approach. *Mutation Research* 682:94–109.

Heron M, Hoyert D, Murphy S, Xu J, Kochanek K, Tejada-Vera B. 2009. Deaths: Final data for 2006. *National Vital Statistics Reports* 57(14):1–80.

Hertzman C, Teschke K, Ostry A, Hershler R, Dimich-Ward H, Kelly S, Spinelli JJ, Gallagher RP, McBride M, Marion SA. 1997. Mortality and cancer incidence among sawmill workers exposed to chlorophenate wood preservatives. *American Journal of Public Health* 87(1):71–79.

Hoar SK, Blair A, Holmes FF, Boysen CD, Robel RJ, Hoover R, Fraumeni JF. 1986. Agricultural herbicide use and risk of lymphoma and soft-tissue sarcoma. *Journal of the American Medical Association* 256(9):1141–1147.

Hobbs CG, Birchall MA. 2004. Human papillomavirus infection in the etiology of laryngeal carcinoma. *Current Opinion in Otolaryngology and Head and Neck Surgery* 12(2):88–92.

Hoffman RE, Stehr-Green PA, Webb KB, Evans RG, Knutsen AP, Schramm WF, Staake JL, Gibson BB, Steinberg KK. 1986. Health effects of long term exposure to 2,3,7,8-tetrachlorodibenzo-*p*-dioxin. *Journal of the American Medical Association* 255(15):2031–2038.

Hohenadel K, Harris SA, McLaughlin JR, Spinelli JJ, Pahwa P, Dosman JA, Demers PA, Blair A. 2011. Exposure to multiple pesticides and risk of non-Hodgkin lymphoma in men from six Canadian provinces. *International Journal of Environmental Research and Public Health* 8:2320–2330.

Holcombe M, Safe S. 1994. Inhibition of 7,12-dimethylbenzanthracene-induced rat mammary tumor growth by 2,3,7,8-tetrachlorodibenzo-*p*-dioxin. *Cancer Letters* 82(1):43–47.

Holford TR, Zheng T, Mayne ST, Zahm SH, Tessari JD, Boyle P. 2000. Joint effects of nine polychlorinated biphenyl (PCB) congeners on breast cancer risk. *International Journal of Epidemiology* 29(6):975–982.

Hollingshead BD, Beischlag TV, Dinatale BC, Ramadoss P, Perdew GH. 2008. Inflammatory signaling and aryl hydrocarbon receptor mediate synergistic induction of interleukin 6 in MCF-7 cells. *Cancer Research* 68(10):3609–3617.

Holmes AP, Bailey C, Baron RC, Bosanac E, Brough J, Conroy C, Haddy L. 1986. *West Virginia Department of Health Vietnam-Era Veterans Mortality Study: Preliminary Report.* Charles Town, WV: West Virginia Health Department.

Hooiveld M, Heederik DJ, Kogevinas M, Boffetta P, Needham LL, Patterson DG Jr, Bueno de Mesquita HB. 1998. Second follow-up of a Dutch cohort occupationally exposed to phenoxy herbicides, chlorophenols, and contaminants. *American Journal of Epidemiology* 147(9):891–901.

Høyer AP, Jørgensen T, Brock JW, Grandjean P. 2000. Organochlorine exposure and breast cancer survival. *Journal of Clinical Epidemiology* 53(3):323–330.

Hruba E, Vondracek J, Libalova H, Topinka J, Bryja V, Soucek K, Machala M. 2011. Gene expression changes in human prostate carcinoma cells exposed to genotoxic and nongenotoxic aryl hydrocarbon receptor ligands. *Toxicology Letters* 206(2):178–188.

Hsu EL, Yoon D, Choi HH, Wang F, Taylor RT, Chen N, Zhang R, Hankinson O. 2007. A proposed mechanism for the protective effect of dioxin against breast cancer. *Toxicological Sciences* 98(2):436–444.

Huang YK, Pu YS, Chung CJ, Shiue HS, Yang MH, Chen CJ, Hsueh YM. 2008. Plasma folate level, urinary arsenic methylation profiles, and urothelial carcinoma susceptibility. *Food and Chemical Toxicology* 46(3):929–938.

Hussein MA, Juturi JV, Lieberman I. 2002. Multiple myeloma: Present and future. *Current Opinions in Oncology* 14(1):31–35.

IARC (International Agency for Research on Cancer). 2001. Pathology and genetics of tumours of the haemopoietic and lymphoid tissues. In: Jaffe NL, Harris H, Stein, Vardiman JW, eds. *World Health Organization*, IARC.

Ikuta T, Namiki T, Fujii-Kuriyama Y, Kawajiri K. 2009. AHR protein trafficking and function in the skin. *Biochemical Pharmacology* 77(4):588–596.

IOM (Institute of Medicine). 1994. *Veterans and Agent Orange: Health Effects of Herbicides Used in Vietnam.* Washington, DC: National Academy Press.

IOM. 1996. *Veterans and Agent Orange: Update 1996.* Washington, DC: National Academy Press.

IOM. 1999. *Veterans and Agent Orange: Update 1998.* Washington, DC: National Academy Press.

IOM. 2001. *Veterans and Agent Orange: Update 2000.* Washington, DC: National Academy Press.

IOM. 2003. *Veterans and Agent Orange: Update 2002.* Washington, DC: The National Academies Press.

IOM. 2005. *Veterans and Agent Orange: Update 2004.* Washington, DC: The National Academies Press.

IOM. 2006. *Asbestos: Selected Cancers.* Washington, DC: The National Academies Press.

IOM. 2007. *Veterans and Agent Orange: Update 2006.* Washington, DC: The National Academies Press.

IOM. 2009. *Veterans and Agent Orange: Update 2008.* Washington, DC: The National Academies Press.

IOM. 2011. *Veterans and Agent Orange: Update 2010.* Washington, DC: The National Academies Press.

Ishida M, Mikami S, Kikuchi E, Kosaka T, Miyajima A, Nakagawa K, Mukai M, Okada Y, Oya M. 2010. Activation of the aryl hydrocarbon receptor pathway enhances cancer cell invasion by upregulating the MMP expression and is associated with poor prognosis in upper urinary tract urothelial cancer. *Carcinogenesis* 31(2):287–295.

Jaffe ES. 2009. The 2008 WHO classification of lymphomas: Implications for clinical practice and translational research. *Hematology* 1:523–531.

Jaffe ES, Harris NL, Stein H, Vardiman JW (eds). 2001. World Health Organization Classification of Tumours. Pathology and Genetics of Tumours of Haematopoietic and Lymphoid Tissues. Lyon, France, IARC Press. 352 pps.

Jaffe ES, Harris NL, Stein H, Isaacson PG. 2008. Classification of lymphoid neoplasms: The microscope as a tool for disease discovery. *Blood* 112(12):4384–4397.

Jenkins S, Rowell C, Wang J, Lamartiniere CA. 2007. Prenatal TCDD exposure predisposes for mammary cancer in rats. *Reproductive Toxicology* 23(3):391–396.

Johnstone SE, Baylin SB. 2010. Stress and the epigenetic landscape: A link to the pathobiology of human diseases? *Nature Reviews Genetics* 11(11):806–812.

Kalmes M, Hennen J, Clemens J, Blömeke B. 2011. Impact of aryl hydrocarbon receptor (AhR) knockdown on cell cycle progression in human HaCaT keratinocytes. *Journal of Biological Chemistry* 392:643–651.

Kang HK, Weatherbee L, Breslin PP, Lee Y, Shepard BM. 1986. Soft tissue sarcomas and military service in Vietnam: A case comparison group analysis of hospital patients. *Journal of Occupational Medicine* 28(12):1215–1218.

Kang HK, Mahan CM, Lee KY, Magee CA, Selvin S. 2000. Prevalence of gynecologic cancers among female Vietnam veterans. *Journal of Occupational and Environmental Medicine* 42(11):1121–1127.

Karunanayake CP, Spinelli JJ, McLaughlin JR, Dosman JA, Pahwa P, McDuffie HH. 2012. Hodgkin lymphoma and pesticides exposure in men: A Canadian case-control study. *Journal of Agromedicine* 17(1):30–39.

Kato H, Kinshita T, Suzuki S, Nagasaka T, Hatano S, Murate T, Saito H, Hotta T. 1998. Production and effects of interleukin–6 and other cytokines in patients with non-Hodgkin's lymphoma. *Leukemia and Lymphoma* 29(1–2):71–79.

Kato I, Watanabe-Meserve H, Koenig KL, Baptiste MS, Lillquist PP, Frizzera G, Burke JS, Moseson M, Shore RE. 2004. Pesticide product use and risk of non-Hodgkin lymphoma in women. *Environmental Health Perspectives* 112(13):1275–1281.

Keller-Byrne JE, Khuder SA, Schaub EA, McAfee O. 1997. A meta-analysis of non-Hodgkin's lymphoma among farmers in the central United States. *American Journal of Industrial Medicine* 31(4):442–444.

Kenborg L, Lassen CF, Lander F, Olsen JH. 2012. Parkinson's disease among gardeners exposed to pesticides—A Danish cohort study. *Scandinavian Journal of Work, Environment and Health* 38 (1):65–69.

Ketchum NS, Michalek JE, Burton JE. 1999. Serum dioxin and cancer in veterans of Operation Ranch Hand. *American Journal of Epidemiology* 149(7):630–639.

Key TJ, Schatzkin A, Willett WC, Allen NE, Spencer EA, Travis RC. 2004. Diet, nutrition and the prevention of cancer. *Public Health Nutrition* 7(1A):187–200.

Kim S, Dere E, Burgoon LD, Chang CC, Zacharewski TR. 2009. Comparative analysis of AHR-mediated TCDD-elicited gene expression in human liver adult stem cells. *Toxicological Sciences* 112(1):229–244.

Knerr S, Schrenk D. 2006. Carcinogenicity of 2,3,7,8-tetrachlorodibenzo-*p*-dioxin in experimental models. *Molecular Nutrition and Food Research* 50(10):897–907.

Kociba RJ, Keys DG, Beyer JE, Careon RM, Wade CE, Dittenber DA, Kalnins RP, Frauson LE, Park CN, Barnar SD, Hummel RA, Humiston CG. 1978. Results of a two-year chronic toxicity and oncogenicity study of 2,3,7,8-tetrachlorodibenzo-*p*-dioxin in rats. *Toxicology and Applied Pharmacology* 46:279–303.

Kogan MD, Clapp RW. 1988. Soft tissue sarcoma mortality among Vietnam veterans in Massachusetts, 1972 to 1983. *International Journal of Epidemiology* 17(1):39–43.

Kogevinas M, Saracci R, Bertazzi PA, Bueno de Mesquita BH, Coggon D, Green LM, Kauppinen T, Littorin M, Lynge E, Mathews JD, Neuberger M, Osman J, Pearce N, Winkelmann R. 1992. Cancer mortality from soft-tissue sarcoma and malignant lymphomas in an international cohort of workers exposed to chlorophenoxy herbicides and chlorophenols. *Chemosphere* 25:1071–1076.

Kogevinas M, Saracci R, Winkelmann R, Johnson ES, Bertazzi PA, Bueno de Mesquita BH, Kauppinen T, Littorin M, Lynge E, Neuberger M. 1993. Cancer incidence and mortality in women occupationally exposed to chlorophenoxy herbicides, chlorophenols, and dioxins. *Cancer Causes and Control* 4(6):547–553.

Kogevinas M, Kauppinen T, Winkelmann R, Becher H, Bertazzi PA, Bas B, Coggon D, Green L, Johnson E, Littorin M, Lynge E, Marlow DA, Mathews JD, Neuberger M, Benn T, Pannett B, Pearce N, Saracci R. 1995. Soft tissue sarcoma and non-Hodgkin's lymphoma in workers exposed to phenoxy herbicides, chlorophenols and dioxins: Two nested case-control studies. *Epidemiology* 6(4):396–402.

Kogevinas M, Becher H, Benn T, Bertazzi PA, Boffetta P, Bueno de Mesquita HB, Coggon D, Colin D, Flesch-Janys D, Fingerhut M, Green L, Kauppinen T, Littorin M, Lynge E, Mathews JD, Neuberger M, Pearce N, Saracci R. 1997. Cancer mortality in workers exposed to phenoxy herbicides, chlorophenols, and dioxins. An expanded and updated international cohort study. *American Journal of Epidemiology* 145(12):1061–1075.

Köhle C, Bock KW. 2007. Coordinate regulation of Phase I and II xenobiotic metabolisms by the Ah receptor and Nrf2. *Biochemical Pharmacology* 73:1853–1862.

Köhle C, Schwarz M, Bock KW. 2008. Promotion of hepatocarcinogenesis in humans and animal models. *Archives of Toxicology* 82:623–631.

Kollara A, Brown TJ. 2009. Modulation of aryl hydrocarbon receptor activity by four and a half LIM domain 2. *International Journal of Biochemistry and Cell Biology* 41(5):1182–1188.

Kollara A, Brown TJ. 2010. Four and a half LIM domain 2 alters the impact of aryl hydrocarbon receptor on androgen receptor transcriptional activity. *Journal of Steroid Biochemistry and Molecular Biology* 118(1-2):51–58.

Korenaga T, Fukusato T, Ohta M, Asaoka K, Murata N, Arima A, Kubota S. 2007. Long-term effects of subcutaneously injected 2,3,7,8-tetrachlorodibenzo-*p*-dioxin on the liver of rhesus monkeys. *Chemosphere* 67(9):S399–S404.

Koutros S, Alavanja MCR, Lubin JH, Sandler DP, Hoppin JA, Lynch CF, Knott C, Blair A, Freeman LEB. 2010a. An update of cancer incidence in the Agricultural Health Study. *Journal of Occupational and Environmental Medicine* 52(11):1098–1105.

Koutros S, Beane Freeman LE, Berndt SI, Andreotti G, Lubin JH, Sandler DP, Hoppin JA, Yu K, Li Q, Burdette LA, Yuenger J, Yeager M, Alavanja MCR. 2010b. Pesticide use modifies the association between genetic variants on chromosome 8q24 and prostate cancer. *Cancer Research* 70(22):9224–9233.

Koutros S, Andreotti G, Berndt SI, Hughes Barry K, Lubin JH, Hoppin JA, Kamel F, Sandler DP, Burdette LA, Yuenger J, Yeager M, Alavanja MCR, Freeman LEB. 2011. Xenobiotic-metabolizing gene variants, pesticide use, and the risk of prostate cancer. *Pharmacogenetics and Genomics* 21(10):615–623.

Kovacs E. 2006. Multiple myeloma and B cell lymphoma: Investigation of IL–6, IL–6 receptor antagonist (IL–6RA), and GP130 antagonist (GP130A) using various parameters in an in vitro model. *The Scientific World Journal* 6:888–898.

Küppers R, Schwering I, Bräuninger A, Rajewsky K, Hansmann M. 2002. Biology of Hodgkin's lymphoma. *Annals of Oncology* 13(Suppl 1):11–18.

La Rocca C, Alivernini S, Badiali M, Cornoldi A, Iacovella N, Silvestroni L, Spera G, Turrio-Baldassarri L. 2008. TEQ(S) and body burden for PCDDs, PCDFs, and dioxin-like PCBs in human adipose tissue. *Chemosphere* 73(1):92–96.

Labrecque MP, Takhar MK, Hollingshead BD, Prefontaine GG, Perdew GH, Beischlag TV. 2012. Distinct roles for aryl hydrocarbon receptor nuclear translocator and ah receptor in estrogen-mediated signaling in human cancer cell lines. *PLoS ONE* 7(1):10 pps.

Laden F, Bertrand KA, Altshul L, Aster JC, Korrick SA, Sagiv SK. 2010. Plasma organochlorine levels and risk of non-Hodgkin lymphoma in the Nurses' Health Study. *Cancer Epidemiology and Biomarkers of Prevention* 19(5):1381–1384.

Lampi P, Hakulinen T, Luostarinen T, Pukkala E, Teppo L. 1992. Cancer incidence following chlorophenol exposure in a community in southern Finland. *Archives of Environmental Health* 47(3):167–175.

Landgren O, Kyle RA, Hoppin JA, Freeman LEB, Cerhan JR, Katzmann JA, Rajkumar SV, Alavanja MC. 2009. Pesticide exposure and risk of monoclonal gammopathy of undetermined significance in the Agricultural Health Study. *Blood* 113(25):6386–6391.

LaVecchia C, Negri E, D'Avanzo B, Franceschi S. 1989. Occupation and lymphoid neoplasms. *British Journal of Cancer* 60(3):385–388.

Lawrence CE, Reilly AA, Quickenton P, Greenwald P, Page WF, Kuntz AJ. 1985. Mortality patterns of New York State Vietnam veterans. *American Journal of Public Health* 75(3):277–279.

Leavy J, Ambrosini G, Fritschi L. 2006. Vietnam military service history and prostate cancer. *BMC Public Health* 6:75.

Lee WJ, Lijinsky W, Heineman EF, Markin RS, Weisenburger DD, Ward MH. 2004a. Agricultural pesticide use and adenocarcinomas of the stomach and oesophagus. *Occupational and Environmental Medicine* 61(9):743–749.

Lee WJ, Cantor KP, Berzofsky JA, Zahm SH, Blair A. 2004b. Non-Hodgkin's lymphoma among asthmatics exposed to pesticides. *International Journal of Cancer* 111(2):298–302.

Lee WJ, Colt JS, Heineman EF, McComb R, Weisenburger DD, Lijinsky W, Ward MH. 2005. Agricultural pesticide use and risk of glioma in Nebraska, United States. *Occupational and Environmental Medicine* 62(11):786–792.

Lee WJ, Sandler DP, Blair A, Samanic C, Cross AJ, Alavanja MC. 2007. Pesticide use and colorectal cancer risk in the Agricultural Health Study. *International Journal of Cancer* 121(2):339–346.

Lew BJ, Manickam R, Lawrence BP. 2011. Activation of the aryl hydrocarbon receptor during pregnancy in the mouse alters mammary development through direct effects on stromal and epithelial tissues. *Biology of Reproduction* 84(6):1094–1102.

Liao Y, Du X, Zou O. 2012. Extranodal natural killer/T-cell lymphoma, nasal type: Epidemiology study. *Chinese-German Journal of Clinical Oncology* 11(5):P290–P293.

Lin PH, Lin CH, Huang CC, Chuang MC, Lin P. 2007. 2,3,7,8-tetrachlorodibenzo-*p*-dioxin (TCDD) induces oxidative stress, DNA strand breaks, and poly(ADP-ribose) polymerase-1 activation in human breast carcinoma cell lines. *Toxicology Letters* 172(3):146–158.

Lin PH, Lin CH, Huang CC, Fang JP, Chuang MC. 2008. 2,3,7,8-tetrachlorodibenzo-*p*-dioxin modulates the induction of DNA strand breaks and poly(ADP-ribose) polymerase-1 activation by 17beta-estradiol in human breast carcinoma cells through alteration of CYP1A1 and CYP1B1 expression. *Chemical Research in Toxicology* 21(7):1337–1347.

Liu J, Singh B, Tallini G, Carlson DL, Katabi N, Shaha A, Tuttle RM, Ghossein RA. 2006. Follicular variant of papillary thyroid carcinoma: A clinicopathologic study of a problematic entity. *Cancer* 107:1255–1264.

Lo AC, Soliman AS, Khaled HM, Aboelyazid A, Greenson JK. 2010. Lifestyle, occupational, and reproductive factors and risk of colorectal cancer. *Diseases of the Colon and Rectum* 53(5):830–837.

Lu C, Wang Y, Sheng Z, Liu G, Fu Z, Zhao J, Zhao J, Yan XZ, Zhu B, Peng S. 2010. NMR-based metabonomic analysis of the hepatotoxicity induced by combined exposure to PCBs and TCDD in rats. *Toxicology and Applied Pharmacology* 248:178–184.

Lu H, Crawford RB, Suarez-Martinez JE, Kaplan BLF, Kaminski NE. 2010. Induction of the aryl hydrocarbon receptor–responsive genes and modulation of the immunoglobulin M response by 2,3,7,8-tetrachlorodibenzo-*p*-dioxin in primary human B cells. *Toxicological Sciences* 118(1):86–97.

Luecke S, Backlund M, Jux B, Esser C, Krutmann J, Rannug A. 2010. The aryl hydrocarbon receptor (AHR), a novel regulator of human melanogenesis. *Pigment Cell and Melanoma Research* 23:828–833.

Lv L, Lin G, Gao X, Wu C, Dai J, Yang Y, Zou H, Sun H, Gu M, Chen X, Fu H, Bao L. 2011. Case-control study of risk factors of myelodysplastic syndromes according to World Health Organization classification in a Chinese population. *American Journal of Hematology* 86:163–169.

Lynge E. 1985. A follow-up study of cancer incidence among workers in manufacture of phenoxy herbicides in Denmark. *British Journal of Cancer* 52(2):259–270.

Lynge E. 1993. Cancer in phenoxy herbicide manufacturing workers in Denmark, 1947–87—An update. *Cancer Causes and Control* 4(3):261–272.

Madak-Erdogan Z, Katzenellenbogen BS. 2012. Aryl hydrocarbon receptor modulation of estrogen receptor alpha-mediated gene regulation by a multimeric chromatin complex involving the two receptors and the coregulator RIP140. *Toxicological Sciences* 125(2):401–411.

Magnani C, Coggon D, Osmond C, Acheson ED. 1987. Occupation and five cancers: A case-control study using death certificates. *British Journal of Industrial Medicine* 44(11):769–776.

Mahan CM, Bullman TA, Kang HK, Selvin S. 1997. A case-control study of lung cancer among Vietnam veterans. *Journal of Occupational and Environmental Medicine* 39(8):740–747.

Maluf E, Hamerschlak N, Cavalcanti AB, Avezum Júnlor A, Eluf-Neto J, Passetto Falcao R, Lorand-Metze IG, Goldenberg D, Leite Santana C, De Oliveira Werneck Rodrigues D, Nascimento Da Motta Passos L, Mange Rosenfeld LG, Pitta M, Loggetto S, Feitosa Ribeiro AA, Velloso ED, Kondo AT, De Miranda Coelho EO, Tostes Pintao MC, Moraes De Souza H, Borbolla JR, Pasquini R. 2009. Incidence and risk factors of aplastic anemia in Latin American countries: The Latin case-control study. *Haematologica* 94(9):1220–1226.

Mantovani A, Allavena P, Sica A, Balkwill F. 2008. Cancer-related inflammation. *Nature* 454:436–444.

Manuwald U, Garrido MV, Berger J, Manz A, Baur X. 2012. Mortality study of chemical workers exposed to dioxins: Follow-up 23 years after chemical plant closure. *Occupational and Environmental Medicine* 69(9):636–642.

Manz A, Berger J, Dwyer JH, Flesch-Janys D, Nagel S, Waltsgott H. 1991. Cancer mortality among workers in chemical plant contaminated with dioxin. *Lancet* 338(8773):959–964.

Marlowe JL, Fan Y, Chang X, Peng L, Knudsen ES, Xia Y, Puga A. 2008. The aryl hydrocarbon receptor binds to E2F1 and inhibits E2F1-induced apoptosis. *Molecular Biology of the Cell* 19:3263–3271.

Marur S, D'Souza G, Westra WH, Forastiere AA. 2010. HPV-associated head and neck cancer: A virus-related cancer epidemic. *Lancet Oncology* 11:781–789.

McBride DI, Collins JJ, Humphry NF, Herbison P, Bodner KM, Aylward LL, Burns CJ, Wilken M. 2009a. Mortality in workers exposed to 2,3,7,8-tetrachlorodibenzo-*p*-dioxin at a trichlorophenol plant in New Zealand. *Journal of Environmental Medicine* 51(9):1049–1056.

McBride DI, Burns CJ, Herbison GP, Humphry NF, Bodner K, Collins JJ. 2009b. Mortality in employees at a New Zealand agrochemical manufacturing site. *Occupational Medicine* 59(4):255–263.

McDuffie HH, Klaassen DJ, Dosman JA. 1990. Is pesticide use related to the risk of primary lung cancer in Saskatchewan? *Journal of Occupational Medicine* 32(10):996–1002.

McDuffie HH, Pahwa P, McLaughlin JR, Spinelli JJ, Fincham S, Dosman JA, Robson D, Skinnider LF, Choi NW. 2001. Non-Hodgkin's lymphoma and specific pesticide exposures in men: Cross-Canada study of pesticides and health. *Cancer Epidemiology, Biomarkers and Prevention* 10(11):1155–1163.

McGee SF, Lanigan F, Gilligan E, Groner B. 2006. Mammary gland biology and breast cancer. Conference on Common Molecular Mechanisms of Mammary Gland Development and Breast Cancer Progression. *EMBO Reports* 7(11):1084–1088.

McLean D, Pearce N, Langseth H, Jäppinen P, Szadkowska-Stanczyk I, Person B, Wild P, Kishi R, Lynge E, Henneberger P, Sala M, Teschke K, Kauppinen T, Colin D, Kogevinas M, Boffetta P. 2006. Cancer mortality in workers exposed to organochlorine compounds in the pulp and paper industry: An international collaborative study. *Environmental Health Perspectives* 114(7):1007–1012.

McNally RJQ, Blakey K, Parslow RC, James PW, Pozo BG, Stiller C, Vincent TJ, Norman P, McKinney PA, Murphy MF, Craft AW, Feltbower RG. 2012. Small-area analyses of bone cancer diagnosed in Great Britain provide clues to aetiology. *BMC Cancer* 12(1):270–279.

Mellemgaard A, Engholm G, McLaughlin JK, Olsen JH. 1994. Occupational risk factors for renal-cell carcinoma in Denmark. *Scandinavian Journal of Work, Environment, and Health* 20(3):160–165.

Merletti F, Richiardi L, Bertoni F, Ahrens W, Buemi A, Costa-Santos C, Eriksson M, Guenel P, Kaerlev L, Jockel KH, Llopis-Gonzalez A, Merler E, Miranda A, Morales-Suarez-Varela MM, Olsson H, Fletcher T, Olsen J. 2005. Occupational factors and risk of adult bone sarcomas: A multicentric case-control study in Europe. *International Journal of Cancer* 118(3):721–727.

Meyer A, Alexandre PCB, de Rezende Chrisman J, Markowitz SB, Koifman RJ, Koifman S. 2011. Esophageal cancer among Brazilian agricultural workers: Case-control study based on death certificates. *International Journal of Hygiene and Environmental Health* 214(2):151–155.

Michalek JE, Pavuk M. 2008. Diabetes and cancer in Veterans of Operation Ranch Hand after adjustment for calendar period, days of sprayings, and time spent in Southeast Asia. *Journal of Occupational and Environmental Medicine* 50(3):330–340.

Michalek JE, Wolfe WH, Miner JC. 1990. Health status of Air Force veterans occupationally exposed to herbicides in Vietnam. II. Mortality. *Journal of the American Medical Association* 264(14):1832–1836.

Miligi L, Costantini AS, Bolejack V, Veraldi A, Benvenuti A, Nanni O, Ramazzotti V, Tumino R, Stagnaro E, Rodella S, Fontana A, Vindigni C, Vineis P. 2003. Non-Hodgkin's lymphoma, leukemia, and exposures in agriculture: Results from the Italian Multicenter Case-control Study. *American Journal of Industrial Medicine* 44:627–636.

Miligi L, Costantini AS, Veraldi A, Benvenuti A, WILL (Italian Working Group Leukemia Lymphomas), Vineis P. 2006. Cancer and pesticides: An overview and some results of the Italian Multicenter Case-control Study on hematolymphopoietic malignancies. *Annals of the New York Academy of Sciences* 1076:366–377.

Miller BA, Kolonel LN, Bernstein L, Young JL Jr, Swanson GM, West D, Key CR, Liff JM, Glover CS, Alexander GA, et al. (eds). 1996. *Racial/Ethnic Patterns of Cancer in the United States 1988–1992*. Bethesda, MD: National Cancer Institute. NIH Pub. No. 96-4104.

Mills PK, Yang R. 2005. Breast cancer risk in Hispanic agricultural workers in California. *International Journal of Occupational and Environmental Health* 11(2):123–131.

Mills PK, Yang RC. 2007. Agricultural exposures and gastric cancer risk in Hispanic farm workers in California. *Environmental Research* 104(2):282–289.

Mills PK, Yang R, Riordan D. 2005. Lymphohematopoietic cancers in the United Farm Workers of America (UFW), 1988–2001. *Cancer Causes and Control* 16(7):823–830.

Mitchell KA, Lockhart CA, Huang G, Elferink CJ. 2006. Sustained aryl hydrocarbon receptor activity attenuates liver regeneration. *Molecular Pharmacology* 70(1):163–170.

Morris PD, Koepsell TD, Daling JR, Taylor JW, Lyon JL, Swanson GM, Child M, Weiss NS. 1986. Toxic substance exposure and multiple myeloma: A case-control study. *Journal of the National Cancer Institute* 76(6):987–994.

Morrison H, Semenciw RM, Morison D, Magwood S, Mao Y. 1992. Brain cancer and farming in western Canada. *Neuroepidemiology* 11(4-6):267–276.

Morrison H, Savitz D, Semenciw RM, Hulka B, Mao Y, Morison D, Wigle D. 1993. Farming and prostate cancer mortality. *American Journal of Epidemiology* 137(3):270–280.

Morrison HI, Semenciw RM, Wilkins K, Mao Y, Wigle DT. 1994. Non-Hodgkin's lymphoma and agricultural practices in the prairie provinces of Canada. *Scandinavian Journal of Work, Environment, and Health* 20(1):42–47.

Morton LM, Wang SS, Cozen W, Linet MS, Chatterjee N, Davis S, Severson RK, Colt JS, Vasef MA, Rothman N, Blair A, Berstein L, Cross AJ, De Roos AJ, Engels EA, Hein DW, Hill DA, Kelemen LE, Lim U, Lynch CF, Schenk M, Wacholder S, Ward MH, Zahm SH, Chanock SJ, Cerhan JR, Hartge P. 2008. Etiology among non-Hodgkin lymphoma subtypes. *Blood* 112(13):5150–5160.

Mulero-Navarro S, Carvajal-Gonzalez JM, Herranz M, Ballestar E, Fraga MF, Ropero S, Esteller M, Fernandez-Salguero PM. 2006. The dioxin receptor is silenced by promoter hypermethylation in human acute lymphoblastic leukemia through inhibition of Sp1 binding. *Carcinogenesis* 27(5):1099–1104.

Musicco M, Sant M, Molinari S, Filippini G, Gatta G, Berrino F. 1988. A case-control study of brain gliomas and occupational exposure to chemical carcinogens: The risks to farmers. *American Journal of Epidemiology* 128:778–785.

Nanni O, Amadori D, Lugaresi C, Falcini F, Scarpi E, Saragoni A, Buiatti E. 1996. Chronic lymphocytic leukaemias and non-Hodgkin's lymphomas by histological type in farming-animal breeding workers: A population case-control study based on a priori exposure matrices. *Occupational and Environmental Medicine* 53(10):652–657.

NCI (National Cancer Institute). 2010. *Surveillance, Epidemiology, and End Results (SEER) Incidence and US Mortality Statistics: SEER Incidence—Crude Rates for White/Black/Other 2004–2008*. http://www.seer.cancer.gov/canques/incidence.html (accessed May 9, 2011).

NCI. 2013. *Surveillance, Epidemiology, and End Results (SEER) Incidence and US Mortality Statistics: SEER Incidence—Crude Rates for White/Black/Other 2005–2009.* http://www.seer.cancer.gov/canques/incidence.html (accessed April 2, 2013).

Nielsen GD, Wolkoff P. 2010. Cancer effects of formaldehyde: A proposal for an indoor air guideline value. *Archives of Toxicology* 84(6):423–446.

Nikiforov YE. 2011. Molecular analysis of thyroid tumors. *Modern Pathology* (Suppl 2):S34–S43.

Nordby KC, Andersen A, Kristensen P. 2004. Incidence of lip cancer in the male Norwegian agricultural population. *Cancer Causes and Control* 15(6):619–626.

NTP (National Toxicology Program). 1982a. *Technical Report Series No. 209. Carcinogenesis Bioassay of 2,3,7,8-Tetrachlorodibenzo-p-dioxin (CAS No. 1746-01-6) in Osborne-Mendel Rats and B6c3F1 Mice (Gavage Study).* NIH Publication No. 82-1765. 195 pps. National Toxicology Program, Research Triangle Park, NC, and Bethesda, MD.

NTP. 1982b. *Technical Report Series No. 201. Carcinogenesis Bioassay of 2,3,7,8-Tetrachlorodibenzo-p-dioxin (CAS No. 1746-01-6) in Swiss-Webster Mice (Dermal Study).* National Toxicology Program, Research Triangle Park, NC, and Bethesda, MD.

NTP. 2006. *NTP Technical Report on the Toxicology and Carcinogenesis Studies of 2,3,7,8-Tetrachlorodibenzo-p-dioxin (TCDD) (CAS No. 1746-01-6) in Female Harlan Sprague-Dawley Rats (Gavage Studies).* Issue 521:4–232. National Toxicology Program, Research Triangle Park, NC, and Bethesda, MD.

NTP. 2011. 2,3,7,8-Tetrachlorodibenzo-*p*-dioxin. *Report on Carcinogens, 12th ed.* Pp. 396–398.

Nyska A, Jokinen MP, Brix AE, Sells DM, Wyde ME, Orzech D, Haseman JK, Flake G, Walker NJ. 2004. Exocrine pancreatic pathology in female Harlan Sprague-Dawley rats after chronic treatment with 2,3,7,8-tetrachlorodibenzo-*p*-dioxin and dioxin-like compounds. *Environmental Health Perspectives* 112(8):903–909.

Nyska A, Yoshizawa K, Jokinen MP, Brix AE, Sells DM, Wyde ME, Orzech DP, Kissling GE, Walker NJ. 2005. Olfactory epithelial metaplasia and hyperplasia in female Harlan Sprague-Dawley rats following chronic treatment with polychlorinated biphenyls. *Toxicologic Pathology* 33(3):371–377.

O'Brien TR, Decoufle P, Boyle CA.1991. Non-Hodgkin's lymphoma in a cohort of Vietnam veterans. *American Journal of Public Health* 81:758–760.

O'Donnell EF, Kopparapu PR, Koch DC, Jang HS, Phillips JL, Tanguay RL, Kerkvliet NI, Kollur SK. 2012. The aryl hydrocarbon receptor mediates leflunomide-induced growth inhibition of melanoma cells. *PLoS ONE* 7(7):13 pps.

Olsson H, Brandt L. 1988. Risk of non-Hodgkin's lymphoma among men occupationally exposed to organic solvents. *Scandinavian Journal of Work, Environment, and Health* 14:246–251.

Orsi L, Delabre L, Monnerau A, Delva P, Berthou C, Fenaux P, Marti G, Soubeyran P, Huguet F, Mipied N, Leporrier M, Hemon D, Troussard X, Clavel J. 2009. Occupational exposure to pesticides and lymphoid neoplasms among men: Results of a French case-control study. *Occupational and Environmental Medicine* 66(5):291–298.

O'Toole BI, Catts SV, Outram S, Pierse KR, Cockburn J. 2009. The physical and mental health of Australian Vietnam veterans 3 decades after the war and its relation to military service, combat, and post-traumatic stress disorder. *American Journal of Epidemiology* 170(3):318–330.

O'Toole BI, Catts SV, Outram S, Pierse KR, Cockburn J. 2010. Factors associated with civilian mortality in Australian Vietnam veterans three decades after the war. *Military Medicine* 175(2):88–95.

Ott MG, Zober A. 1996. Cause specific mortality and cancer incidence among employees exposed to 2,3,7,8-TCDD after a 1953 reactor accident. *Occupational and Environmental Medicine* 53:606–612.

Ovando BJ, Ellison CA, Vezina CM, Olson JR. 2010. Toxicogenomic analysis of exposure to TCDD, PCB126 and PCB153: Identification of genomic biomarkers of exposure to AhR ligands. *BMC Genomics* 11:583.

Pahwa P, McDuffie HH, Dosman JA, Robson D, McLaughlin JR, Spinelli JJ, Fincham S. 2003. Exposure to animals and selected risk factors among Canadian farm residents with Hodgkin's Disease, multiple myeloma, or soft tissue sarcoma. *Journal of Occupational and Environmental Medicine* 45(8):857–868.

Pahwa P, McDuffie HH, Dosman JA, McLaughlin JR, Spinelli JJ, Robson D, Fincham S. 2006. Hodgkin lymphoma, multiple myeloma, soft tissue sarcomas, insect repellents, and phenoxyherbicides. *Journal of Occupational and Environmental Medicine* 48(3):264–274.

Pahwa P, Karunanayake CP, Dosman JA, Spinelli JJ, McLaughlin JR. 2011. Soft-tissue sarcoma and pesticides exposure in men: Results of a Canadian case-control study. *Journal of Occupational and Environmental Medicine* 53(11):1279–1286.

Pahwa P, Karunanayake CP, Dosman JA, Spinelli JJ, McDuffie HH, McLaughlin JR. 2012. Multiple myeloma and exposure to pesticides: A Canadian case-control study. *Journal of Agromedicine* 17(1):40–50.

Park JY, Shigenaga MK, Ames BN. 1996. Induction of cytochrome P4501A1 by 2,3,7,8-tetrachlorodibenzo-*p*-dioxin or indolo(3,2-b)carbazole is associated with oxidative DNA damage. *Proceedings of the National Academy of Sciences of the United States of America* 93(6):2322–2327.

Pavuk M, Michalek JE, Schecter A, Ketchum NS, Akhtar FZ, Fox KA. 2005. Did TCDD exposure or service in Southeast Asia increase the risk of cancer in Air Force Vietnam veterans who did not spray Agent Orange? *Journal of Occupational and Environmental Medicine* 47(4):335–342.

Pavuk M, Michalek JE, Ketchum NS. 2006. Prostate cancer in US Air Force veterans of the Vietnam War. *Journal of Exposure Science and Environmental Epidemiology* 16(2):184–190.

Pearce NE, Smith AH, Fisher DO. 1985. Malignant lymphoma and multiple myeloma linked with agricultural occupations in a New Zealand cancer registry-based study. *American Journal of Epidemiology* 121:225–237.

Pearce NE, Smith AH, Howard JK, Sheppard RA, Giles HJ, Teague CA. 1986. Non-Hodgkin's lymphoma and exposure to phenoxyherbicides, chlorophenols, fencing work, and meat works employment: A case-control study. *British Journal of Industrial Medicine* 43:75–83.

Pearce NE, Sheppard RA, Smith AH, Teague CA. 1987. Non-Hodgkin's lymphoma and farming: An expanded case-control study. *International Journal of Cancer* 39:155–161.

Peng TL, Chen J, Mao W, Liu X, Tao Y, Chen LZ, Chen MH. 2009a. Potential therapeutic significance of increased expression of aryl hydrocarbon receptor in human gastric cancer. *World Journal of Gastroenterology* 15(14):1719–1729.

Peng TL, Chen J, Mao W, Song X, Chen MH. 2009b. Aryl hydrocarbon receptor pathway activation enhances gastric cancer cell invasiveness likely through a c-Jun-dependent induction of matrix metalloproteinase-9. *BMC Cell Biology* 10:27.

Percy C, Ries GL, Van Holten VD. 1990. The accuracy of liver cancer as the underlying cause of death on death certificates. *Public Health Reports* 105:361–368.

Perrotta C, Staines A, Codd M, Kleefeld S, Crowley D, T'Mannetje A, Becker N, Brennan P, De Sanjosé S, Foretova L, Maynadié M, Nieters A, Boffetta P, Cocco P. 2012. Multiple myeloma and lifetime occupation: Results from the EPILYMPH study. *Journal of Occupational Medicine and Technology* 7(1):25.

Persson B, Dahlander AM, Fredriksson M, Brage HN, Ohlson CG, Axelson O. 1989. Malignant lymphomas and occupational exposures. *British Journal of Industrial Medicine* 46:516–520.

Persson B, Fredriksson M, Olsen K, Boeryd B, Axelson O. 1993. Some occupational exposures as risk factors for malignant lymphomas. *Cancer* 72:1773–1778.

Pesatori AC, Consonni D, Tironi A, Landi MT, Zocchetti C, Bertazzi PA. 1992. Cancer morbidity in the Seveso area, 1976–1986. *Chemosphere* 25:209–212.

Pesatori AC, Baccarelli A, Consonni D, Lania A, Beck-Peccoz P, Bertazzi PA, Spada A. 2008. Aryl hydrocarbon receptor-interacting protein and pituitary adenomas: A population-based study on subjects exposed to dioxin after the Seveso, Italy, accident. *European Journal of Endocrinology* 159(6):699–703.

Pesatori AC, Consonni D, Rubagotti M, Grillo P, Bertazzi PA. 2009. Cancer incidence in the population exposed to dioxin after the "Seveso accident": Twenty years of follow-up. *Environmental Health* 8:1–11.

Piaggi S, Novelli M, Martino L, Masini M, Raggi C, Orciuolo E, Masiello P, Casini A, De Tata V. 2007. Cell death and impairment of glucose-stimulated insulin secretion induced by 2,3,7,8-tetrachlorodibenzo-*p*-dioxin (TCDD) in the beta-cell line INS-1e. *Toxicology and Applied Pharmacology* 220(3):333–340.

Prihartono N, Kriebel D, Woskie S, Thetkhathuek A, Sripaung N, Padungtod C, Kaufman D. 2011. Risk of aplastic anemia and pesticide and other chemical exposures. *Asia-Pacific Journal of Public Health* 23(3):369–377.

Prochazka M, Feychting M, Ahlbom A, Edwards CG, Nise G, Plato N, Schwartzbaum JA, Forssen UM. 2010. Occupational exposures and risk of acoustic neuroma. *Occupational and Environmental Medicine* 67(11):766–771.

Pu YS, Yang SM, Huang YK, Chung CJ, Huang SK, Chiu AW, Yang MH, Chen CJ, Hsueh YM. 2007. Urinary arsenic profile affects the risk of urothelial carcinoma even at low arsenic exposure. *Toxicology and Applied Pharmacology* 218(2):99–106.

Rajkumar SV, Dispenzieri A, Kyle RA. 2006. Monoclonal gammopathy of undetermined significance, Waldenstrom macroglobulinemia, AL amyloidosis, and related plasma cell disorders: Diagnosis and treatment. *Mayo Clinic Proceedings* 81(5):693–703.

Ramlow JM, Spadacene NW, Hoag SR, Stafford BA, Cartmill JB, Lerner PJ. 1996. Mortality in a cohort of pentachlorophenol manufacturing workers, 1940–1989. *American Journal of Industrial Medicine* 30:180–194.

Rashid BA, Wani MA, Kirmani AR, Raina TH, Ramzan AU, Alam S, Dhar A, Arif S, Javed S. 2010. Malignant brain tumors (brain cancer) in orchard farmers of Kashmir linked to pesticides. *Current Neurobiology* 1(2):137–150.

Ray S, Swanson HI. 2009. Activation of the aryl hydrocarbon receptor by TCDD inhibits senescence: A tumor promoting event? *Biochemical Pharmacology* 77(4):681–688.

Read D, Wright C, Weinstein P, Borman B. 2007. Cancer incidence and mortality in a New Zealand community potentially exposed to 2,3,7,8-tetrachlorodibenzo-*p*-dioxin from 2,4,5-trichlorophenoxyacetic acid manufacture. *Australian and New Zealand Journal of Public Health* 31(1):13–18.

Reif JS, Pearce N, Fraser J. 1989. Occupational risks of brain cancer: A New Zealand cancer registry-based study. *Journal of Occupational Medicine* 31(10):863–867.

Revich B, Aksel E, Ushakova T, Ivanova I, Zhuchenko N, Klyuev N, Brodsky B, Sotskov Y. 2001. Dioxin exposure and public health in Chapaevsk, Russia. *Chemosphere* 43(4-7):951–966.

Reynolds P, Hurley SE, Petreas M, Goldberg DE, Smith D, Gilliss D, Mahoney ME, Jeffrey SS. 2005. Adipose levels of dioxins and risk of breast cancer. *Cancer Causes and Control* 16(5):525–535.

Richardson DB, Terschuren C, Hoffmann W. 2008. Occupational risk factors for non-Hodgkin's lymphoma: A population-based case-control study in Northern Germany. *American Journal of Industrial Medicine* 51(4):258–268.

Riedel D, Pottern LM, Blattner WA. 1991. Etiology and epidemiology of multiple myeloma. In: Wiernick PH, Camellos G, Kyle RA, Schiffer CA, eds. *Neoplastic Disease of the Blood and Blood Forming Organs*. New York: Churchill Livingstone.

Riihimaki V, Asp S, Hernberg S. 1982. Mortality of 2,4-dichlorophenoxyacetic acid and 2,4,5-trichlorophenoxyacetic acid herbicide applicators in Finland: First report of an ongoing prospective cohort study. *Scandinavian Journal of Work, Environment, and Health* 8:37–42.

Rix BA, Villadsen E, Engholm G, Lynge E. 1998. Hodgkin's disease, pharyngeal cancer, and soft tissue sarcomas in Danish paper mill workers. *Journal of Occupational and Environmental Medicine* 40(1):55–62.

Robinson CF, Waxweiler RJ, Fowler DP. 1986. Mortality among production workers in pulp and paper mills. *Scandinavian Journal of Work, Environment, and Health* 12:552–560.

Rollison DE, Epling-Burnette P, Park JY, Lee JH, Park H, Jonathan K, Cole AL, Painter JS, Guerrier M, Meléndez-Santiago J, Fulp W, Komrokji R, Lancet J, List AF. 2011. Telomere length in myelodysplastic syndromes. *Leukemia and Lymphoma* 52(8):1528–1536.

Ronco G, Costa G, Lynge E. 1992. Cancer risk among Danish and Italian farmers. *British Journal of Industrial Medicine* 49:220–225.

Roth MJ, Wei WQ, Baer J, Abnet CC, Wang GQ, Sternberg LR, Warner AC, Johnson LL, Lu N, Giffen CA, Dawsey SM, Qiao YL, Cherry J. 2009. Aryl hydrocarbon receptor expression is associated with a family history of upper gastrointestinal tract cancer in a high-risk population exposed to aromatic hydrocarbons. *Cancer Epidemiology Biomarkers and Prevention* 18(9):2391–2396.

Roulland S, Lebailly P, Lecluse Y, Briand M, Pottier D, Gauduchon P. 2004. Characterization of the t(14;18) *BCL2-IGH* translocation in farmers occupationally exposed to pesticides. *Cancer Research* 64(6):2264–2269.

Roulland S, Navarro JM, Grenot P, Milili M, Agopian J, Montpellier B, Gauduchon P, Lebailly P, Schiff C, Nadel B. 2006. Follicular lymphoma-like B cell in healthy individuals: A novel intermediate step in early lymphomagenesis. *The Journal of Experimental Medicine* 203(11):2425–2431.

Rowland RE, Edwards LA, Podd JV. 2007. Elevated sister chromatid exchange frequencies in New Zealand Vietnam War veterans. *Cytogenetic and Genome Research* 116(4):248–251.

Rudel RA, Fenton SE, Ackerman JM, Euling SY, Makris SL. 2011. Environmental exposures and mammary gland development: State of the science, public health implications, and research recommendations. *Environmental Health Perspectives* 119(8):1053–1061.

Ruder AM, Yiin JH. 2011. Mortality of US pentachlorophenol production workers through 2005. *Chemosphere* 83(6):851–861.

Ruder AM, Waters MA, Butler MA, Carreon T, Calvert GM, Davis-King KE, Schulte PA, Sanderson WT, Ward EM, Connally LB, Heineman EF, Mandel JS, Morton RF, Reding DJ, Rosenman KD, Talaska G. 2004. Gliomas and farm pesticide exposure in men: The Upper Midwest Health Study. *Archives of Environmental Health* 59(12):650–657.

Salehi F, Turner MC, Phillips KP, Wigle DT, Krewski D, Aronson KJ. 2008. Review of the etiology of breast cancer with special attention to organochlorines as potential endocrine disruptors. *Journal of Toxicology and Environmental Health—Part B: Critical Reviews* 11(3–4):276–300.

Samanic C, Rusiecki J, Dosemeci M, Hou L, Hoppin JA, Sandler DP, Lubin J, Blair A, Alavanja MC. 2006. Cancer incidence among pesticide applicators exposed to dicamba in the Agricultural Health Study. *Environmental Health Perspectives* 114(10):1521–1526.

Samanic CM, De Roos AJ, Stewart PA, Rajaraman P, Waters MA, Inskip PD. 2008. Occupational exposure to pesticides and risk of adult brain tumors. *American Journal of Epidemiology* 167(8):976–985.

Santibañez M, Alguacil J, de la Hera MG, Navarrete-Muñoz EM, Llorca J, Aragonés N, Kauppinen T, Vioque J; PANESOES Study Group. 2012. Occupational exposures and risk of stomach cancer by histological type. *Occupational and Environmental Medicine* 69(4):268–275.

Saracci R, Kogevinas M, Bertazzi PA, Bueno de Mesquita BH, Coggon D, Green LM, Kauppinen T, L'Abbe KA, Littorin M, Lynge E, Mathews JD, Neuberger M, Osman J, Pearce N, Winkelmann R. 1991. Cancer mortality in workers exposed to chlorophenoxy herbicides and chlorophenols. *Lancet* 338:1027–1032.

Schlezinger JJ, Liu D, Farago M, Seldin DC, Belguise K, Sonenshein GE, Sherr DH. 2006. A role for the aryl hydrocarbon receptor in mammary gland tumorigenesis. *Biological Chemistry* 387(9):1175–1187.

Sekeres M. 2011. Epidemiology, natural history, and practice patterns of patients with myelodysplastic syndromes in 2010. *Journal of the National Comprehensive Cancer Network* 9(1):57–63.

Semenciw RM, Morrison HI, Morison D, Mao Y. 1994. Leukemia mortality and farming in the prairie provinces of Canada. *Canadian Journal of Public Health* 85:208–211.

Senft AP, Dalton TP, Nebert DW, Genter MB, Puga A, Hutchinson RJ, Kerzee JK, Uno S, Shertzer HG. 2002. Mitochondrial reactive oxygen production is dependent on the aromatic hydrocarbon receptor. *Free Radical Biology and Medicine* 33(9):1268–1278.

Shah SR, Freedland SJ, Aronson WJ, Kane CJ, Presti JC Jr, Amling CL, Terris MK. 2009. Exposure to Agent Orange is a significant predictor of prostate-specific antigen (PSA)-based recurrence and a rapid PSA doubling time after radical prostatectomy. *BJU International* 103:1168–1172.

Shah I, Houck K, Judson RS, Kavlock RJ, Martin MT, Reif DM, Wambaugh J, Dix DJ. 2011. Using nuclear receptor activity to stratify hepatocarcinogens. *PLoS ONE* 6(2):11 pps.

Sharma-Wagner S, Chokkalingam AP, Malker HS, Stone BJ, McLaughlin JK, Hsing AW. 2000. Occupation and prostate cancer risk in Sweden. *Journal of Occupational and Environmental Medicine* 42(5):517–525.

Shertzer HG, Dalton TP, Talaska G, Nebert DW. 2002. Decrease in 4-aminobiphenyl-induced methemoglobinemia in CYP1A2(-/-) knockout mice. *Toxicology and Applied Pharmacology* 181(1):32–37.

Siegel R, Naishadham D, Jemal A. 2012. Cancer statistics, 2012. *CA: A Cancer Journal for Clinicians* 62(1):10–29.

Siemiatycki J, Wacholder S, Dewar R, Wald L, Bégin D, Richardson L, Rosenman K, Gérin M. 1988. Smoking and degree of occupational exposure: Are internal analyses in cohort studies likely to be confounded by smoking status? *American Journal of Industrial Medicine* 13(1):59–69.

Simanainen U, Haavisto T, Tuomisto JT, Paranko J, Toppari J, Tuomisto J, Peterson RE, Viluksela M. 2004. Pattern of male reproductive system effects after in utero and lactational 2,3,7,8-tetrachlorodibenzo-*p*-dioxin (TCDD) exposure in three differentially TCDD-sensitive rat lines. *Toxicological Sciences* 80(1):101–108.

Singh NP, Nagarkatti M, Nagarkatti P. 2008. Primary peripheral T cells become susceptible to 2,3,7,8-tetrachlorodibenzo-*p*-dioxin-mediated apoptosis in vitro upon activation and in the presence of dendritic cells. *Molecular Pharmacology* 73(6):1722–1735.

Singh KP, Garrett RW, Casado FL, Gasiewicz TA. 2011. Aryl hydrocarbon receptor-null allele mice have hematopoietic stem/progenitor cells with abnormal characteristics and functions. *Stem Cells and Development* 20(5):769–784.

Smith AH, Pearce NE. 1986. Update on soft tissue sarcoma and phenoxyherbicides in New Zealand. *Chemosphere* 15:1795–1798.

Smith AH, Fisher DO, Giles HJ, Pearce NE. 1983. The New Zealand soft tissue sarcoma case-control study: Interview findings concerning phenoxyacetic acid exposure. *Chemosphere* 12:565–571.

Smith AH, Pearce NE, Fisher DO, Giles HJ, Teague CA, Howard JK. 1984. Soft tissue sarcoma and exposure to phenoxyherbicides and chlorophenols in New Zealand. *Journal of the National Cancer Institute* 73:1111–1117.

Smith JG, Christophers AJ. 1992. Phenoxy herbicides and chlorophenols: A case control study on soft tissue sarcoma and malignant lymphoma. *British Journal of Cancer* 65:442–448.

Smith-Warner SA, Spiegelman D, Yaun SS, van den Brandt PA, Folsom AR, Goldbohm RA, Graham S, Holmberg L, Howe GR, Marshall JR, Miller AB, Potter JD, Speizer FE, Willett WC, Wolk A, Hunter DJ. 1998. Alcohol and breast cancer in women: A pooled analysis of cohort studies. *Journal of the American Medical Association* 279(7):535–540.

Solet D, Zoloth SR, Sullivan C, Jewett J, Michaels DM. 1989. Patterns of mortality in pulp and paper workers. *Journal of Occupational Medicine* 31:627–630.

Spinelli JJ, Ng CH, Weber JP, Connors JM, Gascoyne RD, Lai AS, Brooks-Wilson AR, Le ND, Berry BR, Gallagher RP. 2007. Organochlorines and risk of non-Hodgkin lymphoma. *International Journal of Cancer* 121(12):2767–2775.

Steenland K, Piacitelli L, Deddens J, Fingerhut M, Chang LI. 1999. Cancer, heart disease, and diabetes in workers exposed to 2,3,7,8-tetrachlorodibenzo-*p*-dioxin. *Journal of the National Cancer Institute* 91(9):779–786.

Stott WT, Johnson KA, Landry TD, Gorzinski SJ, Cieszlak FS. 1990. Chronic toxicity and oncogenicity of picloram in Fischer 344 rats. *Journal of Toxicology and Environmental Health* 30:91–104.

Svensson BG, Mikoczy Z, Stromberg U, Hagmar L. 1995. Mortality and cancer incidence among Swedish fishermen with a high dietary intake of persistent organochlorine compounds. *Scandinavian Journal of Work, Environmental, and Health* 21(2):106–115.

Swaen GM, van Vliet C, Slangen JJM, Sturmans F. 1992. Cancer mortality among licensed herbicide applicators. *Scandinavian Journal of Work, Environment, and Health* 18:201–204.

Swaen GM, van Amelsvoort LG, Slangen JJ, Mohren DC. 2004. Cancer mortality in a cohort of licensed herbicide applicators. *International Archives of Occupational and Environmental Health* 77(4):293–295.

Szentirmay Z, Polus K, Tamas L, Szentkuti G, Kurcsics J, Csernak E, Toth E, Kasler M. 2005. Human papilomavirus in head and neck cancer: Molecular biology and climicopathological correlations. *Cancer Metastasis Review* 24:19–34.

't Mannetje A, McLean D, Cheng S, Boffetta P, Colin D, Pearce N. 2005. Mortality in New Zealand workers exposed to phenoxy herbicides and dioxins. *Occupational and Environmental Medicine* 62(1):34–40.

Takahashi N, Yoshida T, Ohnuma A, Horiuchi H, Ishitsuka K, Kashimoto Y, Kuwahara M, Nakashima N, Harada T. 2011. The enhancing effect of the antioxidant n-acetylcysteine on urinary bladder injury induced by dimethylarsinic acid. *Toxicologic Pathology* 39(7):1107–1114.

Tarone RE, Hayes HM, Hoover RN, Rosenthal JF, Brown LM, Pottern LM, Javadpour N, O'Connell KJ, Stutzman RE. 1991. Service in Vietnam and risk of testicular cancer. *Journal of the National Cancer Institute* 83:1497–1499.

Teitelbaum SL, Gammon MD, Britton JA, Neugut AI, Levin B, Stellman SD. 2007. Reported residential pesticide use and breast cancer risk on Long Island, New York. *American Journal of Epidemiology* 165(6):643–651.

Thiess AM, Frentzel-Beyme R, Link R. 1982. Mortality study of persons exposed to dioxin in a trichlorophenol-process accident that occurred in the BASF AG on November 17, 1953. *American Journal of Industrial Medicine* 3(2):179–189.

Thomas TL. 1987. Mortality among flavour and fragrance chemical plant workers in the United States. *British Journal of Industrial Medicine* 44:733–737.

Thomas TL, Kang HK. 1990. Mortality and morbidity among Army Chemical Corps Vietnam veterans: A preliminary report. *American Journal of Industrial Medicine* 18:665–673.

Thomas TL, Kang H, Dalager N. 1991. Mortality among women Vietnam veterans, 1973–1987. *American Journal of Epidemiology* 134:973–980.

Thompson IM, Goodman PJ, Tangen CM, Lucia MS, Miller GJ, Ford LG, Lieber MM, Cespedes RD, Atkins JN, Lippman SM, Carlin SM, Ryan A, Szczepanek CM, Crowley JJ, Coltman CA Jr. 2003. The influence of finasteride on the development of prostate cancer. *New England Journal of Medicine* 349(3):215–224.

Thörn Å, Gustavsson P, Sadigh J, Westerlund-Hännerstrand B, Hogstedt C. 2000. Mortality and cancer incidence among Swedish lumberjacks exposed to phenoxy herbicides. *Occupational and Environmental Medicine* 57:718–720.

Torchio P, Lepore AR, Corrao G, Comba P, Settimi L, Belli S, Magnani C, di Orio F. 1994. Mortality study on a cohort of Italian licensed pesticide users. *The Science of the Total Environment* 149(3):183–191.

Toth K, Somfai-Relle S, Sugar J, Bence J. 1979. Carcinogenicity testing of herbicide 2,4,5-trichlorophenoxyethanol containing dioxin and of pure dioxin in Swiss mice. *Nature* 278(5704):548–549.

Tritscher AM, Mahler J, Portier CJ, Lucier GW, Walker NJ. 2000. Induction of lung lesions in female rats following chronic exposure to 2,3,7,8-tetrachlorodibenzo-*p*-dioxin. *Toxicologic Pathology* 28(6):761–769.

Tuomisto JT, Pekkanen J, Kiviranta H, Tukiainen E, Vartiainen T, Tuomisto J. 2004. Soft-tissue sarcoma and dioxin: A case-control study. *International Journal of Cancer* 108(6):893–900.

Turunen AW, Verkasalo PK, Kiviranta H, Pukkala E, Jula A, Mannisto S, Rasanen R, Marniemi J, Vartiainen T. 2008. Mortality in a cohort with high fish consumption. *International Journal of Epidemiology* 37(5):1008–1017.

Van den Berg M, Birnbaum LS, Denison M, De Vito M, Farland W, Feeley M, Fiedler H, Hakansson H, Hanberg A, Haws L, Rose M, Safe S, Schrenk D, Tohyama C, Tritscher A, Tuomisto J, Tysklind M, Walker N, Peterson RE. 2006. The 2005 World Health Organization reevaluation of human and Mammalian toxic equivalency factors for dioxins and dioxin-like compounds. *Toxicological Sciences* 93(2):223–241.

van Grevenynghe J, Bernard M, Langouet S, Le Berre C, Fest T, Fardel O. 2005. Human CD34-positive hematopoietic stem cells constitute targets for carcinogenic polycyclic aromatic hydrocarbons. *Journal of Pharmacology and Experimental Therapeutics* 314(2):693–702.

Van Miller JP, Lalich JJ, Allen JR. 1977. Increased incidence of neoplasms in rats exposed to low levels of 2,3,7,8-tetrachlorodibenzo-*p*-dioxin. *Chemosphere* 9:537–544.

Viel JF, Arveux P, Baverel J, Cahn JY. 2000. Soft-tissue sarcoma and non-Hodgkin's lymphoma clusters around a municipal solid waste incinerator with high dioxin emission levels. *American Journal of Epidemiology* 152(1):13–19.

Viel JF, Clement MC, Hagi M, Grandjean S, Challier B, Danzon A. 2008. Dioxin emissions from a municipal solid waste incinerator and risk of invasive breast cancer: A population-based case-control study with GIS-derived exposure. *International Journal of Health Geographics* 7:4.

Viel JF, Floret N, Deconinck E, Focant JF, De Pauw E, Cahn JY. 2011. Increased risk of non-Hodgkin lymphoma and serum organochlorine concentrations among neighbors of a municipal solid waste incinerator. *Environment International* 37:449–453.

Vineis P, Terracini B, Ciccone G, Cignetti A, Colombo E, Donna A, Maffi L, Pisa R, Ricci P, Zanini E, Comba P. 1986. Phenoxy herbicides and soft-tissue sarcomas in female rice weeders. A population-based case-referent study. *Scandinavian Journal of Work, Environment, and Health* 13:9–17.

Vineis P, Faggiano F, Tedeschi M, Ciccone G. 1991. Incidence rates of lymphomas and soft-tissue sarcomas and environmental measurements of phenoxy herbicides. *Journal of the National Cancer Institute* 83:362–363.

Visintainer PF, Barone M, McGee H, Peterson EL. 1995. Proportionate mortality study of Vietnam-era veterans of Michigan. *Journal of Occupational and Environmental Medicine* 37(4):423–428.

Vogel CF, Li W, Sciullo E, Newman J, Hammock B, Reader JR, Tuscano J, Matsumura F. 2007. Pathogenesis of aryl hydrocarbon receptor-mediated development of lymphoma is associated with increased cyclooxygenase-2 expression. *American Journal of Pathology* 171(5):1538–1548.

Vogel CFA, Li W, Wu D, Miller JK, Sweeney C, Lazennec G, Fujisawa Y, Matsumura F. 2011. Interaction of aryl hydrocarbon receptor and NF-κB subunit RelB in breast cancer is associated with interleukin-8 overexpression. *Archives of Biochemistry and Biophysics* 512 (1):78–86.

Vorderstrasse BA, Fenton SE, Bohn AA, Cundiff JA, Lawrence BP. 2004. A novel effect of dioxin: Exposure during pregnancy severely impairs mammary gland differentiation. *Toxicological Sciences* 78(2):248–257.

Waggoner JK, Kullman GJ, Henneberger PK, Umbach DM, Blair A, Alavanja MCR, Kamel F, Lynch CF, Knott C, London SJ, Hines CJ, Thomas KW, Sandler DP, Lubin JH, Beane Freeman LE, Hoppin JA. 2011. Mortality in the agricultural health study, 1993–2007. *American Journal of Epidemiology* 173(1):71–83.

Walker NJ, Wyde ME, Fischer LJ, Nyska A, Bucher JR. 2006. Comparison of chronic toxicity and carcinogenicity of 2,3,7,8-tetrachlorodibenzo-*p*-dioxin (TCDD) in 2-year bioassays in female Sprague-Dawley rats. *Molecular Nutrition and Food Research* 50(10):934–944.

Walker NJ, Yoshizawa K, Miller RA, Brix AE, Sells DM, Jokinen MP, Wyde ME, Easterling M, Nyska A. 2007. Pulmonary lesions in female Harlan Sprague-Dawley rats following two-year oral treatment with dioxin-like compounds. *Toxicologic Pathology* 35(7):880–889.

Wang A, Kligerman AD, Holladay SD, Wolf DC, Robertson JL. 2009. Arsenate and dimethylarsinic acid in drinking water did not affect DNA damage repair in urinary bladder transitional cells or micronuclei in bone marrow. *Environmental and Molecular Mutagenesis* 50(9):760–770.

Wang SL, Chang YC, Chao HR, Li CM, Li LA, Lin LY, Papke O. 2006. Body burdens of polychlorinated dibenzo-*p*-dioxins, dibenzofurans, and biphenyls and their relations to estrogen metabolism in pregnant women. *Environmental Health Perspectives* 114(5):740–745.

Wang SS, Nieters A. 2010. Unraveling the interactions between environmental factors and genetic polymorphisms in non-Hodgkin lymphoma risk. *Expert Reviews in Anticancer Therapy* 10(3):403–413.

Wang T, Wyrick KL, Meadows GG, Wills TB, Vorderstrasse BA. 2011. Activation of the aryl hydrocarbon receptor by TCDD inhibits mammary tumor metastasis in a syngeneic mouse model of breast cancer. *Toxicological Sciences* 124(2):291–298.

Wanibuchi H, Salim E, Kinoshita A, Shen J, Wei M, Morimura K, Yoshida K, Kuroda K, Endo G, Fukushima S. 2004. Understanding arsenic carcinogenicity by the use of animal models. *Toxicology and Applied Pharmacology* 198(3):366–376.

Warner M, Eskenazi B, Mocarelli P, Gerthoux PM, Samuels S, Needham L, Patterson D, Brambilla P. 2002. Serum dioxin concentrations and breast cancer risk in the Seveso Women's Health Study. *Environmental Health Perspectives* 110(7):625–628.

Warner M, Mocarelli P, Samuels S, Needham L, Brambilla P, Eskenazi B. 2011. Dioxin exposure and cancer risk in the Seveso Women's Health Study. *Environmental Health Perspectives* 119(12):1700–1705.

Watanabe KK, Kang HK. 1995. Military service in Vietnam and the risk of death from trauma and selected cancers. *Annals of Epidemiology* 5:407–412.

Watanabe KK, Kang HK. 1996. Mortality patterns among Vietnam veterans: A 24-year retrospective analysis. *Journal of Occupational and Environmental Medicine* 38(3):272–278.

Watanabe KK, Kang HK, Thomas TL. 1991. Mortality among Vietnam veterans: With methodological considerations. *Journal of Occupational Medicine* 33:780–785.

Waterhouse D, Carman WJ, Schottenfeld D, Gridley G, McLean S. 1996. Cancer incidence in the rural community of Tecumseh, Michigan: A pattern of increased lymphopoietic neoplasms. *Cancer* 77(4):763–770.

Wei M, Wanibuchi H, Morimura K, Iwai S, Yoshida K, Endo G, Nakae D, Fukushima S. 2002. Carcinogenicity of dimethylarsinic acid in make F344 rats and genetic alterations in incuded urinary bladder tumors. *Carcinogenesis* 23(8):1387–1397.

Weiderpass E, Adami HO, Baron JA, Wicklund-Glynn A, Aune M, Atuma S, Persson I. 2000. Organochlorines and endometrial cancer risk. *Cancer Epidemiology, Biomarkers and Prevention* 9:487–493.

Weinberg RA. 2008. Twisted epithelial-mesenchymal transition blocks senescence. *Nature Cell Biology* 10(9):1021–1023.

Weiss C, Faust D, Schreck I, Ruff A, Farwerck T, Melenberg A, Schneider S, Oesch-Bartlomowicz B, Zatloukalova J, Vondracek J, Oesch F, Dietrich C. 2008. TCDD deregulates contact inhibition in rat liver oval cells via Ah receptor, JunD and cyclin A. *Oncogene* 27(15):2198–2207.

Wen S, Yang FX, Gong Y, Zhang XL, Hui Y, Li JG, Liu AIL, Wu YN, Lu WQ, Xu Y. 2008. Elevated levels of urinary 8-hydroxy-2′-deoxyguanosine in male electrical and electronic equipment dismantling workers exposed to high concentrations of polychlorinated dibenzo-*p*-dioxins and dibenzofurans, polybrominated diphenyl ethers, and polychlorinated biphenyls. *Environmental Science and Technology* 42(11):4202–4207.

WHO (World Health Organization). 2008. *WHO Classification of Tumours of Haematopoietic and Lymphoid Tissue* (4th edition). Lyon, France: World Health Organization.

Wigle DT, Semenciw RB, Wilkins K, Riedel D, Ritter L, Morrison HI, Mao Y. 1990. Mortality study of Canadian male farm operators: Non-Hodgkin's lymphoma mortality and agricultural practices in Saskatchewan. *Journal of the National Cancer Institute* 82:575–582.

Wiklund K. 1983. Swedish agricultural workers: A group with a decreased risk of cancer. *Cancer* 51:566–568.

Wiklund K, Holm LE. 1986. Soft tissue sarcoma risk in Swedish agricultural and forestry workers. *Journal of the National Cancer Institute* 76(2):229–234.

Wiklund K, Lindefors BM, Holm LE. 1988. Risk of malignant lymphoma in Swedish agricultural and forestry workers. *British Journal of Industrial Medicine* 45:19–24.

Wiklund K, Dich J, Holm LE, Eklund G. 1989a. Risk of cancer in pesticide applicators in Swedish agriculture. *British Journal of Industrial Medicine* 46:809–814.

Wiklund K, Dich J, Holm LE. 1989b. Risk of soft tissue sarcoma, Hodgkin's disease and non-Hodgkin's lymphoma among Swedish licensed pesticide applicators. *Chemosphere* 18:395–400.

Wolfe WH, Michalek JE, Miner JC, Rahe A, Silva J, Thomas WF, Grubbs WD, Lustik MB, Karrison TG, Roegner RH, Williams DE. 1990. Health status of Air Force veterans occupationally exposed to herbicides in Vietnam. I. Physical health. *Journal of the American Medical Association* 264:1824–1831.

Wong O, Harris F, Armstrong TW, Hua F. 2010. A hospital-based case-control study of non-Hodgkin lymphoid neoplasms in Shanghai: Analysis of environmental and occupational risk factors by subtypes of the WHO classification. *Chemico-Biological Interactions* 184:129–146.

Woods JS, Polissar L, Severson RK, Heuser LS, Kulander BG. 1987. Soft tissue sarcoma and non-Hodgkin's lymphoma in relation to phenoxy herbicide and chlorinated phenol exposure in western Washington. *Journal of the National Cancer Institute* 78:899–910.

Wrensch M, Minn Y, Chew T, Bondy M, Berger MS. 2002. Epidemiology of primary brain tumors: Current concepts and review of the literature. *Neuro-Oncology* 4(4):278–299.

Wyde ME, Braen AP, Hejtmancik M, Johnson JD, Toft JD, Blake JC, Cooper SD, Mahler J, Vallant M, Bucher JR, Walker NJ. 2004. Oral and dermal exposure to 2,3,7,8-tetrachlorodibenzo-*p*-dioxin (TCDD) induces cutaneous papillomas and squamous cell carcinomas in female hemizygous Tg.AC transgenic mice. *Toxicological Sciences* 82(1):34–45.

Xie G, Peng Z, Raufman JP. 2012. Src-mediated aryl hydrocarbon and epidermal growth factor receptor cross talk stimulates colon cancer cell proliferation. *American Journal of Physiology—Gastrointestinal and Liver Physiology* 302(9):G1006–G1015.

Xu JX, Hoshida Y, Yang WI, Inohara H, Kubo T, Kim GE, Yoon JH, Kojya S, Bandoh N, Harabuchi Y, Tsutsumi K, Koizuka I, Jia XS, Kirihata M, Tsukuma H, Aozasa K. 2006. Life-style and environmental factors in the development of nasal NK/T-cell lymphoma: A case-control study in East Asia. *International Journal of Cancer* 120(2):406–410.

Yamamoto S, Konishi Y, Matsuda T, Murai T, Shibata MA, Matsui-Yuasa I, Otani S, Kuroda K, Endo G, Fukushima S. 1995. Cancer incidence by an organic arsenic compound, dimethylarsinic acid (cacodylic acid), in F344/DuCrj rats after pretreatment with five carginogens. *Cancer Research* 55(6):1271–1276.

Yamanaka K, Ohtsubo K, Hasegawa A, Hayashi H, Ohji H, Kanisawa M, Okada S. 1996. Exposure to dimethylarsinic acid, a main metabolite of inorganic arsenics, strongly promotes tumorigenesis initiated by 4-nitroquinoline 1-oxide in the lungs of mice. *Carcinogenesis* 17(4):767–770.

Yang X, Solomon S, Fraser LR, Trombino AF, Liu D, Sonenshein GE, Hestermann EV, Sherr DH. 2008. Constitutive regulation of CYP1B1 by the aryl hydrocarbon receptor (AhR) in pre-malignant and malignant mammary tissue. *Journal of Cellular Biochemistry* 104(2):402–417.

Yiin JH, Ruder AM, Stewart PA, Waters MA, Carreón T, Butler MA, Calvert GM, Davis-King KE, Schulte PA, Mandel JS, Morton RF, Reding DJ, Rosenman KD. 2012. The Upper Midwest Health Study: A case-control study of pesticide applicators and risk of glioma. *Environmental Health: A Global Access Science Source* 11:39.

Yoshizawa K, Walker NJ, Jokinen MP, Brix AE, Sells DM, Marsh T, Wyde ME, Orzech D, Haseman JK, Nyska A. 2005a. Gingival carcinogenicity in female Harlan Sprague-Dawley rats following two-year oral treatment with 2,3,7,8-tetrachlorodibenzo-*p*-dioxin and dioxin-like compounds. *Toxicological Sciences* 83(1):64–77. [erratum appears in *Toxicological Sciences* 2005; 83(2):405–406].

Yoshizawa K, Marsh T, Foley JF, Cai B, Peddada S, Walker NJ, Nyska A. 2005b. Mechanisms of exocrine pancreatic toxicity induced by oral treatment with 2,3,7,8-tetrachlorodibenzo-*p*-dioxin in female Harlan Sprague-Dawley rats. *Toxicological Sciences* 85(1):594–606.

Yoshizawa K, Heatherly A, Malarkey DE, Walker NJ, Nyska A. 2007. A critical comparison of murine pathology and epidemiological data of TCDD, PCB126, and PeCDF. *Toxicologic Pathology* 35(7):865–879.

Yoshizawa K, Brix AE, Sells DM, Jokinen MP, Wyde M, Orzech DP, Kissling GE, Walker NJ, Nyska A. 2009. Reproductive lesions in female Harlan Sprague-Dawley rats following two-year oral treatment with dioxin and dioxin-like compounds. *Toxicologic Pathology* 37(7):921–937.

Yoshizawa K, Walker NJ, Nyska A, Kissling GE, Jokinen MP, Brix AE, Sells DM, Wyde ME. 2010. Thyroid follicular lesions induced by oral treatment for 2 years with 2,3,7,8-tetrachlorodibenzo-*p*-dioxin and dioxin-like compounds in female Harlan Sprague-Dawley rats. *Toxicologic Pathology* 38:1037–1050.

Zack JA, Suskind RR. 1980. The mortality experience of workers exposed to tetrachlorodibenzodioxin in a trichlorophenol process accident. *Journal of Occupational Medicine* 22:11–14.

Zahm SH, Fraumeni JF Jr. 1997. The epidemiology of soft tissue sarcoma. *Seminars in Oncology* 24(5):504–514.

Zahm SH, Weisenburger DD, Babbitt PA, Saal RC, Vaught JB, Cantor KP, Blair A. 1990. A case-control study of non-Hodgkin's lymphoma and the herbicide 2,4-dichlorophenoxyacetic acid (2,4-D) in eastern Nebraska. *Epidemiology* 1:349–356.

Zahm SH, Blair A, Weisenburger DD. 1992. Sex differences in the risk of multiple myeloma associated with agriculture. *British Journal of Industrial Medicine* 49:815–816.

Zahm SH, Weisenburger DD, Saal RC, Vaught JB, Babbitt PA, Blair A. 1993. The role of agricultural pesticide use in the development of non-Hodgkin's lymphoma in women. *Archives of Environmental Health* 48:353–358.

Zakerinia M, Namdari M, Amirghofran S. 2012. The relationship between exposure to pesticides and the occurrence of lymphoid neoplasm. *Iranian Red Crescent Medical Journal* 14(6):337–344.

Zambon P, Ricci P, Bovo E, Casula A, Gattolin M, Fiore AR, Chiosi F, Guzzinati S. 2007. Sarcoma risk and dioxin emissions from incinerators and industrial plants: A population-based case-control study (Italy). *Environmental Health: A Global Access Science Source* 6:19.

Zhang J, Zong H, Li S, Zhang D, Zhang L, Xia Q. 2012. Activation of aryl hydrocarbon receptor suppresses invasion of esophageal squamous cell carcinoma cell lines. *Tumori* 98(1):152–157.

Zhong Y, Rafnsson V. 1996. Cancer incidence among Icelandic pesticide users. *International Journal of Epidemiology* 25(6):1117–1124.

Zober A, Messerer P, Huber P. 1990. Thirty-four-year mortality follow-up of BASF employees exposed to 2,3,7,8-TCDD after the 1953 accident. *International Archives of Occupational and Environmental Health* 62:139–157.

9

Fertility and Gestational Outcomes

Chapter Overview

Based on new evidence and a review of prior studies, the committee for Update 2012 *did not find any new significant associations between the relevant exposures and fertility or gestational outcomes. Current evidence supports the findings of earlier studies that*

- *None of the fertility or gestational outcomes had sufficient evidence of an association with the chemicals of interest.*
- *None of the fertility or gestational outcomes had limited or suggestive evidence of an association between the chemicals of interest.*
- *There is inadequate or insufficient evidence to determine whether there is an association between the chemicals of interest and endometriosis; decreased sperm counts or sperm quality, subfertility, or infertility; spontaneous abortion, stillbirth, neonatal death, or infant death; and low birth weight or preterm delivery.*
- *There is limited or suggestive evidence of* no *association between paternal exposure to 2,3,7,8-tetrachlorodibenzo-*p*-dioxin (TCDD) and spontaneous abortion.*

This chapter summarizes the scientific literature published since *Veterans and Agent Orange: Update 2010*, hereafter referred to as *Update 2010* (IOM, 2011), on the association between exposure to herbicides and adverse effects on fertility and during gestation. (Analogous shortened names are used to refer to the updates for 1996, 1998, 2000, 2002, 2004, 2006, and 2008 [IOM, 1996,

1999, 2001, 2003, 2005, 2007, 2009] of the original report *Veterans and Agent Orange: Health Effects of Herbicides Used in Vietnam* [*VAO*; IOM, 1994].) The literature considered in this chapter includes studies of a broad spectrum of reproductive effects in Vietnam veterans or other populations occupationally or environmentally exposed to the herbicides sprayed in Vietnam or to TCDD. Because some polychlorinated biphenyls (PCBs), some polychlorinated dibenzofurans (PCDFs), and some polychlorinated dibenzodioxins (PCDDs) other than TCDD have dioxin-like biologic activity, studies of populations exposed to PCBs or PCDFs were reviewed if their results were presented in terms of TCDD toxic equivalents (TEQs). Although all studies reporting TEQs based on PCBs were reviewed, studies that reported TEQs based only on mono-ortho PCBs (which are PCBs 105, 114, 118, 123, 156, 157, 167, and 189) were given very limited consideration because mono-ortho PCBs typically contribute less than 10% to total TEQs, based on the World Health Organization's revised toxicity equivalency factors (TEFs) of 2005 (La Rocca et al., 2008; van den Berg et al., 2006).

The adverse outcomes evaluated in this chapter include impaired fertility (in which declines in sperm quality may be involved), endometriosis, increased fetal loss (spontaneous abortion and stillbirth), neonatal and infant mortality, and the adverse gestational outcomes of low birth weight or preterm delivery. In this update, consideration of the possibility of adverse health outcomes at any time during the lives of all progeny of Vietnam veterans has been moved to a separate chapter: Chapter 10, "Effects on Future Generations."

Because the vast majority of Vietnam veterans are men, the primary focus of the VAO series has been on potential adverse effects of herbicide exposure on men, and the etiologic importance of the exposed party's sex does not play the dominant role in nonreproductive outcomes that it does in reproductive outcomes. However, about 8,000 women served in Vietnam (H. Kang, US Department of Veterans Affairs, personal communication, December 14, 2000), so findings relevant to female reproductive health, such as endometriosis, are also included in the present chapter. Whenever the information was available, an attempt was made to evaluate the effects of exposure on adult men and women separately.

The categories of association and the approach to categorizing the health outcomes are discussed in Chapters 1 and 2. To reduce repetition throughout the report, Chapter 6 characterizes study populations and presents design information related to new publications that report findings on multiple health outcomes or that revisit study populations considered in earlier updates.

BIOLOGIC PLAUSIBILITY OF EFFECTS ON FERTILITY AND REPRODUCTION

This chapter opens with a general discussion of factors that influence the plausibility of adverse reproductive effects of TCDD and the four herbicides used in Vietnam. There have been few reproductive studies of the four herbicides in question, particularly picloram and cacodylic acid, and those studies generally have shown toxicity only at very high doses, so the preponderance of the following discussion concerns TCDD, which other than in controlled experimental circumstances usually occurred in a mixture of dioxins (dioxin congeners in addition to TCDD).

TCDD is stored in fat tissue and has a long biologic half-life, so internal exposure at generally constant concentrations may continue after episodic, high-level exposure to external sources ceases. If a person had high exposure, high amounts of dioxins may still be stored in fat tissue and be mobilized, particularly at times of weight loss. That would not be expected to be the case for nonlipophilic chemicals, such as cacodylic acid.

Dioxin exposure has the potential to disrupt male reproductive function by altering gene expression that is pertinent to spermatogenesis and by altering steroidogenesis (Wong and Cheng, 2011) and to disrupt female reproductive function by altering gene expression pertinent to ovarian follicle growth and maturation, uterine function, placental development, and fetal morphogenesis and growth.

A father's direct contribution to a pregnancy is limited to the contents of the sperm that fertilizes an egg; those contents had long been thought to consist of greatly condensed, transcriptionally inert deoxyribonucleic acid (DNA) constituting half the paternal genome (a haploid set of chromosomes). Consequently, it was believed that paternally-derived damage to the embryo or offspring could only result from changes in sperm DNA, but dioxins have not been shown to mutate DNA sequence. More recently, however, it has been recognized that sperm also carry a considerable collection of ribonucleic acid (RNA) fragments (Kramer and Krawetz, 1997; Krawetz et al., 2011). Although ribosomal and messenger RNAs have been detected, as yet, demonstration of an active role has been limited to several of the small RNAs found in mature sperm (Krawetz, 2005), in such functions as fertilization itself (Amanai et al., 2006), early embryonic development (Hamatani, 2012; Suh and Blelloch, 2011), and epigenetic determinations (Kawano et al., 2012). Epigenetic effects are ones that result in permanent (heritable) changes in gene expression without a change in DNA sequence arising from modification to DNA (usually involving methylation) or to other cellular components such as histones and RNAs (Jirtle and Skinner, 2007). Therefore, male infertility or fetal loss associated with exposure to the chemicals of interest (COIs) might be mediated by epigenetic modifications to components of sperm other than their DNA (Krawetz, 2005).

A mother's contribution to a pregnancy is obviously more extensive, and damage to an embryo or offspring can result from epigenetic changes of the egg DNA or from direct effects of exposure on placenta formation and the fetus during gestation. Mobilization of dioxin during pregnancy may be increased because the body is drawing on fat stores to supply nutrients to the developing fetus. TCDD has been measured in human circulating maternal blood, cord blood, and placenta. Thus, dioxin in the mother's bloodstream could cross the placenta and expose the developing embryo and fetus. Data indicate that dioxin can accumulate in placental tissue, but the amount of TCDD that can transfer to the fetus appears to be very limited—TCDD's transfer index was the lowest of 13 environmental toxicants evaluated in perfusion studies of human placentas (Mose et al., 2012).

On the basis of laboratory animal studies, TCDD can affect reproduction, so a connection between TCDD exposure and human reproductive and gestational effects is biologically plausible. However, definitive conclusions based on animal studies about the potential for TCDD to cause reproductive and gestational toxicity in humans are complicated by differences in sensitivity and susceptibility among animals, strains, and species; by the lack of strong evidence of organ-specific effects across species; by differences in route, dose, duration, and timing of exposure in experimental protocols and real-world exposure; and by substantial differences between laboratory animals and humans in the toxicokinetics of TCDD. Experiments with 2,4-dichlorophenoxyacetic acid (2,4-D) and 2,4,5-trichlorophenoxyacetic acid (2,4,5-T) indicate that they have subcellular effects that could constitute a biologically plausible mechanism for reproductive and gestational effects. However, the preponderance of evidence from animal studies indicates that they do not have reproductive effects. There is insufficient information on picloram and cacodylic acid to assess the biologic plausibility of their reproductive or gestational effects.

The sections on biologic plausibility of the specific outcomes considered in this chapter present more detailed toxicologic findings that are of particular relevance to the outcomes discussed.

ENDOMETRIOSIS

Endometriosis (*International Classification of Diseases, Ninth Revision* [ICD-9], code 617) affects 5.5 million women in the United States and Canada at any given time (NICHD, 2007). The endometrium is the tissue that lines the inside of the uterus and is built up and shed each month during menstruation. In endometriosis, endometrial cells are found outside the uterus—usually in other parts of the reproductive system, in the abdomen, or on surfaces near the reproductive organs. The ectopic tissue develops into growths or lesions that continue to respond to hormonal changes in the body and break down and bleed each month in concert with the menstrual cycle. Unlike blood released during normal shedding of the endometrium, blood released from endometrial lesions has no way to leave the body and results in inflammation and internal bleeding. The degeneration of blood and tissue can cause scarring, pain, infertility, adhesions, and intestinal problems.

There are several theories of the etiology of endometriosis, including a genetic contribution, but the cause remains unknown. Estrogen dependence and immune modulation are established features of endometriosis but do not adequately explain its cause. It has been proposed that endometrium is distributed through the body via blood or the lymphatic system; that menstrual tissue backs up into the fallopian tubes, implants in the abdomen, and grows; and that all women experience some form of tissue backup during menstruation but only those who have immune-system or hormonal problems experience the tissue growth associated with endometriosis. Despite numerous symptoms that can indicate endometriosis, diagnosis is possible only through laparoscopy or a more invasive surgical technique. Several treatments for endometriosis are available, but there is no cure.

Conclusions from *VAO* and Previous Updates

Endometriosis was first reviewed in this series of reports in *Update 2002*, which identified two relevant environmental studies. Additional studies considered in later updates have not changed the conclusion that the evidence is inadequate or insufficient to support an association with herbicide exposure. Table 9-1 provides a summary of relevant studies that have been reviewed.

Update of the Epidemiologic Literature

No Vietnam-veteran, occupational, or case-control studies of exposure to the COIs and endometriosis have been published since *Update 2010*.

Environmental Studies

Cai et al. (2011) recruited 17 women who were undergoing diagnostic laparoscopy for infertility in Japan during October 2004–March 2007. Of those women, 10 were found to have endometriosis, and 7 were not. Serum and peritoneal fluid were collected from each participant during her follicular phase and analyzed for 7 PCDDs, 10 PCDFs, and 12 dioxin-like PCBs. Concentrations adjusted for lipids were measured with gas chromatography–mass spectrometry, and from them, TEQs attributable to dioxins, to furans, and to PCBs and an overall total in serum and peritoneal fluid were calculated for each participant. There were no differences in lipid-adjusted TEQ for any of the categories in either serum or peritoneal fluid between women who had endometriosis and women who did not. The authors noted that in women who had high PCDD and PCDF simultaneously in the peritoneal fluid, there was an association with endometriosis (odds ratio [OR] = 2.5, 95% confidence interval [CI] 1.17–5.34). Although this finding achieved statistical significance by usual standards, the sample studied was very small and the biologic importance of this isolated result is unclear.

TABLE 9-1 Selected Epidemiologic Studies—Endometriosis (Shaded Entry Is New to This Update)

Study Population	Study Results	Reference
ENVIRONMENTAL		
Studies Conducted in the United States		
Case-control study of women in Atlanta, Georgia, with endometriosis; 60 cases and 64 controls	Results for cases vs controls: Total TEQ (determined by GC/MS): OR = 01.0 (95% CI 0.9–1.1)	Niskar et al., 2009
Studies Conducted in Belgium		
88 matched triads (264 total); patients with deep endometriotic nodules, pelvic endometriosis, controls matched for age, gynecologic practice in Belgium; routes of exposure to DLCs examined	Results for pelvic endometriosis vs controls: Dietary fat: OR = 1.0 (95% CI 1.0–1.0) BMI: OR = 1.0 (95% CI 0.9–1.0) Occupation: OR = 0.5 (95% CI 0.2–1.1) Traffic: OR = 1.0 (95% CI 0.3–2.8) Incinerator: OR = 1.0 (95% CI 1.0–1.1)	Heilier et al., 2007
Serum DLC and aromatase activity in endometriotic tissue from 47 patients in Belgium	No association between TEQs (determined by GC/MS) of DLCs in serum and aromatase activity by regression analyses p-values = 0.37–0.90 for different endometriosis subgroups	Heilier et al., 2006
Endometriosis in Belgian women with overnight fasting serum levels of PCDD, PCDF, PCB	50 exposed cases, risk of increase of 10 pg/g lipid of TEQ compounds (determined by GC/MS); OR = 2.6 (95% CI 1.3–5.3)	Heilier et al., 2005
Belgian women with environmental exposure to PCDDs, PCDFs; compared analyte concentrations in cases vs controls	Mean concentration of TEQ (determined by GC/MS) Cases (n = 10), 26.2 (95% CI 18.2–37.7) Controls (n = 132), 25.6 (95% CI 24.3–28.9) No significant difference	Fierens et al., 2003
Patients undergoing infertility treatment in Belgium; compared number of women with, without endometriosis who had serum dioxin levels up to 100 pg TEQ/g of serum lipid (determined by CALUX bioassay)	Six exposed cases: OR = 4.6 (95% CI 0.5–43.6)	Pauwels et al., 2001

TABLE 9-1 Endometriosis, continued

Study Population	Study Results	Reference
Studies Conducted in Italy		
Case-control study of Italian women with endometriosis; 80 cases and 78 controls (TEQs determined by CALUX bioassay)	Results for endometriosis vs controls: dl PCB118 compared to ≤ 13.2 ng/g: 13.3–24.2 ng/g; OR = 3.17 (95% CI 1.36–7.37) ≥ 24.3 ng/g; OR = 3.79 (95% CI 1.61–8.91) Total TEQ compared to ≤ 15.6 pgC-TEQ/g fat: 15.7–29.5 pgC-TEQ/g fat; OR = 0.52 (95% CI 0.18–1.48) ≥ 29.6 pgC-TEQ/g fat; OR = 0.73 (95% CI 0.26–2.01)	Porpora et al., 2009
Case-control study of Italian women with endometriosis, measured serum PCBs	Mean total PCBs (ng/g) Cases, 410 ng/g Control, 250 ng/g All PCB congeners: OR = 4.0 (95% CI 1.3–13)	Porpora et al., 2006
Pilot study of Italian, Belgian women of reproductive age; compared concentrations of TCDD, total TEQ (determined by GC/MS) in pooled blood samples from women who had diagnosis of endometriosis with controls	Mean concentration of TCDD (ppt of lipid): Italy: Controls (10 pooled samples), 1.6 Cases (2 sets of 6 pooled samples), 2.1, 1.3 Belgium: Controls (7 pooled samples), 2.5 Cases (Set I, 5 pooled samples; Set II, 6 pooled samples), 2.3, 2.3 Mean concentration of TEQ (ppt of lipid): Italy: Controls (10 pooled samples), 8.9 ± 1.3 (99% CI 7.2–11.0) Cases (2 sets of 6 pooled samples), 10.7 ± 1.6; 10.1 ± 1.5 Belgium: Controls (7 pooled samples), 24.7 ± 3.7 (99% CI 20–29) Cases (Set I, 5 pooled samples; Set II, 6 pooled samples), 18.1 ± 2.7; 27.1 ± 4.0	De Felip et al., 2004

continued

TABLE 9-1 Endometriosis, continued

Study Population	Study Results	Reference
Residents of Seveso Zones A and B up to 30 yrs old in 1976; population-based historical cohort comparing incidence of endometriosis across serum TCDD concentrations	Serum TCDD (ppt): ≤ 20 (n = 2 cases), RR = 1.0 (reference) 20.1–100, (n = 8), RR = 1.2 (90% CI 0.3–4.5) > 100, (n = 9), RR = 2.1 (90% CI 0.5–8.0)	Eskenazi et al., 2002a
Studies Conducted in Israel		
Residents of Jerusalem being evaluated for infertility; compared number of women with high TCDD who had (n = 44), did not have (n = 35) a diagnosis of endometriosis	8 exposed cases: OR = 7.6 (95% CI 0.9–169.7)	Mayani et al., 1997
Studies Conducted in Japan		
17 women undergoing diagnostic laparoscopy for infertility, 10 were found to have endometriosis and 7 were not	TEQ calculated for each person based on PCDDs, PCDFs, and 12 dl-PCBs. No difference in lipid-adjusted exposure levels between those with and without endometriosis. Association was seen with endometriosis and women with high PCDD and PCDF (OR = 2.5, 95% CI 1.2–5.3)	Cai et al., 2011
138 infertility patients in Japan; laproscopically confirmed case-control status, serum dioxin, PCB TEQ (determined by GC/MS); P450 genetic polymorphism	Results for advanced endometriosis: Total TEQ: OR = 0.5 (95% CI 0.2–1.7) Genotype-specific: ORs = 0.3–0.6 No significant interaction between genotype, dioxin TEQ	Tsuchiya et al., 2007

NOTE: BMI, body mass index; CALUX, chemical activated luciferase gene expression; CI, confidence interval; dl, dioxin-like; DLC, dioxin-like compound; GC/MS, gas chromatography/mass spectrometry; OR, odds ratio; PCB, polychlorinated biphenyl; PCDD, polychlorinated dibenzo-*p*-dioxin; PCDF, polychlorinated dibenzofuran; RR, relative risk or risk ratio; TCDD, 2,3,7,8-tetrachlorodibenzo-*p*-dioxin; TEQ, (total) toxic equivalent.

Biologic Plausibility

Laboratory studies that used animal models and examined gene-expression changes associated with human endometriosis provide evidence of the biologic plausibility of a link between TCDD exposure and endometriosis. Genetic polymorphisms in the aryl hydrocarbon receptor (AHR) signaling complex have recently been associated with susceptibility to advanced endometriosis in humans (Wu et al., 2012). The first suggestion that TCDD exposure may be linked to endometriosis came as a secondary finding of a study that exposed female rhesus monkeys (*Macaca mulatta*) chronically to low concentrations of dietary TCDD for 4 years (Rier et al., 1993). Ten years after the exposure ended, the investigators documented an increased incidence of endometriosis in the monkeys that correlated with the TCDD exposure concentration. The sample was too small to yield a definitive conclusion that TCDD was a causal agent of endometriosis, but it led to numerous studies of the ability of TCDD to promote the growth of preexisting endometriotic lesions.

There are a number of mechanisms by which TCDD may promote endometrial lesions, which constitute additional support of biologic plausibility of a link between TCDD and endometriosis. Human endometrial tissue and cultured human endometrial epithelial cells both express the AHR; its dimerization partner, the aryl hydrocarbon nuclear translocator (Khorram et al., 2002); and three AHR target genes—CYP1A1, 1A2, and 1B1 (Bulun et al., 2000; Willing et al., 2011). That suggests that endometrial tissue is responsive to TCDD. Recently, it was shown that CYP1A1 expression is greater in ectopic endometrial tissue than in eutopic uterine tissue in the absence of TCDD exposure; this suggests that CYP1A1 may play a role in disease etiology (Singh et al., 2008). Other mechanisms by which TCDD may promote endometriosis include altering the ratio of progesterone receptor A to B and blocking the ability of progesterone to suppress matrix metalloproteinase expression—actions that promote endometrial-tissue invasion and that are observed in women who have endometriosis (Igarashi et al., 2005).

TCDD also induces changes in gene expression that mirror those observed in endometrial lesions. In addition to the induction of CYP1A1 noted above, TCDD can induce expression of histamine-releasing factor, which is increased in endometrial lesions and accelerates their growth (Oikawa et al., 2002, 2003). Similarly, TCDD stimulates expression of RANTES (*r*egulated on *a*ctivation, *n*ormal *T*-cell–*e*xpressed, and *s*ecreted protein) in endometrial stromal cells, and RANTES concentration and bioactivity are increased in women who have endometriosis (Zhao et al., 2002). The two CC-motif chemokines (chemotactic cytokines), RANTES and macrophage-inflammatory protein 1α (MIP-1α), have been identified as potential contributors to the pathogenesis and progression of endometriosis. Previous studies showed that the combination of 17β-estradiol and TCDD increased the secretion of RANTES and MIP-1α in endometrial stromal cells (Yu et al., 2008), and a more recent study showed that the same combination suppressed the expression of tetraspanin CD82, a tumor-metastasis suppressor, and thus promoted the invasion of endometrial stromal cells (Li et al., 2011). Those results support the idea that TCDD in combination with estradiol may contribute to the development of endometriosis by increasing invasiveness of endometrial cells. Despite that compelling evidence, chronic exposure of rats to TCDD, PCB153, dioxin-like PCB118 or PCB126, or 2,3,4,7,8-PeCDF (the furan congener with the highest TEF) individually or to various mixtures of these chemicals fails to alter endometrial histology in a consistent manner (Yoshizawa et al., 2009). Differences between rodent and human endometrium could account for the lack of observed effects in rats.

In summary, experimental studies, particularly ones that used human eutopic and ectopic endometrial tissue, provide evidence of the biologic plausibility of a link between TCDD exposure and endometriosis.

Synthesis

The studies linking dioxin exposure with endometriosis are few and inconsistent. The single new epidemiologic study since *Update 2010* found no substantive pattern of dioxin-like activity in serum or in peritoneal fluid that would distinguish infertile women who do and do not have endometriosis; however, this study was very small and involved a large number of statistical tests. Although animal studies support the biologic plausibility of an association, contemporary human exposures may be too low to show an association consistently.

Conclusion

On the basis of the evidence reviewed here, in *VAO*, and in the previous VAO updates, the committee concludes that there is inadequate or insufficient evidence to determine whether there is an association between exposure to the COIs and human endometriosis.

FERTILITY

Male reproductive function is under the control of several components whose proper coordination is important for normal fertility. Several of the components and some health outcomes related to male fertility, including reproductive hormones and sperm characteristics, can be studied as indicators of fertility. The reproductive neuroendocrine axis involves the central nervous system, the anterior pituitary gland, and the testis. The hypothalamus integrates neural inputs from the central and peripheral nervous systems and regulates the gonadotropins luteinizing hormone (LH) and follicle-stimulating hormone (FSH). Both are secreted into the circulation in episodic bursts by the anterior pituitary gland and are necessary for normal spermatogenesis. In the testis, LH interacts with receptors on Leydig cells, where it stimulates increased testosterone synthesis. FSH and the testosterone from the Leydig cells interact with Sertoli cells in the seminiferous tubule epithelium to regulate spermatogenesis. More detailed reviews of the male reproductive hormones can be found elsewhere (Knobil et al., 1994; Yen and Jaffe, 1991). Several agents, such as lead and dibromochloropropane, affect the neuroendocrine system and spermatogenesis (for reviews, see Bonde and Giwercman, 1995; Tas et al., 1996). Recent reviews on the effects of various environmental toxicants, including TCDD, on testicular steroidogenesis and spermatogenesis provide insights into potential underlying mechanisms, including reducing testosterone production in Leydig cells and inhibiting the formation of cyclic adenosine monophosphate (Mathur and D'Cruz, 2011; Svechnikov et al., 2010).

Studies of the relationship between chemicals and fertility are less common in women than in men. Some chemicals may disrupt the female hormonal balance necessary for proper functioning. Normal menstrual-cycle functioning is also important in the risk of hormonally related diseases, such as osteopenia, breast cancer, and cardiovascular disease. Chemicals can have multiple effects on the female system, including modulation of hormone concentrations that result in menstrual-cycle or ovarian-cycle irregularities, changes in menarche and menopause, and impairment of fertility (Bretveld et al., 2006a,b).

Conclusions from *VAO* and Previous Updates

The committee responsible for the original *VAO* report (IOM, 1994) concluded that there was inadequate or insufficient evidence of an association between exposure to 2,4-D, 2,4,5-T, TCDD, picloram, or cacodylic acid and alterations in sperm characteristics or infertility. Additional information available to the committees responsible for *Update 1996*, *Update 1998*, *Update 2000*, *Update 2002*, *Update 2004*, *Update 2006*, *Update 2008*, and *Update 2010* did not change the conclusion that exposure to the COIs had not been found to be associated with impaired fertility in either men or women. Reviews of the relevant studies are presented in the earlier reports. Tables 9-2 and 9-3 summarize the studies related to male and female fertility, respectively.

Update of the Epidemiologic Literature

Male Fertility

No new epidemiologic studies of exposure to the COIs and effects on male fertility have been published since *Update 2010*.

Female Fertility

No Vietnam-veteran, occupational, or case-control studies of exposure to the COIs and female fertility have been published since *Update 2010*.

Environmental Studies

The literature searches for *Update 2012* identified several studies relating menstrual-cycle characteristics to exposures that might have included COIs.

TABLE 9-2 Selected Epidemiologic Studies—Male Fertility (Altered Hormone Concentrations, Decreased Sperm Counts or Quality, Subfertility, or Infertility)

Study Population	Exposed Cases[a]	**Exposure of Interest**/Estimated Relative Risk (95% CI)[a]	Reference
VIETNAM VETERANS			
US Air Force Health Study—Ranch Hand veterans vs SEA veterans (unless otherwise noted)		**All COIs**	
AFHS (964 Ranch Hands, 1,259 comparisons)		Coefficient (p-value) for In(Testosterone) vs In(TCDD) in 1987	Gupta et al., 2006
Comparison TCDD quartile I (mean, 2.14 ppt)	nr	0 (referent)	
Comparison TCDD quartile II (mean, 3.54 ppt)	nr	–0.063 (0.004)	
Ranch Hand TCDD quartile I (mean, 4.14 ppt)	nr	0.002 (0.94)	
Comparison TCDD quartile III (mean, 4.74 ppt)	nr	–0.048 (0.03)	
Comparison TCDD quartile IV (mean, 7.87 ppt)	nr	–0.079 (< 0.001)	
Ranch Hand TCDD quartile II (mean, 8.95 ppt)	nr	–0.052 (0.03)	
Ranch Hand TCDD quartile III (mean, 18.40 ppt)	nr	–0.029 (0.22)	
Ranch Hand TCDD quartile IV (mean, 76.16 ppt)	nr	–0.056 (0.02)	
Effects on specific hormone concentrations or sperm count in Ranch Hands			Henriksen et al., 1996
Low testosterone			
High dioxin (1992)	18	1.6 (0.9–2.7)	
High dioxin (1987)	3	0.7 (0.2–2.3)	
Low dioxin (1992)	10	0.9 (0.5–1.8)	
Low dioxin (1987)	10	2.3 (1.1–4.9)	
Background (1992)	9	0.5 (0.3–1.1)	
High FSH			
High dioxin (1992)	8	1.0 (0.5–2.1)	
Low dioxin (1992)	12	1.6 (0.8–3.0)	
Background (1992)	16	1.3 (0.7–2.4)	
High LH			
High dioxin (1992)	5	0.8 (0.3–1.9)	
Low dioxin (1992)	5	0.8 (0.5–3.3)	
Background (1992)	8	0.8 (0.4–1.8)	
Low sperm count			
High dioxin	49	0.9 (0.7–1.2)	
Low dioxin	43	0.8 (0.6–1.0)	
Background	66	0.9 (0.7–1.2)	

TABLE 9-2 Male Fertility (Altered Hormone Concentrations, Decreased Sperm Counts or Quality, Subfertility, or Infertility), continued

Study Population	Exposed Cases[a]	**Exposure of Interest**/Estimated Relative Risk (95% CI)[a]	Reference
US CDC Vietnam Experience Study—Cross-sectional study, with medical examinations, of Army veterans: 9,324 deployed vs 8,989 nondeployed		**All COIs**	
Detailed description of cohort			CDC, 1989a
Lower sperm concentration	42	2.3 (1.2–4.3)	
Proportion of abnormal sperm	51	1.6 (0.9–2.8)	
Reduced sperm motility	83	1.2 (0.8–1.8)	
US American Legion Cohort		**All COIs**	
American Legionnaires who served in SEA			Stellman et al., 1988
Difficulty in having children	349	1.3 ($p < 0.01$)	
OCCUPATIONAL—INDUSTRIAL			
IARC Phenoxy Herbicide Cohort—Workers exposed to any phenoxy herbicide or chlorophenol (production or spraying) vs respective national mortality rates			
NIOSH Cross-sectional Medical Study—248 chemical workers employed at plants in Newark, New Jersey (1951–1969), and Verona, Michigan (1968–1972), vs 231 nonexposed neighborhood referents, measured in 1987		**Dioxins, phenoxy herbicides**	
Testosterone (< 10.4 nmol/L)			Egeland et al., 1994
Referents (TCDD < 20 ppt)	11	1.0	
Workers	25	2.1 (1.0–4.6)	
Quartile I (TCDD < 20 ppt)	2	0.9 (0.2–4.5)	
Quartile II (TCDD 20–75 ppt)	7	3.9 (1.3–11.3)	
Quartile III (TCDD 76–240 ppt)	6	2.7 (0.9–8.2)	
Quartile IV (TCDD 241–3,400 ppt)	10	2.1 (0.8–5.8)	
FSH (> 31 IU/L)	20	1.5 (0.7–3.3)	
LH (> 28 IU/L)	23	1.6 (0.8–3.3)	
OCCUPATIONAL—HERBICIDE-USING WORKERS (*not* related to IARC sprayer cohorts)			
Canada—Sawmill Workers in British Columbia; 26,487 workers for ≥ 1 yr at 14 mills using chlorophenates 1950–1985		**Chlorophenates, not TCDD**	
Workers having a live birth within 1 yr after the initiation of employment			Heacock et al., 1998
Standard fertility ratio	18,016 (births)	0.7 (0.7–0.8)[b]	
Mantel-Haenszel rate-ratio estimator	18,016 (births)	0.9 (0.8–0.9)[b]	

continued

TABLE 9-2 Male Fertility (Altered Hormone Concentrations, Decreased Sperm Counts or Quality, Subfertility, or Infertility), continued

Study Population	Exposed Cases[a]	**Exposure of Interest**/Estimated Relative Risk (95% CI)[a]	Reference
Cumulative exposure (hours)			
120–1,999	7,139	0.8 (0.8–0.9)[b]	
2,000–3,999	4,582	0.9 (0.8–1.0)[b]	
4,000–9,999	4,145	1.0 (0.9–1.1)[b]	
≥ 10,000	1,300	1.1 (1.0–1.2)[b] (p < 0.01 overall)	
Denmark—Danish farmers (n = 1,146), 18–50 yrs of age, who used any potentially spermatotoxic pesticides, including 2,4-D		**Herbicides**	Larsen et al., 1998
Farmers using pesticides vs organic farmers	523	1.0 (0.8–1.4)[c]	
Used three or more pesticides	nr	0.9 (0.7–1.2)[c]	
Used manual sprayer for pesticides	nr	0.8 (0.6–1.1)[c]	
ENVIRONMENTAL			
Seveso, Italy, Residential Cohort—Industrial accident July 10, 1976 (723 residents Zone A; 4,821 Zone B; 31,643 Zone R; 181,574 local reference group) (ICD-9 171)		**TCDD**	
Men exposed in Seveso, Zone A, vs age-matched men residing outside the contamination zone, measured semen characteristics, estradiol, FSH, testosterone, LH, inhibin B		*Author's evaluation (data not shown)*	Mocarelli et al., 2008
Age at 1976 exposure:			
Infant/prepuberty (1–9 yrs), n = 71 vs 176		Sensitive	
Puberty (10–17 yrs), n = 44 vs 136		Intermediate response	
Adult (18–26 yrs), n = 20 vs 60		No associations	
Other International Environmental Studies			
Belgian men in general population		**PCBs, dioxin**	Dhooge et al., 2006
Association with 2-fold increase in CALUX-TEQ		Change (p-value)	
Sperm concentration		25.2% (p = 0.07)	
Semen volume		–16.0% (p = 0.03)	
Total testosterone		–7.1% (p = 0.04)	
Free testosterone		–6.8% (p = 0.04)	
Belgium—Adolescent girls (17 yrs of age) in communities close to industrial sources of heavy metals, PCBs, VOCs, and PAHs—delays in sexual maturity	200	PCBs, DLCs	Staessen et al., 2001
In Hoboken, Belgium	8	4.0 (nr)	
In Wilrik, Belgium	15	1.7 (nr)	
Polish, Greenlandian, Ukranian, Swedish men in general population; AHR binding measured with CALUX assay		**dl activity**	Toft et al., 2007

TABLE 9-2 Male Fertility (Altered Hormone Concentrations, Decreased Sperm Counts or Quality, Subfertility, or Infertility), continued

Study Population	Exposed Cases[a]	**Exposure of Interest**/Estimated Relative Risk (95% CI)[a]	Reference
Measurement of semen quality (concentration, motility, percentage normal)		No consistent associations	
CASE-CONTROL STUDIES			
US Case-Control Studies			
Missouri—men with or without low sperm quality (21–40 yrs of age)		**2,4-D**	Swan et al., 2003
Increased urinary metabolite markers for 2,4-D	5	0.8 (0.2–3.0)	
International Case-Control Studies			
Argentinean farmers exposed to 2,4-D (n = 32) vs 25 nonexposed controls, March–July 1989		**2,4-D**	Lerda and Rizzi, 1991
Sperm count (millions/mL)	exposed: 49.0 vs control: 101.6		
Motility (%)	exposed: 24.8 vs control: 70.4		
Sperm death (%)	exposed: 82.9 vs control: 37.1[d]		
Anomalies (%)	exposed: 72.9 vs control: 33.4		
Canada—study of erectile dysfunction in urology patients in Ontario		**PCBs/**Highest vs lowest PCB groups	Polsky et al., 2007
PCB-118 (TEF = 0.0001)		1.0 (0.5–2.1)	
PCB-118 (TEF = 0.0001)		0.9 (0.5–1.6)	
PCB-170		0.6 (0.3–1.2)	
PCB-180		0.7 (0.4–1.4)	
Greenland Inuit men (n = 53) and European men (n = 247), DNA sperm integrity among Inuit men		**POPs**	Krüger et al., 2008
Median % DNA fragmentation index			
Inuits		6.8	
Europeans		12	
Median % DNA stainability			
Inuits		11	
Europeans		8.9	
Korean male waste incinerator workers (n = 6) vs controls (n = 8), dioxin measured by air monitoring		**Phenoxy herbicides**	Oh et al., 2005
Reduced number of sperm (10^6/ml)		($p = 0.050$)	
Workers		42.9 ± 18.0	
Controls		56.1 ± 44.5	

continued

TABLE 9-2 Male Fertility (Altered Hormone Concentrations, Decreased Sperm Counts or Quality, Subfertility, or Infertility), continued

Study Population	Exposed Cases[a]	**Exposure of Interest**/Estimated Relative Risk (95% CI)[a]	Reference
DNA-damaged sperm (%)		(p = 0.001)	
Workers		1.40 ± 0.08	
Controls		1.26 ± 0.03	
Turkey (Ankara)—Adipose-tissue samples from fertile and infertile men (21–46 yrs of age) assayed for PCB-118, April 2002–June 2007		**DLCs**	Cok et al., 2010
	21 fertile	68.8 ng/g lipid	
	25 infertile	21.7 ng/g lipid (p = 0.003)	
Turkey (Ankara)—Adipose-tissue samples from fertile and infertile men (21–45 yrs of age) assayed for dioxin, furans, dl PCBs, June 2003–September 2005		**DLCs**	Cok et al., 2008
	22 fertile	9.4 TEQ pg/g lipid (p = 0.003)	
	23 infertile	12.5 TEQ pg/g lipid (p = 0.065)	

NOTE: 2,4-D, 2,4-dichlorophenoxyacetic acid; AFHS, Air Force Health Study; AHR, aryl hydrocarbon receptor; CALUX, assay for determination of dioxin-like activity; CDC, Centers for Disease Control and Prevention; CI, confidence interval; COI, chemicals of interest; dl, dioxin-like; DLC, dioxin-like chemical; DNA, deoxyribonucleic acid; FSH, follicle-stimulating hormone; IARC, International Agency for Research in Cancer; ICD-9, *International Classification of Diseases, 9th Revision*; IU, international unit; LH, luteinizing hormone; nr, not reported; NIOSH, National Institute for Occupational Safety and Health; PAH, polycyclic aromatic hydrocarbon; PCB, polychlorinated biphenyl; POP, persistent organic pollutants; ppt, parts per trillion; SEA, Southeast Asia; TCDD, 2,3,7,8-tetrachlorodibenzo-*p*-dioxin; TEF, toxicity equivalency factor; TEQ, (total) toxic equivalent; VOC, volatile organic compound.

[a]Given when available; results other than estimated risk explained individually.

[b]For this study, relative risk has been replaced with standardized fertility ratio, for which value less than 1.0 indicates adverse effect.

[c]For this study, relative risk has been replaced with fecundability ratio, for which value less than 1.0 indicates adverse effect.

[d]Table 1 in reference reverses these figures—control, 82.9%; exposed, 37.1%—but text ("The percentages of asthenospermia, mobility, necrosperma and teratospermia were greater in the exposed group than in controls. . .") suggests that this is a typographical error.

Yang et al. (2011) examined the relation between exposure to PCB and PCDF-contaminated cooking oil ("Yucheng exposure") in Taiwan and self-reported menstrual-cycle characteristics in 197 Yucheng-exposed women and 218 neighborhood referents. There was no association between Yucheng exposure and cycle irregularity or dysmenorrhea, but results based only on group membership without further characterization of exposure with respect to the COIs do not

TABLE 9-3 Selected Epidemiologic Studies—Female Fertility (Altered Hormone Concentrations, Subfertility, or Infertility)

Study Population	Exposed Cases[a]	**Exposure of Interest**/Estimated Relative Risk (95% CI)[a]	Reference
OCCUPATIONAL—HERBICIDE-USING WORKERS (*not* related to IARC sprayer cohorts)			
UNITED STATES			
US Agricultural Health Study—prospective study of licensed pesticide sprayers in Iowa and North Carolina: commercial (n = 4,916), private/farmers (n = 52,395, 97.4% men), and spouses of private sprayers (n = 32,347, 0.007% men), enrolled 1993–1997; followups with CATIs 1999–2003 and 2005–2010		**Phenoxy herbicides**	
8,038 premenopausal women age 30–55 at enrollment			Farr et al., 2006
Pesticide exposure	5,013	0.9 (0.8–1.0)	
Herbicide exposure	3,725	0.9 (0.7–1.1)	
Phenoxy herbicide exposure	1,379	0.9 (0.7–1.1)	
Menstrual-cycle characteristics of 3,103 premenopausal women age 21–40			Farr et al., 2004
Reported at enrollment had used herbicides	1,291		
Short menstrual cycle		0.6 (0.4–1.0)	
Long menstrual cycle		1.0 (0.5–2.0)	
Irregular		0.6 (0.3–0.9)	
Missed period		1.4 (1.0–2.0)	
Intermenstrual bleeding		1.1 (0.8–1.7)	
ENVIRONMENTAL			
Seveso (Italy) Women's Health Study—Industrial accident July 10, 1976; 981 women between infancy and 40 yrs of age at the time of the accident, who resided in Zones A and B		**TCDD**	
Time to pregnancy and infertility in women from Zones A and B who attempted pregnancy after 1976			Eskenazi et al., 2010
20-yr followup to 1996—men and women			
Time to pregnancy (adjusted fecundability OR)			
Log_{10} TCDD	278	0.8 (0.6–1.0)	
Categorical TCDD (ppt)			
≤ 20	52	1.0 (reference)	
20.1–44.4	76	0.8 (0.5–1.3)	
44.5–100	75	0.7 (0.5–1.1)	
> 100	75	0.6 (0.4–1.0)	

continued

TABLE 9-3 Female Fertility (Altered Hormone Concentrations, Subfertility, or Infertility), continued

Study Population	Exposed Cases[a]	**Exposure of Interest**/Estimated Relative Risk (95% CI)[a]	Reference
Infertility (adjusted OR)			
Log_{10} TCDD	49	1.9 (1.1–3.2)	
Categorical TCDD (ppt)			
≤ 20	6	1.0 (reference)	
20.1–44.4	9	1.1 (0.4–3.6)	
44.5–100	16	2.5 (0.8–7.3)	
> 100	18	2.8 (1.0–8.1)	
Fibroids among women from Zones A and B who were newborn to age 40 in 1976			Eskenazi et al., 2007
Uterine fibroids (age-adjusted HR)			
Log_{10} TCDD (ppt)	251	0.8 (0.7–1.1)	
Categorical TCDD (ppt)			
≤ 20	62	1.0 (reference)	
20.1–75.0	110	0.6 (0.4–0.8)	
> 75	79	0.6 (0.4–0.9)	
Ovarian function in women from Zones A and B who were newborn to age 40 in 1976; results are for a 10-fold increase in serum TCDD			Warner at al., 2007
Ovarian follicles (age-adjusted OR):			
in follicular phase	65	1.0 (0.4–2.2)	
Ovulation (age-adjusted OR):			
in luteal phase	87	1.0 (0.5–1.9)	
in midluteal phase	55	1.0 (0.4–2.7)	
Estradiol (age-adjusted ß):		slopes for Log_{10} TCDD	
in luteal phase	87	−1.8 (−10.4–6.8)	
in midluteal phase	55	−3.1 (−14.1–7.8)	
Progesterone (age-adjusted ß):			
in luteal phase	87	−0.7 (−2.4–1.0)	
in midluteal phase	55	−0.8 (−3.7–2.0)	
Age at menopause in women from Zones A and B who were newborn to age 40 in 1976			Eskenazi et al., 2005
Onset of natural menopause (unadjusted HR)			
Log_{10} TCDD	169	1.0 (0.8–1.3)	
Menopause category		Serum TCDD median (IQR)	
Premenopause	260	43.6 (0.2–0.9)	
Natural menopause	169	45.8 (0.3–1.0)	
Surgical menopause	83	43.4 (0.3–1.0)	
Impending menopause	13	43.8 (0.2–1.1)	
Perimenopause	33	36.5 (0.2–0.9)	
Other	58	39.6 (0.2–0.9)	
Age at menarche in women from Zones A and B who were premenarcheal in 1976	282	1.0 (0.8–1.1)	Warner et al., 2004

TABLE 9-3 Female Fertility (Altered Hormone Concentrations, Subfertility, or Infertility), continued

Study Population	Exposed Cases[a]	**Exposure of Interest**/Estimated Relative Risk (95% CI)[a]	Reference
All premenarcheal women in 1976 (unadjusted HR)			
Log_{10} TCDD	282	1.0 (0.8–1.1)	
Women < 8 yrs in 1976 (unadjusted HR)			
Log_{10} TCDD	158	1.1 (0.9–1.3)	
Menstrual-cycle characteristics in women from Zones A and B who were premenopausal, less than age 44, and not recently pregnant, breastfeeding, or using hormonal medications			Eskenazi et al., 2002b
Menstrual-cycle length (adjusted ß)			
Log_{10} TCDD	277	0.4 (−0.1–0.9)	
Premenarcheal at explosion		0.9 (0.0–1.9)	
Postmenarcheal at explosion		0.0 (−0.6–0.5)	
Days of menstrual flow (adjusted ß)			
Log_{10} TCDD	301	0.2 (−0.1–0.4)	
Premenarcheal at explosion		0.2 (−0.2–0.5)	
Postmenarcheal at explosion		0.2 (−0.2–0.5)	
Heaviness of flow (scanty vs moderate/heavy; adjusted OR)			
Log_{10} TCDD	30	0.8 (0.4–1.6)	
Premenarcheal at explosion		0.3 (0.1–1.1)	
Postmenarcheal at explosion		1.4 (0.7–2.6)	
Irregular cycle (vs regular; adjusted OR)			
Log_{10} TCDD	24	0.5 (0.2–1.0)	
Premenarcheal at explosion		0.5 (0.2–1.4)	
Postmenarcheal at explosion		0.4 (0.2–1.2)	
Other International Environmental Studies			
Taiwanese pregnant women (18–40 yrs of age); placental TEQ concentrations of TCDDs, TCDFs, PCBs		**Dioxin/** Regression adjusted for maternal age, BMI, parity	Chao et al., 2007
≥ 18 yrs old, "regular menstrual cycle"			
Dioxin TEQ		p = 0.032	
PCB TEQ		p = 0.077	
Women with "longest menstrual cycle"			
Dioxin TEQ		p = 0.269	
PCB TEQ		p = 0.006	
CASE-CONTROL STUDIES			
US Case-Control Studies			
Women in Wisconsin with or without infertility (maternal exposure)—incidence		**Phenoxy herbicides**	Greenlee et al., 2003

continued

TABLE 9-3 Female Fertility (Altered Hormone Concentrations, Subfertility, or Infertility), continued

Study Population	Exposed Cases[a]	Exposure of **Interest**/Estimated Relative Risk (95% CI)[a]	Reference
Mixed or applied herbicides	21	2.3 (0.9–6.1)	
Used 2,4,5-T	9	9 cases (2.7%) 11 controls (3.4%)	
Used 2,4-D	4	4 cases (1.2%) 4 controls (1.2%)	

NOTE: 2,4-D, 2,4-dichlorophenoxyacetic acid; 2,4,5-T, 2,4,5-trichlorophenoxyacetic acid; BMI, body mass index; CATI, computer-assisted telephone interviewing; CI, confidence interval; HR, hazard ratio; IARC, International Agency for Research on Cancer; IQR, inter-quartile range; OR, odds ratio; PCB, polychlorinated biphenyl; ppt, parts per trillion; TCDD, 2,3,7,8-tetrachlorodibenzo-*p*-dioxin; TCDF, tetrachlorodibenzofuran; TEQ, (total) toxic equivalent.

[a]Given when available; results other than estimated risk explained individually.

meet this committee's criteria for consideration. However, women exposed to contaminated oil who also reported skin manifestations of exposure (chloracne, hyperkeratosis, or abnormal nails)—highly indicative of exposure to dioxin-like chemicals (DLCs)—did report menstrual cycles shorter than those of community referents by about 1.2 days (95% CI 1.7–0.7).

Buck Louis et al. (2011) provided associations in relation to summed concentrations of multiple PCB congeners, only some of which exhibit dioxin-like activity. They reported an association between increased concentrations of estrogenic PCBs (which do not include dioxin-like PCBs) and increased cycle length but no such relationship for the sum of eight anti-estrogenic PCBs (six of which are dioxin-like).

Uterine leiomyomas (fibroids) are also recognized as a contributor to infertility. In 2001–2004, Lambertino et al. (2011) contacted 580 women who had participated in the Great Lakes Fish Consumption Study, which had been initiated in the early 1990s. Updated information on health, reproductive history, and fish consumption was gathered from these subjects and merged with existing data. Blood samples were provided by 197 of them and analyzed for serum concentrations of various persistent organic pollutants, including a number of PCBs. The exposure measure for the category "dioxin-like PCBs" consisted of the summed concentrations of only the mono-ortho PCBs 118 and 167. There was no difference in the concentrations for the exposure category between women who had and had not self-reported the occurrence of these benign tumors, but because this result is based solely on mono-ortho PCBs, which typically contribute only a small percentage to total TEQs, no conclusions can be drawn.

Since *Update 2010*, there have been no additional studies of time to pregnancy (TTP) with sufficient exposure specificity to add to the evidence from the previous literature. Burdorf et al. (2011) examined TTP among 8,880 women enrolled in a prospective birth cohort in the Netherlands (Generation R Study) as part of an assessment of occupational exposures based on a job exposure matrix. They found no association between occupational exposure to "pesticides" and increased TTP, but the exposure classification of "pesticides" is insufficiently specific to determine whether any compounds related to Agent Orange exposure were among those included.

Biologic Plausibility

Although a recent study reported that doses of 2,4-D greater than 50 mg/kg/day produces acute testicular toxicity in male rats (Joshi et al. 2012), there is little evidence that lower doses of either 2,4-D or 2,4,5-T (when free of TCDD contamination) given chronically have substantial effects on reproductive organs or fertility (Charles et al., 2001; Munro et al., 1992) and the no-observed-adverse-effect level for 2,4-D is recognized as 15 mg/kg/day (Gervais et al., 2008). In contrast, many diverse laboratory studies have provided evidence that TCDD can affect reproductive-organ function and reduce fertility in both males and females.

The administration of TCDD to male animals elicits reproductive toxicity by affecting testicular, epididymal, prostate, and seminal vesicle weight and function and by decreasing the rate of sperm production. The mechanisms underlying those effects are not known, but primary hypotheses are that they are mediated through dysregulation of testicular steroidogenesis, altered Sertoli cell function, and increases in oxidative stress. Studies published since *Update 2010* have reinforced those possibilities. Exposure of cultured testicular Leydig cells to 25 nM TCDD markedly alters gene expression (Naville et al., 2011), and exposure of cultured Sertoli cells to 5 nM TCDD decreases viability and increases markers of oxidative stress (Aly and Khafagy, 2011). Exposure of adult rats or mice to TCDD (2–7 μg/kg/week for 45–60 days) reduces testicular and reproductive function, and these effects can be attenuated by co-treatment with various antioxidants (Beytur et al., 2012; Ciftci et al., 2012; Sönmez et al., 2011; Yin et al., 2012). The results of those studies are supported by the transgenic mouse model that harbors a constitutively active AHR in which testicular and ventral prostate weights and sperm number are reduced (Brunnberg et al., 2011).

Many studies have examined the effects of TCDD on the female reproductive system. Two primary mechanisms that probably contribute to abnormal follicle development and decreased numbers of ova after TCDD exposure are "cross-talk" of the AHR with the estrogen receptor and dysregulation of the hypothalamic–pituitary–gonadal axis. Oocytes are directly responsive to TCDD, so TCDD's effects on hormone concentrations, hormone-receptor signaling, and ovarian responsiveness to hormones all probably contribute to TCDD-induced female reproductive toxicity. Since *Update 2008*, additional work addressing TCDD's effects on female reproduction in animal models has been published. The data of Jung et al. (2010) in rats show that a single gavage treatment of 32 μg/kg TCDD reduces the proliferation of granulosa cells and thus attenuates cell-cycle progression and potentially contributes to the reduction in ovulation rates observed in other studies. In contrast, Karman et al. (2012) found that 1 nM TCDD exposure in vitro did not reduce rates of growth of murine antral follicles, but did reduce secretion of progesterone and estradiol by the follicles. Concentrations of those hormones could be restored by the addition of the precursor pregnenolone, and this suggests that TCDD acts upstream of pregnenolone formation. That would be consistent with previous observations in zebrafish that 10, 40, and 100 ppb TCDD in food depressed estradiol biosynthesis (Heiden et al., 2008).

Since *Update 2010*, studies of TCDD in rodents have provided additional evidence that dioxin has effects on early embryo development and effects on placenta formation. A recent study that used a rat in vitro fertilization model demonstrated that 100 nM TCDD perturbs chromatin and cytoskeletal remodeling at the earliest stages of embryo development, but these changes failed to result in any apparent morphologic changes at later stages of development (Petroff et al., 2011). The long-term potential effects of those early changes on pregnancy outcome are unknown. It has previously been shown that TCDD may have direct effects on human trophoblast formation at 0.2–2 nM in vitro and thus the capacity to influence the developing fetus (Chen et al., 2010). That idea is supported by a recent study that showed the ability of 5 nM TCDD to activate the AHR signaling pathway in both rat and human placental trophoblasts (Stejskalova et al., 2011). Finally, a study has demonstrated that TCDD at 0.1, 1, and 10 nM reduces in a dose-dependent fashion the ability of trophoblastic spheroids (which constitute an embryo surrogate) to attach to endometrial epithelial cells (Tsang et al., 2012). The more recent literature continues to support the biologic plausibility of effects of TCDD on male and female reproduction.

Sex Ratio

Although it would not constitute an adverse health outcome in an individual veteran, the perturbations in the sex ratio of children born to an exposed population suggest the exposure has an impact on the reproductive process. As shown in Table 9-4, studies of the sex ratios observed among children born to people exposed during the 1976 Seveso accident (Mocarelli et al., 1996, 2000) suggested that paternal exposure to dioxin may result in a lower sex ratio (that is, a smaller-than-expected proportion of male infants at birth), particularly when the father was exposed early in his life (sex ratio [SR] = 0.382). Consideration all 481 singleton births in 1994–2005 to women who resided in Zones A and B and were less than 28 years old at the time of the Seveso accident (18–46 years old at the beginning of period when births were identified), however, generated crude

TABLE 9-4 Selected Epidemiologic Studies—Sex Ratio[a] (Shaded Entry Is New for This Update)

Study Population	Sex Ratio of Offspring (boys/total)[b]	Comments	Reference
VIETNAM VETERANS			
US Vietnam Veterans			
US Air Force Health Study—Ranch Hand veterans vs SEA veterans (unless otherwise noted)			
Births from service through 1993 in AFHS			Michalek et al., 1998b
Comparison group	0.504	Not formally analyzed	
Dioxin level in Ranch Hand personnel			
Background	0.502		
Low	0.487		
High	0.535		
OCCUPATIONAL—INDUSTRIAL			
NIOSH Cross-Sectional Study			
Workers producing trichlorophenol and derivatives, including 2,4,5-T		No difference on basis of age at first exposure	Schnorr et al., 2001
Serum TCDD in fathers			
Neighborhood controls (< 20 ppt)	0.544	Referent	
Working fathers			
< 20 ppt	0.507	None significantly decreased (or increased)	
20–255 ppt	0.567		
255– < 1,120 ppt	0.568		
≥ 1,120 ppt	0.550		
Other Studies of Industrial Workers (*not* related to NIOSH phenoxy cohort)			
Austrian chloracne cohort—157 men, 2 women; exposed to TCDD during 2,4,5-T production			Moshammer and Neuberger, 2000
Children born after starting TCDD exposure in 1971	0.464 (26 boys: 30 girls)	Fewer sons, especially if father was less than 20 yrs old when exposed: SR = 0.20 (1 boy: 4 girls)	
Children born before 1971	0.613 (19 boys: 12 girls)		
Russian workers manufacturing 2,4,5,-trichlorophenol (1961–1988) or 2,4,5-T (1964–1967)			Ryan et al., 2002
Either parent exposed	0.401 (91 boys: 136 girls)	$p < 0.001$	
Only father exposed	0.378 (71 boys: 117 girls)	$p < 0.001$	

continued

TABLE 9-4 Sex Ratio,[a] continued

Study Population	Sex Ratio of Offspring (boys/total)[b]	Comments	Reference
Only mother exposed	0.513 (20 boys: 19 girls)	ns	
OCCUPATIONAL—PAPER AND PULP WORKERS			
Canada—British Columbian sawmill workers (n = 26,487)			Heacock et al., 1998
Chlorophenate-exposed workers	0.515		
Nonexposed workers	0.519		
Province overall	0.512		
OCCUPATIONAL—HERBICIDE-USING WORKERS (*not* related to IARC sprayer cohorts)			
Canadian OFFHS fathers' exposure during 3 mo before conception:			Savitz et al., 1997
No chemical activity	0.503	Referent	
Crop herbicides (some phenoxy herbicides)	0.500	ns	
Protective equipment used, not used	0.510	ns	
No protective equipment	0.450	ns	
ENVIRONMENTAL			
Seveso, Italy, Residential Cohort—Industrial accident July 10, 1976 (723 residents Zone A; 4,821 Zone B; 31,643 Zone R; 181,574 local reference group)			
Births 1994–2005 in women 0–28 yrs old at time of Seveso accident			Baccarelli et al., 2008
Zone A	0.571		
Zone B	0.508		
Zone R	0.495		
Births 1977–1996 in people from Zones A, B, R, 3–45 yrs old at time of 1976 Seveso accident	0.514	Referent	Mocarelli et al., 2000
Neither parent exposed	0.608	ns	
Father exposed (whether or not mother exposed)	0.440	$p = 0.03$	
Father < 19 yrs old in 1976	0.382	$p = 0.002$	
Father at least 19 yrs old in 1976	0.469	ns	
Only mother exposed	0.545	ns	
Parent (either sex) from Seveso Zone A			Mocarelli et al., 1996
Births 1977–1984	0.351 (26 boys: 48 girls)	$p < 0.001$, related to parental TCDD serum	
Births 1985–1994	0.484 (60 boys: 64 girls)	ns	

TABLE 9-4 Sex Ratio,[a] continued

Study Population	Sex Ratio of Offspring (boys/total)[b]	Comments	Reference
Ecological Study of Residents of Chapaevsk, Russia			
Residents near chemical plant in operation 1967–1987 in Chapaevsk, Russia			Revich et al., 2001
1983–1997	0.507	No clear pattern	
Minimum in 1989	0.401		
Maximum in 1987	0.564		
Maximum in 1995	0.559		
Other International Environmental Studies			
JAPAN—Yusho incident			
Parents (one or both) exposed to PCBs, PCDFs (not TCDD) in 1968			Yoshimura et al., 2001
All Japan in 1967	0.513	Referent	
Births 1967 (before poisoning incident)	0.516	ns	
Births 1968–1971 (after incident)	0.574	ns	
Births 1968–2009			Tsukimori et al., 2012a
Father exposed (whether or not mother exposed)	0.505	$p = 0.74$	
Father < 20 yrs old in 1967	0.465	$p = 0.15$	
Mother exposed (whether or not father exposed)	0.501	$p = 0.62$	
Mother < 20 yrs old in 1967	0.450	$p = 0.06$	
TAIWAN			
Taiwanese pregnant women (18–40 yrs of age); placental TEQ concentrations of TCDDs, TCDFs, PCBs	nr	No association	Chao et al., 2007
Births in individuals exposed to PCBs, PCDFs, PCDDs in 1979 **Yucheng incident**		vs unexposed with same demographics	del Rio Gomez et al., 2002
Father exposed (whether or not mother exposed)	0.490	$p = 0.037$	
Father < 20 yrs old in 1979	0.458	$p = 0.020$	
Father at least 20 yrs old in 1979	0.541	$p = 0.60$	
Mother exposed (whether or not father exposed)	0.504	$p = 0.45$	
Mother < 20 yrs old in 1979	0.501	$p = 0.16$	
Mother at least 20 yrs old in 1979	0.500	$p = 0.40$	
UNITED STATES			
San Francisco Bay area—serum concentrations in pregnant women during 1960s	OR for male birth (not SR)		Hertz-Picciotto et al., 2008
90th percentile vs 10th percentile		SRs all < 0.5	
Total PCBs	0.4 (0.3–0.8)	$p = 0.007$	
dl PCBs			
PCB 105	0.6 (0.4–0.9)	$p = 0.02$	

continued

TABLE 9-4 Sex Ratio,[a] continued

Study Population	Sex Ratio of Offspring (boys/total)[b]	Comments	Reference
PCB 118	0.7 (0.5–1.2)	p = 0.17	
PCB 170	0.6 (0.4–0.9)	p = 0.02	
PCB 180	0.8 (0.5–1.2)	p = 0.32	
Births after 1963 to Michigan fish-eaters with serum PCBs in both parents			Karmaus et al., 2002
Paternal PCBs > 8.1 µg/L	0.571	$p < 0.05$ (but for *more* sons)	
Maternal PCBs > 8.1 µg/L	0.494	ns	

NOTE: 2,4,5-T, 2,4,5-trichlorophenoxyacetic acid; AFHS, Air Force Health Study; dl, dioxin-like; NIOSH, National Institute for Occupational Safety and Health; ns, not significant; nr, not reported; OFFHS, Ontario Farm Family Health Study; OR, odds ratio; PCB, polychlorinated biphenyl; PCDD, polychlorinated dibenzodioxin; PCDF, polychlorinated dibenzofurans; ppt, parts per trillion; SEA, Southeast Asia; SR, sex ratio; TCDD, 2,3,7,8-tetrachlorodibenzo-*p*-dioxin; TCDF, tetrachlorodibenzofuran; TEQ, (total) toxic equivalent.

[a]VAO reports before *Update 1998* did not address association between perturbations in sex ratio of offspring and exposure to chemicals of interest.

[b]Given when available.

SRs showing that male births slightly exceeded female births in Zones A and B (SR = 0.516) and that an increase (SR = 0.571) was more pronounced for the 56 births in Zone A (Baccarelli et al., 2008).

A similar depression in the SR concentrated in fathers who were less than 20 years old at the time of the Yucheng poisoning with oil contaminated with PCBs, PCDFs, and PCDDs was reported by del Rio Gomez et al. (2002). On the other hand, Yoshimura et al. (2001) found a nonsignificant increase in the SR (SR = 0.574) of children born in the 4 years following the similar 1967 Yusho poisoning by rice oil contaminated with PCBs and PCDFs (but not TCDD) when at least 1 parent was exposed. Following up on the Yusho cohort, however, Tsukimori et al. (2012a) did note modest nonsignificant decreases in the SR when either the mother (SR = 0.450) or the father (SR = 0.465) was less than 20 years old at the time of the poisoning. In considering the second generation of Yusho offspring, Tsukimori et al. (2012a) found no effect on SR in the grandchildren of the exposed men, but the daughters of exposed women showed a tendency toward decreased SRs, especially if the grandmother had been young when exposed (results not tabled).

Chao et al. (2007) mentioned that they did not find an association between SR of offspring and the TEQ concentrations of dioxins, furans, or PCBs in the placentas from 119 Taiwanese women. Hertz-Picciotto et al. (2008) found evidence of an effect on SR in an analysis of the serum concentrations of nine PCB congeners (of which the two dioxin-like congeners were the mono-ortho PCBs 105 and 118) in blood gathered during the 1960s from 399 pregnant women in the San Francisco Bay area. The adjusted odds of male birth were significantly decreased when the 90th percentile of the total concentration of all nine PCBs was compared with the 10th percentile (OR = 0.45, 95% CI 0.26–0.80, p = 0.007). The proportion of male births was significantly reduced for only two of the PCBs when analyzed separately: dioxin-like, mono-ortho PCB 105 and non-dioxin-like PCB 170 (p = 0.02 for each).

Reductions in the expected number of male offspring have also been reported in cohorts of men who were occupationally exposed to dioxin (Moshammer and Neuberger, 2000; Ryan et al., 2002), but other such cohorts did not manifest this relationship (Heacock et al., 1998; Savitz et al., 1997; Schnorr et al., 2001). In the single report relevant to this outcome in Vietnam veterans, however, the SR was increased in the Operation Ranch Hand group that had the highest serum dioxin concentrations (Michalek et al., 1998b), but no formal analysis of this outcome was reported.

A population-level finding of a paternally mediated effect would be a strong indicator that dioxin exposure can interfere with the male reproductive process. James (2006) has interpreted perturbation of SRs by dioxins and other agents as being an indicator of parental endocrine disruption. If James's hypothesis were demonstrated to hold, it would be concordant with a reduction in testosterone in exposed men. Another pathway to an altered SR might involve male embryos' experiencing more lethality with induction of mutations due to their unmatched X chromosome. A genotoxic mechanism has not been expected to apply to TCDD, but sex-specific adverse consequences of modified imprinting of gametes might be a possible mechanism leading to observation of altered SRs at birth. To date, however, results regarding the proportion of sons among the children of fathers exposed to dioxin-like chemicals do not present a clear pattern of reduction.

There has been no work with experimental animals that has specifically examined the effects of TCDD on SRs of offspring, nor have any alterations in SR been reported in animal studies that examined developmental effects of TCDD on offspring.

Synthesis

Reproduction is a sensitive toxic endpoint of TCDD and DLCs in rodents. It is clear that the fetal rodent is more sensitive than the adult rodent to adverse effects of TCDD. The sensitivity of those endpoints in humans is less apparent. There is little evidence that exposure to dioxin is associated with a reduction in sperm quality or a reduction in fertility. However, the committee for *Update 2008* noted that the evidence that TCDD exposure reduces serum testosterone in men is consistent across several epidemiologic studies with appropriate consideration of confounders, including one of Vietnam veterans that found a dose–response relationship. The biologic plausibility of such a relationship is supported by concomitant increases observed in gonadotropins and the results of animal studies. Human populations that have shown evidence of reduced testosterone with exposure to DLCs include a general population sample (Dhooge et al., 2006), occupationally exposed people (Egeland et al., 1994), and Vietnam veterans in the Air Force Health Study (Gupta et al., 2006). The evidence that DLCs may modify the SR lends credence to the hypothesis that these chemicals have an effect on male reproductive functioning.

Despite the relative consistency of the finding of a reduction in testosterone, the testosterone concentrations observed even in the highest-exposure groups studied are well within the normal range. The small reduction in testosterone is not expected to have adverse clinical consequences. There is evidence of compensatory physiologic mechanisms. The occupational study by Egeland et al. (1994) found increased gonadotropins in addition to reduced testosterone. Gonadotropins stimulate the production of testosterone in men.

The first published study to examine dioxin exposure in women and association with TTP and infertility was reviewed in *Update 2010*. A dose–response relationship between TCDD exposure and TTP and infertility was observed and is consistent with published observations of the rat model. However, there have been no additional studies of dioxin exposure specifically and TTP since *Update 2010*. Epidemiologic studies have not provided data sufficient to interpret the effects of dioxin specifically on menstrual-cycle function in humans.

Conclusions

On the basis of its evaluation of the evidence reviewed here and in previous VAO reports, the present committee concludes that there is inadequate or insufficient evidence of an association between exposure to the COIs and decreased sperm counts or sperm quality, subfertility, or infertility.

SPONTANEOUS ABORTION, STILLBIRTH, NEONATAL DEATH, AND INFANT DEATH

Spontaneous abortion is the expulsion of a nonviable fetus, generally before 20 weeks of gestation, that is not induced by physical or pharmacologic means. The background risk of recognized spontaneous abortion is generally 7–15% (Hertz-Picciotto and Samuels, 1988), but it is established that many more pregnancies terminate before women become aware of them (Wilcox et al., 1988); such terminations are known as subclinical pregnancy losses and generally are not included in studies of spontaneous abortion. Estimates of the risk of recognized spontaneous abortion vary with the design and method of analysis. Studies have included cohorts of women asked retrospectively about pregnancy history, cohorts of pregnant women (usually those receiving prenatal care), and cohorts of women who are monitored for future pregnancies. The value of retrospective reports can be limited by loss of memory, particularly of spontaneous abortions that took place long before the interview. Studies that enroll women who appear for prenatal care require the use of life tables and specialized statistical techniques to account for differences in the times at which women seek medical care during pregnancy. Enrollment of women before pregnancy provides the theoretically most valid estimate of risk, but it can attract nonrepresentative study groups because the study protocols are demanding for the women.

Countries and US states have different legal definitions of the age of fetal viability and apply these terms differently, but typically *stillbirth* or *late fetal death* refers to the delivery at or after 20 weeks of gestation of a fetus that shows no signs of life, including a fetus that weighs more than 500 g regardless of gestational age (Kline et al., 1989); *neonatal death* refers to the death of a live-born infant within 28 days of birth; and *infant death* to a death that occurs before the first birthday.

The causes of stillbirth and early neonatal death overlap considerably, so they are commonly analyzed together in a category referred to as *perinatal mortality* (Kallen, 1988). Stillbirths make up less than 1% of all births (CDC, 2000). The most common causes of perinatal mortality (Kallen, 1988) in low-birth-weight (500–2,500 g) live-born and stillborn infants are placental and delivery complications—abruptio placenta, placenta previa, malpresentation, and umbilical-cord conditions. The most common causes of perinatal death of infants weighing more than 2,500 g at birth are complications of the cord, placenta, and membranes, and congenital malformations (Kallen, 1988).

Conclusions from *VAO* and Previous Updates

The committee responsible for the original *VAO* report concluded that there was inadequate or insufficient evidence of an association between exposure to 2,4-D, 2,4,5-T, TCDD, picloram, or cacodylic acid and spontaneous abortion or perinatal death. Additional information available to the committees responsible for *Update 1996*, *Update 1998*, and *Update 2000* did not change that conclusion.

The committee responsible for *Update 2002*, however, found that there was enough evidence available concerning paternal exposure specifically to TCDD to conclude that there was suggestive evidence that paternal exposure to TCDD is *not* associated with the risk of spontaneous abortion. That conclusion was based primarily on the National Institute for Occupational Safety and Health study (Schnorr et al., 2001), which investigated a large number of pregnancies fathered by workers whose serum TCDD concentrations were extrapolated back to the time of conception; no association was observed up to the highest-exposure group (1,120 ppt or higher). Indications of positive association were seen in studies of Vietnam veterans (CDC, 1989a,b; Field and Kerr, 1988; Stellman et al., 1988), but the committee for *Update 2002* asserted that these might be due to exposure to phenoxy herbicides rather than to TCDD and concluded that there was insufficient information to determine whether there is an association between maternal exposure to TCDD and the risk of spontaneous abortion or between maternal or paternal exposure to 2,4-D, 2,4,5-T, picloram, or cacodylic acid and the risk of spontaneous abortion.

The additional information (none of which concerned paternal exposure) reviewed by the committees responsible for *Update 2004*, *Update 2006*, *Update 2008*, and *Update 2010* did not change these conclusions.

The relevant studies concerning perinatal death are reviewed in the earlier reports, and Table 9-5 summarizes the findings of studies concerning spontaneous abortion.

Update of the Epidemiologic Literature

No studies of exposure to the COIs and spontaneous abortion or perinatal death have been published since *Update 2010*.

Biologic Plausibility

Laboratory animal studies have demonstrated that TCDD exposure during pregnancy can alter concentrations of circulating steroid hormones and disrupt placental development and function and thus contribute to a reduction in survival of implanted embryos and to fetal death (Huang et al., 2011; Ishimura et al., 2009; Wang et al., 2011). There is no evidence of a relationship between paternal or maternal exposure to TCDD and spontaneous abortion. Exposure to 2,4-D or 2,4,5-T causes fetal toxicity and death after maternal exposure in experimental animals. However, that effect occurs only at high doses and in the presence of maternal toxicity. No fetal toxicity or death has been reported to occur after paternal exposure to 2,4-D.

Laboratory studies of maternal TCDD exposure during pregnancy have demonstrated the induction of fetal death; neonatal death, however, is only rarely observed and is usually the result of cleft palate, which leads to an inability to nurse. Studies addressing the potential for perinatal death as a result of paternal exposure to TCDD or herbicides are inadequate to support conclusions.

Synthesis

No epidemiologic evidence concerning the COIs and spontaneous abortion, stillbirth, neonatal death, or infant death has been published since *Update 2010*, and toxicologic studies do not provide clear evidence of biologic plausibility of an association. Furthermore, given the ages of the Vietnam-veteran cohort, pub-

TABLE 9-5 Selected Epidemiologic Studies—Spontaneous Abortion[a]

Study Population	Exposed Cases[b]	**Exposure of Interest**/Estimated Relative Risk (95% CI)[b]	Reference
VIETNAM VETERANS			
US Vietnam Veterans			
US Air Force Health Study—Ranch Hand veterans vs Southeast Asia veterans (unless otherwise noted)		**All COIs**	
Air Force Ranch Hand veterans	157		Wolfe et al., 1995
Background	57	1.1 (0.8–1.5)	
Low exposure	56	1.3 (1.0–1.7)	
High exposure	44	1.0 (0.7–1.3)	
US CDC Vietnam Experience Study—Cross-sectional study, with medical examinations, of Army veterans: 9,324 deployed vs 8,989 nondeployed		**All COIs**	
Overall	1,566	1.3 (1.2–1.4)	CDC, 1989a
Self-reported low exposure	489	1.2 (1.0–1.4)	
Self-reported medium exposure	406	1.4 (1.2–1.6)	
Self-reported high exposure	113	1.7 (1.3–2.1)	
US VA Cohort of Female Vietnam Veterans		**All COIs**	
Female Vietnam-era veterans (maternal exposure)		1.0 (0.82–1.21)	Kang et al., 2000
Vietnam veterans (1,665 pregnancies)	278	nr	
Vietnam-era veterans who did not serve in Vietnam (1,912 pregnancies)	317	nr	
US National Vietnam Veterans		**All COIs**	
Female Vietnam veterans (maternal exposure)			Schwartz, 1998
Women who served in Vietnam	113	nr	
Women who did not serve in the war zone	124	nr	
Civilian women	86	nr	
US American Legion Cohort		**All COIs**	
American Legionnaires with service 1961–1975			Stellman et al., 1988
Vietnam veterans vs Vietnam-era veterans			
All Vietnam veterans	231	1.4 (1.1–1.6)	
Low exposure	72	1.3 (1.0–1.7)	
Medium exposure	53	1.5 (1.1–2.1)	
High exposure	58	1.7 (1.2–2.4)	
Vietnam-era veterans vs herbicide handlers	9	1.6 (0.7–3.3)	
Vietnam veterans			
Low exposure	72	1.0	
Medium exposure	53	1.2 (0.8–1.7)	
High exposure	58	1.4 (0.9–1.9)	
State Studies of US Vietnam Veterans			

continued

TABLE 9-5 Spontaneous Abortion,[a] continued

Study Population	Exposed Cases[b]	**Exposure of Interest**/Estimated Relative Risk (95% CI)[b]	Reference
Massachusetts—Wives of Vietnam veterans presenting at Boston Hospital for Women			Aschengrau and Monson, 1990
27 weeks of gestation	10	0.9 (0.4–1.9)	
13 weeks of gestation	nr	1.2 (0.6–2.8)	
International Vietnam-Veteran Studies			
Tasmanian Veterans with Service in Vietnam		**All COIs**	
Followup of Australian Vietnam veterans	199	1.6 (1.3–2.0)	Field and Kerr, 1988
OCCUPATIONAL—INDUSTRIAL			
IARC Phenoxy Herbicide Cohort—Workers exposed to any phenoxy herbicide or chlorophenol (production or spraying) vs respective national mortality rates		**Dioxins, phenoxy herbicides**	
NIOSH Mortality Cohort (12 US plants, 5,172 male production and maintenance workers, 1942–1984) (included in IARC cohort as of 1997)		**Dioxins, phenoxy herbicides**	
Wives and partners of men in NIOSH cohort			Schnorr et al., 2001
Estimated paternal TCDD serum at time of conception			
< 20 ppt	29	0.8 (0.5–1.2)	
20 to < 255 ppt	11	0.8 (0.4–1.6)	
255 to < 1120	11	0.7 (0.3–1.6)	
≥ 1120 ppt	8	1.0 (0.4–2.2)	
Dow Workers with Potential TCDD Exposure and reproductive outcomes studied in offspring of 930 men working with chlorophenol, 1939–1975		**Dioxins, phenoxy herbicides**	Townsend et al., 1982
Wives of men employed involved in chlorophenol processing at Dow Chemical Co.	85	1.0 (0.8–1.4)	
Monsanto workers in Nitro, West Virginia, occupationally exposed and potentially exposed after 1949 explosion (1948–1969)		**Dioxins, phenoxy herbicides**	
Followup of current and retired 2,4,5-T production workers (n = 235; 117 with chloracne exposure), 1948–1969	14	0.9 (0.4–1.8)	Moses et al., 1984
Followup of 2,4,5-T production workers (204 exposed, 163 unexposed), 1948–1969	69	0.9 (0.6–1.2)	Suskind and Hertzberg, 1984
OCCUPATIONAL—HERBICIDE-USING WORKERS (*not* related to IARC sprayer cohorts)			
New Zealand—Followup of 2,4,5-T sprayers vs nonsprayers (n = 989)		**Herbicides** *90% CI*	Smith et al., 1982
	43	0.9 (0.6–1.3)	

TABLE 9-5 Spontaneous Abortion,[a] continued

Study Population	Exposed Cases[b]	**Exposure of Interest**/Estimated Relative Risk (95% CI)[b]	Reference
US Forest Service		**Herbicides**	
Women employed by US Forest Service—miscarriages (maternal exposure)	141	2.0 (1.1–3.5)	Driscoll et al., 1998
ENVIRONMENTAL			
Seveso, Italy, Women's Health Study—Industrial accident July 10, 1976; 981 women between infancy and 40 yrs of age at the time of the accident, who resided in Zones A, B)		**TCDD**	
SWHS participants living in Zones A, B in 1976 (maternal exposure)			Eskenazi et al., 2003
Pregnancies 1976–1998	97	0.8 (0.6–1.2)	
Pregnancies 1976–1984	44	1.0 (0.6–1.6)	
Ecological Study of Residents of Chapaevsk, Russia		**TCDD**	
Residents of Samara Region, Russia (maternal and paternal exposure)			Revich et al., 2001
Chapaevsk	nr	24.4% (20.0–29.5%)[c]	
Samara	nr	15.2% (14.3–16.1%)[c]	
Toliatti	nr	10.6% (9.8–11.5%)[c]	
Syzran	nr	15.6% (13.4–18.1%)[c]	
Novokuibyshevsk	nr	16.9% (14.0–20.3%)[c]	
Other small towns	nr	11.3% (9.4–13.8%)[c]	
Ontario Farm Family Health Study		**Phenoxy herbicides**	
Ontario farm families (maternal, paternal exposures)			Arbuckle et al., 2001
Phenoxyacetic acid herbicide exposure in preconception period, spontaneous-abortion risk	48	1.5 (1.1–2.1)	
Other International Environmental Studies			
Japan—Spontaneous abortions among pregnancies (excluding induced abortions) of women in 1968 Yusho incident (maternal exposure)		**PCBs, PCDFs**	Tsukimori et al., 2008
10 yrs after vs 10 yrs before	nr	2.1 (0.8–5.2)	
10-fold increase in maternal blood concentration (drawn 2001–2005) of			
PeCDF	nr	1.6 (1.1–2.3)	
PCB 126 (TEF = 0.1)	nr	2.5 (0.9–6.9)	
PCB 169 (TEF = 0.01)	nr	2.3 (1.1–4.8)	

continued

TABLE 9-5 Spontaneous Abortion,[a] continued

Study Population	Exposed Cases[b]	**Exposure of Interest**/Estimated Relative Risk (95% CI)[b]	Reference
Taiwanese pregnant women (18–40 yrs of age); placental TEQ concentrations of PCDDs, PCDFs, PCBs		**PCDD, PCBs** nr, but reported ns	Chao et al., 2007
Vietnamese women who were, or whose husbands were, exposed to herbicides sprayed during Vietnam War	nr	**COIs**/nr, anecdotal reports of miscarriage in pilot study	Tuyet and Johansson, 2001
CASE-CONTROL STUDIES			
US Case-Control Studies			
Washington, Oregon—wives of men occupationally exposed to 2,4-D; all reported		**2,4-D**	Carmelli et al., 1981
		90% CI	
work exposure to herbicides (high and medium)	63	0.8 (0.6–1.1)	
Farm exposure	32	0.7 (0.4–1.5)	
Forest and commercial exposure	31	0.9 (0.6–1.4)	
Exposure during conception period			
Farm exposure	15	1.0 (0.5–1.8)	
Forest and commercial exposure	16	1.6 (0.9–1.8)	
Fathers 18–25 yrs old			
Farm exposure	1	0.7 (nr)	
Forest and commercial exposure	3	4.3 (nr)	
Fathers 26–30 yrs old			
Farm exposure	4	0.4 (nr)	
Forest and commercial exposure	8	1.6 (nr)	
Fathers 31–35 yrs old			
Farm exposure	10	2.9 (nr)	
Forest and commercial exposure	5	1.0 (nr)	

NOTE: 2,4-D, 2,4-dichlorophenoxyacetic acid; 2,4,5-T, 2,4,5-trichlorophenoxyacetic acid; CDC, Centers for Disease Control and Prevention; CI, confidence interval; COI, chemical of interest; IARC, International Agency for Research on Cancer; NIOSH, National Institute for Occupational Safety and Health; nr, not reported; ns, not significant (usually refers to $p < 0.05$); PeCDF, 2,3,4,7,8-pentachlorodibenzofuran; PCB, polychlorinated biphenyl; PCDF, polychlorinated dibenzofuran; ppt, parts per trillion; SWHS, Seveso Women's Health Study; TCDD, 2,3,7,8-tetrachlorodibenzo-*p*-dioxin; TEF, toxic equivalency factor; TEQ, (total) toxic equivalent; VA, US Department of Veterans Affairs.

[a]Unless otherwise indicated, results are for paternal exposure.

[b]Given when available; results other than estimated risk explained individually.

[c]Spontaneous abortion rate per 100 full-term pregnancies for 1991–1997.

lication of additional information on this outcome in the target population of the VAO series is not likely.

Conclusions

On the basis of the evidence reviewed to date, the committee concludes that paternal exposure to TCDD is *not* associated with risk of spontaneous abortion and that insufficient information is available to determine whether there is an association between maternal exposure to TCDD or either maternal or paternal exposure to 2,4-D, 2,4,5-T, picloram, or cacodylic acid and the risk of spontaneous abortion. The committee concludes that there is inadequate or insufficient evidence to determine whether there is an association between exposure to the COIs and stillbirth, neonatal death, or infant death.

BIRTH WEIGHT AND PRETERM DELIVERY

Birth weight and the length of the gestation period can have important effects on neonatal morbidity and mortality and on health over the life span. Defined by the World Health Organization as a birth weight under 2,500 g (Alberman, 1984), low birth weight (LBW) has two distinct causes. Intrauterine growth retardation (IUGR) occurs when fetal growth is diminished and a fetus or baby fails to attain a normal weight or is small for gestational age (SGA). The concept of IUGR represents birth weight, adjusted for gestational age, that is lower than average according to local or national fetal-growth graphs (Romo et al., 2009). LBW can also be secondary to preterm delivery (PTD), which is delivery at less than 259 days, or 37 completed weeks, of gestation, calculated on the basis of the date of the first day of the last menstrual period (Bryce, 1991). LBW due to either cause occurs in about 7% of live births. When no distinction is made between the causes of LBW (IUGR or PTD), the factors most strongly associated with it are maternal tobacco use during pregnancy, multiple births, and race or ethnicity. Other potential risk factors are low socioeconomic status, malnutrition, maternal weight, birth order, maternal complications during pregnancy (such as severe pre-eclampsia or intrauterine infection) and obstetric history, job stress, and cocaine or caffeine use during pregnancy (Alexander and Slay, 2002; Alexander et al., 2003; Ergaz et al., 2005; Kallen, 1988; Peltier, 2003). Established risk factors for PTD include race (black), marital status (single), low socioeconomic status, previous LBW or PTD, multiple gestations, tobacco use, and cervical, uterine, or placental abnormalities (Berkowitz and Papiernik, 1993).

Birth weight is a strong and consistent predictor of infant mortality and, to a smaller extent, of health problems later in life, including adverse neurodevelopmental outcomes and adult-onset chronic diseases (Wilcox, 2001). However, the importance and interpretation of associations with birth weight or, by extension, with common classifications of birth weight—such as LBW, IUGR, and SGA—

are often unclear and a subject of controversy among researchers. Across populations, the frequency distribution of birth weight is Gaussian, with an extended lower tail, or "residual distribution," that includes preterm and LBW infants. The predominant, normal distribution corresponds largely to term births. In general, shifts in the predominant distribution do not tend to correspond to notable shifts in infant mortality (Wilcox, 2001). A number of factors may result in shifts in the predominant distribution; altitude, race or ethnicity, and maternal smoking are among the better studied, thereby producing a larger (or smaller) percentage of LBW babies. However, populations that have a larger percentage of LBW infants do not always have higher infant mortality (Wilcox, 2001).

Population trends in birth weight are tracked internationally to identify opportunities for intervention and to understand country-specific infant mortality (UNICEF, 2004). Being born at the lower tail of the birth-weight distribution may have significant and immediate health and economic consequences. Pregnancies afflicted by fetal growth restriction incur greater medical expenses in the prenatal and immediate postnatal period and higher risks of hospitalization in the first year of life (NRC, 2003). Thus, although an exogenous factor exerts an effect at all points in the birth-weight growth curve, the economic and clinical consequences of that effect might be borne disproportionately by those at the lower end of the birth-weight distribution.

Conclusions from *VAO* and Previous Updates

The committee responsible for *VAO* concluded that there was inadequate or insufficient evidence to determine whether there is an association between exposure to the COIs and LBW or PTD.

Update 2010 considered three studies of prenatal exposure to DLCs and birth weight. In a prospective cohort study of 514 women in Sapporo, Japan, Konishi et al. (2009) reported that a significant reduction in birth weight was associated with total TEQs (–220.5 g per 10-fold increase in TEQ; 95% CI –399.2 to –41.9) in maternal blood. A significant reduction in birth weight was also observed in connection separately with dioxin-like PCDD TEQs and PCDF TEQs and marginally with TEQs based on all dioxin-like PCBs. When stratified on infant sex, the association remained statistically significant for males but not females. In a coastal area of Japan (where consumption of seafood is common), Tawara et al. (2009) found that the concentrations of several individual dioxin-like PCDD and PCDF congeners and of total TEQs in maternal breast milk were inversely related to newborn length, but none was related to birth weight. Similarly, in a nested study of fatty-fish consumption in the Danish National Birth Cohort, Halldorsson et al. (2009) did not find that total maternal serum TEQs derived with the AHR-CALUX assay were associated with birth weight.

Additional information available to the committees responsible for *Update 1996*, *Update 1998*, *Update 2000*, *Update 2002*, *Update 2004*, *Update 2006*,

Update 2008, and *Update 2010* did not change that conclusion. Reviews of the relevant studies are presented in the earlier reports. The most relevant findings on birth weight after paternal and maternal exposure to the COIs are summarized in Tables 9-6 and 9-7, respectively.

Update of the Epidemiologic Literature

No Vietnam-veteran, occupational, or case-control studies of exposure to the COIs and LBW or PTD have been published since *Update 2010*.

Environmental Studies

Nishijo et al. (2012) examined the association between dioxin exposure and infant growth among 210 mother-infant pairs residing in dioxin-contaminated districts near the Da Nang airbase in Vietnam. Full-term babies from uncomplicated deliveries were recruited in 2008 and 2009. Breast milk was collected 1 month after birth and analyzed for 7 PCDDs and 10 PCDFs. Maternal interviews provided detailed covariate data, and pregnancy and delivery information was obtained from the obstetricians. All infants were breastfed until 4 months after birth. Length of residence in the contaminated districts was directly related to PCDD/F-TEQ exposure quartile and maternal age. However, overall, breast-milk concentrations 1 month after birth were not excessively increased, even given the proximity of the subjects to the contaminated districts. Body weight of 4-month-old boys whose breast-milk PCDDs/F-TEQ (pg/g of fat) was in the fourth quartile (highest exposure) was significantly lower than that of boys whose breast-milk exposure was in the first quartile (lowest exposure) (6,562 g vs 6,927 g), as was their body mass index (15.9 kg/m^2 vs 16.5 kg/m^2). Body weight, however, did not decline linearly with increasing quartile of exposure. No effect was found in girls, and the overall sample of this study was small.

Tsukimori et al. (2012b) examined the association of maternal exposure to PCDDs, PCDFs, and PCBs in relation to birth weight among women who were accidentally exposed to rice oil contaminated with PCBs, PCDDs, or PCDFs in western Japan (in the Yusho incident of 1968). A nationwide health examination of Yusho survivors has been conducted annually since 1986. As of 2009, 737 women were registered with the Study Group for Yusho; to qualify, they had to have signs and symptoms of Yusho oil disease, a history of consumption of contaminated oil, or the characteristic profile of PCBs and polychlorinated quarter-phenyls in their blood. The 2009 mailed questionnaire included questions about maternal and infant outcomes. Date of delivery, gestational age at delivery, and birth weight were obtained from the record of pregnancy care provided by each patient. Of the 737 women registered, 206 gave birth after the Yusho incident. The analysis was based on 190 births after the Yusho incident to 101 women who provided blood samples collected in 2001 or later for measurement of PCDDs,

TABLE 9-6 Selected Epidemiologic Studies—Birth Weight Following Paternal Exposure

Reference	Primary Exposure	Sample Size	Outcome/Main Findings	Adjustment Covariates
VIETNAM VETERANS				
US Air Force Health Study—Ranch Hand veterans vs SEA veterans; births from service through 1993 in AFHS				
Michalek et al., 1998a	Ranch Hands	2,082 births	No association with IUGR	Adjusted by stratification for father's race, mother smoking during pregnancy, mother's alcohol use, mother's age, father's age, father's military occupation
US CDC Vietnam Experience Study—Cross-sectional study, with medical examinations, of Army veterans: 9,324 deployed vs 8,989 nondeployed				
CDC, 1989a,b	Military service in VA	1,771 Vietnam; 1,561 non-Vietnam	LBW/RR 1.1 (0.8–1.4)	Maternal age and gravidity. Also model with smoking history, alcohol use, educational attainment, marital status, illicit drug use in military
US American Legion Cohort—American Legionnaires with service 1961–1975				
Stellman et al., 1988	US men deployed to SEA during Vietnam War, and other deployed men during same time period	2,858 in SEA 3,933 deployed elsewhere (n = 6,081)	"no difference between the birthweight of boys born to servicemen stationed in SEA compared to those born to controls, nor did girls' birthweight differs between two groups"	Sex, age of father at time of child's birth, age of mother, mother smoking during pregnancy, military service in SEA and exposure to combat and AO—these were not multivariate adjusted models, so strong smoking effect might have had an influence. These appear to have all been independent models
Tasmanian Veterans with Service in Vietnam—Followup of Australian Vietnam veterans				
Field and Kerr, 1988	Military service in Vietnam	~550	LBW/RR 1.6 (1.0–2.5)	RR calculated by committee member
OCCUPATIONAL—INDUSTRIAL				
Lawson et al., 2004	Wives of chemical workers highly exposed to TCDD-contaminated chemicals	~500 exposed 600 referents	No association with birth weight overall	Adjusted for sex, education, parity, smoking, length of gestation, no stratification by sex

TABLE 9-6 Birth Weight Following Paternal Exposure, continued

Reference	Primary Exposure	Sample Size	Outcome/Main Findings	Adjustment Covariates
OCCUPATIONAL—HERBICIDE-USING WORKERS				
Dimich-Ward et al., 1996	Chlorophenate, wood preservative in sawmill industry	19,675 births	No association (ORs for SGA ~1)	Sex, maternal and paternal age, birth yr, matching

NOTE: AFHS, Air Force Health Study; AO, Agent Orange; CDC, Centers for Disease Control and Prevention; IUGR, intrauterine growth restriction; LBW, low birth weight; OR, odds ratio; RR, relative risk; SEA, Southeast Asia; SGA, small for gestational age; TCDD, 2,3,7,8-trichlorodibenzo-*p*-dioxin; VA, US Department of Veterans Affairs.

PCDFs, and non-ortho PCBs. A simple decay model was used to estimate chemical concentration at the time of delivery. Models were adjusted for important predictors of fetal growth, including gestational age at delivery. Increased maternal exposure to PCDDs and PCDFs was strongly associated with reduced birth weight overall, which appeared to be driven by strong effects in male infants. For each 10-fold increase in total-PCDDs TEQ, male infant birth weight was decreased by about 200 g (95% CI –33 to –70 g), which was statistically significant (p = 0.003). A similar magnitude of association was found for non-ortho PCBs TEQ, whereas the total-PCDFs TEQ and total TEQ were 130–170 g. All the individual congeners, including 2,3,7,8-TCDD and 1,2,3,7,8-pentachlorodibenzodioxin, were associated with significant decrements in birth weight in males. There were no significant associations in females overall or for individual congeners despite the fact that there were no significant differences in exposure levels between sexes of the infants. In addition, the odds of delivering a LBW infant (birth weight < 2,500 g) increased significantly with each 10-fold increase in total exposure to PCDD TEQ (OR = 8.1, 95% CI 1.67–38.86), total non-ortho PCB TEQ (OR = 9.32, 95% CI 1.40–62.03), and total TEQ (OR = 4.36, 95% CI 1.21–15.72). This study has many strengths, but there was some concern with respect to the accuracy of the exposure extrapolation model, specifically with respect to the treatment of births and breastfeeding events that occurred in the period between the index pregnancy and the blood collection. Using the historical serum samples available, the study did not explicitly measure non-dioxin-like PCBs. Given the complex nature of the Yusho exposure, which was predominantly a PCB exposure with PCDF contaminants, it is not possible with these data to disentangle the effects of the non-dioxin-like PCB exposures. Although the Yusho cohort does have higher TEQs than the general population, the toxic effects of the Yusho exposure were driven predominantly by PCDFs, not TCDD.

TABLE 9-7 Selected Epidemiologic Studies—Birth Weight Following Maternal Exposure (Shaded Entries Are New Information for This Update)

Reference	Primary Exposure	Sample Size	Outcome/Main Findings	Adjustment Covariates
VIETNAM VETERANS				
US VA Cohort of Female Vietnam Veterans				
H. Kang, personal correspondence, February 27, 2013	*Military service*	*2,689*	***BW girls = + 0.5 oz BW boys = –0.8 oz (difference in boys comes to –22.7 g***	*Unadjusted differences and major uncontrolled confounders (smoking, parity, race)*
Kang et al., 2000	Military service	4,140	LBW (OR = 1.06, 95% CI 0.8–1.5)	Maternal age, education, race, marital status, military characteristics, smoking, drinking, average number of hours worked during pregnancy, complications during pregnancy
ENVIRONMENTAL				
Seveso, Italy, Women's Health Study—Industrial accident July 10, 1976 (981 women who were between infancy and 40 yrs old, who resided in Zones A or B)				
Baccarelli et al., 2008	Seveso	51	No association with LBW	None
Eskenazi et al., 2003 *(B. Eskenazi, personal correspondence, January 30, 2013—researchers checked for effect modification by sex but found none)*	Seveso	608 overall	Birth weight (nonsignificant negative coefficients). SGA—ORs between 1.2–1.8; none are technically significant. OR = 1.2, 0.8–1.8 is overall	Gestational age, sex, parity, history of LBW, maternal height, maternal BMI, maternal age, maternal education, smoking

TABLE 9-7 Birth Weight Following Maternal Exposure, continued

Reference	Primary Exposure	Sample Size	Outcome/Main Findings	Adjustment Covariates
Vietnamese Studies				
Nishijo et al., 2012	People living around contaminated airbase in Vietnam	210	**At birth no effect, but birth-weight discrepancy grows with months from delivery. Significant at 4 months.** Effect only seen in boys	Parity, maternal age, weight, educational period, alcohol use, family income, family smoking, gestational weeks, infant age on the day of examination
Times Beach and Quail Run Cohorts				
Stockbauer et al., 1988	TCDD soil contamination in Missouri	Matched sets, ~400 (2:1)	LBW: 1.5 (95% CI 0.2–2.3)	Sex, maternal education, parity, marital status, prepregnancy weight, smoking, history of previous SAB and fetal deaths
Yusho, Japan, Cohort—population exposed to PCDDs, PCDFs, and PCBs in contaminated cooking oil				
Tsukimori et al., 2012b	Yusho	190	**~ –200g birth-weight reduction with PCDD TEQ (p = 0.003) in males, also overall effect but driven by effect in boys**	Gestational age, maternal age, parity, smoking, duration breastfeeding, seafood consumption
Kuratsune et al., 1972	Yusho	11	None calculated	—
Other Environmental Studies				
Japan				
Konishi et al., 2009	Sapporo, Japan; contemporary cohort	514	**BW (–220.5 g per 10-fold increase in TEQ, 95% CI –399.2 to –41.9); effect driven by males**	Gestational age, maternal age, maternal height, maternal weight before pregnancy, parity, smoking, inshore fish intake, blood sampling period, infant sex

continued

TABLE 9-7 Birth Weight Following Maternal Exposure, continued

Reference	Primary Exposure	Sample Size	Outcome/Main Findings	Adjustment Covariates
Tawara et al., 2009	Coastal Japan; contemporary cohort	75	Some weak negative correlations	Unadjusted; Spearman correlations
Nishijo et al., 2008	Breast-milk dioxin levels	42	Negative correlation for TEQ-PCDD and TEQ, PCDF, but not "significant"	Spearman correlations
Finland				
Vartiainen et al., 1998	Random sampling of mother/infant pairs from urban/rural Finland	167	**Birth weight decreased with increasing concentrations of I-TEQ, especially among boys**	Unadjusted; effect goes away when restricted to primiparas
Netherlands				
Patandin et al., 1998	Dutch children—PCB 118 exposure (only total)	207	**Birth weight = –119 (53.7); p = 0.03**	Smoking, alcohol, gestational age, target height, parity
United States				
Kezios et al., 2012	California Child Health and Human Development Study	600	No association with birth weight	Race, age, smoking status, BMI, sex, length of gestation, lipids
Sagiv et al., 2007	PCB 118	722	Negative birth-weight effects with increasing exposure quartile, nonsignificant—0, –18, –72, –69.5	Gestational age, infant size, birth year, maternal age, race parity, height, prepregnancy BMI, smoking, local fish consumption

NOTE: BMI, body mass index; BW, birth weight; CI, confidence interval; I-TEQ, international (total) toxic equivalent; LBW, low birth weight; OR, odds ratio; PCB, polychlorinated biphenyls; PCDD, polychlorinated dibenzo-*p*-dioxin; PCDF, polychlorinated dibenzofurans; SAB, spontaneous abortion; SGA, small for gestational age; TCDD, 2,3,7,8-trichlorodibenzo-*p*-dioxin; TEQ, (total) toxic equivalent; VA, US Department of Veterans Affairs.

It is also noteworthy that serum TCDD was not higher in the Yusho mothers than in the general population. Nonetheless, the results raise concerns and in theory would provide some plausibility of later associations with diseases in offspring, from neurodevelopmental impairment to adult-onset chronic diseases.

Finally, Kezios et al. (2012) examined the association of maternal exposure to PCBs and infant growth measures in 600 infants (born in 1960–1963) participating in the Child Health and Development Studies in northern California. Eleven PCB congeners were measured in postpartum maternal seruma, including dioxin-like, mono-ortho PCB 118. Overall, there was no association between PCB 118 concentration and infant birth weight, and no interaction related to infant sex. There was also no association with length of gestation.

Biologic Plausibility

The available evidence from experimental animal studies indicates that TCDD exposure during pregnancy can reduce body weight at birth but only at high doses. Laboratory studies of the potential male-mediated developmental toxicity of TCDD and herbicides as a result of exposure of adult male animals are inadequate to support conclusions. TCDD and herbicides are known to cross the placenta, and this leads to direct exposure of the fetus. Data from studies of experimental animals also suggest that the preimplantation embryo and developing fetus are sensitive to the toxic effects of 2,4-D and TCDD after maternal exposure.

Synthesis

Three studies provide some evidence of deficit in birth weight in relation to maternal exposure to DLCs—Konishi et al. (2009, reviewed in *Update 2010*), Nishijo et al. (2012), and Tsukimori et al (2012b)—some with notably stronger effects in male infants. LBW itself was examined overall only in the Tsukimori study, in which it was found to be significantly increased in association with exposure. None of the studies found associations with prematurity or gestational length continuously. In Tsukimori et al. (2012b), the magnitude of birth weight decrease associated with a 10-fold increase in total TEQ exposure is comparable with that found for maternal active smoking (about a 200-g birth-weight deficit). The implication of this finding is unclear—animal evidence indicates that in utero TCDD exposure can reduce birth weight at high doses in both male and female pups, but there are insufficient data to support conclusions about any sex-specific effects of TCDD.

Two older studies had addressed this outcome without reporting separate results by infant sex, and the committee asked researchers from each team whether they could make such a comparison. Both responded to the inquiries, but the information they provided did little to support the hypothesis that there tended to be a lowering of birth weight in male infants. The one previous Vietnam-era study (Kang et al., 2000) reported no association with LBW in 4,140 female military veterans, and Kang replied that a reanalysis showed that the average birth weight of the boys was only slightly lower than that of the girls (see Table 9-7) (H. Kang, US Department of Veterans Affairs, personal communication, February 27, 2013). Eskenazi et al. (2003), in their analysis of the Seveso population that had high TCDD exposures, reported no overall association with SGA and birth weight, although they did not report the results of any analyses that considered effect modification by infant sex; Eskenazi replied to the committee's question by reporting that the researchers had made the comparison by infant sex but they found nothing of interest and so did not report details (B. Eskenazi, Seveso Women's Health Study, personal communication, January 30, 2013).

There are a number of challenges in conducting these types of epidemiologic studies in a rigorous way. First, the prenatal and immediate postpartum period is not a stable pharmacokinetic state, involving substantial changes in body volume and fat mobilization. Biomarker measures during pregnancy may be substantially affected by weight change during pregnancy. Moreover, extrapolation of a more recent biomarker measure back many years to a more relevant period is complicated by intervening pregnancy and breastfeeding events, which result in substantial uncertainty in the index exposure level. Overall, although the committee notes that the animal literature does support an effect of TCDD exposure on birth weight, the epidemiologic literature is insufficiently robust to allow a final determination. However, the committee is concerned about a potential association of maternal exposure with birth weight.

Conclusions

On the basis of the evidence reviewed here and in previous VAO reports, the committee concludes that there is inadequate or insufficient evidence to determine whether there is an association between exposure to the COIs and low birth weight or preterm delivery.

REFERENCES[1]

Alberman E. 1984. Low birth weight. In: Bracken MB, ed. *Perinatal Epidemiology*. New York: Oxford University Press. Pp. 86–98.

Alexander GR, Slay M. 2002. Prematurity at birth: Trends, racial disparities, and epidemiology. *Mental Retardation and Developmental Disabilities Research Reviews* 8(4):215–220.

[1]Throughout this report, the same alphabetic indicator after year of publication is used consistently for a given reference when there are multiple citations by the same first author in a given year. The convention of assigning the alphabetic indicators in order of citation in a given chapter is not followed.

Alexander GR, Kogan M, Bader D, Carlo W, Allen M, Mor J. 2003. US birth weight/gestational age-specific neonatal mortality: 1995–1997 rates for whites, Hispanics, and blacks. *Pediatrics* 111(1):e61–e66.

Aly HAA, Khafagy RM. 2011. 2,3,7,8-tetrachlorodibenzo-*p*-dioxin (TCDD)-induced cytotoxicity accompanied by oxidative stress in rat Sertoli cells: Possible role of mitochondrial fractions of Sertoli cells. *Toxicology and Applied Pharmacology* 252:273–280.

Amanai M, Brahmajjosyula M, Perry ACF. 2006. A restricted role for sperm-borne microRNAs in mammalian fertilization. *Biology of Reproduction* 75:877–884.

Arbuckle TE, Lin Z, Mery LS. 2001. An exploratory analysis of the effect of pesticide exposure on the risk of spontaneous abortion in an Ontario farm population. *Environmental Health Perspectives* 109(8):851–857.

Aschengrau A, Monson RR. 1990. Paternal military service in Vietnam and the risk of late adverse pregnancy outcomes. *American Journal of Public Health* 80(10):1218–1224.

Baccarelli A, Giacomini SM, Corbetta C, Landi MT, Bonzini M, Consonni D, Grillo P, Patterson DG Jr, Pesatori AC, Bertazzi PA. 2008. Neonatal thyroid function in Seveso 25 years after maternal exposure to dioxin. *PLoS Medicine* 5(7):1133–1142.

Berkowitz GS, Papiernik E. 1993. Epidemiology of preterm delivery. *Epidemiologic Reviews* 15:414–443.

Beytur A, Ciftci O, Aydin M, Cakir O, Timurkaan N, Yılmaz N. 2012. Protocatechuic acid prevents reproductive damage caused by 2,3,7,8-tetrachlorodibenzo-*p*-dioxin (TCDD) in male rats. *Andrologia* 44:454–461.

Bonde JP, Giwercman A. 1995. Occupational hazards to male fecundity. *Reproductive Medicine Review* 4:59–73.

Bretveld RW, Thomas CMG, Scheepers PTJ, Zielhuis GA, Roeleveld N. 2006a. Pesticide exposure: The hormonal function of the female reproductive system disrupted? *Reproductive Biology and Endocrinology* 4:20.

Bretveld RW, Zielhuis GA, Roeleveld N. 2006b. Time to pregnancy among female greenhouse workers. *Scandinavian Journal of Work, Environment and Health* 32(5):359–367.

Brunnberg S, Andersson P, Poellinger L, Hanberg A. 2011. The constitutively active Ah receptor (CA-AhR) mouse as a model for dioxin exposure—Effects in reproductive organs. *Chemosphere* 85:1701–1706.

Bryce R. 1991. The epidemiology of preterm birth. In: Kiely M, ed. *Reproductive and Perinatal Epidemiology*. Boca Raton, FL: CRC Press. Pp. 437–444.

Buck Louis GM, Rios LI, McLain A, Cooney MA, Kostyniak PJ, Sundaram R. 2011. Persistent organochlorine pollutants and menstrual cycle characteristics. *Chemosphere* 85 (11):1742–1748.

Bulun SE, Zeitoun KM, Kilic G. 2000. Expression of dioxin-related transactivating factors and target genes in human eutopic endometrial and endometriotic tissues. *American Journal of Obstetrics and Gynecology* 182(4):767–775.

Burdorf A, Brand T, Jaddoe VW, Hofman A, Mackenbach JP, Steegers EAP. 2011. The effects of work-related maternal risk factors on time to pregnancy, preterm birth and birth weight: The Generation R study. *Occupational and Environmental Medicine* 68(3):197–204.

Cai LY, Izumi S, Suzuki T, Goya K, Nakamura E, Sugiyama T, Kobayashi H. 2011. Dioxins in ascites and serum of women with endometriosis: A pilot study. *Human Reproduction* 26(1):117–126.

Carmelli D, Hofherr L, Tomsic J, Morgan RW. 1981. *A Case-Control Study of the Relationship Between Exposure to 2,4-D and Spontaneous Abortions in Humans.* SRI International. Prepared for the National Forest Products Association and the US Department of Agriculture, Forest Service.

CDC (Centers for Disease Control and Prevention). 1989a. *Health Status of Vietnam Veterans. Vietnam Experience Study, Vol. V, Reproductive Outcomes and Child Health.* Atlanta, GA: US Department of Health and Human Services.

CDC. 1989b. *Health Status of Vietnam Veterans. Vietnam Experience Study, Vol. V, Reproductive Outcomes and Child Health.* Atlanta, GA: US Department of Health and Human Services.

CDC. 2000. National Center for Health Statistics. National Vital Statistics System. *Vital Statistics of the United States, Vol. II, Mortality, Part A, for Data Years 1950–1993.* Washington, DC: US Government Printing Office. Data for 1994 to 1998. Data are available on the NCHS website at http://www.cdc.gov/nchs/datawh/statab/unpubd/mortabs.htm.

Chao HR, Wang SL,Lin LY, Lee WJ, Päpke O. 2007. Placental transfer of polychlorinated dibenzo-*p*-dioxins, dibenzofurans, and biphenyls in Taiwanese mothers in relation to menstrual cycle characteristics. *Food Chemical Toxicology* 45:259–265.

Charles JM, Hanley TR, Wilson RD, van Ravenzwaay B, Bus JS. 2001. Developmental toxicity studies in rats and rabbits on 2,4-dichlorophenoxyacetic acid and its forms. *Toxicological Sciences* 60:121–131.

Chen SC, Liao TL, Wei YH, Tzeng CR, Kao SH. 2010. Endocrine disruptor, dioxin (TCDD)-induced mitochondrial dysfunction and apoptosis in human trophoblast-like jar cells. *Molecular Human Reproduction* 16(5):361–372.

Ciftci O, Aydin M, Ozdemir I, Vardi N. 2012. Quercetin prevents 2,3,7,8-tetrachlorodibenzo-*p*-dioxin induced testicular damage in rats. *Andrologia* 44:164–173.

Cok I, Donmez MK, Satiroglu MH, Aydinuraz B, Henkelmann B, Shen H, Kotalik J, Schramm KW. 2008. Concentrations of polychlorinated dibenzo-*p*-dioxins (PCDDs), polychlorinated dibenzofurans (PCDFs), and dioxin-like PCBs in adipose tissue of infertile men. *Archives of Environmental Contamination and Toxicology* 55(1):143–152.

Cok I, Durmaz TC, Durmaz E, Satiroglu MH, Kabukcu C. 2010. Determination of organochlorine pesticide and polychlorinated biphenyl levels in adipose tissue of infertile men. *Environmental Monitoring and Assessment* 162(1-4):301–309.

De Felip E, Porpora MG, di Domenico A, Ingelido AM, Cardelli M, Cosmi EV, Donnez J. 2004. Dioxin-like compounds and endometriosis: A study on Italian and Belgian women of reproductive age. *Toxicology Letters* 150(2):203–209.

del Rio Gomez I, Marshall T, Tsai P, Shao YS, Guo YL. 2002. Number of boys born to men exposed to polychlorinated byphenlys [sic]. *Lancet* 360:143–144.

Dhooge W, van Larebeke N, Koppen G, Nelen V, Schoeters G, Vlietinck R, Kaufman JM, Comhaire F, Flemish E, Health Study Group. 2006. Serum dioxin-like activity is associated with reproductive parameters in young men from the general Flemish population. *Environmental Health Perspectives* 114(11):1670–1676.

Dimich-Ward H, Hertzman C, Teschke K, Hershler R, Marion SA, Ostry A, Kelly S. 1996. Reproductive effects of paternal exposure to chlorophenate wood preservatives in the sawmill industry. *Scandinavian Journal of Work, Environment and Health* 22(4):267–273.

Driscoll R, Donovan B, Esswein E, Mattorano D. 1998. Health hazard evaluation report. *US Department of Agriculture* 1–72.

Egeland GM, Sweeney MH, Fingerhut MA, Wille KK, Schnorr TM, Halperin WE. 1994. Total serum testosterone and gonadotropins in workers exposed to dioxin. *American Journal of Epidemiology* 139:272–281.

Ergaz Z, Avgil M, Ornoy A. 2005. Intrauterine growth restriction—etiology and consequences: What do we know about the human situation and experimental animal models? *Reproductive Toxicology* 20(3):301–322.

Eskenazi B, Mocarelli P, Warner M, Samuels S, Vercellini P, Olive D, Needham LL, Patterson DG Jr, Brambilla P, Gavoni N, Casalini S, Panazza S, Turner W, Gerthoux PM. 2002a. Serum dioxin concentrations and endometriosis: A cohort study in Seveso, Italy. *Environmental Health Perspectives* 110(7):629–634.

Eskenazi B, Warner M, Mocarelli P, Samuels S, Needham LL, Patterson DG Jr, Lippman S, Vercellini P, Gerthoux PM, Brambilla P, Olive D. 2002b. Serum dioxin concentrations and menstrual cycle characteristics. *American Journal of Epidemiology* 156(4):383–392.

Eskenazi B, Mocarelli P, Warner M, Chee WY, Gerthoux PM, Samuels S, Needham LL, Patterson DG Jr. 2003. Maternal serum dioxin levels and birth outcomes in women of Seveso, Italy. *Environmental Health Perspectives* 111(7):947–953.

Eskenazi B, Warner M, Marks AR, Samuels S, Gerthoux PM, Vercellini P, Olive DL, Needham L, Patterson D Jr, Mocarelli P. 2005. Serum dioxin concentrations and age at menopause. *Environmental Health Perspectives* 113(7):858–862.

Eskenazi B, Warner M, Samuels S, Young J, Gerthoux PM, Needham L, Patterson D, Olive D, Gavoni N, Vercellini P, Mocarelli P. 2007. Serum dioxin concentrations and risk of uterine leiomyoma in the Seveso Women's Health Study. *American Journal of Epidemiology* 166(1):79–87.

Eskenazi B, Warner M, Marks AR, Samuels S, Needham L, Brambilla P, Mocarelli P. 2010. Serum dioxin concentrations and time to pregnancy. *Epidemiology* 21(2):224–231.

Farr SL, Cooper GS, Cai J, Savitz DA, Sandler DP. 2004. Pesticide use and menstrual cycle characteristics among premenopausal women in the Agricultural Health Study. *American Journal of Epidemiology* 160(12):1194–1204.

Farr SL, Cai J, Savitz DA, Sandler DP, Hoppin JA, Cooper GS. 2006. Pesticide exposure and timing of menopause: The Agricultural Health Study. *American Journal of Epidemiology* 163(8):731–742.

Field B, Kerr C. 1988. Reproductive behaviour and consistent patterns of abnormality in offspring of Vietnam veterans. *Journal of Medical Genetics* 25:819–826.

Fierens S, Mairesse H, Heilier JF, de Burbure C, Focant JF, Eppe G, de Pauw E, Bernard A. 2003. Dioxin/polychlorinated biphenyl body burden, diabetes and endometriosis: Findings in a population-based study in Belgium. *Biomarkers* 8(6):529–534.

Gervais JA, Luukinen B, Buhl K, Stone D. 2008. *2,4-D Technical Fact Sheet.* National Pesticide Information Center, Oregon State University Extension Services.

Greenlee AR, Arbuckle TE, Chyou PH. 2003. Risk factors for female infertility in an agricultural region. *Epidemiology* 14(4):429–436.

Gupta VK, Ali I, Suhas, Saini VK. 2006. Adsorption of 2,4-D and carbofuran pesticides using fertilizer and steel industry wastes. *Journal of Colloid and Interface Science* 299(2):556–563.

Halldorsson TI, Thorsdottir I, Meltzer HM, Strøm M, Olsen SF. 2009. Dioxin-like activity in plasma among Danish pregnant women: Dietary predictors, birth weight and infant development. *Environmental Research* 109(1):22–28.

Hamatani T. 2012. Human spermatozoal RNAs. *Fertility and Sterility* 97(2):275–281.

Heacock H, Hogg R, Marion SA, Hershler R, Teschke K, Dimich-Ward H, Demers P, Kelly S, Ostry A, Hertzman C. 1998. Fertility among a cohort of male sawmill workers exposed to chlorophenate fungicides. *Epidemiology* 9(1):56–60.

Heiden TCK, Struble CA, Rise ML, Hessner MJ, Hutz RJ, Carvan IMJ. 2008. Molecular targets of 2,3,7,8-tetrachlorodibenzo-*p*-dioxin (TCDD) within the zebrafish ovary: Insights into TCDD-induced endocrine disruption and reproductive toxicity. *Reproductive Toxicology* 25(1):47–57.

Heilier JF, Nackers F, Verougstraete V, Tonglet R, Lison D, Donnez J. 2005. Increased dioxin-like compounds in the serum of women with peritoneal endometriosis and deep endometriotic (adenomyotic) nodules. *Fertility and Sterility* 84(2):305–312.

Heilier JF, Donnez J, Defrere S, Van Kerckhove V, Donnez O, Lison D. 2006. Serum dioxin-like compounds and aromatase (CYP19) expression in endometriotic tissues. *Toxicology Letters* 167(3):238–244.

Heilier JF, Donnez J, Nackers F, Rousseau R, Verougstraete V, Rosenkranz K, Donnez O, Grandjean F, Lison D, Tonglet R. 2007. Environmental and host-associated risk factors in endometriosis and deep endometriotic nodules: A matched case-control study. *Environmental Research* 103(1):121–129.

Henriksen GL, Michalek JE, Swaby JA, Rahe AJ. 1996. Serum dioxin, testosterone, and gonadotropins in veterans of Operation Ranch Hand. *Epidemiology* 7(4):352–357.

Hertz-Picciotto I, Samuels SJ. 1988. Incidence of early loss of pregnancy. *New England Journal of Medicine* 319(22):483–484.

Hertz-Picciotto I, Jusko TA, Willman EJ, Baker RJ, Keller JA, Teplin SW, Charles MJ. 2008. A cohort study of in utero polychlorinated biphenyl (PCB) exposures in relation to secondary sex ratio. *Environmental Health: A Global Access Science Source* 7:37.

Huang L, Huang R, Ran XR, Liu HY, Zhang Y, Dai LJ, Li B. 2011. Three-generation experiment showed female C57BL/6J mice drink drainage water containing low level of TCDD-like activity causing high pup mortality. *Journal of Toxicological Sciences* 36(6):713–724.

Igarashi TM, Bruner-Tran KL, Yeaman GR, Lessey BA, Edwards DP, Eisenberg E, Osteen KG. 2005. Reduced expression of progesterone receptor-B in the endometrium of women with endometriosis and in cocultures of endometrial cells exposed to 2,3,7,8-tetrachlorodibenzo-*p*-dioxin. *Fertility and Sterility* 84(1):67–74.

IOM (Institute of Medicine). 1994. *Veterans and Agent Orange: Health Effects of Herbicides Used in Vietnam.* Washington DC: National Academy Press.

IOM. 1996. *Veterans and Agent Orange: Update 1996.* Washington, DC: National Academy Press.

IOM. 1999. *Veterans and Agent Orange: Update 1998.* Washington, DC: National Academy Press.

IOM. 2001. *Veterans and Agent Orange: Update 2000.* Washington, DC: National Academy Press.

IOM. 2003. *Veterans and Agent Orange: Update 2002.* Washington, DC: The National Academies Press.

IOM. 2005. *Veterans and Agent Orange: Update 2004.* Washington, DC: The National Academies Press.

IOM. 2007. *Veterans and Agent Orange: Update 2006.* Washington, DC: The National Academies Press.

IOM. 2009. *Veterans and Agent Orange: Update 2008.* Washington, DC: The National Academies Press.

IOM. 2011. *Veterans and Agent Orange: Update 2010.* Washington, DC: The National Academies Press.

Ishimura R, Kawakami T, Ohsako S, Tohyama C. 2009. Dioxin-induced toxicity on vascular remodeling of the placenta. *Biochemical Pharmacology* 77(4):660–669.

James WH. 2006. Offspring sex ratios at birth as markers of paternal endocrine disruption. *Environmental Research* 100:77–85.

Jirtle RL, Skinner MS. 2007. Environmental epigenomics and disease susceptibility. *Nature Reviews Genetics* 8:253–262.

Joshi SC, Tebrewal P, Sharma A, Sharma P. 2012. Evaluation of toxic effect of 2,4-D (2,4-dichlorophenoxyacetic acid) on fertility and biochemical parameters of male reproductive system of albino rats. *International Journal of Pharmacy and Pharmaceutical Sciences* 4(3):338–342.

Jung NK, Park JY, Park JH, Kim SY, Park JK, Chang WK, Lee HC, Kim SW, Chun SY. 2010. Attenuation of cell cycle progression by 2,3,7,8-tetrachlorodibenzo-*p*-dioxin eliciting ovulatory blockade in gonadotropin-primed immature rats. *Endocrine Journal* 57(10):863–871.

Kallen B. 1988. *Epidemiology of Human Reproduction.* Boca Raton, FL: CRC Press.

Kang HK, Mahan CM, Lee KY, Magee CA, Mather SH, Matanoski G. 2000. Pregnancy outcomes among US women Vietnam veterans. *American Journal of Industrial Medicine* 38(4):447–454.

Karman BN, Basavarajappa MS, Craig ZR, Flaws JA. 2012. 2,3,7,8-Tetrachlorodibenzo-*p*-dioxin activates the aryl hydrocarbon receptor and alters sex steroid hormone secretion without affecting growth of mouse antral follicles in vitro. *Toxicology and Applied Pharmacology* 261:88–96.

Karmaus W, Huang S, Cameron L. 2002. Parental concentration of dichlorodiphenyl dichloroethene and polychlorinated biphenyls in Michigan fish eaters and sex ratio in offspring. *Journal of Occupational and Environmental Medicine* 44(1):8–13.

Kawano M, Kawaji H, Grandjean V, Klani J, Rassoulzadegan M. 2012. Novel small noncoding RNAs in mouse spermatozo, zygotes and early embryos. *PLoS ONE* 7(9):e44542.

Kezios KL, Liu X, Cirillio PM, Kalantzi OI, Wang Y, Petreas MX, Park JS, Bradwin G, Cohn BA, Factor-Litvak P. 2012. Prenatal polychlorinated biphenyl exposure is associated with decreased gestational length but not birth weight: Archived samples from the child health and development studies pregnancy cohort. *Environmental Health: A Global Access Science Source* 11(1):49.

Khorram O, Garthwaite M, Golos T. 2002. Uterine and ovarian aryl hydrocarbon receptor (AHR) and aryl hydrocarbon receptor nuclear translocator (ARNT) mRNA expression in benign and malignant gynaecological conditions. *Molecular Human Reproduction* 8(1):75–80.

Kline J, Stein Z, Susser M. 1989. *Conception to birth: Epidemiology of prenatal development.* New York: Oxford University Press.

Knobil E, Neill JD, Greenwald GS, Markert CL, Pfaff DW, eds. 1994. *The Physiology of Reproduction.* New York: Raven Press.

Konishi K, Sasaki S, Kato S, Ban S, Washino N, Kajiwara J, Todaka T, Hirakawa H, Hori T, Yasutake D, Kishi R. 2009. Prenatal exposure to PCDDs/PCDFs and dioxin-like PCBs in relation to birth weight. *Environmental Research* 109(7):906–913.

Kramer JA, Krawetz SA. 1997. RNA in spermatozoa: Implications for the alternative haploid genome. *Molecular Human Reproduction* 3(6):473–478.

Krawetz SA. 2005. Paternal contribution: New insights and future challenges. *Nature Reviews Genetics* 6:633–642.

Krawetz SA, Kruger A, Lalancette C, Tagett R, Anton E, Draghici S, Diamond MP. 2011. A survey of small RNAs in human sperm. *Human Reproduction* 26(12):3401–3412.

Krüger T, Spanò M, Long M, Eleuteri P, Rescia M, Hjelmborg PS, Manicardi GC, Bizzaro D, Giwercman A, Toft G, Bonde JP, Bonefeld-Jorgensen EC. 2008. Xenobiotic activity in serum and sperm chromatin integrity in European and Inuit populations. *Molecular Reproduction and Development* 75:669–680.

Kuratsune M, Yoshimura T, Matsuzaka J, A. Y. 1972. Epidemiologic study on Yusho, a poisoning caused by ingestion of rice oil contaminated with a commercial brand of polychlorinated biphenyls. *Environmental Health Perspectives* 1:119–128.

La Rocca C, Alivernini S, Badiali M, Cornoldi A, Iacovella N, Silvestroni L, Spera G, Turrio-Baldassarri L. 2008. TEQs and body burden for PCDDs, PCDFs, and dioxin-like PCBs in human adipose tissue. *Chemosphere* 73(1):92–96.

Lambertino A, Turyk M, Anderson H, Freels S, Persky V. 2011. Uterine leiomyomata in a cohort of Great Lakes sport fish consumers. *Environmental Research* 111(4):565–572.

Larsen SB, Joffe M, Bonde JP. 1998. Time to pregnancy and exposure to pesticides in Danish farmers. *Occupational and Environmental Medicine* 55(4):278–283.

Lawson CC, Schnorr TM, Whelan EA, Deddens JA, Dankovic DA, Piacitelli LA, Sweeney MH, Connally LB. 2004. Paternal occupational exposure to 2,3,7,8-tetrachlorodibenzo-*p*-dioxin and birth outcomes of offspring: Birth weight, preterm delivery, and birth defects. *Environmental Health Perspectives* 112(14):1403–1408.

Lerda D, Rizzi R. 1991. Study of reproductive function in persons occupationally exposed to 2,4-dichlorophenoxyacetic acid (2,4-D). *Mutation Research* 262(1):47–50.

Li MQ, Hou XF, Lv SJ, Meng YH, W XQ, Tang, CL, Li DJ. 2011. CD82 gene suppression in endometrial stromal cells leads to increase of the cell invasiveness in the endometriotic milieu. *Journal of Molecular Endocrinology* 47:195–208.

Mathur PM, D'Cruz SC. 2011. The effect of environmental contaminants on testicular function. *Asian Journal of Andrology* 13:585–591.

Mayani A, Barel S, Soback S, Almagor M. 1997. Dioxin concentrations in women with endometriosis. *Human Reproduction* 12(2):373–375.

Michalek JE, Albanese RA, Wolfe WH. 1998a. *Project Ranch Hand II: An Epidemiologic Investigation of Health Effects in Air Force Personnel Following Exposure to Herbicides—Reproductive Outcome Update.* US Department of Commerce, National Technical Information Service. Report number AFRL-HE-BR-TR-1998-0073.

Michalek JE, Rahe AJ, Boyle CA. 1998b. Paternal dioxin, preterm birth, intrauterine growth retardation, and infant death. *Epidemiology* 9(2):161–167.

Mocarelli P, Brambilla P, Gerthoux PM, Patterson DG Jr, Needham LL. 1996. Change in sex ratio with exposure to dioxin. *Lancet* 348(9024):409.

Mocarelli P, Gerthoux PM, Ferrari E, Patterson DG Jr, Kieszak SM, Brambilla P, Vincoli N, Signorini S, Tramacere P, Carreri V, Sampson EJ, Turner WE, Needham LL. 2000. Paternal concentrations of dioxin and sex ratio of offspring. *Lancet* 355:1858–1863.

Mocarelli P, Gerthoux PM, Patterson DG Jr, Milani S, Limonta G, Bertona M, Signorini S, Tramacere P, Colombo L, Crespi C, Brambilla P, Sarto C, Carreri V, Sampson EJ, Turner WE, Needham LL. 2008. Dioxin exposure, from infancy through puberty, produces endocrine disruption and affects human semen quality. *Environmental Health Perspectives* 116(1):70–77.

Mose T, Mathiesen L, Karttunen V, Nielsen JKS, Sieppi E, Kummu M, Mørck TA, Myöhänen K, Partanen H, Vähäkangas K, Knudsen LE, Myllynen P. 2012. Meta-analysis of data from human ex vivo placental perfusion studies on genotoxic and immunotoxic agents within the integrated European project NewGeneris. *Placenta* 33:433–439

Moses M, Lilis R, Crow KD, Thornton J, Fischbein A, Anderson HA, Selikoff IJ. 1984. Health status of workers with past exposure to 2,3,7,8-tetrachlorodibenzo-*p*-dioxin in the manufacture of 2,4,5-trichlorophenoxyacetic acid: Comparison of findings with and without chloracne. *American Journal of Industrial Medicine* 5(3):161–182.

Moshammer H, Neuberger M. 2000. Sex ratio in the children of the Austrian chloracne cohort. *Lancet* 356(9237):1271–1272.

Munro IC, Carlo GL, Orr JC, Sund KG, Wilson RD, Kennepohl E, Lynch BS, Jablinske M, Lee NL. 1992. A comprehensive integrated review and evaluation of the scientific evidence relating to the safety of the herbicide 2,4-D. *American College of Toxicology* 11:559–664.

Naville D, Rebourcet D, Chauvin MA, Vega N, Jalabert A, Vigier M, Loizon E, Bégeot M, Magueresse-Battistoni BL. 2011. Direct and indirect impact of 2,3,7,8-tetrachlorodibenzo-*p*-dioxin (TCDD) on adult mouse Leydig cells: An in vitro study. *Toxicology Letters* 207:251–257.

NICHD (National Institute of Child Health and Human Development). 2007. *Endometriosis.* National Institute of Health. http://www.nichd.nih.gov/health/topics/endometriosis.cfm (accessed December 17, 2008).

Nishijo M, Tawara K, Nakagawa H, Honda R, Kido T, Nishijo H, Saito S. 2008. 2,3,7,8-tetrachlorodibenzo-*p*-dioxin in maternal breast milk and newborn head circumference. *Journal of Exposure Science and Environmental Epidemiology* 18(3):246–251.

Nishijo M, Tai PT, Nakagawa H, Maruzeni S, Anh NTN, van Luong H, Anh TH, Honda R, Morikawa Y, Kido T, Nishijo H. 2012. Impact of perinatal dioxin exposure on infant growth: A cross-sectional and longitudinal studies in dioxin-contaminated areas in Vietnam. *PLoS ONE* 7(7):e40273.

NRC (National Research Council). 2003. *Improving Birth Outcomes: Meeting the Challenge in the Developing World.* Washington, DC: The National Academies Press.

Niskar AS, Needham LL, Rubin C, Turner WE, Martin CA, Patterson DG Jr, Hasty L, Wong LY, Marcus M. 2009. Serum dioxins, polychlorinated biphenyls, and endometriosis: A case-control study in Atlanta. *Chemosphere* 74(7):944–949.

Oh E, Lee E, Im H, Kang HS, Jung WW, Won NH, Kim EM, Sul D. 2005. Evaluation of immuno- and reproductive toxicities and association between immunotoxicological and genotoxicological parameters in waste incineration workers. *Toxicology* 210(1):65–80.

Oikawa K, Ohbayashi T, Mimura J, Fujii-Kuriyama Y, Teshima S, Rokutan K, Mukai K, Kuroda M. 2002. Dioxin stimulates synthesis and secretion of IgE-dependent histamine-releasing factor. *Biochemical and Biophysical Research Communications* 290(3):984–987.

Oikawa K, Kosugi Y, Ohbayashi T, Kameta A, Isaka K, Takayama M, Kuroda M, Mukai K. 2003. Increased expression of IgE-dependent histamine-releasing factor in endometriotic implants. *Journal of Pathology* 199(3):318–323.

Patandin S, Koopman-Esseboom C, de Ridder MA, Weisglas-Kuperus N, Sauer PJ. 1998. Effects of environmental exposure to polychlorinated biphenyls and dioxins on birth size and growth in Dutch children. *Pediatric Research* 44(4):538–545.

Pauwels A, Schepens PJC, Hooghe TD, Delbeke L, Dhont M, Brouwer A, Weyler J. 2001. The risk of endometriosis and exposure to dioxins and polychlorinated biphenyls: A case-control study of infertile women. *Human Reproduction* 16(10):2050–2055.

Peltier MR. 2003. Immunology of term and preterm labor. *Reproductive Biology and Endocrinology* 1:122–132.

Petroff BK, Valdez KE, Brown SB, Piasecka J, Albertini DF. 2011. The aryl hydrocarbon receptor agonist 2,3,7,8-tetrachloro-dibenzo-*p*-dioxin (TCDD) alters early embryonic development in a rat IVF exposure model. *Reproductive Toxicology* 32:286–292.

Polsky JY, Aronson KJ, Heaton JP, Adams MA. 2007. Pesticides and polychlorinated biphenyls as potential risk factors for erectile dysfunction. *Journal of Andrology* 28(1):28–37.

Porpora MG, Ingelido AM, di Domenico A, Ferro A, Crobu M, Pallante D, Cardelli M, Cosmi EV, De Felip E. 2006. Increased levels of polychlorobiphenyls in Italian women with endometriosis. *Chemosphere* 63(8):1361–1367.

Porpora MG, Medda E, Abballe A, Bolli S, De Angelis I, di Domenico A, Ferro A, Ingelido AM, Maggi A, Panici PB, De Felip E. 2009. Endometriosis and organochlorinated environmental pollutants: A case-control study on Italian women of reproductive age. *Environmental Health Perspectives* 117(7):1070–1075.

Revich B, Aksel E, Ushakova T, Ivanova I, Zuchenko N, Lyuev N, Brodsky B, Sotsov Y. 2001. Dioxin exposure and public health in Chapaevsk, Russia. *Chemosphere* 43(4-7):951–966.

Rier SE, Martin DC, Bowman RE, Dmowski WP, Becker JL. 1993. Endometriosis in rhesus monkeys (*Macaca mulatta*) following chronic exposure to 2,3,7,8-tetrachlorodibenzo-*p*-dioxin. *Fundamental and Applied Toxicology* 21(4):433–441.

Romo A, Carceller R, Tobajas J. 2009. Intrauterine growth retardation (IUGR): Epidemiology and etiology. *Pediatric Endocrinology Reviews* 6(Suppl 3):332–336.

Ryan JJ, Amirova Z, Carrier G. 2002. Sex ratios of children of Russian pesticide producers exposed to dioxin. *Environmental Health Perspectives* 110(11):A699–A701.

Sagiv SK, Tolbert PE, Altshul LM, Korrick SA. 2007. Organochlorine exposures during pregnancy and infant size at birth. *Epidemiology* 18(1):120–129.

Savitz DA, Arbuckle A, Kaczor D, Curtis KM. 1997. Male pesticide exposure and pregnancy outcome. *American Journal of Epidemiology* 146(12):1025–1036.

Schnorr TM, Lawson CC, Whelan EA, Dankovic DA, Deddens JA, Piacitelli LA, Reefhuis J, Sweeney MH, Connally LB, Fingerhut MA. 2001. Spontaneous abortion, sex ratio, and paternal occupational exposure to 2,3,7,8-tetrachlorodibenzo-*p*-dioxin. *Environmental Health Perspectives* 109(11):1127–1132.

Schwartz LS. 1998. *Health Problems of Women Veterans of the Vietnam War.* Doctoral dissertation, Yale University.

Singh MN, Stringfellow HF, Taylor SE, Ashton KM, Ahmad M, Abdo KR, El-Agnaf OMA, Martin-Hirsch PL, Martin FL. 2008. Elevated expression of CYP1A1 and gamma–SYNUCLEIN in human ectopic (ovarian) endometriosis compared with eutopic endometrium. *Molecular Human Reproduction* 14(11):655–663.

Smith AH, Fisher DO, Pearce N, Chapman CJ. 1982. Congenital defects and miscarriages among New Zealand 2,4,5-T sprayers. *Archives of Environmental Health* 37:197–200.

Sönmez M, Türk G, Çeribaş AO, Sakin F, Ateşşahin A. 2011. Attenuating effect of lycopene and ellagic acid on 2,3,7, 8-tetrachlorodibenzo-*p*-dioxin-induced spermiotoxicity and testicular apoptosis. *Drug and Chemical Toxicology* 34(4):347–356.

Staessen JA, Nawrot T, Hond ED, Thijs L, Fagard R, Hoppenbrouwers K, Koppen G, Nelen V, Schoeters G, Vanderschueren D, Van Hecke E, Verschaeve L, Vlietinck R, Roels HA. 2001. Renal function, cytogenetic measurements, and sexual development in adolescents in relation to environmental pollutants: A feasibility study of biomarkers. *Lancet* 357(9269):1660–1669. [Comment in *Lancet* 2001. 358(9295):1816–1817.]

Stejskalova L, Vecerova L, Perez LM, Vrzal R, Dvorak Z, Nachtigal P, Pavek P. 2011. Aryl hydrocarbon receptor and aryl hydrocarbon nuclear translocator expression in human and rat placentas and transcription activity in human trophoblast cultures. *Toxicological Sciences* 123(1):26–36.

Stellman SD, Stellman JM, Sommer JF Jr. 1988. Health and reproductive outcomes among American Legionnaires in relation to combat and herbicide exposure in Vietnam. *Environmental Research* 47:150–174.

Stockbauer JW, Hoffman RE, Schramm WF, Edmonds LD. 1988. Reproductive outcomes of mothers with potential exposure to 2,3,7,8-tetrachlorodibenzo-*p*-dioxin. *American Journal of Epidemiology* 128:410–419.

Suh N, Blelloch R. 2011. Small RNAs in early mammalian development: From gametes to gastrulation. *Development* 138:1653–1661.

Suskind RR, Hertzberg VS. 1984. Human health effects of 2,4,5-T and its toxic contaminants. *Journal of the American Medical Association* 251:2372–2380.

Svechnikov K, Izzo G, Landreh L, Weisser J, Söder O. 2010. Endocrine disruptors and Leydig cell function. *Journal of Biomedicine and Biotechnology* (Article ID 684504, 10 pp).

Swan SH, Kruse RL, Liu F, Barr DB, Drobnis EZ, Redmon JB, Wang C, Brazil C, Overstreet JW; Study for Future Families Research Group. 2003. Semen quality in relation to biomarkers of pesticide exposure. *Environmental Health Perspectives* 111(12):1478–1484.

Tas S, Lauwerys R, Lison D. 1996. Occupational hazards for the male reproductive system. *Critical Reviews in Toxicology* 26(3):261–307.

Tawara K, Nishijo M, Honda R, Maruzeni S, Seto T, Kido T, Saito S, Nakagawa H. 2009. Effects of maternal dioxin exposure on newborn size at birth among Japanese mother-infant pairs. *Environmental Health and Preventive Medicine* 14(2):88–95.

Toft G, Long M, Kruger T, Hjelmborg PS, Bonde JP, Rignell-Hydbom A, Tyrkiel E, Hagmar L, Giwercman A, Spano M, Bizzaro D, Pedersen HS, Lesovoy V, Ludwicki JK, Bonefeld-Jorgensen EC. 2007. Semen quality in relation to xenohormone and dioxin-like serum activity among Inuits and three European populations. *Environmental Health Perspectives* 115(Suppl 1):15–20.

Townsend JC, Bodner KM, Van Peenen PFD, Olson RD, Cook RR. 1982. Survey of reproductive events of wives of employees exposed to chlorinated dioxins. *American Journal of Epidemiology* 115:695–713.

Tsang H, Cheung TY, Kodithuwakku SP, Chai J, Yeung WSB, Wong CKC, Lee KF. 2012. 2,3,7,8-tetrachlorodibenzo-*p*-dioxin (TCDD) suppresses spheroids attachment on endometrial epithelial cells through the down-regulation of the Wnt-signaling pathway. *Reproductive Toxicology* 33:60–66.

Tsuchiya M, Tsukino H, Iwasaki M, Sasaki H, Tanaka T, Katoh T, Patterson DG Jr, Turner W, Needham L, Tsugane S. 2007. Interaction between cytochrome P450 gene polymorphisms and serum organochlorine TEQ levels in the risk of endometriosis. *Molecular Human Reproduction* 13(6):399–404.

Tsukimori K, Tokunaga S, Shibata S, Uchi H, Nakayama D, Ishimaru T, Nakano H, Wake N, Yoshimura T, Furue M. 2008. Long-term effects of polychlorinated biphenyls and dioxins on pregnancy outcomes in women affected by the Yusho incident. *Environmental Health Perspectives* 116(5):626–630.

Tsukimori K, Yasukawa F, Uchi H, Furue M, Morokuma S. 2012a. Letter to the editor: Sex ratio in two generations of the Yusho cohort. *Epidemiology* 23(2):349–350.

Tsukimori K, Uchi H, Mitoma C, Yasukawa F, Chiba T, Todaka T, Kajiwara J, Yoshimura T, Hirata T, Fukushima K, Wake N, Furue M. 2012b. Maternal exposure to high levels of dioxins in relation to birth weight in women affected by Yusho disease. *Environment International* 38 (1):79–86.

Tuyet LTN, Johansson A. 2001. Impact of chemical warfare with Agent Orange on women's reproductive lives in Vietnam: A pilot study. *Reproductive Health Matters* 9(18):156–164.

UNICEF (United Nations Children's Fund). 2004. *Low Birthweight: Country, Regional, and Global Estimates.* New York: UNICEF.

van den Berg M, Birnbaum LS, Denison M, De Vito M, Farland W, Feeley M, Fiedler H, Hakansson H, Hanberg A, Haws L, Rose M, Safe S, Schrenk D, Tohyama C, Tritscher A, Tuomisto J, Tysklind M, Walker N, Peterson RE, 2006. The 2005 World Health Organization reevaluation of human and mammalian toxic equivalency factors for dioxins and dioxin-like compounds. *Toxicological Sciences* 93(2):223–241.

Vartiainen T, Jaakkola JJ, Saarikoski S, Tuomisto J. 1998. Birth weight and sex of children and the correlation to the body burden of PCDDs/PCDFs and PCBs of the mother. *Environmental Health Perspectives* 106(2):61–66.

Wang J, Liu X, Li T, Liu C, Zhao Y. 2011. Increased hepatic Igf2 gene expression involves C/EBP in TCDD-induced teratogenesis in rats. *Reproductive Toxicology* 32:313–321.

Warner M, Samuels S, Mocarelli P, Gerthoux PM, Needham L, Patterson DG Jr, Eskenazi B. 2004. Serum dioxin concentrations and age at menarche. *Environmental Health Perspectives* 112(13):1289–1292.

Warner M, Eskenazi B, Olive DL, Samuels S, Quick-Miles S, Vercellini P, Gerthoux PM, Needham L, Patterson DG Jr, Mocarelli P. 2007. Serum dioxin concentrations and quality of ovarian function in women of Seveso. *Environmental Health Perspectives* 115(3):336–340.

Wilcox AJ. 2001. On the importance—and the unimportance—of birthweight. *International Journal of Epidemiology* 30:1233–1241.

Wilcox AJ, Weinberg CR, O'Connor JF, Baird DD, Schlatterer JP, Canfield RE, Armstrong EG, Nisula BC. 1988. Incidence of early pregnancy loss. *New England Journal of Medicine* 319:189–194.

Willing C, Peich M, Danescu A, Kehlen A, Fowler PA, Hombach-Klonisch S. 2011. Estrogen-independent actions of environmentally relevant AhR-agonists in human endometrial epithelial cells. *Molecular Human Reproduction* 17(2):115–126.

Wolfe WH, Michalek JE, Miner JC, Rahe AJ, Moore CA, Needham LL, Patterson DG Jr. 1995. Paternal serum dioxin and reproductive outcomes among veterans of Operation Ranch Hand. *Epidemiology* 6:17–22.

Wong E, Cheng CY. 2011. Impacts of environmental toxicants on male reproductive dysfunction. *Cell Press* 32(5):290–299.

Wu CH, Guo CY, Yang JG, Tsai HD, Chang YJ, Tsai PC, Hsu CC, Kuo PL. 2012. Polymorphisms of dioxin receptor complex components and detoxification-related genes jointly confer susceptibility to advanced-stage endometriosis in the Taiwanese Han population. *American Journal of Reproductive Immunology* 67:160–168.

Yang CY, Huang TS, Lin KC, Kuo P, Tsai PC, Guo YL. 2011. Menstrual effects among women exposed to polychlorinated biphenyls and dibenzofurans. *Environmental Research* 111(2):288–294.

Yen SC, Jaffe RB. 1991. *Reproductive Endocrinology.* Philadelphia: W.B. Saunders Company.

Yin HP, Xu JP, Zhou XQ, Wang Y. 2012. Effects of vitamin E on reproductive hormones and testis structure in chronic dioxin-treated mice. *Toxicology and Industrial Health* 28(2):152–161.

Yoshimura T, Kaneko S, Hayabuchi H. 2001. Sex ratio in offspring of those affected by dioxin and dioxin-like compounds: The Yusho, Seveso, and Yucheng incidents. *Occupational and Environmental Medicine* 58(8):540–541.

Yoshizawa K, Brix AE, Sells DM, Jokinen MP, Wyde M, Orzech DP, Kissling GE, Walker NJ, Nyska A. 2009. Reproductive lesions in female Harlan Sprague-Dawley rats following two-year oral treatment with dioxin and dioxin-like compounds. *Toxicologic Pathology* 37(7):921–937.

Yu J, Wang Y, Zhou WH, Wang L, He YY, Li DJ. 2008. Combination of estrogen and dioxin is involved in the pathogenesis of endometriosis by promoting chemokine secretion and invasion of endometrial stromal cells. *Human Reproduction* 23(7):1614–1626.

Zhao D, Lebovic DI, Taylor RN. 2002. Long-term progestin treatment inhibits RANTES (regulated on activation, normal T cell expressed and secreted) gene expression in human endometrial stromal cells. *Journal of Clinical Endocrinology and Metabolism* 87(6):2514–2519.

10

Effects on Future Generations

Chapter Overview

Based on new evidence and a review of prior studies, the committee for Update 2012 *did not find any new significant associations between the relevant exposures and adverse outcomes in future generations. Current evidence supports the findings of earlier studies that*

- *No adverse outcomes in future generations had sufficient evidence of an association with the chemicals of interest.*
- *There is limited or suggestive evidence of an association between the chemicals of interest and spina bifida.*
- *There is inadequate or insufficient evidence to determine whether there is an association between parental exposure to the chemicals of interest and birth defects other than spina bifida, childhood cancers, or disease in their children as they mature or in later generations.*

The original report in this series, *Veterans and Agent Orange: Health Effects of Herbicides Used in Vietnam* (*VAO*; IOM, 1994) contained a single chapter devoted to reproductive outcomes, as was the case through the publication of *Veterans and Agent Orange: Update 2000*, hereafter referred to as *Update 2000* (IOM, 2001). (Analogous shortened names are used to refer to the updates for 1996, 1998, 2002, 2004, 2006, 2008, and 2010 [IOM, 1996, 1999, 2003, 2005, 2007, 2009, 2011]). In *Update 2002*, the chapter's concerns were extended to include consideration of developmental effects. In *Update 2008*, the chapter also addressed the possibility that adverse effects of exposure to the chemicals in the herbicides used by the military in Vietnam might extend beyond the children of exposed people and affect future generations.

The committee for the current update decided to divide the material into two separate chapters. Chapter 9 contains information on reproductive outcomes affecting the parental generation and the course of gestation. The current chapter focuses and expands on issues related to possible adverse effects in future generations—both the children of Vietnam veterans and their offspring in turn. Since its inception, the VAO series has considered birth defects (primarily limited to problems detectable at birth or within the first year of life) and childhood cancers (usually restricted to particular cancers that characteristically appear in infants and children and are diagnosed before the age of 18 years). Because of concerns increasingly expressed by veterans and corresponding interest in the Department of Veterans Affairs, in *Update 2010* the attention of VAO committees was extended to include all types of medical issues occurring in the veterans' children regardless of age and to include such problems in successive generations. It is hoped that by devoting a separate chapter to the possible "post-birth" problems of the progeny of Vietnam veterans, we can more clearly present the evidence for maternally and paternally mediated effects separately because the underlying biology is quite distinct in the two cases.

This chapter summarizes the scientific literature published since *Update 2010* that investigated associations between parental exposure to herbicides and adverse effects on offspring, including future generations, throughout their life spans. The epidemiologic literature considered in this chapter includes studies of a broad spectrum of effects in children of Vietnam veterans or other populations occupationally or environmentally exposed to the herbicides sprayed in Vietnam or to the contaminant 2,3,7,8-tetrachlorodibenzo-*p*-dioxin (TCDD). Because some polychlorinated biphenyls (PCBs), some polychlorinated dibenzofurans (PCDFs), and some polychlorinated dibenzodioxins (PCDDs) other than TCDD have dioxin-like biologic activity, studies of populations exposed to PCBs or PCDFs were reviewed if their results were presented in terms of TCDD toxic equivalents (TEQs). Although all studies reporting TEQs based on PCBs were reviewed, studies that reported TEQs based only on mono-ortho PCBs (which are PCBs 105, 114, 118, 123, 156, 157, 167, and 189) were given very limited consideration because mono-ortho PCBs typically contribute less than 10% to total TEQs, based on the World Health Organization (WHO) revised toxicity equivalency factors of 2005 (La Rocca et al., 2008; van den Berg et al., 2006). Although some multigenerational studies have been conducted on laboratory animals, to date there have not been human studies of descendants beyond the first generation for the chemicals of interest (COIs).

Because most Vietnam veterans are men, the primary focus of the VAO series has been on potential adverse effects of herbicide exposure on men. For non-reproductive outcomes, the etiologic importance of the exposed person's sex does not play a dominant role; but for the possible transmission of adverse effects to future generations, it is critically important, from the perspective of the biologic mechanism, which parent experienced the exposure in question. About 8,000 women served in Vietnam (H. Kang, US Department of Veterans Affairs, personal communication, December 14, 2000), so adverse outcomes in the offspring of female Vietnam veterans are a concern. Exposure scenarios in human populations and experimental animals studied differ in their applicability to our population of concern according to whether the exposed parent was male or female, and it is necessary to evaluate the effects of maternal and paternal exposure separately. As will be noted repeatedly, however, almost all Vietnam veterans were men, but the amount of research providing reliable information on the consequences of paternal exposure is extremely sparse not only for the COIs in the VAO report series but also for the full array of environmental agents that may pose threats to the health of future generations.

In addition, for published epidemiologic or experimental results to be fully relevant to evaluation of the plausibility of reproductive effects in Vietnam veterans, whether female or male, the veterans' exposure needs to have occurred before conception. With the possible exception of female veterans who became pregnant while serving in Vietnam, pregnancies that might have been affected occurred after deployment, when primary exposure had ceased. In the case of pregnancies of women who have previously been substantially exposed to the lipophilic dioxins, direct exposure of the fetus throughout gestation is possible owing to mobilization of toxicants from the mother's adipose tissue. The chapter also addresses the biologic plausibility of adverse effects on offspring mediated by male veterans through semen transmission during pregnancies that occurred after deployment.

The categories of association and the approach to categorizing the health outcomes are discussed in Chapters 1 and 2. To reduce repetition throughout the report, Chapter 6 characterizes the study population and presents design information on new publications that report findings on multiple health outcomes or that revisit study populations considered in earlier updates.

BIOLOGIC PLAUSIBILITY OF EFFECTS IN FUTURE GENERATIONS

There have been few offspring studies of the four herbicides in question, particularly picloram and cacodylic acid, and those studies generally have shown toxicity only at very high doses, so the preponderance of the following discussion concerns TCDD, which outside controlled experimental circumstances usually occurred in a mixture of dioxins (dioxin congeners in addition to TCDD).

Because TCDD is stored in fat tissue and has a long biologic half-life, internal exposure at generally constant concentrations may continue after episodic, high-level exposure to external sources has ceased. If a person had high exposure, there may still be large amounts of dioxins stored in fat tissue, which may be mobilized, particularly at times of weight loss. That would not be expected to be the case for nonlipophilic chemicals, such as cacodylic acid.

The mechanisms of possible effects on offspring differ greatly for men and women exposed to the COIs during their service in Vietnam. A father's (paternal) contribution to adverse effects in his offspring is limited mainly to the contents of the fertilizing sperm, which had long been believed to consist almost exclusively of greatly condensed, transcriptionally inert deoxyribonucleic acid (DNA) for half the paternal genome (a haploid set of chromosomes). As a result, it was thought that any paternally-derived damage to the embryo or offspring would have to arise from changes in sequence or arrangement of the sperm's DNA; the fact that dioxins have not been shown to be genotoxic fostered skepticism that adverse outcomes in offspring could arise from paternal exposure to the COIs. More recently, however, it has been recognized that sperm also carry a considerable collection of ribonucleic acid (RNA) fragments (Kramer and Krawetz, 1997; Krawetz et al., 2011). Although ribosomal (rRNAs) and messenger RNAs (mRNAs) have been detected in mature sperm, as yet, any roles they may play in fertilization or development have not been delineated. Functionality has been demonstrated for several of the small RNAs found in mature sperm (Krawetz, 2005); they have been found to play critical roles in early embryonic development (Hamatani, 2012; Suh and Blelloch, 2011) and epigenetic determinations (Kawano et al., 2012). Epigenetic effects are ones that result in permanent (heritable) changes in gene expression without a change in DNA sequence arising from modification to DNA (usually involving methylation) or to other cellular components such as histones and RNAs (Jirtle and Skinner, 2007). Alterations in DNA expression arising from epigenetic modification of an individual's somatic cell lines may not be manifested for long periods of time. In epigenetic transgenerational inheritance, an alteration in the germ line must be maintained for at least three generations following in utero exposures and for at least two generations after adult exposures (Jirtle and Skinner, 2007), so this process requires exposure precisely at the time in germline development when epigenetic programming is being established (Skinner et al., 2010). Therefore, paternally-derived adverse outcomes in offspring associated with exposure to the COIs could be mediated not just by genetic alterations of DNA, but also by epigenetic modifications to components of sperm in addition to their DNA (Krawetz, 2005). There is also a more remote possibility, if body burden were sufficiently high, that TCDD exposure might occur through absorption of seminal plasma through the vaginal wall, which could affect gestating offspring in an otherwise unexposed mother.

A mother's (maternal) contribution to a pregnancy and offspring is obviously more extensive, and any damage to the resulting offspring or later generations can result from epigenetic changes in the egg or from direct effects of exposure on the fetus during gestation and on the neonate during lactation. Herein, we review biologic plausibility and relevant data on female veterans and male veterans separately because the underlying pathways for adverse effects in offspring are so different.

Paternal Preconception and Postconception Exposure

There is particular interest in the possibility of paternally-mediated effects on offspring and later generations because the vast majority of Vietnam veterans are male. There are two feasible pathways through which TCDD and other COIs from paternal exposures could lead to developmental and later life effects in offspring and potentially future generations. One involves direct alterations in the paternal fertilizing sperm cells that transmit adverse effects to resulting offspring through genetic or epigenetic mechanisms as delineated in Chapter 4. Those effects would occur before conception. The other involves transmission of the contaminants to a female partner through seminal fluid during an established pregnancy, that is, after conception.

Preconception Exposure

There is no evidence that dioxins can mutate DNA sequences; thus, genetic changes in sperm genes—as has been shown in connection with irradiation or the anticancer drug cyclophosphamide (Codrington et al., 2004)—due to preconception exposures to TCDD are not likely. There is potential for TCDD to alter sperm cells of adults before fertilization through epigenetic pathways. The sperm epigenome is distinct from that of the egg (oocyte) or somatic cells (all other nongamete cells in the body). The mature sperm cell has less global methylation than somatic cells and unique DNA methylation marks (particularly on paternally imprinted genes) that put the gametes in a pluripotent state before fertilization (Hales et al., 2011). Chemical alterations of methylation foci in DNA of adult sperm have the potential to contribute to permanent effects in offspring, as demonstrated in fetal alcohol syndrome (Jenkins and Carrell, 2012a; Ouko et al., 2009). During spermatogenesis in the adult, most sperm histones are replaced by protamines, which render the sperm transcriptionally quiescent and permit extensive DNA compaction. But recent evidence has shown that some core histones are retained in human sperm at sites that are important during embryo development, so their perturbation by exogenous chemicals remains a possibility (Hammoud, et al., 2009). That is particularly important because although genome-wide DNA demethylation occurs in paternal DNA after-fertilization and would erase most sites that have been reprogrammed by chemicals, histone modification patterns are retained and thus may transmit chemical-induced alterations across generations (Puri et al., 2010). Finally, despite the exclusion of almost all cytoplasm, mature sperm have been found to carry a diverse spectrum of RNAs, including mRNAs, rRNAs, and noncoding RNAs, which may affect the developing embryo (Hamatani, 2012; Krawetz, 2005; Krawetz et al., 2011; Suh and Blelloch, 2011). It has recently been demonstrated that small RNAs of paternal origin may direct epigenetic modifications during embryo development and lead to changes in phenotype later in life (Hales et al., 2011). Heavy metals have been shown to interact with sperm's nuclear proteins, and this mechanism is suspected to be a basis of paternally-mediated lead toxicity (Quintanilla-Vega et al., 2000). Disturbances in the establishment of the epigenetic marks in mature sperm may change cell fate in the early embryo and have effects throughout development and postnatal life (Jenkins and Carrell, 2012b). Direct evidence of dioxin-mediated changes in the epigenome of mature sperm is not available, but dioxins have been shown to modify DNA methylation in microRNAs in somatic cells (Hou et al., 2011), so the pathway is biologically plausible.

Postconception Exposure

Contaminants such as TCDD that are present in the tissues and blood of exposed males can be transported as parent compounds or metabolites into seminal fluid, the noncellular component of the ejaculate. Typically, concentrations of contaminants in seminal fluid are lower than those in serum, but direct assessments of ratios of serum to seminal fluid in TCDD have not been reported. Seminal-fluid contaminants can be transmitted to a female during sexual intercourse and be absorbed through the vaginal wall; if concentrations are high, they will potentially affect a current pregnancy (Chapin et al, 2004; Klemmt and Scialli, 2005). TCDD and other persistent organic pollutants have been identified and quantified in seminal plasma of exposed men, including Vietnam veterans (Schecter et al., 1996; Schlebusch et al., 1989; Stachel et al., 1989); thus, this transmission route is theoretically possible. In the Schecter (1996) study, serum TCDD was measured in 50 Vietnam veterans from Michigan who had confirmed or self-reported potential for Agent Orange exposure and had blood drawn an average of 26 years after the possible exposure. Of those, 6 had TCDD greater than 20 parts per trillion (ppt) on a lipid-adjusted basis, and this supports the idea that some veterans did have high initial exposures. A subgroup of 17 men contributed semen at the time of blood draw, and dioxin congeners were analyzed in three randomly pooled samples—a process necessary to provide sufficient volume for chemical analysis. Although measured concentrations were very low, the results documented the existence of dioxins and dibenzofurans in seminal plasma of the veterans long after possible Agent Orange exposure. Because results on serum and semen concentrations could not be linked for individual veterans and because it is unknown whether any of the subjects who had high serum dioxin concentrations after 26 years contributed semen for the seminal-fluid measurements, the value of this information is slight. Seminal-fluid concentrations of TCDD and related chemicals closer to the period of exposure in Vietnam have not been determined, so it is not possible to assess the clinical consequences of this exposure route for female partners and gestating offspring. Banked Operation Ranch Hand specimens, however, might provide a valuable resource for comparing TCDD concentrations in serum and seminal fluid.

Furthermore, despite the potential for a seminal-fluid route of exposure, the critical question of dose sufficiency remains unanswered, that is, Could absorbed TCDD concentrations be high enough to transmit adverse effects in the fetus? To that end, one must take into account several factors: the volume of seminal plasma is relatively low (1–5 mL); because of leakage, only a fraction of seminal constituents are absorbed across the vaginal wall; and dilution of absorbed chemicals in the female bloodstream (that is, in a high volume) before transmission across the placenta is estimated at 3 orders of magnitude or more (Klemmt and Scially, 2005), and this reduces a serum concentration of 20 ppt to a scale of parts per quadrillion (10^{-15}). Although studies to address the issue directly have not been undertaken, the dilution factor makes adverse fetal and offspring outcomes as a consequence of seminal plasma exposures to TCDD during pregnancy extremely unlikely.

Empirical Epidemiologic Evidence on Paternal Transmission

The idea that exposure of either parent to a toxicant before conception could result in an adverse outcome in offspring is not new and remains a topic of much interest. Epidemiologic studies have reported occasional findings of paternally transmitted adverse outcomes associated with paternal exposures to certain agents, but none has been replicated convincingly. Even in instances in which an agent is recognized as mutagenic or potentially carcinogenic for exposed men, adverse consequences have not been demonstrated in offspring. For example, the hypothesis was extensively investigated in the early 1990s in relation to fathers' exposure to ionizing radiation before conception and an increase in leukemia in their offspring. The initial study (Gardner et al., 1990) was conducted in men who worked at the Sellafield nuclear facility in West Cumbria, United Kingdom. It was presumed that the men were exposed to radiation as a result of working at Sellafield. An association was found between fathers' radiation exposures before conception and an increase in leukemia among their children. However, later studies have failed to confirm that finding (Draper et al., 1997; Kinlen, 1993; Kinlen et al., 1993; Parker et al., 1993). Similarly, rigorous followup of children of atomic-bomb survivors has not demonstrated increased risks of cancer or birth defects (Izumi et al., 2003; Schull, 2003), and other studies of effects (birth defects and cancer) in the children of male cancer survivors after chemotherapy or radiation treatment have found little support for paternal transmission (Chow et al., 2009; Dohle, 2010; Howell and Shalet, 2005; Madanat-Harjuoja et al., 2010), although sperm and fertility clearly are adversely effected (Green et al., 2010).

The committee was unable to find a single instance of epidemiologic evidence that convincingly demonstrated that paternal exposure to any particular chemical before conception resulted in cancer or birth defects in offspring. However, there are few data for addressing the hypothesis of paternal exposure and adverse effects in human offspring in which the exposure occurred before conception only to the father and was measured with an objective dosimeter. Thus, it is difficult to assert conclusively that the available epidemiologic evidence supports or does not support paternal transmission; considerable uncertainty remains on many fronts and would presumably vary by agent and mode of exposure. Several systematic reviews of the topic have been conducted (Chia and Shi, 2002; Weselak et al., 2007, 2008; Wigle et al., 2007, 2008) and have not established firm relationships between specific agents and particular effects in offspring. Paternal occupation (by job title or job–exposure matrices) has been linked to increased risk of selected birth defects (Desrosiers et al., 2012; Fear et al., 2007; Shaw et al., 2002), and neuroblastoma (De Roos et al., 2001a,b). Moreover, increased risks of childhood brain cancer have been reported in relation to paternal exposure to selected pesticides, particularly herbicides and fungicides (van Wijngaarden et al., 2003), although the authors noted considerable uncertainty in the robustness of the findings. Therefore, the hypothesis that paternal preconception exposure to toxic agents may result in harm to their children remains unresolved in part because of the sparseness of epidemiologic research on the subject.

Maternal Exposure

A mother's exposures can affect a pregnancy and the resulting offspring far more extensively than paternal exposures. Because of the long half-life of TCDD and its bioaccumulation in adipose tissues, women exposed to Agent Orange in Vietnam would have potential to expose their offspring to TCDD directly during later pregnancies. Thus, damage to the resulting offspring or future generations could result from epigenetic changes in an egg before conception or from direct effects of exposure on the fetus during gestation and on the neonate during lactation. Dioxin in the mother's bloodstream can cross the placenta and expose the developing embryo and fetus. Furthermore, mobilization of dioxin during pregnancy or lactation may be increased because the body is drawing on fat stores to supply nutrients to the developing fetus or nursing infant. TCDD has been measured in circulating human maternal blood, cord blood, placenta, and breast milk (Suzuki et al., 2005), and it is estimated that an infant breastfed for 1 year accumulates a dose of TCDD that is 6 times as high as an infant not breastfed (Lorber and Phillips, 2002). Offspring effects of maternal exposures may not be manifested immediately and could be a result of dioxin-mediated reprogramming of developing organs and lead to disease onset later in life.

An emerging field of research referred to as the developmental basis of adult disease (Barker et al., 2012) has been investigating maternal nutritional exposures, stress, and alcohol exposure, and more recent studies have involved exposures to TCDD and other environmental toxicants. The molecular basis of the later-life effects is believed to be primarily epigenetic. Maladies that may be manifested later in life include neurologic and reproductive disorders, thyroid changes, and adult-onset cancers. Furthermore, germ cells (eggs and spermatogonia) in offspring undergo critical developmental stages during fetal life, and emerging evidence demonstrates that fetal exposures are capable of altering the germ cells epigenetically and of resulting in transmission of adverse effects to future generations (transgenerational inheritance).

Laboratory animal studies have established that TCDD can affect development, so a connection between TCDD exposure and effects on offspring, including developmental disruption and disease onset in later life, is biologically plausible. It has been established in several animal studies that TCDD at high doses is a potent teratogen. However, definitive conclusions based on animal studies about the potential for TCDD to cause later-life toxicity in human offspring are complicated by differences in sensitivity and susceptibility among individual animals, strains, and species; by differences in route, dose, duration, and timing of exposure in experimental protocols and real-world exposure; and by differences in the toxicokinetics of TCDD between laboratory animals and humans. Experiments with 2,4-dichlorophenoxyacetic acid (2,4-D) and 2,4,5-trichlorophenoxyacetic acid (2,4,5-T) indicate that they have subcellular effects that could constitute a biologically plausible mechanism for developmental effects, but only at very high doses. There is insufficient information on picloram and cacodylic acid to assess the biologic plausibility of their developmental or delayed effects in offspring.

Chapter 4 presents more detailed toxicologic findings that are relevant to the biologic plausibility of the outcomes discussed here.

BIRTH DEFECTS

March of Dimes defines a birth defect as an abnormality of structure, function, or metabolism, whether genetically determined or resulting from an environmental influence during embryonic or fetal life (Bloom, 1981). Other terms, often used interchangeably, are *congenital anomaly* and *congenital malformation*. Major birth defects, which occur in 2–3% of live births, are abnormalities that are present at birth and are severe enough to interfere with viability or physical well-being. Birth defects are detected in another 5% of babies through the first year of life. The causes of most birth defects are unknown. Genetic factors, exposure to some medications, exposure to environmental contaminants, occupational exposures, and lifestyle factors have been implicated in the etiology of birth defects (Kalter and Warkany, 1983). Most etiologic research has focused on the effects of maternal and fetal exposures, but as discussed in the beginning of this chapter, it is theoretically possible that epigenetic alterations of the paternal gamete caused by preconception exposures could result in paternally-mediated effects. It should be noted that a substantial amount of epidemiologic research on suspect toxic agents has been conducted, but has not definitively established paternal preconception exposures as a contributing factor to the occurrence of birth defects (Chow et al., 2009; Desrosiers et al., 2012; Dohle, 2010; Schull, 2003).

Conclusions from *VAO* and Previous Updates

The committee responsible for *VAO* concluded that there was inadequate or insufficient evidence to determine whether there is an association between exposure to 2,4-D, 2,4,5-T or its contaminant TCDD, picloram, or cacodylic acid and birth defects in offspring. Additional information available to the committee responsible for *Update 1996* led it to conclude that there was limited or suggestive evidence of an association between at least one of the COIs and spina bifida in the children of veterans; there was no change in the conclusions regarding other birth defects. The committee for *Update 2002*, which reviewed the study of female Vietnam veterans (Kang et al., 2000) that reported significant increases in birth defects in their offspring, did not find those results adequate to modify prior conclusions, although Congress did mandate service-related status to a number of birth defects in the children of female Vietnam veterans. Later VAO committees have not encountered enough additional data to merit changing the conclusion that the evidence is inadequate to support an association between exposure to the COIs and birth defects (aside from spina bifida) in the offspring of either male or female veterans.

Summaries of the results of studies of birth defects and specifically of neural-tube defects that were reviewed in the current report and in earlier VAO reports are in Tables 10-1 and 10-2, respectively.

Update of the Epidemiologic Literature

No Vietnam-veteran, occupational, or case-control studies of exposure to the COIs and birth defects have been published since *Update 2010*.

Environmental Studies

Since *Update 2010*, three studies have examined maternal exposure to the COIs in relation to congenital cryptorchidism or hypospadias; two based on a Danish–Finnish joint prospective cohort (Krysiak-Baltyn et al., 2012; Virtanen et al., 2012) and one that used the US National Birth Defects Prevention Study (NBDPS), a population-based case-control study of congenital malformations that uses a multistate surveillance systems (Rocheleau et al., 2011).

Virtanen et al. (2012) examined placental concentrations of dioxins and PCBs in relation to congenital cryptorchidism in a nested case-control study within the joint prospective Danish–Finnish cohort study of the incidence of and risk factors for congenital cryptorchidism and hypospadias. Boys born in 1997–2001 in Copenhagen were examined for cryptorchidism at birth and at the age of 3 months. In preterm boys who had undescended testis, cryptorchidism was diagnosed only if the testis remained undescended at the expected date of delivery. Midwives collected and froze placentas immediately after birth. The

TABLE 10-1 Selected Epidemiologic Studies—Birth Defects in Offspring of Subjects[a] (Shaded Entries Are New Information for This Update)

Study Population	Exposed Cases[b]	**Exposure of Interest**/Estimated Relative Risk (95% CI)[b]	Reference
VIETNAM VETERANS			
US Vietnam Veterans			
US Air Force Health Study—Ranch Hand veterans vs SEA veterans (unless otherwise noted)		**All COIs**	
Verified birth defects in children born to AFHS veterans			Michalek et al., 1998a
Before service in SEA	nr	0.7 (nr)	
After service in SEA	nr	1.5 (nr)	
High-exposure Ranch Hands relative to comparisons			Wolfe et al.,1995
All anomalies	57	1.0 (0.8–1.3)	
Nervous system	3	nr	
Eye	3	1.6 (0.4–6.0)	
Ear, face, neck	5	1.7 (0.6–4.7)	
Circulatory system, heart	4	0.9 (0.3–2.7)	
Respiratory system	2	nr	
Digestive system	5	0.8 (0.3–2.0)	
Genital system	6	1.2 (0.5–3.0)	
Urinary system	7	2.1 (0.8–5.4)	
Musculoskeletal	31	0.9 (0.6–1.2)	
Skin	3	0.5 (0.2–1.7)	
Chromosomal anomalies	1	nr	
CDC Birth Defects Study—Hospital records reviewed for offspring of 7,924 Vietnam veterans and 7,364 non–Vietnam veterans		**All COIs**	
General Birth Defects Study—hospital records	130	1.0 (0.8–1.3)	CDC, 1989b
Major birth defects	51	1.2 (0.8–1.9)	
Digestive system defects	18	2.0 (0.9–4.6)	
Birth defects—black Vietnam veterans only	21	3.4 (1.5–7.6)	
Vietnam veterans identified through CDC Metropolitan Atlanta Congenital Defects Program			Erikson et al., 1984a
Any major birth defects	428	1.0 (0.8–1.1)	
Multiple birth defects with reported exposure	25	1.1 (0.7–1.7)	
EOI-5: spina bifida	1	2.7 (1.2–6.2)	
EOI-5: cleft lip with or without cleft palate	5	2.2 (1.0–4.9)	

TABLE 10-1 Birth Defects in Offspring of Subjects,[a] continued

Study Population	Exposed Cases[b]	**Exposure of Interest**/Estimated Relative Risk (95% CI)[b]	Reference
US CDC Vietnam Experience Study—Cross-sectional study, with medical examinations, of Army veterans: 9,324 deployed vs 8,989 nondeployed		**All COIs**	
Reproductive outcomes—interview data			CDC, 1989a
Total anomalies	826	1.3 (1.2–1.4)	
Nervous-system defects	33	2.3 (1.2–4.5)	
Ear, face, neck defects	37	1.6 (0.9–2.8)	
Integument	41	2.2 (1.2–4.0)	
Musculoskeletal defects	426	1.2 (1.1–1.5)	
Hydrocephalus	11	5.1 (1.1–23.1)	
Spina bifida	9	1.7 (0.6–5.0)	
Hypospadias	10	3.1 (0.9–11.3)	
Multiple defects	71	1.6 (1.1–2.5)	
Children of veterans reporting high exposure	46	1.7 (1.2–2.4)	
US VA Cohort of Female Vietnam Veterans		**All COIs**	
Female Vietnam-era veterans—deployed vs nondeployed (maternal exposure)			Kang et al., 2000
"Likely" birth defects	nr	1.7 (1.2–2.2)	
"Moderate-to-severe" birth defects	nr	1.5 (1.1–2.0)	
State Studies of US Vietnam Veterans			
Massachusetts Vietnam-era veterans		**All COIs**	
Vietnam veterans whose children were born at Boston Hospital for Women			Aschengrau and Monson, 1990
All congenital anomalies (crude OR)			
vs men without known military service	55	1.3 (0.9–1.9)	
vs non–Vietnam veterans	55	1.2 (0.8–1.9)	
One or more major malformations (crude OR)			
vs men without known military service	18	1.8 (1.0–3.1)	
vs non–Vietnam veterans	18	1.3 (0.7–2.4)	
International Vietnam-Veteran Studies			
Australian Vietnam Veterans—58,077 men and 153 women who served on land or in Vietnamese waters during 5/23/1962–7/1/1973 vs Australian population		**All COIs**	
Validation Study		*Expected number of exposed cases*	AIHW, 1999
Down syndrome	67	92 expected (73–111)	

continued

TABLE 10-1 Birth Defects in Offspring of Subjects,[a] continued

Study Population	Exposed Cases[b]	**Exposure of Interest**/Estimated Relative Risk (95% CI)[b]	Reference
Tracheo-esophageal fistula	10	23 expected (14–32)	
Anencephaly	13	16 expected (8–24)	
Cleft lip or palate	94	64 expected (48–80)	
Absent external body part	22	34 expected (23–45)	
Extra body part	74	74 expected (nr)	
Vietnam veterans vs all other men	127	1.0 (0.8–1.3)	Donovan et al., 1984
National service veterans—Vietnam service vs no Vietnam service	69	1.3 (0.9–2.0)	
OCCUPATIONAL—INDUSTRIAL			
IARC Phenoxy Herbicide Cohort—Workers exposed to any phenoxy herbicide or chlorophenol (production or spraying) vs respective national mortality rates			
NIOSH Mortality Cohort (12 US plants, 5,172 male production and maintenance workers 1942–1984) (included in IARC cohort as of 1997)		**Dioxins, phenoxy herbicides**	
Wives of workers with measured serum TCDD in NIOSH cohort	14	nr	Lawson et al., 2004
Dow Workers with Potential TCDD Exposure and reproductive outcomes in offspring of 930 men working with chlorophenol 1939–1975	30	0.9 (0.5–1.4)	Townsend et al., 1982
Monsanto workers in Nitro, West Virginia, occupationally exposed and potentially exposed after 1949 explosion (1948–1969)		**Dioxins, phenoxy herbicides**	
Followup of current and retired 2,4,5-T production workers (n = 235; 117 with chloracne exposure), 1948–1969	11	1.3 (0.5–3.4)	Moses et al., 1984
Followup of 2,4,5-T production workers (204 exposed, 163 unexposed), 1948–1969	18	1.1 (0.5–2.2)	Suskind and Hertzberg, 1984
OCCUPATIONAL—HERBICIDE-USING WORKERS (*not* related to IARC sprayer cohorts)			
Canada—Pregnancies with one or more birth defects in OFFHS	108	**Herbicides**	Weselak et al., 2008
Use on farm, during 3 months before conception, of			

TABLE 10-1 Birth Defects in Offspring of Subjects,[a] continued

Study Population	Exposed Cases[b]	**Exposure of Interest**/Estimated Relative Risk (95% CI)[b]	Reference
Herbicides	24	0.7 (0.4–1.1)	
Male offspring	19	0.9 (0.5–1.6)	
Direct paternal use	19	0.5 (0.3–1.0)	
Phenoxy herbicides	12	0.6 (0.3–1.1)	
Male offspring	9	0.8 (0.4–1.7)	
Direct paternal use	8	0.4 (0.2–0.9)	
2,4-D	10	1.1 (0.6–2.1)	
Male offspring	7	1.3 (0.6–2.8)	
Direct paternal use	6	0.6 (0.3–1.5)	
Dicamba	8	1.7 (0.8–3.5)	
Male offspring	7	2.4 (1.1–5.5)	
Use on farm, during 3 months after conception, of			
Herbicides	7	0.5 (0.2–1.2)	
Phenoxy herbicides	9	0.8 (0.4–1.5)	
2,4-D	7	1.0 (0.4–2.3)	
Canadian sawmill workers with exposure in upper 3 quartiles for any job held up to 3 months before conception			Dimich-Ward et al., 1996
Cataracts	11	5.7 (1.4–22.6)	
Genital organs	105	1.3 (0.9–1.5)	
New Zealand—Followup of 2,4,5-T sprayers vs nonsprayers (n = 989)		**Herbicides** *90% CI*	Smith et al., 1982
	13	1.2 (0.6–2.5)	
Norway—farmers (maternal, paternal exposure)	4,189	1.0 (1.0–1.1)	Kristensen et al., 1997
United States—Minnesota private pesticide appliers		**Pesticides**	Garry et al., 1996
All births with anomalies	125	1.4 (1.2–1.7)	
Circulatory, respiratory	17	1.7 (1.0–2.8)	
Gastrointestinal	6	1.7 (0.8–3.8)	
Urogenital	20	1.7 (1.1–2.6)	
Musculoskeletal, integumental	30		
Maternal age < 30 years	11	0.9 (0.5–1.7)	
Maternal age > 30 years	19	2.5 (1.6–4.0)	
Chromosomal	8	1.1 (0.5–2.1)	
Other	48		
Maternal age < 35 years	36	1.1 (0.8–1.6)	
Maternal age > 35 years	12	3.0 (1.6–5.3)	

continued

TABLE 10-1 Birth Defects in Offspring of Subjects,[a] continued

Study Population	Exposed Cases[b]	**Exposure of Interest**/Estimated Relative Risk (95% CI)[b]	Reference
ENVIRONMENTAL			
Seveso, Italy, Residential Cohort—Industrial accident July 10, 1976 (723 residents Zone A; 4,821 Zone B; 31,643 Zone R; 181,574 local reference group)		**TCDD**	
Maternal, paternal, in utero exposure		*90% CI*	Mastroiacovo et al., 1988
Zones A, B, R—total defects	137	1.0 (0.8–1.1)	
Zones A and B—total defects	27	1.2 (0.9–1.6)	
Zones A and B—mild defects	14	1.4 (0.9–2.2)	
Ecological Study of Residents of Chapaevsk, Russia		**Dioxin**	Revich et al., 2001
Congenital malformations	nr	nr, but ns	
Times Beach/Quail Run Cohorts		**Dioxin**	
Persons in Missouri with documented TCDD soil contamination near residence (maternal, paternal, in utero exposure)		**TCDD**	Stockbauer et al., 1988
Total birth defects	17	0.8 (0.4–1.5)	
Major defects	15	0.8 (0.4–1.7)	
Midline defects	4	0.7 (0.2–2.3)	
Other International Environmental Studies			
France—Case-control study (2001–2003 births) of urinary tract defects (n = 304) vs regional controls (n = 226) (same population as Cordier et al., 2004)		**Dioxin**	Cordier et al., 2010
Maternal exposure to			
Atmospheric dioxin	63	2.0 (1.2–3.4)	
Above median	33	2.8 (1.3–6.1)	
Below median	30	1.4 (0.7–2.9)	
Dioxin deposits	75	1.8 (1.1–3.0)	
Above median	41	3.0 (1.5–5.9)	
Below median	34	1.2 (0.6–2.2)	
France—Births (1988–1997): maternal residence in municipality with solid-waste incinerator vs not		**Dioxin**	Cordier et al., 2004
Minor anomalies	518	0.9 (0.8–1.1)	
Chromosomal anomalies	204	1.0 (0.9–1.2)	
Monogenic anomalies	83	1.1 (0.8–1.4)	
Unknown or multifactoral etiology	964	1.1 (1.0–1.2)	
Specific major anomalies with significant increases reported (of 23 categories reported)			
Facial clefts	152	1.3 (1.1–1.6)	
Renal dysplasia	60	1.6 (1.1–2.2)	
Turkey—Cross-sectional study of MIH in Turkey; n = 109 from industrialized community with high levels of PCDDs and n = 44 from low-industrialized community		**PCDDs** Prevalence of MIH 4/44 and 10/109, no difference	Kuscu et al., 2009

TABLE 10-1 Birth Defects in Offspring of Subjects,[a] continued

Study Population	Exposed Cases[b]	**Exposure of Interest**/Estimated Relative Risk (95% CI)[b]	Reference
United States—Rural or farm residents of Minnesota, Montana, North Dakota, South Dakota (maternal, paternal exposure)		2,4-D, MCPA	Schreinemachers, 2003
Any birth anomaly	213	1.1 (0.9–1.3)	
Central-nervous-system anomalies	12	0.8 (0.5–1.4)	
Circulatory, respiratory anomalies	39	1.7 (1.1–2.6)	
Digestive-system anomalies	24	0.9 (0.6–1.5)	
Urogenital anomalies	44	1.0 (0.7–1.5)	
Musculoskeletal, integumental anomalies	70	1.5 (1.1–2.1)	
Chromosomal anomalies	17	0.9 (0.6–1.6)	
United States—Persons exposed to an electric-transformer fire in Binghamton, New York—total birth defects (maternal, paternal exposure)	1	**Chlorophenols** 2.1 (0.1–11.9)	Fitzgerald et al., 1989
CASE-CONTROL STUDIES			
US Case-Control Studies			
US National Birth Defects Prevention Study—Hypospadias and maternal herbicide exposure; JEM to determine exposure from conception through first trimester of pregnancy (647 cases vs 1,496 controls)		**Herbicides, pesticides**	Rocheleau et al., 2011
Second- or third-degree hypospadias	36	1.0 (0.5–2.1)	
Arkansas—hypospadias as function of mother's residence within 500 m of agricultural pesticide use during gestation weeks 6–16		Dicamba	Meyer et al., 2006
Dicamba (lb)			
0	nr	1.0	
> 0– < 0.04	nr	0.5 (0.3–1.0)	
≥ 0.04	nr	0.9 (0.4–2.1)	
Baltimore mothers in the BWIS exposed to herbicides during first trimester (maternal exposure)	8	**Herbicides** 2.8 (1.2–6.9)	Loffredo et al., 2001
International Case-Control Studies			
Denmark/Finland—Relationship between congenital cryptorchidism and PCBs and dioxins in breast milk (130 samples)		**Dioxin, PCBs** ns	Krysiak-Baltyn et al., 2012
Denmark/Finland—Relationship between congenital cryptorchidism and PCBs and dioxins in placentas; 112 Finnish subjects (56 cases, 56 controls) and 168 Danish subjects (39 cases, 129 controls)		**Dioxin, PCBs** ns	Virtanen et al., 2012

continued

TABLE 10-1 Birth Defects in Offspring of Subjects,[a] continued

Study Population	Exposed Cases[b]	**Exposure of Interest**/Estimated Relative Risk (95% CI)[b]	Reference
Finland—Followup of participants from previous case-control study of cleft lip and palate, n = 167 placenta tissue analyzed for PCDD/Fs and children assessed for MIH		**PCDDs, PCDFs** 24/167 with MIH TEQ of PCDDs not associated with MIH; duration of breastfeeding not association with MIH	Laisi et al., 2008
Japan—Investigated multiple pregnancy outcomes in Japanese-infant deaths from congenital defects		**Dioxin**	Tango et al., 2004
	42	nr, but ns	
New Zealand—Residents of areas subject to aerial 2,4,5-T spraying		**2,4,5-T** *90% CI*	Hanify et al., 1981
All birth malformations excluding dislocated or dislocatable hip	164	1.7 (1.4–2.1)	
All heart malformations	20	3.9 (2.1–7.4)	
Hypospadias, epispadias	18	5.6 (2.7–11.7)	
Talipes	52	1.7 (1.2–2.3)	
Cleft lip	6	0.6 (0.3–1.3)	
Isolated cleft palate	7	1.4 (0.6–3.2)	
Spain—Residents of agricultural areas—at least median score on chlorophenoxy-herbicide exposure duration (months) index		**Herbicides**	García et al., 1998
	14	3.1 (0.6–16.9)	
The Netherlands—Infants born in Zeeburg, Amsterdam, clinics 1963–1965 with orofacial cleft (maternal exposure)		**Dioxin**	ten Tusscher et al., 2000
Births in 1963	5	nr, but said to be significant	
Births in 1964	7	nr, but said to be significant	

NOTE: 2,4-D, 2,4-dichlorophenoxyacetic acid; 2,4,5-T, 2,4,5-trichlorophenoxyacetic acid; AFHS, Air Force Health Study; BWIS, Baltimore–Washington Infant Study; CDC, Centers for Disease Control and Prevention; CI, confidence interval; COI, chemical of interest; EOI, exposure opportunity index; IARC, International Agency for Research on Cancer; JEM, job-exposure matrix; MCPA, 4-chloro-2-methylphenoxyacetic acid; MIH, molar incisor hypomineralization; NIOSH, National Institute for Occupational Safety and Health; nr, not reported; ns, not significant; OFFHS, Ontario Farm Family Health Study; OR, odds ratio; PCB, polychlorinated biphenyl; PCDD, polychlorinated dibenzodioxins; PCDF, polychlorinated dibenzofurans; SEA, Southeast Asia; TCDD, 2,3,7,8-tetrachlorodibenzo-*p*-dioxin; TEQ, (total) toxic equivalent; VA, US Department of Veterans Affairs.

[a]Unless otherwise indicated, studies show paternal exposure.

[b]Given when available; results other than estimated risk explained individually.

TABLE 10-2 Selected Epidemiologic Studies—Neural-Tube Defects in Offspring of Subjects[a]

Study Population	Exposed Cases[b]	**Exposure of Interest**/Estimated Relative Risk (95% CI)[b]	Reference
VIETNAM VETERANS			
US Vietnam Veterans			
US Air Force Health Study—Ranch Hand veterans vs SEA veterans (unless otherwise noted)		**All COIs**	
Air Force Operation Ranch Hand personnel—neural-tube defects	4[c]	nr	Wolfe et al., 1995
CDC Birth Defects Study—Hospital records reviewed for offspring of 7,924 Vietnam veterans and 7,364 non–Vietnam veterans		**All COIs**	
Vietnam veterans identified through CDC Metropolitan Atlanta Congenital Defects Program			Erickson et al., 1984a,b
Service in Vietnam			
Spina bifida	19	1.1 (0.6–1.7)	
Anencephaly	12	0.9 (0.5–1.7)	
Military records indicate opportunity for exposure			
Spina bifida	20	2.7 (1.2–6.2)	
Anencephaly	7	0.7 (0.2–2.8)	
US CDC Vietnam Experience Study—Cross-sectional study, with medical examinations, of Army veterans: 9,324 deployed vs 8,989 nondeployed		**All COIs**	
VES cohort—reproductive outcomes			CDC, 1989b
Spina bifida			
Vietnam veterans' children	9	1.7 (0.6–5.0)	
Non–Vietnam veterans' children	5	1.0	
Anencephaly			
Vietnam veterans' children	3	nr	
Non–Vietnam veterans' children	0	1.0	
International Vietnam-Veteran Studies			
Australian Vietnam Veterans—58,077 men and 153 women who served on land or in Vietnamese waters during 5/23/1962–7/1/1973 vs Australian population		**All COIs**	
Validation Study		*Expected number of exposed cases*	AIHW, 1999
Spina bifida—maximums	50	33 expected (22–44)	

continued

TABLE 10-2 Neural-Tube Defects in Offspring of Subjects,[a] continued

Study Population	Exposed Cases[b]	**Exposure of Interest**/Estimated Relative Risk (95% CI)[b]	Reference
Anencephaly	13	16 expected (8–24)	
Australian Vietnam veterans—neural-tube defects	16	**All COIs** 0.9 (nr)	ADVA, 1983
OCCUPATIONAL—HERBICIDE-USING WORKERS			
Norwegian farmers—spina bifida (maternal, paternal exposures)		**Herbicides**	Kristensen et al., 1997
Tractor spraying equipment	28	1.6 (0.9–2.7)	
Tractor spraying equipment, orchards, greenhouses[d]	5	2.8 (1.1–7.1)	
United States—birth defects in children born to licensed pesticide appliers in Minnesota linked to state birth registries		**Herbicides, pesticides**	Garry et al., 1996
Central-nervous-system defects	6	1.1 (0.5–2.4)	
ENVIRONMENTAL			
Times Beach/Quail Run Cohorts		**Dioxin**	
Persons in Missouri with documented TCDD soil contamination near residence (maternal, paternal, in utero exposure)		**TCDD**	Stockbauer et al., 1988
Central-nervous-system defects	3	3.0 (0.3–35.9)	
Other International Environmental Studies			
France—Population-based birth defects registry in Rhône-Alpes region (1988–1997): maternal residence in municipality with solid-waste incinerator vs not	49	**Dioxin** 0.9 (0.6–1.2)	Cordier et al., 2004
CASE-CONTROL STUDIES			
Canada—British Columbian sawmill workers with exposure in upper 3 quartiles for any job held up to 3 months before conception		**Herbicides**	Dimich-Ward et al., 1996
Spina bifida, anencephaly	22	2.4 (1.1–5.3)	
Spina bifida only	18	1.8 (0.8–4.1)	
New Zealand—Residents of areas subject to aerial 2,4,5-T spraying		**2,4,5-T** *90% CI*	Hanify et al., 1981
Anencephaly	10	1.4 (0.7–2.9)	
Spina bifida	13	1.1 (0.6–2.1)	

TABLE 10-2 Neural-Tube Defects in Offspring of Subjects,[a] continued

Study Population	Exposed Cases[b]	**Exposure of Interest**/Estimated Relative Risk (95% CI)[b]	Reference
The Netherlands—Children of Dutch farmers who were born with spina bifida (1980–1992), 470 cases vs 456 healthy controls		**Herbicides, pesticides**	Blatter et al., 1997
Spina bifida—moderate, heavy exposure			
Pesticide use	8	1.7 (0.7–4.0)	
Herbicide use	7	1.6 (0.6–4.0)[e]	

NOTE: 2,4,5-T, 2,4,5-trichlorophenoxyacetic acid; CDC, Centers for Disease Control and Prevention; CI, confidence interval; COI, chemical of interest; nr, not reported; SEA, Southeast Asia; TCDD, 2,3,7,8-tetrachlorodibenzo-*p*-dioxin; VES, Vietnam Experience Study.

[a]Unless otherwise indicated, studies show paternal exposure.

[b]Given when available; results other than estimated risk explained individually.

[c]Of four neural-tube defects reported in Operation Ranch Hand offspring, two were spina bifida (high dioxin exposure), one spina bifida (low dioxin), one anencephaly (low dioxin); no neural-tube defects reported in comparison cohort; 454 postservice births studied in Ranch Hand veterans; 570 in comparison cohort.

[d]Greenhouse workers would not have been exposed to chemicals of interest.

[e]Calculated from data presented in the paper.

study included 56 Finnish cases and 56 controls that were individually matched on date of birth (± 2 weeks), parity, gestational age (± 1 week), smoking during pregnancy, and maternal diabetes. It also included 39 Danish subjects and 129 controls that were not matched on the above factors. Concentrations of 17 PCDD or PCDFs and 37 PCBs were measured and presented as total TEQs and as individual congeners. There were no significant differences between cases and controls in either the Finnish or Danish samples with respect to dioxin TEQs. Although there were some isolated and country-specific significant associations, none was replicated in all the countries, and concentrations of some congeners in controls exceeded those in cases. In a similarly designed study, Krysiak-Baltyn et al. (2012) examined breast-milk concentrations of PCBs and dioxins in relation to congenital cryptorchidism. Of the COIs measured, only dioxin-like OctoCDF concentrations in cases exceeded those in controls, and only in the Danish subset.

Using a job–exposure matrix to estimate maternal herbicide exposure from conception through the first trimester of pregnancy, Rocheleau et al. (2011) examined the association of herbicide exposure with hypospadias in the NBDPS. Affected children and fetuses were identified through active case ascertainment by each surveillance program. Controls (1,496) were a random sample of all unaffected live births in the areas covered by the state-based surveillance systems, and cases (647) had a diagnosis of second- or third-degree hypospadias.

Maternal interviews were conducted no later than 24 months after delivery. The following covariates were examined for evidence of confounding: maternal age; parity; history of miscarriage, singleton, or multiple pregnancy; gestational age and birth weight of the index infant; maternal alcohol consumption or smoking during or before the first trimester; use of a folic acid–containing supplement; prepregnancy body mass index; and several sociodemographic characteristics. The overall participation rate was about 70%. In general, participants exposed to herbicides were also exposed to insecticides or fungicides. In a model adjusted for all other pesticide classes, periconception herbicide exposure was not associated with second- or third-degree hypospadias (odds ratio [OR] = 0.99, 95% confidence interval [CI] 0.47–2.10), but there were very few exposed cases (36).

Ren et al. (2011) conducted a case-control study of neural-tube defects (NTDs) in subjects recruited from four rural counties of the Shanxi Province in China in 2005–2007. Cases were identified through a population-based birth-defects surveillance program. Healthy controls were individually matched to cases on sex, hospital of birth, mother's county of residence, and date of the mother's last menstrual period ("as close as possible"). Maternal interviews were conducted within 1 week of pregnancy termination or delivery to ascertain information on periconception use of folic-acid supplements; smoking exposure; exposure to pesticides, solvents, and heavy metals; other environmental exposures; and a variety of demographic, lifestyle, and reproductive history information. Placentas were collected at delivery or termination of NTD-affected pregnancies and measured for concentrations of polycyclic aromatic hydrocarbons, organochlorine pesticides, PCBs, and lipids. Models were adjusted for matching factors, in addition to maternal occupation, age, educational level, parity, folic-acid supplementation, passive smoking, and fever or influenza during pregnancy. Of the eight PCB congeners measured, six exhibited some dioxin-like activity (mono-ortho PCBs 105, 118, 156, 157, 167, and 189), but the measures of association were provided only as a sum, including also 206 and 209. Overall, there were no differences in the median placental concentrations of the total PCB sum between NTD cases (0.90 ng/g of lipid) and controls (0.87 ng/g of lipid).

Biologic Plausibility

2,4-D has been previously shown to be a teratogen, although at exposures that exceed maternal renal clearance, which are not relevant to Agent Orange exposure. A new study has shown for the first time that late in utero and early postnatal 2,4-D exposure can result in nephrotoxicity in offspring, although at one-sixth of the LD_{50} (Troudi et al., 2011). Other herbicides of interest can induce fetal malformations but typically only at high doses that are toxic to pregnant women. It is well established that TCDD is a potent teratogen in all laboratory species that have been studied, although the pattern of birth defects that are produced is often species-specific. Since *Update 2010*, studies have investigated the mechanisms underlying various TCDD-induced birth defects in rodents and other animal models, including hydronephrosis, cleft palate, reproductive organ anomalies, neurogenesis, and perturbed heart, kidney, and lung development (Dong et al., 2010; Falahatpisheh et al., 2011; Jacobs et al., 2011; Lanham et al., 2012; Latchney et al., 2011; Neri et al., 2011; Tait et al., 2011; Yoshioka et al., 2012; Yuan et al., 2012). Those mechanisms have not been fully elucidated, but it has been demonstrated that TCDD-induced birth defects require the aryl hydrocarbon receptor (AHR) but do not require induction of cytochrome P4501A1 (Dragin et al., 2006; Jang et al., 2007; Mimura et al., 1997). When pregnant AHR-null mice are exposed to TCDD, the fetuses do not exhibit any of the typical developmental malformations associated with TCDD exposure, but fetuses of TCDD-exposed pregnant CYP1A1 null mice do. In addition, an AHR antagonist can attenuate TCDD-induced birth defects in mice. Thus, activation of the AHR by TCDD during development appears to be a key first step in mediating TCDD's developmental toxicity. Although structural differences in the AHR have been identified among species, it functions similarly in animals and humans. Therefore, a common mechanism mediated by the AHR in which tissue growth and differentiation processes are affected probably underlies the developmental toxicity of TCDD in humans and animals. It has been shown that antioxidant treatment provides protection against some TCDD-induced teratogenicity; this suggests that reactive oxygen species might be involved in the pathways that lead to these structural changes (Jang et al., 2008). A few new studies indicate that stem cells and organ-specific progenitor cells may be direct targets and that maternal TCDD exposures interfer with proliferation and cell differentiation through the AHR and result in defects in organ morphogenesis (Latchney, 2011; Neri, 2011). Few laboratory studies of potential male-mediated developmental toxicity (and, specifically, birth defects) attributable to exposure to TCDD and herbicides have been conducted. Feeding of simulated Agent Orange mixtures to male mice produced no adverse effects in offspring (Lamb et al., 1981).

Synthesis

Embryonic and fetal development in rodents is sensitive to toxic effects of exposure to TCDD and dioxin-like chemicals. It is clear that the fetal rodent is more sensitive to adverse effects of TCDD than the adult rodent. Human data are generally lacking, however, and the sensitivity to developmental disruption in humans is less apparent, in part because contemporary studies of environmental dioxin exposure and birth defects have used extremely low exposures. The four studies since *Update 2010* that have assessed exposure to relevant chemicals and congenital malformations all examined only maternal exposure, which is of little relevance to the majority of Agent Orange–exposed veterans. Furthermore, those environmental studies were conducted in populations exposed to contemporary concentrations, which may be too low for adverse fetal effects to be observed.

The studies were well designed and adjusted for important confounders, but they do not provide evidence of an association at these exposure levels.

Conclusions

There was one new study of the relationship between maternal exposure to dioxin-like, mono-ortho PCBs and NTDs in offspring, which found no association, and there were no new studies of parental exposure to 2,4-D, 2,4,5-T, TCDD, cacodylic acid, or picloram and spina bifida in offspring. The committee concludes that the evidence of an association between exposure to the COIs and spina bifida is still limited or suggestive. The evidence of an association between exposure to the COIs and other birth defects is inadequate or insufficient.

CANCERS IN OFFSPRING

The American Cancer Society (ACS) estimated that 11,630 children less than 15 years old will receive a diagnosis of cancer in the United States in 2013 (ACS, 2013). Treatment and supportive care of children who have cancer have continued to improve. The 5-year survival rate for children who receive a cancer diagnosis has increased from less than 60% in the 1970s to more than 80% in 2013. Despite those advances, cancer remains the leading cause of death from disease in children less than 15 years old, and 1,310 deaths were projected for 2013 (ACS, 2013).

Leukemia is the most common cancer in children, accounting for about one-third of all childhood cancer cases. In 2010, ACS anticipated that almost 3,317 children would receive a leukemia diagnosis (ACS, 2010). Of those, almost 2,000 would have acute lymphocytic leukemia (ALL); most of the rest would have acute myeloid leukemia (AML). AML (*International Classification of Diseases, Ninth Revision* [ICD-9] 205) is also referred to as acute myelogenous leukemia or acute nonlymphocytic leukemia. For consistency, this report uses *acute myeloid leukemia*, or AML, regardless of usage in the source materials. ALL is most common in early childhood, peaking at the ages of 2–3 years, and AML is most common during the first 2 years of life. ALL incidence is consistently higher in boys than in girls; AML incidence is similar in boys and girls (NCI, 2001). Through early adulthood, ALL rates are about twice as high in whites as in blacks; AML exhibits no consistent pattern in this respect. Chapter 8 contains additional information on leukemia as part of the discussion of adult cancer.

The second-most common group of cancers in children are those of the central nervous system—the brain and the spinal cord. Other cancers in children include lymphomas, bone cancers, soft-tissue sarcomas, renal cancers, eye cancers, and adrenal cancers. In contrast with adult cancers, relatively little is known about the etiology of most childhood cancers, especially about potential environmental risk factors and the effects of parental exposures.

Conclusions from *VAO* and Previous Updates

The committee responsible for *VAO* concluded that there was inadequate or insufficient evidence to determine whether there is an association between exposure to 2,4-D, 2,4,5-T, TCDD, picloram, or cacodylic acid and childhood cancers. Additional information available to the committees responsible for *Update 1996* and *Update 1998* did not change that conclusion. The committee responsible for *Update 2000* reviewed the material in earlier VAO reports and newly available published literature and concluded that there was limited or suggestive evidence of an association between exposure to at least one of the COIs and AML. After the release of *Update 2000*, investigators involved in one study discovered an error in their published data. The *Update 2000* committee reconvened to evaluate the previously-reviewed and new literature regarding AML, and it produced *Acute Myelogenous Leukemia* (IOM, 2002). It reclassified AML from "limited/suggestive evidence of an association" to "inadequate evidence to determine whether an association exists."

Table 10-3 summarizes the results of the relevant studies. The committees responsible for *Update 2002*, *Update 2004*, *Update 2006*, *Update 2008*, and *Update 2010* reviewed the material in earlier VAO reports and in newly-available published literature and agreed that there remained inadequate or insufficient evidence to determine whether there is an association between exposure to the COIs and childhood cancers.

Update of Epidemiologic Literature

No Vietnam-veteran, occupational, or environmental studies of exposure to the COIs and childhood cancer have been published since *Update 2010*.

Case-Control Studies

Two childhood-leukemia studies examined the relationship of herbicide exposures and leukemia risk. Chokkalingam et al. (2012) conducted a population-based epidemiologic study of 377 ALL cases and 448 controls in the Northern California Childhood Leukemia Study and examined association with self-reported exposure to indoor and outdoor household pesticides overall and in subgroups that had hypothesized susceptibility genotypes in 42 xenobiotic transport and metabolism genes. With no adjustment for confounders indicated, they found a borderline-significantly-increased risk of ALL with outdoor herbicide use before birth (OR = 1.46, 95% CI 1.04–2.04) and with indoor insecticide use (OR = 1.29, 95% CI 0.97–1.72).

Slater et al. (2011) examined infant leukemia risk in the Children's Oncology Group study associated with maternal exposure to herbicides at any time during the period from 1 month before conception throughout pregnancy, during only the

TABLE 10-3 Selected Epidemiologic Studies—Childhood Cancer[a]

Study Population	Exposed Cases[b]	**Exposure of Interest**/Estimated Relative Risk (95% CI)[b]	Reference
VIETNAM VETERANS			
US Vietnam Veterans			
CDC Birth Defects Study—Hospital records reviewed for offspring of 7,924 Vietnam veterans and 7,364 non–Vietnam veterans		**All COIs**	
Vietnam veterans identified through CDC Metropolitan Atlanta Congenital Defects Program			Erickson et al., 1984b
"Other" neoplasms	87	1.8 (1.0–3.3)	
US CDC Vietnam Experience Study—Cross-sectional study, with medical examinations, of Army veterans: 9,324 deployed vs 8,989 nondeployed		**All COIs**	
VES cohort—reproductive outcomes			CDC, 1989b
Cancer	25	1.5 (0.7–2.8)	
Leukemia	12	1.6 (0.6–4.0)	
US veterans—case-control study of children's leukemia			Wen et al., 2000
AML, ALL			
Father ever served in Vietnam, Cambodia	117	1.2 (0.9–1.6)	
< 1 year in Vietnam or Cambodia	61	1.4 (0.9–2.0)	
> 1 year in Vietnam or Cambodia	49	1.2 (0.8–1.7)	
AML only			
Father ever served in Vietnam, Cambodia	40	1.7 (1.0–2.9)	
< 1 year in Vietnam or Cambodia	13	2.4 (1.1–5.4)	
> 1 year in Vietnam or Cambodia	16	1.5 (0.7–3.2)	
International Vietnam-Veteran Studies			
Australian Vietnam Veterans' children—revised validation study		**All COIs**	
AML	12[c]	1.3 (0.8–4.0)	AIHW, 2001
Australian Vietnam veterans' children—validation study—AML			*AIHW, 2000*
This study, which incorrectly calculated expected number of AML cases, is updated by AIHW (2001) above			
Tasmanian Veterans with Service in Vietnam		**All COIs**	
Cancer in children of Australian Vietnam veterans	4	nr	Field and Kerr, 1988
OCCUPATIONAL—HERBICIDE-USING WORKERS			
Canada—Sawmill Workers in British Columbia; 26,487 workers for ≥ 1 year at 14 mills using chlorophenates 1950–1985		**Chlorophenates, not TCDD**	

TABLE 10-3 Childhood Cancer,[a] continued

Study Population	Exposed Cases[b]	**Exposure of Interest**/Estimated Relative Risk (95% CI)[b]	Reference
Workers having a live birth within 1 yr after the initiation of employment			Heacock et al., 1998
Leukemia			
All workers' offspring—incidence	11	1.0 (0.5–1.8)	
Chlorophenate exposure: high- vs low-exposure subjects	5	0.8 (0.2–3.6)	
Brain cancer			
All workers' offspring—incidence	9	1.3 (0.6–2.5)	
Chlorophenate exposure: high- vs low-exposure subjects	5	1.5 (0.4–6.9)	
United States—US Agricultural Health Study—prospective study of licensed pesticide sprayers in Iowa and North Carolina: commercial (n = 4,916), private/farmers (n = 52,395, 97.4% men), and spouses of private sprayers (n = 32,347, 0.007% men), enrolled 1993–1997; followups with CATIs 1999–2003 and 2005–2010		**Phenoxy herbicides**	
Offspring of male pesticide applicators in Iowa from AHS			Flower et al., 2004
Maternal exposure to chlorophenoxy herbicides	7	0.7 (0.3–1.5)	
Paternal exposure to chlorophenoxy herbicides	28	1.3 (0.6–2.6)	
Maternal exposure to 2,4-D	7	0.7 (0.3–1.6)	
Paternal exposure to 2,4-D	26	1.3 (0.7–2.4)	
ENVIRONMENTAL			
Seveso, Italy, Residential Cohort—Industrial accident July 10, 1976 (723 residents Zone A; 4,821 Zone B; 31,643 Zone R; 181,574 local reference group) (ICD-9 171)		**TCDD**	
Seveso residents 0–19 yrs old—10-yr followup, morbidity, all exposure zones			Pesatori et al., 1993
All cancers	17	1.2 (0.7–2.1)	
Ovary, uterine adnexa	2	nr (0 cases expected)	
Brain	3	1.1 (0.3–4.1)	
Thyroid	2	4.6 (0.6–32.7)	
HL	3	2.0 (0.5–7.6)	
Lymphatic leukemia	2	1.3 (0.3–6.2)	
Myeloid leukemia	3	2.7 (0.7–11.4)	
Seveso residents 0–19 yrs old—10-yr followup, mortality, all exposure zones			Bertazzi et al., 1992

continued

TABLE 10-3 Childhood Cancer,[a] continued

Study Population	Exposed Cases[b]	**Exposure of Interest**/Estimated Relative Risk (95% CI)[b]	Reference
All cancers	10	7.9 (3.8–13.6)	
Leukemias	5	3.9 (1.2–1.8)	
Lymphatic leukemia	2	1.6 (0.1–4.5)	
Myeloid leukemia	1	0.8 (0.0–3.1)	
Leukemia, others	2	1.6 (0.1–4.6)	
Central-nervous-system tumors	2	1.6 (0.1–4.6)	
Other International Environmental Studies			
Canada—ALL in children (0–9 yrs old) in households using herbicides (1980–1993)		**Herbicides**	Infante-Rivard et al., 1999
Exposure during pregnancy	118	1.8 (1.3–2.6)	
Exposure during childhood	178	1.4 (1.1–1.9)	
England—Renal cancer in subjects (1–15 yrs of age) with paternal occupation in agriculture		**Herbicides, pesticides**	Pearce and Parker, 2000
	21	0.9 (0.2–3.8)	
Norway—Cancer in children of agricultural workers (n = 1,275) identified in cancer registries (1965–1991)		**Pesticides**	Kristensen et al., 1996
Children with AML whose parents purchased pesticides	12	1.4 (0.6–2.9)	
CASE-CONTROL STUDIES			
US Case-Control Studies			
Children's Oncology Group—Studies association between infant leukemia and maternal herbicide exposure (443 cases vs 324 population controls)		**Herbicides** ns	Slater et al., 2011
Children's Oncology Group—Childhood GCTs residential exposure to herbicides 6 months before conception, during gestation, through breastfeeding period		**Pesticides**	Chen et al., 2006
Maternal exposure	47	1.3 (0.9–1.7)	
Daughters	36	1.4 (1.0–2.0)	
Sons	11	1.0 (0.5–1.8)	
Paternal exposure	90	1.0 (0.7–1.3)	
Daughters	32	1.2 (0.7–2.0)	
Sons	58	1.0 (0.7–1.4)	
Children's Oncology Group—Parental occupational exposure to pesticide and GCTs, 1993–2001 (253 cases vs 394 controls)		**Pesticides**	Chen et al., 2005
Maternal	32	1.1 (0.7–1.6)	
Paternal	39	0.9 (0.6–1.3)	
Children's Cancer Group—exposure to pesticides, weed killers—AML		**Pesticides**	Buckley et al., 1989
Any paternal exposure	27	2.3 (p = 0.5)	
Paternal exposure > 1,000 days	17	2.7 (1.0–7.0)	
Maternal exposure > 1,000 days	7	undefined	

TABLE 10-3 Childhood Cancer,[a] continued

Study Population	Exposed Cases[b]	**Exposure of Interest**/Estimated Relative Risk (95% CI)[b]	Reference
California (Northern California Childhood Leukemia Study)—Exposure to "outdoor herbicides" and ALL (and variants in metabolic genes) (377 cases vs 448 controls)		**Herbicides**	Chokkalingam at al., 2012
Outdoor herbicide use before birth		1.5 (1.0–2.0)	
California—Maternal exposure to agricultural pesticide in class of "probable human carcinogens" (including cacodylic acid) during 9 months before delivery		**Pesticides**	Reynolds et al., 2005b
All sites	223	1.0 (0.9–1.2)	
Leukemias	179	1.2 (0.9–1.5)	
Central-nervous-system tumors	31	0.9 (0.5–1.4)	
New York State—Neuroblastoma risk in children, age ≤ 14 yrs of age (1976–1987)		**Pesticides**	Kerr et al., 2000
Maternal occupational exposure to insecticides	40	2.3 (1.4–3.7)	
Paternal exposure to dioxin	7	6.9 (1.3–68.4)	
International Case-Control Studies			
Canada and United States—Study of Wilm's tumor		**Herbicides**	Cooney et al., 2007
Maternal report of household use of herbicides from month before conception through child's diagnosis	112	1.0 (0.7–1.4)	
Canada and United States—Neuroblastoma risk in children (538 cases, 504 controls) from 139 hospitals in US and Canada (exposures as reported by both parents)		**Herbicides, pesticides**	Daniels et al., 2001
Pesticides in home (used ever)	nr	1.6 (1.0–2.3)	
Herbicides in garden	nr	1.9 (1.1–3.2)	
Pesticides in garden	nr	2.2 (1.3–3.6)	
Costa Rica—parental occupational exposure to pesticide, childhood leukemia		**Herbicides**	Monge et al., 2007
Parental exposures in yr before conception to			
Herbicides	53	1.2 (0.8–1.7)	
Phenoxyacetic acids	28	1.0 (0.6–1.6)	
Picloram (all ALL)	11	1.6 (0.7–3.4)	
High vs low	8	6.3 (1.0–38.6)	
Maternal exposures to			
Herbicides			
In yr before conception	9	2.0 (0.8–5.0)	
In 1st trimester	8	5.3 (1.4–20.0)	
In 2nd trimester	8	5.3 (1.4–20.0)	
In 3rd trimester	7	2.3 (0.8–6.8)	
Phenoxyacetic acids in yr before conception	4	1.3 (0.4–4.8)	

continued

TABLE 10-3 Childhood Cancer,[a] continued

Study Population	Exposed Cases[b]	**Exposure of Interest**/Estimated Relative Risk (95% CI)[b]	Reference
West Germany—population-based study of childhood cancer (1993–1997) (2,358 cases vs 2,588 controls)		**Pesticides**	Meinert et al., 2000
Leukemia			
Paternal exposure yr before pregnancy	62	1.5 (1.1–2.2)	
Paternal exposure during pregnancy	57	1.6 (1.1–2.3)	
Maternal exposure yr before pregnancy	19	2.1 (1.1–4.2)	
Maternal exposure during pregnancy	15	3.6 (1.5–8.8)	
Lymphomas			
Paternal exposure yr before pregnancy	11	1.5 (0.7–3.1)	
Paternal exposure during pregnancy	10	1.6 (0.7–3.6)	
Maternal exposure yr before pregnancy	3	2.9 (0.7–13.0)	
Maternal exposure during pregnancy	4	11.8 (2.2–64.0)	
France—Hematopoietic malignancies in children < 15 yrs of age (2003–2004)		**Herbicides**	Rudant et al., 2007
Maternal household herbicide use during pregnancy			
Acute leukemia	53	1.5 (1.0–2.2)	
Without paternal exposure	4	5.0 (1.3–19.0)	
All ALL	nr	1.7 (1.2–2.5)	
Common B-cell ALL	nr	1.9 (1.3–2.9)	
Mature B-cell ALL	nr	1.5 (0.3–6.4)	
T-cell ALL	nr	0.5 (0.1–2.0)	
AML	nr	1.2 (0.5–2.8)	
HL	9	1.1 (0.5–2.4)	
Without paternal exposure	0	nr	
Nodular sclerosis	nr	1.3 (0.5–3.1)	
Mixed cell	nr	0.8 (0.1–6.6)	
NHL	14	1.5 (0.8–2.7)	
Without paternal exposure	0	nr	
Burkitt's lymphoma	nr	1.7 (0.7–4.0)	
B-cell lymphoblastic	nr	0.7 (0.2–3.0)	
T-cell lymphoblastic	nr	2.6 (0.7–9.0)	
Anaplastic large cell	nr	1.4 (0.3–2.8)	

NOTE: 2,4-D, 2,4-dichlorophenoxyacetic acid; AHS, Agricultural Health Study; AIHW, Australian Institute for Health and Welfare; ALL, acute lymphocytic leukemia; AML, acute myeloid leukemia; CATI, computer-assisted telephone interviewing; CDC, Centers for Disease Control and Prevention; CI, confidence interval; COI, chemical of interest; GCT, germ-cell tumor; HL, Hodgkin lymphoma; ICD, *International Classification of Diseases*; NHL, non-Hodgkin lymphoma; nr, not reported; ns, not significant; TCDD, 2,3,7,8-tetrachlorodibenzo-*p*-dioxin; VES, Vietnam Experience Study.

[a]Unless otherwise indicated, studies show paternal exposure.

[b]Given when available; results other than estimated risk explained individually.

[c]Of the 12, 9 were observed, 3 additional cases estimated to have occurred in portion of cohort whose data were not validated.

preconception period, and during only the pregnancy. They found no significant associations.

Biologic Plausibility

Paternal or maternal exposure to xenobiotics potentially could increase the susceptibility of offspring to cancer through multiple mechanisms. Susceptibility could be increased by inheriting a genetic predisposition, which by itself could increase the development of cancer or the likelihood of developing cancer after future exposure to a carcinogen; the mother or father would transmit either an acquired genetic defect or an epigenetic alteration that predisposed the child to cancer. Alternatively, a maternally-mediated increase in susceptibility to childhood cancer could result from direct exposure of a child in utero or via lactation to a xenobiotic that induces epigenetic alterations that increase cancer susceptibility or is itself carcinogenic.

It has been shown that prenatal TCDD exposure of rats is associated with altered mammary-gland differentiation and an increase in the number of mammary adenocarcinomas (Brown et al., 1998). The demonstration that *early postnatal* TCDD exposure does not increase mammary-cancer risk (Desaulniers et al., 2004) does not contradict the finding that TCDD-induced changes in utero mediate the increase in cancer susceptibility (Fenton et al., 2000, 2002). Developmental epigenetic alterations may be involved in the prenatal effects. TCDD has been shown to suppress the expression of two tumor-suppressor genes, $p16^{Ink4a}$ and p53, via an epigenetic mechanism that appears to involve DNA methylation (Ray and Swanson, 2004). Similarly, it was reported that prenatal TCDD exposure increases methylation of two growth-related imprinted genes, H19 and Igf2, in the developing fetus (Wu et al., 2004).

Although there is no direct evidence from animal models that TCDD increases the risk of childhood cancers, such as acute leukemia and germ-cell tumors, emerging research suggests that prenatal TCDD exposure can disrupt epigenetic imprinting patterns and alter organ differentiation and thus could contribute to an increased susceptibility to cancer later in life. Smith et al. (2005) showed that chromosomal rearrangements associated with childhood ALL are evident in the neonatal blood spots; this suggests that childhood leukemias begin before birth, perhaps due to maternal exposures to genotoxic xenobiotics.

Synthesis

Two case-control studies considered childhood leukemias and herbicide use. One found a marginally significantly increased risk of ALL in association with maternal herbicide use before conception, and the other saw no increases in childhood leukemias related to maternal herbicide exposure shortly before or during pregnancy. No new epidemiologic evidence specifically concerning the COIs and childhood cancers has been published since *Update 2010*.

Conclusions

On the basis of the evidence reviewed here and in previous VAO reports, the committee concludes that there is inadequate or insufficient evidence to determine whether there is an association between exposure to the COIs and childhood cancers.

EFFECTS OCCURRING LATER IN OFFSPRING'S LIFE OR IN LATER GENERATIONS

In response to a special request from the Department of Veterans Affairs, continuing inquiries from veterans and their families, and increasing attention in research efforts, the committee for *Update 2010* addressed whether it is feasible to assess associations between exposure to the herbicides sprayed in Vietnam and health effects that occur later in the lives of children of Vietnam veterans and even in their grandchildren; such associations had not been formally reviewed in prior VAO updates. The previously-considered outcomes of birth defects observable within the first year of life and childhood cancer (diagnosis before the age of 18 years) were augmented to include all cancers and physical and neurobehavioral problems that might be manifested at any age. In addition, for the first time, the committee for *Update 2010* explored the possibility of transgenerational effects resulting from exposure-related epigenetic changes in the parents or exposed fetuses that would lead to adverse health effects in later generations, such as grandchildren.

Conclusions from *VAO* and Previous Updates

The potential effect of maternal and paternal exposure of Vietnam veterans to herbicides on the development of disease other than cancer in their children after the first year of life or in later generations had not been considered in updates before *Update 2010*.

For *Update 2010*, epidemiologic studies that evaluated the potential for effects of maternal or paternal exposure to the COIs in offspring were identified. Rather than identifying specific diseases in offspring, much of the research involved the measurement of physiologic biomarkers that might indicate a potential for disease development later in life. The committee for *Update 2010* therefore cautioned strongly that the *clinical consequences* of any observed changes are highly uncertain. The committee maintained its standard requirement for exposure specific to components of the herbicides sprayed in Vietnam. Although it may be physiologically possible for paternal exposure to cause changes in offspring that are manifested later in life, none of the published epidemiologic studies assessed such potential. Thus, the observation of any changes reported in the studies discussed in this section of *Update 2010* would be applicable only to children born to female Vietnam veterans during or after their deployment in Vietnam.

Changes Detected in Children After Parental Exposure

Thyroid Hormone Concentrations

Since *Update 2010*, there has been one additional epidemiologic study of childhood thyroid hormone concentrations associated with perinatal exposure to dioxins and dioxin-like PCBs. Leijs et al. (2012) conducted a followup study of 33 children 14–19 years old in whose mothers' breast milk PCDD or PCDF exposure was determined. All children were born in the Amsterdam–Zaandam region. Spearman's correlations were calculated by comparing PCDD, PCDF, and dioxin-like PCB TEQs with childhood triiodothyronine (T3), thyroxine (T4), free thyroxine (FT4), thyroxine-binding globulin (TBG), and thyroid-stimulating hormone (TSH) concentrations. Laboratory methods for measuring thyroid hormone were not provided. There was no correlation between perinatal dioxin exposure and T3, T4, FT4, TBG, or TSH. There was a significant correlation between dioxin-like PCB TEQs and childhood T3, but the magnitude was not provided; the significance level was $p = 0.047$. Those results conflict with the results of the Nagayama et al. (1998) study; however, the Leijs et al. (2012) study was small, and no covariate adjustment was performed for potentially-important factors, such as the child's age and sex, the mother's age, and the mother's smoking or alcohol consumption during pregnancy.

Cognitive or Motor Development

Since *Update 2010*, there has been one additional study of infant neurobehavioral development in relation to prenatal dioxin exposure. Nishijo et al. (2012) examined the association between dioxin exposure and infant growth and development in 210 mother–infant pairs that resided in dioxin-contaminated districts near the Da Nang airbase in Vietnam. Full-term babies from uncomplicated deliveries were recruited in 2008–2009. Breast milk was collected 1 month after birth and analyzed for 7 PCDDs and 10 PCDFs. Maternal interviews provided detailed covariate data, and pregnancy and delivery information was obtained from the obstetricians. All infants were breastfed until 4 months after birth. The duration of residence in the contaminated districts was directly related to PCDD and PCDF TEQ exposure quartile and maternal age. In boys, statistically-significant decrements in expressive communication skills as measured by the Bayley Scales of Infant and Toddler Development III (BSID-III) at the age of 4 months were noted in the 4th quartile of exposure relative to the 1st. Although the differences were not statistically significant, infants of both sexes in the highest quartile of prenatal exposure exhibited lower cognitive scores on the BSID-III (about 6 points than the 1st quartile in boys and 4 points in girls) and lower total motor scores (about 4 points in boys and 3 points in girls). However, measures of neurodevelopment in very early life are generally unstable.

Immune-Cell Populations and Prevalence of Allergies or Asthma in Children

Since *Update 2010*, there has been one additional study of allergies and infections during infancy in relation to prenatal exposure to dioxin-like compounds. Miyashita et al. (2011) examined allergies and infections in 364 mother–infant pairs enrolled during 2002–2005 in the Hokkaido Study on Environment and Children's Health (Sapporo, Japan). Third-trimester maternal blood concentrations of PCDDs, PCDFs, and dioxin-like PCBs were measured, and total maternal dioxin TEQs were calculated. Covariates (including exposure to environmental tobacco smoke, maternal education, annual household income, and maternal dietary intake of fish and meat during pregnancy) were assessed through maternal interviews. Maternal interviews also provided information about hospitalization or medical treatment of infants for asthma, eczema, other allergic diseases, otitis media, febrile seizures, respiratory syncytial virus infection, and other diseases from birth to the age of 18 months. A modified version of the International Study of Asthma and Allergies in Childhood (ISAAC) questionnaire was administered. Development of allergies or infections in infants was defined as having had a doctor's diagnosis, hospitalization, or medical treatment between birth and the age of 18 months. Asthma was expanded to include cases in which the mother gave positive responses to all questions on the modified ISAAC questionnaire. There were no associations between maternal exposure and childhood food allergy, eczema, or asthma, although there was a weak positive trend of increased risk of asthma with increasing exposure to PCDFs ($p = 0.059$). There was also a weak positive association of third trimester PCDF concentrations and increased risk of otitis media (overall trend $p = 0.027$); compared with the children of women in the lowest quartile of exposure, the children of those in the highest quartile had 2.5 times the risk of having a confirmed case of otitis media (95% CI 1.07–5.88) in multivariate adjusted models. The effect was more pronounced in male infants, who showed an indication of a dose–response relationship, with an increase in risk in the highest quartile for dioxin activity from furans (OR = 3.80, 95% CI 1.09–13.18) and for total dioxin activity (OR = 4.44, 95% CI 1.20–16.45). There were also significant congener-specific associations with otitis media for octachlorodienzo-*p*-dioxin (OCDD) (all quartiles relative to the 1st quartile), 2,3,4,7,8-pentachlorodibenzofuran (4th quartile relative to 1st quartile), dioxin-like non-ortho PCB 77 (4th quartile relative to 1st quartile), and dioxin-like mono-ortho PCB 157 (2nd quartile and 4th quartile relative to 1st quartile). Those findings provide some support for immunotoxic effects of dioxin-like compounds when the mother is exposed.

Jusko et al. (2011) reported on PCB exposures in Eastern Slovakia, examining concentrations in maternal and cord serum and immunoglobulin concentrations in offspring. No association between immunoglobulin concentrations and exposure was noted.

Offspring Reproductive Function

Since *Update 2010*, there have been three epidemiologic studies of maternal or perinatal exposure to dioxins and dioxin-like PCBs in relation to child reproductive development. Humblet et al. (2011) examined the association with maternal dioxin exposure in the highly-contaminated region of Chapaevsk, Russia, which until 2003 was the site of chlorinated-chemical production at the Middle Volga Chemical Plant. A mother's serum concentration 8–9 years after pregnancy served as a surrogate measure of her son's in utero and lactational exposure. The study investigated 444 mother–son pairs (89% of the 499 peripubertal boys in the entire cohort) that were recruited when the boys were 8–9 years old by using the townwide health-insurance information system in 2003–2005. At study entry, a physical examination was conducted on each boy, maternal and child blood samples were drawn for measurement of TEQs and total PCB concentrations, and an extensive interview was administered. One of the study investigators (blinded to the subjects' dioxin concentrations) conducted all pubertal staging at study entry and annually thereafter. A carefully-considered covariate adjustment plan was implemented in this high-quality study. No association of maternal serum total TEQs was seen in any of the three indexes of pubertal onset measured. In a subset of boys who breastfed for at least 6 months, a dose-related delay (relative to those who breastfed less) in pubertal onset was seen with increasing quartiles of maternal TEQs. Overall, the study does not provide particularly strong or consistent evidence of an association between perinatal TEQ exposure and pubertal onset among boys.

Reproductive function in sons was also investigated by Mocarelli et al. (2011); 78 men 18–26 years old who were born to women living in the most dioxin-polluted areas near Seveso, Italy, were eligible for the study. After refusals and exclusion for varicoceles, only 39 subjects (50%) remained, but previously-gathered information on all the mothers demonstrated that nonparticipation was not associated with the mothers' serum concentrations or with whether the sons were breastfed. Of the 39, 21 were breastfed (and so received both in utero and postnatal exposure via their mothers), and 18 were formula-fed (and so received only in utero exposure from their mothers). At-home semen samples were collected from the sons and graded according to the WHO (WHO, 1999) recommendations. At the same visit, fasting blood samples were obtained, and they were measured for follicle-stimulating hormone (FSH), inhibin B, serum 17-β-estradiol, luteinizing hormone, and testosterone. Maternal serum TCDD measurements were taken from maternal serum frozen since 1976–1977. Of consecutive blood donors, 123 men matched for age and socioeconomic status whose mothers had not resided in the contaminated area were asked to be controls, and 58 (47%) participated. Hormone data were adjusted for body mass index (BMI), smoking behavior, age at the time of test, chemical exposure, and alcohol use. Sperm-function models were also adjusted for educational level, employment status, and abstinence time. Seveso-exposed men had a lower adjusted mean sperm concentration than the comparison population (46.2×10^6/mL vs 81.0×10^6/mL, p = 0.01), lower total sperm count (139.2×10^6 vs 229.9×10^6; p = 0.03), and lower progressive motile sperm count (50.6×10^6 vs 90.5×10^6; p = 0.05). These and other associations (sperm progressive motility, FSH, and inhibin B) appeared to be substantially modified by whether the man had been breastfed in childhood; the effects were strongest in, and to some degree limited to, men who had been breastfed. This indicates that early-life exposure via breast milk had more of an impact on these fertility-related outcomes in the later lives of the sons than did in utero exposure, but breastfeeding is a relevant mode of maternal exposure for the children of female Vietnam veterans. Those results suggest an effect of early-life exposure on adult reproductive function. Their reliability depends on the assumption that the Seveso-exposed and comparison populations are similar on all factors other than exposure, but the data provided indicate moderate differences in the sons' ages and duration of breastfeeding, while the covariate data provided are too limited for a full evaluation of the similarity of the groups. The results might have been enhanced by analyses using the mothers' measured dioxin concentrations.

Finally, Su et al. (2012) followed up 56 children (23 boys and 33 girls) from the Taiwanese mother–child birth cohort previously described (Chao et al., 2004; Wang et al., 2004, 2005). Children were stratified into low and high median placental PCDD, PCDF, and PCB exposure groups according to their mother's overall median exposure. The children's 8-hour fasting blood samples were obtained at followup and analyzed for testosterone, estradiol, luteinizing hormone, FSH, triglyceride, cholesterol, and insulin. There were few associations overall between dioxins and dioxin-like PCBs and hormone concentrations, other than higher median estradiol concentrations (3.0 ng/dL vs 1.8 ng/dL) in children whose mothers had lower total TEQs than in children whose mothers had higher total TEQs (p = 0.003). However, the comparisons were not adjusted for plausible confounders.

Biologic Plausibility

As reported in *Update 2010*, results of studies in rodent models provide support for the idea that prenatal exposure to TCDD can result in adverse effects in offspring later in life, including immune disorders, behavioral disturbances, reproductive impairment, kidney disease, and cancers (Foster et al., 2011; Prescott, 2011; Puga, 2011; Takeda et al., 2012). Results of several new studies also support the idea. Using two mouse models, investigators showed that prenatal TCDD (2.5–5.0 mg/kg of body weight) modified multiple immune signatures in adult offspring that were indicative of adult-onset autoimmunity (Holladay et al., 2011). Adult-onset inflammatory disease and lupus-like autoimmunity were also observed in mice at 36 weeks of age after high-dose prenatal TCDD exposures (Mustafa et al., 2011). A single prenatal exposure of rats to TCDD (0.7 μg/kg of body weight) reduced brain developmental myelination and compromised remyelination potential in adults (Fernández et al., 2010), and in utero TCDD in mice alters neural progenitor differentiation (Mitsuhashi et al., 2010). However, a recent study suggested that, unlike murine neurospheres (which represent neural progenitor cells), human neurospheres were nonresponsive to TCDD because of lack of the AHR receptor—an indication of species specificity in response (Gassmann et al., 2010). Perinatal TCDD (0.2–0.4 μg/kg of body weight) in rats perturbed neuroendocrine function as measured by thyrotropin and growth hormone concentrations in exposed offspring through peripubertal postnatal day 30, and this supports the idea of continued later-life thyroid hormone disturbances (Ahmed, 2011). As discussed below, a few animal studies have provided evidence of transmission of adverse effects to later generations.

Mechanisms that could underlie later-life effects in offspring and effects in later generations (transgenerational inheritance) could involve epigenetic processes as described at the beginning of this chapter. Research into dioxin's potential as an epigenetic agent is in its early stages, but a few studies have suggested that dioxin has such properties. Direct evidence, however, is limited to maternal exposures of the developing embryo or fetus during in utero growth, and there have been no reports on paternal TCDD exposure and later-life effects in offspring or paternally-mediated transgenerational effects. As reported in *Update 2010*, Wu et al. (2004) demonstrated that TCDD exposure of mouse embryos before implantation in unexposed females resulted in epigenetic changes, including increased methylation and reduced expression of imprinted genes, which implied that early embryonic exposure alone was sufficient to alter gene expression in the resulting offspring. Transmission of effects to later generations would involve epigenetic alterations in the developing germ cells of a fetus that was directly exposed to maternal TCDD in utero. The germ-line epigenome modified either through altered DNA methylation or through core histone modifications would be permanent (that is, would escape the normal erasure of an imprinted gene) and would be transmitted over several generations.

Results of a few recent studies support a transgenerational inheritance due to in utero exposure to TCDD. Exposure of pregnant mice to TCDD (at 10 μg/kg) reduced fertility and increased premature birth in three later generations (Bruner-Tran and Osteen, 2011); effects were transmitted through both male and female offspring (Ding et al., 2011; McConaha et al., 2011). Exposure of gestating female rats (F0) to dioxin (TCDD) at 100 ng/kg was recently shown to result in earlier puberty in the offspring (F1) and two later generations (F2 and F3) and to reduce ovarian follicle numbers in females of the F3 generation; this implies transgenerational inheritance (Manikkam et al., 2012a). The F3 effects appear to be transmitted through the sperm that were initially exposed to maternal dioxin in utero. In a second paper by the same research team, additional diseases appeared later in life in the first generation (directly-exposed offspring), including prostate disease in males and ovarian follicle loss and polycystic ovarian disease in females (Manikkan et al., 2012b). Further third-generation effects were noted, including kidney disease in males and polycystic ovarian disease in females, and imply transgenerational inheritance. The latter appear to be transmitted through the sperm originally exposed to maternal dioxin in utero inasmuch as sperm DNA methylation changes were observed at 50 chromosomal sites in generations F1–F3.

Another mode of epigenetic change is modification of the spatial arrangement of chromosomes, which can influence gene expression and cell differentiation. Oikawa et al. (2008) have found that TCDD, through the AHR, modifies the positions of chromosomes in the interphase nuclei of human preadipocytes.

The studies discussed above suggest that TCDD has the potential to influence the epigenome and therefore could promote changes in offspring that lead to disease later in life.

Synthesis

The epidemiologic studies designed to examine effects of the COIs in more-mature offspring have evaluated a variety of biomarkers pertaining to the neurologic, immunologic, and endocrine systems. Most have not examined defined clinical conditions, although data on associations with otitis media (Miyashita et al., 2011; Weisglas-Kuperus et al., 2000) and impaired fertility in adult sons of exposed females (Mocarelli et al., 2011) are emerging. More studies that examine those and other end points are required. In particular, it would be of interest to obtain information on neuropsychiatric conditions in children who were exposed in utero, such as attention-deficit hyperactivity disorder and other clinically-defined neurodevelopmental outcomes. The animal literature contains evidence that environmental agents mediated by maternal exposure affect later generations through fetal and germ-line modifications, but, in the case of adult male exposures before conception of the next generation, there is insufficient evidence of transgenerational affects.

Conclusions

There is inadequate or insufficient evidence to determine whether there is an association between exposure of men and women to 2,4-D, 2,4,5-T, TCDD, picloram, or cacodylic acid before conception or during pregnancy and disease in their children as they mature or in later generations. Although results of laboratory research support the plausibility of transgenerational clinical conditions, the body of human data is insufficient to support an association between the COIs and such disease states in human offspring.

REFERENCES[1]

ACS (American Cancer Society). 2010. *Cancer Facts and Figures 2010*. http://www.cancer.org/acs/groups/content/@nho/documents/document/acspc–024113.pdf (accessed May 16, 2011).

ACS. 2013. *Cancer Facts and Figures 2013*. Atlanta, GA: American Cancer Society.

ADVA (Australia Department of Veterans Affairs). 1983. *Case-Control Study of Congenital Anomalies and Vietnam Service*. Canberra, Australia: ADVA.

Ahmed RG. 2011. Perinatal TCDD exposure alters developmental neuroendocrine system. *Food and Chemical Toxicology* 49:1276–1284.

AIHW (Australian Institute of Health and Welfare). 1999. *Morbidity of Vietnam Veterans: A Study of the Health of Australia's Vietnam Veteran Community: Volume 3: Validation Study*. Canberra, Australia.

AIHW. 2000. *Morbidity of Vietnam Veterans. Adrenal Gland Cancer, Leukaemia and Non-Hodgkin's Lymphoma: Supplementary Report No. 2*. (AIHW cat. no. PHE 28). Canberra, Australia: AIHW.

AIHW. 2001. *Morbidity of Vietnam Veterans. Adrenal Gland Cancer, Leukaemia and Non-Hodgkin's Lymphoma: Supplementary Report No. 2*. Revised edition (AIHW cat. No. PHE 34). Canberra, Australia: AIHW.

Aschengrau A, Monson RR. 1990. Paternal military service in Vietnam and the risk of late adverse pregnancy outcomes. *American Journal of Public Health* 80(10):1218–1224.

Barker DJP, Lampl M, Roseboom T, Winder N. 2012. Resource allocation in utero and health in later life. *Placenta* 33:e30–e34.

Bertazzi PA, Zocchetti C, Pesatori AC, Guercilena S, Consonni D, Tironi A, Landi MT. 1992. Mortality of a young population after accidental exposure to 2,3,7,8-tetrachlorodibenzodioxin. *International Journal of Epidemiology* 21(1):118–123.

Blatter BM, Hermens R, Bakker M, Roeleveld N, Verbeek AL, Zielhuis GA. 1997. Paternal occupational exposure around conception and spina bifida in offspring. *American Journal of Industrial Medicine* 32(3):283–291.

Bloom AD, ed. 1981. *Guidelines for Studies of Human Populations Exposed to Mutagenic and Reproductive Hazards*. White Plains, NY: March of Dimes Foundation.

Brown NM, Manzolillo PA, Zhang JX, Wang J, Lamartiniere CA. 1998. Prenatal TCDD and predisposition to mammary cancer in the rat. *Carcinogenesis* 19(9):1623–1629.

Bruner-Tran KL, Osteen KG. 2011. Developmental exposure to TCDD reduces fertility and negatively affects pregnancy outcomes across multiple generations. *Reproductive Toxicology* 31:344–350.

[1]Throughout this report, the same alphabetic indicator after year of publication is used consistently for a given reference when there are multiple citations by the same first author in a given year. The convention of assigning the alphabetic indicators in order of citation in a given chapter is not followed.

Buckley JD, Robison LL, Swotinsky R, Garabrant DH, LeBeau M, Manchester P, Nesbit ME, Odom L, Peters JM, Woods WG, Hammond GD. 1989. Occupational exposures of parents of children with acute nonlymphocytic leukemia: A report from the Childrens' Cancer Study Group. *Cancer Research* 49(14):4030–4037.

CDC (Centers for Disease Control and Prevention). 1989a. *Health Status of Vietnam Veterans. Vietnam Experience Study, Vol. V, Reproductive Outcomes and Child Health.* Atlanta, GA: US Department of Health and Human Services.

CDC. 1989b. *Health Status of Vietnam Veterans. Vietnam Experience Study, Vol. V, Reproductive Outcomes and Child Health.* Atlanta, GA: US Department of Health and Human Services.

Chao HR, Wang SL, Lee CC, Yu HY, Lu YK, Päpke O. 2004. Level of polychlorinated dibenzo-*p*-dioxins, dibenzofurans and biphenyls (PCDD/Fs, PCBs) in human milk and the input to infant body burden. *Food and Chemical Toxicology* 42:1299–1308.

Chapin RE, Robbins WA, Schieve LA, Sweeney AM, Tabacova SA, Tomashek KM. 2004. Off to a good start: The influence of pre- and periconceptional exposures, parental fertility, and nutrition on children's health. *Environmental Health Perspectives* 112(1):69–78.

Chen Z, Stewart PA, Davies S, Giller R, Krailo M, Davis M, Robison L, Shu XO. 2005. Parental occupational exposure to pesticides and childhood germ-cell tumors. *American Journal of Epidemiology* 162(9):858–867.

Chen Z, Robison L, Giller R, Krailo M, Davis M, Davies S, Shu XO. 2006. Environmental exposure to residential pesticides, chemicals, dusts, fumes, and metals, and risk of childhood germ cell tumors. *International Journal of Hygiene and Environmental Health* 209(1):31–40.

Chia SE, Shi LM. 2002. Review of recent epidemiological studies on paternal occupations and birth defects. *Occupational and Environmental Medicine* 59(3):149–155.

Chokkalingam AP, Metayer C, Scelo GA, Chang JS, Urayama KY, Aldrich MC, Guha N, Hansen HM, Dahl GV, Barcellos LF, Wiencke JK, Wiemels JL, Buffler PA. 2012. Variation in xenobiotic transport and metabolism genes, household chemical exposures, and risk of childhood acute lymphoblastic leukemia. *Cancer Causes and Control* 23(8):1367–1375.

Chow EJ, Kamineni A, Daling, JR, Fraser A, Wiggins CL, Mineau GP, Hamre MR, Severson RK, Drews-Botsch C, Mueller BA. 2009. Reproductive outcomes in male cancer survivors: A linked cancer-birth registry analysis. *Archives of Pediatric and Adolescent Medicine* 163(10):887–894.

Codrington AM, Hales BF, Robaire B. 2004. Spermiogenic germ cell phase-specific DNA damage following cyclophosphamide exposure. *Journal of Andrology* 25(3):354–362.

Cooney MA, Daniels JL, Ross JA, Breslow NE, Pollock BH, Olshan AF. 2007. Household pesticides and the risk of Wilms tumor. *Environmental Health Perspectives* 115(1):134–137.

Cordier S, Chevrier C, Robert-Gnansia E, Lorente C, Brula P, Hours M. 2004. Risk of congenital anomalies in the vicinity of municipal solid waste incinerators. *Occupational and Environmental Medicine* 61(1):8–15.

Cordier S, Lehebel A, Amar E, Anzivino-Viricel L, Hours M, Monfort C, Chevrier C, Chiron M, Robert-Gnansia E. 2010. Maternal residence near municipal waste incinerators and the risk of urinary tract birth defects. *Occupational and Environmental Medicine* 67(7):493–499.

Daniels JL, Olshan AF, Teschke K, Herz-Picciotto I, Savitz DA, Blatt J, Bondy ML, Neglia JP, Pollock BH, Cohn SL, Look AT, Seeger RC, Castleberry RP. 2001. Residential pesticide exposure and neuroblastoma. *Epidemiology* 12:20–27.

De Roos AJ, Olshan AF, Teschke K, Poole C, Savitz DA, Blatt J, Bondy ML, Pollock BH. 2001a. Parental occupational exposures to chemicals and incidence of neuroblastoma in offspring. *American Journal of Epidemiology* 154(2):106–114.

De Roos AJ, Teschke K, Savitz DA, Poole C, Grufferman S, Pollock BH, Olshan AF. 2001b. Parental occupational exposures to electromagnetic fields and radiation and incidence of neuroblastoma in offspring. *Epidemiology* 12(5):508–517.

Desaulniers D, Leingartner K, Musicki B, Cole J, Li M, Charboneau M, Tsang BK. 2004. Lack of effects of postnatal exposure to a mixture of aryl hydrocarbon-receptor agonists on the development of methylnitrosourea-induced mammary tumors in Sprague-Dawley rats. *Journal of Toxicology and Environmental Health Part A* 67(18):1457–1475.

Desrosiers TA, Herring AH, Shapira SK, Hooiveld M, Luben TJ, Herdt-Losavio ML, Olshan AF; National Birth Defects Prevention Study. 2012. Paternal occupation and birth defects: Findings from the National Birth Defects Prevention Study. *Occupational and Environmental Medicine* 69(8):534–542.

Dimich-Ward H, Hertzman C, Teschke K, Hershler R, Marion SA, Ostry A, Kelly S. 1996. Reproductive effects of paternal exposure to chlorophenate wood preservatives in the sawmill industry. *Scandinavian Journal of Work, Environment and Health* 22(4):267–273.

Ding T, McConaha M, Boyd KL, Osteen KG, Bruner-Tran KL. 2011. Developmental dioxin exposure of either parent is associated with an increased risk of preterm birth in adult mice. *Reproductive Toxicology* 31:351–358.

Dohle GR. 2010. Male infertility in cancer patients: Review of the literature. *International Journal of Urology* 17:327–331.

Dong B, Nishimura N, Vogel CF, Tohyama C, Matsumura F. 2010. TCDD-induced cyclooxygenase-2 expression is mediated by the nongenomic pathway in mouse MMDD1 macula densa cells and kidneys. *Biochemical Pharmacology* 79(3):487–497.

Donovan JW, MacLennan R, Adena M. 1984. Vietnam service and the risk of cogenital anomalies: A case-control study. *Medical Journal of Australia* 140(7):394–397.

Dragin N, Dalton TP, Miller ML, Shertzer HG, Nebert DW. 2006. For dioxin-induced birth defects, mouse or human CYP1A2 in maternal liver protects whereas mouse CYP1A1 and CYP1b1 are inconsequential. *Journal of Biological Chemistry* 281(27):18591–18600.

Draper GJ, Little MP, Sorahan T, Kinlen LJ, Bunch KJ, Conquest AJ, Kendall GM, Kneale GW, Lancashire RJ, Muirhead CR, O'Connor CM, Vincent TJ. 1997. Cancer in the offspring of radiation workers: A record linkage study. *British Medical Journal* 315(7117):1181–1188.

Erickson JD, Mulinare J, Mcclain P, Fitch T, James L, McClearn A, Adams M. 1984a. *Vietnam Veterans' Risks for Fathering Babies with Birth Defects.* Atlanta, GA: US Department of Health and Human Services, Centers for Disease Control.

Erickson JD, Mulinare J, McClain PW, Fitch TG, James LM, McClearn AB, Adams MJ. 1984b. Vietnam veterans' risks for fathering babies with birth defects. *Journal of the American Medical Association* 252(7):903–912.

Falahatpisheh MH, Nanez A, Ramos KS. 2011. AHR regulates WT1 genetic programming during murine nephrogenesis. *Molecular Medicine* 17(11–12):1275–1284.

Fear NT, Hey HK, Vincent T, Murphy M. 2007. Paternal occupation and neural tube defects: A case-control study based on the Oxford Record Linkage Study register. *Paediatric and Perinatal Epidemiology* 21(2):163–168.

Fenton SE, Hamm JT, Birnbaum LS, Youngblood GL. 2000. Adverse effects of TCDD on mammary gland development in Long Evans rats: A two generational study. *Organohalogen Compounds* 48:157–160.

Fenton SE, Hamm JT, Birnbaum LS, Youngblood GL. 2002. Persistent abnormalities in the rat mammary gland following gestational and lactational exposure to 2,3,7,8–tetrachlorodibenzo-*p*-dioxin (TCDD). *Toxicological Sciences* 67(1):63–74.

Fernández M, Paradisi M, D'Intino G, Del Vecchio G, Sivilia S, Giardino L, Calzà L. 2010. A single prenatal exposure to the endocrine disruptor 2,3,7,8-tetrachlorodibenzo-*p*-dioxin alters developmental myelination and remyelination potential in the rat brain. *Journal of Neurochemistry* 115(4):897–909.

Field B, Kerr C. 1988. Reproductive behaviour and consistent patterns of abnormality in offspring of Vietnam veterans. *Journal of Medical Genetics* 25:819–826.

Fitzgerald EF, Weinstein AL, Youngblood LG, Standfast SJ, Melius JM. 1989. Health effects three years after potential exposure to the toxic contaminants of an electrical transformer fire. *Archives of Environmental Health* 44:214–221.

Flower KB, Hoppin JA, Lynch CF, Blair A, Knott C, Shore DL, Sandler DP. 2004. Cancer risk and parental pesticide application in children of Agricultural Health Study participants. *Environmental Health Perspectives* 112(5):631–635.

Foster WG, Maharaj-Briceño S, Cyr DG. 2011. Dioxin-induced changes in epididymal sperm count and spermatogenesis. *Ciência and Saúde Coletiva* 16(6):2893–2905.

García AM, Benavides FG, Fletcher T, Orts E. 1998. Paternal exposure to pesticides and congenital malformations. *Scandinavian Journal of Work, Environment and Health* 24(6):473–480.

Gardner MJ, Snee MP, Hall AJ, Powell CA, Downes S, Terrell JD. 1990. Results of case-control study of leukaemia and lymphoma among young people near Sellafield nuclear plant in West Cumbria. *British Medical Journal* 300(6722):423–429.

Garry VF, Schreinemachers D, Harkins ME, Griffith J. 1996. Pesticide appliers, biocides, and birth defects in rural Minnesota. *Environmental Health Perspectives* 104(4):394–399.

Gassmann K, Abel J, Bothe H, Haarmann-Stemmann T, Merk HF, Quasthoff KN, Rockel TD, Schreiber T, Fritsche E. 2010. Species-specific differential AHR expression protects human neural progenitor cells against developmental neurotoxicity of PAHs. *Environmental Health Perspectives* 118(11):1571–1577.

Green DM, Kawashima T, Stovall M, Leisenring W, Sklar CA, Mertens AC, Donaldson SS, Byrne J, Robison LL. 2010. Fertility of male surviviors of childhood cancer: A report from the Childhood Cancer Survivor Study. *Journal of Clinical Oncology* 28(2):332–339.

Hales BF, Grenier L, Lalancette C, Robaire B. 2011. Epigenetic programming: From gametes to blasatocyst. *Birth Defects Research (Part A)* 91:652–665.

Hamatani T. 2012. Human spermatozoal RNAs. *Fertility and Sterility* (9792):275–281.

Hammoud SS, Nix DA, Zhang H, Purwar J, Carrell DT, Cairns BR. 2009. Distinctive chromatin in human sperm packages genes for embryo development. *Nature* 460:473–478.

Hanify JA, Metcalf P, Nobbs CL, Worsley KJ. 1981. Aerial spraying of 2,4,5-T and human birth malformations: An epidemiological investigation. *Science* 212:349–351.

Heacock H, Hogg R, Marion SA, Hershler R, Teschke K, Dimich-Ward H, Demers P, Kelly S, Ostry A, Hertzman C. 1998. Fertility among a cohort of male sawmill workers exposed to chlorophenate fungicides. *Epidemiology* 9(1):56–60.

Holladay SD, Mustafa A, Gogal RM Jr. 2011. Prenatal TCDD in mice increases adult autoimmunity. *Reproductive Toxicology* 31:312–318.

Hou L, Zhang X, Wang D, Baccarelli A. 2011. Environmental chemical exposures and human epigenetics. *International Journal of Epidemiology* 41(1):79–105.

Howell SJ, Shalet SM. 2005. Spermatogenesis after cancer treatment: Damage and recovery. *Journal of the National Cancer Institute Monographs* 34:12–17.

Humblet O, Williams PL, Korrick SA, Sergeyev O, Emond C, Birnbaum LS, Burns JS, Altshul L, Patterson DG Jr, Turner WE, Lee MM, Revich B, Hauser R. 2011. Dioxin and polychlorinated biphenyl concentrations in mother's serum and the timing of pubertal onset in sons. *Epidemiology* 22(6):827–835.

Infante-Rivard C, Labuda D, Krajinovic M, Sinnett D. 1999. Risk of childhood leukemia associated with exposure to pesticides and with gene polymorphisms. *Epidemiology* 10:481–487.

IOM (Institute of Medicine). 1994. *Veterans and Agent Orange: Health Effects of Herbicides Used in Vietnam.* Washington DC: National Academy Press.

IOM. 1996. *Veterans and Agent Orange: Update 1996.* Washington, DC: National Academy Press.

IOM. 1999. *Veterans and Agent Orange: Update 1998.* Washington, DC: National Academy Press.

IOM. 2001. *Veterans and Agent Orange: Update 2000.* Washington, DC: National Academy Press.

IOM. 2002. *Veterans and Agent Orange: Herbicide/Dioxin Exposure and Acute Myelogenous Leukemia in the Children of Vietnam Veterans.* Washington, DC: National Academy Press.

IOM. 2003. *Veterans and Agent Orange: Update 2002.* Washington, DC: The National Academies Press.

IOM. 2005. *Veterans and Agent Orange: Update 2004.* Washington, DC: The National Academies Press.

IOM. 2007. *Veterans and Agent Orange: Update 2006.* Washington, DC: The National Academies Press.

IOM. 2009. *Veterans and Agent Orange: Update 2008.* Washington, DC: The National Academies Press.

IOM. 2011. *Veterans and Agent Orange: Update 2010.* Washington, DC: The National Academies Press.

Izumi S, Koyama K, Soda M, Suyama A. 2003. Cancer incidence in children and young adults did not increase relative to parental exposure to atomic bombs. *British Journal of Cancer* 89:1709–1713.

Jacobs H, Dennefeld C, Féret B, Viluksela M, Håkansson H, Mark M, Ghyselinck NB. 2011. Retinoic acid drives aryl hydrocarbon receptor expression and is instrumental to dioxin-induced toxicity during palate development. *Environmental Health Perspectives* 119(11):1590–1595.

Jang JY, Shin S, Choi BI, Park D, Jeon JH, Hwang SY, Kim JC, Kim YB, Nahm SS. 2007. Antiteratogenic effects of alpha-naphthoflavone on 2,3,7,8-tetrachlorodibenzo-*p*-dioxin (TCDD) exposed mice in utero. *Reproductive Toxicology* 24(3-4):303–309.

Jang JY, Park D, Shin S, Jeon JH, Choi Bi, Joo SS, Hwang SY, Nahm SS, Kim YB. 2008. Antiteratogenic effect of resveratrol in mice exposed in utero to 2,3,7,8-tetrachlorodibenzo-*p*-dioxin. *European Journal of Pharmacology* 591(1–3):280–283.

Jenkins TG, Carrell DT. 2012a. Dynamic alterations in the paternal epigenetic landscape following fertilization. *Frontiers in Genetics* 3:1–8.

Jenkins TG, Carrell DT. 2012b. The sperm epigenome and potential implications for the developing embryo. *Reproduction* 143:727–734.

Jirtle RL, Skinner MS. 2007. Environmental epigenomics and disease susceptibility. *Nature Reviews Genetics* 8:253–262.

Jusko TA, De Roos AJ, Schwartz SM, Lawrence BP, Palkovicova L, Nemessanyi T, Drobna B, Fabisikova A, Kocan A, Jahnova E, Kavanagh TJ, Trnovec T, Hertz-Picciotto I. 2011. Maternal and early postnatal polychlorinated biphenyl exposure in relation to total serum immunoglobulin concentrations in 6-month-old infants. *Journal of Immunotoxicology* 8(1):95–100.

Kalter H, Warkany J. 1983. Congenital malformations. Etiologic factors and their role in prevention (first of two parts). *New England Journal of Medicine* 308:424–431.

Kang HK, Mahan CM, Lee KY, Magee CA, Mather SH, Matanoski G. 2000. Pregnancy outcomes among US women Vietnam veterans. *American Journal of Industrial Medicine* 38(4):447–454.

Kawano M, Kawaji H, Grandjean V, Klani J, Rassoulzadegan M. 2012. Novel small noncoding RNAs in mouse spermatozo, zygotes and early embryos. *PLOS ONE* 7(9):e44542.

Kerr M, Nasca PC, Mundt KA, Michalek AM, Baptiste MS, Mahoney MC. 2000. Parental occupational exposures and risk of neuroblastoma: A case-control study (United States). *Cancer Causes and Control* 11:635–643.

Kinlen LJ. 1993. Can paternal preconceptional radiation account for the increase of leukaemia and non-Hodgkin's lymphoma in Seacale. *British Medical Journal* 306(6894):1718–1721.

Kinlen LJ, Clarke K, Balkwaill A. 1993. Paternal preconceptional radiation exposure in the nuclear industry and leukaemia and non-Hodgkin's lymphoma in young people in Scotland. *British Medical Journal* 306(6886):1153–1158.

Klemmt L, Scialli AR. 2005. The transport of chemicals in semen. *Birth Defects Research (Part B)* 74:119–131.

Kramer JA, Krawetz SA. 1997. RNA in spermatozoa: Implications for the alternative haploid genome. *Molecular Human Reproduction* 3(6):473–478.

Krawetz SA. 2005. Paternal contribution: New insights and future challenges. *Nature Reviews Genetics* 6:633–642.

Krawetz SA, Kruger A, Lalancette C, Tagett R, Anton E, Draghici S, Diamond MP. 2011. A survey of small RNAs in human sperm. *Human Reproduction* 26(12):3401–3412.

Kristensen P, Andersen A, Irgens LM, Bye AS, Sundheim L. 1996. Cancer in offspring of parents engaged in agricultural activities in Norway: Incidence and risk factors in the farm environment. *International Journal of Cancer* 65(1):39–50.

Kristensen P, Irgens LM, Andersen A, Bye AS, Sundheim L. 1997. Birth defects among offspring of Norwegian farmers, 1967–1991. *Epidemiology* 8(5):537–544.

Kuscu OO, Caglar E, Aslan S, Durmusoglu E, Karademir A, Sandalli N. 2009. The prevalence of molar incisor hypomineralization (MIH) in a group of children in a highly polluted urban region and a windfarm–green energy island. *International Journal of Paediatric Dentistry* 19(3):176–185.

Krysiak-Baltyn K, Toppari J, Skakkebaek NE, Jensen TS, Virtanen HE, Schramm KW, Shen H, Vartiainen T, Kiviranta H, Taboureau O, Audouze K, Brunak S, Main KM. 2012. Association between chemical pattern in breast milk and congenital cryptorchidism: Modelling of complex human exposures. *International Journal of Andrology* 35:294–302.

Laisi S, Kiviranta H, Lukinmaa PL, Vartiainen T, Alaluusua S. 2008. Molar–incisor–hypomineralisation and dioxins: New findings. *European Archives of Paediatric Dentistry: Official Journal of the European Academy of Paediatric Dentistry* 9(4):224–227.

Lamb JC 4th, Moore JA, Marks TA, Haseman JK. 1981. Development and viability of offspring of male mice treated with chlorinated phenoxy acids and 2,3,7,8-tetrachlorodibenzo-*p*-dioxin. *Journal of Toxicology and Environmental Health* 8(5-6):835–844.

Lanham KA, Peterson RE, Heideman W. 2012. Sensitivity to dioxin decreases as zebrafish mature. *Toxicological Sciences* 127(2):360–370.

La Rocca C, Alivernini S, Badiali M, Cornoldi A, Iacovella N, Silvestroni L, Spera G, Turrio-Baldassarri L. 2008. TEQs and body burden for PCDDs, PCDFs, and dioxin-like PCBs in human adipose tissue. *Chemosphere* 73(1):92–96.

Latchney SE, Lioy DT, Henry EC, Gasiewicz TA, Strathmann FG, Mayer-Pröschel M, Opanashuk LA. 2011. Neural precursor cell proliferation is disrupted through activation of the aryl hydrocarbon receptor by 2,3,7,8-tetrachlorodibenzo-*p*-dioxin. *Stem Cells and Development* 20(2):313–326.

Lawson CC, Schnorr TM, Whelan EA, Deddens JA, Dankovic DA, Piacitelli LA, Sweeney MH, Connally LB. 2004. Paternal occupational exposure to 2,3,7,8-tetrachlorodibenzo-*p*-dioxin and birth outcomes of offspring: Birth weight, preterm delivery, and birth defects. *Environmental Health Perspectives* 112(14):1403–1408.

Leijs MM, ten Tusscher GW, Olie K, van Teunenbroek T, van Aalderen WM, de Voogt P, Vulsma T, Bartonova A, Krayer von Krauss M, Mosoiu C, Riojas-Rodriguez H, Calamandrei G, Koppe JG. 2012. Thyroid hormone metabolism and environmental chemical exposure. *Environmental Health* 11(Suppl 1):S1–S10.

Loffredo CA, Silbergeld EK, Ferencz C, Zhang J. 2001. Association of transposition of the great arteries in infants with maternal exposures to herbicides and rodenticides. *American Journal of Epidemiology* 153(6):529–536.

Lorber M, Phillips L. 2002. Infant exposure to dioxin-like compounds in breast milk. *Environmental Health Perspectives* 110(6):A325–A332.

Madanat-Harjuoja LS, Malila N, Lahteenmaki P, Pukkula E, Mulviihill JJ, Boise JD Jr, Sankila R. 2010. Risk of cancer among children of cancer patients: A nationwide study in Finland. *International Journal of Cancer* 126:1196–1205.

Manikkam M, Guerrero-Bosagna C, Tracey R, Haque MM, Skinner MK. 2012a. Transgenerational actions of environmental compounds on reproductive disease and identification of epigenetic biomarkers of ancestral exposures. *PLoS ONE* 7(2):12 pps.

Manikkam M, Tracey R, Guerrero-Bosagna C, Skinner MK. 2012b. Dioxin (TCDD) induces epigenetic transgenerational inheritance of adult onset disease and sperm epimutations. *PLoS ONE* 7(9):15 pps.

Mastroiacovo P, Spagnolo A, Marni E, Meazza L, Betrollini R, Segni G, Brogna-Pignatti C. 1988. Birth defects in Seveso area after TCDD contamination. *Journal of the American Medical Association* 259:1668–1672 (published erratum appears in *JAMA* 1988, 260:792).

McConaha ME, Ding T, Lucas JA, Arosh JA, Osteen KG, Bruner-Tran KL. 2011. Preconception omega-3 fatty acid supplementation of adult male mice with a history of developmental 2,3,7,8-tetrachlorodibenzo-*p*-dioxin exposure prevents preterm birth in unexposed female partners. *Reproduction* 142:235–241.

Meinert R, Schüz J, Kaletsch U, Kaatsch P, Michaelis J. 2000. Leukemia and non-Hodgkin's lymphoma in childhood and exposure to pesticides: Results of a register-based case-control study in Germany. *American Journal of Epidemiology* 151(7):639–646.

Meyer KJ, Reif JS, Veeramachaneni DN, Luben TJ, Mosley BS, Nuckols JR. 2006. Agricultural pesticide use and hypospadias in eastern Arkansas. *Environmental Health Perspectives* 114(10):1589–1595.

Michalek JE, Albanese RA, Wolfe WH. 1998a. *Project Ranch Hand II: An Epidemiologic Investigation of Health Effects in Air Force Personnel Following Exposure to Herbicides—Reproductive Outcome Update.* US Department of Commerce, National Technical Information Service. Report number AFRL-HE-BR-TR-1998-0073.

Mimura J, Yamashita K, Nakamura K, Morita M, Takagi TN, Nakao K, Ema M, Sogawa K, Yasuda M, Katsuki M, Fujii-Kuriyama Y. 1997. Loss of teratogenic response to 2,3,7,8-tetrachlorodibenzo-*p*-dioxin (TCDD) in mice lacking the Ah (dioxin) receptor. *Genes to Cells* 2(10):645–654.

Mitsuhashi T, Yonemotob J, Soneb H, Kosugea Y, Kosakia K, Takahashi T. 2010. In utero exposure to dioxin causes neocortical dysgenesis through the actions of p27Kip1. *Proceedings of the National Academy of Sciences of the United States of America* 107(37):16331–16335.

Miyashita C, Sasaki S, Saijo Y, Washino N, Okada E, Kobayashi S, Konishi K, Kajiwara J, Todaka T, Kishi R. 2011. Effects of prenatal exposure to dioxin-like compounds on allergies and infections during infancy. *Environmental Research* 111:551–558.

Mocarelli P, Gerthoux PM, Needham LL, Patterson DG Jr, Limonta G, Falbo R, Signorini S, Bertona M, Crespi C, Sarto C, Scott PK, Turner WE, Brambilla P. 2011. Perinatal exposure to low doses of dioxin can permanently impair human semen quality. *Environmental Health Perspectives* 119(5):713–718.

Monge P, Wesseling C, Guardado J, Lundberg I, Ahlbom A, Cantor KP, Weiderpass E, Partanen T. 2007. Parental occupational exposure to pesticides and the risk of childhood leukemia in Costa Rica. *Scandinavian Journal of Work, Environment and Health* 33(4):293–303.

Moses M, Lilis R, Crow KD, Thornton J, Fischbein A, Anderson HA, Selikoff IJ. 1984. Health status of workers with past exposure to 2,3,7,8-tetrachlorodibenzo-*p*-dioxin in the manufacture of 2,4,5-trichlorophenoxyacetic acid: Comparison of findings with and without chloracne. *American Journal of Industrial Medicine* 5(3):161–182.

Mustafa A, Holladay S, Witonsky S, Zimmerman K, Manari A, Countermarsh S, Karpuzoglu E, Gogal R. 2011. Prenatal TCDD causes persistent modulation of the postnatal immune response, and exacerbates inflammatory disease, in 36-week-old lupus-like autoimmune SNF1 mice. *Birth Defects Research (Part B)* 92:82–94.

Nagayama J, Okamura K, Iida T, Hirakawa H, Matsueda T, Tsuji H, Hasegawa M, Sato K, Ma HY, Yanagawa T, Igarashi H, Fukushige J, Watanabe T. 1998. Postnatal exposure to chlorinated dioxins and related chemicals on thyroid hormone status in Japanese breast-fed infants. *Chemosphere* 37(9-12):1789–1793.

NCI (National Cancer Institute). 2001. *Surveillance, Epidemiology, and End Results (SEER) database.* http://seer.cancer.gov/ScientificSystems/CanQues (accessed March 19).

Neri T, Merico V, Fiordaliso F, Salio M, Rebuzzini P, Sacchi L, Bellazzi R, Redi CA, Zuccotti M, Garagna S. 2011. The differentiation of cardiomyocytes from mouse embryonic stem cells is altered by dioxin. *Toxicology Letters* 202:226–236.

Nishijo M, Tai PT, Nakagawa H, Maruzeni S, Anh NT, Luong HV, Anh TH, Honda R, Morikawa Y, Kido T, Nishijo H. 2012. Impact of perinatal dioxin exposure on infant growth: A cross-sectional and longitudinal studies in dioxin-contaminated areas in Vietnam. *PLoS ONE* 7(7):10 pps.

Oikawa K, Yoshida K, Takanashi M, Tanabe H, Kiyuna T, Ogura M, Saito A, Umezawa A, Kuroda M. 2008. Dioxin interferes in chromosomal positioning through the aryl hydrocarbon receptor. *Biochemical and Biophysical Research Communications* 374(2):361–364.

Ouko LA, Shantikumar K, Knezovich J, Haycock P, Schnugh DJ, Ramsay M. 2009. Effect of alcohol consumption on CpG methylation in the differentially methylated regions of *H19* and *IG-DMR* in male gametes: Implications for fetal alcohol spectrum disorders. *Alcoholism: Clinical and Experimental Research* 33(9):1615–1627.

Parker L, Craft AW, Smith J, Dickinson H, Wakeford R, Binks K, McElvenny D, Scott L, Slovak A. 1993. Geographical distribution of preconceptional radiation doses to fathers employed at the Sellafield nuclear installation, West Cumbria. *British Medical Journal* 307:966–971.

Pearce MS, Parker L. 2000. Paternal employment in agriculture and childhood kidney cancer. *Pediatric Hematology and Oncology* 17(3):223–230.

Pesatori AC, Consonni D, Tironi A, Zocchetti C, Fini A, Bertazzi PA. 1993. Cancer in a young population in a dioxin-contaminated area. *International Journal of Epidemiology* 22(6):1010–1013.

Prescott SL. 2011. The influence of early environmental exposures on immune development and subsequent risk of allergic disease. *Allergy* 66(Suppl 95):4–6.

Puga A. 2011. Perspectives on the potential involvement of the AH receptor-dioxin axis in cardiovascular disease. *Toxicological Sciences* 120(2):256–261.

Puri D, Dhawan J, Mishra RK. 2010. The paternal hidden agenda: Epigenetic inheritance through sperm chromatin. *Epigenetics* 5(5):386–391.

Quintanilla-Vega B, Hoover DJ, Bal W, Silbergeld EK, Waalkes MP, Anderson LD. 2000. Lead interaction with human protamine (HP2) as a mechanism of male reproductive toxicity. *Chemical Research in Toxicology* 13:594–600.

Ray SS, Swanson HI. 2004. Dioxin-induced immortalization of normal human keratinocytes and silencing of p53 and p16INK4a. *Journal of Biological Chemistry* 279(26):27187–27193.

Ren A, Qiu X, Jin L, Ma J, Li Z, Zhang L, Zhu H, Finnell RH, Zhu T. 2011. Association of selected persistent organic pollutants in the placenta with the risk of neural tube defects. *Proceedings of the National Academy of Sciences of the United States of America* 108(31):12770–12775.

Revich B, Aksel E, Ushakova T, Ivanova I, Zuchenko N, Lyuev N, Brodsky B, Sotsov Y. 2001. Dioxin exposure and public health in Chapaevsk, Russia. *Chemosphere* 43(4-7):951–966.

Reynolds P, Von Behren J, Gunier RB, Goldberg DE, Harnly M, Hertz A. 2005b. Agricultural pesticide use and childhood cancer in California. *Epidemiology* 16(1):93–100.

Rocheleau CM, Romitti PA, Sanderson WT, Sun L, Lawson CC, Waters MA, Stewart PA, Olney RS, Reefhuis J. 2011. Maternal occupational pesticide exposure and risk of hypospadias in the National Birth Defects Prevention Study. *Birth Defects Research (Part A)* 91(11):927–936.

Rudant J, Menegaux F, Leverger G, Baruchel A, Nelken B, Bertrand Y, Patte C, Pacquement H, Verite C, Robert A, Michel G, Margueritte G, Gandemer V, Hemon D, Clavel J. 2007. Household exposure to pesticides and risk of childhood hematopoietic malignancies: The ESCALE study (SFCE). *Environmental Health Perspectives* 115(12):1787–1793.

Schecter A, McGee H, Stanley JS, Boggess K, Brandt-Rauf P. 1996. Dioxins and dioxin-like chemicals in blood and semen of American Vietnam veterans from the state of Michigan. *American Journal of Industrial Medicine* 30(6):647–654.

Schlebusch H, Wagner U, van der Ven H, al-Hasani S, Diedrich K, Krebs D. 1989. Polychlorinated biphenyls: The occurrence of the main congeners in follicular and sperm fluids. *Journal of Clinical Chemistry and Clinical Biochemistry* 27(9):663–667.

Schreinemachers DM. 2003. Birth malformations and other adverse perinatal outcomes in four US wheat-producing states. *Environmental Health Perspectives* 111(9):1259–1264.

Schull WJ. 2003. The children of atomic bomb survivors. A synopsis. *Journal of Radiological Protection* 23(4):369–384.

Shaw GM, Nelson V, Olshan AF. 2002. Paternal occupational group and risk of offspring with neural tube defects. *Paediatric and Perinatal Epidemiology* 16(4):328–333.

Skinner MK, Manikkam M, Guerrero-Bosagna C. 2010. Epigenetic transgenerational actions of environmental factors in disease etiology. *Trends Endocrinology and Metabolism* 21(4):214–222.

Slater ME, Linabery AM, Spector LG, Johnson KJ, Hilden JM, Heerema NA, Robison LL, Ross JA. 2011. Maternal exposure to household chemicals and risk of infant leukemia: A report from the Children's Oncology Group. *Cancer Causes and Control* 22(8):1197–1204.

Smith AH, Fisher DO, Pearce N, Chapman CJ. 1982. Congenital defects and miscarriages among New Zealand 2,4,5-T sprayers. *Archives of Environmental Health* 37:197–200.

Smith MT, McHale CM, Wiemels JL, Zhang L, Wiencke JK, Zheng S, Gunn L, Skibola CF, Ma X, Buffler PA. 2005. Molecular biomarkers for the study of childhood leukemia. *Toxicology and Applied Pharmacology* 206(2):237–245.

Stachel B, Dougherty RC, Lahl U, Schlösser M, Zeschmar B. 1989. Toxic environmental chemicals in human semen: Analytical method and case studies. *Andrologia* 21(3):282–291.

Stockbauer JW, Hoffman RE, Schramm WF, Edmonds LD. 1988. Reproductive outcomes of mothers with potential exposure to 2,3,7,8-tetrachlorodibenzo-*p*-dioxin. *American Journal of Epidemiology* 128:410–419.

Su PH, Huang PC, Lin CY, Ying TH, Chen JY, Wang SL. 2012. The effect of in utero exposure to dioxins and polychlorinated biphenyls on reproductive development in eight year-old children. *Environment International* 39:181–187.

Suh N, Blelloch R. 2011. Small RNAs in early mammalian development: From gametes to gastrulation. *Development* 138:1653–1661.

Suskind RR, Hertzberg VS. 1984. Human health effects of 2,4,5-T and its toxic contaminants. *Journal of the American Medical Association* 251:2372–2380.

Suzuki G, Nakano M, Nakano S. 2005. Distribution of PCDDs/PCDFs and co-PCBs in human maternal blood, cord blood, placenta, milk, and adipose tissue: Dioxins showing high toxic equivalency factor accumulate in the placenta. *Bioscience, Biotechnology and Biochemistry* 69(10):1836–1847.

Tait S, La Rocca C, Mantovani A. 2011. Exposure of human fetal penile cells to different PCB mixtures: Transcriptome analysis points to diverse modes of interference on external genitalia programming. *Reproductive Toxicology* 32:1–14.

Takeda T, Fujii M, Taura J, Ishii Y, Yamada H. 2012. Dioxin silences gonadotropin expression in perinatal pups by inducing histone deacetylases: A new insight into the mechanism for the imprinting of sexual immaturity by dioxin. *Journal of Biological Chemistry* 287(22):18440–18450.

Tango T, Fujita T, Tanihata T, Minowa M, Doi Y, Kato N, Kunikane S, Uchiyama I, Tanaka M, Uehata T. 2004. Risk of adverse reproductive outcomes associated with proximity to municipal solid waste incinerators with high dioxin emission levels in Japan. *Journal of Epidemiology* 14(3):83–93.

ten Tusscher GW, Stam GA, Koppe JG. 2000. Open chemical combustions resulting in a local increased incidence of orofacial clefts. *Chemosphere* 40(9-11):1263–1270.

Townsend JC, Bodner KM, Van Peenen PFD, Olson RD, Cook RR. 1982. Survey of reproductive events of wives of employees exposed to chlorinated dioxins. *American Journal of Epidemiology* 115:695–713.

Troudi A, Soudani N, Samet AM, Amara IB, Zeghal N. 2011. 2,4-dichlorophenoxyacetic acid effects on nephrotoxicity in rats during late pregnancy and early postnatal periods. *Ecotoxicology and Environmental Safety* 74:2316–2323.

van den Berg M, Birnbaum LS, Denison M, De Vito M, Farland W, Feeley M, Fiedler H, Hakansson H, Hanberg A, Haws L, Rose M, Safe S, Schrenk D, Tohyama C, Tritscher A, Tuomisto J, Tysklind M, Walker N, Peterson RE, 2006. The 2005 World Health Organization reevaluation of human and mammalian toxic equivalency factors for dioxins and dioxin-like compounds. *Toxicological Sciences.* 93(2):223–241.

van Wijngaarden E, Stewart PA, Olshan AF, Savitz DA, Bunin GR. 2003. Parental occupational exposure to pesticides and childhood brain cancer. *American Journal of Epidemiology* 157(11):989–997.

Virtanen HE, Koskenniemi JJ, Sundqvist E, Main KM, Kiviranta H, Tuomisto JT, Tuomisto J, Viluksela M, Vartiainen T, Skakkebaek NE, Toppari J. 2012. Associations between congenital cryptorchidism in newborn boys and levels of dioxins and PCBs in placenta. *International Journal of Andrology* 35(3):283–293.

Wang SL, Lin CY, Guo YL, Lin LY, Chou WL, Chang LW. 2004. Infant exposure to polychlorinated dibenzo-*p*-dioxins, dibenzofurans and biphenyls (PCDD/Fs, PCBs)—correlation between prenatal and postnatal exposure. *Chemosphere* 54:1459–1473.

Wang SL, Su PH, Jong SB, Guo YL, Chou WL, Päpke O. 2005. In utero exposure to dioxins and polychlorinated biphenyls and its relations to thyroid function and growth hormone in newborns. *Environmental Health Perspectives* 113:1645–1650.

Weisglas-Kuperus N, Patandin S, Berbers GAM, Sas TCJ, Mulder PGH, Sauer PJJ, Hooijkaas H. 2000. Immunologic effects of background exposure to polychlorinated biphenyls and dioxins in Dutch preschool children. *Environmental Health Perspectives* 108(12):1203–1207.

Wen WQ, Shu XO, Steinbuch M, Severson RK, Reaman GH, Buckley JD, Robison LL. 2000. Paternal military service and risk for childhood leukemia in offspring. *American Journal of Epidemiology* 151(3):231–240.

Weselak M, Arbuckle TE, Foster W. 2007. Pesticide exposures and developmental outcomes: The epidemiological evidence. *Journal of Toxicology and Environmental Health (Part B)* 10:41–80.

Weselak M, Arbuckle TE, Wigle DT, Walker MC, Krewski D. 2008. Pre-and post-conception pesticide exposure and the risk of birth defects in an Ontario farm population. *Reproductive Toxicology* 25(4):472–480.

WHO (World Health Organization). 1999. *Laboratory Manual for the Examination of Human Semen and Sperm-Cervical Mucus Interaction.* 4th ed. Cambridge, UK: Cambridge University Press.

Wigle DT, Arbuckle TE, Walker M, Wade MG, Liu S, Krewski D. 2007. Environmental hazards: Evidence for effects on child health. *Journal of Toxicology and Environmental Health (Part B)* 10:3–39.

Wigle DT, Arbuckle TE, Turner MC, Berube A, Yang Q, Liu S, Krewski D. 2008. Epidemiologic evidence of relationships between reproductive and child health outcomes and environmental chemical contaminants. *Journal of Toxicology and Environmental Health (Part B)* 11:373–517.

Wolfe WH, Michalek JE, Miner JC, Rahe AJ, Moore CA, Needham LL, Patterson DG Jr. 1995. Paternal serum dioxin and reproductive outcomes among veterans of Operation Ranch Hand. *Epidemiology* 6:17–22.

Wu Q, Ohsako S, Ishimura R, Suzuki JS, Tohyama C. 2004. Exposure of mouse preimplantation embryos to 2,3,7,8-tetrachlorodibenzo-*p*-dioxin (TCDD) alters the methylation status of imprinted genes H19 and Igf2. *Biological Reproduction* 70(6):1790–1797.

Yoshioka W, Aida-Yasuoka K, Fujisawa N, Kawaguchi T, Ohsako S, Hara S, Uematsu S, Akira S, Tohyama C. 2012. Critical role of microsomal prostaglandin E synthase-1 in the hydronephrosis caused by lactational exposure to dioxin in mice. *Toxicological Sciences* 127(2):547–554.

Yuan X, Liu L, Pu Y, Zhang X, He X, Fu Y. 2012. 2,3,7,8-Tetrachlorodibenzo-*p*-dioxin induces a proteomic pattern that defines cleft palate formation in mice. *Food and Chemical Toxicology* 50:2270–2274.

11

Neurologic Disorders

Chapter Overview

Based on new evidence and a review of prior studies, the committee for Update 2012 *did not find any new significant associations between the relevant exposures and neurological disorders. Current evidence supports the findings of earlier studies that*

- *No adverse cardiovascular or metabolic outcome has sufficient evidence of an association with the chemicals of interest.*
- *There is limited or suggestive evidence of an association between the chemicals of interest and Parkinson disease.*
- *There is inadequate or insufficient evidence to determine whether there is an association between the chemicals of interest and for all other adverse neurologic outcomes.*

Immediate effects of toxicants may involve all aspects of the nervous system, whereas delayed effects are likely to produce more focal problems. Diffuse damage to the central nervous system (CNS) may cause alterations in thinking, consciousness, or attention, often in combination with abnormalities in movement. Focal dysfunction can cause myriad syndromes, depending on which area is damaged. Neurologic disorders can cause problems with thinking and emotional dysregulation, but for the purpose of this review they are distinguished from psychiatric conditions—such as posttraumatic stress disorder, depression, and anxiety—and from systemic conditions of uncertain cause, such as chronic fatigue syndrome, although either type of condition may actually have some neurophysiologic contributing factors. In this chapter, we will consider possible diffuse CNS effects of toxic exposure and specific clinical conditions that result from focal dysfunction. Examples of diseases that result from degeneration of specific brain areas are Parkinson disease (PD), Alzheimer disease (AD), spinocerebellar degeneration, and amyotrophic lateral sclerosis (ALS); these diseases can occur in the absence of any toxicant exposure, but all may be triggered by aspects of the environment, including toxicant exposure.

Disorders of the peripheral nervous system (PNS) are generally referred to as neuropathies. Neuropathies may be purely motor and affect only movement or purely sensory; most often, however, both motor and sensory fibers are affected. Neuropathies usually are symmetric and start with symptoms related to dysfunction of fibers that travel the greatest distance to their target organ. For that reason, symptoms of neuropathy generally start in the digits and travel toward the torso. Most neuropathies also affect autonomic fibers and thus can result in changes in blood pressure and heart rate and in symptoms related to the control of digestion. Toxicant exposure can induce immediate damage to peripheral nerves, and previous updates found limited or suggestive evidence that dioxin exposure caused such short-term effects. Evidence related to rapid onset of these conditions is presented in Appendix B, which deals with short-term adverse health effects. Previously undistilled information concerning persistence of symptoms after early effects is also evaluated in Appendix B. The overall focus of this chapter is on *delayed* adverse effects on the PNS and the CNS.

Timing is important in assessing the effects of chemical exposure on neurologic function and must be considered in the design and critique of epidemiologic studies. In the original *Veterans and Agent Orange: Health Effects of Herbicides Used in Vietnam* report, hereafter referred to as *VAO* (IOM, 1994), attention was focused on persistent neurobehavioral disorders. That focus was maintained in *Update 1996* (IOM, 1996), *Update 1998* (IOM, 1999), *Update 2000* (IOM, 2001), and *Update 2002* (IOM, 2003). A slight change in emphasis toward chronic neurodegenerative disorders was reflected in the change in the name of this chapter to "Neurologic Disorders" in *Update 2004* (IOM, 2005), which was carried forward in *Update 2006* (IOM, 2007), *Update 2008* (IOM, 2009), and *Update 2010* (IOM, 2012). The present chapter reviews data pertinent to persistent neurologic disorders of all types.

Case identification in neurologic disorders is often difficult because there are few disorders for which there are specific diagnostic tests. Many disorders involve cellular or molecular biochemical effects, so even the most advanced imaging techniques can miss an abnormality. Because the nervous system is not readily accessible for biopsy, pathologic confirmation usually is not feasible. However, identifiable neurologic disorders always result in objective abnormalities that are reflected in anatomic or functional tests or discovered via clinical examination.

Many studies have addressed the possible contribution of various chemical exposures to neurologic disorders, but the committee's focus is on the health effects of a particular set of chemicals: four herbicides—2,4-dichlorophenoxyacetic acid (2,4-D), 2,4,5-trichlorophenoxyacetic acid (2,4,5-T), picloram (4-amino-3,5,6-trichloropicolinic acid), and cacodylic acid (dimethyl arsenic acid)—and 2,3,7,8-tetrachlorodibenzo-*p*-dioxin (TCDD), a contaminant of 2,4,5-T. The committee also considers studies of exposure to polychlorinated biphenyls (PCBs) and other dioxin-like chemicals to be informative if their results were reported in terms of TCDD toxic equivalents (TEQs) or concentrations of specific congeners. Although all studies reporting TEQs based on PCBs were reviewed, studies that reported TEQs based only on mono-ortho PCBs (which are PCBs 105, 114, 118, 123, 156, 157, 167, and 189) were given very limited consideration because mono-ortho PCBs typically contribute less than 10% to total TEQs, based on the World Health Organization revised toxicity equivalency factors of 2005 (La Rocca et al., 2008; van den Berg et al., 2006). The specificity of exposure assessment is an important consideration in weighing evidence relevant to the committee's charge.

This chapter reviews the association between exposure to the chemicals of interest (COIs) and neurobehavioral disorders, neurodegenerative disorders, and chronic peripheral system disorders. The scientific evidence supporting biologic plausibility is also reviewed here. More complete discussions of the categories of association and of this committee's approach to categorizing health outcomes are presented in Chapters 1 and 2. For citations new to this update that revisit previously studied populations, design information can be found in Chapter 5.

BIOLOGIC PLAUSIBILITY

Experimental data regarding the biologic plausibility of a connection between exposure to the COIs and various neurologic disorders continue to accrue. This section summarizes in a general way some of the information reviewed in the current update and, for completeness, includes information from prior updates.

Several studies have dealt with mechanisms of neurotoxicity that might be ascribed to the COIs, notably 2,4-D and TCDD. Molecular effects of the COIs are described in detail in Chapter 4. Some aspects of the biochemical activity they induce suggest pathways by which there could be effects on the neural systems. A number of the studies suggest that the COIs, primarily 2,4-D, have neurologic effects, both neurochemical and behavioral, in animal models if exposure occurs during development or in cultured nerve cells (Konjuh et al., 2008; Rosso et al., 2000a,b; Sturtz et al., 2008); older references described behavioral effects of developmental exposure of rodents to a 2,4-D–2,4,5-T mixture (Mohammad and St. Omer, 1986; St. Omer and Mohammad, 1987). Perinatal exposures to TCDD and coplanar, dioxin-like PCBs have reportedly caused deficits in learning behavior in rats (Curran et al., 2011; Haijima et al., 2010; Hojo et al., 2008). However, caution in interpreting the significance of those studies is warranted because the developing nervous system is different from the mature nervous system and may not be an appropriate model for the possible consequences of exposure of adults to the COIs.

Some studies further support suggestions that the concentration of reactive oxygen species could alter the functions of specific signaling cascades and be involved in neurodegeneration (Drechsel and Patel, 2008). Such studies do not specifically concern the COIs but are potentially relevant to these chemicals inasmuch as TCDD and herbicides have been reported to elicit oxidative stress (Byers et al., 2006; Celik et al., 2006; Shen et al., 2005). In addition, TCDD has been shown to affect phosphokinase C biochemistry in nerve cells and so could affect the integrity and physiology of nerve cells (Kim et al., 2007; Lee et al., 2007). Cytochrome P450 1A1, the aryl hydrocarbon receptor (AHR), and the AHR nuclear transporter occur in the brain, so TCDD might be likely to exert effects in the brain (Huang et al., 2000). In addition, although they dealt with hepatocytes and not cells of the nervous system, earlier studies have indicated that 2,4-D affected aspects of mitochondrial energetics and mitochondrial calcium flux (Palmeira et al., 1994a,b, 1995a,b); if these effects can also occur in nervous-system cell mitochondria, which is feasible, the energy balance and pathways of cells in the nervous system could be affected, and there could be later damage to nervous-system function. Those mechanistic studies, although they did not produce convincing evidence of specific effects of the COIs in the neurologic outcomes of concern, suggest possible avenues to pursue to determine linkages between the COIs and the neurologic outcomes that could occur in adult humans.

Basic scientific studies have emphasized the importance of alterations in neurotransmitter systems as potential mechanisms that underlie TCDD-induced neurobehavioral disorders. Neuronal cultures treated with 2,4-D exhibited decreased neurite extension associated with intracellular changes, including a decrease in microtubules, inhibition of the polymerization of tubulin, disorganization of the Golgi apparatus, and inhibition of ganglioside synthesis. Those mechanisms are important for maintaining the connections among nerve cells that are necessary for neuronal function and that are involved in axon regeneration and recovery from peripheral neuropathy. Animal experiments have demonstrated that TCDD treatments affect the fundamental molecular events that underlie neurotransmission initiated by calcium uptake. And mechanistic studies have demonstrated that 2,4,5-T can alter cellular metabolism and the cholinergic transmission necessary for neuromuscular transmission.

TCDD treatment of rats at doses that do not cause general systemic illness or wasting disease produces electrodiagnostic changes in peripheral nerve function and pathologic findings that are characteristic of toxicant-induced axonal peripheral neuropathy.

As discussed in Chapter 4, extrapolation of observations of cells in culture or animal models to humans is complicated by differences in sensitivity and susceptibility among animals, strains, and species; by the lack of strong evidence of organ-specific effects occurring consistently across species; and by differences in route, dose, duration, and timing of chemical exposures. Thus, although the toxicologic observations themselves cannot establish a conclusion that the COIs produced neurotoxic effects in humans, they do suggest the biologic plausibility of an association and point to potential mechanisms that might have come into play.

NEUROBEHAVIORAL (COGNITIVE OR NEUROPSYCHIATRIC) DISORDERS

This section summarizes the findings of *VAO* and previous updates on neurobehavioral disorders and incorporates information published in the past 2 years into the evidence database.

Conclusions from *VAO* and Previous Updates

On the basis of the data available at the time, the committees responsible for *VAO*, *Update 1996*, *Update 1998*, *Update 2000*, *Update 2002*, *Update 2004*, *Update 2006*, *Update 2008*, and *Update 2010* concluded that there was inadequate or insufficient evidence to determine whether there is an association between exposure to the COIs and neurobehavioral disorders. Many of the data that informed that conclusion came from the Air Force Health Study (AFHS; AFHS, 1991, 1995, 2000; Barrett et al., 2001, 2003). Urban et al. (2007) confirmed that acute neurologic symptoms experienced shortly after an acute exposure to TCDD could be sustained more than 30 years after the exposure, but this study did not address delayed effects. For other studies (Kamel et al., 2007a; Solomon et al., 2007), no relationship was found with diverse neurologic outcomes and exposure to unspecified herbicides. Many of the studies reviewed were found to be methodologically flawed (Dahlgren et al., 2003; Pazderova-Vejlupkova et al., 1981; Pelclová et al., 2001, 2002) or uninformative (ADVA, 2005c; Decoufle et al., 1992; Park et al., 2005; Visintainer et al., 1995). *VAO* and the updates offer more complete discussions of the studies considered.

Update of the Epidemiologic Literature

One environmental study explored the association between pesticides and rapid-eye-movement (REM) sleep disorder. Postuma et al. (2012) conducted a case-control study of REM sleep disorder in 347 cases and 347 age- and sex-matched controls. Data on occupation and occupational exposures were captured by questionnaire. Significantly increased odds ratios (ORs) for REM sleep behavior disorder (RBD) were found in farmers and in those reporting occupational exposure to herbicides (OR = 2.54, 95% confidence interval [CI] 1.05–6.16) but not nonoccupational herbicide exposure (OR = 1.30, 95% CI 0.56–2.99).

Baldi et al. (2011) examined French vineyard workers' performance on nine neurobehavioral tests. The adjusted odds of scoring in the worst 25% were higher in exposed than unexposed workers on all tests, and the differences were significant on all but one. Exposure was determined from job and task histories, but it was exposure only to the general category of "pesticides" and so did not satisfy the committee's criteria for adequate exposure specificity.

Biologic Plausibility

Some animal studies have suggested possible involvement of the COIs in the occurrence of neurobehavioral effects. Akahoshi et al. (2009) produced a mouse neuroblastoma cell line that overexpressed the AHR, which is important in dopamine synthesis. Treating the line with TCDD increased tyrosine hydroxylase activity and led to increased dopamine expression. The implication of that finding is not clear, but changes in dopamine regulation have been implicated in a number of neurobehavioral syndromes. In vitro exposure of human CD34+ cells to TCDD induced modulation in gene expression involving the GABAergic pathway, which may be associated with altered synaptic transmission, visual perception, and other neurologic conditions (Fracchiolla et al., 2011).

Other recent studies have focused on neurobehavioral outcomes following perinatal exposure, which is of concern for the offspring of Vietnam veterans as discussed in Chapter 10. Haijima et al. (2010) found that perinatal exposure to TCDD impaired memory in male offspring. Mitsui et al. (2006) reported that hippocampus-dependent learning could be impaired in male rats exposed to TCDD in utero and that impairment could affect fear conditioning. Curran et al. (2011) assessed the effect of CYP1A2 and the AHR genotype on altered learning and memory in mice exposed to an environmentally relevant mixture of dioxin-like (coplanar) and non-dioxin-like PCBs in utero and during lactation. They observed the most significant deficits in response to PCB treatment in *Ahrb1_Cyp1a2*(–/–) mice, including impaired novel-object recognition and increased failure rate in the Morris water maze. Lensu et al. (2006) examined areas in the hypothalamus for possible involvement in TCDD effects on food consumption, potentially related to wasting syndrome, and suggested that their results were not consistent with a primary role of the hypothalamus. Studies in rodents have also detected molecular effects in cerebellar granule cells and neuroblasts, which are involved in cognitive and motor processes (Kim and Yang, 2005; Williamson et al., 2005). Sturtz et al. (2008) found that 2,4-D affected rat maternal behavior. The specific relevance of those studies and studies cited in earlier updates to neurobehavioral effects is unclear.

A summary of the biologic plausibility of neurologic effects arising from exposure to the COIs is presented at the beginning of this chapter.

Synthesis

There is not consistent epidemiologic evidence of an association between exposure to the COIs and neurobehavioral (cognitive or neuropsychiatric) disorders. More research on the COIs and RBD is warranted.

Conclusion

On the basis of the evidence reviewed here and in previous VAO reports, the committee concludes that there is inadequate or insufficient evidence to determine whether there is an association between exposure to the COIs and neurobehavioral (cognitive or neuropsychiatric) disorders.

NEURODEGENERATIVE DISEASES

This section summarizes the findings of previous VAO reports on neurodegenerative diseases—specifically PD and ALS—and incorporates information published in the past 2 years into the evidence database. Also, a section on AD has been added in this update.

Parkinson Disease and Parkinsonism

PD is a progressive neurodegenerative disorder that affects millions of people worldwide. Its primary clinical manifestations are bradykinesia, resting tremor, cogwheel rigidity, and gait instability. Those signs were first described in 1817 as a single entity by James Parkinson. In recent years, many nonmotor manifestations of PD have been described, and they can be the presenting symptoms of the disease. They include cognitive dysfunction that often progresses to frank dementia, sleep disturbances, hallucinations, psychosis, mood disorders, fatigue, and autonomic dysfunction (Langston, 2006).

In the almost two centuries since the initial description, much has been learned about the genetic predisposition and pathophysiology of the disease, but its etiology in most patients is unknown, and specific environmental risk factors remain largely unproved. The diagnosis of PD is based primarily on clinical examination; in recent years, magnetic resonance imaging and functional brain imaging have been increasingly useful. PD must be distinguished from a variety of Parkinsonian syndromes, including drug-induced Parkinsonism, and neurodegenerative diseases, such as atrophy of multiple systems, that have Parkinsonian features combined with other abnormalities. Ultimately, a diagnosis of PD can be confirmed with postmortem pathologic examination of brain tissue for the characteristic loss of neurons from the substantia nigra and telltale Lewy body intracellular inclusions. Pathologic findings in other causes of Parkinsonism show different patterns of brain injury.

Estimates of incidence of PD range from 2 to 22 per 100,000 person-years, and estimates of prevalence range from 18 to 182 per 100,000 persons. It affects about 1% of all persons more than 60 years old and up to 5 million people worldwide. PD is the second-most common neurodegenerative disease (after AD). Age is a risk factor for PD; the peak incidence and prevalence are consistently found in people 60–80 years old. A consensus statement from a 2007 meeting of PD experts (Bronstein et al., 2009) concluded that, in addition to firm evidence that the toxicant 1-methyl-4-phenyl-1,2,4,6-tetrahydropyridine (MPTP) can induce PD, there is substantial evidence that men are at greater risk and that smoking and coffee consumption are associated with reduced risk.

Heredity has long been suspected of being an important risk factor for PD; as many as 25% of all PD patients have at least one first-degree relative who has PD. At least 13 gene mutations have been identified in autosomal-dominant PD, including mutations in parkin and α-synuclein (Klein and Lohmann-Hedrich, 2007). Mutations associated with an autosomal recessive inheritance pattern have also been described. Complex genetics may be found to account for an increasing number of PD cases in coming years, but environmental risk factors clearly are also important.

Conclusions from *VAO* and Previous Updates

The committees responsible for *VAO*, *Update 1996*, *Update 1998*, *Update 2000*, *Update 2002*, *Update 2004*, and *Update 2006* concluded that there was inadequate or insufficient information to determine whether there was an association between exposure to the COIs and PD. Several studies of PD were reviewed by those committees and are described briefly here.

In addition to two new case-control studies examining association specifically with chlorophenoxy acid or esters (Brighina et al., 2008; Hancock et al., 2008), the committee responsible for *Update 2008* considered five earlier case-control studies that examined the association between exposure to the COIs and PD. Two of these did not find associations with herbicide exposure (Stern et al., 1991; Taylor et al., 1999), but they may have been limited by little actual herbicide exposure, particularly occupational exposure. Three found significant associations with herbicide exposure (Butterfield et al., 1993; Gorell et al., 1998; Semchuk et al., 1992), and two found increased ORs specifically with chlorophenoxy acid or esters (Brighina et al., 2008; Hancock et al., 2008). In the new case-control studies, the doubling in risk observed by Hancock et al. (2008) did not achieve statistical significance (OR = 2.07, 95% CI 0.69–6.23), while the increase for chlorophenoxy acids or esters chemical class noted by Brighina et al. (2008) was significant only in the quartile of cases who were youngest at diagnosis (OR = 1.52, 95% CI 1.04–2.22). In the prospective Agricultural Health Study (AHS), incident PD was related in a dose–response manner to increasing days of pesticide use (Kamel et al., 2007b). On the basis of the evidence summarized above, *Update 2008* concluded that there was limited/suggestive evidence relating exposure to the COIs and PD.

Update 2010 reviewed four more epidemiologic studies related to PD risk and the COIs. Two did not find associations with 2,4-D and other phenoxy herbicides (Dhillon et al., 2008; Firestone et al., 2010). Two others did find significant associations. In an analysis of 519 cases and 511 controls, Tanner et al. (2009) found an OR of 2.59 (95% CI 1.03–6.48) for 2,4-D exposure. Elbaz et al. (2009) conducted extensive job or task history evaluations among 224 PD cases and 557 controls, all of whom were agricultural workers in France, and found a suggestive increase in odds of PD (OR = 1.8, 95% CI 0.9–3.3) associated with the use of phenoxy herbicides, and this result was statistically significant when the analyses were restricted to people more than 65 years old (OR = 2.9, 95% CI 1.1–7.3), in contrast to the significant increase reported by Brighina et al. (2008) only in the youngest subjects. The analysis of phenoxy herbicides, however, was not adjusted for use of other types of pesticides. Another study found no association between herbicide exposure and progressive supranuclear palsy (Vidal et al., 2009), which is a distinct disease that has many similar symptoms. The committee responsible for *Update 2010* affirmed the conclusion of the previous committee.

Those findings are summarized in Table 11-1.

Update of the Epidemiologic Literature

Vietnam-Veteran and Case-Control Studies No Vietnam-veteran studies or case-control studies addressing exposure to the COIs and PD have been published since *Update 2010*.

Occupational Studies Since the previous update, Kenborg et al. (2012) compared hospitalization for PD among 3,124 male members of the Danish Union of Gardeners with that among the general Danish population. With more than 68,323 person-years of followup, 28 gardeners were hospitalized for PD, which did not differ significantly from the rate in the general population (standardized hospitalization ratio [SHR] = 1.14, 95% CI 0.76–1.65). Year of birth was used as a surrogate for intensity of exposure, and high exposure was assumed for those born before 1915 (11 cases, SHR = 1.55, 95% CI 0.77–2.77), intermediate exposure for those born in 1915–1934 (16 cases, SHR = 1.15, 95% CI 0.66–1.87), and low exposure for those born in 1935 or later (1 case, SHR = 0.28, 95% CI 0.00–1.58). Although the specific pesticides to which individuals were exposed are not known, Danish gardeners have been found to have much higher exposures to pesticides—primarily herbicides, including phenoxy herbicides—than the general Danish population (Hansen et al., 1992, 2007).

Two other occupational studies were published since the previous update, but the exposure assessments lacked specificity for the COIs. One study of agricultural workers in France considered only type of farming (Moisan et al., 2011),

TABLE 11-1 Epidemiologic Studies of Herbicide[a] Exposure and Parkinson Disease (Shaded Entries Are New Information for This Update)

Reference and Country	Cases in Study Group	Comparison Group	Exposure Assessment	Exposure(s):[a]	n	OR (95% CI)	Diagnosis of Neurologic Dysfunction
Kenborg et al., 2012; Denmark	28 PD cases from male members of Danish Union of Gardeners (n = 3,124)	Incidence of PD in general population of Denmark	Hospital diagnosis of PD, 1977–2008	Pesticides (including phenoxy herbicides)		Hospitalization:	Not specified
					28	1.1 (0.8–1.7)	
						Born before 1915:	
					11	1.6 (0.8–2.8)	
						Born 1915–1934:	
					16	1.2 (0.7–1.9)	
						Born 1935 or later:	
					1	0.3 (0.0–1.6)	
Rugbjerg et al., 2011; Canada	403 PD cases from pharmacy database	405 matched controls	Initial screening phone interview followed by an in-person physical assessment employing a checklist and record of symptoms, reviewed by a neurologist specializing in movement disorders	Herbicides	33	1.8 (0.97–3.4)	Parkinsonian tremor, rigidity, bradykinesia, masked facies, micrographia, or postural imbalance
				Neurotoxic pesticides (including 2,4-D, 2,4,5-T)	35	1.8 (0.95–3.3)	
Firestone et al., 2010 (updates and expands Firestone et al. [2005]); Washington, United	Enrolled cases increased from 250 (in original study) to 404	526 unrelated controls	Structured face-to-face interviews; demographic information collected, job descriptions (if held for more than 6 months) and workplace exposures to various industrial toxicants identified from	2,4-D	8	0.8 (0.3–2.0)	≥ 2 of 4 cardinal signs; must have bradykinesia or resting tremor, may have cogwheel rigidity, or postural reflex impairment

Dhillon et al., 2008; United States (University of Texas)	100 PD cases recruited from a medical center's neurological institute in East Texas	84 controls without PD recruited from the same medical center	Professionally-administered questionnaire used to determine military history (including spraying herbicides/pesticides), personal use/mixing and average duration of exposure to herbicides and specific pesticides, among other exposures	Ever personally used/mixed or applied:			PD diagnosed by neurologist specializing in movement disorders using standard clinical/lab diagnostic criteria
				Herbicide use—home or agricultural	34	0.8 (0.4–1.4)	
				2,4-D	17	1.2 (0.6–2.8)	
				2,4,5-T	4	0.5 (0.1–1.6)	
				Silvex or other 2,4,5-TP products	1	0.3 (0.0–2.7)	
Elbaz et al., 2009; France	224 PD cases	557 controls	Initial self-assessment, plus individual interview with occupational specialist	Phenoxy herbicides	na	1.8 (0.9–3.3)	≥ 2 cardinal signs (resting tremor, bradykinesia, rigidity, impaired postural reflexes)
				Age of onset > 65 yrs	na	2.9 (1.1–7.3)	
Tanner et al., 2009; United States	519 cases; consecutively eligible subjects between July 1, 2004, and May 31, 2007	521 controls frequency matched to cases by age, sex, and location	Telephone interviewers collected information about exposures before the reference age; employment history—industry, location, processes, materials, and job tasks. Toxicant exposure collected for some jobs.	2,4-D	16	2.6 (1.0–6.5)	Enrolling investigator determined diagnosis and type of Parkinsonism, Unified Parkinson Disease Rating Scale score, and clinical features

continued

TABLE 11-1 Epidemiologic Studies of Herbicide[a] Exposure and Parkinson Disease, continued

Reference and Country	Cases in Study Group	Comparison Group	Exposure Assessment	Exposure(s):[a]	n	OR (95% CI)	Diagnosis of Neurologic Dysfunction
Brighina et al., 2008; United States (Mayo Clinic)	833 PD sequential cases from clinic; median age = 67.7 yrs, 208 cases ≤ 59.8 yrs	472 unaffected siblings and 361 unrelated controls	Self-report down to specific herbicides; 2,4-D said to be most prevalent in cases, but published analysis not that detailed	For *youngest quartile* at diagnosis:			PD diagnosed by movement disorder specialist
				Pesticides (ever):	87	1.8 (1.1–2.9)	
				Herbicides (ever):		2.5 (1.3–4.5)	
				Phenoxy herbicides		1.5 (1.0–2.2)	
				Insecticides (ever):		1.0 (0.6–1.7)	
				Fungicides (ever):		1.0 (0.3–3.2)	
Hancock et al., 2008; United States (Duke)	319 cases	296 unaffected relatives and others	All comparisons referent to those who never applied any pesticide	Pesticide application:	200	1.6 (1.1–2.3)	
				Insecticides:		1.8 (1.2–2.8)	
				Botanical:	7	5.9 (0.6–56)	
				Organophosphate:	53	1.9 (1.1–3.6)	
				Herbicides:		1.6 (1.0–2.5)	
				Chlorophenoxy:	15	2.1 (0.7–6.2)	
				Phosophonoglycine:	57	1.5 (0.9–2.5)	
				Triazine:	5	1.1 (0.3–3.6)	
Kamel et al., 2007b; United States (Agricultural Health Study) (Updates Kamel et al., [2005])	83 prevalent cases at enrollment; 78 incident cases during followup among private applicators and spouses	79,557 without PD at enrollment; 55,931 without PD followed up	Self-report of individual herbicides (2,4-D; 2,4,5-T; 2,4,5-TP) on detailed self-administered questionnaires at enrollment or telephone interview for followup	For incident cases:			
				2,4-D:	49	1.0 (0.5–2.1)	
				2,4,5-T:	24	1.8 (1.0–3.3)	
				2,4,5-TP:	7	0.9 (0.4–1.8)	
				Dicamba:	32	1.5 (0.8–2.8)	
				Paraquat:	11	1.0 (0.5–1.9)	
				Trifuralin:	32	1.7 (1.0–3.2)	
				Cyanazine	26	1.0 (0.5–1.8)	
				For prevalent cases:			
				2,4-D:	47	0.9 (0.5–1.8)	
				2,4,5-T:	16	0.9 (0.5–1.7)	
				2,4,5-TP:	4	0.8 (0.3–1.9)	

				Dicamba:	26	0.9 (0.5–1.6)	
				Paraquat:	14	1.8 (1.0–3.4)	
				Trifuralin:	31	0.9 (0.5–1.6)	
				Cyanazine	30	2.6 (1.4–4.9	
Firestone et al., 2005; Washington, United States (Updated by Firestone et al. [2010])	250 (156 men) newly diagnosed 1992–2002 at Group Health Cooperative	388 (241 men)	Interview determining occupational and home-based pesticide exposure characterized by chemical name or brand, duration, and frequency	Occupational, men only			Controlled for age, sex, smoking
				Pesticides:	19	1.0 (0.5–1.9)	
				Insecticides:	15	0.9 (0.4–1.8)	
				Fungicides:	2	0.4 (0.1–3.9)	
				Herbicides:	9	1.4 (0.5–3.9)	
				Paraquat:	2	1.7 (0.2–12.8)	
				Home use, all subjects			
				Pesticides:	178	1.0 (0.7–1.4)	
				Insecticides:	141	0.8 (0.6–1.1)	
				Fungicides:	14	0.6 (0.3–1.1)	
				Herbicides:	116	1.1 (0.8–1.5)	
Behari et al., 2001; India	377 (301 men, 76 women)	377 matched for age (± 3 yrs), but not sex	Structured interview	McNemar chi-square:			
				Herbicides:		p = 0.010	
				(protective effect—*not confirmed* by multivariate analysis)			
				Insecticide:		p = 0.169	
				Rodenticide:		p = 0.662	
Engel et al., 2001; United States (cross-sectional, but otherwise fairly high-quality design)	238	72	Self-administered questionnaire for occupational exposure	[prevalence ratios]			
				Any pesticide:		0.8 (0.5–1.2)	Neurologic exam by trained nurse
				Herbicides:		0.9 (0.6–1.3)	
				Insecticides:		0.9 (0.6–1.5)	
				Fungicides:		0.8 (0.6–1.3)	

continued

TABLE 11-1 Epidemiologic Studies of Herbicide[a] Exposure and Parkinson Disease, continued

Reference and Country	Cases in Study Group	Comparison Group	Exposure Assessment	Exposure(s):[a]	n	OR (95% CI)	Diagnosis of Neurologic Dysfunction
Kuopio et al., 1999; Finland	123 (onset of PD before 1984; 63 men, 60 women)	246 matched on sex, age (± 2 yrs), and urban/rural	Interview—pesticides or herbicides regularly or occasionally used	Pesticide use:	39	1.0 (0.6–1.7)	Neurologic exam
				Occasional use:	26	1.2 (0.7–2.0)	
				Regular use:	13	0.7 (0.3–1.3)	
				Herbicide use:	33	1.4 (0.8–2.5)	
				Occasional use:	20	1.7 (0.9–3.2)	
				Regular use:	13	0.8 (0.4–1.7)	
Taylor et al., 1999; Boston Medical Center	140	147 controls referred by cases	Interview—exposure recorded as total days for lifetime	Logistic analysis adjusted for age, sex, family history, education, smoking, water source, head injury, depression			Neurologic exam
				Pesticides:		1.0 (0.9–1.2)	
				Herbicides:		1.1 (0.7–1.7)	
Gorell et al., 1998; United States	144 (age > 50 yrs)	464	Interview—herbicide and insecticide use while working on a farm or gardening	All occupations contributing exposure to			Standard criteria of PD by history
				Herbicides:		4.1 (1.4–12.2)	
				Insecticides:		3.6 (1.8–7.2)	
				Fungicides:		1.6 (0.5–5.5)	
Liou et al., 1997; Taiwan	120	240 hospital controls matched for age (± 2 yrs) and sex	Interview—occupational exposures to herbicides or pesticides	Pesticides vs no pesticides:		2.9 (2.3–3.7)	Neurologic exam
				But no Paraquat use:		2.2 (0.9–5.6)	
				Paraquat use:		4.7 (2.0–12))	
				Paraquat use vs no Paraquat:		3.2 (2.4–4.3)	
Seidler et al., 1996; Germany	380 (age < 66 yrs with PD after 1987)	755 (379 neighborhood, 376 regional; neighborhood controls may be overmatched)	Interview—dose-years = years of application weighted by use	Pesticides:		2.1 (1.6–2.6)	Neurologic exam
				Herbicides—high dose:		2.4 (1.0–6.0)	
				Dose trend			
				vs neighbor controls		$p = 0.06$	
				vs regional controls		$p < 0.001$	
				Insecticides—high dose:		2.1 (0.9–4.8)	
				Dose trend			

				vs neighbor controls		p = 0.12	
				vs regional controls		p < 0.001	
Hertzman et al., 1994; Canada	127 (71 men, 56 women)	245 (121 with cardiac disease; 124 voters)	Interview—occupation with probable pesticide exposure	Cases vs voters—among men			Neurologic exam
				Pesticides:			
				Herbicides:		2.3 (1.1–4.9)	
				Chlorophenoxys:		1.2 (0.6–2.5)	
				Paraquat:		1.2 (0.6–2.4)	
				Insecticides:		1.3 (0.3–4.6)	
				Fungicides:		0.3 (0.1–0.9)	
Butterfield et al., 1993; United States	63 young onset cases (age < 50 yrs)	68	Questionnaire—pesticide or insecticide use 10 times in any year	Herbicides:		3.2 p = 0.033	Standard criteria of PD by history
				Insecticides:		5.8 p < 0.001	
				Dwelling fumigated:		5.3 p = 0.45	
Semchuk et al., 1992; Calgary, Alberta, Canada	130 living cases from register of Calgary residents (population-based)	260 community controls matched for age (± 2.5 yrs) and sex, identified by RDD	Interview—self-report of exposure for each job held > 1 mo	Pesticides:	32	2.3 (1.3–4.0)	Neurologic exam confirming idiopathic PD without dementia (average 7.8 yrs from diagnosis)
				Herbicides:	17	3.1 (1.3–7.0)	
				Exposed during age interval:			
				16–25 yrs		1.4 (0.5–4.3)	
				26–35 yrs		4.8 (1.5–15.0)	
				36–45 yrs		3.8 (1.2–13.0)	
				46–55 yrs		4.9 (1.3–19.0)	
				Insecticides:	17	2.1 (1.0–4.1)	
				Fungicides:	16	1.6 (0.8–3.3)	

continued

TABLE 11-1 Epidemiologic Studies of Herbicide[a] Exposure and Parkinson Disease, continued

Reference and Country	Cases in Study Group	Comparison Group	Exposure Assessment	Exposure(s):[a]	n	OR (95% CI)	Diagnosis of Neurologic Dysfunction
Stern et al., 1991; New Jersey and Pennsylvania, United States	69—all young-onset cases identified (age < 40 yrs); 80—random selection of old onset cases (age > 59 yrs)	149 nominated by each case or picked from hospital; matched by age (± 6 yrs), sex, and race	Interview—self-report of insecticide and pesticide use by self or others in home or garden	Insecticides:		0.7 (0.3–1.4)	Review of medical records, responsive to PD medication (under treatment average of 8.2 yrs), without major cognitive impairment
				Onset < 40 yrs:		0.6 (0.2–1.7)	
				Onset > 59 yrs:		0.8 (0.3–2.1)	
				Herbicides:		1.1 (0.7–1.7)	
				Onset < 40 yrs:		0.9 (0.5–1.7)	
				Onset > 59 yrs:		1.3 (0.7–2.4)	
				Adjusted for smoking, head injury, rural residence:			
				Insecticides:		0.5 (0.2–1.1)	
				Herbicides:		0.9 (0.6–1.5)	
Hertzman et al., 1990; British Columbia, Canada	57 prevalent PD patients (age < 79 yrs) (50–54 had confirmed PD, not clear exactly how many)	122 age 50–79 who responded from electoral rolls	Questionnaire—ever worked in an orchard	Work in orchards:		3.7 (1.3–10.3)	Neurologic exam confirmed diagnostic criteria in 55 of 69 cases identified by asking physicians in area
				Paraquat:	4/57	(p = 0.01)	

NOTE: 2,4-D, 2,4-dichlorophenoxyacetic acid; 2,4,5-T, 2,4,5-trichlorophenoxyacetic acid; 2,4,5-TP, 2-(2,4,5-trichlorophenoxy) propionic acid or Silvex; CI, confidence interval; OR, odds ratio; PD, Parkinson disease; RDD, random-digit dialing.

[a]For the objective of the VAO review series, only associations with herbicides are of possible relevance; only the phenoxy herbicides, cacodylic acid, and picloram are of specific interest.

and another of pesticide users in Great Britain did not specify which pesticides were used (Frost et al., 2011).

The committee also noted the publication of Ruder and Yiin (2011), but that analysis examined mortality from all neurologic disorders together and so is unhelpful in light of the great heterogeneity of conditions in this rubric.

Environmental Studies Sanyal et al. (2010) conducted a case-control study of 175 PD cases at a movement-disorder clinic and 350 age- and sex-matched controls recruited from among relatives of patients attending the clinic. Whether they were relatives of the 175 PD patients was not made clear, nor were specifics of control recruitment, such as the participation rate. Participation among cases was reported as 100% of those still alive and who had not moved out of the area. Exposure was determined with a structured interview and questionnaire. Subjects who had at least 5 years of exposure to herbicides were considered to be exposed. Herbicide exposure was reported three times more frequently among cases than controls, but only six cases and four controls reported such exposure. In multivariate analysis, the authors did not find a significant association with exposure to herbicides, but an effect estimate was not reported so whether the lack of significance resulted from adjustments or small numbers cannot be determined. Thus, this study cannot be considered evidence either for or against an association with herbicides.

Rugbjerg et al. (2011) conducted a case-control study in British Columbia, Canada, for which 403 PD patients, 40–69 years old, were recruited from a pharmacy database that managed reimbursements for PD medications and 405 controls matched on birth-year, sex, and geography. Pesticide exposure was self-reported and based on job history, which was used by industrial hygienists to determine whether pesticide exposure was likely to have been greater than background. Self-reported exposure to herbicides (OR = 1.82, 95% CI 0.97–3.40) and to neurotoxic pesticides, including 2,4-D and 2,4,5-T (OR = 1.76, 95% CI 0.95–3.25), were increased, although both results were substantially reduced in analyses of exposures based on industrial hygienists' review.

Several other papers examined the association between pesticides and PD, but the exposure assessments were not more detailed than "pesticide" exposure (Das et al., 2011; Kiyohara et al., 2010; Lin et al., 2011; Pereira and Garrett, 2010). In addition, an ecologic study in Spain examined prevalence of PD by areas of high and low pesticide use, but the use of pesticides was dominated by nonherbicide pesticides, so whether the analysis contrast reflects herbicide exposure differences is unclear (Parron et al., 2011).

Biologic Plausibility

Several reviews of the literature have addressed the possible involvement of environmental chemicals in the etiology of PD. Recently, van der Mark et al.

(2012) conducted a systematic review and meta-analysis of the epidemiologic literature published on PD and exposure to pesticides. The results suggest that exposure to pesticides, and to herbicides or insecticides in particular, increases the risk of developing PD. Most studies reviewed relied solely on self-report (yes or no), and none of the specific COIs was identified in the reviewed studies. McDowell and Chesselet (2012) recently reviewed the literature on the ability of both toxin-induced (6-hydroxydopamine, MPTP, rotenone, cycad) and genetically-based animal models to reproduce the nonmotor symptoms of PD. Gao and Hong (2011) and Kwok (2010) reviewed research on the genetic, epigenetic, and environmental causes of PD, which suggests that PD develops from multiple risk factors, including age, genetic predisposition, and environmental exposure. However, exposures to none of the COIs have been linked with development of PD.

The very clear PD-like toxicity resulting from human exposure to MPTP has indicated that select chemicals can result in the same type of damage to dopaminergic neurons as PD does, and MPTP has become an important toxicant in studies that use animal and in vitro models. It is notable that MPTP's bioactive metabolite, MPP+, is similar in chemical structure to Paraquat (a commonly-used herbicide, but not one used in Vietnam), but different from the COIs in this report. Pesticides that have been shown to produce PD-like toxicity in animal models include Paraquat, rotenone, maneb, and dieldrin; and substantial research has gone into understanding the molecular mechanisms responsible for the toxicity, especially in connection with Paraquat and rotenone, as reviewed recently by Blandini and Armentero (2012) and Duty and Jenner (2011) and in the past by others, including Di Monte et al. (2002), Drechsel and Patel (2008), Hatcher et al. (2008), Nunomura et al. (2007), and Sherer et al. (2002a). The damage done to dopaminergic neurons in PD is probably caused by oxidative stress and inflammation and may well also involve damage to mitochondria in the target cells (Liang et al., 2007; Littlejohn et al., 2011; Sarnico et al., 2008). In that regard, Bongiovanni et al. (2007) found that rat cerebellar granule cells in culture produce increased concentrations of reactive oxygen species when exposed to 2,4-D. The COIs for this committee are known to be distributed to the CNS, but they have not been investigated in similar experimental systems, so there is no evidence that they could cause inflammation or oxidative stress similar to those caused by the compounds, such as Paraquat, that have been investigated.

Research on the neurotoxicity of 2,4-D has been going on for a number of years, but most of it has focused on its effects on the developing rodent nervous system. The studies have often used high doses of 2,4-D that have resulted in adverse changes in the developing nervous system—both neurochemical (such as changes in D2 receptors, tyrosine hydroxylase, and dopamine beta-hydroxylase) and behavioral (for example, Bortolozzi et al., 1999, 2002, 2003, 2004; Duffard et al., 1996; Evangelista de Duffard et al., 1990, 1995; Garcia et al., 2004, 2006; Rosso et al., 2000a,b). Injection of 2,4-D directly into the rat brain yielded toxicity in the basal ganglia (Bortolozzi et al., 2001), but this route of administration is highly artificial. Recent studies showed that postpartum dietary exposure of females to 2,4-D resulted in adverse alterations in maternal behavior and neurochemical changes, including increases in dopamine and its metabolites 3,4-dihydroxyphenylacetic acid and homovanillic acid (Sturtz et al., 2008). Such an increase in dopamine is the reverse of what is seen in PD, in which degradation of the dopaminergic system occurs. In addition, a study of mice and 2,4-D yielded no evidence of neurochemical damage to the dopaminergic system (Thiffault et al., 2001). One study indicated that 2,4-D, among a variety of pesticides and metals, caused fibrillation of α-synuclein in vitro, but it used purified protein and did not report data on 2,4-D but rather a generalized result (Uversky et al., 2002), so little confidence can be placed in it. Because most of the studies were on the developing nervous system, not the mature nervous system, and some studies yielded evidence of a lack of a role of 2,4-D in the development of PD, the existing studies are of little use in addressing the question of the etiology of PD.

A summary of the biologic plausibility of neurologic effects arising from exposure to the COIs is presented at the end of this chapter.

Synthesis

The committee responsible for *Update 2012* reviewed epidemiologic studies published since *Update 2010* that examined the association between herbicides—possibly including the COIs—and PD, but they lacked the exposure specificity of earlier studies. A new case-control study, by Rugbjerg et al. (2011) found a positive association between herbicide exposure and PD, although only when exposure was determined by questionnaire, not by industrial hygienist review of occupational history. The followup study by Kenborg et al. (2012) of Danish gardeners who had individually-uncharacterized pesticide exposures that were known to have been primarily to herbicides, including the phenoxys, was also consistent with an association. The committee also noted that the study by Postuma et al. (2012) described in the neurobehavioral disorders section above found a significant association between the COIs and REM sleep disorder, which may be an early symptom of PD, but the association between smoking and RBD was opposite to what is expected for PD. The committee reviewed several other studies that lacked exposure specificity adequate to be useful for this review. There continues to be a dearth of investigation of veterans, and biologic plausibility is still lacking. We continue to urge the performance of studies relating PD incidence to exposure in the Vietnam-veteran population. We are also concerned that a biologic mechanism by which the COIs may cause PD has not been demonstrated. Nevertheless, the epidemiologic evidence continues to support an association between herbicide exposure and PD and to be consistent with an association with exposure to the phenoxy herbicides (and perhaps to other specific herbicides).

Conclusions

On the basis of the evidence reviewed here and in previous VAO reports, the committee concludes that there is limited or suggestive evidence of an association between exposure to the COIs and PD.

Amyotrophic Lateral Sclerosis

ALS is a progressive, adult-onset, motor neuron disease that presents with muscle atrophy, weakness, and fasciculations and with signs that imply involvement of motor pathways in the CNS. The cause of most cases of ALS is unknown, but about 10% of cases reportedly show an autosomal-dominant pattern of inheritance. Several environmental exposures, including military service, have been investigated as potential risk factors for ALS, but no studies have found conclusive evidence of an association. One-fifth of familial-ALS patients have mutations in the gene that encodes superoxide dismutase-1 (Rosen et al., 1993). The incidence of sporadic ALS is 1–2 per 100,000 person-years, and the incidence of ALS peaks at the ages of 55–75 years (Brooks, 1996). The diagnosis of ALS is made through clinical examination and electrodiagnostic testing and has a high degree of accuracy when performed by experienced neurologists (Rowland, 1998; Rowland and Shneider, 2001).

Summary of Previous Updates

ALS was first considered by the committee for *Update 2002*. Although multiple potential etiologic factors have been investigated (Breland and Currier, 1967; Deapen and Henderson, 1986; Gallagher and Sander, 1987; Hanisch et al., 1976; Kurtzke and Beebe, 1980; McGuire et al., 1997; Mitchell and Borasio, 2007; Roelofs-Iverson et al., 1984; Savettieri et al. 1991; Sutedja et al., 2009a,b), associations have not been consistently identified.

Pesticide or herbicide exposure has been associated with increased risk of ALS, including a doubling of the risk after long-term occupational exposure to pesticides (Deapen and Henderson, 1986) and a tripling after exposure to agricultural chemical products (Savettieri et al., 1991) and after exposure to herbicides (McGuire et al., 1997), but none of the risk estimates was statistically significant. A population-based case-control study demonstrated associations between exposure to agricultural chemical products and ALS in men, with an OR of 2.4 and a trend with duration of exposure that were both statistically significant (McGuire et al., 1997). A mortality study of Dow Chemical Company employees exposed to 2,4-D found three deaths from ALS with a significant positive association (relative risk, 3.45, 95% CI 1.10–11.11) (Burns et al., 2001).

In *Update 2006*, three additional studies were reviewed. Morahan and Pamphlett (2006) published an Australian case-control study in which the cases were self-reported and the controls chosen in nonrandom fashion. The authors found an increased risk of ALS after exposure to pesticides or herbicides, but the lack of appropriate case and control ascertainment and the fact that specific COIs were not asked about make the results of this study difficult to interpret. Weisskopf et al. (2005) followed vital status of subjects in the American Cancer Society's (ACS's) cohort for the Cancer Prevention Study II and demonstrated an increased risk of ALS in those who served in any of the armed services during times of conflict. They adjusted for a variety of confounding variables in their model, including exposure to herbicides, and found that none of them significantly altered their conclusions; thus, this large study indirectly suggests the lack of a strong effect of herbicide exposure on ALS risk. Finally, a case-control study of Australian Vietnam veterans reported an association between deployment in Vietnam and ALS (ADVA, 2005c) but did not specifically study exposure to pesticides or herbicides.

No additional studies concerning exposure to the COIs and ALS were found for review in *Update 2008*, and *Update 2010* considered one additional study (Weisskopf et al., 2009). No association was seen between self-reported pesticide or herbicide exposure in the ACS Cancer Prevention Study II, but the lack of exposure specificity and the possibility of exposure estimation error limit the weight of this evidence.

Table 11-2 summarizes the results of the relevant studies.

Update of the Epidemiologic Literature

Vietnam-Veteran or Case-Control Studies No Vietnam-veteran studies or case-control studies addressing exposure to the COIs and ALS have been published since *Update 2010*.

Occupational Studies Since *Update 2010*, Kamel et al. (2012) have evaluated the relationship between a variety of chemical exposures and death from ALS in the AHS. In the AHS, private pesticide applicators and their spouses in Iowa and North Carolina reported on their use of specific pesticides when enrolled in 1993–1997. Among 84,739 pesticide applicators and their spouses, 41 ALS deaths were identified via linkage with the National Death Index in followup through February 7, 2010. Exposure to herbicides—which included exposure to the COIs—had somewhat-increased odds of ALS (OR = 1.6, 95% CI 0.7–3.7) in analyses adjusted for age and sex. A weaker association was seen in analyses specifically of 2,4-D (OR = 1.00, 95% CI 0.5–2.1) and 2,4,5-T (OR = 1.3, 95% CI 0.5–3.2).

Frost et al. (2011) examined ALS mortality in pesticide users in Great Britain compared with the general population. The standard mortality ratio (SMR) for ALS was not increased, but details on what specific pesticides—or types—this

TABLE 11-2 Epidemiologic Studies of Pesticide[a] Exposure and Amyotrophic Lateral Sclerosis (Shaded Entries Are New Information for This Update)

Reference; Country	Study Group	Comparison Group	Exposure Assessment	Significant Association with Pesticides[a]	Exposure of Interest/ Estimated Risk (95% CI)	Neurologic Dysfunction
Kamel et al., 2012; United States (AHS)	41	84,698	Self-administered questionnaire		Herbicides: 1.6 (0.7–3.7) 2,4-D: 1.0 (0.5–2.1) 2,4,5-T: 1.3 (0.5–3.2)	ALS cases identified via linkage with National Death Index
Pamphlett, 2012; Australia (followup to Morahan and Pamphlett [2006])	614	778	Questionnaire	+	Herbicide/pesticide exposure: Men: 1.8 (1.3–2.4) Women: 1.4 (1.0–2.0)	Self-reported and fulfilled probable or definite revised El Escorial criteria
Morahan and Pamphlett, 2006; Australia	179	179	Questionnaire—exposure to environmental toxicants	+	Herbicide, pesticide exposure: 1.6 (1.0–2.4); industrial exposure: 5.6 (2.1–15.1)	Self-reported
ADVA, 2005c; Australia	nr	nr	Deployment to Vietnam	+	4.7 (1.0–22.8)	
Weisskopf et al., 2005	nr	nr	Self-administered questionnaire	+	1.5 (1.1–2.1); $p = 0.007$	Self-reported military services, death certificates
Burns et al., 2001; United States	1,567	40,600	Industrial hygienist ranked jobs for exposure to 2,4-D to derive years of exposure and cumulative exposure	+	3.45 (1.1–11.1)	Death certificates

McGuire et al., 1997; United States	174	348	Self-reported lifetime job history, workplace exposures reviewed by panel of four industrial hygienists	+	Herbicide exposure: 2.4 (1.2–4.8); significant trend analysis for dose–effect relationship with agricultural chemicals: $p = 0.03$	New diagnosis of ALS 1990–1994 in western Washington state
Chancellor et al., 1993; Scotland	103	103	Required regular occupational exposure to pesticides for 12 months or more		1.4 (0.6–3.1)	Scottish Motor Neuron Register
Savettieri et al., 1991; Italy	46	92	Continual exposure to agricultural chemicals		3.0 (0.4–20.3)	Cases reviewed by neurologists
Deapen and Henderson, 1986; United States	518	518	Ever worked in presence of pesticides		2.0 (0.8–5.4)	ALS Society of America

NOTE: 2,4-D, 2,4-dichlorophenoxyacetic acid; 2,4,5-T, 2,4,5-trichlorophenoxyacetic acid; ADVA, Australian Department of Veterans Affairs; AHS, Agricultural Health Study; ALS, amyotrophic lateral sclerosis; CI, confidence interval; nr, not reported.

[a]For the objective of the VAO review series, only associations with herbicides are of possible relevance; only phenoxy herbicides, cacodylic acid, and picloram are of specific interest.

group was exposed to were not known, so the results of the study do not contribute to the evidentiary database according to VAO criteria.

Environmental Studies Pamphlett (2012) followed up on the prior report in Australia (Morahan and Pamphlett [2006], reviewed in *Update 2006*) and included additional cases and controls from the original report. Among 614 ALS cases and 778 controls, increased odds of ALS were found for herbicide or pesticide exposure in both men (OR = 1.77, 95% CI 1.30–2.39) and women (OR = 1.43, 95% CI 1.03–1.99). However, those results appear unadjusted, and the limitations described in *Update 2006* persist in the newer report, limiting the interpretability of the results.

Two other environmental studies were published since *Update 2010*, each of which found a statistically-significantly-increased risk of ALS, but the exposures occurred in agricultural work or other pesticide-related professional activities (Bonvicini et al., 2010) or were self-reported pesticide or insecticide exposures (Das et al., 2012). Thus, the studies are of little use in assessing the association with the COIs.

Biologic Plausibility

Several studies have addressed mechanisms of neurotoxicity that might be ascribed to COIs, notably 2,4-D and TCDD. Molecular effects of the COIs are described in Chapter 4. Some of those effects suggest possible pathways by which there could be effects on the neural systems. A number of the studies suggest that the COIs have had neurologic effects in animal models when exposure occurred during development. There also are some studies that further support suggestions that the concentrations of reactive oxygen species could alter the functions of specific signaling cascades and may be involved in neurodegeneration. Although they do not specifically concern the COIs, such studies are potentially relevant to them inasmuch as TCDD and herbicides have been reported to elicit oxidative stress (Celik et al., 2006; Shen et al., 2005). The mechanistic studies suggest avenues to pursue to determine linkages between the COIs and the neurologic outcomes that could result in adult humans. No toxicology studies concerning exposure to the COIs and ALS have been published since *Update 2006*.

A summary of the biologic plausibility of neurologic effects of exposure to the COIs is presented at the beginning of this chapter.

Synthesis

One well-designed study was published since *Update 2010* (Kamel et al., 2012) that suggested an association between herbicides as a class, but not specifically 2,4-D or 2,4,5-T, and ALS.

Conclusions

On the basis of the evidence reviewed here and in previous VAO reports, the committee concludes that the evidence of an association between exposure to the COIs and ALS remains inadequate or insufficient.

Alzheimer Disease

AD (*International Classification of Diseases, Ninth Revision* 331.0) is a progressive, neurodegenerative form of dementia that is characterized by memory loss, confusion, mood changes, social withdrawal, and deteriorating speech and judgment. The course of the disease is divided into four stages—predementia, early, moderate, and advanced—depending on the level of cognitive and functional impairment. Diagnosis typically occurs in people more than 60 years old as symptoms develop, although predementia and early AD are occasionally seen in people as young as 30 years old. AD is the sixth-leading cause of death in the United States and the fifth-leading cause of death in people more than 65 years old (Singh et al., 2012). In 2012, an estimated 5.4 million Americans were living with the diagnosis. Mean life expectancy is 7 years after an AD diagnosis; about 3% of people who receive the diagnosis live 14 years or more (Alzheimer's Association, 2012). Although the etiology of the disease remains elusive, suspected risk factors for AD include diet, exposure to aluminum or solvents, and genetics.

Summary of Previous Updates

This is the first VAO update to address AD directly. Although literature searches have not identified epidemiologic studies of possible association of AD with exposure to the specific COIs, association with exposure to the broad classification of "pesticides" has been investigated. Because AD is a condition of considerable interest to aging Vietnam veterans, the committee for this update thought it appropriate to present the small amount of peripherally-related available information. In doing so, we revisit below two publications that include inadequately specific exposure characterization that were mentioned briefly in *Update 2002* (Gauthier et al., 2001) and *Update 2004* (Baldi et al., 2003).

Update of the Epidemiologic Literature

Vietnam-Veterans Studies No Vietnam-veteran studies addressing exposure to the COIs and AD have been published since *Update 2010*.

Occupational Studies Frost et al. (2011) studied 62,960 pesticide users (median age at start of followup was about 30, followed for 829,709 person-years) in Great Britain and found only three AD cases, all in men. There was no difference in SMR for AD between the pesticide users and the general male population (SMR = 0.95, 95% CI 0.31–2.94). However, all-cause mortality in men was significantly lower in pesticide users (SMR = 0.58, 95% CI 0.55–0.60). The specific pesticides that this group used were not stated, so these results cannot be regarded as sufficiently well characterized to contribute to the evidentiary database concerning the COIs and the occurrence of AD.

Environmental Studies In 1992, Baldi et al. (2003) sought out 2,792 people in France who had been 65 years old or older in 1987 when they participated in an earlier study. Of these, 1,507 were alive and agreed to participate at a 5-year followup point. From 1992 through 1998, 96 incident AD cases were identified, 25 of which were in men. Pesticide exposure (including herbicides, insecticides, and fungicides together) was determined on the basis of job histories. A significant association between pesticide exposure and AD was found in men (RR = 2.39, 95% CI 1.02–5.63) but not in women (RR = 0.89, 95% CI 0.49–1.62). Actual exposures are likely to be different between men and women because of differences in tasks performed that involve pesticide exposure.

An ecologic study in Spain examined prevalence of AD by high- and low-pesticide-use areas (Parron et al., 2011). The age- and sex-adjusted prevalence ratio (PR) for AD was significantly higher in the high-pesticide-use areas (PR = 1.65, 95% CI 1.52–1.80), but this pesticide use was dominated by nonherbicide pesticides, so whether the analysis contrast reflects herbicide exposure differences is unclear.

Case-Control Studies Gauthier et al. (2001) found that long-term exposure to herbicides and insecticides was not significantly related to the development of AD. About 67 cases of probable and possible AD diagnosed according to criteria of the National Institute of Neurological and Communicative Disorders and Strokes and the Alzheimer's Disease and Related Disorders Association (now the Alzheimer's Association) were matched for age and sex with nondemented controls. Exposure data on each municipality were examined to establish the area sprayed with herbicides and insecticides in 1971, 1976, 1981, 1986, and 1991. The results were combined with the subjects' residential histories to establish potential environmental pesticide exposure. Logistic regression with adjustment for confounders found that long-term exposure to herbicides and insecticides did not have a significant effect on the development of AD. Occupational exposure to neurotoxic substances, including pesticides, was also not significantly related to AD.

Biologic Plausibility

Some animal studies have suggested involvement of the COIs in the occurrence of neurobehavioral effects. Akahoshi et al. (2009) produced a mouse neuroblastoma cell line that overexpressed the AHR, which is important in dopamine synthesis. Treating the line with TCDD increased tyrosine hydroxylase activity and led to increased dopamine expression. The implication of that finding is not clear, but changes in dopamine regulation have been implicated in a number of neurobehavioral syndromes. Other recent studies have focused on perinatal exposure. Haijima et al. (2010) found that perinatal exposure to TCDD impaired memory in male offspring. Mitsui et al. (2006) reported that hippocampus-dependent learning could be impaired in male rats exposed in utero to TCDD and that impairment could have affected fear conditioning. Lensu et al. (2006) examined areas in the hypothalamus for possible involvement in TCDD's effects on food consumption, potentially related to wasting syndrome, and suggested that their results were not consistent with a primary role of the hypothalamus. Studies in rodents have also detected molecular effects in cerebellar granule cells or neuroblasts, which are involved in cognitive and motor processes (Kim and Yang, 2005; Williamson et al., 2005).

Bongiovanni et al. (2011) reported that in vitro exposure of rat cerebellar granule cell cultures to 2,4-D produced a drastic decrease in cell viability, in association with an increased incidence of necrosis and apoptosis, and an increased concentration of reactive oxygen species, a decrease in glutathione content, and an abnormal activity of some enzymes relative to that in the control group. Earlier, Sturtz et al. (2008) found that 2,4-D affected rat maternal behavior. The specific neurobehavioral relevance of those studies and studies cited in earlier updates is unclear.

A general summary of the biologic plausibility of neurologic effects of exposure to the COIs is presented at the beginning of this chapter.

Synthesis

There is no epidemiologic evidence on an association between exposure to the specific COIs and AD. Findings with respect to broader categories of pesticides are inconsistent. The data on AD are limited to exposure measures that are too nonspecific to implicate the COIs.

Conclusion

On the basis of the evidence reviewed here and in previous VAO reports, the committee concludes that there is inadequate or insufficient evidence to determine whether there is an association between exposure to the COIs and AD.

CHRONIC PERIPHERAL SYSTEM DISORDERS

The peripheral neuropathies are an array of disorders caused by damage to nerve fibers (axonal neuropathies) or to the myelin sheath that surrounds many fibers (demyelinating neuropathies). Manifestations of neuropathy can include a combination of sensory changes, motor weakness, and autonomic instability. Clinically, various forms of peripheral neuropathy can be characterized by the distribution of nerve abnormalities and their patterns of progression.

Peripheral neuropathy resulting from toxic exposure usually affects nerve fibers in a symmetric pattern, beginning distally in the longest fibers (in the toes) and moving proximally (toward the spine). This kind of neuropathy is called symmetric axonal sensorimotor polyneuropathy. Sensory deficits begin at the toes, progress above the ankles, and only later affect the hands. Motor symptoms show the same general pattern. Physiologically, various forms of peripheral neuropathy can be characterized by results of electrodiagnostic testing to indicate which neural structures are affected. Most toxicant-induced neuropathies involve injury to the nerve-cell bodies (neurons) or nerve fibers (axons) that produces changes in the amplitude of a nerve's response to an electric stimulus.

The clinical appearances of most symmetric axonal neuropathies are similar except for variation in rates of progression and in whether pain is prominent. No specific signature distinguishes a toxicant-related neuropathy from one induced by other causes. As many as 30% of neuropathies are "idiopathic"; that is, no etiology is determined despite exhaustive clinical evaluation.

The most common toxicant-induced neuropathy occurs as a result of chronic alcohol exposure. Peripheral neuropathy also occurs commonly as a complication of diabetes; its reported prevalence in people who have chronic diabetes is up to 50%. It is important to include assessment of alcohol use and diabetes as covariates in epidemiologic studies, because the neuropathies that are related to these conditions are clinically and physiologically indistinguishable from other toxicant-induced neuropathies.

Toxicant exposure can result in early-onset (immediate) peripheral neuropathy or delayed-onset peripheral neuropathy that occurs years after the external exposure has ended. The committee considers a neuropathy to be of early onset if abnormalities appear within 1 year after external exposure ends and to be of delayed onset if abnormalities appear more than 1 year after external exposure ends. A review of the data supporting the association of exposure with early-onset peripheral neuropathy is presented in Appendix B, and will not be recapitulated here. Because the exposures of interest for Vietnam veterans are long past, immediate effects of the COIs are no longer pertinent for this cohort. The focus of this section will be on data related to delayed-onset peripheral neuropathy.

Summary from *VAO* and Previous Updates

The committee for *Update 2010* decided to move health outcomes that are manifested shortly after exposure to the COIs (TCDD in particular) to an appendix because they are no longer of interest for Vietnam veterans whose exposure occurred decades ago. Early-onset peripheral neuropathy was in this group with chloracne and porphyria cutanea tarda (PCT). That committee did, however, note that early-onset peripheral neuropathy is not necessarily a transient condition, as had been the previous judgment.

Henceforth, this section will address only studies of delayed-onset peripheral neuropathy.

A study by the Centers for Disease Control (now the Centers for Disease Control and Prevention [CDC]) (CDC, 1988); focused on service in Vietnam, not on exposure to the COIs, and therefore provided no evidence of the possible effects of specific exposures. Decoufle et al. (1992) reported no association between self-reported exposure to herbicides in Vietnam and peripheral neuropathy.

There was no indication of an increased incidence of peripheral neuropathy in the first examination, which established the baseline for Operation Ranch Hand veterans (AFHS, 1984). A peer-reviewed article described the peripheral-neuropathy data on the AFHS cohort (Michalek et al., 2001). In a primary analysis, the investigators had included diabetes as a potential confounder in the statistical model. In a secondary analysis, subjects who had conditions that were known to be associated with neuropathy were excluded, and subjects who had diabetes were enumerated. In both analyses, there were strong and significant associations between dioxin concentrations and possible and probable neuropathy, and significant trends were found with increasing concentrations of dioxin. However, there were too few nondiabetic subjects to produce useful estimates of risk in the absence of the contribution of diabetes. Thus, questions remained about the specific association between exposure to the COIs and peripheral neuropathy in the absence of any effect of diabetes. The large veteran studies are limited by the confounding nature of concurrent diabetes and alcohol exposure, both of which also are related to neuropathy.

Lee et al. (2008) evaluated the association of exposure to a variety of toxicants to the presence of neuropathy in subjects who had either frank diabetes or impaired glucose tolerance. Concentrations of dioxin-like PCBs were ranked, and subjects who had hemoglobin A1C levels of greater or less than 7 were compared separately. In neither group was there evidence of an increased incidence of neuropathy or of a dose–response relationship that suggested a concentration-dependent risk of neuropathy. Given the underlying risk of neuropathy inherent in patients who have diabetes, the lack of information regarding duration of diabetes and the small subject numbers render this study difficult to evaluate.

Update of the Epidemiologic Literature

No new studies of exposure to the COIs and chronic peripheral neuropathy have been published since *Update 2010*.

Biologic Plausibility

No new studies directly pertinent to peripheral neuropathy were identified in the present update. However, it is worth reiterating findings from earlier updates.

Neuronal cell cultures treated with 2,4-D showed decreased neurite extension associated with intracellular changes, including a decrease in microtubules, inhibition of the polymerization of tubulin, disorganization of the Golgi apparatus, and inhibition of ganglioside synthesis (Rosso et al., 2000a,b). Normal activity of those target processes is important for maintaining synaptic connections between nerve cells and supporting the mechanisms involved in axon regeneration during recovery from peripheral neuropathy. Grahmann et al. (1993) and Grehl et al. (1993) reported observation of electrophysiologic and pathologic abnormalities, respectively, in the peripheral nerves of rats treated with TCDD. When the animals were sacrificed 8 months after exposure, there were pathologic evidence of persistent axonal nerve damage and histologic findings typical of toxicant-induced injury. Those results constitute evidence of the biologic plausibility of an association between exposure to the COIs and peripheral neuropathy.

A summary of the biologic plausibility of neurologic effects arising from exposure to the COIs is presented at the end of this chapter.

Synthesis

The epidemiologic studies relating industrial or individual exposure to acute neuropathy were judged by the committee for *Update 1996* and later updates to constitute limited or suggestive evidence of an association between exposure to the COIs and early-onset transient peripheral neuropathy. As summarized above, results of further studies of the long-term sequelae of the exposures also suggest persistence of symptoms either permanently or over years. However, no data suggest that exposure to COIs can lead to the development of delayed-onset chronic neuropathy many years after termination of exposure of those who did not originally complain of early-onset neuropathy.

Conclusions

The committee for *Update 2010* concluded that, in addition to evidence supporting an association for transient early-onset peripheral neuropathy, there is limited or suggestive evidence of an association between exposure to the COIs and early-onset peripheral neuropathy that may be persistent.

On the basis of the evidence reviewed to date, however, the present committee concludes that there is inadequate or insufficient evidence to determine whether there is an association between exposure to the COIs and delayed-onset chronic neuropathy.

HEARING LOSS

Hearing loss increases markedly with age; about one-fourth of people more than 70 years old are affected (NCHS, 2010). Its prevalence is somewhat higher in men than in women (NCHS, 1994). The most common forms of hearing impairment in adults are presbycusis and tinnitus. Heritable factors may influence susceptibility to hearing loss, but external agents can also contribute. Aspirin at high doses can cause reversible tinnitus, and permanent hearing loss may be induced by pharmaceuticals (particularly antibiotics and antineoplastic drugs) and by some environmental and industrial chemicals (primarily solvents and metals). In occupational medicine, hearing loss is most often considered as being noise-induced. Cochlear development has been found to be impaired by hypothyroidism induced by endocrine disruptors (Howdeshell, 2002), but such a gestational effect would not pertain to Vietnam veterans exposed to herbicides as adults.

Summary from *VAO* and Previous Updates

Epidemiologic results on hearing loss in relation to service in Vietnam or to herbicide exposure more generally were first discussed in *Update 2010*; the literature searches for that report found two citations that addressed this health outcome. O'Toole et al. (2009) reexamined the health status of a cohort of Australian Vietnam veterans; as for almost every health endpoint surveyed in that group, the incidences of self-reported complete or partial deafness and of tinnitus showed statistically significant increases compared to the general population, and the committee for *Update 2010* had serious concerns that the results reported in O'Toole et al. (2009) were compromised by recall bias and other methodologic problems. Excesses in self-reported hearing loss were also found among licensed pesticide applicators in the AHS at the time of the 5-year followup interview (Crawford et al., 2008), but this effect was associated with insecticide exposure, not with herbicide use.

Update of the Epidemiologic Literature

No epidemiologic studies addressing herbicide exposure and hearing loss have been published since *Update 2010*.

Biologic Plausibility

Although no studies of hearing loss in adult animals directly exposed to the COIs were found, Crofton and Rice (1999) reported that perinatal maternal PCB126 exposure resulted in low-frequency hearing deficits in offspring of exposed maternal rats. Increased auditory thresholds occurred in the group treated at 1.0 μg/kg/day for 0.5- and 1-kHz tones, but higher frequencies were not significantly affected. The frequency-specific deficit was hypothesized to be caused by postnatal hypothyroxinemia that occurred during a sensitive period for development of the low-frequency regions of the cochlea. It was consistent with that hypothesis that pups from the study were found to have decreased serum

T4 concentrations on postnatal day 21. It is important to note that PCB126 is a potent dioxin-like compound, having one-tenth the toxic potency of TCDD (see Chapter 4).

A summary of the biologic plausibility of neurologic effects arising from exposure to the COIs is presented at the end of this chapter.

Synthesis

Two prior studies observed increased risk of hearing loss in Vietnam veterans and pesticide applicators, but neither was able to examine the specific COIs for the committee or to confirm hearing loss clinically. Furthermore, the report from the AHS (Crawford et al., 2008) observed an association only in insecticide applicators, not in herbicide applicators. The O'Toole et al. (2009) study evaluated Vietnam veterans, but it used a comparison group that was limited to the general population, not veterans from the same era who were not deployed to Vietnam, so it could not distinguish between hearing loss that may be associated with noise related to military service and hearing loss potentially associated with exposures to toxic chemicals. In the absence of new studies, the synthesis remains unchanged since *Update 2010*.

Conclusion

On the basis of the evidence reviewed here, the committee concludes that there is inadequate or insufficient evidence to determine whether there is an association between exposure to the COIs and hearing loss.

REFERENCES[1]

ADVA (Australian Department of Veteran's Affairs). 2005c. *Australian National Service Vietnam Veterans Mortality and Cancer Incidence Study.* Canberra, Australia: Department of Veterans' Affairs.

AFHS (Air Force Health Study). 1984. *An Epidemiological Investigation of Health Effects in Air Force Personnel Following Exposure to Herbicides. Baseline Morbidity Study Results.* Brooks AFB, TX: USAF School of Aerospace Medicine. NTIS AD-A138 340.

AFHS. 1991. *An Epidemiological Investigation of Health Effects in Air Force Personnel Following Exposure to Herbicides. Serum Dioxin Analysis of 1987 Examination Results.* Brooks AFB, TX: USAF School of Aerospace Medicine.

AFHS. 1995. *An Epidemiological Investigation of Health Effects in Air Force Personnel Following Exposure to Herbicides. 1992 Follow-Up Examination Results.* Brooks AFB, TX: Epidemiological Research Division. Armstrong Laboratory.

[1]Throughout this report, the same alphabetic indicator after year of publication is used consistently for a given reference when there are multiple citations by the same first author in a given year. The convention of assigning the alphabetic indicators in order of citation in a given chapter is not followed.

AFHS. 2000. *An Epidemiological Investigation of Health Effects in Air Force Personnel Following Exposure to Herbicides. 1997 Follow-Up Examination Results.* Brooks AFB, TX: Epidemiologic Research Division, Armstrong Laboratory. AFRL-HE-BR-TR-2000-02.

Akahoshi E, Yoshimura S, Uruno S, Ishihara-Sugano M. 2009. Effect of dioxins on regulation of tyrosine hydroxylase gene expression by aryl hydrocarbon receptor: A neurotoxicology study. *Environmental Health: A Global Access Science Source* 8(1):24.

Alzheimer's Association. 2012. Alzheimer's disease facts and figures. *Alzheimer's and Dementia* 8(2):1–72.

Baldi I, Lebailly P, Mohammed-Brahim B, Letenneur L, Dartigues JF, Brochard P. 2003. Neurodegenerative diseases and exposure to pesticides in the elderly. *American Journal of Epidemiology* 157(5):409–414.

Baldi I, Gruber A, Rondeau V, Lebailly P, Brochard P, Fabrigoule C. 2011. Neurobehavioral effects of long-term exposure to pesticides: Results from the 4-year follow-up of the PHYTONER study. *Occupational and Environmental Medicine* 68:108–115.

Barrett DH, Morriss RD, Akhtar FZ, Michalek JE. 2001. Serum dioxin and cognitive functioning among veterans of Operation Ranch Hand. *NeuroToxicology* 22:491–502.

Barrett DH, Morris RD, Jackson WG Jr, Stat M, Michalek JE. 2003. Serum dioxin and psychological functioning in US Air Force veterans of the Vietnam War. *Military Medicine* 168:153–159.

Behari M, Srivastava AK, Das RR, Pandey RM. 2001. Risk factors of Parkinson's disease in Indian patients. *Journal of Neurological Sciences* 190(1-2):49–55.

Blandini F, Armentero MT. 2012. Animal models of Parkinson's disease. *FEBS Journal* 279:1156–1166.

Bongiovanni B, De Lorenzi P, Ferri A, Konjuh C, Rassetto M, Duffard AME, Cardinali DP, Duffard R. 2007. Melatonin decreases the oxidative stress produced by 2,4-dichlorophenoxyacetic acid in rat cerebellar granule cells. *Neurotoxicity Research* 11(2):93–99.

Bongiovanni B, Ferri A, Brusco A, Rassetto M, Lopez LM, de Duffard AME, Duffard R. 2011. Adverse effects of 2,4-dichlorophenoxyacetic acid on rat cerebellar granule cell cultures were attenuated by amphetamine. *Neurotoxicity Research* 19:544–555.

Bonvicini F, Marcello N, Mandrioli J, Pietrini V, Vinceti M. 2010. Exposure to pesticides and risk of amyotrophic lateral sclerosis: A population-based case-control study. *Annali Dell'istituto Superiore Di Sanità* 46(3):284–287.

Bortolozzi AA, Duffard RO, Evangelista de Duffard AM. 1999. Behavioral alterations induced in rats by a pre- and postnatal exposure to 2,4-dichlorophenoxyacetic acid. *Neurotoxicology and Teratology* 21(4):451–465.

Bortolozzi A, de Duffard AME, Dajas F, Duffard R, Silveira R. 2001. Intracerebral administration of 2,4-dichlorophenoxyacetic acid induces behavioral and neurochemical alterations in the rat brain. *NeuroToxicology* 22(2):221–232.

Bortolozzi A, Duffard R, Antonelli M, Evangelista de Duffard AM. 2002. Increased sensitivity in dopamine D(2)-like brain receptors from 2,4-dichlorophenoxyacetic acid (2,4-D)-exposed and amphetamine-challenged rats. *Annals of the New York Academy of Sciences* 965:314–323.

Bortolozzi A, Duffard R, de Duffard AM. 2003. Asymmetrical development of the monoamine systems in 2,4-dichlorophenoxyacetic acid treated rats. *NeuroToxicology* 24(1):149–157.

Bortolozzi AA, Evangelista de Duffard AM, Duffard RO, Antonelli MC. 2004. Effects of 2,4-dichlorophenoxyacetic acid exposure on dopamine D2-like receptors in rat brain. *Neurotoxicology and Teratology* 26(4):599–605.

Breland AE, Currier RD. 1967. Multiple sclerosis and amyotrophic lateral sclerosis in Mississippi. *Neurology* 17:1011–1016.

Brighina L, Frigerio R, Schneider NK, Lesnick TG, de Andrade M, Cunningham JM, Farrer MJ, Lincoln SJ, Checkoway H, Rocca WA, Maraganore DM. 2008. Alpha-synuclein, pesticides, and Parkinson disease: A case-control study. *Neurology* 70(16 pt 2):1461–1469.

Bronstein J, Carvey P, Chen H, Cory-Slechta DA, DiMonte D, Duda J, English PB, Goldman S, Grate S, Hansen ,J, Hoppin J, Jewell S, Kamel F, Koroshetz W, Langston J, Logroscino G, Nelson L, Ravina B, Rocca WA, Ross G, Schettler T, Schwarzschild M, Scott B, Seegal R, Singleton A, Steenland, K, Tanner C, Eeden, S, Weisskopf M. 2009. Meeting report: Consensus statement—Parkinson's disease and the environment: Collaborative on Health and the Environment and Parkinson's Action Network (CHE PAN) Conference 26–28 June 2007. *Environmental Health Perspectives* 117(1):117–121.

Brooks BR. 1996. Clinical epidemiology of amyotrophic lateral sclerosis. *Neurological Clinics* 14(2):399–420.

Burns CJ, Beard KK, Cartmill JB. 2001. Mortality in chemical workers potentially exposed to 2,4-dichlorophenoxyacetic acid (2,4-D) 1945–94: An update. *Occupational and Environmental Medicine* 58:24–30.

Butterfield PG, Valanis BG, Spencer PS, Lindeman CA, Nutt JG. 1993. Environmental antecedents of young-onset Parkinson's disease. *Neurology* 43:1150–1158.

Byers JP, Masters K, Sarver JG, Hassoun EA. 2006. Association between the levels of biogenic amines and superoxide anion production in brain regions of rats after subchronic exposure to TCDD. *Toxicology* 228(2-3):291–298.

CDC (Centers for Disease Control). 1988. Health status of Vietnam veterans. II. Physical health. *Journal of the American Medical Association* 259:2708–2714.

Celik I, Tuluce Y, Isik I. 2006. Influence of subacute treatment of some plant growth regulators on serum marker enzymes and erythrocyte and tissue antioxidant defense and lipid peroxidation in rats. *Journal of Biochemical and Molecular Toxicology* 20(4):174–182.

Chancellor AM, Slattery JM, Fraser H. 1993. Risk factors for motor neuron disease: A case-control study based on patients from the Scottish motor neuron disease register. *Journal of Neurology, Neurosurgery, and Psychiatry* 56:1200–1206.

Crawford JM, Hoppin JA, Alavanja MCR, Blair A, Sandler DP, Kamel F. 2008. Hearing loss among licensed pesticide applicators in the Agricultural Health Study. *Journal of Occupational and Environmental Medicine* 50(7):817–826.

Crofton KM, Rice DC. 1999. Low-frequency hearing loss following perinatal exposure to 3,3′,4,4′,5-pentachlorobiphenyl (PCB 126) in rats. *Neurotoxicology and Teratology* 21(3): 299–301.

Curran CP, Nebert DW, Genter MB, Patel KV, Schaefer TL, Skelton MR, Williams MT, Vorhees CV. 2011. In utero and lactational exposure to PCBs in mice: Adult offspring show altered learning and memory depending on CYP1a2 and Ahr genotypes. *Environmental Health Perspectives* 119(9):1286–1293.

Dahlgren J, Warshaw R, Horsak RD, Parker FM 3rd, Takhar H. 2003. Exposure assessment of residents living near a wood treatment plant. *Environmental Research* 92(2):99–109.

Das K, Ghosh M, Nag C, Nandy SP, Banerjee M, Datta M, Devi G, Chaterjee G. 2011. Role of familial, environmental and occupational factors in the development of Parkinson's disease. *Neurodegenerative Diseases* 8:345–351.

Das K, Nag C, Ghosh M. 2012. Familial, environmental, and occuational risk factors in development of amyotrophic lateral sclerosis. *North American Journal of Medical Sciences* 4(8):350–355.

Deapen DM, Henderson BE. 1986. A case-control study of amyotrophic lateral sclerosis. *American Journal of Epidemiology* 123:790–799.

Decoufle P, Holmgreen P, Boyle CA, Stroup NE. 1992. Self-reported health status of Vietnam veterans in relation to perceived exposed to herbicides and combat. *American Journal of Epidemiology* 135:312–323.

Dhillon AS, Tarbutton GL, Levin JL, Plotkin GM, Lowry LK, Nalbone JT, Shepherd S. 2008. Pesticide/environmental exposures and Parkinson's disease in east Texas. *Journal of Agromedicine* 13(1):37–48.

Di Monte D, Lavasani M, Manning-Bog A. 2002. Environmental factors in Parkinson's disease. *NeuroToxicology* 23(4-5):487–502.

Drechsel DA, Patel M. 2008. Role of reactive oxygen species in the neurotoxicity of environmental agents implicated in Parkinson's disease. *Free Radical Biology and Medicine* 44(11):1873–1886.

Duffard R, Garcia G, Rosso S, Bortolozzi A, Madariaga M, Di Paolo O, Evangelista De Duffard A. 1996. Central nervous system myelin deficit in rats exposed to 2,4-dichlorophenoxyacetic acid throughout lactation. *Neurotoxicology and Teratology* 18(6):691–696.

Duty S, Jenner P. 2011. Animal models of Parkinson's disease: A source of novel treatments and clues to the cause of the disease. *British Journal of Pharmacology* 164:1357–1391.

Elbaz A, Clavel J, Rathouz PJ, Moisan F, Galanaud JP, Delemotte B, Alperovitch A, Tzourio C. 2009. Professional exposure to pesticides and Parkinson disease. *Annals of Neurology* 66(4):494–504.

Engel LS, Checkoway H, Keifer MC, Seixas NS, Longstreth WT, Scott KC, Hudnell K, Anger WK, Camicioli R. 2001. Parkinsonism and occupational exposure to pesticides. *Occupational and Environmental Medicine* 58:582–589.

Evangelista de Duffard AM, Orta C, Duffard RO. 1990. Behavioral changes in rats fed a diet containing 2,4-dichlorophenoxyacetic butyl ester. *Neurotoxicology* 11:563–572.

Evangelista de Duffard AM, Bortolozzi A, Duffard RO. 1995. Altered behavioral responses in 2,4-dichlorophenoxyacetic acid treated and amphetamine challenged rats. *Neurotoxicology* 16(3):479–488.

Firestone JA, Smith-Weller T, Franklin G, Swanson P, Longstreth WT Jr, Checkoway H. 2005. Pesticides and risk of Parkinson disease: A population-based case-control study. *Archives of Neurology* 62(1):91–95.

Firestone JA, Lundin JI, Powers KM, Smith-Weller T, Franklin GM, Swanson PD, Longstreth WT Jr, Checkoway H. 2010. Occupational factors and risk of Parkinson's disease: A population-based case-control study. *American Journal of Industrial Medicine* 53(3):217–223.

Fracchiolla NS, Todoerti K, Bertazzi PA, Servida F, Corradini P, Carniti C, Colombi A, Pesatori AC, Neri A, Deliliers GL. 2011. Dioxin exposure of human CD34+ hemopoietic cells induces gene expression modulation that recapitulates its in vivo clinical and biological effects. *Toxicology* 283:18–23.

Frost G, Brown T, Harding AH. 2011. Mortality and cancer incidence among British agricultural pesticide users. *Occupational Medicine* 61:303–310.

Gallagher JP, Sander M. 1987. Trauma and amyotrophic lateral sclerosis: A report of 78 patients. *Acta Neurologica Scandinavia* 75:1041–1043.

Gao HM, Hong JS. 2011. Gene–environment interactions: Key to unraveling the mystery of Parkinson's disease. *Progress in Neurobiology* 94:1–19.

Garcia C, Pascual JA, Mena E, Hernandez T. 2004. Influence of the stabilisation of organic materials on their biopesticide effect in soils. *Bioresource Technology* 95(2):215–221.

Garcia GB, Konjuh C, Duffard RO, de Duffard AME. 2006. Dopamine-beta-hydroxylase immunohistochemical study in the locus coeruleus of neonate rats exposed to 2,4-dichlorophenoxyacetic acid through mother's milk. *Drug and Chemical Toxicology* 29(4):435–442.

Gauthier E, Fortier I, Courchcesne F, Pepin P, Mortimer J, Gauvreau D. 2001. Environmental pesticide exposure as a risk factor for Alzheimer's disease: A case-control study. *Environmental Research* 86:37–45.

Gorell JM, Johnson CC, Rybicki BA, Peterson EL, Richardson RJ. 1998. The risk of Parkinson's disease with exposure to pesticides, farming, well water, and rural living. *Neurology* 50:1346–1350.

Grahmann F, Claus D, Grehl H, Neundoerfer B. 1993. Electrophysiologic evidence for a toxic polyneuropathy in rats after exposure to 2,3,7,8-tetrachlorodibenzo-*p*-dioxin (TCDD). *Journal of Neurological Sciences* 115(1):71–75.

Grehl H, Grahmann F, Claus D, Neundorfer B. 1993. Histologic evidence for a toxic polyneuropathy due to exposure to 2,3,7,8-tetrachlorodibenzo-*p*-dioxin (TCDD) in rats. *Acta Neurologica Scandinavica* 88(5):354–357.

Haijima A, Endo T, Zhang Y, Miyazaki W, Kakeyama M, Tohyama C. 2010. In utero and lactational exposure to low doses of chlorinated and brominated dioxins induces deficits in the fear memory of male mice. *NeuroToxicology* 31(4):385–390.

Hancock DB, Martin ER, Mayhew GM, Stajich JM, Jewett R, Stacy MA, Scott BL, Vance JM, Scott WK. 2008. Pesticide exposure and risk of Parkinson's disease: A family-based case-control study. *BMC Neurology* 8(6):1–12.

Hanisch R, Dworsky RL, Henderson BE. 1976. A search for clues to the cause of amyotrophic lateral sclerosis. *Archives of Neurology* 33:456–457.

Hansen ES, Hasle H, Lander F. 1992. A cohort study on cancer incidence among Danish gardeners. *American Journal of Industrial Medicine* 21:651–660.

Hansen ES, Lander F, Lauritsen JM. 2007. Time trends in cancer risk and pesticide exposure, a long-term follow-up of Danish gardeners. *Scandinavian Journal of Work, Environment and Health* 33(6):465–469.

Hatcher JM, Pennell KD, Miller GW. 2008. Parkinson's disease and pesticides: A toxicological perspective. *Trends in Pharmacological Sciences* 29(6):322–329.

Hertzman C, Wiens M, Bowering D, Snow B, Calne D. 1990. Parkinson's disease: A case-control study of occupational and environmental risk factors. *American Journal of Industrial Medicine* 17:349–355.

Hertzman C, Wiens M, Snow B, Kelly S, Calne D. 1994. A case-control study of Parkinson's disease in a horticultural region of British Columbia. *Movement Disorders* 9:69–75.

Hojo R, Kakeyama M, Kurokawa Y, Aoki Y, Yonemoto J, Tohyama C. 2008. Learning behavior in rat offspring after in utero and lactational exposure to either TCDD or PCB126. *Environmental Health and Preventive Medicine* 13(3):169–180.

Howdeshell KL. 2002. A model of the development of the brain as a construct of the thyroid system. *Environmental Health Perspectives* 110(Suppl 3):337–348.

Huang P, Rannug A, Ahlbom E, Haakansson H, Ceccatelli S. 2000. Effect of 2,3,7,8-tetrachlorodibenzo-*p*-dioxin on the expression of cytochrome P450 1A1, the aryl hydrocarbon receptor, and the aryl hydrocarbon receptor nuclear translocator in rat brain and pituitary. *Toxicology and Applied Pharmacology* 169(2):159–167.

IOM (Institute of Medicine). 1994. *Veterans and Agent Orange: Health Effects of Herbicides Used in Vietnam.* Washington, DC: National Academy Press.

IOM. 1996. *Veterans and Agent Orange: Update 1996.* Washington, DC: National Academy Press.

IOM. 1999. *Veterans and Agent Orange: Update 1998.* Washington, DC: National Academy Press.

IOM. 2001. *Veterans and Agent Orange: Update 2000.* Washington, DC: National Academy Press.

IOM. 2003. *Veterans and Agent Orange: Update 2002.* Washington, DC: The National Academies Press.

IOM. 2005. *Veterans and Agent Orange: Update 2004.* Washington, DC: The National Academies Press.

IOM. 2007. *Veterans and Agent Orange: Update 2006.* Washington, DC: The National Academies Press.

IOM. 2009. *Veterans and Agent Orange: Update 2008.* Washington, DC: The National Academies Press.

IOM. 2012. *Veterans and Agent Orange: Update 2010.* Washington, DC: The National Academies Press.

Kamel F, Engel LS, Gladen BC, Hoppin JA, Alavanja MC, Sandler DP. 2005. Neurologic symptoms in licensed private pesticide applicators in the Agricultural Health Study. *Environmental Health Perspectives* 113(7):877–882.

Kamel F, Engel LS, Gladen BC, Hoppin JA, Alavanja MC, Sandler DP. 2007a. Neurologic symptoms in licensed pesticide applicators in the Agricultural Health Study. *Human and Experimental Toxicology* 26(3):243–250.

Kamel F, Tanner C, Umbach D, Hoppin J, Alavanja M, Blair A, Comyns K, Goldman S, Korell M, Langston J, Ross G, Sandler D. 2007b. Pesticide exposure and self-reported Parkinson's disease in the Agricultural Health Study. *American Journal of Epidemiology* 165(4):364–374.

Kamel F, Umbach DM, Bedlack RS, Richards M, Watson M, Alavanja MC, Blair A, Hoppin JA, Schmidt S, Sandler DP. 2012. Pesticide exposure and amyotrophic lateral sclerosis. *Neurotoxicology* 33(3):457–462.

Kenborg L, Lassen CF, Lander F, Olsen JH. 2012. Parkinson's disease among gardeners exposed to pesticides—a Danish cohort study. *Scandinavian Journal of Work, Environment and Health* 38(1):65–69.

Kim JS, Lim HS, Cho SI, Cheong HK, Lim MK. 2003. Impact of Agent Orange exposure among Korean Vietnam veterans. *Industrial Health* 41(3):149–157.

Kim SY, Yang JH. 2005. Neurotoxic effects of 2,3,7,8-tetrachlorodibenzo-*p*-dioxin in cerebellar granule cells. *Experimental and Molecular Medicine* 37:58–64.

Kim SY, Lee HG, Choi EJ, Park KY, Yang JH. 2007. TCDD alters PKC signaling pathways in developing neuronal cells in culture. *Chemosphere* 67(9):S421–S427.

Kiyohara C, Miyake Y, Koyanagi M, Fujimoto T, Shirasawa S, Tanaka K, Fukushima W, Sasaki S, Tsuboi Y, Yamada T, Oeda T, Miki T, Kawamura N, Sakae N, Fukuyama H, Hirota Y, Nagai M; Fukuoka Kinki Parkinson's Disease Study Group. 2010. GST polymorphisms, interaction with smoking and pesticide use, and risk for Parkinson's disease in a Japanese population. *Parkinsonism and Related Disorders* 16:447–452.

Klein C, Lohmann-Hedrich K. 2007. Impact of recent genetic findings in Parkinson's disease. *Current Opinion in Neurology* 20(4):453–464.

Konjuh C, Garcia G, Lopez L, de Duffard AME, Brusco A, Duffard R. 2008. Neonatal hypomyelination by the herbicide 2,4-dichlorophenoxyacetic acid. Chemical and ultrastructural studies in rats. *Toxicological Sciences* 104(2):332–340.

Kuopio A, Marttila RJ, Helenius H, Rinne UK. 1999. Environmental risk factors in Parkinson's disease. *Movement Disorders* 14:928–939.

Kurtzke JF, Beebe GW. 1980. Epidemiology of amyotrophic lateral sclerosis: 1. A case-control comparison based on ALS deaths. *Neurology* 30:453–462.

Kwok JBJ. 2012. Role of epigenetics in Alzheimer's and Parkinson's disease. *Epigenomics* 2(5):671–682.

Langston JW. 2006. The Parkinson's complex: Parkinsonism is just the tip of the iceberg. *Annals of Neurology* 59(4):591–596.

La Rocca C, Alivernini S, Badiali M, Cornoldi A, Iacovella N, Silvestroni L, Spera G, Turrio-Baldassarri L. 2008. TEQs and body burden for PCDDs, PCDFs, and dioxin-like PCBs in human adipose tissue. *Chemosphere* 73(1):92–96.

Lee DH, Jacobs DR Jr, Steffes M. 2008. Association of organochlorine pesticides with peripheral neuropathy in patients with diabetes or impaired fasting glucose. *Diabetes* 57(11):3108–3111.

Lee HG, Kim SY, Choi EJ, Park KY, Yang JH. 2007. Translocation of PKC-betaII is mediated via RACK-1 in the neuronal cells following dioxin exposure. *NeuroToxicology* 28(2):408–414.

Lensu S, Miettinen R, Pohjanvirta R, Lindén J, Tuomisto J. 2006. Assessment by c-Fos immunostaining of changes in brain neural activity induced by 2,3,7,8-tetrachlorodibenzo-*p*-dioxin (TCDD) and leptin in rats. *Basic and Clinical Pharmacology and Toxicology* 98:363–371.

Liang CL, Wang TT, Luby-Phelps K, German DC. 2007. Mitochondria mass is low in mouse substantia nigra dopamine neurons: Implications for Parkinson's disease. *Experimental Neurology* 203(2):370–380.

Lin CH, Wu RM, Tai CH, Chen ML, Hu FC. 2011. Hippocampal metabolomics reveals 2,3,7,8-tetrachlorodibenzo-*p*-dioxin toxicity associated with ageing in Sprague-Dawley rats. *Talanta* 85:1007–1012.

Liou HH, Tsai MC, Chen CJ, Jeng JS, Chang YC, Chen SY, Chen RC. 1997. Environmental risk factors and Parkinson's disease: A case-control study in Taiwan. *Neurology* 48:1583–1588.

Littlejohn D, Mangano E, Clarke M, Bobyn J, Moloney K, Hayley S. 2011. Inflammatory mechanisms of neurodegeneration in toxin-based models of Parkinson's disease. *SAGE-Hindawi Access to Research* 2011:18 pps.

McDowell K, Chesselet MF. 2012. Animal models of the non-motor features of Parkinson's disease. *Neurobiology of Disease* 46:597–606.

McGuire V, Longstreth WT, Nelson LM, Koepsell TD, Checkoway H, Morgan MS, van Belle G. 1997. Occupational exposure and amyotrophic lateral sclerosis: A population-based case-control study. *American Journal of Epidemiology* 145:1076–1088.

Michalek JE, Akhtar FZ, Arezzo JC, Garabrant DH, Albers JW. 2001. Serum dioxin and peripheral neuropathy in veterans of Operation Ranch Hand. *Neurotoxicology* 22:479–490.

Mitchell JD, Borasio GD. 2007. Amyotrophic lateral sclerosis. *Lancet* 369:2031–2041.

Mitsui T, Sugiyama N, Maeda S, Tohyama C, Arita J. 2006. Perinatal exposure to 2,3,7,8-tetrachlorodibenzo-*p*-dioxin suppresses contextual fear conditioning—accompanied activation of cyclic AMP response element-binding protein in the hippocampal CA1 region of male rats. *Neuroscience Letters* 398(3):206–210.

Mohammad FK, St. Omer VE. 1986. Behavioral and developmental effects in rats following in utero exposure to 2,4-D/2,4,5-T mixture. *Neurobehavioral Toxicology and Teratology* 8(5):551–560.

Moisan F, Spinosi J, Dupupet JL, Delabre L, Mazurie JL, Goldberg M, Imbernon E, Tzourio C, Elbaz A. 2011. The relation between type of farming and prevalence of Parkinson's disease among agricultural workers in five French districts. *Movement Disorders* 26(2):271–279.

Morahan JM, Pamphlett R. 2006. Amyotrophic lateral sclerosis and exposure to environmental toxins: An Australian case-control study. *Neuroepidemiology* 27(3):130–135.

NCHS (National Center for Health Statistics). 1994. *Vital and Health Statistics: Prevalence and Characteristics of Persons with Hearing Trouble: United States, 1990–91.* Series 10: Data from the National Health Survey, Number 188. Hyattsville, MD.

NCHS. 2010. *Vision, hearing, balance, and sensory impairment in Americans aged 70 years and over: United States, 1999–2006.* NCHS Data Brief, Number 31. Hyattsville, MD.

Nunomura A, Moreira PI, Lee HG, Zhu X, Castellani RJ, Smith MA, Perry G. 2007. Neuronal death and survival under oxidative stress in Alzheimer and Parkinson diseases. *CNS and Neurological Disorders—Drug Targets* 6(6):411–423.

O'Toole BI, Catts SV, Outram S, Pierse KR, Cockburn J. 2009. The physical and mental health of Australian Vietnam veterans 3 decades after the war and its relation to military service, combat, and post-traumatic stress disorder. *American Journal of Epidemiology* 170(3):318–330.

Palmeira CM, Moreno AJ, Madeira VM. 1994a. Interactions of herbicides 2,4-D and dinoseb with liver mitochondrial bioenergetics. *Toxicology and Applied Pharmacology* 127:50–57.

Palmeira CM, Moreno AJ, Madeira VMC. 1994b. Metabolic alterations in hepatocytes promoted by the herbicides paraquat, dinoseb and 2,4-D. *Archives of Toxicology* 68:24–31.

Palmeira CM, Moreno AJ, Madeira VM. 1995a. Effects of paraquat, dinoseb and 2,4-D on intracellular calcium and on vasopressin-induced calcium mobilization in isolated hepatocytes. *Archives of Toxicology* 69:460–466.

Palmeira CM, Moreno AJ, Madeira VM. 1995b. Thiols metabolism is altered by the herbicides paraquat, dinoseb and 2,4-D: A study in isolated hepatocytes. *Toxicology Letters* 81:115–123.

Pamphlett R. 2012. Exposure to environmental toxins and the risk of sporadic motor neuron disease: An expanded Australian case-control study. *European Journal of Neurology* 19:1343–1348.

Park RM, Schulte PA, Bowman JD, Walker JT, Bondy SC, Yost MG, Touchstone JA, Dosemeci M. 2005. Potential occupational risks for neurodegenerative diseases. *American Journal of Industrial Medicine* 48(1):63–77.

Parron T, Alarcon R, Requena M, Hernandez AF. 2011. An ecological study of pesticide exposure and different health conditions in Andalusia (south Spain). *Toxicology Letters* 205:S126–S127.

Pazderova-Vejlupkova J, Lukas E, Nemcova M, Pickova J, Jirasek L. 1981. The development and prognosis of chronic intoxication by tetrachlorodibenzo-*p*-dioxin in men. *Archives of Environmental Health* 36:5–11.

Pelclová D, Fenclová Z, Dlasková Z, Urban P, Lukás E, Procházka B, Rappe C, Preiss J, Kocan A, Vejlupková J. 2001. Biochemical, neuropsychological, and neurological abnormalities following 2,3,7,8-tetrachlorodibenzo-*p*-dioxin (TCDD) exposure. *Archives of Environmental Health* 56(6):493–500.

Pelclová D, Fenclová Z, Preiss J, Prochazka B, Spacil J, Dubska Z, Okrouhlik B, Lukás E, Urban P. 2002. Lipid metabolism and neuropsychological follow-up study of workers exposed to 2,3,7,8- tetrachlordibenzo-*p*-dioxin. *International Archives of Occupational and Environmental Health* 75:S60–S66.

Pereira D, Garrett C. 2010. Factores de risco da doença de Parkinson: Um estudo epidemiológico. *Acta Medica Portuguesa* 23:15–24.

Postuma RB, Montplaisir JY, Pelletier A, Dauvilliers Y, Oertel W, Iranzo A, Ferini-Strambi L, Arnulf I, Hogl B, Manni R, Miyamoto T, Mayer G, Stiasny-Kolster K, Puligheddu M, Ju Y, Jennum P, Sonka K, Santamaria J, Fantini ML, Zucconi M, Leu-Semenescu S, Frauscher B, Terzaghi M, Miyamoto M, Unger MM, Cochen De Cock V, Wolfson C. 2012. Environmental risk factors for REM sleep behavior disorder: A multicenter case-control study. *Neurology* 79(5):428–434.

Roelofs-Iverson RA, Mulder DW, Elverback LR, Kurland LT, Craig AM. 1984. ALS and heavy metals: A pilot case-control study. *Neurology* 34:393–395.

Rosen DR, Siddique T, Patterson D, Figlewicz DA, Sapp P, Hentati A, Donaldson D, Goto J, O'Regan JP, Deng HX, Rahmani Z, Krizus A, McKenna-Yasek D, Cayabyab A, Gaston S, Tanzi R, Halperin JJ, Herzfeldt B, Van den Berg R, Hung WY, Bird T, Deng G, Mulder DW, Smith C, Laing NG, Soriano E, Pericak-Vance MA, Haines J, Rouleau GA, Gusella J, Horvitz HR, Brown RH. 1993. Mutations in Cu/Zn superoxide dismutase gene are associated with familial amyotrophic lateral sclerosis. *Nature* 362(6415):59–62.

Rosso SB, Caceres AO, Evangelista de Duffard AM, Duffard RO, Quiroga S. 2000a. 2,4-dichlorophenoxyacetic acid disrupts the cytoskeleton and disorganizes the Golgi apparatus of cultured neurons. *Toxicological Sciences* 56:133–140.

Rosso SB, Garcia GB, Madariaga MJ, De Duffard AME, Duffard RO. 2000b. 2,4-dichlorophenoxyacetic acid in developing rats alters behaviour, myelination and regions brain gangliosides pattern. *NeuroToxicology* 21(1-2):155–164.

Rowland LP. 1998. Diagnosis of amyotrophic lateral sclerosis. *Journal of the Neurological Sciences* 160(Suppl 1):S6–S24.

Rowland LP, Shneider NA. 2001. Amyotrophic lateral sclerosis. *New England Journal of Medicine* 344(22):1688–1700.

Ruder AM, Yiin JH. 2011. Mortality of US pentachlorophenol production workers through 2005. *Chemosphere* 83:851–861.

Rugbjerg K, Harris MA, Shen H, Marion SA, Tsui JKC, Teschke K. 2011. Pesticide exposure and risk of Parkinson's disease—a population-based case-control study evaluating the potential for recall bias. *Scandinavian Journal of Work, Environment and Health* 37(5):427–436.

Sanyal J, Chakraborty DP, Sarkar B, Banerjee TK, Mukherjee SC, Ray BC, Rao VR. 2010. Environmental and familial risk factors of Parkinsons disease: Case-control study. *Canadian Journal of Neurological Sciences* 37:637–642.

Sarnico I, Boroni F, Benarese M, Sigala S, Lanzillotta A, Battistin L, Spano P, Pizzi M. 2008. Activation of NF-kappaB p65/c-Rel dimer is associated with neuroprotection elicited by mGlu5 receptor agonists against MPP(+) toxicity in SK-N-SH cells. *Journal of Neural Transmission* 115(5):669–676.

Savettieri G, Salemi G, Arcara A, Cassata M, Castiglione MG, Fierro B. 1991. A case-control study of amyotrophic lateral sclerosis. *Neuroepidemiology* 10:242–245.

Seidler A, Hellenbrand W, Robra BP, Vieregge P, Nischan P, Joerg J, Oertel WH, Ulm G, Schneider E. 1996. Possible environmental, occupational, and other etiologic factors for Parkinson's disease: A case-control study in Germany. *Neurology* 46:1275–1284.

Semchuk KM, Love EJ, Lee RG. 1992. Parkinson's disease and exposure to agricultural work and pesticide chemicals. *Neurology* 42:1328–1335.

Shen D, Dalton TP, Nebert DW, Shertzer HG. 2005. Glutathione redox state regulates mitochondrial reactive oxygen production. *Journal of Biological Chemistry* 280(27):25305–25312.

Sherer T, Betarbet R, Stout A, Lund S, Baptista M, Panov A, Cookson M, Greenamyre J. 2002a. An in vitro model of Parkinson's disease: Linking mitochondrial impairment to altered alpha-synuclein metabolism and oxidative damage. *Journal of Neuroscience: The Official Journal of the Society for Neuroscience* 22(16):7006–7015.

Singh S, Kushwah AS, Singh R, Farswan M, Kaur R. 2012. Current therapeutic strategy in Alzheimer's disease. *European Review for Medical and Pharmacological Sciences* 16(12):1651–1664.

Solomon C, Poole J, Palmer KT, Peveler R, Coggon D. 2007. Neuropsychiatric symptoms in past users of sheep dip and other pesticides. *Occupational and Environmental Medicine* 64(4):259–266.

St. Omer VEV, Mohammad FF. 1987. Ontogeny of swimming behavior and brain catecholamine turnover in rats prenatally exposed to a mixture of 2,4-dichlorophenoxyacetic and 2,4,5-trichlorophenoxyacetic acids. *Neuropharmacology* 9:1351–1358.

Stern M, Dulaney E, Gruber SB, Golbe L, Bergen M, Hurtig H, Gollomp S, Stolley P. 1991. The epidemiology of Parkinson's disease: A case-control study of young-onset and old-onset patients. *Archives of Neurology* 48:903–907.

Sturtz N, Deis RP, Jahn GA, Duffard R, Evangelista de Duffard AM. 2008. Effect of 2,4-dichlorophenoxyacetic acid on rat maternal behavior. *Toxicology* 247(2-3):73–79.

Sutedja NA, Fischer K, Veldink JH, van der Heijdem GJ, Kromhout H, Heederik D, Huisman MH, Wokke JJ, van den Berg LH. 2009a. What we truly know about occupation as a risk factor for ALS: A critical and systematic review. *Amyotrophic Lateral Sclerosis* 10:295–301.

Sutedja NA, Fischer K, Veldink JH, van der Heijdem GJ, Kromhout H, Heederik D, Huisman MH, Wokke JJ, van den Berg LH. 2009b. Exposure to chemicals and metals and risk of amyotrophic lateral sclerosis: A systematic review. *Amyotrophic Lateral Sclerosis* 10:302–309.

Tanner CM, Ross GW, Jewell SA, Hauser RA, Jankovic J, Factor SA, Bressman S, Deligtisch A, Marras C, Lyons KE, Bhudhikanok GS, Roucoux DF, Meng C, Abbott RD, Langston JW. 2009. Occupation and risk of Parkinsonism: A multicenter case-control study. *Archives of Neurology* 66(9):1106–1113.

Taylor CA, Saint-Hilaire MH, Cupples LA, Thomas CA, Burchard AE, Feldman RG, Myers RH. 1999. Environmental, medical, and family history risk factors for Parkinson's disease: A New England-based case-control study. *American Journal of Medical Genetics (Neuropsychiatric Genetics)* 88:742–749.

Thiffault C, Langston WJ, Di Monte DA. 2001. Acute exposure to organochlorine pesticides does not affect striatal dopamine in mice. *Neurotoxicity Research* 3(6):537–543.

Urban P, Pelclová D, Lukas E, Kupka K, Preiss J, Fenclová Z, Smerhovsky Z. 2007. Neurological and neurophysiological examinations on workers with chronic poisoning by 2,3,7,8-TCDD: Follow-up 35 years after exposure. *European Journal of Neurology* 14(2):213–218.

Uversky V, Kiowa Bower JL, Fink AL. 2002. Synergistic effects of pesticides and metals on the fibrillation of α-synuclein: Implications for Parkinson's disease. *NeuroToxicology* 23:527–536.

van den Berg M, Birnbaum LS, Denison M, De Vito M, Farland W, Feeley M, Fiedler H, Hakansson H, Hanberg A, Haws L, Rose M, Safe S, Schrenk D, Tohyama C, Tritscher A, Tuomisto J, Tysklind M, Walker N, Peterson RE. 2006. The 2005 World Health Organization reevaluation of human and mammalian toxic equivalency factors for dioxins and dioxin-like compounds. *Toxicological Sciences* 93(2):223–241.

van der Mark M, Brouwer M, Kromhout H, Nijssen P, Huss A, Vermeulen R. 2012. Is pesticide use related to Parkinson disease? Some clues to heterogeneity in study results. *Environmental Health Perspectives* 120(3):340–347.

Vidal JS, Vidailhet P, Derkinderen P, Dubard de Gaillarbois T, Tzourio C, Alperovitch A. 2009. Risk factors for progressive supranuclear palsy: A case-control study in France. *Journal of Neurology, Neurosurgery and Psychiartry* 80:1271–1274.

Visintainer PF, Barone M, McGee H, Peterson EL. 1995. Proportionate mortality study of Vietnam-era veterans of Michigan. *Journal of Occupational and Environmental Medicine* 37:423–428.

Weisskopf MG, O'Reilly EJ, McCullough ML, Calle EE, Thun MJ, Cudkowicz M, Ascherio A. 2005. Prospective study of military service and mortality from ALS. *Neurology* 64(1):32–37.

Weisskopf MG, Morozova N, O'Reilly EJ, McCullough ML, Calle EE, Thun MJ, Ascherio A. 2009. Prospective study of chemical exposures and amyotrophic lateral sclerosis. *Journal of Neurology, Neurosurgery and Psychiatry* 80(5):558–561.

Williamson MA, Gasiewicz TA, Opanashuk LA. 2005. Aryl hydrocarbon receptor expression and activity in cerebellar granule neuroblasts: Implications for development and dioxin neurotoxicity. *Toxicological Sciences* 83:340–348.

12

Cardiovascular and Metabolic Outcomes

Chapter Overview

Based on new evidence and a review of prior studies, the committee for Update 2012 *found one new association: limited or suggestive evidence of association between the relevant exposures and stroke. Current evidence supports the findings of earlier studies concerning cardiovascular and metabolic outcomes:*

- *No adverse cardiovascular or metabolic outcome has sufficient evidence of an association with the chemicals of interest.*
- *There is limited or suggestive evidence of an association between the chemicals of interest and type 2 diabetes, hypertension, ischemic heart disease, and now stroke.*
- *There is inadequate or insufficient evidence to determine whether there is an association between the chemicals of interest and for all other adverse cardiovascular or metabolic outcomes.*

This chapter summarizes and presents conclusions about the strength of the evidence from epidemiologic studies regarding an association between exposure to the chemicals of interest (COIs)—2,4-dichlorophenoxyacetic acid (2,4-D), 2,4,5-trichlorophenoxyacetic acid (2,4,5-T) and its contaminant 2,3,7,8-tetrachlorodibenzo-*p*-dioxin (TCDD), picloram, and cacodylic acid—and type 2 diabetes and circulatory disorders. The committee also considers studies of exposure to polychlorinated biphenyls (PCBs) and other dioxin-like chemicals to be informative if their results were reported in terms of TCDD toxic equivalents (TEQs) or concentrations of specific congeners. Although all studies reporting

TEQs based on PCBs were reviewed, studies that reported TEQs based only on mono-ortho PCBs (which are PCBs 105, 114, 118, 123, 156, 157, 167, and 189) were given very limited consideration because mono-ortho PCBs typically contribute less than 10% to total TEQs, based on the World Health Organization revised toxicity equivalency factors (TEFs) of 2005 (La Rocca et al., 2008; van den Berg et al., 2006).

TYPE 2 DIABETES

Diabetes mellitus is a group of heterogeneous metabolic disorders characterized by hyperglycemia and quantitative or qualitative deficiency of insulin action (Orchard et al., 1992). Although all forms share hyperglycemia, the pathogenic processes involved in its development differ. Most cases of diabetes mellitus are in one of two categories: type 1 diabetes is characterized by a lack of insulin caused by the destruction of insulin-producing cells in the pancreas (β cells), and type 2 diabetes is characterized by a combination of resistance to the actions of insulin and inadequate secretion of insulin (called relative insulin deficiency). In old classification systems, type 1 diabetes was called insulin-dependent diabetes mellitus or juvenile-onset diabetes mellitus, and type 2 was called non–insulin-dependent diabetes mellitus or adult-onset diabetes mellitus. Type 1 diabetes occurs as a result of immunologically-mediated destruction of β cells in the pancreas, which often occurs during childhood but can occur at any age. As in many autoimmune diseases, genetic and environmental factors influence pathogenesis. Some viral infections are believed to be important environmental factors that can trigger the autoimmunity associated with type 1 diabetes. The modern classification system recognizes that type 2 diabetes can occur in children and can require insulin treatment. Long-term complications of both types can include cardiovascular disease (CVD), nephropathy, retinopathy, neuropathy, and increased vulnerability to infections. Keeping blood sugar concentrations within the normal range is crucial for preventing complications.

About 90% of all cases of diabetes mellitus are of type 2, and type 2 has been the type of diabetes that epidemiologic investigations relevant to Vietnam veterans have addressed. Onset can occur before the age of 30 years, and incidence increases steadily with age. The main risk factors are age, obesity, abdominal fat deposition, a history of gestational diabetes (in women), physical inactivity, ethnicity (prevalence is greater in blacks and Hispanics than in whites), and family history. The relative contributions of those features are not known. Prevalence and mortality statistics in the US population for 2006 are presented in Table 12-1.

The etiology of type 2 diabetes is unknown, but three major components have been identified: peripheral insulin resistance (thought by many to be primary) in target tissues (muscle, adipose tissue, and liver), a defect in β-cell secretion of insulin, and overproduction of glucose by the liver. In states of insulin resistance, insulin secretion is initially higher for each concentration of glucose

TABLE 12-1 Prevalence of and Mortality from Diabetes, Lipid Disorders, and Circulatory Disorders in the United States, 2009/2010

ICD-9 Range	Diseases of Circulatory System	Prevalence (% of Americans 20 years old and older)		Mortality (number of deaths, all ages)	
		Men	Women	Men	Women
250	Diabetes	nr	nr	35,100	33,700
	Physician-diagnosed	8.7[a]	7.9[a]	nr	nr
	Undiagnosed	4.7[a]	2.3[a]	nr	nr
	Prediabetes	46.0[a]	30.5[a]	nr	nr
	Lipid disorders				
	Total cholesterol ≥ 200 mg/dL	41.3	44.9	nr	nr
	Total cholesterol ≥ 240 mg/dL	12.7	14.7	nr	nr
	LDL cholesterol ≥ 130 mg/dL	31.9	30.0	nr	nr
	HDL cholesterol < 40 mg/dL	31.8	12.3	nr	nr
390–459	All circulatory disorders	36.7	34.0	386,400	401,500
390–398	Rheumatic fever and rheumatic heart disease	nr	nr	nr	nr
401–404[b]	Hypertensive disease	33.6	32.2	27,700	34,100
401	Essential hypertension	nr	nr	nr	nr
402	Hypertensive heart disease	nr	nr	nr	nr
403	Hypertensive renal disease	nr	nr	nr	nr
404	Hypertensive heart and renal disease	nr	nr	nr	nr
410–414, 429.2	Ischemic, coronary heart disease	7.9	5.1	210,100	176,300
410, 412	Acute, old myocardial infarction	4.2	1.7	68,800	56,700
411	Other acute, subacute forms of ischemic heart disease	nr	nr	nr	nr
413	Angina pectoris	3.3	3.2	nr	nr
414	Other forms of chronic ischemic heart disease	nr	nr	nr	nr
429.2	Cardiovascular disease, unspecified	nr	nr	nr	nr
415–417[b]	Diseases of pulmonary circulation	nr	nr	nr	nr
420–429	Other forms of heart disease (such as pericarditis, endocarditis, myocarditis, cardiomyopathy)	nr	nr	nr	nr
426–427	Arrhythmias	nr	nr	nr	nr
428	Heart failure	2.5	1.8	23,600	32,800
430–438[b]	Cerebrovascular disease (such as hemorrhage, occlusion, transient cerebral ischemia; includes mention of hypertension in ICD-401)	2.6	3.0	52,100	76,800
440–448[b]	Diseases of arteries, arterioles, capillaries	nr	nr	nr	nr

TABLE 12-1 Continued

ICD-9 Range	Diseases of Circulatory System	Prevalence (% of Americans 20 years old and older)		Mortality (number of deaths, all ages)	
		Men	Women	Men	Women
451–459	Diseases of veins, lymphatics, other diseases of circulatory system	nr	nr	nr	nr

NOTE: ICD, International Classification of Diseases; nr, not reported.
[a]For all ages.
[b]Gap in ICD-9 sequence follows.
SOURCE: AHA, 2012, pps. e6–e245.

than in people who do not have diabetes. That hyperinsulinemic state is a compensation for peripheral resistance and in many cases keeps glucose concentrations normal for years. Eventually, β-cell compensation becomes inadequate, and there is progression to overt diabetes with concomitant hyperglycemia. Why the β cells cease to produce sufficient insulin is not known.

Pathogenetic diversity and diagnostic uncertainty are among the important problems associated with epidemiologic study of diabetes mellitus. Multiple likely pathogenetic mechanisms lead to diabetes mellitus, which include diverse genetic susceptibilities (as varied as autoimmunity and obesity) and all sorts of potential environmental and behavioral factors (such as viruses, nutrition, and activity level). The multiplicity of contributing factors can lead to various responses to particular exposures. Because up to half of the cases of diabetes are undiagnosed, the potential for ascertainment bias in population-based surveys is high (more intensively-followed groups or those with more frequent health-care contact are more likely to get the diagnosis); this emphasizes the need for formal standardized testing (to detect undiagnosed cases) in epidemiologic studies.

Scientists have named a clustering of cardiovascular risk factors—including hypertension, hyperglycemia, high triglycerides, abdominal obesity, and low high-density lipoprotein—metabolic syndrome. Although it is not a disease entity itself, metabolic syndrome is associated with a fivefold increased risk of type 2 diabetes and a doubling of the risk of cardiovascular disease (Alberti et al., 2009). There is a growing literature on the association between the COIs and metabolic syndrome and its components. Given its strong linkage with type 2 diabetes, new literature that deals with metabolic syndrome as an outcome will be discussed primarily in this section.

Conclusions from *VAO* and Previous Updates

The committee responsible for *Veterans and Agent Orange: Health Effects of Herbicides Used in Vietnam* (*VAO*; IOM, 1994) concluded that there was inadequate or insufficient information to determine whether there is an association between exposure to the COIs and diabetes mellitus. Additional information available to the committees responsible for *Update 1996* (IOM, 1996) and *Update 1998* (IOM, 1999) did not change that conclusion.

In 1999, in response to a request from the Department of Veterans Affairs, the Institute of Medicine called together a committee to conduct an interim review of the scientific evidence regarding type 2 diabetes. That review focused on information published after the deliberations of the *Update 1998* committee and resulted in the report *Veterans and Agent Orange: Herbicide/Dioxin Exposure and Type 2 Diabetes* (*Type 2 Diabetes*; IOM, 2000). The committee responsible for that report determined that there was limited or suggestive evidence of an association between exposure to at least one COI and type 2 diabetes. The committees responsible for *Update 2000* (IOM, 2001), *Update 2002* (IOM, 2003), *Update 2004* (IOM, 2005), *Update 2006* (IOM, 2007), *Update 2008* (IOM, 2009), and *Update 2010* (IOM, 2012) upheld that finding. Reviews of the pertinent studies are found in the earlier reports. Table 12-2 presents a summary.

Update of the Epidemiologic Literature

Vietnam-Veteran Studies

No Vietnam-veteran studies addressing exposure to the COIs and diabetes have been published since *Update 2010*.

Occupational Studies

Ruder and Yiin (2011) reported the mortality experience of 2,122 workers involved in the production of 2,3,4,5,6-pentachlorophenol (PCP) at four plants in the United States through 2005. One-third of the cohort also worked in departments that used tricholorophenol (TCP) or its derivatives that were contaminated with TCCD. The mortality experience of the workers was compared with that of the US general population. Diabetes mortality was not higher in the 720 workers exposed to both PCP and TCP, among whom only 8 deaths were ascertained (standardized mortality ratio [SMR] = 1.14, 95% confidence interval [CI] 0.49–2.24).

Waggoner et al. (2011) reported that the risks of mortality from diabetes from 1993 to 2007 among both the applicators and spouses in the Agricultural Health Study (AHS) (without consideration of specific exposures) were significantly decreased in comparison to the general public. The AHS has been generating

TABLE 12-2 Selected Epidemiologic Studies—Diabetes and Related Health Outcomes (Shaded Entries Are New Information for This Update)

Study Population	Exposed Cases[a]	**Exposure of Interest**/Estimated Relative Risk (95% CI)[a]	Reference
VIETNAM VETERANS			
US Vietnam Veterans			
US Air Force Health Study—Ranch Hand veterans vs SEA veterans (unless otherwise noted)		**All COIs**	
AFHS—followup through 2004			Michalek and Pavuk, 2008
Calendar period in Vietnam			
During or before 1969	130	1.7 (p = 0.005)	
Background (serum TCDD ≤ 10 ppt)	39	1.3 (0.8–2.0)	
Low (10–91 ppt)	40	1.9 (1.2–2.9)	
High (> 91 ppt)	51	2.0 (1.3–3.1)	
After 1969	50	0.9 (p = 0.45)	
Spraying during tour			
≥ 90 days	170	1.3 (p = 0.04)	
Background (serum TCDD ≤ 10 ppt)	42	1.0 (0.7–1.4)	
Low (10–91 ppt)	60	1.5 (1.0–2.0)	
High (> 91 ppt)	68	1.6 (1.1–2.2)	
< 90 days	10	0.6 (p = 0.12)	
AFHS—Ranch Hand–comparison subject pairs—within-pair differences; lower Ranch Hand insulin sensitivity with greater TCDD levels			Kern et al., 2004
1997 examination (29 pairs)		(p = 0.01)	
2002 examination (71 pairs)		(p = 0.02)	
Air Force Ranch Hand veterans (n = 343)	92	ns	
AFHS—comparison veterans only, OR by quartiles of serum dioxin concentration			Longnecker and Michalek, 2000[b]
Quartile 1: < 2.8 ng/kg	26	1.0	
Quartile 2: 2.8– < 4.0 ng/kg	25	0.9 (0.5–1.7)	
Quartile 3: 4.0– < 5.2 ng/kg	57	1.8 (1.0–3.0)	
Quartile 4: ³ 5.2 ng/kg	61	1.6 (0.9–2.7)	
AFHS—through 1992 examination cycle Ranch Hand veterans—high-exposure group			Henriksen et al., 1997[b]
Glucose abnormalities	60	1.4 (1.1–1.8)	
Diabetes prevalence	57	1.5 (1.2–2.0)	
Use of oral medications for diabetes	19	2.3 (1.3–3.9)	
Serum insulin abnormalities	18	3.4 (1.9–6.1)	
US VA Cohort of Army Chemical Corps—Expanded as of 1997 to include all Army men with chemical MOS (2,872 deployed vs 2,737 nondeployed) serving during Vietnam era (7/1/1965–3/28/1973)		**All COIs**	
Incidence—Self-reported diabetes diagnosed by doctor			

continued

TABLE 12-2 Diabetes and Related Health Outcomes, continued

Study Population	Exposed Cases[a]	**Exposure of Interest**/Estimated Relative Risk (95% CI)[a]	Reference
CATI survey of stratified sample: 1,499 deployed (795 with TCDD measured) vs 1,428 nondeployed (102 with TCDD measured)			Kang et al., 2006
Deployed vs nondeployed	226	1.2 (0.9–1.5)	
Sprayed herbicides in Vietnam (n = 662) vs never (n = 811)	123	1.5 (1.1–2.0)	
Mortality—diabetes			
Through 2005			Cypel and Kang, 2010
Deployed veterans (2,872) vs nondeployed (2,737)	27	1.8 (0.7–4.4)	
ACC deployed men in Kang et al. (2006) reported sprayed herbicide vs did not spray	ns	2.2 (0.6–8.0)	
US CDC Vietnam Experience Study—Cross-sectional study, with medical examinations, of Army veterans: 9,324 deployed vs 8,989 nondeployed		**All COIs**	
Followup—deployed vs nondeployed			CDC, 1988
Interviewed—self-reported diabetes	155	1.2 (p > 0.05)	
Subset with physical examinations			
Self-reported diabetes	42	1.1 (p > 0.05)	
Fasting serum glucose		Geometric means 93.4 vs 92.4 mg/dl p < 0.05)	
International Vietnam-Veteran Studies			
Australian Vietnam Veterans—58,077 men and 153 women served on land or in Vietnamese waters during 5/23/1962–7/1/1973 vs Australian population		**All COIs**	
Incidence			
Validation study (expected number of exposed cases (95% CI)			
Men		*Cases expected*	CDVA, 1998a[b]
Self-report of doctor's diagnosis	2,391		
(proportion of respondents)	(6%)	1,780 (1,558–2,003)	
Women		*Cases expected*	CDVA, 1998b[b]
Self-report of doctor's diagnosis	5		
(proportion of respondents)	(2%)	10 (9–11)	
Mortality			
All branches, return–2001	55	0.5 (0.4–0.7)	ADVA, 2005b
Navy	12	0.5 (0.3–0.9)	
Army	37	0.5 (0.4–0.7)	
Air Force	6	0.5 (0.2–1.0)	

TABLE 12-2 Diabetes and Related Health Outcomes, continued

Study Population	Exposed Cases[a]	**Exposure of Interest**/Estimated Relative Risk (95% CI)[a]	Reference
1980–1994			CDVA, 1997a
Sample of 1,000 Male Australian Vietnam Veterans—prevalence		**All COIs**	
450 interviewed 2005–2006 vs respondents to 2004–2005 national survey	55	1.0 (0.8–1.3)	O'Toole et al., 2009
641 interviewed 1990–1993 vs respondents to 1989–1990 national survey (self-report of doctor diagnosis)	12	1.6 (0.4–2.7)	O'Toole et al., 1996
Australian Conscripted Army National Service (18,940 deployed vs 24,642 nondeployed)		**All COIs**	
Mortality 1966–2001	6	0.3 (0.1–0.7)	ADVA, 2005c
Korean Vietnam Veterans		**All COIs**	
Korean veterans of Vietnam era: 1,224 deployed vs 154 nondeployed—incidence	154	2.7 (1.1–6.7)	Kim JS et al., 2003
OCCUPATIONAL—INDUSTRIAL			
IARC Phenoxy Herbicide Cohort—Workers exposed to any phenoxy herbicide or chlorophenol (production or spraying) vs respective national mortality rates			
Diabetes—mortality	33	2.3 (0.5–9.5)	Vena et al., 1998
German Production Workers at BASF Ludwigshafen Plant (680 men working > 1 mo in 1957–1987) (in IARC cohort as of 1997) and women—no results		**Dioxins; 2,4-D; 2,4,5-T; MCPA; MCPP; 2,4-DP**	
BASF Cleanup Workers from 1953 accident (n = 247); 114 with chloracne, 13 more with erythema; serum TCDD levels (*not* part of IARC)		**Focus on TCDD**	
Incidence			
BASF workers potentially exposed to TCDD following an accident involving trichlorophenol		p = 0.06	Ott et al., 1994
Through 1989 (n = 158 men exposed within 1 yr of accident vs 161 other BASF employees 1953–1969)	10	0.5 (0.2–1.0)	Zober et al., 1994
New Zealand Phenoxy Herbicide Production Workers and Sprayers (1,599 men and women working any time in 1969–1988 at Dow plant in New Plymouth) (in IARC cohort)		**Dioxins; 2,4-D; 2,4,5-T; MCPA; MCPB; 2,4,5-TCP; Picloram**	

continued

TABLE 12-2 Diabetes and Related Health Outcomes, continued

Study Population	Exposed Cases[a]	**Exposure of Interest**/Estimated Relative Risk (95% CI)[a]	Reference
Mortality 1969–2004			McBride et al., 2009
TCP production workers			
(Preliminary) NIOSH Cross-Sectional Medical Study		**Dioxin/phenoxy herbicides**	
Workers exposed to 2,4,5-T, derivatives			Calvert et al., 1999[b]
Serum TCDD pg/g of liquid			
< 20	7	2.1 (0.8–5.8)	
20–75	6	1.5 (0.5–4.3)	
75–238	3	0.7 (0.2–2.6)	
238–3,400	10	2.0 (0.8–4.9)	
Dioxin-exposed workers in two chemical plants		1.1, p = < 0.003	Sweeney et al., 1997/98
NIOSH/Ranch Hand Comparison—Ranch Hand veterans, workers exposed to TCDD-contaminated products compared with nonexposed comparison cohorts		**Dioxin/phenoxy herbicides**	
Ranch Hands	147	1.2 (0.9–1.5)	Steenland et al., 2001
Workers	28	1.2 (0.7–2.3)	
NIOSH Mortality Cohort (12 US plants, 5,172 male production and maintenance workers 1942–1984) (included in IARC cohort as of 1997)		**Dioxins, phenoxy herbicides**	
Highly-exposed industrial cohort (n = 5,132)			Steenland et al., 1999[b]
Diabetes as underlying cause	26	1.2 (0.8–1.7)	
Diabetes among multiple causes	89	1.1 (0.9–1.3)	
Chloracne subcohort (n = 608)	4	1.1 (0.3–2.7)	
Dioxin-exposed workers—mortality[c]			Steenland et al., 1992[b]
Diabetes as underlying cause	16	1.1 (0.6–1.8)	
Diabetes among multiple causes	58	1.1 (0.8–1.4)	Sweeney et al., 1992
NIOSH production workers	26	1.6 (0.9–3.0)	
Monsanto Plant—Nitro, WV		**Dioxin/phenoxy herbicides**	
2.4.5-T, TCP production workers with chloracne	22	2.3 (1.1–4.8)	
All Dow TCP-Exposed Workers (TCP production 1942–1979 or 2,4,5-T production 1948–1982 in Midland, Michigan) (in IARC and NIOSH cohorts)		**2,4,5-T; 2,4,5-TCP**	
1942–2003 (n = 1,615)	16	1.1 (0.6–1.8)	Collins et al., 2009a
1940–1982 (n = 2,187 men)	4	0.7 (0.2–1.9)	Cook et al., 1987

TABLE 12-2 Diabetes and Related Health Outcomes, continued

Study Population	Exposed Cases[a]	**Exposure of Interest**/Estimated Relative Risk (95% CI)[a]	Reference
All Dow PCP-Exposed Workers—all workers from the two plants that only made PCP (in Tacoma, Washington, and Wichita, Kansas) and workers who made PCP and TCP at two additional plants (in Midland, Michigan, and Sauget, Illinios)		**2,4,5-T; 2,4,5-TCP**	Ruder and Yiin, 2011
1940–2005 (n = 2,122)	18	0.8 (0.5–1.2)	
PCP and TCP (n = 720)	8	1.1 (0.5–2.2)	
PCP (no TCP) (n = 1,402)	10	0.6 (0.3–1.2)	
Dow PCP Production Workers (1937–1989 in Midland, Michigan) (*not* in IARC and NIOSH cohorts)		**Low chlorinated dioxins; 2,4-D**	
Mortality 1940–2004 (n = 577, excluding 196 also having exposure to TCP)	8	1.1 (0.5–2.2)	Collins et al., 2009b
Mortality 1940–1989 (n = 770)	4	1.2 (0.3–3.0)	Ramlow et al., 1996
Other Studies of Industrial Workers (*not* related to IARC or NIOSH phenoxy cohorts)			
Czechoslovakia Production Workers—Production workers admitted to hospital in Prague	11	**2,4,5-T, TCP** nr	Pazderova-Vejlupkova et al., 1981
German Production Workers—West German chemical-production workers		**Dioxin, phenoxy herbicides**	Von Benner et al., 1994
	nr	nr	
Japanese Waste-Incinerator Workers—Workers exposed to PCDD at municipal waste incinerator		**Dioxin, phenoxy herbicides**	Kitamura et al., 2000
	8	nr, but ns	
United Kingdom Production Workers—TCP production workers		**Dioxin, phenoxy herbicides**	May, 1982
	2	nr	
OCCUPATIONAL—PAPER AND PULP WORKERS		**TCDD**	
New Hampshire pulp and paper workers, 883 white men working ≥ 1 yr, mortality through July 1985	9	1.4 (0.7–2.7)	Henneberger et al., 1989
OCCUPATIONAL—HERBICIDE-USING WORKERS (*not* related to IARC sprayer cohorts)			
UNITED STATES			
US Agricultural Health Study—prospective study of licensed pesticide sprayers in Iowa and North Carolina: commercial (n = 4,916 men), private/farmers (n = 52,395, 97.4% men), and spouses of private sprayers (n = 32,347, 0.007% men), enrolled 1993–1997; followups with CATIs 1999–2003 and 2005–2010		**Phenoxy herbicides**	

continued

TABLE 12-2 Diabetes and Related Health Outcomes, continued

Study Population	Exposed Cases[a]	**Exposure of Interest**/Estimated Relative Risk (95% CI)[a]	Reference
Incidence			
Self-reported incidence diabetes (1999–2003) in licensed applicators			Montgomery et al., 2008
2,4-D	73	0.9 (0.8–1.1)	
2,4,5-T	28	1.0 (0.9–1.2)	
Self-reported gestational diabetes in wives of licensed applicators			Saldana et al., 2007
Documented exposure during 1st trimester		*ORs read from graph*	
2,4-D	10	~1.0 (ns)	
2,4,5-T	3	~5 ($p < 0.05$)	
2,4,5-TP	2	~7 ($p < 0.05$)	
Dicamba	7	~3 ($p \sim 0.06$)	
Mortality			
Enrollment through 2007, vs state rates			Waggoner et al., 2011
Applicators (n = 1,641)	98	0.5 (0.3–0.5)	
Spouses (n = 676)	42	0.4 (0.3–0.6)	
Enrollment through 2000, vs state rates			Blair et al., 2005
Private applicators (men and women)	26	0.3 (0.2–0.5)	
Spouses of private applicators (> 99% women)	18	0.6 (0.4–1.0)	
ENVIRONMENTAL			
Seveso, Italy, Residential Cohort—Industrial accident July 10, 1976 (723 residents Zone A; 4,821 Zone B; 31,643 Zone R; 181,574 local reference group) (ICD-9 171)		**TCDD**	
Incidence			
Children residing in Seveso at time of incident—development of diabetes			Baccarelli et al., 2005b
101 with chloracne	1	nr	
211 without chloracne	2	nr	
Mortality			
25-yr followup to 2001—men and women			Consonni et al., 2008
Zone A	3	1.0 (0.3–3.1)	
Zone B	26	1.3 (0.9–1.9)	
Zone R	192	1.3 (1.1–1.5)	
20-yr followup to 1996			Bertazzi et al., 2001
Zones A and B—men	6	0.8 (0.3–1.7)	
Zones A and B—women	20	1.7 (0.1–2.7)	
15-yr followup to 1991—men			Bertazzi et al., 1998[b]
Zone B	6	1.2 (0.5–2.7)	
15-yr followup to 1991—women			Bertazzi et al., 1998[b]
Zone A	2	1.8 (0.4–7.0)	
Zone B	13	1.8 (1.0–3.0)	

TABLE 12-2 Diabetes and Related Health Outcomes, continued

Study Population	Exposed Cases[a]	**Exposure of Interest**/Estimated Relative Risk (95% CI)[a]	Reference
15-yr followup to 1991			Pesatori et al., 1998[b]
Zone R men	37	1.1 (0.8–1.6)	
Zone R women	74	1.2 (1.0–1.6)	
National Health and Nutrition Examination Survey		**Dioxin, dl PCBs**	
NHANES 1999–2002 participants			Everett et al., 2007
Total diabetes (self-report or HbA1c > 6.1%)			
HxCDD (TEF = 0.1)			
> 42.0–99.1 pg/g		1.8 (1.1–2.8)	
> 99.1 pg/g		2.0 (0.9–4.4)	
PCB 126 (TEF = 0.1)			
> 31.3–83.8 pg/g		1.7 (1.0–2.7)	
> 83.8 pg/g		3.7 (2.1–6.5)	
NHANES 1999–2002 participants			Lee et al., 2006
HpCDD > 90th percentile vs nondetectable	46	2.7 (1.3–5.5)	
OCDD > 90th percentile vs nondetectable	31	2.1 (0.9–5.2)	
Anniston (AL) Community Health Survey—774 residents of Anniston, Alabama, an area with high level of PCBs		**PCBs**	
Association between diabetes and PCB levels in serum	202		Silverstone et al., 2012
Dioxin TEQs		1.2 (0.9–2.0)	
Prospective Investigation of the Vasculature in Uppsala Seniors (PIVUS)—Prospective (cross-sectional) study of residents (≥ 70 yrs of age) living in Uppsala, Sweden, between April 2001 and June 2004 (n = 989; 725 in diabetes analysis)		**Polychlorinated biphenyls, PCBs**	
Risk elevations compared to the lowest exposure quintiles:			Lee et al., 2011b
Second quintile, PCB 105		5.2 (1.3–84.4)	
Fourth quintile, PCB 118		10.7 (1.1–25.5)	
Fourth quintile, PCB 157		3.5 (1.0–12.4)	
Third quintile, PCB 189		3.5 (1.0–11.9)	
Coronary Artery Risk Development in Young Adults (CARDIA) Study		**Pesticides, PCBs**	
Nested case-control study within CARDIA study, relationship between persistent organic pollutants and type 2 diabetes (nested cases = 90 of 116 study participants who provided blood samples in 1987/88 exam and later developed diabetes)			Lee et al., 2010
Quartile 1 of PCB 156 (model 2, adjusted)		Referent	
Quartile 2		1.3 (0.5–3.5)	
Quartile 3		0.9 (0.3–2.6)	
Quartile 4		0.8 (0.2–2.9)	

continued

TABLE 12-2 Diabetes and Related Health Outcomes, continued

Study Population	Exposed Cases[a]	**Exposure of Interest**/Estimated Relative Risk (95% CI)[a]	Reference
Quartile 1 of PCB 157 (model 2, adjusted)		Referent	
Quartile 2		1.0 (0.4–2.5)	
Quartile 3		0.5 (0.2–1.5)	
Quartile 4		0.5 (0.1–1.7)	
Quartile 1 of PCB 167 (model 2, adjusted)		Referent	
Quartile 2		0.9 (0.4–2.2)	
Quartile 3		1.0 (0.4–2.5)	
Quartile 4		0.5 (0.2–1.3)	
Other Environmental Studies			
BELGIUM			
Belgium residents (142 women, 115 men) exposed to dioxin, PCBs		**Dioxin, PCBs**	Fierens et al., 2003
Subjects in top decile for dioxin		5.1 (1.2–21.7)	
CANADA			
Population-based survey in Saskatchewan		**Herbicides**	Masley et al., 2000
	28	nr	
FINLAND			
Finnish fishermen (n = 6,410) and spouses (n = 4,260) registered between 1980 and 2002 compared to national statistics		**Serum dioxin**	Turunen et al., 2008
Fishermen	5	0.7 (0.1–1.0)	
Spouses	5	0.8 (0.3–1.9)	
GREENLAND			
Survey of Greenland Inuit—cross-sectional study		**dl PCBs**	Jørgensen et al., 2008
Quartile of dl PCBs (compared to Quartile 1)		*Adjusted prevalence OR*	
Quartile 2		1.6 (0.6–4.1)	
Quartile 3		1.9 (0.7–5.1)	
Quartile 4		1.2 (0.4–3.2)	
JAPAN			
Association between PCB congener levels and definite diabetes in participants in the Saku Control Obesity Program (n = 15)		**PCBs**	Tanaka et al., 2011
PCB 118 and definite diabetes (total lipids)		1.0 (0.9–1.1)	
PCB 156 and definite diabetes (total lipids)		1.5 (0.9–2.7)	
Total dioxin (pg TEQ/g lipid)		**Dioxin**	Uemura et al., 2008
≥ 20.00–31.00	17	2.1 (0.9–5.4)	
≥ 31.00	39	3.8 (1.6–10.1)	

TABLE 12-2 Diabetes and Related Health Outcomes, continued

Study Population	Exposed Cases[a]	**Exposure of Interest**/Estimated Relative Risk (95% CI)[a]	Reference
TAIWAN		**Dioxin, phenoxy herbicides**	
Residents around 12 municipal waste incinerators—prevalence of physician-diagnosed diabetes with TEQs for serum PCDD/Fs in logistic model adjusted for age, sex, smoking, BMI	29	2.4 (0.2–31.9)	Chen et al., 2006
UNITED STATES		**dl PCBs**	
Great Lakes sport fish consumers—cross-sectional study		*Adjusted prevalence OR*	
Sum of dl-PCBs			
< limit of detection		Reference	
0.2–0.3 ng/g lipid		1.2	
0.3–1.6 ng/g lipid		2.1 ($p < 0.05$) p-trend = 0.03	
Vertac/Hercules Superfund site residents (n = 62)—OR for high insulin in nondiabetic subjects at various times, levels for TCDD > 15 ppt compared with persons with TCDD < 15 ppt		**TCDD**	Cranmer et al., 2000[b]
Fasting (insulin > 4.5 μIU/mL)	3	8.5 (1.5–49.4)	
30-min (insulin > 177 μIU/mL)	3	7.0 (1.3–39.0)	
60-min (insulin > 228 μIU/mL)	4	12 (2.2–70.1)	
120-min (insulin > 97.7 μIU/mL)	6	56 (5.7–556)	

NOTE: 2,4-D, 2,4-dichlorophenoxyacetic acid; 2,4-DP, 2,4-dichlorophenoxypropanoic acid; 2,4,5-T, 2,4,5-trichlorophenoxyacetic acid; 2,4,5-TCP, 2,4,5-trichlorophenol; 2,4,5-TP, 2-(2,4,5-trichlorophenoxy) propionic acid; ACC, Army Chemical Corps; AFHS, Air Force Health Study; BMI, body-mass index; CARDIA, Coronary Artery Risk Development in Young Adults; CATI, computer-assisted telephone interviewing; CDC, Centers for Disease Control and Prevention; CI, confidence interval; COI, chemical of interest; dl, dioxin-like; HbA1c, hemoglobin A1c; HpCDD, 1,2,3,4,6,7,8-heptachlorodibenzo-*p*-dioxin; HxCDD, 1,2,3,6,7,9-hexachlorodibenzo-*p*-dioxin; IARC, International Agency for Research on Cancer; ICD, *International Classification of Diseases*; IU, international unit; MCPA, 2 methyl-4-chlorophenoxyacetic acid; MCPB, 4-(4-chloro-2-methylphenoxy)butanoic acid; MCPP, methylchlorophenoxypropionic acid; MOS, military occupational specialty; NHANES, National Health and Nutrition Examination Survey; NIOSH, National Institute for Occupational Safety and Health; nr, not reported; ns, not significant; OCDD, 1,2,3,4,6,7,8,9-octachlorodibenzo-*p*-dioxin; OR, odds ratio; PCB, polychlorinated biphenyl; PCDD, polychlorinated dibenzo-*p*-dioxin; PCDD/Fs, chlorinated dioxins and furans combined; PCP, pentachlorophenol; PIVUS, Prospective Investigation of the Vasculature in Uppsala Seniors; ppt, parts per trillion; SEA, Southeast Asia; TCDD, 2,3,7,8-tetrachlorodibenzo-*p*-dioxin; TCDF, tetrachlorodibenzofuran; TCP, trichlorophenol; TEF, toxicity equivalency factor; TEQ, (total) toxic equivalent; VA, US Department of Veterans Affairs.

[a]Given when available; results other than estimated risk explained individually.

[b]Study is discussed in greater detail in *Veterans and Agent Orange: Herbicide/Dioxin Exposure and Type 2 Diabetes* (IOM, 2000).

[c]Includes some subjects covered in other references cited in the category occupational cohorts.

valuable information on the COIs for a number of years, but these results, like those in Alavanja et al. (2005) and Blair et al. (2005), are not herbicide-specific and so are not regarded as being fully informative for the committee's task.

Boers et al. (2012) reported an updated mortality analysis of workers exposed to TCDD at two Dutch chlorophenoxy-herbicide production facilities. The analysis did not distinguish diabetes deaths within the category "disease of endocrine system and blood."

Environmental Studies

Lee et al. (2010) reported the results of a nested case-control study within the Coronary Artery Risk Development in Young Adults (CARDIA) cohort study that looked for a relationship between several persistent organic pollutants (POPs) and type 2 diabetes. The investigators identified 116 CARDIA participants who were free of diabetes when they provided a blood sample in the 1987–1988 examination but developed diabetes during the next 18 years. Of the 116, 90 cases were randomly selected for further analysis. Controls (90) were randomly selected from all participants who had a fasting glucose concentration below 100 mg/dL at all CARDIA examinations in which glucose was measured. After adjustment for age, race, sex, and body-mass index (BMI), none of the three measured PCBs that had dioxin-like activity (mono-ortho PCBs 156, 157, and 167) was associated with incident diabetes.

Lee et al. (2011b) studied the association between plasma concentrations of PCBs and the development of type 2 diabetes in participants in the Prospective Investigation of the Vasculature in Uppsala Seniors (PIVUS). PIVUS participants were residents of Uppsala, Sweden, who were 70 years old in the period April 2001–June 2004. Of the 2,205 selected, 1,106 chose to participate in the baseline examination. The final analytic sample included 989 participants for the cross-sectional baseline analyses: 112 who had type 2 diabetes at baseline, 152 who were not available at followup 5 years later, and 725 who participated in the analysis of diabetes incidence. On the basis of either a high fasting plasma glucose concentration or the use of hypoglycemic medication, 36 incident cases were ascertained. In addition to 3 lipophilic organochlorine pesticides, 14 PCBs were measured, including 5 dioxin-like, mono-ortho PCBs (PCBs 105, 118, 156, 157, and 189). Estimates of the relative risk of diabetes associated with exposure were adjusted for various risk factors: BMI, exercise, alcohol consumption, triglyceride and total cholesterol concentrations, cigarette-smoking, and sex. For the total concentration of all 14 PCBs, the diabetes risks for the top three quintiles were significantly elevated compared with that of the lowest quintile, and there was a strongly significant increasing trend in risk with rising quintile ($p \leq 0.001$). Every measured PCB was associated with elevated diabetes risk comparing high to low quintiles. For the 5 dioxin-like, mono-ortho PCBs, the highest quintile odds ratios (ORs) ranged from 2.6 to 8.0, but none of their risk elevations compared to the lowest exposure quintiles was statistically significant with the exceptions of the second quintile for PCB 105 (adjusted OR = 10.7, 95% CI 1.3–84.4), the third quintile for PCB 189 (adjusted OR = 3.5, 95% CI 1.0–11.9), and the fourth quintile for PCB 118 (adjusted OR = 5.2, 95% CI 1.1–25.5), PCB 157 (adjusted OR = 3.5, 95% CI 1.0–12.4); also, none of their tests for a linear trend was statistically significant. For the 9 PCBs without dioxin-like activity, however, there were 16 significant results for paired comparisons with the lowest quintile and four modestly significant dose–responses, so the mono-ortho dioxin-like PCBs do not appear to be driving the overall observed association with diabetes risk.

Anniston, Alabama, is a location with substantial environmental PCB contamination. Silverstone et al. (2012) gathered survey results from 1,110 participants recruited from a targeted sample of 1,823 households in the community (61% participation); 774 of them (70%) also had clinical examinations. Diabetes (202 cases) was defined on the basis of a physician diagnosis of diabetes or a fasting glucose concentration greater than 125 mg/dL. Concentrations of 35 PCBs were measured. Analyses by logistic regression adjusted for BMI, family history, age, ethnicity, sex, education, marital status, and duration of residence in Anniston and excluded 171 individuals with prediabetes. The total PCB burden was associated with increased diabetes prevalence (OR per standard deviation increase in blood concentrations = 1.23, 95% CI 0.88–1.72). The prevalence of diabetes also increased with increasing TEQs based only on mono-ortho PCBs (OR per standard deviation increase in blood concentrations = 1.20, 95% CI 0.87–2.02). Neither increase was significant, and they were of similar magnitude.

The association between prevalent diabetes and PCB burden was also assessed in the Saku Control Obesity Program (Tanaka et al., 2011). Subjects were 235 participants in an obesity-treatment trial. Diabetes was determined on the basis of blood measures or a prescription for a hypoglycemic medication. Fifteen participants had definite diabetes. There were no statistically-significant associations between the two dioxin-like mono-ortho PCBs measured (PCBs 118 and 156) and diabetes prevalence.

Case-Control Studies

No case-control studies of exposure to the COIs and type 2 diabetes have been published since *Update 2010*.

Other Reviewed Studies That Address Metabolic Syndrome and Risk Factors for Diabetes

Chang et al. (2010b, 2011a) report findings from a cross-sectional sample of Taiwanese living in an area with a high level of industrial contamination updating and extending an earlier report that was discussed in *Update 2010* (Chang et al., 2010a). The updated report extended the survey period for an additional 7 months

(July 2005–December 2007), increasing from 1,478 to 1,812 the number of area residents who were surveyed and from whom blood was collected and analyzed for dioxins, furans, and mercury. Metabolic syndrome and its components were examined in 1,490 non-diabetic residents (Chang et al., 2010b). The prevalence of metabolic syndrome increased steeply and monotonically with dioxin TEQs based on congener analysis of polychlorinated dibenzo-*p*-dioxins (PCDDs) and polychlorinated dibenzofurans (PCDFs). For those in the 90th percentile of TEQs (≥ 62.2 pg/g lipid), the prevalence of metabolic syndrome was about 37%, compared with less than 5% for those in the 10th percentile. The odds of having metabolic syndrome in the highest TEQ quintile were 2.3-fold higher than in the lowest quintile (95% CI 1.3–3.9) after adjustment for age, sex, smoking, alcohol use, obesity, and family history of diabetes or hypertension. Of the metabolic syndrome components, dioxin TEQ was most strongly related to diastolic blood pressure, fasting glucose, and waist circumference. There were strong associations between most individual congeners concentrations and metabolic syndrome prevalence; TCDD, 2,3,4,7,8-pentachlorodibenzofuran, and 1,2,3,6,7,8-hexachlorodibenzofuran showed the strongest associations. This population was also coexposed to environmental mercury, which was explored in a subsequent paper on a subset of this study population (n = 1,449). Chang et al. (2011a) showed that TEQs, based on congener analysis of PCDDs and PCDFs, were strongly associated with insulin resistance, but not defective pancreatic β-cell function, for which the results was independent of mercury exposure.

Chang et al. (2012) surveyed 156 employees 50 years old or older from a closed Taiwanese plant that had manufactured sodium pentachlorophenol (Na-PCP). The process had involved very high exposure to COIs for the committee. Clinical-chemistry values of the workers were compared with those of residents of similar ages in the general population. It should be noted that the workers lived in the community mentioned in the preceding paragraph that was exposed to dioxin through the accidental release of Na-PCP. Previous employment at the plant was associated with much higher concentrations of dioxin-like PCDDs and PCDFs (109.6 ± 94.5 pg/g of lipid) than the general population (22.9 ± 10.0). After adjustment for age, sex, smoking, and drinking, the employees had high odds of having increased glucose concentrations (> 100 mg/dL, OR = 7.22, 95% CI 4.04–12.90); and high odds of having increased triglyceride concentrations (> 150 mg/dL, OR = 4.31, 95% CI 2.57–7.22). There was not an increased prevalence of elevated serum cholesterol (≥ 200 mg/dL, OR = 0.95, 95% CI 0.64–1.41).

Obesity is a strong risk factor for diabetes. Rönn et al. (2011) examined the cross-sectional relationship between POPs and fat mass determined by dual-energy X-ray absorptiometry in 890 participants in the PIVUS study. They calculated the differences in total fat mass among categories of PCB exposure and adjusted for sex, height, lean mass, smoking, exercise habits, education, daily energy intake, and alcohol consumption. Of the 16 PCBs measured, 7 were dioxin-like; 2 were not mono-ortho (PCBs 126 and 169) with higher dioxin-equivalency factors (TEFs) than the mono-ortho PCBs (PCBs 105, 118, 156, 157, and 189). Fat mass was 0.672 kg lower for each log-unit increase in circulating dioxin-like PCB 126 ($p = 0.003$) and 3.4 kg lower for each log-unit increase in circulating dioxin-like PCB 169 ($p = 0.0001$). Those in the highest quintile of PCB 126 and PCB 169 exposure had 2.2 and 6.9 kg less fat mass, respectively, than those in the lowest quintile. Although dioxin-like mono-ortho PCBs 126, 156, 157, and 189 also showed strong inverse associations with fat mass, paradoxically, two other dioxin-like mono-ortho PCBs, 105 and 118, showed strong positive associations with fat mass. Further, non-dioxin-like PCBs also showed strong inverse associations (such as PCBs 116, 138, 170, 180, 206, and 209). When all congeners were modeled simultaneously, the dioxin-like mono-ortho PCB 118, non-dioxin-like PCB 138, and octachlorobenzene-*p*-dioxin (OCDD) were positively associated with fat mass, and non-dioxin-like PCB 180 was inversely associated with fat mass. A significant sex interaction was detected for several of the associations with both dioxin-like mono-ortho PCBs and non-dioxin-like PCBs. The directions of the associations were similar in men and women but much stronger in the women.

The PIVUS study investigators also examined the association between organic pollutants and abdominal obesity (Lee et al., 2012a), which is more strongly linked to diabetes and cardiovascular disease risk than is overall adiposity. Abdominal obesity was defined as a waist circumference greater than 102 cm in men or greater than 88 cm in women. The study examined both the cross-sectional and longitudinal associations between waist circumference and the analyzed pollutants. At baseline, plasma concentrations of dioxin-like PCB 126 (the measured chemical with the highest dioxin-equivalent activity) were associated with a significantly higher prevalence of abdominal obesity in men. Some other dioxin-like mono-ortho PCBs (105 and 118) were also associated with abdominal obesity, but other mono-ortho PCBs (156, 157, and 189) were not, nor was OCDD. In both men and women, it appeared that the association depended on the number of chlorine atoms on the molecules regardless of dioxin activity.

Lee et al. (2011a) examined the associations between blood concentrations of POPs and the trajectories of change in obesity, dyslipidemia, and insulin resistance in the 90 controls who were selected for the CARDIA diabetes analysis discussed above. The study participants were young adults (mean age, 27.2 years) at the time of exposure assessment during the study's year-2 examination. Metabolic measures were reassessed in the year-20 examination. The paper reports the year-20 values by quintile of each pollutant adjusted for age, sex, race, baseline value of the measure, triglycerides, and total cholesterol at year 2. The measured congeners that had dioxin-like activity were mono-ortho PCBs 105, 118, 156, 157, and 167. Of those, PCB 156 concentration was associated with significantly lower BMI at year 20 (p for linear trend = 0.02). The mean BMI of those who had the highest PCB 156 concentrations was 29.7; it was 34.3 in those who had the lowest concentrations. No significant associations were seen with year-20 plasma triglyceride, high-density lipoprotein (HDL) cholesterol, low-density lipoprotein (LDL) cholesterol levels, or HOMA-IR (an index of insulin resistance).

Biologic Plausibility

Several biologic mechanisms that have been studied in cell culture and animal models may explain the potential diabetogenic effects of TCDD in humans. TCDD is known to modify expression of genes related to insulin transport and signaling and to inflammation (Kim MJ et al., 2012). The present committee's literature review included two new studies that increased mechanistic biologic plausibility. Wang et al. (2011) found that mice that lacked the aryl hydrocarbon receptor (AHR) (AHR knockouts) had enhanced insulin sensitivity and glucose tolerance; this suggested that the AHR has a physiologic function in glucose metabolism and supported the speculation that sustained activation of the AHR by dioxin-like chemicals could contribute to diabetes. That would be consistent with results of a previous study by Kurita et al. (2009), who found that exposure of mice to dioxin significantly reduced insulin secretion after a glucose challenge. In an in vitro study of differentiated adipocytes, TCDD significantly reduced insulin-stimulated glucose uptake (Hsu et al., 2010). Thus, mechanisms associated with insulin signaling and glucose uptake may contribute to the diabetogenic effects of TCDD observed in humans.

Synthesis

The new epidemiologic evidence on diabetes reviewed in this update includes followup on three occupationally-exposed study populations and several new studies of environmental exposure. The studies of Boers et al. (2012), Ruder and Yiin (2011), and Waggoner et al. (2011) all analyzed the mortality experience of workers. Diabetes mortality is not a useful endpoint because complications of diabetes, rather than diabetes itself, are most often listed as the cause of death of those who have the disease, so most cases of diabetes would be missed if mortality data were used. In addition, the workers are compared with the US population, which is likely to have a worse mortality experience than the workers studied because workers had to have some level of health to be employed.

The retrospective comparisons of Korean Vietnam-era veterans with acute coronary syndrome on the basis of whether they did or did not service in Vietnam (Kim JB et al., 2012) are not helpful in assessing whether herbicide exposure played a role in the development of diabetes. Two new informative prospective epidemiologic studies of exposure to some COIs and incident diabetes appeared since the last update (Lee et al., 2010, 2011b). The prospective design is helpful because it ensures that an exposure to a chemical occurred before disease onset, a requirement for any causal relationship. That is an important consideration for exposures that are measured in blood, in that the disease process or the treatment of the disease may affect the magnitude of the exposure, and the measured value might not represent an exposure before disease onset. Both studies were able to include many potential confounding variables, such as obesity and physical activity, and this helps to reduce the risk of bias. In spite of those strengths, both studies are difficult to interpret with respect to exposures of Vietnam veterans. In the CARDIA study (Lee et al., 2010), the investigators measured only three mono-ortho PCBs, and they had only weak dioxin-like activity. In addition, the exposures were small. Thus, the putative dioxin burden would be expected to be much lower than that of veterans, and the lack of association might be due to an insufficient dose. The PIVUS investigators (Lee et al., 2011b) measured many more COIs, but the exposures were also small. Only 36 new cases were ascertained, so the results are imprecise. Nevertheless, there was an association between the highest concentrations of the chemicals and diabetes risk. The results were not specific for pollutants that had dioxin activity, and many PCBs that lack dioxin activity were also found to be associated with diabetes risk. Although the positive association is consistent with an association between dioxin and diabetes onset, the lack of exposure specificity implies that the basis of the association might not be related to a dioxin-specific pathway.

In addition to those prospective studies, two surveys were considered. One included residents of a community in Alabama that had substantial environmental contamination. Some evidence suggested a higher prevalence of diabetes in residents that had increased dioxin TEQs, but the association was not specific for PCBs that had dioxin-like activity. In addition, the participation rate of sampled persons was only 61%, so selection bias introduced by differential nonparticipation cannot be ruled out. The other survey was based on a convenience sample of residents of Saku, Japan, who were enrolled in the obesity-control program. The small number of cases (15) and the small number of relevant compounds (mono-ortho PCBs 118 and 156) prevent definitive interpretation.

Several studies looked at COIs and risk factors for diabetes. The PIVUS investigators related PCBs and OCDD to both total fat mass and abdominal obesity. The cross-sectional results suggest that, if anything, blood concentrations of PCB 126 and PCB 169 with the highest level of dioxin-like activity were associated with lower levels of obesity, although OCDD with no dioxin activity also was associated with increased body fat. The relationship between PCBs and abdominal obesity seemed to involve the number of chlorine atoms in the molecule rather than any dioxin-like activity. Lee et al. (2011a) looked at the 20-year changes in diabetes-related risk factors in the 90 CARDIA participants selected as controls for their nested case-control study of diabetes. Only mono-ortho PCB 156 was associated with BMI over the 20 years; those who had higher PCB 156 concentrations at baseline had lower BMIs 20 years later. Measures of glucose homeostasis over 20 years were unrelated to PCB concentrations at baseline. Again, the studies involved populations that had low absolute exposure, and their results suggest nonspecific effects based on chemical attributes other than dioxin-like activity.

Chang et al. (2010b, 2011a) showed that in Taiwanese who lived in a heavily-contaminated area there was a strong association between TEQs based on PCDDs and PCDFs and the prevalence of metabolic syndrome and insulin resistance, strong risk factors for diabetes. Chang et al. (2012) also showed that workers in the plant making the pesticide had higher fasting glucose concentrations than the general population. Those reports are of interest because of the high exposures to TCDD and related chemicals that had very strong dioxin activities. The studies also adjusted for many relevant risk factors. The strong associations support a link between exposure to the COIs and diabetes. Nevertheless, the cross-sectional design limits the strength of conclusions that can be drawn.

In the aggregate, the newly added studies support prior VAO committees' inclusion of diabetes in the limited and suggestive category. The negative studies either examined suboptimal endpoints or were conducted in populations that had very low exposure to relevant chemicals. The new study from the PIVUS cohort does show an association with dioxin-like compounds, but the association was not specific to compounds that have dioxin-like properties. Its interpretation is further limited by the small number of cases, which impedes the ability to explore exposure specificity. The survey of a highly-exposed Taiwanese population shows a strong association with the diabetes risk factor metabolic syndrome. However, because of its cross-sectional design, it is not possible to prove that the exposure to the putative cause preceded the onset of the outcome.

Conclusion

On the basis of the evidence reviewed here and in previous VAO reports, the committee reaffirms its conclusion that there is limited or suggestive evidence of an association between exposure to at least one COIs and diabetes.

CIRCULATORY DISORDERS

This section covers a variety of conditions encompassed by the 9th revision of the *International Classification of Diseases, Ninth Revision* (ICD-9), codes 390–459, such as acute and chronic rheumatic fever (ICD-9 390–398), hypertension (ICD-9 401–404), ischemic heart disease (IHD; ICD-9 410–414), heart failure (ICD-9 428), cerebrovascular disease (ICD-9 430–438), and peripheral vascular disease (ICD-9 443). *Coronary heart disease* is related specifically to atherosclerosis; *ischemic heart disease* is broader and typically includes atherosclerosis and its symptoms. The American Heart Association reports mortality related to coronary heart disease, not to its symptoms, which include angina and myocardial infarction (MI). Table 12-1 contains estimates of prevalence of and mortality from individual disorders of the circulatory system in the US population in 2009.

Circulatory diseases are a group of diverse conditions, of which hypertension, coronary heart disease, and stroke are the most prevalent and account for 75% of deaths from circulatory diseases in the United States. In addition to family history, the major risk factors for circulatory diseases include age, race, smoking, serum cholesterol, BMI or percentage of body fat, and diabetes. Ideally, epidemiologic investigations of circulatory diseases would consider the conditions in this category separately rather than together because they have different patterns of occurrence, and many have different etiologies. However, many mortality studies follow the ICD-9 rubric and report deaths from circulatory diseases together. Deaths from coronary or IHD, heart failure, and, to a lesser extent, stroke predominate. Many of the reports also break out subcategories (such as cerebrovascular disease and hypertension). The relative importance of heart failure would be determined by the age of the cohort. In younger cohorts, most of the deaths in this category would be expected to be from IHD. Cerebrovascular deaths are deaths from strokes, which can be classified as either ischemic or hemorrhagic. In the US population, the great majority of strokes are of the ischemic type.

The methods used in morbidity studies can involve the direct assessment of the circulatory system, including analysis of symptoms or history, physical examination of the heart and peripheral arteries, ultrasound measurements of the heart and arteries, electrocardiography (ECG), chest radiography, cardiac computed tomography (CT), and more recently cardiac magnetic resonance imaging (MRI). Ultrasonography, CT, and MRI can be used to visualize the heart and related vasculature directly. ECG can be used to detect heart conditions and abnormalities, such as arrhythmias (abnormal heart rhythms), heart enlargement, and heart attacks (myocardial infarctions). Chest radiography can be used to assess the consequences of IHD and hypertension, such as the enlargement of the heart seen in heart failure. It is sometimes difficult to determine the time of onset of clinical findings, so the temporal relationship between exposure and disease occurrence may be uncertain. Cardiovascular-disease epidemiologists prefer to observe cohorts over time for the incidence of discrete clinical events, such as acute myocardial infarction (ideally verified on the basis of changes in ECG readings and enzyme concentrations) and death due to heart disease. The onset of new angina symptoms or the performance of a revascularization procedure in a person who has no history of disease is also used as evidence of incident disease. In many occupational studies, only mortality information is available. The attribution of death to a vascular cause is often based on a death certificate, whose accuracy can be uncertain.

The practice of evaluating the evidence on hypertension separately from that on other circulatory diseases was established in *Update 2006*; separate consideration of IHD began in *Update 2008*. The number of studies with data on stroke and cerebrovascular disease is increasing, so this endpoint can be considered in its own right in this report separately from discussions of "other circulatory diseases."

Conclusions from *VAO* and Previous Updates

The committee responsible for *VAO* concluded that there was inadequate or insufficient information to determine whether there is an association between exposure to the COIs and circulatory disorders. Additional information available to the committees responsible for *Update 1996*, *Update 1998*, *Update 2000*, *Update 2002*, and *Update 2004* did not change that conclusion.

The committee responsible for *Update 2006* reviewed new studies and intensively revisited all the studies related to IHD and hypertension that had been discussed in previous updates and concluded that there is limited or suggestive evidence to support an association between exposure to the herbicides used in Vietnam and hypertension. That committee was unable to reach a consensus as to whether that was also the case for IHD, so that outcome remained in the category of inadequate evidence.

After consideration of the relative strengths and weaknesses of the evidence regarding the COIs and IHD (ICD-9 410–414) and the relevant toxicologic literature, the committee responsible for *Update 2008* judged that the evidence was adequate to advance this health outcome from the "inadequate or insufficient" category into the "limited or suggestive" category, again acknowledging that bias and confounding could not be entirely ruled out. That conclusion was not changed in *Update 2010*. The committee for *Update 2010* also reaffirmed the *Update 2006* conclusion of limited or suggestive evidence of an association between herbicide exposure and hypertension.

The previous studies and studies published since *Update 2010* are all summarized in Table 12-3.

Update of the Epidemiologic Literature

Hypertension

Vietnam-Veteran Studies No Vietnam-veteran studies addressing exposure to the COIs and hypertension have been published since *Update 2010*.

Occupational Studies No occupational studies addressing exposure to the COIs and hypertension have been published since *Update 2010*.

Environmental Studies The survey of residents of an area of high dioxin contamination in Taiwan was introduced above (Chang et al., 2010b). The authors used factor analysis to determine which components of metabolic syndrome appeared to be most strongly associated with dioxin TEQ concentrations, based on serum PCDDs and PCDFs. Dioxin TEQs were more strongly associated with blood pressure than other syndrome components. In multivariate models, they found a highly-statistically-significant association between TEQ concentrations

TABLE 12-3 Selected Epidemiologic Studies—Circulatory Disorders (Shaded Entries Are New Information for This Update)

Study Population	Exposed Cases[a]	**Exposure of Interest**/Estimated Relative Risk (95% CI)[b]	*Reference*/ Comments
VIETNAM VETERANS			
US Vietnam Veterans			
US Air Force Health Study—Ranch Hand veterans vs SEA veterans (unless otherwise noted)		**All COIs**	
Through 1999—Ranch Hand personnel (n = 1,262) vs SEA veterans (19,078)—circulatory disease—mortality			*Ketchum and Michalek, 2005*
Ranch Hand subjects vs all SEA veterans			
Pilots and navigators	18	1.1 (0.7–1.8)	Not adjusted for known risk factors
Administrative officers	2	1.8 (0.4–7.8)	
Enlisted flight engineers	6	0.5 (0.2–1.1)	
Ground crew	40	1.7 (1.2–2.4)	
Atherosclerosis	28	1.7 (1.1–2.5)	
Hypertensive disease	2	2.5 (0.6–10.8)	
Stroke	5	2.3 (0.9–6.0)	
Subjects with serum TCDD measures			Adjusted for smoking and family history of heart disease
SEA comparison group	31	1.0	
Background (0.6–10.0 ppt)	8	0.8 (0.4–1.8)	
Low (10.0–29.2 ppt)	12	1.8 (0.9–3.5)	
High (18.0–617.8 ppt)	9	1.5 (0.7–3.3)	
US VA Cohort of Army Chemical Corps—Expanded as of 1997 to include all Army men with chemical MOS (2,872 deployed vs 2,737 nondeployed) serving during Vietnam era (07/01/1965–03/28/1973)		**All COIs**	
Incidence—Self-reported circulatory disorders diagnosed by doctor			
CATI survey of stratified sample: 1,499 deployed (795 with TCDD measured) vs 1,428 nondeployed (102 with TCDD measured)			*Kang et al., 2006* Diagnoses not confirmed by medical record review. Adjusted for age, race, rank, BMI, and smoking. Serum TCDD levels measured in subset of subjects; self-reported
Vietnam veterans vs non–Vietnam veterans			
Hypertension requiring medication	496	1.1 (0.9–1.3)	
Heart disease diagnosed by physician	243	1.1 (0.9–1.4)	
Sprayers vs nonsprayers			
All (diabetics, nondiabetics)			
Hypertension requiring medication	247	1.3 (1.0–1.6)	
Heart disease diagnosed by physician	129	1.4 (1.1–1.9)	

continued

TABLE 12-3 Circulatory Disorders, continued

Study Population	Exposed Cases[a]	**Exposure of Interest**/Estimated Relative Risk (95% CI)[b]	*Reference*/ Comments
All veterans, contribution of spraying to logistic regression model			sprayers had significantly higher concentrations than others, so that category regarded as valid surrogate for elevated exposure
All (diabetics, nondiabetics)			
Hypertension requiring medication		1.3 (1.1–1.6)	
Heart disease diagnosed by physician		1.5 (1.2–1.9)	
Nondiabetics only			
Hypertension requiring medication		1.2 (1.0–1.5)	
Heart disease diagnosed by physician		1.5 (1.1–2.0)	
Controlling for diabetic status			
Hypertension requiring medication		1.3 (1.0–1.6)	
Heart disease diagnosed by physician		1.5 (1.1–1.9)	
Mortality—Circulatory disorders			
Vietnam veterans vs non–Vietnam veterans—through 2005			*Cypel and Kang, 2010* Deaths, causes of deaths from national death registries. Adjustment for race, rank duration of service, and age
Circulatory system disease	184	1.2 (0.9–1.6)	
Hypertension	5	0.9 (0.2–3.9)	
Cerebrovascular disease	27	1.5 (0.7–3.3)	
Sprayers vs nonsprayers (subset studied in Kang et al. [2006])			
Circulatory system disease	ns	1.2 (0.6–2.3)	
Hypertension	ns	2.4 (0.2–28.5)	
Cerebrovascular disease	ns	2.1 (0.4–12.3)	
894 ACC members assigned to Vietnam in 1966–1971—			*Thomas and Kang, 1990* Not adjusted for known risk factors
Through 1987 (vs US male population)			
Circulatory diseases (ICD 390–458)	6	0.6	
US CDC Vietnam Experience Study—Cross-sectional study, with medical examinations, of Army veterans: 9,324 deployed vs 8,989 nondeployed		**All COIs**	
Incidence			
Deployed vs nondeployed			*CDC, 1988* Not adjusted for known risk factors
Hypertension after discharge			
Interviewed	2,013	1.3 ($p < 0.05$)	
Examined	623	1.2 ($p < 0.05$)	
Mortality			
Deployed vs nondeployed (1965–2000)	185	1.0 (0.8–1.2)	*Boehmer et al., 2004*
Circulatory disease			
Yr of death			

TABLE 12-3 Circulatory Disorders, continued

Study Population	Exposed Cases[a]	**Exposure of Interest**/Estimated Relative Risk (95% CI)[b]	*Reference/* Comments
1970–1984	nr	0.6 (0.3–1.2)	Adjusted for age, race, military occupation
1985–2000 (partition at 1970 arbitrary)	nr	1.1 (0.9–1.3)	
Discharged before 1970	nr	0.8 (0.6–1.1)	
Discharged after 1970	125	1.4 (1.0–2.0)	
Ischemic heart disease			
0–15 yrs since discharge	8	0.8 (0.3–1.6)	
> 15 yrs since discharge	117	1.1 (0.9–1.5)	
US VA Proportionate Mortality Study—sample of deceased male Vietnam-era Army and Marine veterans who served 7/4/1965–3/1/1973		**All COIs**	
1965–1988—mortality (PMR)			*Watanabe and Kang, 1996*
Served in Vietnam vs never deployed to SEA			
Circulatory disease			Not adjusted for known risk factors
Army	5,756	0.97 ($p > 0.05$)	
Marine Corps	1,048	0.92 ($p < 0.05$)	
US VA Study of Male Vietnam Veterans Wounded in Combat		**All COIs**	
Mortality through 1981—US wounded Vietnam veterans vs US men (focus on suicide)			*Bullman and Kang, 1996*
Circulatory disease	246	0.7 (0.6–0.9)	
US VA Cohort of Female Vietnam Veterans		**All COIs**	
Through 2004—mortality			*Cypel and Kang, 2008*
Circulatory system diseases			
Vietnam vs non-SEA veterans	129	0.8 (0.6–1.0)	Adjusted for duration of service, yr of birth, race
Nurses only	102	0.8 (0.6–1.0)	
US American Legion Cohort		**All COIs**	
American Legionnaires serving during Vietnam era—morbidity			*Stellman et al., 1988*
Service in SEA vs not, with medically-diagnosed			Not age-adjusted
High blood pressure	592	1.1 ($p > 0.05$)	
Heart disease	97	1.5 ($p < 0.05$)	Age-adjusted
State Studies of US Vietnam Veterans			
Massachusetts Vietnam-era veterans—(1958–1973)—mortality (1972–1983); deployed vs nondeployed			*Kogan and Clapp, 1985* (state report)

continued

TABLE 12-3 Circulatory Disorders, continued

Study Population	Exposed Cases[a]	**Exposure of Interest**/Estimated Relative Risk (95% CI)[b]	*Reference*/ Comments
Deaths 1972–1983 (PMR)			Not adjusted for age; VVs thought to be younger
Circulatory system (except cerebrovascular)	139	0.9 ($p > 0.05$)	
Cerebrovascular	28	1.1 ($p > 0.05$)	
Deaths 1978–1983 (PMR)			Expected less "diluted" effect for later time
Circulatory system (except cerebrovascular)	85	0.8 ($p < 0.05$)	
Cerebrovascular	19	1.6 ($p < 0.05$)	
Wisconsin Vietnam-era veterans—923 white male Vietnam veterans with **Wisconsin** death certificate (1968–1978) vs proportions for Vietnam-era veterans (all diseases of circulatory system)			*Anderson et al., 1986*
White male Vietnam veterans vs:	100		
National population		0.69 ($p < 0.05$)	
State population		0.62 ($p < 0.05$)	
Nonveterans		0.58 ($p < 0.05$)	
All veterans		0.86 ($p > 0.05$)	
Vietnam-era veterans		1.0 (0.8–1.2)	
International Vietnam-Veteran Studies			
Australian Vietnam Veterans—58,077 men and 153 women served on land or in Vietnamese waters during 5/23/1962–7/1/1973 vs Australian population		**All COIs**	
Mortality—All branches, return–2001			
Circulatory disease	1,767	0.9 (0.8–0.9)	*ADVA, 2005b*
1963–1979	186	0.7 (0.6–0.8)	
1980–1990	546	0.9 (0.8–1.0)	Pattern of increasing risks with time could indicate dissipation of healthy warrior effect
1991–2001	1,035	0.9 (0.9–1.0)	
Ischemic heart disease	1,297	0.9 (0.9–1.0)	
1963–1979	124	0.7 (0.6–0.8)	
1980–1990	421	1.0 (0.9–1.0)	
1991–2001	753	1.0 (0.9–1.1)	
Stroke	223	0.8 (0.7–0.9)	
1963–1979	35	0.8 (0.5–1.1)	
1980–1990	59	0.7 (0.5–0.9)	
1991–2001	129	0.8 (0.7–1.0)	
1980–1994			*CDVA, 1997a*
Circulatory disease		1.0 (0.9–1.1)	Not adjusted for known risk factors
Ischemic heart disease		1.0 (0.9–1.1)	
Cerebral hemorrhage		0.8 (0.5–1.2)	

TABLE 12-3 Circulatory Disorders, continued

Study Population	Exposed Cases[a]	**Exposure of Interest**/Estimated Relative Risk (95% CI)[b]	*Reference/* Comments
Sample of 1,000 Male Australian Vietnam Veterans—prevalence		**All COIs**	
450 interviewed 2005–2006 vs respondents to 2004–2005 national survey			*O'Toole et al., 2009*
Hypertensive disease	192	1.1 (1.0–1.3)	
Ischemic heart disease			Prevalence ratios calculated with age adjustment
Angina	44	2.3 (1.7–3.0)	
Without angina	59	4.1 (3.1–5.0)	
Cerebrovascular disease	12	2.4 (1.2–3.5)	
Hemorrhoids	81	7.7 (6.1–9.2)	
641 interviewed 1990–1993 vs respondents to 1989–1990 national survey			*O'Toole et al., 1996*
Hypertensive disease	nr	2.2 (1.7–2.6)	
Heart disease	nr	2.0 (0.9–3.1)	
Hemorrhoids	nr	7.4 (5.5–9.3)	
Other circulatory diseases	nr	2.4 (1.6–3.2)	
Australian Conscripted Army National Service (18,940 deployed vs 24,642 nondeployed)		**All COIs**	
Mortality			
1966–2001			*ADVA, 2005c*
Circulatory disease	208	1.1 (0.9–1.3)	
Ischemic heart disease	159	1.2 (0.9–1.5)	
Stroke	15	0.6 (0.3–1.2)	
1982–1994 (deployed vs nondeployed)			*CDVA, 1997b*
Circulatory disease	77	1.0 (0.7–1.3)	Not adjusted for known risk factors
Ischemic heart disease	57	1.0 (0.7–1.4)	
Cerebral hemorrhage	3	1.0 (0.1–5.7)	
Other	17	0.9 (0.4–1.7)	
Korean Vietnam Veterans—morbidity		**All COIs**	*Kim JS et al., 2003*
Deployed vs nondeployed (unadjusted)			Concerns: selection bias, diagnosis quality, low participation, sample pooling made TCDD concentrations useless
Valvular heart disease	8	$p = 0.0019$	
Congestive heart failure	5	$p = 0.5018$	
Ischemic heart disease	34	$p = 0.0143$	
Hypertension	383	2.3 (1.3–4.0)	
Adjusted for age, smoking, alcohol, BMI, education, marital status			

continued

TABLE 12-3 Circulatory Disorders, continued

Study Population	Exposed Cases[a]	**Exposure of Interest**/Estimated Relative Risk (95% CI)[b]	*Reference/* Comments
OCCUPATIONAL—INDUSTRIAL			
IARC Phenoxy Herbicide Cohort—Workers exposed to any phenoxy herbicide or chlorophenol (production or spraying) vs respective national mortality rates		**Dioxin, phenoxy herbicides**	
Mortality 1939–1992			*Vena et al., 1998* (same dataset as *Kogevinas et al. [1997]* [emphasis on cancer])
All male phenoxy herbicide workers			
All circulatory disease (ICD 390–459)	1,738	0.9 (0.9–1.0)	
Ischemic heart disease (ICD 410–414)	1,179	0.9 (0.9–1.0)	
Cerebrovascular disease (ICD 430–438)	254	0.9 (0.8–1.0)	
Other diseases of the heart (ICD 415–429)	166	1.1 (1.0–1.3)	
All female phenoxy herbicide workers			
All circulatory disease (ICD 390–459)	48	1.0 (0.7–1.3)	Not adjusted for known risk factors
Ischemic heart disease (ICD 410–414)	24	1.1 (0.7–1.6)	
Cerebrovascular disease (ICD 430–438)	9	0.7 (0.3–1.4)	
Other diseases of the heart (ICD 415–429)	6	0.9 (0.3–2.0)	
Workers with phenoxy herbicide exposure only			
All circulatory disease (ICD 390–459)	588	0.9 (0.8–0.9)	
Ischemic heart disease (ICD 410–414)	394	0.9 (0.8–0.9)	
Cerebrovascular disease (ICD 430–438)	96	0.9 (0.7–1.1)	
Other diseases of the heart (ICD 415–429)	32	0.9 (0.8–0.9)	
TCDD-exposed workers			
All circulatory disease (ICD 390–459)	1,170	0.9 (0.9–1.0)	
Ischemic heart disease (ICD 410–414)	789	1.0 (0.9–1.0)	
Cerebrovascular disease (ICD 430–438)	162	0.8 (0.7–1.0)	
Other diseases of the heart (ICD 415–429)	138	1.2 (1.0–1.4)	
Contribution of TCDD exposure to Poisson regression analysis			Adjusted for age, timing of exposure
All circulatory disease (ICD 390–459)	1,151	1.5 (1.2–2.0)	
Ischemic heart disease (ICD 410–414)	775	1.7 (1.2–2.3)	
Cerebrovascular disease (ICD 430–438)	161	1.5 (0.8–2.9)	
British MCPA Plant—Production 1947–1982 (n = 1,545) (included in IARC cohort) and spraying 1947–1972 (n = 2,561) (*not* included in IARC cohort)		**MCPA**	

TABLE 12-3 Circulatory Disorders, continued

Study Population	Exposed Cases[a]	**Exposure of Interest**/Estimated Relative Risk (95% CI)[b]	*Reference/* Comments
Mortality through 1983 (hypertensive, ischemic heart disease (ICD 401–414, 428–429)	337		*Coggon et al., 1986*
vs national rates		0.8 (0.7–0.9)	
vs rural adjustment		0.9 (0.8–1.0)	
British Production Workers at four plants (included in IARC cohort)		**Dioxins, but TCDD unlikely; MCPA**	*Coggon et al., 1991*
Mortality—circulatory disease	74	1.2 (0.9–1.5)	
Plant A (1975–1987)	34	1.7 (adjusted = 1.4, p ≈ 0.05)	
Plant B (1969–1987)	5	0.95	
Plant C (1963–1987)	12	0.84	
Plant D (1969–1987)	23	0.97	
Danish Production Workers (3,390 men and 1,069 women involved in production of phenoxy herbicides unlikely to contain TCDD at 2 plants in 1947–1987) (in IARC cohort)		**Dioxins, but TCDD unlikely; 2,4-D, 2,4-DP, MCPA, MCPP**	
Incidence			
Incidence 1943–1987 (men only)			*Lynge, 1993*
Incidence 1943–1982			*Lynge, 1985*
Men			
Women			
Mortality			
Mortality 1955–2006			*Boers et al., 2012*
TCDD plasma level (HRs, by tertile)	93	1.2 (1.1–1.3)	
Background (≤ 0.4)	33	—	
Low (0.4–4.1)	6	0.9 (0.4–2.5)	
Medium (4.1–20.1)	6	1.5 (0.6–4.0)	
High (≥ 20.1)	7	2.7 (1.0–7.2)	
Dutch production workers in Plant A (549 men exposed during production 1955–1985; 594 unexposed) (in IARC cohort)		**Dioxins, 2,4,5-T, 2,4,5-TCP**	
Mortality 1955–2006 (HRs for lagged TCDD plasma levels)			*Boers et al., 2012*
Ischemic heart disease (ICD-9 120–125)	60	1.2 (1.1–1.4)	
Cerebrovascular disease (ICD-9 160–167)	24	0.9 (0.7–1.1)	
Mortality 1955–2006			*Boers et al., 2010*
Ischemic heart disease	43	1.2 (0.7–2.0)	

continued

TABLE 12-3 Circulatory Disorders, continued

Study Population	Exposed Cases[a]	**Exposure of Interest**/Estimated Relative Risk (95% CI)[b]	*Reference*/ Comments
Accident 1963	17	1.6 (0.7–3.6)	HRs adjusted
Main production workers	9	1.0 (0.5–2.2)	for age,
Occasionally-exposed	17	1.1 (0.6–2.1)	yr of first
Cerebrovascular disease	17	1.2 (0.4–3.6)	employment.
Accident 1963	2	0.3 (0.1–1.4)	Referent group
Main production workers	5	1.3 (0.4–4.7)	are unexposed workers
Occasionally-exposed	10	1.5 (0.5–4.3)	
Mortality 1955–1991 (549 exposed vs 482 nonexposed male workers)			*Hooiveld et al., 1998*
All circulatory disease (ICD 390–459)	45	1.4 (0.8–2.5)	
TCDD > 124 ng/kg	nr	1.5 (0.8–2.9)	Adjusted for
Ischemic heart disease (ICD 410–414)	33	1.8 (0.9–3.6)	age, timing of
TCDD > 124 ng/kg	nr	2.3 (1.0–5.0)	exposure
Cerebrovascular disease (ICD 430–438)	9	1.4 (0.4–5.1)	
TCDD > 124 ng/kg	nr	0.8 (0.2–4.1)	
Other heart disease (ICD 415–429)	3	0.7 (0.1–4.3)	
TCDD > 124 ng/kg	nr	0.4 (0.0–4.9)	
Dutch production workers in Plant B (414 men exposed during production 1965–1986; 723 unexposed) (in IARC cohort)		**2,4-D; MCPA; MCPP; highly-chlorinated dioxins unlikely**	
Mortality 1965–2006			*Boers et al., 2010*
Ischemic heart disease	18	1.6 (0.8–3.1)	HRs adjusted
Main production workers	5	1.7 (0.6–4.6)	for age,
Occasionally-exposed	13	1.6 (0.7–3.3)	yr of first
Cerebrovascular disease	7	1.0 (0.4–2.8)	employment.
Main production workers	1	0.9 (0.1–7.1)	Referent group
Occasionally-exposed	6	1.1 (0.4–3.2)	are unexposed workers
German Production Workers at Bayer Plant in Uerdingen (135 men working > 1 mo in 1951–1976) (in IARC cohort as of 1997) and women—no results		**Dioxins; 2,4,5-TCP**	
Mortality 1951–1992 (circulatory diseases, ICD 390–458)	12	0.7 (0.4–1.3)	*Becher et al., 1996*
German Production Workers at Bayer Plant in Dormagen (520 men working > 1 mo in 1965–1989) (in IARC cohort as of 1997) and women—no results		**Dioxins; 2,4-D; 2,4,5-T; MCPA; MCPP; 2,4-DP**	
Mortality 1965–1989 (circulatory diseases, ICD 390–458)	3	0.3 (0.1–1.0)	*Becher et al., 1996*

TABLE 12-3 Circulatory Disorders, continued

Study Population	Exposed Cases[a]	**Exposure of Interest**/Estimated Relative Risk (95% CI)[b]	*Reference/* Comments
German Production Workers at BASF Ludwigshafen Plant (680 men working > 1 mo in 1957–1987) (in IARC cohort as of 1997) and women—no results		**Dioxins; 2,4-D; 2,4,5-T; MCPA; MCPP; 2,4-DP**	
Mortality 1956–1989 (circulatory diseases, ICD 390–458)	32	0.8 (0.5–1.1)	*Becher et al., 1996*
BASF Cleanup Workers from 1953 Accident (n = 247); 114 with chloracne, 13 more with erythema; serum TCDD levels (*not* part of IARC)		**Focus on TCDD**	
Mortality—1953–1992			*Ott and Zober, 1996*
Circulatory diseases	37	0.8 (0.6–1.2)	
< 0.1 estimated TCDD µg/kg bw	13	0.8 (0.4–1.4)	
0.1–0.99	11	1.0 (0.5–1.7)	Reliability of estimated body burden is questionable
≥ 1.0	13	0.8 (0.4–1.3)	
Ischemic heart disease	16	0.7 (0.4–1.1)	
< 0.1 estimated TCDD µg/kg bw	7	0.9 (0.3–1.8)	
0.1–0.99	4	0.7 (0.2–1.7)	
≥ 1.0	5	0.6 (0.2–1.3)	
German Production Workers at Boehringer–Ingelheim Plant in Hamburg (1,144 men working > 1 mo in 1952–1984; generation of TCDD reduced after chloracne outbreak in 1954) and women—no results (in IARC cohort as of 1997)		**Dioxins; 2,4,5-T; 2,5-DCP; 2,4,5-TCP**	
Mortality 1952–2007			*Manuwald et al., 2012*
Men			
Circulatory system disease		1.2 (1.0–1.3)	
Women			
Circulatory system disease		0.7 (0.6–0.9)	
Mortality 1952–1992; estimated blood PCDD, PCDF, TCDD from work history, measured in 190 of 1,189 men, divided into 4 lowest quintiles, top 2 deciles			*Flesch-Janys et al., 1995*
Estimated final PCDD, PCDF, TEQs (ng/kg)			

continued

TABLE 12-3 Circulatory Disorders, continued

Study Population	Exposed Cases[a]	**Exposure of Interest**/Estimated Relative Risk (95% CI)[b]	*Reference*/ Comments
Circulatory disease (ICD 390–459)	156		Gas workers provide a more appropriate comparison group for the data on production workers than the national population data used in *Flesch-Janys, 1997/98; Flesch-Janys et al., 1998*
1.0–12.2		0.9 (0.6–1.5)	
12.3–39.5		0.9 (0.6–1.5)	
39.6–98.9		1.5 (1.0–2.2)	
99.0–278.5		1.6 (1.1–2.2)	
278.6–545.0		1.6 (1.0–2.6)	
545.1–4,361.9		2.1 (1.2–3.5)	
		p-trend < 0.01	
Ischemic heart disease (ICD 410–414)	76		
1.0–12.2		1.0 (0.5–2.0)	
12.3–39.5		1.0 (0.5–1.8)	
39.6–98.9		1.0 (0.5–1.8)	
99.0–278.5		1.1 (0.6–2.0)	
278.6–545.0		1.7 (0.9–3.3)	
545.1–4,361.9		2.7 (1.5–5.0)	
		p-trend < 0.01	
Estimated final TCDD (ng/kg)			
Circulatory disease (ICD 390–459)	156		
0–2.8		1.2 (0.8–1.8)	Not adjusted for known risk factors
2.81–14.4		0.9 (0.5–1.4)	
14.5–49.2		1.4 (0.9–2.0)	
49.3–156.7		1.6 (1.1–2.4)	
156.8–344.6		1.5 (1.0–2.4)	
344.7–3,890.2		2.0 (1.2–3.3)	
		p-trend = 0.01	
Ischemic heart disease (ICD 410–414)	76		
0–2.8		1.4 (0.8–2.4)	Potential for exposure misclassification
2.81–14.4		0.8 (0.4–1.6)	
14.5–49.2		1.2 (0.7–2.2)	
49.3–156.7		0.9 (0.5–1.8)	
156.8–344.6		1.6 (0.9–3.0)	
344.7–3,890.2		2.5 (1.3–4.7)	
		p-trend < 0.01	
New Zealand Phenoxy Herbicide Production Workers and Sprayers (1,599 men and women working any time in 1969–1988 at Dow plant in New Plymouth) (in IARC cohort)		**Dioxins; 2,4-D; 2,4,5-T; MCPA; MCPB; 2,4,5-TCP; Picloram**	
Mortality 1969–2004			*McBride et al., 2009*
Ever-exposed workers—stroke	15	1.1 (0.6–1.9)	
Ever-exposed workers—ischemic heart disease	61	1.1 (0.9–1.5)	

TABLE 12-3 Circulatory Disorders, continued

Study Population	Exposed Cases[a]	**Exposure of Interest**/Estimated Relative Risk (95% CI)[b]	*Reference/* Comments
Ischemic heart disease:			Adjusted for age, sex, hire yr, birth yr
TCDD exposure ppt-months			
0–68.3	14	1.0 (reference group)	
68.4–475.0	18	1.2 (0.6–2.6)	
475.1–2,088.7	15	1.3 (0.6–2.9)	
2,088.7+	14	0.9 (0.4–2.4)	
Production Workers (713 men and 100 women worked > 1 mo in 1969–1984)			
Mortality 1969–2000			*'t Mannetje et al., 2005*
Circulatory disease	51	1.0 (0.7–1.3)	Not adjusted for known risk factors
Hypertensive disease	0	0.0 (0.0–3.5)	
Ischemic heart disease	38	1.0 (0.7–1.4)	
All-causes (SMR)	nr	1.0 (0.8–1.2)	
Sprayers (697 men and 2 women on register of New Zealand applicators, 1973–1984)			
Mortality 1973–2000			*'t Mannetje et al., 2005*
Circulatory disease	33	0.5 (0.4–0.7)	Not adjusted for known risk factors
Hypertensive disease	1	0.8 (0.0–4.5)	
Ischemic heart disease	22	0.5 (0.3–0.8)	
All-causes (SMR)	nr	0.6 (0.5–0.8)	
(Preliminary) NIOSH Cross-Sectional Medical Study—490 workers from chemical plants in Newark, New Jersey and Verona, Missouri, 1951–1969 (morbidity)		**Dioxin/phenoxy herbicides**	*Calvert et al., 1998*
Verified conditions			
TCDD-exposed (281) vs nonexposed (260)			Not adjusted for known risk factors
Myocardial infarction	17	1.3 (0.6–2.8)	
Current systolic hypertension	64	1.1 (0.7–1.6)	
Current diastolic hypertension	77	1.2 (0.8–1.8)	
TCDD effect vs nonexposed in logistic model. Self-reported, verified conditions combined			

continued

TABLE 12-3 Circulatory Disorders, continued

Study Population	Exposed Cases[a]	**Exposure of Interest**/Estimated Relative Risk (95% CI)[b]	*Reference*/ Comments
Myocardial infarction			Adjusted for age, sex, BMI, smoking, drinking, diabetes, triglycerides, total cholesterol, HDL, family history of heart disease, and chemical plant
Serum TCDD < 238 pg/g of lipid	nr	1.1 (0.3–4.5)	
Serum TCDD ≥ 238 pg/g of lipid	nr	1.1 (0.2–5.1)	
Hypertension			
Serum TCDD < 238 pg/g of lipid	nr	1.3 (0.9–2.0)	
Serum TCDD ≥ 238 pg/g of lipid	nr	1.1 (0.6–1.9)	
Verified conditions			
Current systolic hypertension			
Serum TCDD < 238 pg/g of lipid	nr	1.1 (0.7–1.8)	
Serum TCDD ≥ 238 pg/g of lipid	nr	1.2 (0.6–2.3)	
Current diastolic hypertension			
Serum TCDD < 238 pg/g of lipid	nr	1.4 (0.9–2.1)	
Serum TCDD ≥ 238 pg/g of lipid	nr	1.0 (0.5–1.9)	
NIOSH Mortality Cohort (12 US plants, 5,172 male production and maintenance workers 1942–1984) (included in IARC cohort as of 1997)		**Dioxins, phenoxy herbicides**	
Through 1993			*Steenland et al., 1999*
Cerebrovascular disease (ICD 430–438)	69	1.0 (0.7–1.2)	Not adjusted for known risk factors
Ischemic heart disease (ICD 410–414)	456	1.1 (1.0–1.2)	
Chloracne subcohort (n = 608) vs US population; exposure subcohort (n = 3,538)	92		Adjusted for age
< 19 cumulative TCDD	nr	1.0	
19–138	nr	1.2 (0.8–2.0)	
139–580	nr	1.3 (0.8–2.2)	No units given for exposure derived from job–exposure matrix
581–1,649	nr	1.3 (0.8–2.1)	
1,650–5,739	nr	1.4 (0.9–2.2)	
5,740–20,199	nr	1.6 (1.0–2.6)	
≥ 20,200	nr	1.8 (1.1–2.9) p-trend = 0.05 p-trend log < 0.001	
Monsanto workers (n = 240) involved in 2,4,5-T production (1948–1969) and 163 unexposed workers, results of clinical examination July 1979—morbidity		**Dioxin, phenoxy herbicides**	*Suskind and Hertzberg, 1984*
Hypertension	70	(p > 0.05)	Adjusted for age
Coronary artery disease	22	(p > 0.05)	

TABLE 12-3 Circulatory Disorders, continued

Study Population	Exposed Cases[a]	**Exposure of Interest**/Estimated Relative Risk (95% CI)[b]	*Reference/* Comments
All Dow TCP-Exposed Workers (TCP production 1942–1979 or 2,4,5-T production 1948–1982 in Midland, Michigan) (in IARC and NIOSH cohorts)		**2,4,5-T; 2,4,5-TCP**	
1942–2003 (n = 1,615)			*Collins et al., 2009a*
Ischemic heart disease	218	1.1 (0.9–1.2)	No adjustment discussed
Cerebrovascular disease	37	1.0 (0.7–1.4)	
March 1955–1977 (n = 884 workers); mortality			*Zack and Gaffey, 1983*
Circulatory disease (ICD 390–458)	92	1.11 ($p > 0.05$)	Not adjusted for known risk factors
Atherosclerosis and CHD (ICD 410–413)	79	1.33 ($p > 0.05$)	
March 1949–1978 (n = 121); mortality—121 TCP workers with chloracne			*Zack and Suskind, 1980*
Circulatory disease (ICD 390–458)	17	0.68 ($p > 0.05$)	Not adjusted for known risk factors
Atherosclerosis and CHD (ICD 410–413)	13	0.73 ($p > 0.05$)	
All Dow PCP-Exposed Workers—all workers from the two plants that only made PCP (in Tacoma, Washington, and Wichita, Kansas) and workers who made PCP and TCP at two additional plants (in Midland, Michigan, and Sauget, Illinois)		**2,4,5-T; 2,4,5-TCP**	*Ruder and Yiin, 2011*
1940–2005 (n = 2,122)			
Rheumatic heart disease (ICD-9 390–398)	4	0.6 (0.2–1.6)	
Ischemic heart disease (ICD-9 410–414)	350	1.0 (0.9–1.2)	
Hypertension with heart disease ICD-9 402, 404)	6	0.4 (0.2–1.0)	
Cerebrovascular disease (ICD-9 430–438)	64	1.0 (0.7–1.2)	
PCP and TCP (n = 720)			
Rheumatic heart disease (ICD-9 390–398)	0	0.0 (0.0–1.9)	
Ischemic heart disease (ICD-9 410–414)	120	1.1 (0.9–1.3)	
Hypertension with heart disease ICD-9 402, 404)	0	0.0 (0.0–1.0)	
Cerebrovascular disease (ICD-9 430–438)	20	1.0 (0.6–1.5)	
PCP (no TCP) (n = 1,402)			

continued

TABLE 12-3 Circulatory Disorders, continued

Study Population	Exposed Cases[a]	**Exposure of Interest**/Estimated Relative Risk (95% CI)[b]	*Reference*/ Comments
Rheumatic heart disease (ICD-9 390–398)	4	0.9 (0.3–2.3)	
Ischemic heart disease (ICD-9 410–414)	230	1.0 (0.9–1.1)	
Hypertension with heart disease ICD-9 402, 404)	6	0.6 (0.2–1.3)	
Cerebrovascular disease (ICD-9 430–438)	44	0.9 (0.7–1.2)	
Dow 2,4-D Production Workers (1945–1982 in Midland, Michigan) (subset of all TCP-exposed workers)		**2,4-D, lower chlorinated dioxins**	
Through 1994 (n = 1,517), circulatory disease			*Burns et al., 2001*
0 yrs latency	158	1.0 (0.8–1.1)	
≥ 20 yrs latency	130	1.1 (0.9–1.2)	
Dow PCP Production Workers (1937–1989 in Midland, Michigan) (*not* in IARC and NIOSH cohorts)		**Low chlorinated dioxins, 2,4-D**	
Mortality 1940–2004 (n = 577, excluding 196 also having exposure to TCP)			*Collins et al., 2009b*
Ischemic heart disease	99	1.0 (0.8–1.3)	No adjustment discussed
Cerebrovascular disease	17	0.9 (0.5–1.2)	
Mortality 1940–1989 (n = 770)			*Ramlow et al., 1996*
Circulatory disease (ICD 390–458)	115	1.0 (0.8–1.1)	
Arteriosclerotic heart disease (ICD 410–413)	86	1.0 (0.8–1.3)	
Cerebrovascular disease (ICD 430–438)	15	1.0 (0.6–1.7)	
Other Studies of Industrial Workers (*not* related to IARC or NIOSH phenoxy cohorts)			
Japanese Waste-Incinerator Workers—Workers exposed to PCDD at municipal waste incinerator		**Dioxin, phenoxy herbicides**	*Kitamura et al., 2000*
Hypertension by PCDD, PCDF	14 of 94	No increases observed	Adjusted for age, BMI, smoking
OCCUPATIONAL—PAPER AND PULP WORKERS		**TCDD**	
IARC cohort of pulp and paper workers—60,468 workers from 11 countries, TCDD among 27 agents assessed by JEM			*McLean et al., 2006*
Exposure to nonvolatile organochlorine compounds—circulatory disease (mortality)			Not adjusted for known riskfactors
Never	2,727	0.9 (0.8–1.0)	
Ever	2,157	1.0 (1.0–1.0)	

TABLE 12-3 Circulatory Disorders, continued

Study Population	Exposed Cases[a]	**Exposure of Interest**/Estimated Relative Risk (95% CI)[b]	*Reference/* Comments
OCCUPATIONAL—HERBICIDE-USING WORKERS (*not* related to IARC sprayer cohorts)			
ITALIAN Licensed Pesticide Users—male farmers in southern Piedmont licensed 1970–1974			
Italian rice growers with documented phenoxy use, 1960–1980)—mortality (1957–1992) (n = 1,487)		**Phenoxy herbicides**	*Gambini et al., 1997*
Myocardial infarction	67	0.7 (0.6–0.9)	
Other ischemic heart diseases	72	0.4 (0.3–0.5)	
Stroke	155	1.0 (0.8–1.1)	
THE NETHERLANDS			
Dutch Licensed Herbicide Sprayers—1,341 certified before 1980		**Herbicides**	
Through 2000			*Swaen et al., 2004*
Circulatory disease	70	0.7 (0.5–0.9)	
UNITED STATES			
US Agricultural Health Study—prospective study of licensed pesticide sprayers in Iowa and North Carolina: commercial (n = 4,916 men), private/farmers (n = 52,395, 97.4% men), and spouses of private sprayers (n = 32,347, 0.007% men), enrolled 1993–1997; followups with CATIs 1999–2003 and 2005–2010		**Phenoxy herbicides**	
Study of myocardial infarction			*Mills et al., 2009*
Mortality among 54,069 male applicators			
2,4-D	73	0.9 (0.7–1.1)	Adjusted for age, state, smoking. Incidence analysis further adjusted for BMI
2,4,5-T	32	1.0 (0.8–1.2)	
2,4,5-TP	14	1.1 (0.8–1.4)	
Dicamba	42	0.9 (0.8–1.2)	
Non-fatal incidence among 32,024 male applicators—yr-5 survey			
2,4-D	78	1.2 (1.0–1.4)	
2,4,5-T	37	1.2 (1.0–1.4)	
2,4,5-TP	14	1.1 (0.9–1.4)	
Dicamba	47	1.1 (0.9–1.3)	

continued

TABLE 12-3 Circulatory Disorders, continued

Study Population	Exposed Cases[a]	**Exposure of Interest**/Estimated Relative Risk (95% CI)[b]	*Reference/* Comments
Enrollment through 2001—mortality			*Blair et al., 2005*
Private applicators (farmers), spouses			Adjusted for
Circulatory disease	619	0.5 (0.5–0.6)	age, race, state, sex, and calendar yr of death
Enrollment through 2007, vs state rates			*Waggoner et al., 2011*
Applicators (n = 1,641)			
Rheumatic heart disease	8	0.7 (0.3–1.4)	
Hypertension with heart disease	40	0.5 (0.4–0.7)	
Hypertension without heart disease	15	0.4 (0.2–0.6)	
Ischemic heart disease	1,099	0.5 (0.5–0.6)	
Cerebrovascular disease	236	0.5 (0.5–0.6)	
Spouses (n = 676)			
Rheumatic heart disease	7	0.7 (0.3–1.5)	
Hypertension with heart disease	7	0.3 (0.1–0.6)	
Hypertension without heart disease	6	0.3 (0.1–0.7)	
Ischemic heart disease	211	0.5 (0.4–0.5)	
Cerebrovascular disease	105	0.6 (0.5–0.7)	
US Department of Agriculture Workers—nested case-control study of white men dying 1970–1979		**Herbicides**	
Forest conservationists		p-trend < over yrs worked	*Alavanja et al., 1989*
Ischemic heart disease (ICD 410–414)	543	1.0 (0.9–1.1)	Not adjusted
Cerebrovascular disease (ICD 430–438)	99	0.9 (0.8–1.1)	for known risk factors
Florida Licensed Pesticide Applicators		**Herbicides**	*Blair et al., 1983*
Pesticide applicators in Florida licensed 1965–1966 (n = 3,827)—mortality through 1976			Not adjusted for known risk
Circulatory diseases (ICD 390–458)			factors
ENVIRONMENTAL			
Seveso, Italy, Residential Cohort—Industrial accident July 10, 1976 (723 residents Zone A; 4,821 Zone B; 31,643 Zone R; 181,574 local reference group) (ICD-9 171)		**TCDD**	
25-yr followup to 2001			*Consonni et al., 2008*
Zone A, sexes combined			

TABLE 12-3 Circulatory Disorders, continued

Study Population	Exposed Cases[a]	**Exposure of Interest**/Estimated Relative Risk (95% CI)[b]	*Reference/* Comments
All circulatory diseases (ICD 390–459)	45	1.1 (0.8–1.4)	Adjusted for gender, age, period
Chronic rheumatic heart diseases (ICD 393–398)	3	5.7 (1.8–18.0)	
Hypertension (ICD 400–405)	5	2.2 (0.9–5.3)	
Ischemic heart diseases (ICD 410–414)	13	0.8 (0.5–1.4)	
Acute myocardial infarction (ICD 410)	6	0.6 (0.3–1.4)	
Chronic ischemic heart diseases (ICD 412, 414)	7	1.1 (0.5–2.3)	
Cerebrovascular diseases (ICD 430–438)	11	0.9 (0.5–1.6)	
Zone B, sexes combined			
All circulatory diseases (ICD 390–459)	289	1.0 (0.9–1.1)	
Chronic rheumatic heart diseases (ICD 393–398)	1	0.3 (0.0–2.2)	
Hypertension (ICD 400–405)	11	0.7 (0.4–1.3)	
Ischemic heart diseases (ICD 410–414)	102	1.0 (0.8–1.2)	
Acute myocardial infarction (ICD 410)	54	0.9 (0.7–1.1)	
Chronic ischemic heart diseases (ICD 412, 414)	47	1.1 (0.8–1.4)	
Cerebrovascular diseases (ICD 430–438)	101	1.2 (1.0–1.5)	
Zone R, sexes combined			
All circulatory diseases (ICD 390–459)	2,357	1.1 (1.0–1.1)	
Chronic rheumatic heart diseases (ICD 393–398)	24	1.0 (0.6–1.5)	
Hypertension (ICD 400–405)	144	1.2 (1.0–1.4)	
Ischemic heart diseases (ICD 410–414)	842	1.1 (1.0–1.1)	
Acute myocardial infarction (ICD 410)	447	1.0 (0.9–1.1)	
Chronic ischemic heart diseases (ICD 412, 414)	390	1.2 (1.0–1.3)	
Cerebrovascular diseases (ICD 430–438)	695	1.1 (1.0–1.2)	
National Health and Nutrition Examination Survey		**Dioxin, dl PCBs**	
NHANES 1999–2002—newly-diagnosed hypertension; 524 adults (≥ 40 yrs of age) excluding treated hypertensives		≥ 75th percentile vs < 25th percentile	*Ha et al., 2009*
Men			
PCDDs	23	2.3 (0.7–7.8) p-trend = 0.15	
PCDFs	21	1.9 (0.7–4.9) p-trend = 0.17	

continued

TABLE 12-3 Circulatory Disorders, continued

Study Population	Exposed Cases[a]	**Exposure of Interest**/Estimated Relative Risk (95% CI)[b]	*Reference/* Comments
dl PCBs	27	1.7 (0.8–6.6) p-trend = 0.11	Adjusted for age, race, income, BMI, cigarette-smoking, serum cotinine, alcohol, exercise
Women			
PCDDs	33	5.0 (1.2–21.5) p-trend = 0.08	
PCDFs	30	4.2 (1.3–14.3) p-trend = 0.01	
dl PCBs	28	1.1 (0.3–3.5) p-trend = 0.93	
26.1–59.1		1.1 (0.9–1.4)	
> 59.1		1.8 (1.2–2.6)	
PCB 156 (ng/g of lipid) (TEF = 0.0005)			
≤ 12.5		1.0	
12.6–15.4		1.3 (0.9–1.9)	
> 15.4		1.2 (0.8–1.9)	
PCB 169 (pg/g of lipid) (TEF = 0.01)			
≤ 27.0		1.0	
27.1–46.4		1.1 (0.9–1.5)	
> 46.4		1.3 (0.9–1.9)	
NHANES 1999–2002—self-reported cardiovascular disease (excluding hypertension)—889 nondiabetics ≥ 40 yrs of age		≥ 75th percentile vs < 25th percentile	*Ha et al., 2007*
Men			
HxCDD	18	2.5 (0.8–7.7)	Adjusted for age, race, income, BMI, cigarette-smoking, serum cotinine, alcohol, exercise, HDL, total cholesterol, triglycerides hypertension, C-reactive protein
HpCDD	18	2.4 (0.5–10.3)	
OCDD	16	2.1 (0.6–7.7)	
PCDDs	23	2.2 (0.8–6.1)	
PCDFs	19	0.7 (0.3–1.7)	
dl PCBs	22	1.7 (0.6–5.5)	
Women			
HxCDD	21	2.8 (0.9–8.6)	
HpCDD	14	1.9 (0.3–10.8)	
OCDD	17	0.7 (0.2–2.8)	
PCDDs	19	2.0 (0.7–6.4)	
PCDFs	15	1.0 (0.3–2.8)	
dl PCBs	23	5.0 (1.2–20.4)	
NHANES 1999–2004—prevalent hypertension (self-report told by doctor, ≥ 140/90 mmHg or antihypertensive medications)—3,398–3,712 individuals depending on congener			*Everett et al., 2008*
PCB 118 (ng/g of lipid) (TEF = 0.0001)			

TABLE 12-3 Circulatory Disorders, continued

Study Population	Exposed Cases[a]	**Exposure of Interest**/Estimated Relative Risk (95% CI)[b]	*Reference*/ Comments
≤ 12.5		1.0	Adjusted for age, sex, race, smoking status, BMI, exercise, total cholesterol, family history of myocardial infarction
12.6–27.5		1.4 (1.1–1.8)	
> 27.5		2.0 (1.3–3.0)	
PCB 126 (ng/g of lipid) (TEF = 0.1)			
≤ 26.1		1.0	
26.2–59.1		1.1 (0.9–1.4)	
> 59.1		1.8 (1.2–2.6)	
PCB 156 (ng/g of lipid) (TEF = 0.0005)			
≤ 12.5		1.0	
12.6–15.4		1.3 (0.9–1.9)	
> 15.4		1.2 (0.8–1.9)	
PCB 169 (ng/g of lipid) (TEF = 0.01)			
≤ 27.0		1.0	
27.1–46.4		1.1 (0.9–1.5)	
> 46.4		1.3 (0.9–1.9)	
NHANES 1999–2002—721 nondiabetics ≥ 20 with fasting blood samples and measured POPs high blood pressure (≥ 130/85 hg)	nr	≥ 75th percentile vs those with nondetectable level	*Lee et al., 2007c*
PCDDs		1.7 (1.0–3.1)	
HxCDD		1.2 (0.7–2.2)	Adjusted for age, race, sex, income, cigarette-smoking, serum cotinine, alcohol consumption, exercise
HpCDD		2.6 (1.3–5.0)	
OCDD		1.1 (0.6–2.0)	
PCDFs		1.9 (1.2–3.3)	
PeCDF		1.3 (0.7–2.4)	
HxCDF		2.3 (1.3–4.0)	
HpCDF		1.4 (0.8–2.3)	
Dioxin-like PCBs		1.4 (0.8–2.7)	
PCB 74		1.2 (0.6–2.4)	
PCB 118		1.8 (1.0–3.5)	
PCB 126		2.1 (1.2–3.7)	
PCB 169		0.6 (0.3–1.1)	
Other International Environmental Studies			
FINLAND			
Finnish fishermen (n = 6,410) and spouses (n = 4,260) registered between 1980 and 2002 compared to national statistics		**TCDD, PCBs, TEQs**	*Turunen et al., 2008*
Ischemic heart disease			Standardized mortality analysis—age-adjusted
Men	269	0.7 (0.7–0.8)	
Women	62	0.7 (0.5–0.8)	
Cerebrovascular disease			
Men	67	0.7 (0.5–0.9)	
Women	46	1.0 (0.7–11.3)	

continued

TABLE 12-3 Circulatory Disorders, continued

Study Population	Exposed Cases[a]	**Exposure of Interest**/Estimated Relative Risk (95% CI)[b]	*Reference/* Comments
TAIWAN			
Residents around 12 municipal waste incinerators in Taiwan—prevalence		**Dioxin/phenoxy herbicides**	*Chen et al., 2006*
Hypertension diagnosed by a physician	118	5.6 (1.6–19.6)	
Serum PCDD/F (TEQs in logistic model)		0.9 (0.2–3.7)	
UNITED STATES			
Superfund site caused by wood-treatment facility in Pensacola, Florida—47 workers, residents—prevalence		**Dioxin/phenoxy herbicides**	*Karouna-Renier et al., 2007*
Hypertension defined by self-report, medication use, or 2 readings of systolic blood pressure greater than 140 mmHg or diastolic blood pressure greater than 90 mmHg		1.1 (1.1–1.2) [error likely; published OR, lower confidence limit identical to 3 decimal places]	Adjusted for age, race, sex, BMI, tobacco and alcohol use, worker status
Serum PCDD/F (TEQs in logistic model)			

NOTE: 2,4-D, 2,4-dichlorophenoxyacetic acid; 2,4-DP, dichlorprop; 2,4,5-T, 2,4,5-trichlorophenoxyacetic acid; 2,4,5-TCP, 2,4,5-trichlorophenol; 2,4,5-TP, 2-(2,4,5-trichlorophenoxy) propionic acid; 2,5-DCP, 2,5-dichlorophenol; ACC, Army Chemical Corps; BMI, body mass index; bw, body weight; CATI, computer-assisted telephone interviewing; CDC, Centers for Disease Control and Prevention; CHD, coronary heart disease; CI, confidence interval; COI, chemical of interest; dl, dioxin-like; HDL, high-density lipoprotein; HpCDD, 1,2,3,4,6,7,8-heptachlorodibenzo-*p*-dioxin; HpCDF, 1,2,3,4,6,7,8-heptachlorodibenzofuran; HR, hazard ratio; HxCDD, 1,2,3,6,7,8-hexachlorodibenzo-*p*-dixion; HxCDF, 1,2,3,4,7,8-hexachlorodibenzofuran; IARC, International Agency for Research on Cancer; ICD, *International Classification of Diseases*; JEM, job–exposure matrix; MCPA, 2-methyl-4-chlorophenoxyacetic acid; MCPB, 4-(4-chloro-2-methylphenoxy)butanoic acid; MCPP, methylchlorophenoxypropionic acid; MOS, months of service; NHANES, National Health and Nutrition Examination Survey; NIOSH, National Institute for Occupational Safety and Health; nr, not reported; ns, not significant; OCDD, 1,2,3,4,6,7,8,9-octachlorodibenzo-*p*-dioxin; OR, odds ratio; PCB, polychlorinated biphenyl; PCDD, polychlorinated dibenzo-*p*-dioxin; PCDD/F, dioxins and furans combined; PCDF, polychlorinated dibenzofuran; PCP, pentachlorophenol; PeCDF, 2,3,4,7,8-pentachlorodibenzofuran; PMR, proportional mortality ratio; POP, persistent organic pollutant; ppt, parts per trillion; SEA, Southeast Asia; SMR, standardized mortality ratio; TCDD, 2,3,7,8-tetrachlorodibenzo-*p*-dixoin; TCP, trichlorophenol; TEF, toxicity equivalency factor for individual congener; TEQ, (total) toxic equivalent; VA, US Department of Veterans Affairs; VV, Vietnam veterans.

[a]Subjects male unless otherwise noted.

[b]Given when available; results other than estimated risk explained individually.

and diastolic blood pressure (p = 0.006) but not systolic blood pressure after adjustment for age, sex, obesity, smoking status, alcohol use, and family history of hypertension or diabetes. That finding was also reported in a further analysis of the sample by Chang et al. (2011b), who examined the associations between dioxin and related chemicals and CVD risk by using the Framingham risk score and its components.

Goncharov et al. (2011) examined data on the 394 residents of Anniston, Alabama, to determine the relationship between blood pressure and serum concentrations of 35 PCBs and 9 chlorinated pesticides. Persons taking antihypertensive medications were excluded. Other than age, total serum PCB concentrations were the strongest correlate of blood pressure after adjustment for age, BMI, sex, race, smoking status, and exercise. The authors saw a weak association between blood pressure and mono-ortho PCBs, but it was not statistically significant. PCBs that had more potent dioxin-like activity were not measurable within the limits of the assay used.

Jones et al. (2011) examined urinary arsenic concentrations and hypertension in the 2003–2008 National Health and Nutrition Examination Survey and observed no statistically significant association.

Case-Control Studies No case-control studies of exposure to the COIs and hypertension have been published since *Update 2010*.

Ischemic Heart Disease

Vietnam-Veteran Studies Kim JB et al. (2012) studied outcomes of Vietnam-era South Korean veterans undergoing coronary angiography because of acute coronary syndrome (chest pain arising from unstable angina, ST-segment myocardial infarction, or non-ST-segment myocardial infarction) according to whether they served in Vietnam (121) or did not serve (130). This study examines whether a history of Vietnam service is associated with the clinical course of coronary disease, not the occurrence of coronary disease itself. Thus, its findings are not relevant to the question of whether the COIs cause ischemic coronary disease.

Occupational Studies Boers et al. (2012) reported an updated mortality analysis of workers exposed to TCDD at two Dutch chlorophenoxy-herbicide production facilities. Results of that cohort have been included in previous VAO reports. The new analysis advances previous reports by using semiquantitative dose estimates derived by back-extrapolating exposures on the basis of blood TCDD concentrations measured in blood of 197 former employees. Workers in plant A were exposed to high concentrations of dioxin both as a contaminant of 2,4,5-T production and through accidental exposure after the explosion of a kiln. Plant B was involved in 2,4-D production, but TCDD exposure was assumed to be minimal. The study followed all male employees of either factory during their years of operation, which lasted until 1985 for plant A and 1986 for plant B. Mortality was ascertained through the end of 2006. There were 339 deaths among the 1,020 workers included from plant A and 202 deaths among the 1,036 workers from plant B. No risk factors for heart disease other than age were available. About 93 deaths were due to IHD. There was a significant association between death from IHD and dioxin exposure (hazard ratio [HR] for natural log-transformed TCDD exposure = 1.19, 95% CI 1.08–1.32). The estimated association was slightly higher when the analysis was restricted to plant A (HR = 1.24, 95% CI 1.09–1.43). The authors examined dioxin exposure as a categoric variable and found that the higher mortality was evident only in those who had the highest putative TCDD exposure, ^{3}9.9 parts per trillion (ppt) (HR = 2.60, 95% CI 1.57–4.31).

Manuwald et al. (2012) reported the 23-year followup of workers exposed to dioxins in a chemical plant in Hamburg, Germany, that manufactured herbicides and pesticides, including 2,4,5-T. Results on that cohort have been included in previous VAO reports. The study included 1,191 men and 398 women who were employed full-time at the plant for at least 3 months during 1952–1984. The mortality experience of employees was compared with that of the populations of Hamburg and the Federal Republic of Germany over the same period. Worker exposure was estimated on the basis of the putative intensity of exposure in different work areas in the plant. About 695 deaths were reported through the end of followup on December 31, 2007. Mortality from diseases of the circulatory system was significantly higher than expected in men (SMR = 1.16, 95% CI 1.02–1.31) but significantly lower than expected in women (SMR = 0.74, 95% CI 0.56–0.94). Estimated exposure to TCDD was substantially higher in male workers (median = 77.4 ppt) than in female workers (median = 19.5 ppt). When workers were categorized in quartiles by estimated exposure, there was no evidence that the standardized mortality ratio from circulatory diseases increased with higher estimated dose.

Ruder and Yiin (2011) reported the mortality experience of 2,122 workers involved in the production of PCP in four plants in the United States through 2005. Details are reported above. In comparison to the general US population, IHD was not significantly elevated in the 720 workers exposed to both PCP and TCP; 131 deaths were ascertained (SMR = 1.11, 95% CI 0.92–1.54). Workers in two of the four plants had TCDD exposures sufficient to cause chloracne. Workers in these two plants had higher SMRs for IHD than workers in the other two plants, but these elevations were not higher than those expected based on the US population rates.

Waggoner et al. (2011) reported on mortality in the Agricultural Health Study from 1993 to 2007. Previous reports on the cohort have documented that most of its members have been exposed to COIs (2,4-D and 2,4,5-T), but this report describes the mortality experience of only the cohort as a whole without consideration of pesticide-specific exposures. Therefore, the information presented cannot be used either to confirm or to refute associations between the COIs and cardiovascular-disease mortality.

Environmental Studies Lind et al. (2012) studied the relationship between exposure to POPs and the prevalence of carotid artery plaque in the PIVUS study by using ultrasonography. Sonography can be used to obtain images of atherosclerotic lesions (plaques) in the arterial wall and to measure arterial wall thickness (intima-media thickness, IMT). Thickness is a measure of the extent of the atherosclerotic process, correlates with atherosclerosis in the coronary arteries, and predicts acute coronary events. The technique also provides a measure of the extent to which the arterial walls reflect sound (echogenicity)—poor echogenicity is an indication of lipid content, and high echogenicity is an indication of calcification and collagen. Low echogenicity also predicts cardiovascular events but does not correlate well with IMT and thus provides complementary information. Echogenicity may be more strongly related to inflammatory and lipid factors, whereas IMT is more strongly related to blood pressure and smoking history. The investigators measured serum concentrations of 16 PCB congeners and other POPs in 990 participants, all 70 years old. The evaluated PCBs were detectable in more than 90% of the study population. The authors analyzed individual congeners and a summary score based on dioxin TEQs. Statistical models adjusted for sex, waist circumference, BMI, blood glucose, systolic and diastolic blood pressure, HDL and LDL cholesterol, serum triglycerides, smoking, and use of antihypertensive drugs and HMG CoA reductase inhibitors. Concentrations of seven POPs were associated with the presence of plaque, but there was no clear correspondence with dioxin activity. Plaque presence was most strongly associated with pollutants that have six or more chlorine atoms. Total dioxin TEQs were not associated with plaque, but TEQs of mono-ortho-substituted PCBs were. The prevalence of plaque increased by 67% for every natural-log increase in the serum concentration of these substances (OR = 1.67, 95% CI 1.20–2.32). Total TEQs were significantly associated with IMT (p = 0.009). Among the substances measured, TEQs from dioxin-like coplanar non-ortho-substituted PCBs were more strongly related to IMT than those of mono-ortho-substituted PCBs. Echogenicity was inversely associated with the concentrations of PCB 126, a PCB that has strong dioxin-like properties, and of the highly-chlorinated PCBs. Total TEQs were also strongly and inversely associated with echogenicity (p = 0.001). The association was restricted to TEQs of dioxin-like coplanar non-ortho-substituted PCBs.

Case-Control Studies No case-control studies of exposure to the COIs and ischemic heart disease have been published since *Update 2010*.

Other Reviewed Studies In a further analysis of the survey of Taiwanese residents of an area that had heavy dioxin contamination, Chang et al. (2011b) related serum dioxin TEQs, based on PCDDs and PCDFs, to future cardiovascular disease risk by examining relationships with individual risk factors and with the Framingham risk score, which is used in the United States to estimate 10-year risk of CVD. Compared with those who had dioxin TEQs in the lowest 25th percentile, those in the 75th percentile had more than 6 times the odds of being at high cardiovascular risk (OR = 6.22, 95% CI 2.47–15.63). However, there did not appear to be an increase in serum cholesterol, compared with the general population, in Taiwanese workers who were exposed to very high dioxin TEQ concentrations (Chang et al., 2012).

Obesity, blood pressure, and diabetes are all risk factors for IHD, and findings related to their associations with the COIs have been summarized in the previous sections (Chang et al. 2010, 2011a, 2012; Goncharov et al., 2011; Lee et al., 2011a, 2012a; Rönn et al., 2011).

Cerebrovascular Disease and Stroke

Vietnam-Veteran Studies No Vietnam-veteran studies addressing exposure to the COIs and cerebrovascular disease and stroke have been published since *Update 2010*.

Occupational Studies Several of the occupational studies summarized above also presented data on cerebrovascular-disease mortality, which is due primarily to stroke. Neither Ruder and Yiin (2011) nor Boers et al. (2012) observed an increase in cerebrovascular deaths among the workers compared to the general population (SMR = 1.00, 95% CI 0.61–1.54; SMR = 0.98, 95% CI 0.83–1.16, respectively). Manuwald et al. (2012), however, observed a significantly higher-than-expected mortality from cerebrovascular disease in 1,149 male workers (54 deaths, SMR = 1.57, 95% CI 1.19–2.05)—but not in the 388 female workers (11 deaths, SMR = 0.64. 95% CI 0.32–1.15).

Environmental Studies The PIVUS investigators (Lee et al., 2012b) examined the relationship between POPs in 898 70-year-old residents of Uppsala, Sweden, and their incidence of stroke 5 years later. The investigators measured 16 PCBs, OCDD, and 4 other pollutants. Thirty-five participants developed stroke; stroke subtype was not determined. All ORs discussed below were adjusted for gender, BMI, cigarette-smoking, exercise, alcohol consumption, hypertension, diabetes, triglycerides, and serum cholesterol. Plasma concentrations of OCDD and of most PCBs with fewer than seven chlorine atoms were positively related to stroke risk. Participants in the highest 25th percentile of OCDD had 3.5 times the odds of developing stroke compared with those in the lowest 25th percentile (95% CI 1.1–11.7). Both chemicals that had dioxin-like properties and those that did not were positively associated with stroke. Total TEQs, however, were strongly associated with stroke risk. Participants in the highest 25th percentile of TEQs had

3.8 times the odds of developing stroke compared with those in the lowest 25th percentile (95% CI 1.2–12.2). Those with TEQs at or above the 90th percentile had 4.2 times the odds of developing stroke (95% CI 1.1–15.8). Stroke risk was also greater in participants that had higher concentrations of chlorine-containing pesticides.

Sergeev and Carpenter (2010) examined the rates of hospitalization for stroke with comorbid diabetes in New York state during a 12-year period. Rates were analyzed according to proximity to environmental sources of POPs. No specific exposure to the COIs was documented, and the committee did not consider the paper further.

Case-Control Studies No case-control studies of exposure to the COIs and cerebrovascular disease or stroke have been published since *Update 2010*.

Biologic Plausibility

Studies have demonstrated that both the vasculature and adipose tissue are targets of TCDD toxicity and provided a mechanistic understanding of how TCDD exposure increases the risk of circulatory diseases, such as hypertension, IHD, and stroke. TCDD exposure of cultured endothelial cells or cultured adipocytes induces major changes in gene expression and leads to substantial increases in oxidative stress and inflammatory markers (Andersson et al., 2011; Han et al., 2012; Ishimura et al., 2009; Kerley-Hamilton et al., 2012a; Kim MJ et al., 2012; Kopf and Walker, 2010; Majkova et al., 2009; Puga et al., 2004). Notably, loss of the AHR, as in AHR knockout mice, is associated with decreases in blood pressure (modeling hypotension), while sustained activation of the AHR resulting from dioxin exposure leads to increases in blood pressure. Agbor et al. (2011). Zhang et al. (2010) showed that the genetic loss of AHR from all tissues or solely from endothelial cells, respectively, results in hypotension. In contrast, Kopf et al. (2010) demonstrated that chronic exposure of mice to TCDD induces hypertension associated with significant increases in vascular oxidative stress and decreases in vascular relaxation. Those changes in vascular function and blood pressure could be mediated in part by increases in metabolism of arachidonic acid to vasoconstrictive and inflammatory eicosanoids (Bui et al., 2012). Studies have also demonstrated that exposure to AHR agonists, including TCDD and benzo[a]pyrene, increases the incidence, severity, and progression of atherosclerosis, a primary cause of IHD and stroke (Dalton et al., 2001; Kerley-Hamilton et al., 2012a; Wu et al., 2011). Furthermore, Wu et al. (2011) demonstrated that TCDD mediates those affects in part by increasing vascular inflammation. In addition to the vasculature, studies have suggested that the heart is a target of TCDD. TCDD exposure increases hypertrophy of rat cardiac cells in culture (Zordoky and El-Kadi, 2010) and impairs the differentiation of mouse embryonic stem cells into cardiomyocytes (Neri et al., 2011).

In addition to direct effects of TCDD on the vasculature and heart, there is evidence that TCDD influences other CVD risk factors, for example, promoting obesity (Kerley-Hamilton et al., 2012b), accumulating macrophage lipid, inducing lipid mobilization, and altering lipid metabolism. Thus, on the basis of animal models, there appear to be several overlapping and potentially contributing pathways that link TCDD exposure and increased CVD risk.

Synthesis

In this section, the committee synthesizes information on circulatory disorders from the new studies described above and reconsiders studies that were reviewed in previous updates. Because circulatory diseases constitute a broad group of diverse conditions, hypertension, IHD, and stroke are discussed separately so that the new studies can be adequately synthesized and integrated with the earlier studies.

Hypertension

Hypertension, typically defined as blood pressure above 140/90 mmHg, affects more than 70 million adult Americans and is a major risk factor for coronary heart disease, myocardial infarction, stroke, and heart and renal failure. The major quantifiable risk factors for hypertension are well established and include age, race, BMI or percentage of body fat, and diabetes; the strongest conclusions regarding a potential increase in the incidence of hypertension come from studies that have controlled for these risk factors. The committee responsible for *Update 2006* concluded that the available evidence was consistent with the placement of hypertension in the limited or suggestive category. Additional evidence reviewed in *Updates 2008* and *2010* reaffirmed this conclusion.

The retrospective comparisons of Korean Vietnam-era veterans with acute coronary syndrome on the basis of whether they did or did not serve in Vietnam (Kim JB et al., 2012) are not helpful in assessing whether herbicide exposure played a role in the development of hypertension. Only two relevant and informative publications have appeared since *Update 2010*. Chang et al. (2010) showed a strong relationship between dioxin TEQ in the blood and diastolic blood pressure. The strengths of the study are the large number of potential confounding variables addressed and the clear exposure to the COIs. Its weaknesses are that it is a cross-sectional survey that precludes strong causal inference because the temporal relationship between the exposure and the outcome is not known. Furthermore, surveys are prone to selection factors that may bias relationships between exposures and outcomes. Goncharov et al. (2011) examined a survey of residents of Anniston, Alabama, and found relationships between blood pressure and concentrations of many PCBs, including three dioxin-like mono-ortho PCBs. The study shares strengths and weaknesses with the Taiwanese survey, but exposures to COIs and specifically TCDD were lower in the Alabama sample. The committee did not consider a recent paper by Jones et al. (2011), because the relationship between urinary arsenic and the arsenic-containing chemical that the veterans were exposed to, cacodylic acid, is unclear.

The new relevant data are consistent with a relationship between the COIs and blood pressure. The additional supporting evidence and the strong biologic rationale affirm the present committee's placement of hypertension in the limited and suggestive category.

Ischemic Heart Disease

The committee responsible for *Update 2008* revisited the entire body of evidence on TCDD exposure and heart disease and concluded that the evidence supported moving IHD to the limited and suggestive category. That conclusion was based on evidence of a dose–response relationship in the occupational cohorts, evidence of increased risk of MI in Vietnam veterans, supporting cross-sectional survey data, and a strong biologic rationale. Evidence reviewed for *Update 2010* supported that classification.

Relevant epidemiologic findings published since *Update 2010* are sparse. The occupational studies reviewed are from studies that have been factored into the committee's previous recommendations. It is reassuring that the reanalysis of data on the Dutch chemical workers with improved exposure data confirmed earlier findings (Boers et al., 2012). The study of Korean Vietnam-era veterans having coronary angiography due to acute coronary syndrome (Kim JB et al., 2012) is not helpful in assessing whether herbicide exposure played a role in the development of IHD.

The consideration of carotid atherosclerosis in the PIVUS study (Lind et al., 2012) yielded important new information. The study was cross-sectional; in such studies, there is a concern that a subject's awareness of his disease or the disease process itself may have led to changes in behavior, treatment effects, or the pathologic process itself that modified the measure of exposure gathered at the time of the study. Thus, the exposure measured may not reflect the exposure status when the pathologic process under study started. That concern is reduced in ultrasonographic studies because carotid IMT and plaque are symptomless and not routinely assessed in clinical practice, so it is unlikely that greater IMT would cause changes that would alter serum PCB. In addition, carotid ultrasonography has been used in other cross-sectional studies of the atherosclerotic process, and risk factors identified in cross-sectional studies have been confirmed in longitudinal studies. The investigators were able to control statistically for many potential confounding factors, and this increases confidence in their results. Exposure quantified in terms of dioxin TEQs was found to have a statistically-significant relationship with increased IMT and with decreased echogenicity, both of which are independent risk factors for clinical cardiovascular disease. It is not entirely clear that the observed relationships were specific to PCBs that had dioxin-like activity inasmuch as some other PCBs were also associated with these outcomes. Nevertheless, the new data provide limited support of a link between the COIs and the atherosclerotic process.

The results of the PIVUS study support the continued placement of IHD in the limited and suggestive category. The other available studies that addressed IHD directly either are not informative or replicate earlier findings. New findings relating the COIs to blood pressure, metabolic syndrome, and possibly abdominal obesity constitute further evidence of an association. The present committee therefore decided to retain IHD in the limited and suggestive category.

Cerebrovascular Disease and Stroke

A new study linking COIs to incident stroke was reviewed by the committee for the current update (Lee et al., 2012b). Given that the committee has previously determined that major risk factors for stroke—including type 2 diabetes, hypertension, and IHD—fall into the limited and suggestive category, it decided to reexamine the total body of literature related to stroke and cerebrovascular disease. To assist in the discussion of cerebrovascular disease and stroke, which are being considered separately for the first time in this update, the studies in Table 12-3 providing the best evidence on this endpoint (in terms of design, sample size, and relevance) have been abstracted in Table 12-4.

In the PIVUS study, Lee et al. (2012b) examined the relationship between several of the chemicals that have dioxin-like activity and stroke incidence. Contrasting high and low quartiles, this study found a strong (relative risk [RR] = 3.8) and statistically-significant, albeit imprecise (95% CI 1.2–12.2) relationship between TEQs, based on coplanar and mono-ortho PCBs, and stroke after adjustment for relevant potentially-confounding factors. A statistically-significant dose–response relationship was also seen across exposure quartiles. The association was stronger for TEQ than for total PCB exposure or organochlorine pesticide exposure. The study was well designed, and the measurement of important stroke risk factors allowed appropriate statistical adjustments to be made, but it was limited by the small number of incident stroke cases (35). The authors performed their analyses on exposure measures expressed simply as the concentration of the particular PCB in serum. It is preferred to analyze concentrations on a lipid-adjusted basis because these lipophilic compounds are found in association with serum lipids. Failure to analyze the data in this fashion may theoretically have led to some exposure misclassification. Followup for the incidence of stroke was incomplete (about 80%), and this theoretically could bias the results if the exposure–outcome association differed in people not included in the followup. The TEQ values derived from the serum PCBs were much lower than those experienced by TCDD-exposed people. This low level of exposure and the concern about lack of exposure specificity might suggest the presence of confounding by

TABLE 12-4 Epidemiologic Studies Providing Best Evidence in Terms of Design, Sample Size, and Relevance—Cerebrovascular Disorders/Stroke (Shaded Entries Are New Information for This Update)

Reference	Population	Cases/N	Finding (maximally adjusted OR/RRs shown)	Strengths	Weaknesses
VIETNAM VETERANS					
US Air Force Health Study—Ranch Hand veterans vs SEA veterans					
Ketchum and Michalek, 2005	Ranch Hands, through 1999	5/1,262 RH 34/19,078 SEA	RH vs SEA: 2.3 (0.9–6.0)	• Prospective design • Population of interest • Exposure to COIs documented	• Small number of cases • Mortality, not incidence • Case ascertainment based on reported cause of death • Subtype not determined • Adjusted only for military occupation, yr of birth, smoking, and family history of heart disease
US VA Cohort of Army Chemical Corps—Expanded as of 1997 to include all Army men with chemical MOS (2,872 deployed vs 2,737 nondeployed) serving during Vietnam era (07/01/1965–03/28/1973)					
Cypel and Kang, 2010	Army Chemical Corp, 32 yrs of followup	36/4661 27/2872 6/1473	Vietnam service: Yes/No: 1.48 (0.67–3.62) Vietnam service vs US population 1.47 (0.97–2.13) Sprayers: Yes/No: 2.12 (0.37–12.3)	• Prospective design • Population of interest • Sprayers were exposed to COIs • Sprayer association adjusted for age, duration of service, rank, BMI, race, smoking status	• Small number of cases • Mortality, not incidence • No direct exposure measurement • Case ascertainment based on reported cause of death • Subtype not determined

continued

TABLE 12-4 Cerebrovascular Disorders/Stroke, continued

OCCUPATIONAL					
IARC Phenoxy Herbicide Cohort—Workers exposed to any phenoxy herbicide or chlorophenol (production or spraying) vs respective national mortality rates					
Vena et al., 1998	IARC cohort, variable followup	263/26,976; Internal comparison	TCDD exposure: Yes/No: 1.54 (0.83–2.66)	• Prospective design • Exposure to COIs documented • Evidence of increased risk with increased duration of exposure	• Mortality, not incidence • Case ascertainment based on reported cause of death • Subtype not determined • Adjusted only for age, gender, country, calendar period, employment status, age at first exposure, duration of exposure
ENVIRONMENTAL					
Seveso, Italy, Residential Cohort—Industrial accident July 10, 1976 (723 residents Zone A; 4,821 Zone B; 31,643 Zone R; 181,574 local reference group)					
Consonni et al., 2008	Seveso cohort, 25-yr followup	Zone A: 11/723 Zone B: 101/4821 Zone R: 695/31,643	Zone A vs Ref: 0.9 (0.5–1.63) Zone B vs Ref: 1.21 (0.99–1.48) Zone R vs Ref: 1.09 (1.0–1.38)	• Prospective design • Exposure to TCDD documented	• Dose extrapolated from geography • Mortality • Subtype not determined • Only adjusted for gender, age, presence at time of accident, and time period
Other Environmental					
Lee et al., 2012b	PIVUS, 5-yr incidence	35/898	$TEQ_{(75\%/25\%)}$: 3.8 (1.2–12.22)	• Prospective design • Stroke incidence • Direct exposure assessment • TEQ used • Adjustment for multiple confounders • Dose–response • Stronger effect for TEQ than all PCBs	• Small sample size • No measureable TCDD exposure (all TEQs for DLCs) • Subtype not determined • “metabolic” confounding cannot be ruled out

NOTE: BMI, body mass index; COI, chemical of interest; DLC, dioxin-like chemical; IARC, International Agency for Research on Cancer; MOS, months of service; OR, odds ratio; PCB, polychlorinated biphenyl; PIVUS, Prospective Investigation of the Vasculature in Uppsala Seniors; RH, Ranch Hand; RR, relative risk; SEA, Southeast Asia (Air Force Health Study subjects servicing elsewhere in SEA than Vietnam); TCDD, 2,3,7,8-tetrachlorodibenzo-*p*-dixoin; TEQ, some metabolic factor that is related to both the retention of POPs and stroke risk. However, no such factor is known to exist, so this is only a theoretical possibility.

It is well established that increased carotid IMT, discussed above, is a strong risk factor for stroke (Chambless et al., 2000). Biologic plausibility supporting the link between dioxin exposure and stroke is provided by a number of studies that show that exposure to dioxin or dioxin-like chemicals is associated with increased carotid IMT. Exposure to dioxin-like PCBs in the PIVUS cohort was related both to stroke incidence and to carotid IMT (Lind et al., 2012). Similarly, occupational exposure to TCDD during the production of trichlorophenoxyacetic acid was associated with increased carotid IMT (Pelclová et al., 2009). Although this specific endpoint has not been studied in animal models, it has been shown that rats chronically exposed to TCDD exhibit substantial arterial remodeling characterized by endothelial cell hypertrophy and extensive smooth muscle proliferation and inflammation (Jokinen et al., 2003), which are the same vascular changes associated with increased carotid IMT (Choi et al., 2009).

Consonni et al. (2008) reported on the 25-year mortality experience of residents exposed to dioxin through an accidental industrial release in Seveso, Italy. The mortality from cerebrovascular disease was assessed in residents of areas of high, medium, and low exposure to TCDD compared with residents of nonexposed areas in this region of Italy. The numbers of deaths by exposure zone were 11, 101, and 695, respectively, with corresponding SMRs of 0.9 (95% CI 0.5–1.63), 1.21 (95% CI 0.99–1.48), and 1.09 (95% CI 1.00–1.38). Because of the relatively small number of residents in the high-exposure zone and the rarity of stroke, the precision of the estimate for that zone is quite low; there is, however, evidence related to both the medium-exposure and low-exposure zones of an increase in stroke mortality. The strengths of this study are the documented exposure to a COI and measured TCDD concentrations that support the geographic exposure classification. The associations were adjusted for age, sex, and time but not for other stroke risk factors.

The occurrence of stroke is strongly related to age and is a rare event in populations of younger employed people. Because statistical power is related to the number of observed events, studies of any single factory or collection of factories are relatively unreliable. Under the auspices of the International Agency for Research on Cancer (IARC), Vena et al. (1998) pooled data on 36 populations of workers involved in the manufacture of chemicals associated with dioxin contamination. There were 263 stroke deaths among the 21,863 included phenoxy herbicide or chlorophenol workers. Workers who were exposed to dioxin had 54% higher cerebrovascular-disease mortality than workers who were not (RR = 1.54, 95% CI 0.83–2.66). The present committee reviewed data that updated results from several of the populations included in the IARC report. The Dutch chemical-worker study (Boers et al., 2012) has good exposure measurement, used nonexposed workers in the same plants as the referent population, and 39 total stroke deaths were observed; no association with cerebrovascular death was observed (SMR = 0.98, 95% CI 0.83-1.16). The study of Hamburg chemical workers (Manuwald et al., 2012) did find a statistically-significant 57% higher risk of cerebrovascular-disease mortality than expected in men (54 deaths, SMR = 1.57, 95% CI 1.19–2.05), but not in women (11 deaths, SMR = 0.64. 95% CI 0.32–1.15). The cohort of PCP production workers (not a component of the IARC cohort) considered in this update showed no association, but Ruder and Yiin (2011) used the US population as a referent group, which would tend to understate associations because of confounding by the healthy-worker effect. In addition to the Dutch and Hamburg chemical-worker studies, two articles published before *Update 2010* (Steenland et al., 1999; 't Mannetje et al., 2005) provided updated information on stroke mortality in cohorts that had been included in the IARC analysis. Neither publication reported a significant increase in stroke mortality in exposed workers compared with the general population; however, as noted previously, the healthy-worker effect makes the interpretation of these results difficult. None of the studies could adjust for relevant risk factors, such as smoking and BMI.

Cypel and Kang (2010) reported a 48% (RR = 1.48, 95% CI 0.67–3.62) excess of cerebrovascular-disease deaths over 32 years of followup in the Army Chemical Corps (ACC) veterans who served in Vietnam compared with those who did not. An excess in mortality (RR 2.12, 95% CI 0.3–12.3) was observed in the herbicide-exposed cohort, relative to ACC veterans who had other duties, but the estimate is imprecise due, in part, to the relatively young age of the group and the small number of deaths (36). The associations were not statistically significant, and important potential confounders were not measured. Ketchum and Michalek (2005) reported on the 20-year mortality experience of the 1,262 Operation Ranch Hand veterans who were directly involved in the spraying of Agent Orange. Their mortality experience was compared with that in almost 20,000 other Air Force veterans who were stationed in Southeast Asia during the Vietnam War. The Ranch Hand veterans had a risk of dying from cerebrovascular disease 2.3 times that of the comparison group (RR = 2.3, 95% CI 0.9–6.0, p = 0.08). Only 5 cerebrovascular deaths were observed in the Ranch Hand veterans, compared with 34 in the comparison population. The results were adjusted for age and smoking status but did not achieve the traditional 0.05 level of statistical significance. No new results on Vietnam veterans have been published since *Update 2010*.

The committee was cognizant of the limitations in the literature, including the low overall exposure of the PIVUS cohort to dioxin-like substances and questions about exposure specificity, the relative imprecision in the estimates of effect due to the rarity of stroke as a result of the age of the cohorts, and the often-incomplete control for confounding. Nevertheless—after (1) a careful review of the new evidence of a statistically-significant association in the PIVUS cohort; (2) a careful consideration of the most appropriate prior literature, which shows an overall increase in stroke and cerebrovascular disease associated with exposure to the COIs in environmental, occupational, and Vietnam-veteran populations;

(3) demonstration of biologic plausibility in human and animal studies; and (4) the strong connection between stroke and hypertension, cardiovascular disease, and diabetes, three conditions already in the limited and suggestive category—the committee voted to move stroke to the limited and suggestive category. The published data did not permit the committee to distinguish hemorrhagic from ischemic stroke, but given that only a small percentage of strokes are of the hemorrhagic type in Western populations, this was not seen to be an impediment.

Conclusion

After carefully examining the new evidence, the present committee deemed the new information to justify the continued placement of both hypertension and IHD in the limited or suggestive category. The committee concluded that there is now sufficient evidence to include stroke in the limited or suggestive category but that other forms of circulatory disease should remain in the inadequate or insufficient category.

REFERENCES[1]

ADVA (Australian Department of Veterans Affairs). 2005b. *The Third Australian Vietnam Veterans Mortality Study 2005.* Canberra, Australia: Department of Veterans' Affairs.

ADVA. 2005c. *Australian National Service Vietnam Veterans: Mortality and Cancer Incidence 2005.* Canberra, Australia: Department of Veterans' Affairs.

Agbor LN, Elased KM, Walker MK. 2011. Endothelial cell-specific aryl hydrocarbon receptor knockout mice exhibit hypotension mediated, in part, by an attenuated angiotensin II responsiveness. *Biochemical Pharmacology* 82:514–523.

AHA (American Heart Association). 2012. Heart disease and stroke statistics—2013 update: A report from the American Heart Association. *Circulation* 127:e6–e246.

Alavanja MC, Merkle S, Teske J, Eaton B, Reed B. 1989. Mortality among forest and soil conservationists. *Archives of Environmental Health* 44(2):94–101.

Alavanja MC, Sandler DP, Lynch CF, Knott C, Lubin JH, Tarone R, Thomas K, Dosemeci M, Barker J, Hoppin JA, Blair A. 2005. Cancer incidence in the Agricultural Health Study. *Scandinavian Journal of Work, Environment and Health* 31(Suppl 1):39–45.

Alberti KG, Eckel RH, Grundy SM, Zimmet PZ, Cleeman JI, Donato KA, Fruchart JC, James WP, Loria CM, Smith SC Jr. 2009. International Diabetes Federation Task Force on Epidemiology and Prevention; National Heart, Lung, and Blood Institute; American Heart Association; World Heart Federation; International Atherosclerosis Society; International Association for the Study of Obesity. Harmonizing the metabolic syndrome: A joint interim statement of the International Diabetes Federation Task Force on Epidemiology and Prevention; National Heart, Lung, and Blood Institute; American Heart Association; World Heart Federation; International Atherosclerosis Society; and International Association for the Study of Obesity. *Circulation* 120(16):1640–1645.

---

[1]Throughout this report, the same alphabetic indicator after year of publication is used consistently for a given reference when there are multiple citations by the same first author in a given year. The convention of assigning the alphabetic indicators in order of citation in a given chapter is not followed.

Anderson H, Hanrahan L, Jensen M, Laurin D, Yick W, Wiegman P. 1986. *Wisconsin Vietnam Veteran Mortality Study: Proportionate Mortality Ratio Study Results*. Madison: Wisconsin Division of Health.

Andersson H, Garscha U, Brittebo E. 2011. Effects of PCB126 and 17β-oestradiol on endothelium-derived vasoactive factors in human endothelial cells. *Toxicology* 285:46–56.

Baccarelli A, Pesatori AC, Consonni D, Mocarelli P, Patterson DG Jr, Caporaso NE, Bertazzi PA, Landi MT. 2005b. Health status and plasma dioxin levels in chloracne cases 20 years after the Seveso, Italy accident. *British Journal of Dermatology* 152(3):459–465.

Becher H, Flesch-Janys D, Kauppinen T, Kogevinas M, Steindorf K, Manz A, Wahrendorf J. 1996. Cancer mortality in German male workers exposed to phenoxy herbicides and dioxins. *Cancer Causes and Control* 7(3):312–321.

Bertazzi PA, Bernucci I, Brambilla G, Consonni D, Pesatori AC. 1998. The Seveso studies on early and long-term effects of dioxin exposure: A review. *Environmental Health Perspectives* 106(Suppl 2):625–633.

Bertazzi PA, Consonni D, Bachetti S, Rubagotti M, Baccarelli A, Zocchetti C, Pesatori AC. 2001. Health effects of dioxin exposure: A 20-year mortality study. *American Journal of Epidemiology* 153(11):1031–1044.

Blair A, Grauman D, Lubin J, Fraumeni JJ. 1983. Lung cancer and other causes of death among licensed pesticide applicators. *Journal of the National Cancer Institute* 71:31–37.

Blair A, Sandler DP, Tarone R, Lubin J, Thomas K, Hoppin JA, Samanic C, Coble J, Kamel F, Knott C, Dosemeci M, Zahm SH, Lynch CF, Rothman N, Alavanja MC. 2005. Mortality among participants in the Agricultural Health Study. *Annals of Epidemiology* 15(4):279–285.

Boehmer TK, Flanders WD, McGeehin MA, Boyle C, Barrett DH. 2004. Postservice mortality in Vietnam veterans: 30-year followup. *Archives of Internal Medicine* 164(17):1908–1916.

Boers D, Portengen L, Bueno de Mesquita HB, Heederik D, Vermeulen R. 2010. Cause-specific mortality of Dutch chlorophenoxy herbicide manufacturing workers. *Occupational and Environmental Medicine* 67(1):24–31.

Boers D, Portengen L, Turner WE, Bueno de Mesquita HB, Heederik D, Vermeulen R. 2012. Plasma dioxin levels and cause-specific mortality in an occupational cohort of workers exposed to chlorophenoxy herbicides, chlorophenols and contaminants. *Occupational and Environmental Medicine* 69(2):113–118.

Bui P, Solaimani P, Wu X, Hankinson O. 2012. 2,3,7,8-tetrachlorodibenzo-*p*-dioxin treatment alters eicosanoid levels in several organs of the mouse in an aryl hydrocarbon receptor-dependent fashion. *Toxicology and Applied Pharmacology* 259:143–151.

Bullman T, Kang H. 1996. The risk of suicide among wounded Vietnam veterans. *American Journal of Public Health* 86(5):662–667.

Burns C, Beard K, Cartmill J. 2001. Mortality in chemical workers potentially exposed to 2,4-dichlorophenoxyacetic acid (2,4-D) 1945–94: An update. *Occupational and Environmental Medicine* 58:24–30.

Calvert GM, Wall DK, Sweeney MH, Fingerhut MA. 1998. Evaluation of cardiovascular outcomes among US workers exposed to 2,3,7,8-tetrachlorodibenzo-*p*-dioxin. *Environmental Health Perspectives* 106(Suppl 2):635–643.

Calvert GM, Sweeney MH, Deddens J, Wall DK. 1999. Evaluation of diabetes mellitus, serum glucose, and thyroid function among United States workers exposed to 2,3,7,8-tetrachlorodibenzo-*p*-dioxin. *Occupational and Environmental Medicine* 56(4):270–276.

CDC (Centers for Disease Control). 1988. Centers for Disease Control Vietnam Experience Study. Health status of Vietnam veterans. II: Physical health. *Journal of the American Medical Association* 259(18):2708–2714.

CDVA (Commonwealth Department of Veterans' Affairs). 1997a. *Mortality of Vietnam Veterans: The Veteran Cohort Study. A Report of the 1996 Retrospective Cohort Study of Australian Vietnam Veterans*. Canberra, Australia: Department of Veterans' Affairs.

CDVA. 1997b. *Mortality of National Service Vietnam Veterans: A Report of the 1996 Retrospective Cohort Study of Australian Vietnam Veterans.* Canberra, Australia: Department of Veterans' Affairs.

CDVA. 1998a. *Morbidity of Vietnam Veterans: A Study of the Health of Australia's Vietnam Veteran Community. Volume 1: Male Vietnam Veterans Survey and Community Comparison Outcomes.* Canberra, Australia: Department of Veterans' Affairs.

CDVA. 1998b. *Morbidity of Vietnam Veterans: A Study of the Health of Australia's Vietnam Veteran Community. Volume 2: Female Vietnam Veterans Survey and Community Comparison Outcomes.* Canberra, Australia: Department of Veterans' Affairs.

Chambless LE, Folsom AR, Clegg LX, Sharrett AR, Shahar E, Nieto FJ, Rosamond, WD, Evans G. 2000. Carotid wall thickness is predictive of incident clinical stroke: The Atherosclerosis Risk in Communities (ARIC) study. *American Journal of Epidemiology* 151(5):478–487.

Chang JW, Chen HL, Su HJ, Liao PC, Guo HR, Lee CC. 2010a. Dioxin exposure and insulin resistance in Taiwanese living near a highly contaminated area. *Epidemiology* 21(1):56–61.

Chang JW, Ou HY, Chen HL, Guo HR, Liao PC, Lee CC. 2010b. Interrelationship between exposure to PCDD/Fs and hypertension in metabolic syndrome in Taiwanese living near a highly contaminated area. *Chemosphere* 81(8):1027–1032.

Chang JW, Chen HL, Su HJ, Liao PC, Guo HR, Lee CC. 2011a. Simultaneous exposure of non-diabetics to high levels of dioxins and mercury increases their risk of insulin resistance. *Journal of Hazardous Materials* 185(2-3):749–755.

Chang JW, Chen HL, Chang CC, Su HJ, Liao PC, Lee CC. 2011b. Predicting the risk of cardiovascular disease in people exposed to moderate to high levels of dioxin. *Journal of Hazardous Materials* 198:317–322.

Chang JW, Chen HL, Su HJ, Liao PC, Lee CC. 2012. Biochemical study of retired pentachlorophenol workers with and without following dietary exposure to PCDD/Fs. *Chemosphere* 88(7):813–819.

Chen HL, Su HJ, Guo YL, Liao PC, Hung CF, Lee CC. 2006. Biochemistry examinations and health disorder evaluation of Taiwanese living near incinerators and with low serum PCDD/Fs levels. *Science of the Total Environment* 366:538–548.

Choi YS, Youn HJ, Youn JS, Park CS, Oh YS, Chung WS. 2009. Measurement of the intimal thickness of the carotid artery: Comparison between 40 MHz ultrasound and histology in rats. *Ultrasound Medicine and Biology* 35(6):962–966.

Coggon D, Pannett B, Winter P, Acheson E, Bonsall J. 1986. Mortality of workers exposed to 2-methyl-4-chlorophenoxyacetic acid. *Scandinavian Journal of Work, Environment, and Health* 12:448–454.

Coggon D, Pannett B, Winter P. 1991. Mortality and incidence of cancer at four factories making phenoxy herbicides. *British Journal of Industrial Medicine* 48:173–178.

Collins JJ, Bodner K, Aylward LL, Wilken M, Bodner CM. 2009a. Mortality rates among trichlorophenol workers with exposure to 2,3,7,8-tetrachlorodibenzo-*p*-dioxin. *American Journal of Epidemiology* 170(4):501–506.

Collins JJ, Bodner K, Aylward LL, Wilken M, Swaen G, Budinsky R, Rowlands C, Bodnar CM. 2009b. Mortality rates among workers exposed to dioxins in the manufacture of pentachlorophenol. *Journal of Occupational and Environmental Medicine* 51(10):1212–1219.

Consonni D, Pesatori AC, Zocchetti C, Sindaco R, D'Oro LC, Rubagotti M, Bertazzi PA. 2008. Mortality in a population exposed to dioxin after the Seveso, Italy, accident in 1976: 25 years of follow-up. *American Journal of Epidemiology* 167(7):847–858.

Cook RR, Bond GG, Olson RA, Ott MG. 1987. Update of the mortality experience of workers exposed to chlorinated dioxins. *Chemosphere* 16:2111–2116.

Cranmer M, Louie S, Kennedy RH, Kern PA, Fonseca VA. 2000. Exposure to 2,3,7,8-tetrachlorodibenzo-*p*-dioxin (TCDD) is associated with hyperinsulinemia and insulin resistance. *Toxicological Sciences* 56(2):431–436.

Cypel Y, Kang H. 2008. Mortality patterns among women Vietnam-era veterans: Results of a retrospective cohort study. *Annals of Epidemiology* 18(3):244–252.

Cypel Y, Kang H. 2010. Mortality patterns of Army Chemical Corps veterans who were occupationally exposed to herbicides in Vietnam. *Annals of Epidemiology* 20(5):339–346.

Dalton TP, Kerzee JK, Wang B, Miller M, Dieter MZ, Lorenz JN, Shertzer HG, Nerbert DW, Puga A. 2001. Dioxin exposure is an environmental risk factor for ischemic heart disease. *Cardiovascular Toxicology* 1(4):285–298.

Everett CJ, Frithsen IL, Diaz VA, Koopman RJ, Simpson WM Jr, Mainous AG 3rd. 2007. Association of a polychlorinated dibenzo-*p*-dioxin, a polychlorinated biphenyl, and DDT with diabetes in the 1999–2002 National Health and Nutrition Examination Survey. *Environmental Research* 103(3):413–418.

Everett CJ, Mainous AG 3rd, Frithsen IL, Player MS, Matheson EM. 2008. Commentary on the associaton of polychlorinated biphenyls with hypertension. *Environmental Research* 108(3):428–429.

Fierens S, Mairesse H, Heilier JF, De Burbure C, Focant JF, Eppe G, De Pauw E, Bernard A. 2003. Dioxin/polychlorinated biphenyl body burden, diabetes and endometriosis: Findings in a population-based study in Belgium. *Biomarkers* 8(6):529–534.

Flesch-Janys D. 1997/98. Analyses of exposure to polychlorinated dibenzo-*p*-dioxins, furans, and hexachlorocyclohexane and different health outcomes in a cohort of former herbicide-producing workers in Hamburg, Germany. *Teratogenesis Carcinogenesis and Mutagenesis* 17(4-5):257–264.

Flesch-Janys D, Berger J, Gurn P, Manz A, Nagel S, Waltsgott H, Dwyer. 1995. Exposure to polychlorinated dioxins and furans (PCDD/F) and mortality in a cohort of workers from a herbicide-producing plant in Hamburg, Federal Republic of Germany. *American Journal of Epidemiology* 142:1165–1175.

Flesch-Janys D, Becher H, Berger J, Dwyer JH, Gurn P, Manz A, Nagel S, Steindorf K, Waltsgott H. 1998. [Aspects of dose-response relationship of mortality due to malignant regeneration and cardiovascular diseases and exposure to polychlorinated dibenzodioxins and furans (PCDD/F) in an occupational cohort study—German]. *Arbeitsmedizin Sozialmedizin Umweltmedizin* 24:54–59.

Gambini G, Mantovani C, Pira E, Piolatto P, Negri E. 1997. Cancer mortality among rice growers in Novara Province, Northern Italy. *American Journal of Industrial Medicine* 31:435–441.

Goncharov A, Pavuk M, Foushee HR, Carpenter DO. 2011. Blood pressure in relation to concentrations of PCB congeners and chlorinated pesticides. *Environmental Health Perspectives* 119(3):319–325.

Ha MH, Lee DH, Jacobs DR Jr. 2007. Association between serum concentrations of persistent organic pollutants and self-reported cardiovascular disease prevalence: Results from the National Health and Nutrition Examination Survey, 1999–2002. *Environmental Health Perspectives* 115(8):1204–1209.

Ha MH, Lee DH, Son HK, Park SK, Jacobs DR. 2009. Association between serum concentrations of persistent organic pollutants and prevalence of newly diagnosed hypertension: Results from the National Health and Nutrition Examination Survey 1999–2002. *Journal of Human Hypertension* 23(4):274–286.

Han SG, Han SS, Toborek M, Hennig B. 2012. EGCG protects endothelial cells against PCB 126-induced inflammation through inhibition of AhR and induction of Nrf2-regulated genes. *Toxicology and Applied Pharmacology* 261:181–188.

Henneberger PK, Ferris BG Jr, Monson RR. 1989. Mortality among pulp and paper workers in Berlin, New Hampshire. *British Journal of Industrial Medicine* 46:658–664.

Henriksen GL, Ketchum NS, Michalek JE, Swaby JA. 1997. Serum dioxin and diabetes mellitus in veterans of Operation Ranch Hand. *Epidemiology* 8(3):252–258.

Hooiveld M, Heederik DJ, Kogevinas M, Boffetta P, Needham LL, Patterson DG Jr, Bueno de Mesquita HB. 1998. Second follow-up of a Dutch cohort occupationally exposed to phenoxy herbicides, chlorophenols, and contaminants. *American Journal of Epidemiology* 147(9):891–901.

Hsu HF, Tsou TC, Chao HR, Kuo YT, Tsai FY, Yeh SC. 2010. Effects of 2,3,7,8-tetrachlorodibenzo-*p*-dioxin on adipogenic differentiation and insulin-induced glucose uptake in 3T3-L1 cells. *Journal of Hazardous Materials* 182(1-3):649–655.

IOM (Institute of Medicine). 1994. *Veterans and Agent Orange: Health Effects of Herbicides Used in Vietnam.* Washington, DC: National Academy Press.

IOM. 1996. *Veterans and Agent Orange: Update 1996.* Washington, DC: National Academy Press.

IOM. 1999. *Veterans and Agent Orange: Update 1998.* Washington, DC: National Academy Press.

IOM. 2000. *Veterans and Agent Orange: Herbicide/Dioxin Exposure and Type 2 Diabetes.* Washington, DC: National Academy Press.

IOM. 2001. *Veterans and Agent Orange: Update 2000.* Washington, DC: National Academy Press.

IOM. 2003. *Veterans and Agent Orange: Update 2002.* Washington, DC: The National Academies Press.

IOM. 2005. *Veterans and Agent Orange: Update 2004.* Washington, DC: The National Academies Press.

IOM. 2007. *Veterans and Agent Orange: Update 2006.* Washington, DC: The National Academies Press.

IOM. 2009. *Veterans and Agent Orange: Update 2008.* Washington, DC: The National Academies Press.

IOM. 2012. *Veterans and Agent Orange: Update 2010.* Washington, DC: The National Academies Press.

Ishimura R, Kawakami T, Ohsako S, Tohyama C. 2009. Dioxin-induced toxicity on vascular remodeling of the placenta. *Biochemical Pharmacology* 77(4):660–669.

Jokinen MP, Walker NJ, Brix AE, Sells DM, Haseman JK, Nyska A. 2003. Increase in cardiovascular pathology in female Sprague-Dawley rats following chronic treatment with 2,3,7,8-tetrachlorodibenzo-*p*-dioxin and 3,3',4,4',5-pentachlorobiphenyl. *Cardiovascular Toxicology* 3(4):299–310.

Jones MR, Tellez-Plaza M, Sharrett AR, Guallar E, Navas-Acien A. 2011. Urine arsenic and hypertension in US adults. The 2003–2008 National Health and Nutrition Examination Survey. *Epidemiology* 22:153–161.

Jørgensen ME, Borch-Johnsen K, Bjerregaard P. 2008. A cross-sectional study of the association between persistent organic pollutants and glucose intolerance among Greenland Inuit. *Diabetologia* 51(8):1416–1422.

Kang HK, Dalager NA, Needham LL, Patterson DG, Lees PSJ, Yates K, Matanoski GM. 2006. Health status of Army Chemical Corps Vietnam veterans who sprayed defoliant in Vietnam. *American Journal of Industrial Medicine* 49(11):875–884.

Karouna-Renier NK, Rao KR, Lanza JJ, Davis DA, Wilson PA. 2007. Serum profiles of PCDDs and PCDFs, in individuals near the escambia wood treatment company superfund site in Pensacola, FL. *Chemosphere* 69(8):1312–1319.

Kerley-Hamilton JS, Trask HW, Ridley CJ, Dufour E, Lesseur C, Ringelberg CS, Moodie KL, Shipman SL, Korc M, Gui J, Shworak NW, Tomlinson CR. 2012a. Inherent and benzo[a]pyrene-induced differential aryl hydrocarbon receptor signaling greatly affects life span, atherosclerosis, cardiac gene expression, and body and heart growth in mice. *Toxicological Sciences* 126(2):391–404.

Kerley-Hamilton JS, Trask HW, Ridley CJ, Dufour E, Ringelberg CS, Nurinova N, Wong D, Moodie KL, Shipman SL, Moore JH, Korc M, Shworak NW, Tomlinson CR. 2012b. Obesity is mediated by differential aryl hydrocarbon receptor signaling in mice fed a Western diet. *Environmental Health Perspectives* 120(9):1252–1259.

Kern PA, Said S, Jackson WG Jr, Michalek JE. 2004. Insulin sensitivity following Agent Orange exposure in Vietnam veterans with high blood levels of 2,3,7,8-tetrachlorodibenzo-*p*-dioxin. *Journal of Clinical Endocrinology and Metabolism* 89(9):4665–4672.

Ketchum NS, Michalek JE. 2005. Postservice mortality of Air Force veterans occupationally exposed to herbicides during the Vietnam War: 20-year follow-up results. *Military Medicine* 170(5):406–413.

Kim JB, Kang WY, Moon SG, Kim HJ, Kim KH, Kim YH, Hwang SH, Hwang SH, Kim W. 2012. Clinical outcome of veterans with acute coronary syndrome who had been exposed to Agent Orange. *Chonnam Medical Journal* 48(1):47–51.

Kim JS, Lim HS, Cho SI, Cheong HK, Lim MK. 2003. Impact of Agent Orange exposure among Korean Vietnam veterans. *Industrial Health* 41(3):149–157.

Kim MJ, Pelloux V, Guyot E, Tordjman J, Bui LC, Chevallier A, Forest C, Benelli C, Clément K, Robert Barouki. 2012. Inflammatory pathway genes belong to major targets of persistent organic pollutants in adipose cells. *Environmental Health Perspectives* 120(4):501–514.

Kitamura K, Kikuchi Y, Watanabe S, Waechter G, Sakurai H, Takada T. 2000. Health effects of chronic exposure to polychlorinated dibenzo-*p*-dioxins (PCDD), dibenzofurans (PCDF) and coplanar PCB (Co-PCB) of municipal waste incinerator workers. *Journal of Epidemiology* 10(4):262–270.

Kogan M, Clapp R. 1985. *Mortality Among Vietnam Veterans in Massachusetts, 1972–1983*. Boston, MA: Massachusetts Office of the Commissioner of Veterans Services, Agent Orange Program.

Kogevinas M, Becher H, Benn T, Bertazzi P, Boffetta P, Bueno de Mesquita H, Coggon D, Colin D, Flesch-Janys D, Fingerhut M, Green L, Kauppinen T, Littorin M, Lynge E, Mathews J, Neuberger M, Pearce N, Saracci R. 1997. Cancer mortality in workers exposed to phenoxy herbicides, chlorophenols, and dioxins: An expanded and updated international cohort study. *American Journal of Epidemiology* 145(12):1061–1075.

Kopf PG, Walker MK. 2010. 2,3,7,8-tetrachlorodibenzo-*p*-dioxin increases reactive oxygen species production in human endothelial cells via induction of cytochrome P4501A1. *Toxicology and Applied Pharmacology* 245(1):91–99.

Kopf PG, Scott JA, Agbor LN, Boberg JR, Elased KM, Huwe JK, Walker MK. 2010. Cytochrome P4501A1 is required for vascular dysfunction and hypertension induced by 2,3,7,8-tetrachlorodibenzo-*p*-dioxin. *Toxicological Sciences* 117(2):537–546.

Kurita H, Yoshioka W, Nishimura N, Kubota N, Kadowaki T, Tohyama C. 2009. Aryl hydrocarbon receptor-mediated effects of 2,3,7,8-tetrachlorodibenzo-*p*-dioxin on glucose-stimulated insulin secretion in mice. *Journal of Applied Toxicology* 29(8):689–694.

La Rocca C, Alivernini S, Badiali M, Cornoldi A, Iacovella N, Silvestroni L, Spera G, Turrio-Baldassarri L. 2008. TEQs and body burden for PCDDs, PCDFs, and dioxin-like PCBs in human adipose tissue. *Chemosphere* 73(1):92–96.

Lee DH, Lee IK, Song K, Steffes M, Toscano W, Baker BA, Jacobs DR Jr. 2006. A strong dose-response relation between serum concentrations of persistent organic pollutants and diabetes: Results from the National Health and Examination Survey 1999–2002. *Diabetes Care* 29(7):1638–1644.

Lee DH, Lee IK, Porta M, Steffes M, Jacobs DR Jr. 2007c. Relationship between serum concentrations of persistent organic pollutants and the prevalence of metabolic syndrome among non-diabetic adults: Results from the National Health and Nutrition Examination Survey 1999–2002. *Diabetologia* 50(9):1841–1851.

Lee DH, Steffes MW, Sjödin A, Jones RS, Needham LL, Jacobs DR Jr. 2010. Low dose of some persistent organic pollutants predicts type 2 diabetes: A nested case-control study. *Environmental Health Perspectives* 118(9):1235–1242.

Lee DH, Steffes MW, Sjödin A, Jones RS, Needham LL, Jacobs DR Jr. 2011a. Low dose organochlorine pesticides and polychlorinated biphenyls predict obesity, dyslipidemia, and insulin resistance among people free of diabetes. *PLoS ONE* 6(1):e15977.

Lee DH, Lind PM, Jacobs DR Jr, Salihovic S, van Bavel B, Lind L. 2011b. Polychlorinated biphenyls and organochlorine pesticides in plasma predict development of type 2 diabetes in the elderly: The Prospective Investigation of the Vasculature in Uppsala Seniors (PIVUS) study. *Diabetes Care* 34(8):1778–1784.

Lee DH, Lind L, Jacobs DR Jr, Salihovic S, van Bavel B, Lind PM. 2012a. Associations of persistent organic pollutants with abdominal obesity in the elderly: The prospective investigation of the vasculature in Uppsala seniors (PIVUS) study. *Environment International* 40:170–178.

Lee DH, Lind PM, Jacobs DR, Salihovic S, van Bavel B, Lind L. 2012b. Background exposure to persistent organic pollutants predicts stroke in the elderly. *Environment International* 47:115–120.

Lind PM, van Bavel B, Salihovic S, Lind L. 2012. Circulating levels of persistent organic pollutants (POPs) and carotid atherosclerosis in the elderly. *Environmental Health Perspectives* 120(1):38–43.

Longnecker MP, Michalek JE. 2000. Serum dioxin level in relation to diabetes mellitus among Air Force veterans with background levels of exposure. *Epidemiology* 11(1):44–48.

Lynge E. 1985. A follow-up study of cancer incidence among workers in manufacture of phenoxy herbicides in Denmark. *British Journal of Cancer* 52:259–270.

Lynge E. 1993. Cancer in phenoxy herbicide manufacturing workers in Denmark, 1947–87—an update. *Cancer Causes and Control* 4:261–272.

Majkova Z, Smart E, Toborek M, Hennig B. 2009. Up-regulation of endothelial monocyte chemoattractant protein-1 by coplanar PCB77 is caveolin-1-dependent. *Toxicology and Applied Pharmacology* 237(1):1–7.

Manuwald U, Garrido MV, Berger J, Manz A, Baur X. 2012. Mortality study of chemical workers exposed to dioxins: Follow-up 23 years after chemical plant closure. *Occupational and Environmental Medicine* 69(9):636–642.

Masley ML, Semchuk KM, Senthilselvan A, McDuffie HH, Hanke P, Dosman JA, Cessna AJ, Crossley MFO, Irvine DG, Rosenberg AM, Hagel LM. 2000. Health and environment of rural families: Results of a community canvass survey in the Prairie Ecosystem Study (PECOS). *Journal of Agricultural Safety and Health* 6(2):103–115.

May G. 1982. Tetrachlorodibenzodioxin: A survey of subjects ten years after exposure. *British Journal of Industrial Medicine* 39(2):128–135.

McBride DI, Collins JJ, Humphry NF, Herbison P, Bodner KM, Aylward LL, Burns CJ, Wilken M. 2009. Mortality in workers exposed to 2,3,7,8-tetrachlorodibenzo-*p*-dioxin at a trichlorophenol plant in New Zealand. *Journal of Environmental Medicine* 51(9):1049–1056.

McLean D, Pearce N, Langseth H, Jappinen P, Szadkowska-Stanczyk I, Persson B, Wild P, Kishi R, Lynge E, Henneberger P, Sala M, Teschke K, Kauppinen T, Colin D, Kogevinas M, Boffetta P. 2006. Cancer mortality in workers exposed to organochlorine compounds in the pulp and paper industry: An international collaborative study. *Environmental Health Perspectives* 114(7):1007–1012.

Michalek J, Pavuk M. 2008. Diabetes and cancer in veterans of operation Ranch Hand after adjustment for calendar period, days of spraying, and time spent in Southeast Asia. *Journal of Occupational and Environmental Medicine* 50(3):330–340.

Mills KT, Blair A, Freeman LEB, Sandler DP, Hoppin JA. 2009. Pesticides and myocardial infarction incidence and mortality among male pesticide applicators in the Agricultural Health Study. *American Journal of Epidemiology* 170(7):892–900.

Montgomery MP, Kamel F, Saldana TM, Alavanja MC, Sandler DP. 2008. Incident diabetes and pesticide exposure among licensed pesticide applicators: Agricultural Health Study, 1993–2003. *American Journal of Epidemiology* 167(10):1235–1246.

Neri T, Merico V, Fiordaliso F, Salio M, Rebuzzini P, Sacchi L, Bellazzi R, Redi CA, Zuccotti M, Garagna S. 2011. The differentiation of cardiomyocytes from mouse embryonic stem cells is altered by dioxin. *Toxicology Letters* 202:226–236.

Orchard TJ, LaPorte RE, Dorman JS. 1992. Diabetes. In: Last JM, Wallace RB, eds, *Public Health and Preventive Medicine*, 13th Ed., Norwalk, CT: Appleton and Lange. Pp. 873–883.

O'Toole BI, Marshall RP, Grayson DA, Schureck RJ, Dobson M, Ffrench M, Pulvertaft B, Meldrum L, Bolton J, Vennard J. 1996. The Australian Vietnam Veterans Health Study: II. Self-reported health of veterans compared with the Australian population. *International Journal of Epidemiology* 25(2):319–330.

O'Toole BI, Catts SV, Outram S, Pierse KR, Cockburn J. 2009. The physical and mental health of Australian Vietnam veterans 3 decades after the war and its relation to military service, combat, and post-traumatic stress disorder. *American Journal of Epidemiology* 170(3):318–330.

Ott MG, Zober A. 1996. Morbidity study of extruder personnel with potential exposure to brominated dioxins and furans. II. Results of clinical laboratory studies. *Occupational and Environmental Medicine* 53(12):844–846.

Ott MG, Zober A, Germann C. 1994. Laboratory results for selected target organs in 138 individuals occupationally exposed to TCDD. *Chemosphere* 29:2423–2437.

Pazderova-Vejlupkova J, Lukáš E, Nemcova M, Pickova J, Jirasek L. 1981. The development and prognosis of chronic intoxication by tetrachlorodibenzo-*p*-dioxin in men. *Archives of Environmental Health* 36:5–11.

Pelclová D, Fenclova Z, Urban P, Ridzon P, Preiss J, Kupka K, Malik J, Dubska Z, Navratil T. 2009. Chronic health impairment due to 2,3,7,8-tetrachloro-dibenzo-*p*-dioxin exposure. *Neuroendocrinology Letters* 30(Suppl 1):219–224.

Pesatori AC, Zocchetti C, Guercilena S, Consonni D, Turrini D, Bertazzi PA. 1998. Dioxin exposure and non-malignant health effects: A mortality study. *Occupational and Environmental Medicine* 55:126–131.

Puga A, Sartor MA, Huang MY, Kerzee JK, Wei YD, Tomlinson CR, Baxter CS, Medvedovic M. 2004. Gene expression profiles of mouse aorta and cultured vascular smooth muscle cells differ widely, yet show common responses to dioxin exposure. *Cardiovascular Toxicology* 4(4):385–404.

Ramlow JM, Spadacene NW, Hoag SR, Stafford BA, Cartmill JB, Lerner PJ. 1996. Mortality in a cohort of pentachlorophenol manufacturing workers, 1940–1989. *American Journal of Industrial Medicine* 30(2):180–194.

Rönn M, Lind L, Bavel BV, Salihovic S, Michaelsson K, Lind PM. 2011. Circulating levels of persistent organic pollutants associate in divergent ways to fat mass measured by DXA in humans. *Chemosphere* 85(3):335–343.

Ruder AM, Yiin JH. 2011. Mortality of US pentachlorophenol production workers through 2005. *Chemosphere* 83(6):851–861.

Saldana TM, Basso O, Hoppin JA, Baird DD, Knott C, Blair A, Alavanja MC, Sandler DP. 2007. Pesticide exposure and self-reported gestational diabetes mellitus in the Agricultural Health Study. *Diabetes Care* 30(3):529–534.

Sergeev AV, Carpenter DO. 2010. Increased hospitalizations for ischemic stroke with comorbid diabetes and residential proximity to sources of organic pollutants: A 12-year population-based study. *Neuroepidemiology* 35:196–201.

Silverstone AE, Rosenbaum PF, Weinstock RS, Bartell SM, Foushee HR, Shelton C, Pavuk M. 2012. Polychlorinated biphenyl (PCB) exposure and diabetes: Results from the Anniston community health survey. *Environmental Health Perspectives* 120(5):727–732.

Steenland K, Nowlin S, Ryan B, Adams S. 1992. Use of multiple-cause mortality data in epidemiologic analyses: US rate and proportion files developed by the National Institute for Occupational Safety and Health and the National Cancer Institute. *American Journal of Epidemiology* 136(7):855–862.

Steenland K, Piacitelli L, Deddens J, Fingerhut M, Chang LI. 1999. Cancer, heart disease, and diabetes in workers exposed to 2,3,7,8-tetrachlorodibenzo-*p*-dioxin. *Journal of the National Cancer Institute* 91(9):779–786.

Steenland K, Calvert G, Ketchum N, Michalek J. 2001. Dioxin and diabetes mellitus: An analysis of combined NIOSH and Ranch Hand data. *Occupational and Environmental Medicine* 58(10):641–648.

Stellman S, Stellman J, Sommer JJ. 1988. Health and reproductive outcomes among American Legionnaires in relation to combat and herbicide exposure in Vietnam. *Environmental Research* 47:150–174.

Suskind RR, Hertzberg VS. 1984. Human health effects of 2,4,5-T and its toxic contaminants. *Journal of the American Medical Association* 251(18):2372–2380.

Swaen GM, van Amelsvoort LG, Slangen JJ, Mohren DC. 2004. Cancer mortality in a cohort of licensed herbicide applicators. *International Archives of Occupational and Environmental Health* 77(4):293–295.

Sweeney MH, Hornung RW, Wall DK, Fingerhut MA, Halperin WE. 1992. *Diabetes and serum glucose levels in TCDD-exposed workers.* Abstract of a paper presented at the 12th International Symposium on Chlorinated Dioxins (Dioxin '92), Tampere, Finland, August 24–28.

Sweeney MH, Calvert GM, Egeland GA, Fingerhut MA, Halperin WE, Piacitelli LA. 1997/98. Review and update of the results of the NIOSH medical study of workers exposed to chemicals contaminated with 2,3,7,8-tetrachlorodibenzodioxin. *Teratogenesis, Carcinogenesis, and Mutagenesis* 17(4–5):241–247.

't Mannetje A, McLean D, Cheng S, Boffetta P, Colin D, Pearce N. 2005. Mortality in New Zealand workers exposed to phenoxy herbicides and dioxins. *Occupational and Environmental Medicine* 62(1):34–40.

Tanaka T, Morita A, Kato M, Hirai T, Mizoue T, Terauchi Y, Watanabe S, Noda M; SCOP Study Group. 2011. Congener-specific polychlorinated biphenyls and the prevalence of diabetes in the Saku Control Obesity Program (SCOP). *Endocrine Journal* 58(7):589–596.

Thomas TL, Kang H. 1990. Mortality and morbidity among Army Chemical Corps Vietnam veterans: A preliminary report. *American Journal of Industrial Medicine* 18:665–673.

Turunen AW, Verkasalo PK, Kiviranta H, Pukkala E, Jula A, Mannisto S, Rasanen R, Marniemi J, Vartiainen T. 2008. Mortality in a cohort with high fish consumption. *International Journal of Epidemiology* 37(5):1008–1017.

Uemura H, Arisawa K, Hiyoshi M, Satoh H, Sumiyoshi Y, Morinaga K, Kodama K, Suzuki TI, Nagai M, Suzuki T. 2008. Associations of environmental exposure to dioxins with prevalent diabetes among general inhabitants in Japan. *Environmental Research* 108(1):63–68.

van den Berg M, Birnbaum LS, Denison M, De Vito M, Farland W, Feeley M, Fiedler H, Hakansson H, Hanberg A, Haws L, Rose M, Safe S, Schrenk D, Tohyama C, Tritscher A, Tuomisto J, Tysklind M, Walker N, Peterson RE. 2006. The 2005 World Health Organization reevaluation of human and mammalian toxic equivalency factors for dioxins and dioxin-like compounds. *Toxicological Sciences* 93(2):223–241.

Vena J, Boffeta P, Becher H, Benn T, Bueno de Mesquita HB, Coggon D, Colin D, Flesch-Janys D, Green L, Kauppinen T, Littorin M, Lynge E, Mathews JD, Neuberger M, Pearce N, Pesatori AC, Saracci R, Steenland K, Kogevinas M. 1998. Exposure to dioxin and nonneoplastic mortality in the expanded IARC international cohort study of phenoxy herbicide and chlorophenol production workers and sprayers. *Environmental Health Perspectives* 106(Suppl 2):645–653.

Von Benner A, Edler L, Mayer K, Zober A. 1994. "Dioxin" investigation program of the chemical industry professional association. *Arbeitsmedizin Sozialmedizin Praventivmedizin* 29:11–16.

Waggoner JK, Kullman GJ, Henneberger PK, Umbach DM, Blair A, Alavanja MCR, Kamel F, Lynch CF, Knott C, London SJ, Hines CJ, Thomas KW, Sandler DP, Lubin JH, Beane Freeman LE, Hoppin JA. 2011. Mortality in the Agricultural Health Study, 1993–2007. *American Journal of Epidemiology* 173(1):71–83.

Wang C, Xu CX, Krager SL, Bottum KM, Liao DF, Tischkau SA. 2011. Aryl hydrocarbon receptor deficiency enhances insulin sensitivity and reduces PPAR-α pathway activity in mice. *Environmental Health Perspectives* 119(12):1739–1744.

Watanabe K, Kang H. 1996. Mortality patterns among Vietnam veterans: A 24-year retrospective analysis. *Journal of Occupational and Environmental Medicine* 38(3):272–278.

Wu D, Nishimura N, Kuo V, Fiehn O, Shahbaz S, Van Winkle L, Matsumura F, Vogel CF. 2011. Activation of aryl hydrocarbon receptor induces vascular inflammation and promotes atherosclerosis in apolipoprotein E-/- mice. *Arteriosclerosis, Thrombosis, and Vascular Biology* 31(6):1260–1267.

Zack J, Gaffey W. 1983. A mortality study of workers employed at the Monsanto company plant in Nitro, West Virginia. *Environmental Science Research* 26:575–591.

Zack J, Suskind R. 1980. The mortality experience of workers exposed to tetrachlorodibenzodioxin in a trichlorophenol process accident. *Journal of Occupational Medicine* 22:11–14.

Zhang L, Ma J, Takeuchi M, Usui Y, Hattori T, Okunuki Y, Yamakawa N, Kezuka T, Kuroda M, Goto H. 2010. Suppression of experimental autoimmune uveoretinitis by inducing differentiation of regulatory T cells via activation of aryl hydrocarbon receptor. *Investigative Ophthalmology and Visual Science* 51(4):2109–2117.

Zober A, Ott MG, Messerer P. 1994. Morbidity follow up study of BASF employees exposed to 2,3,7,8-tetrachlorodibenzo-*p*-dioxin (TCDD) after a 1953 chemical reactor incident. *Occupational and Environmental Medicine* 51:479–486.

Zordoky B, El-Kadi A. 2010. 2,3,7,8-tetrachlorodibenzo-*p*-dioxin and beta-naphthoflavone induce cellular hypertrophy in H9c2 cells by an aryl hydrocarbon receptor-dependant mechanism. *Toxicology in Vitro* 24(3):863–871.

13

Other Chronic Health Outcomes

Chapter Overview

Based on new evidence and a review of prior studies, the committee for Update 2012 *did not find any new significant associations between the relevant exposures and adverse chronic health outcomes other than those addressed in earlier chapters. Current evidence supports the findings of earlier studies that:*

- *No other adverse outcomes had sufficient evidence of an association with the chemicals of interest.*
- *No other adverse outcomes had limited or suggestive evidence of an association with the chemicals of interest.*
- *There is inadequate or insufficient evidence to determine whether there is an association between the chemicals of interest and respiratory disorders, gastrointestinal and digestive diseases (including liver toxicity), adverse effects on thyroid homeostasis, eye problems, or bone conditions.*

In previous updates that considered short-term adverse outcomes (see Appendix B), committees found

- *There is sufficient evidence of an association between the chemicals of interest and chloracne.*
- *There is limited or suggestive evidence of an association between the chemicals of interest with early onset peripheral neuropathy and porphyria cutanea tarda.*

This chapter discusses data on the possible association between exposure to the herbicides used in Vietnam—2,4-dichlorophenoxyacetic acid (2,4-D), 2,4,5-trichlorophenoxyacetic acid (2,4,5-T) and its contaminant 2,3,7,8-tetrachlorodibenzo-*p*-dioxin (TCDD), picloram, and cacodylic acid and several noncancer health outcomes: respiratory disorders, gastrointestinal and digestive diseases (including liver toxicity), adverse effects on thyroid homeostasis, eye problems, and bone conditions. The committee also considers results of studies of exposure to polychlorinated biphenyls (PCBs) and other dioxin-like chemicals to be informative if they were reported in terms of TCDD toxic equivalents (TEQs) or concentrations of specific congeners. While all studies reporting TEQs based on PCBs were reviewed, those studies that reported TEQs based only on mono-ortho PCBs (which are PCBs 105, 114, 118, 123, 156, 157, 167, and 189) were given very limited consideration since mono-ortho PCBs typically contribute less than 10% to total TEQs, based on the World Health Organization (WHO) revised toxicity equivalency factors (TEFs) of 2005 (La Rocca et al., 2008; van den Berg et al., 2006).

In previous updates, chloracne and porphyria cutanea tarda were considered with the chronic noncancer conditions. They are accepted as being associated with dioxin exposure, but when they occur it happens within a matter of months of the exposure. In *Update 2010*, the two health outcomes were moved to an appendix on short-term effects along with transient early-onset peripheral neuropathy, which had previously been discussed in the chapter on neurologic disorders.

For each type of health outcome, background information is followed by a brief summary of the findings described in earlier reports by the Institute of Medicine Committee to Review the Health Effects in Vietnam Veterans of Exposure to Herbicides. In the discussion of the most recent scientific literature, studies are grouped by exposure type (Vietnam-veteran, occupational, or environmental). For articles that report on only a single health outcome and are not revisiting a previously studied population, design information is summarized with the results; design information on other studies can be found in Chapter 6. A synopsis of toxicologic and clinical information related to the biologic plausibility that the chemicals of interest (COIs) can influence the occurrence of a health outcome is presented next and followed by a synthesis of all the material reviewed. Each health outcome section ends with the present committee's conclusions regarding the strength of the evidence that supports an association with the COIs. The categories of association and the committee's approach to categorizing the health outcomes are discussed in Chapters 1 and 2.

RESPIRATORY DISORDERS

For the purposes of this report, noncancerous respiratory disorders comprise acute and chronic lung diseases other than cancer. Acute noncancerous respiratory disorders include pneumonia and other respiratory infections; they can increase in frequency and severity when the normal defense mechanisms of the lower respiratory tract are compromised. Chronic noncancerous respiratory disorders generally take two forms: airways disease and parenchymal disease. Airways disease encompasses disorders—among them asthma and chronic obstructive pulmonary disease (COPD)—characterized by obstruction of the flow of air out of the lungs. COPD is also known as chronic obstructive airways disease and includes emphysema and chronic bronchitis. Parenchymal disease, or interstitial disease, generally includes disorders that cause inflammation and scarring of the deep lung tissue, including the air sacs and supporting structures. Parenchymal disease is less common than airways disease and is characterized by reductions in lung capacity, although it can include a component of airway obstruction. Some severe chronic lung disorders, such as cystic fibrosis, are hereditary; because Vietnam veterans received health screenings before entering military service, few severe hereditary chronic lung disorders are expected in that population.

The most important risk factor for many noncancerous respiratory disorders is inhalation of cigarette smoke. Although exposure to cigarette smoke is not associated with all diseases of the lungs, it is the major cause of many airways disorders, especially COPD; it contributes to some interstitial disease; and it compromises host defenses in such a way that people who smoke are generally more susceptible to some types of pneumonia. Cigarette-smoking also makes almost every respiratory disorder more severe and symptomatic than it would otherwise be. The frequency of habitual cigarette-smoking varies with occupation, socioeconomic status, and generation. For those reasons, cigarette-smoking can be a major confounding factor in interpreting the literature on risk factors for respiratory disease. Vietnam veterans are reported to smoke more heavily than do non-Vietnam veterans (Kang et al., 2006; McKinney et al., 1997).

It is well known that causes of death from respiratory diseases, especially chronic diseases, are often misclassified on death certificates. Grouping various respiratory diseases for analysis, unless they all are associated with a given exposure, will lead to attenuation of the estimates of relative risk (RR) and to a diminution of statistical power. Moreover, diagnosis of the primary cause of death from respiratory and cardiovascular diseases is often inconsistent. In particular, when a person had both conditions concurrently and both contributed to death, there may be some uncertainty about which cause should be selected as the primary underlying cause. In other instances, errors may arise in selecting one underlying cause in a complex chain of health events (for example, if COPD leads to congestive heart failure and then to respiratory failure).

Many study populations are small, so investigators group deaths from all noncancerous respiratory diseases into one category that combines pneumonia, influenza, and other diseases with COPD and asthma. The committee notes that an association between the group of all noncancerous respiratory diseases with any of the COIs would be too nonspecific to be clinically meaningful; at most, such a pattern would be an indication that within this broad classification the incidence of some particular disease entity might be affected by an exposure to a COI.

Conclusions from *VAO* and Previous Updates

The committee responsible for *Veterans and Agent Orange: Health Effects of Herbicides Used in Vietnam*, hereafter referred to as *VAO* (IOM, 1994), concluded that there was inadequate or insufficient information to determine whether there is an association between exposure to the COIs and the respiratory disorders specified above. Additional information available to the committees responsible for *Veterans and Agent Orange: Update 1996* (IOM, 1996) and *Update 1998* (IOM, 1999) did not change that finding.

Update 2000 (IOM, 2001) drew attention to findings in the Seveso cohort that suggested a higher mortality from noncancerous respiratory disorders in study subjects, particularly males, who were more heavily exposed to TCDD. Those findings were not replicated in several other relevant studies, although one showed an increase that did not attain statistical significance. The committee responsible for *Update 2000* concluded that although new evidence suggested an increased risk of noncancerous respiratory disorders, particularly COPD, in people exposed to TCDD, the observation was tentative and the information insufficient to determine whether there is an association between exposures to the COIs and respiratory disorders. Additional information available to the committee responsible for *Update 2002* (IOM, 2003) did not change that finding.

Update 2004 (IOM, 2005) included a new cross-sectional study of people who lived near a wood-treatment plant (Dahlgren et al., 2003). Soil and sediment samples from a ditch in the neighborhood contained dioxins and furans. Although exposed residents reported a greater frequency of chronic bronchitis by history (17.8% vs 5.7%; $p < 0.0001$) and asthma by history (40.5% vs 11.0%; $p < 0.0001$) than a "non-exposed" control group, the committee concluded that selection bias and recall bias limited the utility of the results and that there was a possibility of confounding in that history of tobacco use was not accounted for adequately.

Update 2006 (IOM, 2007) reviewed a number of studies of veterans of the Vietnam War. Mortality from respiratory diseases was not found to be higher than expected in the Centers for Disease Control and Prevention Vietnam Experience Study (Boehmer et al., 2004), in the Air Force Health Study (AFHS) (Ketchum and Michalek, 2005), and in two Australian studies of Vietnam veterans (ADVA, 2005b,c). In contrast, in the US Army Chemical Corps (ACC) cohort of Vietnam veterans, Kang et al. (2006) found that the prevalence of self-reported noncancerous respiratory problems diagnosed by a doctor was significantly increased by about 40–60%, although no differences in the prevalence of respiratory problems was found in the subset of veterans whose serum TCDD was above 2.5 parts per trillion (ppt).

In addition, *Update 2006* addressed new studies of potentially exposed occupational cohorts. No associations with respiratory mortality were found in a small subcohort of New Zealand phenoxy-herbicide sprayers included in the International Agency for Research on Cancer cohort ('t Mannetje et al., 2005). In the Agricultural Health Study (AHS), no associations between the herbicide and mortality from COPD were found in private applicators or their spouses (Blair et al., 2005). There was also an AHS analysis (Hoppin et al., 2006a) of specific pesticide exposures and the self-reported prevalence of wheeze that showed an association with "current" exposure to 2,4-D.

Several additional new AHS publications were reviewed in *Update 2008* (IOM, 2009) concerning morbidity from particular self-reported respiratory health problems: analyses concerning wheeze (Hoppin et al., 2006b), asthma (Hoppin et al., 2008), "farmer's lung" or hypersensitivity pneumonitis (Hoppin et al., 2007a), and chronic bronchitis (Hoppin et al., 2007b; Valcin et al., 2007). The 25-year followup of mortality in the Seveso population through 2001 (Consonni et al., 2008) was also considered in *Update 2008*; again there was some increase in mortality from COPD as had been seen in the earlier mortality followup reviewed in *Update 2000*.

New literature considered in *Update 2010* raised considerable concern that a pattern of COPD might be coming into focus. Cypel and Kang (2010) reported cause-specific mortality through 2005 in an ACC cohort of deployed and nondeployed Vietnam-era veterans and in a subset of the original deployed ACC veterans who reported in a morbidity study whether they had sprayed herbicide (Kang et al., 2006). Cypel and Kang (2010) reported a statistically significant excess mortality from COPD (RR = 4.82, 95% confidence interval [CI] 1.10–21.18) when comparing the deployed and nondeployed groups. A similar pattern in the deployed ACC veterans was observed when they were compared with the US male population (SMR = 1.62, 95% CI 0.99–2.51). When the subgroups of deployed ACC veterans who had and had not reported spraying herbicides were compared, the sprayers had an elevated risk for death due to the less specific category of "noncancerous respiratory system disease" (RR = 2.24, 95% CI 0.42–11.83); this was the only one of these comparisons able to control for self-reported herbicide exposure, body-mass index, and smoking status. Deaths due to CODP were lower in non-deployed ACC veterans relative to males in the US population (standardized mortality ratio [SMR] = 0.3, 95% CI 0.04–1.07); this is noteworthy because the prevalence of smoking in the nondeployed ACC veterans was about twice that in men in the US population (Kang et al., 2006). Publications evaluated in *Update 2010* that studied industrial cohorts did not report on COPD but did not find increased mortality from noncancerous respiratory diseases overall (Boers et al., 2010; Collins et al., 2009a,b; McBride et al., 2009a). In the AHS cohort, Hoppin et al. (2009) did not find increased morbidity from asthma associated with 2,4-D or 2,4,5-T use; Slager et al. (2009) found current use of 2,4-D to be associated with an increase in current rhinitis.

Table 13-1 summarizes the results of the relevant studies.

TABLE 13-1 Selected Epidemiologic Studies—Noncancer Respiratory Disease (Shaded Entries Are New Information for This Update)

Study Population	Exposed Cases[a]	**Exposure of Interest**/Estimated Relative Risk (95% CI)[a]	Reference
VIETNAM VETERANS			
US Vietnam Veterans			
US Air Force Health Study—Ranch Hand veterans vs SEA veterans (unless otherwise noted)		**All COIs**	
Mortality			
Through 1999—Ranch Hand personnel (n =1,262) vs SEA veterans (19,078) (respiratory disease, ICD-9 460–519)	8	1.2 (0.6–2.5)	Ketchum and Michalek, 2005
US VA Cohort of Army Chemical Corps—Expanded as of 1997 to include all Army men with chemical MOS (2,872 deployed vs 2,737 nondeployed) serving during Vietnam era (07/01/1965–03/28/1973)		**All COIs**	
Incidence—Self-reported respiratory disease diagnosed by doctor			
CATI survey of stratified sample: 1,499 deployed (795 with TCDD measured) vs 1,428 nondeployed (102 with TCDD measured)			Kang et al., 2006
Deployed vs nondeployed	267	1.4 (1.1–1.8)	
Sprayed herbicides in Vietnam (n = 662) vs never (n = 811)	140	1.6 (1.2–2.1)	
Mortality—respiratory disease			
Through 2005			Cypel and Kang, 2010
Deployed veterans (2,872) vs nondeployed (2,737)			
Respiratory system disease	32 vs 8	2.2 (1.0–4.9)	
Pneumonia, influenza	12 vs 6	1.3 (0.5–3.6)	
COPD	20 vs 2	4.8 (1.1–21.2)	
ACC deployed men in Kang et al. (2006) reported sprayed herbicide vs did not spray			
Respiratory system disease	8	2.2 (0.4–11.8)	
Pulmonary disease (COPD)	6	3.6 (0.4–32.1)	
Through 1991 (respiratory system disease)	11 vs 2	2.6 (0.5–12.2)	Dalager and Kang, 1997
US CDC Vietnam Experience Study—Cross-sectional study, with medical examinations, of Army veterans: 9,324 deployed vs 8,989 nondeployed		**All COIs**	
Incidence			
Physical health— ORs from pulmonary-function tests (case definition: ≥ 80% predicted value)			CDC, 1988
FEV_1	254	0.9 (0.7–1.1)	

TABLE 13-1 Noncancer Respiratory Disease, continued

Study Population	Exposed Cases[a]	**Exposure of Interest**/Estimated Relative Risk (95% CI)[a]	Reference
FVC	177	1.0 (0.8–1.3)	
FEV_1/FVC	152	1.0 (0.8–1.3)	
Mortality			
1965–2000 (noncancerous respiratory mortality, ICD-9 460–519)	20	0.8 (0.5–1.5)	Boehmer et al., 2004
US VA Proportionate Mortality Study—sample of deceased male Vietnam-era Army and Marine veterans who served 7/4/1965–3/1/1973		**All COIs**	
1965–1988			Watanabe and Kang, 1996
Army, deployed (n = 27,596) vs nondeployed (n = 31,757)	648	0.8 ($p < 0.05$)	
Marine Corps, deployed (n = 6,237) vs nondeployed (n = 5,040)	111	0.7 ($p < 0.05$)	
US VA Study of Male Vietnam Veterans Wounded in Combat		**All COIs**	
Mortality through December 1991			Bullman and Kang, 1996
Noncancerous respiratory mortality (ICD-9 460–519)	43	0.9 (0.7–1.2)	
US VA Cohort of Monozygotic Twins—Vietnam-era		**All COIs**	
Incidence of respiratory conditions, deployed vs undeployed			Eisen et al., 1991
Present at time of survey	nr	1.4 (0.8–2.4)	
At any time since service	nr	1.4 (0.9–2.0)	
Required hospitalization	nr	1.8 (0.7–4.2)	
State Studies of US Vietnam Veterans			
923 White male Vietnam veterans with **Wisconsin** death certificate (1968–1978) vs proportions for Vietnam-era veterans (mortality from noncancerous respiratory disease, ICD-8 460–519)			Anderson et al., 1986
Vietnam veterans vs expected deaths calculated from proportions for:	10		
Nonveterans		0.5 (0.3–0.8)	
All veterans		0.8 (0.4–1.5)	
Vietnam-era veterans		1.0 (0.5–1.8)	
International Vietnam-Veteran Studies			
Australian Vietnam Veterans—58,077 men and 153 women served on land or in Vietnamese waters during 5/23/1962–7/1/1973 vs Australian population		**All COIs**	
Mortality			
All branches, return–2001			ADVA, 2005b
Respiratory system disease	239	0.8 (0.7–0.9)	

continued

TABLE 13-1 Noncancer Respiratory Disease, continued

Study Population	Exposed Cases[a]	**Exposure of Interest**/Estimated Relative Risk (95% CI)[a]	Reference
COPD	128	0.9 (0.7–1.0)	
Navy			
Respiratory system disease	50	0.8 (0.6–1.0)	
COPD	28	0.9 (0.6–1.3)	
Army			
Respiratory system disease	162	0.8 (0.7–0.9)	
COPD	81	0.9 (0.7–1.0)	
Air Force			
Respiratory system disease	28	0.6 (0.4–0.9)	
COPD	18	0.8 (0.4–1.2)	
1980–1994			CDVA, 1997a
Noncancerous respiratory mortality (ICD-9 460–519)			
1964–1979	3	0.1 (0.0–0.3)	
1980–1994	92	0.9 (0.7–1.1)	
Chronic obstructive airways disease (ICD-9 460–496)	47	0.9 (0.7–1.2)	
Sample of 1,000 Male Australian Vietnam Veterans—prevalence		**All COIs**	
450 interviewed 2005–2006 vs respondents to 2004–2005 national survey			O'Toole et al., 2009
Chronic lower respiratory disease	nr		
Bronchitis	nr	2.9 (2.2–3.6)	
Emphysema	nr	2.0 (1.3–2.7)	
Asthma	nr	1.3 (1.0–1.6)	
Hay fever, allergic rhinitis	nr	1.2 (0.96–1.4)	
Chronic sinusitis	nr	1.7 (1.5–2.0)	
Other diseases of respiratory system	nr	15.4 (11.7–19.1)	
641 interviewed 1990–1993 vs respondents to 1989–1990 national survey			O'Toole et al., 1996
Asthma	nr	0.9 (0.5–1.4)	
Bronchitis, emphysema	nr	4.1 (2.8–5.5)	
Other	nr	4.0 (2.2–5.9)	
Australian Conscripted Army National Service (18,940 deployed vs 24,642 nondeployed)		**All COIs**	
Mortality			
1966–2001			ADVA, 2005c
Respiratory diseases	18	1.1 (0.6–2.2)	
COPD	8	1.0 (0.3–2.8)	
1982–1994			CDVA, 1997b
1965–1982	2	2.6 (0.2–30.0)	
1982–1994	6	0.9 (0.3–2.7)	

TABLE 13-1 Noncancer Respiratory Disease, continued

Study Population	Exposed Cases[a]	**Exposure of Interest**/Estimated Relative Risk (95% CI)[a]	Reference
OCCUPATIONAL—INDUSTRIAL			
IARC Phenoxy Herbicide Cohort—Workers exposed to any phenoxy herbicide or chlorophenol (production or spraying) vs respective national mortality rates			
Mortality 1939–1992		**Phenoxy herbicides, chlorophenols**	Kogevinas et al., 1997
21,863 exposed workers			
Men	252	0.8 (0.7–0.9)	
Women	7	1.1 (0.4–2.2)	
British MCPA Plant—Production 1947–1982 (n = 1,545) (included in IARC cohort) and spraying 1947–1972 (n = 2,561) (*not* included in IARC cohort)		**MCPA**	
Mortality through 1983 (noncancerous respiratory diseases, ICD-9 460–519)	93	0.6 (0.5–0.8)	Coggon et al., 1986
British Production Workers at 4 plants (included in IARC cohort)		**Dioxins, but TCDD unlikely; MCPA**	Coggon et al., 1991
Mortality 1963–1985 (noncancerous respiratory diseases, ICD-9 460–519)	8	0.7 (0.3–1.3)	
Dutch production workers in Plant A and Plant B, combined (Plant A, 1,020 workers; Plant B, 1,036 workers) (in IARC cohort)		**Dioxins; 2,4-D, 2,4-DP; 2,4,5-T; 2,4,5-TCP MCPA; MCPP**	
Mortality 1955–2006 (diseases of the respiratory system)	52	1.0 (0.8–1.2)	Boers et al., 2012
Dutch production workers in Plant A (549 men exposed during production 1955–1985; 594 unexposed) (in IARC cohort)		**Dioxins, 2,4,5-T, 2,4,5-TCP**	
Mortality 1955–2006 (HRs for lagged TCDD plasma levels)			Boers et al., 2012
Diseases of the respiratory system	31	1.0 (0.8–1.3)	
Mortality 1955–2006	19 vs 12	1.0 (0.4–2.3)	Boers et al., 2010
Dutch production workers in Plant B (414 men exposed during production 1965–1986; 723 unexposed) (in IARC cohort)		**2,4-D; MCPA; MCPP; highly chlorinated dioxins unlikely**	

continued

TABLE 13-1 Noncancer Respiratory Disease, continued

Study Population	Exposed Cases[a]	Exposure of Interest/Estimated Relative Risk (95% CI)[a]	Reference
Mortality 1965–2006	6 vs 15	0.5 (0.2–1.2)	Boers et al., 2010
German Production Workers at Bayer Plant in Uerdingen (135 men working > 1 month in 1951–1976) (in IARC cohort as of 1997) and women—no results		**Dioxins; 2,4,5-TCP**	
Mortality 1951–1992 (ICD-9 460–519)	2	0.9 (0.1–3.1)	Becher et al., 1996
German Production Workers at Bayer Plant in Dormagen (520 men working > 1 month in 1965–1989) (in IARC cohort as of 1997) and women—no results		**Dioxins; 2,4-D; 2,4,5-T; MCPA; MCPP; 2,4-DP**	
Mortality 1965–1989 (ICD-9 460–519)	0	0.0	Becher et al., 1996
German Production Workers at BASF Ludwigshafen Plant (680 men working > 1 month in 1957–1987) (in IARC cohort as of 1997) and women—no results		**Dioxins; 2,4-D; 2,4,5-T; MCPA; MCPP; 2,4-DP**	
Mortality 1956–1989 (ICD-9 460–519)	4	0.6 (0.2–1.6)	Becher et al., 1996
BASF Cleanup Workers from 1953 accident (n = 247); 114 with chloracne, 13 more with erythema; serum TCDD levels (*not* part of IARC)		**Focus on TCDD**	
Incidence			
Through 1989 (n = 158 men exposed within 1 yr of accident vs 161 other BASF employees 1953–1969)			Zober et al., 1994
All noncancerous respiratory diseases (ICD-9 460–419)	nr	33.7/31.0 (p = 0.22)	
Upper respiratory tract infections (ICD-9 460–478)	nr	12.0/9.0 (p = 0.00)	
Pneumonia, influenza (ICD-9 480–487)	nr	17.4/18.8 (p = 0.08)	
COPD (ICD-9 490–496)	nr	8.0/7.5 (p = 0.31)	
Mortality			
1953–1992 (noncancerous respiratory)	1	0.1 (0.0–0.8)	Ott and Zober, 1996
German Production Workers at Boehringer–Ingelheim Plant in Hamburg (1,144 men working > 1 month in 1952–1984; generation of TCDD reduced after chloracne outbreak in 1954) and women—no results (some additions to observed cancers over Manz et al., 1991) (in IARC cohort as of 1997)		**Dioxins; 2,4,5-T; 2,5-DCP; 2,4,5-TCP**	

TABLE 13-1 Noncancer Respiratory Disease, continued

Study Population	Exposed Cases[a]	**Exposure of Interest**/Estimated Relative Risk (95% CI)[a]	Reference
Mortality 1952–2007 (ICD-9 codes 460–519)	33	0.6 (0.4–0.9)	Manuwald et al., 2012
Men	25	0.6 (0.4–0.9)	
Women	8	0.7 (0.3–1.4)	
Mortalilty 1952–1989 (ICD-9 460–519)	10	0.5 (0.3–1.0)	Becher et al., 1996
New Zealand Phenoxy Herbicide Production Workers and Sprayers (1,599 men and women working any time in 1969–1988 at Dow plant in New Plymouth) (in IARC cohort)		**Dioxins; 2,4-D; 2,4,5-T; MCPA; MCPB; 2,4,5-TCP; Picloram**	
Mortality 1969–2004			McBride et al., 2009a
Ever-exposed workers	12	0.8 (0.4–1.4)	
Never-exposed workers	2	0.4 (0.0–1.5)	
Production Workers (713 men and 100 women worked > 1 month in 1969–1984)			
Mortality 1969–2000	9	0.9 (0.4–1.8)	't Mannetje et al., 2005
Sprayers (697 men and 2 women on register of New Zealand applicators, 1973–1984)			
Mortality 1973–2000	6	0.7 (0.2–1.2)	't Mannetje et al., 2005
NIOSH Mortality Cohort (12 US plants, 5,172 male production and maintenance workers 1942–1984) (included in IARC cohort as of 1997)		**Dioxins, phenoxy herbicides**	
Through 1993 (noncancerous respiratory, ICD-9 460–519)	86	0.9 (0.7–1.1)	Steenland et al., 1999
Monsanto workers (n = 240) involved in 2,4,5-T production (1948–1969) and 163 unexposed workers, results of clinical examination July 1979—morbidity			Suskind and Hertzberg, 1984
"Abnormal" outcome on pulmonary-functions tests:			
FEV_1 (< 80% predicted)	32	2.81 ($p = 0.02$)	
FVC (< 80% predicted)	35	2.25 ($p = 0.03$)	
FEV_1/FVC (< 70%)	32	2.97 ($p = 0.01$)	
FEF_{25-75} (< 80% predicted)	47	1.86 ($p = 0.05$)	
All Dow TCP-Exposed Workers (TCP production 1942–1979 or 2,4,5-T production 1948–1982 in Midland, Michigan) (in IARC and NIOSH cohorts)		**2,4,5-T; 2,4,5-TCP**	
1942–2003 (n = 1,615)	44	0.8 (0.6–1.0)	Collins et al., 2009a

continued

TABLE 13-1 Noncancer Respiratory Disease, continued

Study Population	Exposed Cases[a]	**Exposure of Interest**/Estimated Relative Risk (95% CI)[a]	Reference
All Dow PCP-Exposed Workers—all workers from the two plants that only made PCP (in Tacoma, Washington, and Wichita, Kansas) and workers who made PCP and TCP at two additional plants (in Midland, Michigan, and Sauget, Illinois)		**2,4,5-T; 2,4,5-TCP**	Ruder and Yiin, 2011
Respiratory disorders (ICD-9 codes 460–466, 470–478, 480–487, 490–519)			
1940–2005 (n = 2,122)	94	1.0 (0.8–1.3)	
PCP and TCP (n = 720)	21	0.7 (0.5–1.1)	
PCP (no TCP) (n = 1,402)	73	1.2 (0.9–1.5)	
Pneumonia (ICD-9 codes 480–486)			
1940–2005 (n = 2,122)	19	0.7 (0.4–1.0)	
PCP and TCP (n = 720)	8	0.9 (0.4–1.8)	
PCP (no TCP) (n = 1,402)	11	0.5 (0.3–1.0)	
COPD (ICD-9 codes 490–492, 496)			
1940–2005 (n = 2,122)	63	1.4 (1.1–1.8)	
PCP and TCP (n = 720)	10	0.7 (0.3–1.3)	
PCP (no TCP) (n = 1,402)	53	1.7 (1.3–2.2)	
Dow 2,4-D Production Workers (1945–1982 in Midland, Michigan) (subset of all TCP-exposed workers) excluded		**2,4-D, lower chlorinated dioxins**	
Through 1994 (n = 1,517)			Burns et al., 2001
Noncancerous respiratory (ICD-8 460–519)	8	0.4 (0.2–0.7)	
Pneumonia	4	0.6 (0.2–1.4)	
Dow PCP Production Workers (1937–1989 in Midland, Michigan) (*not* in IARC and NIOSH cohorts)		**Low chlorinated dioxins, 2,4-D**	
Mortality 1940–2004 (n = 577, excluding 196 also having exposure to TCP)	19	0.7 (0.4–1.2)	Collins et al., 2009b
Mortality 1940–1989 (n = 770)			Ramlow et al., 1996
Noncancerous respiratory mortality (ICD-8 460–519)	14	0.9 (0.5–1.5)	
Cumulative PCP exposure			
< 1 unit	3	0.6 (0.2–1.9)	
≥ 1 unit	11	0.4 (0.8–2.5)	
Pneumonia (ICD-8 480–486)	6	1.1 (0.4–2.4)	
Emphysema (ICD-8 492)	4	1.3 (0.4–3.3)	
Preliminary NIOSH Cross-Sectional Medical Study—workers in production of sodium trichlorophenol, 2,4,5-T ester contaminated with TCDD—morbidity			
Chronic bronchitis and COPD	2	nr	Sweeney et al., 1997/98

TABLE 13-1 Noncancer Respiratory Disease, continued

Study Population	Exposed Cases[a]	**Exposure of Interest**/Estimated Relative Risk (95% CI)[a]	Reference
ORs for increase in 1 ppt of serum TCDD compared to unexposed workers			Calvert et al., 1991
Chronic bronchitis	nr	0.5 (0.1–2.6)	
COPD	nr	1.2 (0.5–2.8)	
OCCUPATIONAL—HERBICIDE-USING WORKERS (*not* related to IARC sprayer cohorts)			
CANADA—cross-sectional study of self-reported prevalence of self-reported asthma (n = 83) in male farmers (n = 1,939) in Saskatchewan (1982–1983)		**Phenoxy herbicides** *Asthmatics vs nonasthmatics*	Senthilselvan et al., 1992
Phenoxyacetic herbicide use	71	85.5% vs 88.5%	
UNITED STATES			
US Agricultural Health Study—prospective study of licensed pesticide sprayers in Iowa and North Carolina: commercial (n = 4,916 men), private/farmers (n = 52,395, 97.4% men), and spouses of private sprayers (n = 32,347, 0.007% men), enrolled 1993–1997; followups with CATIs 1999–2003 and 2005–2010		**Phenoxy herbicides**	
Incidence			
Prevalence of allergic (n = 127) and nonallergic (n = 314) asthma in male farmers and commercial applicators			Hoppin et al., 2009
Men with allergic asthma exposed to:			
2,4,5-T	38	1.4 (1.0–2.2)	
2,4-D	110	1.6 (0.9–2.7)	
Men with nonallergic asthma exposed to:			
2,4,5-T	88	1.2 (0.9–1.6)	
2,4-D	264	1.2 (0.9–1.6)	
Prevalence of atopic (n = 282) or nonatopic asthma (n = 420) reported by women (> 19 yrs of age) at enrollment (1993–1997)			Hoppin et al., 2008
Women reporting atopic asthma exposed to:			
2,4-D	52	1.5 (1.1–2.1)	
Dicamba	11	1.1 (0.6–2.1)	
Women reporting nonatopic asthma exposed to:			
2,4-D	66	1.1 (0.8–1.4)	
Dicamba	13	0.7 (0.4–1.3)	
Prevalence of chronic bronchitis at enrollment (n = 654) in private applicators exposed to:			Hoppin et al., 2007b

continued

TABLE 13-1 Noncancer Respiratory Disease, continued

Study Population	Exposed Cases[a]	**Exposure of Interest**/Estimated Relative Risk (95% CI)[a]	Reference
2,4-D	78	1.1 (0.9–1.4)	
2,4,5-T	28	1.5 (1.3–1.8)	
2,4,5-TP	9	1.7 (1.3–2.3)	
Dicamba	48	1.0 (0.8–1.2)	
Prevalence of chronic bronchitis at enrollment in nonsmoking farm women (n = 21,541) exposed to:		0.9 (0.7–1.1)	Valcin et al., 2007
2,4-D	16	1.2 (0.9–1.6)	
2,4,5-T	1	1.0 (0.4–2.5)	
Dicamba	5	1.1 (0.6–2.0)	
Mortality			
Enrollment through 2007, vs state rates			Waggoner et al., 2011
Respiratory system diseases			
Applicators (n = 1,641)	346	0.4 (0.3–0.4)	
Spouses (n = 676)	92	0.3 (0.2–0.4)	
Pneumonia			
Applicators (n = 1,641)	76	0.4 (0.3–0.5)	
Spouses (n = 676)	17	0.3 (0.2–0.5)	
COPD			
Applicators (n = 1,641)	165	0.3 (0.3–0.4)	
Spouses (n = 676)	50	0.3 (0.2–0.4)	
Asthma			
Applicators (n = 1,641)	8	0.8 (0.3–1.6)	
Other respiratory diseases			
Applicators (n = 1,641)	97	0.6 (0.5–0.7)	
Spouses (n = 676)	21	0.4 (0.3–0.6)	
Enrollment through 2000, vs state rates			Blair et al., 2005
Private applicators (men and women)	50	0.2 (0.2–0.3)	
Spouses of private applicators (> 99% women)	15	0.3 (0.2–0.7)	
US Department of Agriculture Workers—nested case-control study of white men dying 1970–1979 of noncancerous respiratory diseases (ICD-8 460–519)		**Herbicides**	
Forest conservationists	80	0.8 (0.6–1.0)	Alavanja et al., 1989
Florida Licensed Pesticide Applicators (common phenoxy use assumed but not documented; had been listed by Blair et al., 1983)		**Herbicides**	
Pesticide applicators in Florida licensed 1965–1966 (n = 3,827)—mortality through 1976 from noncancerous respiratory diseases (ICD-8 460–519)	2	**Herbicides** 0.9 (nr)	Blair et al., 1983

TABLE 13-1 Noncancer Respiratory Disease, continued

Study Population	Exposed Cases[a]	**Exposure of Interest**/Estimated Relative Risk (95% CI)[a]	Reference
Any pesticide (dose-response by length of licensure)	8	0.6 (nr)	
< 10 yrs	8	1.5 (nr)	
10–19 yrs	4	1.7 (nr)	
≥ 20 yrs			
ENVIRONMENTAL			
Seveso, Italy Residential Cohort—Industrial accident July 10, 1976 (723 residents Zone A; 4,821 Zone B; 31,643 Zone R; 181,574 local reference group) (ICD-9 171)		**TCDD**	
Mortality			
25-yr followup to 2001—men and women			Consonni et al., 2008
Respiratory disease (ICD-9 460–519)			
Zone A	9	1.4 (0.7–2.7)	
Zone B	48	1.0 (0.8–1.4)	
Zone R	341	1.0 (0.9–1.1)	
COPD (ICD-9 490–493)			
Zone A	7	2.5 (1.2–5.3)	
Zone B	26	1.3 (0.9–1.9)	
Zone R	175	1.2 (1.0–1.4)	
20-yr followup to 1996			Bertazzi et al., 2001
Respiratory disease (ICD-9 460–519)	44	1.0 (0.8–1.4)	
Zone A	9	1.9 (1.0–3.6)	
Zone B	35	1.3 (0.9–2.0)	
COPD (ICD-9 490–493)	29	1.5 (1.1–2.2)	
Zone A	7	3.3 (1.6–6.9)	
Zone B	22	1.3 (0.9–2.0)	
15-yr followup to 1991—men			Bertazzi et al., 1998
Respiratory disease (ICD-9 460–519)			
Zone A	5	2.4 (1.0–5.7)	
Zone B	13	0.7 (0.4–1.2)	
Zone R	133	1.1 (0.9–1.3)	
COPD (ICD-9 490–493)			
Zone A	4	3.7 (1.4–9.8)	
Zone B	9	1.0 (0.5–1.9)	
Zone R	74	1.2 (0.9–1.5)	
15-yr followup to 1991—women			Bertazzi et al., 1998
Respiratory disease (ICD-9 460–519)			
Zone A	2	1.3 (0.3–5.3)	
Zone B	10	1.0 (0.5–1.9)	
Zone R	84	1.0 (0.8–1.2)	
COPD (ICD-9 490–493)			
Zone A	1	2.1 (0.3–14.9)	

continued

TABLE 13-1 Noncancer Respiratory Disease, continued

Study Population	Exposed Cases[a]	**Exposure of Interest**/Estimated Relative Risk (95% CI)[a]	Reference
Zone B	8	2.5 (1.2–5.0)	
Zone R	37	1.3 (0.9–1.9)	
10-yr followup to 1986—men (Zones A, B, R)			Bertazzi et al., 1989a
Respiratory disease (ICD-9 460–519)	55	1.0 (0.7–1.3)	
Pneumonia (ICD-9 480–486)	14	0.9 (0.5–1.5)	
COPD (ICD-9 490–493)	31	1.1 (0.8–1.7)	
10-yr followup to 1986—women (Zones A, B, R)			Bertazzi et al., 1989a
Respiratory disease (ICD-9 460–519)	24	1.0 (0.7–1.6)	
Pneumonia (ICD-9 480–486)	9	0.8 (0.4–1.6)	
COPD (ICD-9 490–493)	8	1.0 (0.5–2.2)	
Cross-sectional study of residents near wood treatment plant (creosote, PCP) in Mississippi, who were plaintiffs (n = 199) in lawsuit vs subjects in comparable area (n = 115) without known exposures		**Dioxin, furans** Prevalence in exposed vs nonexposed	Dahlgren et al., 2003
Chronic bronchitis			
By history		21.7% vs 4.3% ($p < 0.0001$)	
Diagnosed by physician		17.8% vs 5.8% ($p < 0.0001$)	
Chronic bronchitis			
By history		40.5% vs 11.0% ($p < 0.0001$)	
Diagnosed by physician		13.1% vs 12.0% ns	
Other International Environmental Studies			
SWEDEN			
Swedish fishermen (high consumption of fish with persistent organochlorines)		**Organochlorine compounds**	Svensson et al., 1995
Mortality			
East Coast	4	0.5 (0.1–1.2)	
West Coast	43	0.8 (0.6–1.1)	

NOTE: 2,4-D, 2,4-dichlorophenoxyacetic acid; 2,4-DP, dichlorprop; 2,4,5-T, 2,4,5-trichlorophenoxyacetic acid; 2,4,5-TCP, 2,4,5-trichlorophenol; 2,4,5-TP, 2-(2,4,5-trichlorophenoxy) propionic acid; 2,5-DCP, 2,5-dichlorophenol; CATI, computer-assisted telephone interviewing; CI, confidence interval; COI, chemical of interest; COPD, chronic obstructive pulmonary disease; FEF_{25-75}, forced midexpiratory flow; FEV_1, forced expiratory volume in 1 second; FVC, forced vital capacity; HR, hazard ratio; IARC, International Agency for Research on Cancer; ICD-8, *International Classification of Diseases, Eighth Revision*; ICD-9, *International Classification of Diseases, Ninth Revision*; MCPA, 2-methyl-4-chlorophenoxyacetic acid; MCPB, 4-(4-chloro-2-methylphenoxy)butanoic acid; MCPP, methylchlorophenoxypropionic acid; MOS, months of service; NIOSH, National Institute for Occupational Safety and Health; nr, not reported; ns, not significant; OR, odds ratio; PCP, pentachlorophenol; SEA, Southeast Asia; TCDD, 2,3,7,8-tetrachlorodibenzo-*p*-dioxin; TCP, trichlorophenol; VA, US Department of Veterans Affairs.

[a]Given when available; results other than estimated risk explained individually.

Update of the Epidemiologic Literature

Vietnam-Veteran, Environmental, and Case-Control Studies

No Vietnam-veteran studies, environmental studies, or case-control studies of exposure to the COIs and respiratory disorders have been published since *Update 2010*.

Occupational Studies

Ruder and Yiin (2011) reported COPD mortality from 1940 to 2005, relative to US referent rates, in a cohort of 2,122 US pentachlorophenol (PCP) production workers in four plants in the National Institute for Occupational Safety and Health (NIOSH) dioxin cohort. The workers in all four plants were exposed to PCP and to its contaminating polychlorinated dibenzo-*p*-dioxins and dibenzofurans (PCDDs and PCDFs). An all-male subcohort of 720 in two plants was also exposed to TCDD, a contaminant of trichlorophenol (TCP) used in production processes in the plants. Deaths from all nonmalignant respiratory diseases did not differ from US rates in the PCP-only group (21 deaths, SMR = 0.73, 95% CI 0.45–1.11) or for the PCP-plus-TCDD group (73 deaths, SMR = 1.15, 95% CI 0.90–1.45). In the PCP-plus-TCDD group, no increase was reported in COPD (10 deaths, SMR = 0.68, 95% CI 0.33–1.25) or in pneumonia (8 deaths, SMR = 0.90, 95% CI 0.39–1.77). In the PCP-only group, there were excess deaths due to COPD (53 deaths, SMR = 1.71, 95% CI 1.28–2.24) but a decrease of marginal significance in deaths from pneumonia (11 deaths, SMR = 0.54, 95% CI 0.27–0.96). COPD mortality in the combined subcohorts was elevated (63 deaths, SMR = 1.38, 95% CI 1.06–1.77) and generally increased with duration of employment, but reached the level of statistical significance only in the third quartile of duration (182–650 days) of work in any PCP operation (21 deaths, SMR = 1.78, 95% CI 1.10–2.72). The completeness and maturity of this cohort of US PCP workers are strengths of the study. A major limitation is that no information on smoking was available, and this greatly limits conclusions regarding the contribution of these agents to the increase in mortality from COPD. Furthermore, although there was potential for occupational exposure to TEQs in the entire cohort, the subcohort that had potential TCDD exposure did not have increased mortality from COPD. As found earlier by Bodner et al. (2003), the authors noted that there was no difference in mortality between the 236 workers who had diagnoses of chloracne and other workers.

Boers et al. (2012) reported on the mortality experience of workers in two chlorophenoxy-herbicide plants in the Netherlands by using semi-quantitative measures of TCDD exposure. Factory A had 1,167 workers from 1955 to 1985 and produced 2,4,5-T and 2,4,5-TCP, which can be contaminated with TCDD. Factory B had 1,143 workers from 1965 to 1986 and produced 2,4-D, which was contaminated with dioxin congeners other than TCDD. Plasma concentrations of TCDD in 187 workers were used to develop a predictive model for TCDD exposure at the end of employment for each worker, and a Cox proportional-hazards model was used to investigate associations between time-varying TCDD exposure and cause-specific mortality. No relationship was found between TCDD exposure and respiratory diseases. Hazard ratios (HRs) for predicted TCDD concentrations and diseases of the respiratory system were not increased in the entire cohort (HR = 0.97, 95% CI 0.81–1.15 for each unit increase in TCDD exposure on the log scale) and in workers in Factory A (HR = 1.04, 95% CI 0.84–1.28). This publication was a followup of an earlier article on this updated cohort (Boers et al., 2010); it used exposed versus nonexposed exposure categories based on job classification and found that the exposed did not have significantly increased risks of nonmalignant diseases of the respiratory system.

Manuwald et al. (2012) updated mortality though 2007 in a cohort of 1,589 male and female workers employed for at least 3 months during 1952–1984 in a factory in Hamburg, Germany, that produced various herbicides and insecticides, including 2,4,5-T contaminated with TCDD and other higher-chlorinated dioxins and furans. SMRs were calculated by using the population of Hamburg as a reference group. Death due to nonmalignant respiratory diseases was decreased in men (SMR = 0.60, 95% CI 0.39–0.89) and in the total cohort (SMR = 0.62, 95% CI 0.43–0.87), but the smaller group of women did not differ from the referent (n = 389, SMR = 0.70, 95% CI 0.30–1.37). The prevalence of smoking was not controlled for in this study but is suggested not to differ from that in the general population (Flesch-Janys et al., 1995). The results are in contrast with the significant increase in the SMR for respiratory cancer, cancer of the larynx, and cancers of the trachea, bronchus, and lung reported in the cohort.

Waggoner et al. (2011) reported mortality in the AHS from the time of enrollment (1993–1997) through 2007. SMRs in pesticide applicators and their spouses (89,656) in Iowa and North Carolina were calculated from state-specific rates. Death due to COPD was significantly decreased in applicators (165 deaths, SMR = 0.31, 95% CI 0.26–0.36) and their spouses (50 deaths, SMR = 0.27, 95% CI 0.20–0.35). Waggoner et al. (2011) also examined deaths due to pneumonia, asthma, and other respiratory diseases. As was the case with COPD, deaths due to pneumonia and other respiratory disease were significantly decreased in applicators (76 deaths from pneumonia, SMR = 0.40, 95% CI 0.31–0.50; 97 deaths from other causes, SMR = 0.60, 95% CI 0.49–0.73) and were null for asthma (8 deaths, SMR = 0.79, 95% CI 0.34–1.56). The AHS has been generating valuable information on the COIs for a number of years, but these results, like those in Alavanja et al. (2005) and Blair et al. (2005), are not herbicide-specific and so are not regarded as being fully informative for the committee's task.

Biologic Plausibility

Evaluation of the biologic plausibility of induction of or contribution to the development of lung diseases by COIs is hampered by the lack of animal models for studying such endpoints as COPD or asthma because these diseases usually develop in humans in response to additional co-factors (smoking and air pollution). Activation of the aryl hydrocarbon receptor (AHR) by TCDD, however, has been shown to modify expression of genes in the lung that code for inflammatory cytokines, matrix metalloproteases, and mucin production (Wong et al., 2010). These results are consistent with changes associated with a variety of lung diseases—such as bronchitis, asthma, small-airways disease, and lung remodeling (fibrosis)—and support the role of AHR activation in the development of lung injury. AHR activation in vitro in NCI H441 in the Clara cells also activates an IL-1b–to–COX-2–mediated process, which leads to increased mucin production. That process might be facilitated via differentiation of the Clara cell to a mucin-producing, goblet-like cell phenotype. One of the major clinical characteristics of COPD is mucous-cell or goblet-cell hyperplasia in the airways. MUC5AC is a major gel-forming mucin that is frequently elevated in various airway diseases (Rose and Voynow, 2006; Voynow et al., 2006). Lee et al. (2010) reported that TCDD induced time-dependent increases in MUC5AC mRNA and protein synthesis in primary normal human bronchial epithelial cells and in an immortalized normal human bronchial epithelial cell line (HBE1). Recently, Lee et al. (2011) reported that TCDD induced the expression of MUC5AC mRNA and protein and the expression of CYP1A1 in both primary normal human bronchial epithelial cells and the immortalized cell line HBE1. TCDD-induced expression of the mucin gene is consistent with mucous–cell or goblet-cell hyperplasia, which in turn is an element of the pathogenesis of COPD. It is also plausible that the induction of CYP1A1 and CYP1B1 enzymes in the lung by TCDD could result in the metabolism of several chemicals found in tobacco smoke to more toxic intermediates. Exposure to TCDD could thus increase the toxic effects of tobacco smoke and increase respiratory disease. In practice, however, this is not necessarily true, as demonstrated by Uno et al. (2006).

Acute noncancerous respiratory disorders, including pneumonia and other respiratory infections, also can be increased in frequency and severity when the normal defense mechanisms of the lower respiratory tract are compromised. Thus, exposure to chemicals that affect those mechanisms could exacerbate respiratory disorders. There is no evidence that the herbicides used in Vietnam alter such defense mechanisms. However, several laboratory studies have shown that treatment of mice with TCDD increases their mortality after infection with influenza virus (Burleson et al., 1996; Warren et al., 2000). Treatment with TCDD also suppressed the animals' ability to generate an immune response to the virus (Mitchell and Lawrence, 2003). The mechanism underlying increased influenza mortality was not related to the suppression of the immune response to influenza by TCDD but appeared to involve an increase in the inflammatory response associated with an increased flow of neutrophils into the lung (Mitchell and Lawrence, 2003). Teske et al. (2008) investigated the mechanism by which AHR activation influences the pulmonary immune response to viral infection. They demonstrated that the enhanced migration of neutrophils to the infected lung is caused by AHR-driven events extrinsic to the immune system; this suggests that AHR-mediated events within the lung influence neutrophil recruitment, and thereby alter the outcome of respiratory viral infection. Neutrophils produce several toxic products (which kill pathogens), so it is possible that excess neutrophils in the lung produce excess collateral damage and pathologic changes that increase mortality.

Chiba et al. (2012) recently reviewed the role of the AHR in the pathology of asthma and COPD. The authors suggest that AHR activation by TCDD and dioxin-like compounds in cigarette smoke promotes inflammation and the exacerbation of asthma and COPD through the arachidonic acid cascade, cell differentiation, cell–cell adhesion interactions, cytokine expression, and mucin production. Thus, it is biologically plausible that exposure to TCDD results in exacerbation of acute lung disease that is associated with reduced immune responses or of chronic lung diseases, including COPD, that are associated with increased inflammatory responses.

Synthesis

Noncancerous Respiratory Disease (Without Further Specification)

Results of the studies of mortality from noncancerous respiratory diseases reported in *Update 2008* and earlier VAO reports (ADVA, 2005b,c; Anderson et al., 1986; Becher et al., 1996; Blair et al., 1983, 2005; Boehmer et al., 2004; Bullman and Kang, 1996; Burns et al., 2001; Coggon et al., 1986, 1991; Consonni et al., 2008; Crane et al., 1997a; Ketchum and Michalek, 2005; Kogevinas et al., 1997; Ott and Zober, 1996; Ramlow et al., 1996; Steenland et al., 1999; Svensson et al., 1995; 't Mannetje et al., 2005; Zober et al., 1994) did not support the hypothesis that exposures to herbicides or TCDD are associated with the general category of noncancerous respiratory diseases.

A study of the prevalence of self-reported physician-confirmed respiratory problems in a subset of ACC personnel (Kang et al., 2006) was reviewed in *Update 2006*. Comparison of deployed with nondeployed veterans indicated an association (odds ratio [OR] = 1.41, 95% CI 1.13–1.76), as did comparison of those who reported spraying herbicides in Vietnam with those who did not (OR = 1.62, 95% CI 1.26–2.05). In the subset of subjects whose serum TCDD concentrations had been determined, however, people who had respiratory problems were evenly distributed above and below the median, and this argues against the association with herbicide exposure.

Another study of the ACC cohort (Cypel and Kang, 2010) that addressed the mortality experience of the entire cohort was considered in *Update 2010*. An increase in mortality due to respiratory disease was statistically significant when the deployed veterans were compared with men in the US population (SMR = 1.58, 95% CI 1.08–2.23). That observation contrasts with four occupational studies that did not report an association of death due to noncancerous respiratory disease with exposures to herbicides or TCDD (Boers et al., 2010; Collins et al., 2009a,b; McBride et al., 2009a). Similarly, a study of Finnish fishermen found that an increase in serum dioxin TEQs was not associated with mortality from noncancerous respiratory disorders (Turunen et al., 2008).

In the current update, four occupational studies of exposures to the COIs were consistent in reporting no increase in mortality due to pneumonia and the broad category of non-malignant diseases of the respiratory system (Boers et al., 2012; Manuwald et al., 2012; Ruder and Yiin, 2011; Waggoner et al., 2011).

The committee does not believe that scientific conclusions (other than that the evidence is inadequate) can be reached with regard to health outcomes that are defined vaguely, for example, by combining a wide array of disparate respiratory health outcomes into one large category of noncancerous respiratory disease. The nonspecificity of the respiratory conditions reported in these studies makes it exceedingly difficult to draw any conclusions regarding specific respiratory conditions.

Chronic Obstructive Pulmonary Disease

Ruder and Yiin (2011) reported a significant increase in COPD mortality, relative to US referent rates, in a cohort of 2,122 US PCP production workers in four plants in the NIOSH Dioxin Registry. The workers in all four plants were exposed to PCP and to its contaminating PCDDs and PCDFs. That no information on smoking was available, however, greatly limits conclusions regarding the contribution of these agents to the increase in mortality due to COPD. Table 13-2 summarizes the findings with the relevant information from previous studies.

In an earlier study of mortality in a cohort of Vietnam-era veterans who had served in the ACC, as of 1991, the deployed ACC veterans had a nonsignificant adjusted RR of 2.59 for death due to noncancerous respiratory diseases compared with their nondeployed peers (Dalager and Kang, 1997). The study by Cypel and Kang (2010) added 14 years of observation and found an increased risk of death from noncancerous respiratory diseases on the cusp of statistical significance (RR = 2.20, 95% CI 0.99–4.91). For COPD in particular, they reported a statistically significant excess mortality in deployed ACC veterans (RR = 4.82, 95% CI 1.10–21.18) compared with nondeployed ACC veterans. A similar pattern of excess COPD mortality in the deployed veterans persisted when comparisons were made with the US male population (SMR = 1.58, 95% CI 1.08–2.23). In accord with those mortality data, a morbidity survey of 2,927 of the ACC veterans

TABLE 13-2 Selected Epidemiologic Studies—COPD and Pulmonary Function (Shaded Entries Are New Information for This Update)

Study Population	Exposed Cases[a]	**Exposure of Interest**/Estimated Relative Risk (95% CI)[a]	Reference
VIETNAM VETERANS			
US Vietnam Veterans			
US VA Cohort of Army Chemical Corps—Expanded as of 1997 to include all Army men with chemical MOS (2,872 deployed vs 2,737 nondeployed) serving during Vietnam era (07/01/1965–03/28/1973)		**All COIs**	
Through 2005—Mortality			Cypel and Kang, 2010
Deployed veterans (2,872) vs nondeployed (2,737)			
Respiratory system disease	32 vs 8	2.2 (1.0–4.9)	
COPD	20 vs 2	4.8 (1.1–21.2)	
ACC deployed men in Kang et al. (2006) reported sprayed herbicide vs did not spray			
Respiratory system disease	8	2.2 (0.4–11.8)	
Pulmonary disease (COPD)	6	3.6 (0.4–32.1)	
US CDC Vietnam Experience Study—Cross-sectional study, with medical examinations, of Army veterans: 9,324 deployed vs 8,989 nondeployed		**All COIs**	
Incidence			
Physical health—ORs from pulmonary-function tests (case definition: ≥ 80% predicted value)			CDC, 1988
FEV_1	254	0.9 (0.7–1.1)	
FVC	177	1.0 (0.8–1.3)	
FEV_1/FVC	152	1.0 (0.8–1.3)	
International Vietnam-Veteran Studies			
Australian Vietnam Veterans—58,077 men and 153 women served on land or in Vietnamese waters during 5/23/1962–7/1/1973 vs Australian population		**All COIs**	
Mortality			
All branches, return–2001			ADVA, 2005b
Respiratory system disease	239	0.8 (0.7–0.9)	
COPD	128	0.9 (0.7–1.0)	
Navy			
Respiratory system disease	50	0.8 (0.6–1.0)	
COPD	28	0.9 (0.6–1.3)	
Army			
Respiratory system disease	162	0.8 (0.7–0.9)	
COPD	81	0.9 (0.7–1.0)	
Air Force			
Respiratory system disease	28	0.6 (0.4–0.9)	
COPD	18	0.8 (0.4–1.2)	

TABLE 13-2 COPD and Pulmonary Function, continued

Study Population	Exposed Cases[a]	**Exposure of Interest**/Estimated Relative Risk (95% CI)[a]	Reference
1980–1994			CDVA, 1997a
Noncancerous respiratory mortality (ICD-9 460–519)			
Chronic obstructive airways disease (ICD-9 460–496)	47	0.9 (0.7–1.2)	
Australian Conscripted Army National Service (18,940 deployed vs 24,642 nondeployed)		**All COIs**	
Mortality			
1966–2001			ADVA, 2005c
Respiratory diseases	18	1.1 (0.6–2.2)	
COPD	8	1.0 (0.3–2.8)	
OCCUPATIONAL—INDUSTRIAL			
IARC Phenoxy Herbicide Cohort—Workers exposed to any phenoxy herbicide or chlorophenol (production or spraying) vs respective national mortality rates			
BASF Cleanup Workers from 1953 accident (n = 247); 114 with chloracne, 13 more with erythema; serum TCDD levels (*not* part of IARC)		**Focus on TCDD**	
Incidence			
Through 1989 (n = 158 men exposed within 1 yr of accident vs 161 other BASF employees 1953–1969)			Zober et al., 1994
All noncancerous respiratory diseases (ICD-9 460–419)	nr	33.7/31.0 (p = 0.22)	
COPD (ICD-9 490–496)	nr	8.0/7.5 (p = 0.31)	
NIOSH Mortality Cohort (12 US plants, 5,172 male production and maintenance workers 1942–1984) (included in IARC cohort as of 1997)		**Dioxins, phenoxy herbicides**	
Monsanto workers (n = 240) involved in 2,4,5-T production (1948–1969) and 163 unexposed workers, results of clinical examination July, 1979—morbidity			Suskind and Hertzberg, 1984
"Abnormal" outcome on pulmonary-functions tests:			
FEV_1 (< 80% predicted)	32	2.81 (p = 0.02)	
FVC (< 80% predicted)	35	2.25 (p = 0.03)	
FEV_1/FVC (< 70%)	32	2.97 (p = 0.01)	
FEF_{25-75} (< 80% predicted)	47	1.86 (p = 0.05)	

continued

TABLE 13-2 COPD and Pulmonary Function, continued

Study Population	Exposed Cases[a]	**Exposure of Interest**/Estimated Relative Risk (95% CI)[a]	Reference
All Dow PCP-Exposed Workers—all workers from the two plants that only made PCP (in Tacoma, Washington, and Wichita, Kansas) and workers who made PCP and TCP at two additional plants (in Midland, Michigan, and Sauget, Illinois)		**2,4,5-T; 2,4,5-TCP**	Ruder and Yiin, 2011
1940–2005 (n = 2,122)	63	1.4 (0.1–1.8)	
PCP and TCP (n = 720)	10	0.7 (0.3–1.3)	
PCP (no TCP) (n = 1,402)	53	0.7 (0.3–2.2)	
Preliminary NIOSH Cross-sectional Medical Study—workers in production of sodium trichlorophenol, 2,4,5-T ester contaminated with TCDD—morbidity			
Chronic bronchitis and COPD	2	nr	Sweeney et al., 1997/98
ORs for increase in 1 ppt of serum TCDD compared to unexposed workers			Calvert et al., 1991
Chronic bronchitis	nr	0.5 (0.1–2.6)	
COPD	nr	1.2 (0.5–2.8)	
OCCUPATIONAL—HERBICIDE-USING WORKERS (*not* related to IARC sprayer cohorts)			
UNITED STATES			
US Agricultural Health Study—prospective study of licensed pesticide sprayers in Iowa and North Carolina: commercial (n = 4,916 men), private/farmers (n = 52,395, 97.4% men), and spouses of private sprayers (n = 32,347, 0.007% men), enrolled 1993–1997; followups with CATIs 1999–2003 and 2005–2010 *Mortality* (COPD)		**Phenoxy herbicides**	
Enrollment through 2007, vs state rates		SMR	Waggoner et al., 2011
Applicators (n = 1,641)	165	0.3 (0.3–0.4)	
Spouses (n = 676)	50	0.3 (0.2–0.4)	
Enrollment through 2000, vs state rates			Blair et al., 2005
Private applicators (men and women)	50	0.2 (0.2–0.3)	
Spouses of private applicators (> 99% women)	15	0.3 (0.2–0.7)	
ENVIRONMENTAL			
Seveso, Italy, Residential Cohort—Industrial accident July 10, 1976 (723 residents Zone A; 4,821 Zone B; 31,643 Zone R; 181,574 local reference group) (ICD-9 171)		**TCDD**	

TABLE 13-2 COPD and Pulmonary Function, continued

Study Population	Exposed Cases[a]	**Exposure of Interest**/Estimated Relative Risk (95% CI)[a]	Reference
Mortality			
25-yr followup to 2001—men and women			Consonni et al., 2008
COPD (ICD-9 490–493)			
Zone A	7	2.5 (1.2–5.3)	
Zone B	26	1.3 (0.9–1.9)	
Zone R	175	1.2 (1.0–1.4)	
20-yr followup to 1996			Bertazzi et al., 2001
COPD (ICD-9 490–493)	29	1.5 (1.1–2.2)	
Zone A	7	3.3 (1.6–6.9)	
Zone B	22	1.3 (0.9–2.0)	
15-yr followup to 1991—men			Bertazzi et al., 1998
COPD (ICD-9 490–493)			
Zone A	4	3.7 (1.4–9.8)	
Zone B	9	1.0 (0.5–1.9)	
Zone R	74	1.2 (0.9–1.5)	
15-yr followup to 1991—women			Bertazzi et al., 1998
COPD (ICD-9 490–493)			
Zone A	1	2.1 (0.3–14.9)	
Zone B	8	2.5 (1.2–5.0)	
Zone R	37	1.3 (0.9–1.9)	
10-yr followup to 1986—men (Zones A, B, R)			Bertazzi et al., 1989a
COPD (ICD-9 490–493)	31	1.1 (0.8–1.7)	
10-yr followup to 1986—women (Zones A, B, R)			Bertazzi et al., 1989a
COPD (ICD-9 490–493)	8	1.0 (0.5–2.2)	

NOTE: 2,4,5-T, 2,4,5-trichlorophenoxyacetic acid; 2,4,5-TCP, 2,4,5-trichlorophenol; CDC, Centers for Disease Control and Prevention; CI, confidence interval; COI, chemical of interest; COPD, chronic obstructive pulmonary disease; FEF_{25-75}, forced midexpiratory flow; FEV_1, forced expiratory volume in 1 second; FVC, forced vital capacity; IARC, International Agency for Research on Cancer; ICD-9, *International Classification of Diseases, Ninth Revision*; MOS, months of service; NIOSH, National Institute for Occupational Safety and Health; nr, not reported; OR, odds ratio; PCP, pentachlorophenol; SMR, standardized mortality ratio; TCDD, 2,3,7,8-tetrachlorodibenzo-*p*-dioxin; TCP, trichlorophenol; VA, US Department of Veterans Affairs.

[a]Given when available; results other than estimated risk explained individually.

(deployed and nondeployed) conducted in 1999–2000 (Kang et al., 2006) found a significant increase in the broader category of self-reported noncancerous respiratory conditions in deployed ACC veterans (OR = 1.41, 95% CI 1.13–1.76), which was also significantly related to reported use of herbicides in Vietnam (OR = 1.62, 95% CI 1.28–2.05); it used a multiple logistic regression model with adjustments for age, race, body-mass index, rank, and smoking. Among the deployed ACC veterans who had participated in the morbidity study, only 120 deaths had occurred by the end of 2005, so when Cypel and Kang (2010) assessed mortality associated with self-reported herbicide use, adjusted for smoking status, the estimated increase in COPD (adjusted RR = 3.55) had a 95% CI spanning 2 orders of magnitude (0.39–32).

Other studies of US Vietnam veterans, including the Operation Ranch Hand cohort, have found no significant increase in mortality due to the broader classification of noncancerous respiratory mortality (Anderson et al., 1986; Boehmer et al., 2004; Ketchum and Michalek, 2005) but have not addressed causes of death as specific as COPD. The Vietnam Experience Study (CDC, 1988) did not find evidence of compromised lung function; there have been no integrated publications on specific aspects of respiratory morbidity in the Ranch Hand cohort. Studies of the full cohort of male Australian Vietnam veterans vs the general population (ADVA, 2005b; CDVA, 1997a) and of deployed vs nondeployed Australian Army National Service (conscripted) veterans (ADVA, 2005c; CDVA, 1997b) also showed no suggestion of increased mortality from COPD or noncancerous respiratory disorders.

Almost all the studies of mortality in industrial cohorts considered in the VAO updates assessed only the nonspecific category of mortality due to noncancerous respiratory disease, and no significant excesses were reported (Becher et al., 1996; Burns et al., 2001; Kogevinas et al., 1997; Ott and Zober, 1996; Steenland et al., 1999; 't Mannetje et al., 2005). Only an earlier mortality study of Dow Chemical Company TCP workers (Ramlow et al., 1996) reported on a more specific type of respiratory death, emphysema, which was not significantly increased. Only three studies of morbidity related to COPD in industrial populations have been considered in the VAO updates. Increases in the ORs for measures of abnormal pulmonary function were reported in workers at a 2,4,5-T plant in Nitro, West Virginia (Suskind and Hertzberg, 1984), but the other two cross-sectional studies of COPD prevalence had negative findings. Zober et al. (1994) found that episodes of COPD in workers at a BASF plant in Germany were not associated with TCDD exposure. The NIOSH cross-sectional study of production workers exposed to TCDD (Calvert et al., 1991) did not show an increase in COPD or chronic bronchitis or in altered pulmonary function measures associated with increased serum TCDD concentration in workers compared with a community-based referent population.

Waggoner et al. (2011) reported mortality in the AHS from the time of enrollment (1993–1997) through 2007. Death due to COPD was significantly decreased in applicators and their spouses. An early agricultural study (Senthilselvan et al., 1992) found no relationship between self-reported asthma and the use of phenoxy herbicides. Recently, the AHS has generated a number of publications with COPD-related findings. First, Blair et al. (2005) found significant *decreases* in mortality due to COPD in private applicators and their spouses compared with state rates, which may be due to the healthy-worker effect and the inability to adjust for low tobacco use. Analyses, with adjustment for smoking, of self-reported prevalence at enrollment (1993–1997) and prior exposure to phenoxy herbicides found indications of associations with chronic bronchitis in farmers (mostly men) that were significant for 2,4,5-T and 2,4,5-TP (Hoppin et al., 2007b) but only a 20% nonsignificant increase in nonsmoking farm women (Valcin et al., 2007); some association of phenoxy herbicide exposure with allergic asthma was evident (significant for 2,4-D in women and 2,4,5-T in men), but the association with nonallergic asthma in men (Hoppin et al., 2009) or women (Hoppin et al., 2008) was not so clear. The AHS has been generating valuable information on the COIs for a number of years, but these results, like those in Alavanja et al. (2005) and Blair et al. (2005), are not herbicide-specific and so are not regarded as being fully informative for the committee's task.

Mortality studies of the Seveso incident have reported an emerging picture of increased risk of death from COPD (Bertazzi et al., 1998, 2001; Consonni et al., 2008; Pesatori et al., 1998) with higher and significant RRs found in the zone (A) closest to the accident and somewhat lower RRs in the outlying zones. Adjustment for smoking has not been possible for the Seveso cohort. In the only other relevant environmental study, Svensson et al. (1995) assumed that TCDD exposure was higher because of fish consumption by Swedish fishermen but found no increase in mortality from bronchitis or emphysema. Dahlgren et al. (2003) reported that the prevelance of chronic bronchitis was positively associated with environmental exposure to creosote and PCP emissions from a wood-processing plant, but strong concerns about bias are raised by the fact that the study sample was composed of plaintiffs in a lawsuit. There have been no other studies of environmental exposure to the COIs and COPD-related morbidity.

The large increase in relative risk of mortality from COPD in the ACC cohort that served in Vietnam (Cypel and Kang, 2010) motivated the committee to request additional information from Cypel and Kang (March 3, 2011, reply is available on request from the VAO public-access file). The committee learned that the six deaths from "pulmonary disease" among deployed ACC veterans in the morbidity study (Table 5 in the 2010 paper) were indeed COPD cases; among the nondeployed ACC veterans in the morbidity study, there had been only one death from respiratory disease, and it had not been from COPD; and all the respiratory deaths had been in smokers. Conclusions from analysis of COPD mortality in the ACC morbidity-study subset are limited by the very small number of deaths that had occurred by the end of 2005 and by the fact that this subset cannot be considered representative of the entire ACC cohort in that its members were all alive in 1999. Information on smoking status is available only on the people who participated in the 1999–2000 morbidity survey (of the 2,972 subjects, 71.5% of the deployed vs 60.1% of the nondeployed smoked), so the researchers lacked the ability to adjust the RR of COPD mortality in the entire ACC cohort (5,609). Because cigarette-smoking is the major cause of COPD, the committee viewed this as strongly constraining the conclusions that could be drawn from the ACC data overall.

The committee for *Update 2010* consulted with Paul Enright, of the University of Arizona, a medical expert on COPD. That consultation increased concern (as delineated at the beginning of this section on respiratory diseases) that causes of death from COPD are frequently misclassified on death certificates. The common presence of comorbid conditions in people who have COPD makes it difficult to deduce a single contributing cause of death. Furthermore, it was emphasized that COPD is often incorrectly diagnosed in prevalence investigations, and there is considerable debate about the appropriate diagnosic criteria for COPD, particularly in relation to the normal decrease in capacity with age (Celli and Halbert, 2010a,b; Enright and Brusasco et al., 2010a,b).

Thus, the committee for *Update 2010* concluded that it could not base a conclusion about an association with COPD on mortality data, given the questionable nature of death-certificate information on COPD and the routine inability to adjust for smoking. That committee said that additional studies of the incidence of COPD, based on rigorous criteria for its diagnosis and adjustment for smoking, would be particularly valuable in resolving whether there is evidence to support an association with exposure to the COIs.

The small amount of new data provided to the current committee did not alter its concurrence with the conclusions of the *Update 2010* committee. The Department of Veterans Affairs informed the present committee that it has undertaken a morbidity followup on the ACC cohort, taking heed of the previous committee's suggestions, but it will be more than a year before results are released.

Other Specific Respiratory Diseases

There is still not a coherent body of epidemiology evidence to support conclusions as to whether the risks of other particular respiratory problems are associated with exposure to the COIs.

Conclusion

On the basis of the evidence reviewed here and in previous VAO reports, the committee concludes that there is inadequate or insufficient evidence of an association between exposure to the COIs and mortality from all noncancerous respiratory diseases or from COPD specifically. There is also inadequate or insufficient evidence of an association between exposure to the COIs and the prevalence of respiratory diseases, such as wheeze or asthma, COPD, and farmer's lung.

GASTROINTESTINAL AND DIGESTIVE DISEASES, INCLUDING LIVER TOXICITY

This section discusses a variety of conditions encompassed by the *International Classification of Diseases, Ninth Revision* (ICD-9, codes 520–579): diseases of the esophagus, stomach, intestines, rectum, liver, and pancreas. Details on peptic ulcer and liver disease, the two conditions most often discussed in the literature reviewed, are provided below. The symptoms and signs of gastrointestinal disease and liver toxicity are highly varied and often vague.

The essential functions of the gastrointestinal tract are to absorb nutrients and eliminate waste. Those complex tasks involve numerous chemical and molecular interactions on the mucosal surface and complex local and distant neural and endocrine activity. One common condition of the gastrointestinal tract is motility disorder, which might be present in 15% of adults. The most convenient way to categorize diseases that affect the gastrointestinal system is according to the effected anatomic segment. Esophageal disorders predominantly affect swallowing; gastric disorders are related to acid secretion; and conditions that affect the small and large intestines are reflected in alterations in nutrition, mucosal integrity, and motility. Some systemic disorders (inflammatory, vascular, infectious, and neoplastic conditions) also affect the gastrointestinal system.

Peptic-Ulcer Disease

Peptic-ulcer disease refers to ulcerative disorders of the gastrointestinal tract that are caused by the action of acid and pepsin on the stomach or duodenal mucosa. Peptic-ulcer disease is characterized as gastric or duodenal ulcer, depending on the site of origin. Peptic-ulcer disease occurs when the corrosive action of gastric acid and pepsin overcomes the normal mucosal defense mechanisms that protect against ulceration. About 10% of the population has clinical evidence of duodenal ulcer at some time in life; a similar percentage is affected by gastric ulcer. The incidence of duodenal ulcer peaks in the fifth decade, and the incidence of gastric ulcer about 10 years later.

Evidence increasingly indicates that the bacterium *Helicobacter pylori* is linked to peptic-ulcer disease (both duodenal and gastric). *H. pylori* colonizes the gastric mucosa in 95–100% of patients who have duodenal ulcer and in 75–80% of patients who have gastric ulcer. Healthy people in the United States under 30 years old have gastric colonization rates of about 10%. Over the age of 60 years, colonization rates exceed 60%. Colonization alone, however, is not sufficient for the development of ulcer disease; only 15–20% of subjects who have *H. pylori* colonization will develop ulcers in their lifetimes. Other risk factors include genetic predisposition (such as some blood and human leukocyte antigen [HLA] types), cigarette-smoking, and psychologic factors (chronic anxiety and stress).

Liver Disease

Blood tests that reflect liver function are the mainstay of diagnosis of liver disease. Increases in serum bilirubin and in the serum concentrations of some hepatic enzymes—aspartate aminotransferase, alanine aminotransferase, alkaline phosphatase, and γ-glutamyltransferase (GGT)—are commonly noted in liver disorders. The relative sensitivity and specificity of those enzymes for diagnosing liver disease vary, and diagnosis can require several tests. The only regularly reported abnormality in liver function associated with TCDD exposure in humans is an increase in GGT. Estimated serum activity of that enzyme is a sensitive indicator of a variety of conditions, including alcohol and drug hepatotoxicity, infiltrative lesions of the liver, parenchymal liver disease, and biliary tract obstruction. Increases are noted after many chemical and drug exposures that are not followed by evidence of liver injury. The confounding effects of alcohol use (often associated with increased GGT) make interpretation of changes in GGT in exposed people difficult (Calvert et al., 1992). An increase in GGT can be considered a normal biologic adaptation to chemical, drug, or hormone exposure.

Cirrhosis is the most commonly reported liver disease in epidemiologic studies of herbicide or TCDD exposure. Cirrhosis is irreversible chronic injury of the liver with extensive scarring and resulting loss of function. Clinical symptoms and signs include jaundice, edema, abnormalities in blood clotting, and metabolic disturbances. Cirrhosis can lead to portal hypertension with associated gastroesophageal varices, enlarged spleen, abdominal swelling attributable to ascites, and ultimately hepatic encephalopathy that can progress to coma. It generally is impossible to distinguish the various causes of cirrhosis by using clinical signs and symptoms or pathologic characteristics. The most common cause of cirrhosis in North America and many parts of western Europe and South America is excessive alcohol consumption. Other causes are chronic viral infection (hepatitis B or hepatitis C), the poorly understood condition primary biliary cirrhosis, chronic right-sided heart failure, and a variety of less common metabolic and drug-related conditions.

Conclusions from *VAO* and Previous Updates

Some studies that have been reviewed by previous VAO committees focused on liver enzymes, and others reported specific liver diseases. Evaluation of the effects of herbicide and TCDD exposure on noncancer gastrointestinal ailments is challenging in that clinical experience suggests that medical history and physical examination are undependable diagnostic tools for some ailments, so incidence data are sometimes problematic. The strong interdependence among the characteristics of a given person (such as weight and laboratory indexes of hepatic function and health) and TCDD body burden complicates the already difficult task of assessing association.

Most of the analyses of occupational or environmental cohorts have had insufficient numbers of cases to support confident conclusions. Study of the International Agency for Research on Cancer cohort of phenoxy-herbicide and chlorophenol production workers and sprayers (Vena et al., 1998), the only study that had a relatively large number of observations, found less digestive system disease and cirrhosis mortality in exposed workers than in nonexposed controls. A study that compared Australian veterans with the general population (O'Toole et al., 1996) suggested a higher incidence of stomach and duodenal ulcers in both men and women, but the information was self-reported and the analyses were not controlled for confounding influences.

A report from the AFHS (2000) found a significantly higher percentage of other liver disorders in the Ranch Hand veterans in the high-dioxin category than in the Southeast Asia comparison subjects. The excesses were primarily of transaminase and other nonspecific liver abnormalities. Data were consistent with an interpretation of a dose–response relationship, but other explanations were also plausible. There have been later reports (AFHS, 2005) of some abnormalities in liver enzymes in the Ranch Hand cohort, including decreasing C4 complement as dioxin increased; abnormal triglyceride concentrations also increased as the 1987 dioxin concentration increased. Mortality studies of the Ranch Hand cohort, however, have not found increased mortality related to gastrointestinal or liver disease (Ketchum and Michalek, 2005).

A study of ACC Vietnam veterans reported in *Update 2006* found an increased rate of hepatitis associated with Vietnam service but not with a history of spraying herbicide (Kang et al., 2006). Likewise, the Australian Vietnam-veterans study (ADVA, 2005b) did not find an increase in liver disease in military personnel who served in Vietnam compared with the general population of Australia.

Update 2008 reviewed the mortality results through 2001 for the Seveso cohort in Italy (Consonni et al., 2008) and found no excess of deaths related to digestive diseases or related specifically to cirrhosis.

Additional analyses of the mortality experience of the ACC veterans were reviewed in *Update 2010* (Cypel and Kang, 2010). There was about an 80% excess of digestive system or cirrhosis deaths observed in veterans who handled or sprayed herbicides in Vietnam compared with non-Vietnam veteran peers, but chance could not be excluded as an explanation. A survey of self-reported health problems of Australian veterans indicated an excess of a variety of gastrointestinal problems, including diseases of the esophagus, ulcer, and irritable bowel syndrome but not gallstones (O'Toole et al., 2009); however, multiple methodologic weaknesses—including a low response rate, lack of specific exposure information, and the inherent problems associated with self-reported health conditions—make the findings of this study unpersuasive. Several mortality studies of various occupational cohorts exposed to COIs were reviewed (Boers et al., 2010; Collins et al., 2010a,b; McBride et al., 2009a,b). Those studies have been inconsistent but generally found no statistically significance increases in deaths from either ulcers or cirrhosis, although Collins et al. (2009b) found an increase in stomach and duodenal ulcer deaths in 773 workers who were exposed to chlorinated dioxins other than TCDD in the production of PCP.

Thus, the reports have been inconsistent, and interpretation of individual studies is difficult because of a lack of information on alcohol consumption and other risk factors. In the studies that showed the strongest association between potential exposure and gastrointestinal disease (specifically cirrhosis), there was strong evidence that excess alcohol consumption was the cause of the cirrhosis.

The committee responsible for *VAO* concluded that there was inadequate or insufficient information to determine whether there is an association between exposure to the COIs and gastrointestinal and digestive disease, including liver toxicity. Additional information available to the committees responsible for *Update 1996*, *Update 1998*, *Update 2000*, *Update 2002*, *Update 2004*, *Update 2006*, *Update 2008*, and *Update 2010* did not change that conclusion.

Update of the Epidemiologic Literature

Vietnam-Veteran, Environmental, and Case-Control Studies

No Vietnam-veterans studies, environmental studies, or case-control studies of exposure to the COIs and gastrointestinal and digestive disease have been published since *Update 2010*.

Occupational Studies

Four updated mortality analyses of occupational cohorts exposed to COIs with information on gastrointestinal and digestive disease have been published since *Update 2010*.

Boers et al. (2012) reanalyzed mortality data from two Dutch chemical manufacturing plants focusing on TCDD exposure. Exposure estimates were derived by using blood TCDD concentrations measured in a subsample of workers in the two plants and back-extrapolating to exposures in different departments in the plants. No TCDD was generated during the manufacturing of 2,4-D in plant B, so TCDD exposure was limited to workers in plant A, which manufactured 2,4,5-T and other chemicals. The study included all workers employed from 1955 through 1985 with mortality followup until December 31, 2006. Causes of 12 deaths were attributed to the digestive system (ICD-10 codes K00-K92). There was no evidence of an increase in mortality with increasing TCDD exposure. For workers in plant A, the HR for each log-unit increase in TCDD concentration was 0.74 (95% CI 0.48–1.15) after adjustment only for age.

Ruder and Yiin (2011) examined the mortality experience of 2,122 workers who had been employed at plants manufacturing PCP from 1940 to 2005. In the total cohort, 46 deaths were attributed to diseases of the digestive system; this was consistent with the mortality experience of the US population generally (SMR = 0.98, 95% CI 0.72–1.30). There were 15 digestive system deaths in the 720 workers who were exposed to both PCP and TCP; this also was not more than expected (SMR = 0.96, 95% CI 0.54–1.58). The results were effectively the same for those who had not had any opportunity for occupational exposure to TCDD (SMR = 0.99, 95% CI 0.68–1.39).

Manuwald et al. (2012) reported on the mortality experience of 1,191 men and 398 women who were employed full-time for at least 3 months at a German plant that manufactured 2,4,5-T. Deaths were ascertained through 2007, 23 years after the plant's closure. The report updates several previous reports (Becher et al., 1996; Flesch-Janys et al., 1995; Manz et al., 1991). For each worker, total cumulative exposure to TCDD was calculated as the sum of the cumulative exposures in each of the workplaces where the worker had been employed. In neither men nor women were deaths from digestive system causes significantly increased on the basis of the expected mortality pattern derived from regional administrative data (SMR_{men} = 1.09, 95% CI 0.76–1.51; SMR_{women} = 0.59, 95% CI 0.21–1.28). Deaths from liver cirrhosis were 22 of 36 deaths from diseases of the digestive system in men and three of six in women. The number of cirrhosis deaths in men was somewhat higher than expected, but chance could not be ruled out (SMR = 1.26, 95% CI 0.79–1.90).

Waggoner et al. (2011) reported on the mortality experience in 1993–2005 of pesticide applicators and their spouses in the AHS and found no evidence of an association between status as an applicator or an applicator's spouse with mortality from digestive causes. In fact, the applicators had significantly fewer than expected deaths from digestive system diseases overall and from cirrhosis and other liver diseases. The AHS has been generating valuable information on the COIs for a number of years, but these results are not herbicide-specific and so are not regarded as being fully informative for the committee's task.

Biologic Plausibility

The liver is a primary target for the toxicity of many chemicals. It is the first organ that encounters chemicals absorbed from the gastrointestinal tract and is responsible for metabolizing them to water-soluble chemicals that can be excreted in the urine. Because the liver has many detoxifying enzymes that efficiently metabolize many chemicals, liver toxicity is usually associated only with high-dose acute exposure or lower-dose chronic exposure. The liver can be damaged if metabolism of a chemical results in the production of a reactive intermediate that is more toxic than the parent chemical. Changes in serum concentrations of liver enzymes are biomarkers of liver toxicity, and their magnitude correlates with the degree of liver damage. Exposure of laboratory animals to high doses of 2,4-D, 2,4,5-T, and TCDD is known to cause liver damage. The mechanisms by which the phenoxy herbicides damage the liver is based on inhibition of mitochondrial function by blocking of oxidative phosphorylation; this leads to loss of generation of adenosine triphosphate, death of cells, and hepatic necrosis and fibrosis. TCDD-induced hepatotoxicity is mediated by activation of the AHR, which leads to changes in gene transcription and associated changes in cell function. Changes in gene expression are associated with several physiologic processes, oxidative stress, and apoptosis (Boverhof et al., 2005, 2006). TCDD-mediated hepatic steatosis is characterized by the accumulation of triglyceride due to the combined up-regulation of CD36/fatty acid translocase and fatty acid transport proteins, suppression of fatty acid oxidation, inhibition of hepatic export of triglycerides, increase in peripheral fat mobilization, and increased hepatic oxidative stress (Lee et al., 2010). Exposure of rats to TCDD over a 2-year period (NTP, 2004) also produced several changes in the liver, including hepatocyte hypertrophy, multinucleated hepatocytes, inflammation, pigmentation, diffuse fatty change, necrosis, bile duct hyperplasia, bile duct cyst, nodular hyperplasia, portal fibrosis, and cholangiofibrosis.

The AHR displays species differences; for example, the human and mouse AHR C-terminal region sequences share only 58% of amino acid sequence identity. Compared with the mouse AHR (mAHR), the human AHR (hAHR) has about 10-fold lower relative affinity for TCDD; the difference has been attributed to the amino acid residue valine 381 in the ligand-binding domain of the hAHR (Flaveny et al., 2009; Ramadoss and Perdew, 2004). Species differences associated with AHR activation are supported by the divergence in the transcriptomic responses to TCDD in mouse, rat, and human liver (Boutros et al., 2008, 2009; Carlson et al., 2009; Kim et al., 2009). In a recent study, gene-expression changes were compared in adult female primary human and rat hepatocytes exposed to TCDD in vitro (Black et al., 2012). Whole-genome microarrays found that TCDD produced divergent gene-expression profiles in rat and human hepatocytes, both on an ortholog basis (conserved gene in different species) and on a pathway basis. For commonly affected orthologs or signaling pathways, the human hepatocytes were about 15-fold less sensitive than rat hepatocytes. Such findings are consistent with epidemiologic studies that have shown humans to be less sensitive to TCDD-induced hepatotoxicity. However, it should be noted that those in vitro human hepatocyte studies may not reflect the in vivo response of human liver to TCDD.

Few health-relevant effects of phenoxy herbicides or TCDD on the gastrointestinal tract, even after high exposure, have been reported. Thus, the animal data do not support a plausible link between herbicide exposure and gastrointestinal toxicity in Vietnam veterans.

Synthesis

Reports of increased risk of abnormal liver-function tests have been mixed, but evidence is lacking that Vietnam veterans are at greatly increased risk for serious liver disease, peptic ulcers, or other specific gastrointestinal diseases. Data on other populations exposed to COIs also do not suggest a strong connection. The studies are limited primarily to analyses of mortality. The possibility of a relationship between dioxin exposure and subtle alterations in the liver and in lipid metabolism cannot be ruled out, but clinically important effects on the gastrointestinal system have not been demonstrated.

Conclusion

On the basis of the evidence reviewed here and in previous VAO reports, the committee concludes that there is inadequate or insufficient evidence to determine whether there is an association between exposure to the COIs and gastrointestinal and digestive diseases.

THYROID HOMEOSTASIS

Clinical disruptions of thyroid function include various disorders grouped in ICD-9 as codes 242.8 and 246.8. The thyroid secretes the hormones thyroxine (T4) and triiodothyronine (T3), which stimulate and help to regulate metabolism throughout the body. The thyroid also secretes calcitonin, a hormone that controls calcium concentration in the blood and storage of calcium in bones. Secretion of T4 and T3 is under the control of thyroid-stimulating hormone (TSH), which is secreted by the anterior pituitary. Iodine operates in thyroid physiology both as a constituent of thyroid hormones and as a regulator of glandular function. Concentrations of those circulating hormones are regulated primarily by a negative-feedback pathway that involves three organs: the thyroid, the pituitary, and the hypothalamus. In the hypothalamus–pituitary–thyroid feedback scheme, the hypothalamus releases thyrotropin-releasing hormone (TRH), which stimulates the pituitary to produce TSH, which triggers the thyroid to produce T4 and T3. Cells in the hypothalamus and pituitary respond to concentrations of circulating T4 and T3. When T4 and T3 are low, the pituitary is stimulated to deliver more TSH to the thyroid, which increases T4 and T3 output. When circulating T4 and T3 are high, they signal to reduce the output of TRH and TSH. The negative-feedback loop maintains hormone homeostasis.

Disruption of thyroid homeostasis can be stimulatory (hyperthyroidism) or suppressive (hypothyroidism). Both conditions are diagnosed on the basis of blood concentrations of thyroid hormones, TSH, and other proteins (antithyroid antibodies). The prevalence of thyroid dysfunction in adults in the general population ranges from 1% to 10%, depending on the group, the testing setting, sex, age, method of assessment, and the presence of conditions that affect thyroid function. People who have subclinical (biochemical) conditions may or may not show other evidence (signs or symptoms) of thyroid dysfunction.

In *hypothyroidism*, the body lacks sufficient thyroid hormone. Overt hypothyroidism is seen as a high serum concentration of TSH and a low serum concentration of free T4. Subclinical hypothyroidism is defined as a high serum concentration of TSH and a normal serum concentration of free T4. People who have hypothyroidism typically have symptoms of low metabolism. Studies consistently show that subclinical hypothyroidism is common and occurs more frequently in women than in men (Canaris et al., 2000; Hollowell et al., 2002; Sawin et al., 1985). In the Framingham study, for example, among 2,139 people 60 years old or older, 14% of women and 6% of men had subclinical hypothyroidism (Sawin et al., 1985). Subclinical hypothyroidism is a risk factor for overt hypothyroidism. Studies have reported association of hypothyroidism with a wide variety of other conditions.

The term *hyperthyroidism* may involve any disease that results in overabundance of thyroid hormone. Clinical or overt hyperthyroidism is characterized as a low serum concentration of TSH and high serum concentration of free T4. Subclinical hyperthyroidism is defined as a low serum concentration of TSH and a normal serum concentration of free T4. The prevalence of subclinical hyperthyroidism was estimated at about 1% in men and 1.5% in women over 60 years old (Helfand and Redfern, 1998). Conditions associated with hyperthyroidism include Graves disease and diffuse toxic goiter. Like hypothyroidism, hyperthyroidism is more common in women than in men, and although it occurs at all ages, it is most likely to occur in people more than 15 years old. A form of hyperthyroidism called neonatal Graves disease occurs in infants born to mothers who have Graves disease. Occult hyperthyroidism may occur in patients more than 65 years old and is characterized by a distinct lack of typical symptoms.

It is important to distinguish between potential effects on adults and effects that may occur during development. In adults, the thyroid is able to compensate, within reason, for mild or moderate disruption (such as that caused by hyperplasia or goiter). In contrast, the fetus is highly sensitive to alterations in thyroid hormones, and alterations in thyroid homeostasis can hamper the development of many organ systems, including the nervous and reproductive systems; such findings are discussed in Chapter 10, which addresses potential effects of Vietnam veterans' exposure to herbicides on their offspring. Only observations on adults are considered here.

Summary of Previous Updates

Koopman-Esseboom et al. (1994) found an association between dioxin-like congeners and markers of disrupted thyroid homeostasis. The report focused on TCDD and maternal thyroid function during pregnancy and therefore is less relevant to the experience of the predominantly male Vietnam veterans.

Extensive assessment of endocrine function, including a series of thyroid-function tests, was carried out in connection with the Operation Ranch Hand study (AFHS, 1991b). It failed to show any difference in thyroid function between exposed and control veterans. When individual TCDD readings had been obtained for subjects in the AFHS, however, Pavuk et al. (2003) found statistically significantly increased TSH measures from the 1985 and 1987 examinations in the high-exposure category and a significant increasing trend across the three TCDD categories in data gathered during the 1982, 1985, 1987, and 1992 examinations. Other studies of veterans of the Vietnam War have not documented an increased risk of thyroid disease.

Calvert et al. (1999) provided evidence of higher adjusted mean free-T4 concentrations in TCDD-exposed workers, but there was no dose–response relationship with serum TCDD. Bloom et al. (2006) found indications of an inverse relationship between the sum of dioxin-like chemicals and the concentration of free T4 in anglers in New York State but no association between the sum of dioxin-like chemicals and TSH or T3. Abdelouahab et al. (2008) described thyroid function in adult freshwater-fish consumers in Canada; dioxin-like congeners were associated with an increase in TSH and a decrease in T4 but below the threshold at which clinical symptoms would be present. An analysis of 1999–2002 National Health and Nutrition Examination Survey (NHANES) data (Turyk et al., 2007) found total T4 to have a weak inverse relationship with serum TEQs; the effect was somewhat stronger in people over 60 years old and in women compared with men.

The committee for *Update 2008* concurred with previous committees that there was inadequate or insufficient evidence of an association between exposure to the COIs and clinical or overt adverse effects on thyroid homeostasis. Prior committees had also noted increasing evidence of an association between exposure to some COIs and changes in markers of thyroid function below the threshold of clinical symptoms, perhaps because of the adaptive capacity of the adult system to accommodate such variation.

Several studies of thyroid disease were considered in *Update 2010*. Goldner et al. (2010) published negative results for an association between phenoxy herbicide exposures and self-reported history of physician-diagnosed thyroid disease in women in the AHS. Clear effects of dioxin-like chemicals on thyroid function were not apparent in Inuit adults (Dallaire et al., 2009), in a cross-sectional study of a Chinese community exposed to an electronic-waste recycling plant (Zhang et al., 2010), or in women enrolled at the Center for the Health Assessment of Mothers and Children of Salinas in California (CHAMACOS; Chevrier et al., 2008). Schreinemachers (2010) did not find associations of recent exposure to 2,4-D with T4 and TSH concentrations in subjects in NHANES III (1988–1994).

Table 13-3 summarizes findings of studies that have examined the association between dioxin-like congeners and markers of thyroid function.

There has been considerable study of maternal exposure and perinatal effects on thyroid function, which is not directly applicable to the adult exposure of the Vietnam veterans whose own health is the primary concern of these updates. A discussion of that material can be found in Chapter 10, on possible adverse effects on the offspring of Vietnam veterans.

TABLE 13-3 Selected Epidemiologic Studies—Thyroid Homeostasis

Study Population	Exposed Cases[a]	**Exposure of Interest**/Reported Results[a]	Reference
VIETNAM VETERANS			
US Vietnam Veterans			
US Air Force Health Study—Ranch Hand veterans vs SEA veterans (unless otherwise noted)		**All COIs**	
Incidence			
Cross-sectional analysis of Ranch Hand personnel (n = 1,009) and SEA veterans (n = 1,429); THS, total T4, T3%			Pavuk et al., 2003
THS uptake by TCDD category			
Comparisons (SEA veterans—no TCDD spraying)	1,247	Normal = 0–3 μIU/ml	
RH background (TCDD ≤ 10 ppt	409	0.84 (p = 0.88)	
RH low (TCDD > 10 ppt, ≤ 94 ppt)	273	0.87 (p = 0.16)	
RH high (TCDD > 94 ppt)	275	0.90 (p = 0.04)	
T4 (thyroxine) means by TCDD category		Normal = 4.5–11.5 μg/dl	
Comparisons (SEA veterans—no TCDD spraying)	1,247	7.47	
RH background (TCDD ≤ 10 ppt	409	7.56 (p = 0.19)	
RH low (TCDD > 10 ppt, ≤ 94 ppt)	273	7.54 (p = 0.38)	
RH high (TCDD > 94 ppt)	275	7.56 (p = 0.28)	
T3% (triiodothyronin) uptake by TCDD category		Normal 25%–35%	
Comparisons (SEA veterans—no TCDD spraying)	1,247	30.7	
RH background (TCDD ≤ 10 ppt	409	30.7 (p = 0.19)	
RH low (TCDD > 10 ppt, ≤ 94 ppt)	273	30.7 (p = 0.98)	
RH high (TCDD > 94 ppt)	275	30.5 (p = 0.24)	
International Vietnam-Veteran Study			
Sample of 1,000 Male Australian Vietnam Veterans—prevalence		**All COIs**	
450 interviewed 2005–2006 vs respondents to 2004–2005 national survey (disorders of the thyroid gland)	450	1.4 (95% CI 0.5–2.2)	O'Toole et al., 2009
OCCUPATIONAL—INDUSTRIAL			
IARC Phenoxy Herbicide Cohort—Workers exposed to any phenoxy herbicide or chlorophenol (production or spraying) vs respective national mortality rates			
NIOSH Cohort—TCDD-exposed workers from 2,4,5-T plants in Newark, New Jersey, and Verona, Missouri, employed > 15 yrs earlier and matched controls (n = 260)			Calvert et al., 1999

TABLE 13-3 Thyroid Homeostasis, continued

Study Population	Exposed Cases[a]	**Exposure of Interest**/Reported Results[a]	Reference
TSH mU/l		Adjusted mean (SE)	
All workers	278	2.0 (0.1) p = 0.66	
TCDD < 20	75	2.2 (0.3) p = 0.28	
20 ≤ TCDD < 75	66	2.0 (0.3) p = 0.88	
75 ≤ TCDD < 238	66	1.9 (0.3) p = 0.94	
238 ≤ TCDD < 3,400	64	1.8 (0.3) p = 0.65	
Referents (< 20)	257	1.9 (0.1)	
T4 nmol/l		Adjusted mean (SE)	
All workers	278	101.4 (1.0) p = 0.07	
TCDD < 20	75	102.7 (2.0) p = 0.08	
20 ≤ TCDD < 75	66	99.4 (2.1) p = 0.79	
75 ≤ TCDD < 238	66	102.7 (2.1) p = 0.09	
238 ≤ TCDD < 3,400	64	100.1 (2.2) p = 0.58	
Referents (< 20)	257	98.8 (1.1)	
Free T4 index nmol/l		Adjusted mean (SE)	
All workers	278	27.8 (0.3) p = 0.02	
TCDD < 20	75	2.7.7 (0.5) p = 0.15	
20 ≤ TCDD < 75	66	27.4 (0.6) p = 0.36	
75 ≤ TCDD < 238	66	28.2 (0.6) p = 0.03	
238 ≤ TCDD < 3,400	64	27.7 (0.6) p = 0.19	
Referents (< 20)	257	26.8 (0.3)	
OCCUPATIONAL—HERBICIDE-USING WORKERS (*not* related to IARC sprayer cohorts)			
AUSTRALIAN 2,4,5-T in Victoria, Australia (n = 37)		**2,4-D; 2,4,5-T**	Johnson et al., 2001
TSH vs estimated serum TCDD level	32	Normal = 0.3–5.0μIU/ml	
Based on local levels		0.2	
Based on individual sampling LDs		–.03	
Based on back extrapolation		–1.4 (p < 0.05)	

continued

TABLE 13-3 Thyroid Homeostasis, continued

Study Population	Exposed Cases[a]	**Exposure of Interest**/Reported Results[a]	Reference
T4 vs estimated serum TCDD level	32	Normal = 0.045–2.125µg/ml	
Based on local levels		0.1	
Based on individual sampling LDs		–0.0	
Based on back extrapolation		–0.0	
T3 vs estimated serum TCDD level	32	Normal = 0.9–1.9µg/ml	
Based on local levels		–0.1	
Based on individual sampling LDs		–0.4 ($p < 0.05$)	
Based on back extrapolation		–0.5 ($p < 0.01$)	
UNITED STATES			
US Agricultural Health Study—prospective study of licensed pesticide sprayers in Iowa and North Carolina: commercial (n = 4,916 men), private/ farmers (n = 52,395, 97.4% men), and spouses of private sprayers (n = 32,347, 0.007% men), enrolled 1993–1997; followups with CATIs 1999–2003 and 2005–2010		**Phenoxy herbicides**	
Incidence			
Thyroid disease among female spouses (n = 19,529) in Iowa and North Carolina (1993–2003)			Goldner et al., 2010
Hyperthyroid			
Self-reported 2,4-D exposure	46	0.9 (95% CI 0.7–1.3)	
Self-reported 2,4,5-T exposure	3	NA	
Self-reported dicamba exposure	17	0.8 (95% CI 0.8–2.1)	
Hypothyroid			
Self-reported 2,4-D exposure	147	0.96 (95% CI 0.8–1.1)	
Self-reported 2,4,5-T exposure	7	1.0 (95% CI 0.5–2.2)	
Self-reported dicamba exposure	27	0.7 (95% CI 0.5–0.98)	
Other thyroid conditions			
Self-reported 2,4-D exposure	87	1.2 (95% CI 0.95–1.5)	
Self-reported 2,4,5-T exposure	4	NA	
Self-reported dicamba exposure	19	0.96 (95% CI 0.6–1.5)	

TABLE 13-3 Thyroid Homeostasis, continued

Study Population	Exposed Cases[a]	**Exposure of Interest**/Reported Results[a]	Reference
ENVIRONMENTAL			
National Health and Nutrition Examination Survey		2,4-D	
NHANES III—analysis of data from subjects with detectable limits of urinary 2,4-D			Schreinemachers, 2010
TSH			
Detectable 2,4-D	102	1.6 mU/L	
Non-detectable 2,4-D	625	1.7 mU/L	
T4			
Detectable 2,4-D	102	8.5 μg/dl	
Non-detectable 2,4-D	625	8.6 μg/dl	
NHANES (1999–2002, 2001–2002)—Associations with TEQs in individuals without thyroid disease			Turyk et al., 2007
Men (1999–2000)			
T4	402	–0.12 (–0.61 to 0.37)	
TSH	402	–0.09 (–0.38 to 0.20)	
Men (2000–2001)			
T4	497	–0.47 (–0.97 to 0.04)	
TSH	497	–0.02 (–0.20 to 0.16)	
Women (1999–2000)			
T4	310	–0.19 (–0.70 to 0.33)	
TSH	309	–0.15 (–0.14 to 0.44)	
Men (1999–2000)			
T4	386	–0.58 (–1.26 to 0.10)	
TSH	385	–0.06 (–0.15 to 0.35)	
Other Environmental Studies			
CANADA			
Cross-sectional study of Inuit residents (≥ 18 yrs of age) of Nunavik (Québec, Canada)	607	**dl PCBs/** correlation of dl-congeners (adjusted)	Dallaire et al., 2009
TSH		0.02	
fT4		–0.01	
fT3		–0.03 ($p < 0.05$)	

continued

TABLE 13-3 Thyroid Homeostasis, continued

Study Population	Exposed Cases[a]	**Exposure of Interest**/Reported Results[a]	Reference
Cross-sectional study of freshwater fish consumers from two Canadian communities		**dl PCBs**/dl-PCB congeners ß estimates	Abdelouahab et al., 2008
Men	124		
TSH		0.55 ($p < 0.001$)	
T4		–2.19 ($p < 0.05$)	
T3		–0.01	
Women	87		
TSH		0.04	
T4		0.04	
T3		–0.01	
Cross-sectional examination of serum from pregnant women attending Canadian prenatal diagnosis clinic	150	**dl compounds**	Foster et al., 2005
TSH correlation coefficient		ns (value nr)	
T4 correlation coefficient		ns (value nr)	
CHINA—cross-sectional study of a Chinese community in the vicinity of an electronic-waste recycling plant—maternal serum T4 levels at 16 weeks gestation (correlations with contaminant levels in cord blood)		**PCDDs, PCDFs, dl PCBs**	Zhang et al., 2010
dl PCBs		r = –0.413 (p = 0.01)	
PCDD/Fs		r = –0.198 (p = 0.21)	
JAPANESE patients exposed in 1968 during Yusho incident; blood collection from participants 1996 and 1997	16	**PCDDs, PCDFs, dl PCBS**	Nagayama et al., 2001
TSH correlation coefficient		0.01 (p = 0.97)	
T4 correlation coefficient		0.03 (p = 0.9)	
T3 correlation coefficient		–0.09 (p = 0.74)	
THE NETHERLANDS—Part of the prospective longitudinal Dutch PCB/Dioxin study; 105 health mother-infant pairs living in or around Rotterdam, recruited June 1990–February 1992		**Dioxins, PCBs**	Koopman-Esseboom et al., 1994
Maternal serum correlations with dioxin TEQs	78		
T4		–0.4 ($p \leq 0.001$)	
T3		–0.5 ($p \leq 0.001$)	
UNITED STATES			
CHAMACOS Study—334 pregnant women from Salinas Valley, California, providing blood at 26 wks gestation		**dl PCBs** ß (95% CI)	Chevrier et al., 2008
Free T4 vs:			

TABLE 13-3 Thyroid Homeostasis, continued

Study Population	Exposed Cases[a]	**Exposure of Interest**/Reported Results[a]	Reference
PCB TEQs (pg/g)		–0.05 (–0.16 to 0.06)	
Mono-ortho PCBs (ng/g)		–0.09 (–0.19 to 0.01)	
PCB 118 (ng/g)		–0.05 (–0.15 to 0.06)	
PCB 156 (ng/g)		–0.06 (–0.13 to 0.01)	
Total T4 vs:			
PCB TEQs (pg/g)		0.26 (–0.45 to 0.96)	
Mono-ortho PCBs (ng/g)		–0.13 (–0.78 to 0.53)	
PCB 118 (ng/g)		–0.26 (–0.43 to 0.95)	
PCB 156 (ng/g)		–0.05 (–0.52 to 0.42)	
Adult men recruited from Massachusetts infertility clinic (2000–2003)	341	**dl PCBs** Estimated risk (95% CI)	Meeker et al., 2007
T3		0.02 (0.05–0.01)[a]	
fT4		0.01 (0.01–0.05)[a]	
fTSH		0.93 (0.84–1.03)[a]	
Sportfish anglers from New York exposed to dioxin-like compounds in diet	38	**PCDDs, PCDFs, dl PCBs** mean/median (range)	Bloom et al., 2006
TSH µUL/mL		2.0/1.4 (0.2–15.7)	
T4 µg/dL		6.3/6.4 (3.2–10.0)	
Free T4 ng/mL		1.1/1.1 (0.9–1.6)	
T3 ng/dL		92.6/87.5 (56.0–181.0)	

NOTE: 2,4-D, 2,4-dichlorophenoxyacetic acid; 2,4,5-T, 2,4,5-trichlorophenol; CATI, computer-assisted telephone interviewing; CI, confidence interval; COI, chemical of interest; dl, dioxin-like; IARC, International Agency for Research on Cancer; LD, level of detection; NA, not available; NHANES, National Health and Nutrition Examination Survey; nr, no relationship; ns, nonsignificant; PCB, polychlorinated biphenyls; PCDD, polychlorinated dibenzo-*p*-dioxins; PCDD/Fs, chlorinated dioxins and furans combined; PCDF, polychlorinated dibenzofurans; ppt, parts per trillion; SE, standard error; SEA, Southeast Asia; RH, Ranch Hand; T3, triiodothyronine; T4, tetraiodothyronine; TCDD, tetrachlorodibenzo-*p*-dioxin; TEQ, (total) toxic equivalent; TSH, thyroid stimulating hormone.

[a]Adjusted coefficients for change in thyroid hormone level associated with an interquartile range increase in serum dioxin-like congeners.

Update of the Epidemiologic Literature

No new epidemiologic studies of occupational or environmental exposure to the COIs or of Vietnam veterans and effects on thyroid homeostasis have been published since *Update 2010*. Mass media coverage of conference presentations in 2010 created an expectation of results of a study of Graves disease, an autoimmune thyroid condition, but the study had not passed peer review during the publication interval for the present update (Spaulding, 2011).

Biologic Plausibility

The influence of TCDD on thyroid-hormone homeostasis has been measured in numerous animal studies, and exposure has been associated with changes in serum concentrations of T4, T3, and TSH. In most studies, TCDD exposure is associated with a hypothyroid state, including reduced circulating T3 and T4 and increased TSH, especially after chronic exposure. Reduction in circulating T4 concentrations is robust and has recently been proposed as a biomarker of effect of dioxin-like chemicals (Yang et al., 2010). Female rats exposed chronically to TCDD showed follicular-cell hyperplasia and hypertrophy of thyroid follicles that were consistent with overstimulation of the thyroid by TSH (TSH increases as a homeostatic response to low T4 levels) (Yoshizawa et al., 2010). TCDD enhances the metabolism of thyroid hormones primarily through an AHR-dependent induction of glucuronyl transferase activity (Gessner et al., 2012; Kato et al., 2010; Martin et al., 2012; Nishimura et al., 2005). Enhanced accumulation of T4 in hepatic tissue of TCDD-treated mice may also contribute to the reduction circulating T4 (Kato et al., 2010).

Synthesis

Numerous animal experiments and several epidemiologic studies have shown that TCDD and dioxin-like chemicals appear to exert some influence on thyroid homeostasis. The effects of those substances on thyroid hormone and TSH concentrations in humans remain to be definitively elucidated (Langer, 2008). Most of the literature has focused on the correlations between exposure to dioxin-like PCB congeners in environmentally exposed populations, and many of the studies have been limited to women and infants. Few studies of thyroid metabolism in the primarily male Vietnam veterans have been published. In the AFHS study considered in *Update 2004*, Pavuk et al. (2003) reported a trend toward an increasing concentration of TSH that was not accompanied by changes in circulating T4 or T3 in Vietnam veterans. In comparison, T4 has been shown to be susceptible to an influence of dioxin-like chemicals in epidemiologic studies. Notably, in Vietnam-veteran studies, there has been no evidence of changes in clinical thyroid disease. Although an overall assessment of the studies suggests some variation in thyroid-hormone concentrations in relation to TCDD exposure, the functional importance of the changes remains unclear because adaptive capacity should be adequate to accommodate them. It should be noted, however, that although biomarkers of perturbation may be subclinical in most people they may be associated with clear adversity in others.

Conclusions

There is inadequate or insufficient evidence of an association between exposure to the COIs and clinical or overt adverse effects on thyroid homeostasis. Some effects have been observed in humans, but the functional importance of the changes reported in the studies reviewed remains unclear because adaptive capacity could be adequate to accommodate them.

EYE PROBLEMS

Loss of vision is increasingly common with advanced age, and about one-sixth of people over 70 years old have substantial impairment, men and women being similarly affected (NCHS, 2010). The most prevalent ocular problems in the current age range of Vietnam veterans are age-related macular degeneration, cataracts, glaucoma, and diabetic retinopathy. Ocular problems involving chemical agents most often arise from acute, direct contact with caustic or corrosive substances that may have permanent consequences. Ocular impairment arising from systemic exposure to toxic agents may be mediated by nerve damage. Cataracts can be induced by chronic internal exposure of the lens to such chemicals as 2,4-dinitrophenol, corticosteroids, and thallium; glaucoma may be secondary to any toxic inflammation and from topical or systemic treatment with anti-inflammatory corticosteroids (Casarett and Doull, 1995).

Conclusions from *VAO* and Previous Updates

Update 2010 considered one study of Australian Vietnam veterans that found they had a higher prevalence of all the eye conditions assessed—cataracts, presbyopia, color blindness, and other diseases of the eye—than the Australian population (O'Toole et al., 2009). However, the committee noted a lack of information on exposure to the COIs and a lack of clinical confirmation of the eye conditions, and it had serious concerns about the possibility that recall bias played a role in the findings. On the basis of the evidence reviewed, *Update 2010* concluded that there was inadequate or insufficient evidence to determine whether there is an association between exposure to the COIs and eye conditions.

Update of Epidemiologic Evidence

No epidemiologic studies of exposure to the COIs and eye problems have been published since *Update 2010*.

Biologic Plausibility

There have been several recent reports of ocular activity associated with AHR induction in or TCDD exposure of rats (Sugamo et al., 2009), mice (Takeuchi et al., 2009), and human nonpigmented ciliary epithelial cells (Volotinen et al., 2009).

Synthesis

Since *Update 2010*, no additional epidemiologic results have supported the increase in risk of several eye conditions in the Australian Vietnam veterans reported by O'Toole et al. (2009). The reliability of those findings had been of concern to the committee for *Update 2010* because of the lack of information on exposure to the COIs, the lack of clinical confirmation of the eye conditions, and the considerable likelihood of recall bias.

Conclusion

Given the lack of additional evidence, the committee concludes that there is inadequate or insufficient evidence to determine whether there is an association between exposure to the COIs and eye conditions.

BONE CONDITIONS

This section discusses conditions encompassed by ICD-9 code 733.0: osteoporosis, or decreased bone density. Osteoporosis is a skeletal disorder characterized by a decrease in bone mineral density (BMD) and loss of structural and biomechanical properties of the skeleton, which lead to an increased risk of fractures. Although there are no practical methods for assessing overall bone strength, BMD correlates closely with skeletal load-bearing capacity and fracture risk (Lash et al., 2009). WHO has developed definitions of osteoporosis based on BMD measurements. The dual energy X-ray absorptiometry (DEXA) T score is the number of standard deviations from the mean BMD in young women, for whom osteoporosis is defined as T score at any site of –5 or lower, whereas osteopenia is defined as a T score between –1 and –2.5. Although there are no standardized diagnostic criteria for osteoporosis in men, most authorities use the WHO criterion of a T score less than –2.5 relative to normal young women.

Although men have much higher baseline BMD than women have, they seem to have a similar fracture risk for a given BMD (Lash et al., 2009).

Sex is an important risk factor for osteoporosis; about 56% of postmenopausal women have decreased BMD, and 6% have osteoporosis (CDC, 2002). Data on the effects of aging on bone loss in women are well known, but many health care providers and patients are less familiar with the prevalence and effects of bone changes in older men (Orwoll et al., 2010). Individual patients have genetic and acquired risks of osteoporosis, and the osteoporosis disease process can be without symptoms for decades. It is well known that hormones, vitamins, and pharmaceuticals can have adverse effects on bone. Drug-induced osteoporosis occurs primarily in postmenopausal women, but premenopausal women and men are also significantly affected. Glucocorticoids are the most common cause of drug-induced osteoporosis (Mazziotti et al., 2010). Other risk factors for loss of BMD include use of long-acting benzodiazepine or anticonvulsant drugs, previous hyperthyroidism, excessive caffeine intake, and standing for 4 hours a day or less (Lash et al., 2009).

Several studies have described a link between organochlorine exposure and effects on bone growth, most notably reports of infants exposed in utero to high concentration of PCBs and PCDFs who developed irregular calcifications of their skulls (Miller, 1985) and reports of accidental organochlorine poisoning that resulted in osteoporosis (Cripps et al., 1984; Gocmen et al., 1989). However; the epidemiologic studies of the association between environmental exposures to organochlorine compounds and bone disorder have been inconsistent.

Summary of Previous Updates

Update 2010 was the first VAO update that reviewed studies of the association between exposures to the COIs and decrease in BMD. Results from Hodgson et al. (2008) motivated the inclusion of this health outcome. They studied the relationship between environmental exposures and BMD in a set of 325 members of the Osteoporosis Cadmium as a Risk Factor (OSCAR) cohort who were at least 60 years old. Forearm BMD was measured, and blood samples were analyzed for the five dioxin-like mono-ortho PCB congeners (PCB 105, 118, 156, 157, and 167) and TEQs calculated. In men, PCB 118 had a marginally significant negative association with BMD, but the TEQ for all five dioxin-like mono-ortho PCBs did not show an association. In women, PCB 118 alone and the TEQ for all five dioxin-like mono-ortho PCBs were positively associated with BMD (slope $\beta = 0.00008$, $p = 0.045$; $\beta = 1.652$, $p = 0.057$, respectively). When the risk of low BMD (more than 1 standard deviation below the mean) was treated as a binary variable in an adjusted logistic model, there was a significant association with PCB 118 in men, but none of the measured compounds (also including non-dioxin-like PCBs 138, 153, and 180) was predictive in women.

Update of the Epidemiologic Literature

Vietnam-Veteran and Case-Control Studies

No Vietnam veteran or case-control studies of exposure to the COIs and BMD or osteoporosis have been published since *Update 2010*.

Occupational Studies

The recent update of the AHS (Waggoner et al., 2011) reported an inverse association of death with musculoskeletal and connective tissue diseases. This category is difficult to interpret and may be subject to a healthy-worker effect bias. The AHS has been generating valuable information on the COIs for a number of years, but these results, like those in Alavanja et al. (2005) and Blair et al. (2005), are not herbicide-specific and so are not regarded as being fully informative for the committee's task.

Environmental Studies

Cho et al. (2011) recently reported that persistent organic pollutants can interact biologically with fat mass and lean mass and affect BMD. The study involved the NHANES population (2,769 participants).

Biologic Plausibility

Animal studies suggest that TCDD may have some influence on bone formation and maintenance. It is known that TCDD can induce chondrocyte apoptosis in culture, which could be an initial event leading to cartilage degradation as observed in arthritis (Yang and Lee, 2010); Lee and Yang (2012) recently demonstrated that this is mediated by reactive oxygen species. In addition, TCDD exposure via the dam's milk impaired bone mineralization during postnatal development in mice because of a reduction in osteoblastic activity as a result of TCDD-induced up-regulation in the active form of vitamin D in serum (Nishimura et al., 2009). TCDD altered osteogenesis (bone formation) in an in vitro osteoblast model and led to alterations in proteins associated with cytoskeleton organization and biogenesis, a decrease in the expression of calcium-binding proteins, and a decrease in osteoblast calcium deposition (Carpi et al., 2009). In adult rats, TCDD exposure reduced trabecular bone cross-sectional area, but significantly increased total BMD; it was further noted that TCDD decreased expression of the bone-formation marker procollagen type I *N*-terminal propeptide and increased expression of the bone-resorption marker carboxy-terminal collagen cross-link, suggesting a net loss of bone tissue (Lind et al., 2009). It is also known that exposure to polyaromatic hydrocarbons (such as those in tobacco smoke) can affect bone health, and some of these alterations have been shown to be mediated, at least in part by the AHR. That implies that TCDD may alter or modify the effects (Kung et al., 2012; Yan et al., 2011).

Synthesis

The small amount of available epidemiologic information on possible adverse effects of exposure to the COIs on bone structure is based entirely on dioxin-like mono-ortho PCBs, which contribute a small percentage to total TEQs based on all dioxin-like PCBs. The findings of Hodgson et al. (2008) do not constitute a strong or consistent pattern. The alteration in BMD associated with persistent pollutants in the NHANES participants suggests that additional studies of this affect are warranted.

Conclusion

There is inadequate or insufficient evidence of an association between exposure to the COIs and clinical or overt adverse effects of osteoporosis or loss of BMD.

REFERENCES[1]

Abdelouahab N, Mergler D, Takser L, Vanier C, St-Jean M, Baldwin M, Spear PA, Chan HM. 2008. Gender differences in the effects of organochlorines, mercury, and lead on thyroid hormone levels in lakeside communities of Quebec (Canada). *Environmental Research* 107(3):380–392.

ADVA (Australian Department of Veterans Affairs). 2005b. *The Third Australian Vietnam Veterans Mortality Study 2005.* Canberra, Australia: Department of Veterans' Affairs.

ADVA. 2005c. *Australian National Service Vietnam Veterans: Mortality and Cancer Incidence 2005.* Canberra, Australia: Department of Veterans' Affairs.

AFHS (Air Force Health Study). 1991b. *An Epidemiologic Investigation of Health Effects in Air Force Personnel Following Exposure to Herbicides. Mortality Update: 1991.* Brooks AFB, TX: Armstrong Laboratory. AL-TR-1991-0132.

AFHS. 2000. *An Epidemiologic Investigation of Health Effects in Air Force Personnel Following Exposure to Herbicides. 1997 Followup Examination Results.* Brooks AFB, TX: Epidemiologic Research Division, Armstrong Laboratory. AFRL-HE-BR-TR-2000-02.

AFHS. 2005. *An Epidemiologic Investigation of Health Effects in Air Force Personnel Following Exposure to Herbicides. 2002 Followup Examination Results.* Brooks AFB, TX: Epidemiologic Research Division, Armstrong Laboratory. AFRL-HE-BR-SR-2005-0003.

Alavanja M, Merkle S, Teske J, Eaton B, Reed B. 1989. Mortality among forest and soil conservationists. *Archives of Environmental Health* 44:94–101.

[1]Throughout this report, the same alphabetic indicator after year of publication is used consistently for a given reference when there are multiple citations by the same first author in a given year. The convention of assigning the alphabetic indicators in order of citation in a given chapter is not followed.

Anderson H, Hanrahan L, Jensen M, Laurin D, Yick W, Wiegman P. 1986. *Wisconsin Vietnam Veteran Mortality Study: Proportionate Mortality Ratio Study Results.* Madison: Wisconsin Division of Health.

Becher H, Flesch-Janys D, Kauppinen T, Kogevinas M, Steindorf K, Manz A, Wahrendorf J. 1996. Cancer mortality in German male workers exposed to phenoxy herbicides and dioxins. *Cancer Causes and Control* 7(3):312–321.

Bertazzi P, Zocchetti C, Pesatori A, Guercilena S, Sanarico M, Radice L. 1989a. Mortality in an area contaminated by TCDD following an industrial incident. *Medicina Del Lavoro* 80:316–329.

Bertazzi PA, Bernucci I, Brambilla G, Consonni D, Pesatori AC. 1998. The Seveso studies on early and long-term effects of dioxin exposure: A review. *Environmental Health Perspectives* 106(Suppl 2):625–633.

Bertazzi PA, Consonni D, Bachetti S, Rubagotti M, Baccarelli A, Zocchetti C, Pesatori AC. 2001. Health effects of dioxin exposure: A 20-year mortality study. *American Journal of Epidemiology* 153(11):1031–1044.

Black MB, Budinsky RA, Dombkowski A, Cukovic D, LeCluyse EL, Ferguson SS, Thomas RS, Rowlands JC. 2012. Cross-species comparisons of transcriptomic alterations in human and rat primary hepatocytes exposed to 2,3,7,8-tetrachlorodibenzo-*p*-dioxin. *Toxicological Sciences* 127(1):199–215.

Blair A, Grauman D, Lubin J, Fraumeni JJ. 1983. Lung cancer and other causes of death among licensed pesticide applicators. *Journal of the National Cancer Institute* 71:31–37.

Blair A, Sandler DP, Tarone R, Lubin J, Thomas K, Hoppin JA, Samanic C, Coble J, Kamel F, Knott C, Dosemeci M, Zahm SH, Lynch CF, Rothman N, Alavanja MC. 2005. Mortality among participants in the Agricultural Health Study. *Annals of Epidemiology* 15(4):279–285.

Bloom M, Vena J, Olson J, Moysich K. 2006. Chronic exposure to dioxin-like compounds and thyroid function among New York anglers. *Environmental Toxicology and Pharmacology* 21(3):260–267.

Bodner KM, Collins JJ, Bloemen LJ, Carson ML. 2003. Cancer risk for chemical workers exposed to 2,3,7,8-tetrachlorodibenzo-*p*-dioxin. *Occupational and Environmental Medicine* 60:672–675.

Boehmer TK, Flanders WD, McGeehin MA, Boyle C, Barrett DH. 2004. Postservice mortality in Vietnam veterans: 30–year followup. *Archives of Internal Medicine* 164(17):1908–1916.

Boers D, Portengen L, Bueno de Mesquita HB, Heederik D, Vermeulen R. 2010. Cause-specific mortality of Dutch chlorophenoxy herbicide manufacturing workers. *Occupational and Environmental Medicine* 67(1):24–31.

Boers D, Portengen L, Turner WE, Bueno de Mesquita HB, Heederik D, Vermeulen R. 2012. Plasma dioxin levels and cause–specific mortality in an occupational cohort of workers exposed to chlorophenoxy herbicides, chlorophenols and contaminants. *Occupational and Environmental Medicine* 69(2):113–118.

Boutros P, Yan R, Moffat I, Pohjanvirta R, Okey A. 2008. Transcriptomic responses to 2,3,7,8-tetrachlorodibenzo-*p*-dioxin (TCDD) in liver: Comparison of rat and mouse. *BMC Genomics* 9:419.

Boutros P, Bielefeld KA, Pohjanvirta R, Harper PA. 2009. Dioxin-dependent and dioxin-independent gene batteries: Comparison of liver and kidney in AHR-null mice. *Toxicological Sciences* 112(1):245–256.

Boverhof DR, Burgoon LD, Tashiro C, Chittim B, Harkema JR, Jump DB, Zacharewski TR. 2005. Temporal and dose-dependent hepatic gene expression patterns in mice provide new insights into TCDD-mediated hepatotoxicity. *Toxicological Sciences* 85(2):1048–1063.

Boverhof DR, Burgoon LD, Tashiro C, Sharratt B, Chittim B, Harkema JR, Mendrick DL, Zacharewski TR. 2006. Comparative toxicogenomic analysis of the hepatotoxic effects of TCDD in Sprague Dawley rats and C57BL/6 mice. *Toxicological Sciences* 94(2):398–416.

Bullman T, Kang H. 1996. The risk of suicide among wounded Vietnam veterans. *American Journal of Public Health* 86(5):662–667.

Burleson GR, Lebrec H, Yang YG, Ibanes JD, Pennington KN, Birnbaum LS. 1996. Effect of 2,3,7,8-tetrachlorodibenzo-*p*-dioxin (TCDD) on influenza virus host resistance in mice. *Fundamental and Applied Toxicology* 29(1):40–47.

Burns C, Beard K, Cartmill J. 2001. Mortality in chemical workers potentially exposed to 2,4-dichlorophenoxyacetic acid (2,4-D) 1945–94: An update. *Occupational and Environmental Medicine* 58:24–30.

Calvert GM, Sweeney MH, Morris JA, Fingerhut MA, Hornung RW, Halperin WE. 1991. Evaluation of chronic bronchitis, chronic obstructive pulmonary disease, and ventilatory function among workers exposed to 2,3,7,8-tetrachlorodibenzo-*p*-dioxin. *The American Review of Respiratory Disease* 144(6):1302–1306.

Calvert GM, Hornung RV, Sweeney MH, Fingerhut MA, Halperin WE. 1992. Hepatic and gastrointestinal effects in an occupational cohort exposed to 2,3,7,8-tetrachlorodibenzo-*para*-dioxin. *Journal of the American Medical Association* 267:2209–2214.

Calvert GM, Sweeney MH, Deddens J, Wall DK. 1999. Evaluation of diabetes mellitus, serum glucose, and thyroid function among United States workers exposed to 2,3,7,8-tetrachlorodibenzo-*p*-dioxin. *Occupational and Environmental Medicine* 56(4):270–276.

Canaris GJ, Manowitz NR, Mayor G, Ridgway EC. 2000. The Colorado thyroid disease prevalence study. *Archives of Internal Medicine* 160(4):526–534.

Carlson E, McCulloch C, Koganti A, Goodwin S, Sutter T, Silkworth J. 2009. Divergent transcriptomic responses to aryl hydrocarbon receptor agonists between rat and human primary hepatocytes. *Toxicological Sciences* 112(1):257–272.

Carpi D, Korkalainen M, Airoldi L, Fanelli R, Hakansson H, Muhonen V, Tuukkanen J, Viluksela M, Pastorelli R. 2009. Dioxin-sensitive proteins in differentiating osteoblasts: Effects on bone formation in vitro. *Toxicological Sciences* 108(2):330–343.

Casarett L, Doull J. 1995. *Casarett and Doull's Toxicology. The Basic Science of Poisons. 5th ed.* New York, NY: McGraw-Hill.

CDC (Centers for Disease Control and Prevention). 1988. Centers for Disease Control Vietnam Experience Study. Health status of Vietnam veterans. II: Physical health. *Journal of the American Medical Association* 259(18):2708–2714.

CDC. 2002. *National health and nutrition examination survey: Osteoporosis.* http://www.cdc.gov/nchs/data/nhanes/databriefs/osteoporosis.pdf (accessed April 1, 2011).

CDVA. 1997a. *Mortality of Vietnam Veterans: The Veteran Cohort Study. A Report of the 1996 Retrospective Cohort Study of Australian Vietnam Veterans.* Canberra, Australia: Department of Veterans' Affairs.

CDVA. 1997b. *Mortality of National Service Vietnam Veterans: A Report of the 1996 Retrospective Cohort Study of Australian Vietnam Veterans.* Canberra, Australia: Department of Veterans' Affairs.

Celli BR, Halbert, RJ. 2010a. Point: Should we abandon $FEV_1/FEC < 0.70$ to detect airway obstruction? No. *Chest* 138(5):1037–1039.

Celli BR, Halbert, RJ. 2010b. Rebuttal from Drs Celli and Halbert. *Chest* 138(5):1042–1043.

Chevrier J, Eskenazi B, Holland N, Bradman A, Barr DB. 2008. Effects of exposure to polychlorinated biphenyls and organochlorine pesticides on thyroid function during pregnancy. *American Journal of Epidemiology* 168:298–310.

Chiba T, Chihara J, Furue M. 2012. Role of the arylhydrocarbon receptor (AhR) in the pathology of asthma and COPD. *Journal of Allergy* 2012:8 pps.

Cho MR, Shin JY, Hwang JH, Jacobs DR Jr, Kim SY, Lee DH. 2011. Associations of fat mass and lean mass with bone mineral density differ by levels of persistent organic pollutants: National Health and Nutrition Examination Survey 1999–2004. *Chemosphere* 82:1268–1276.

Coggon D, Pannett B, Winter P, Acheson E, Bonsall J. 1986. Mortality of workers exposed to 2-methyl-4-chlorophenoxyacetic acid. *Scandinavian Journal of Work, Environment, and Health* 12:448–454.

Coggon D, Pannett B, Winter P. 1991. Mortality and incidence of cancer at four factories making phenoxy herbicides. *British Journal of Industrial Medicine* 48:173–178.

Collins JJ, Bodner K, Aylward LL, Wilken M, Bodner CM. 2009a. Mortality rates among trichlorophenol workers with exposure to 2,3,7,8-tetrachlorodibenzo-*p*-dioxin. *American Journal of Epidemiology* 170(4):501–506.

Collins JJ, Bodner K, Aylward LL, Wilken M, Swaen G, Budinsky R, Rowlands C, Bodnar CM. 2009b. Mortality rates among workers exposed to dioxins in the manufacture of pentachlorophenol. *Journal of Occupational and Environmental Medicine* 51(10):1212–1219.

Collins JJ, Bodner K, Aylward LL. 2010a. Letter to editors. *American Journal of Epidemiology* 171:129–133.

Collins JJ, Bodner K, Aylward LL. 2010b. Three authors reply. *American Journal of Epidemiology* 171(1):130–131.

Consonni D, Pesatori AC, Zocchetti C, Sindaco R, D'Oro LC, Rubagotti M, Bertazzi PA. 2008. Mortality in a population exposed to dioxin after the Seveso, Italy, accident in 1976: 25 years of followup. *American Journal of Epidemiology* 167(7):847–858.

Crane PJ, Barnard DL, Horsley KW, Adena MA. 1997a. *Mortality of Vietnam Veterans: The Veteran Cohort Study. A Report of the 1996 Retrospective Cohort Study of Australian Vietnam Veterans.* Canberra, Australia: Department of Veterans' Affairs.

Cripps DJ, Peters HA, Gocmen A, Dogramici I. 1984. Porphyria turcica due to hexachlorobenzene: A 20 to 30 year followup study on 204 patients. *British Journal of Dermatology* 111(4):413–422.

Cypel Y, Kang H. 2010. Mortality patterns of Army Chemical Corps veterans who were occupationally exposed to herbicides in Vietnam. *Annals of Epidemiology* 20(5):339–346.

Dahlgren J, Warshaw R, Thornton J, Anderson-Mahoney CP, Takhar H. 2003. Health effects on nearby residents of a wood treatment plant. *Environmental Research* 92(2):92–98.

Dalager NA, Kang HK. 1997. Mortality among Army Chemical Corps Vietnam veterans. *American Journal of Industrial Medicine* 31(6):719–726.

Dallaire R, Dewailly E, Pereg D, Dery S, Ayotte P. 2009. Thyroid function and plasma concentrations of polyhalogenated compounds in Inuit adults. *Environmental Health Perspectives* 117(9):1380–1386.

Eisen S, Goldberg J, True W, Henderson W. 1991. A co-twin control study of the effects of the Vietnam War on the self-reported physical health of veterans. *American Journal of Epidemiology* 134:49–58.

Enright P, Brusasco V. 2010a. Counterpoint: Should we abandon FEV_1/FEC < 0.70 to detect airway obstruction? Yes. *Chest* 138(5):1040–1042.

Enright P, Brusasco V. 2010b. Rebuttal from Drs Enright and Brusasco. *Chest* 138(5):1043–1044.

Flaveny CA, Murray IA, Chiaro CR, Perdew GH. 2009. Ligand selectivity and gene regulation by the human aryl hydrocarbon receptor in transgenic mice. *Molecular Pharmacology* 75(6):1412–1420.

Flesch-Janys D, Berger J, Gurn P, Manz A, Nagel S, Waltsgott H, Dwyer JH. 1995. Exposure to polychlorinated dioxins and furans (PCDD/F) and mortality in a cohort of workers from a herbicide-producing plant in Hamburg, Federal Republic of Germany. *American Journal of Epidemiology* 142(11):1165–1175.

Foster WG, Holloway AC, Hughes CL Jr. 2005. Dioxin-like activity and maternal thyroid hormone levels in second trimester maternal serum. *American Journal of Obstetrics and Gynecology* 193(6):1900–1907.

Gessner DK, Ringseis R, Möller C, Eder K. 2012. Increased plasma thyroid hormone concentrations in LDL receptor deficient mice may be explained by inhibition of aryl hydrocarbon receptor-dependent expression of hepatic UDP-glucuronosyltransferases. *Biochimica et Biophysica Acta* 1820:495–502.

Gocmen A, Peters HA, Cripps DJ, Bryan GT, Morris CR. 1989. Hexachlorobenzene episode in Turkey. *Biomedical and Environmental Sciences* 2(1):36–43.

Goldner WS, Sandler DP, Yu F, Hoppin JA, Kamel F, Levan TD. 2010. Pesticide use and thyroid disease among women in the Agricultural Health Study. *American Journal of Epidemiology* 171(4):455–464.

Helfand M, Redfern CC. 1998. Clinical guidelines part 2. Screening for thyroid disease. *Annals of Internal Medicine* 129:144–158.

Hodgson S, Thomas L, Fattore E, Lind PM, Alfven T, Hellstrom L, Hakansson H, Carubelli G, Fanelli R, Jarup L. 2008. Bone mineral density changes in relation to environmental PCB exposure. *Environmental Health Perspectives* 116(9):1162–1166.

Hollowell JG, Staehling NW, Flanders WD, Hannon WH, Gunter EW, Spencer CA, Braverman LE. 2002. Serum TSH, T(4), and thyroid antibodies in the United States population (1988 to 1994): National Health and Nutrition Examination Survey (NHANES III). *The Journal of Clinical Endocrinology and Metabolism* 87(2):489–499.

Hoppin JA, Umbach DM, London SJ, Lynch CF, Alavanja MC, Sandler DP. 2006a. Pesticides associated with wheeze among commercial pesticide applicators in the Agricultural Health Study. *American Journal of Epidemiology* 163(12):1129–1137.

Hoppin JA, Umbach DM, London SJ, Lynch CF, Alavanja MC, Sandler DP. 2006b. Pesticides and adult respiratory outcomes in the Agricultural Health Study. *Annals of the New York Academy of Sciences* 1076:343–354.

Hoppin JA, Umbach DM, Kullman GJ, Henneberger PK, London SJ, Alavanja MC, Sandler DP. 2007a. Pesticides and other agricultural factors associated with self-reported farmer's lung among farm residents in the Agricultural Health Study. *Occupational and Environmental Medicine* 64(5):334–341.

Hoppin JA, Valcin M, Henneberger PK, Kullman GJ, Limbach DM, London SJ, Alavanja MCR, Sandler DP. 2007b. Pesticide use and chronic bronchitis among farmers in the Agricultural Health Study. *American Journal of Industrial Medicine* 50(12):969–979.

Hoppin JA, Umbach DM, London SJ, Henneberger PK, Kullman GJ, Alavanja MC, Sandler DP. 2008. Pesticides and atopic and nonatopic asthma among farm women in the Agricultural Health Study. *American Journal of Respiratory and Critical Care Medicine* 177(1):11–18.

Hoppin JA, Umbach DM, London SJ, Henneberger PK, Kullman GJ, Coble J, Alavanja MCR, Beane Freeman LE, Sandler DP. 2009. Pesticide use and adult-onset asthma among male farmers in the Agricultural Health Study. *European Respiratory Journal* 34(6):1296–1303.

IOM (Institute of Medicine). 1994. *Veterans and Agent Orange: Health Effects of Herbicides Used in Vietnam.* Washington, DC: National Academy Press.

IOM. 1996. *Veterans and Agent Orange: Update 1996.* Washington, DC: National Academy Press.

IOM. 1999. *Veterans and Agent Orange: Update 1998.* Washington, DC: National Academy Press.

IOM. 2001. *Veterans and Agent Orange: Update 2000.* Washington, DC: National Academy Press.

IOM. 2003. *Veterans and Agent Orange: Update 2002.* Washington, DC: The National Academies Press.

IOM. 2005. *Veterans and Agent Orange: Update 2004.* Washington, DC: The National Academies Press.

IOM. 2007. *Veterans and Agent Orange: Update 2006.* Washington, DC: The National Academies Press.

IOM. 2009. *Veterans and Agent Orange: Update 2008.* Washington, DC: The National Academies Press.

Johnson ES, Shorter C, Bestervelt LL, Patterson DG, Needham LL, Piper WN, Lucier G, Nolan CJ. 2001. Serum hormone levels in humans with low serum concentrations of 2,3,7,8-TCDD. *Toxicology and Industrial Health* 17(4):105–112.

Kang HK, Dalager NA, Needham LL, Patterson DG, Lees PSJ, Yates K, Matanoski GM. 2006. Health status of Army Chemical Corps Vietnam veterans who sprayed defoliant in Vietnam. *American Journal of Industrial Medicine* 49(11):875–884.

Kato Y, Haraguchi K, Kubota M, Seto Y, Okura T, Ikushiro SI, Koga N, Yamada S, Degawa M. 2010. A possible mechanism for the decrease in serum thyroxine level by a 2,3,7,8-tetrachlorodibenzo-*p*-dioxin-like polychlorinated biphenyl congener, 3,3′,4,4′,5-pentachlorobiphenyl in mice. *Drug Metabolism and Disposition* 38(1):150–156.

Ketchum NS, Michalek JE. 2005. Postservice mortality of Air Force veterans occupationally exposed to herbicides during the Vietnam War: 20-year followup results. *Military Medicine* 170(5):406–413.

Kim S, Dere E, Burgoon LD, Chang CC, Zacharewski TR. 2009. Comparative analysis of AHR-mediated TCDD-elicited gene expression in human liver adult stem cells. *Toxicological Sciences* 112(1):229–244.

Kogevinas M, Becher H, Benn T, Bertazzi P, Boffetta P, Bueno de Mesquita H, Coggon D, Colin D, Flesch-Janys D, Fingerhut M, Green L, Kauppinen T, Littorin M, Lynge E, Mathews J, Neuberger M, Pearce N, Saracci R. 1997. Cancer mortality in workers exposed to phenoxy herbicides, chlorophenols, and dioxins. An expanded and updated international cohort study. *American Journal of Epidemiology* 145(12):1061–1075.

Koopman-Esseboom C, Morse D, Weisglas-Kuperus N, Lutkeschipholt I, van der Paauw C, Tuinstra LGMT, Brouwer A, Sauer P. 1994. Effects of dioxins and polychlorinated biphenyls on thyroid hormone status of pregnant women and their infants. *Pediatric Research* 36(4):468–476.

Kung M, Yukata K, O'Keefe RJ, Zuscik MJ. 2012. Aryl hydrocarbon receptor-mediated impairment of chondrogenesis and fracture healing by cigarette smoke and benzo(α)pyrene. *Journal of Cellular Physiology* 227:1062–1070.

La Rocca C, Alivernini S, Badiali M, Cornoldi A, Iacovella N, Silvestroni L, Spera G, Turrio-Baldassarri L. 2008. TEQs and body burden for PCDDs, PCDFs, and dioxin-like PCBs in human adipose tissue. *Chemosphere* 73(1):92–96.

Langer P. 2008. Persistent organochlorinated pollutants (PCB, DDE, HCB, dioxins, furans) and the thyroid—review 2008. *Endocrine Regulations* 42(1):79–104.

Lash RW, Nicholson JM, Velez L, Van Harrison R, McCort J. 2009. Diagnosis and management of osteoporosis. *Primary Care* 36(1):181–198.

Lee HG, Yang JH. 2012. PCB126 induces apoptosis of chondrocytes via ROS-dependent pathways. *Osteoarthritis and Cartilage* 20:1179–1185.

Lee JH, Wada T, Febbraio M, He J, Matsubara T, Lee MJ, Gonzalez FJ, Xie W. 2010. A novel role for the dioxin receptor in fatty acid metabolism and hepatic steatosis. *Gastroenterology* 139(2):653–663.

Lee YC, Oslund KL, Thai P, Velichko S, Fujisawa T, Duong T, Denison MS, Wu R. 2011. 2,3,7,8-Tetrachlorodibenzo-*p*-dioxin–induced MUC5AC expression. *American Journal of Respiratory Cell and Molecular Biology* 45:270–276.

Lind PM, Wejheden C, Lundberg R, Alvarez-Lloret P, Hermsen SA, Rodriguez-Navarro AB, Larsson S, Rannug A. 2009. Short-term exposure to dioxin impairs bone tissue in male rats. *Chemosphere* 75(5):680–684.

Manuwald U, Garrido MV, Berger J, Manz A, Baur X. 2012. Mortality study of chemical workers exposed to dioxins: Followup 23 years after chemical plant closure. *Occupational and Environmental Medicine* 69(9):636–642.

Manz A, Berger J, Dwyer JH, Flesch-Janys D, Nagel S, Waltsgott H. 1991. Cancer mortality among workers in chemical plant contaminated with dioxin. *Lancet* 338:959–964.

Martin LA, Wilson DT, Reuhl KR, Gallo MA, Klaassen CD. 2012. Polychlorinated biphenyl congeners that increase the glucuronidation and biliary excretion of thyroxine are distinct from the congeners that enhance the serum disappearance of thyroxine. *Drug Metabolism and Disposition* 40(3):588–595.

Mazziotti G, Canalis E, Giustina A. 2010. Drug-induced osteoporosis: Mechanisms and clinical implications. *American Journal of Medicine* 123(10):877–884.

McBride DI, Collins JJ, Humphry NF, Herbison P, Bodner KM, Aylward LL, Burns CJ, Wilken M. 2009a. Mortality in workers exposed to 2,3,7,8-tetrachlorodibenzo-*p*-dioxin at a trichlorophenol plant in New Zealand. *Journal of Environmental Medicine* 51(9):1049–1056.

McBride DI, Burns CJ, Herbison GP, Humphry NF, Bodner K, Collins JJ. 2009b. Mortality in employees at a New Zealand agrochemical manufacturing site. *Occupational Medicine* 59(4):255–263.

McKinney WP, McIntire DD, Carmody TJ, Joseph A. 1997. Comparing the smoking behavior of veterans and nonveterans. *Public Health Reports* 112(3):212–217.

Meeker JD, Altshul LM, Hauser R. 2007. Serum PCBs, p,p′-DDE and HCB predict thyroid hormone levels in men. *Environmental Research* 104(2):296–304.

Miller RW. 1985. Cogential PCB poisoning: A reevaluation. *Environmental Health Perspectives* 60:211–214.

Mitchell KA, Lawrence BP. 2003. Exposure to 2,3,7,8-tetrachlorodibenzo-*p*-dioxin (TCDD) renders influenza virus-specific $CD8^+$ T cells hyporesponsive to antigen. *Toxicological Sciences* 74:74–84.

Nagayama J, Tsuji H, Iida T, Hirakawa H, Matsueda T, Ohki M. 2001. Effects of contamination level of dioxins and related chemicals on thyroid hormone and immune response systems in patients with "Yusho." *Chemosphere* 43(4-7):1005–1010.

NCHS (National Center for Health Statistics). 2010. Vision, hearing, balance, and sensory impairment in Americans aged 70 years and over: United States, 1999–2006. *NCHS Data Brief*, Number 31.

Nishimura N, Yonemoto J, Miyabara Y, Fujii-Kuriyama Y, Tohyama C. 2005. Altered thyroxin and retinoid metabolic response to 2,3,7,8-tetrachlorodibenzo-*p*-dioxin in aryl hydrocarbon receptor-null mice. *Archives of Toxicology* 79(5):260–267.

Nishimura N, Nishimura H, Ito T, Miyata C, Izumi K, Fujimaki H, Matsumura F. 2009. Dioxin-induced up-regulation of the active form of vitamin D is the main cause for its inhibitory action on osteoblast activities, leading to developmental bone toxicity. *Toxicology and Applied Pharmacology* 236(3):301–309.

NTP (National Toxicology Program). 2004. *NTP Technical Report on the Toxicology and Carcinogenesis Studies of 2,3,7,8-Tetrachlorodibenzo-[rho]-dioxin (TCDD) (CAS No. 1746-01-6) in Female Harlan Sprague-Dawley Rats (Gavage Studies).* National Toxicology Program, Research Triangle Park, NC, and US Department of Health and Human Services, Public Health Service, National Institutes of Health.

Orwoll E, Bilezikian JP, Vanderschueren D. 2010. *Osteoporosis in Men: The Effects of Gender on Skeletal Health*, 2nd Ed., Oxford, UK: Elsevier, Inc. Pp. 207–219.

O'Toole BI, Marshall RP, Grayson DA, Schureck RJ, Dobson M, Ffrench M, Pulvertaft B, Meldrum L, Bolton J, Vennard J. 1996. The Australian Vietnam Veterans Health Study: II. Self-reported health of veterans compared with the Australian population. *International Journal of Epidemiology* 25(2):319–330.

O'Toole BI, Catts SV, Outram S, Pierse KR, Cockburn J. 2009. The physical and mental health of Australian Vietnam veterans 3 decades after the war and its relation to military service, combat, and post-traumatic stress disorder. *American Journal of Epidemiology* 170(3):318–330.

Ott MG, Zober A. 1996. Cause specific mortality and cancer incidence among employees exposed to 2,3,7,8-TCDD after a 1953 reactor accident. *Occupational and Environmental Medicine* 53:606–612.

Pavuk M, Schecter AJ, Akhtar FZ, Michalek JE. 2003. Serum 2,3,7,8-tetrachlorodibenzo-*p*-dioxin (TCDD) levels and thyroid function in Air Force veterans of the Vietnam War. *Annals of Epidemiology* 13(5):335–343.

Pesatori AC, Zocchetti C, Guercilena S, Consonni D, Turrini D, Bertazzi PA. 1998. Dioxin exposure and non-malignant health effects: A mortality study. *Occupational and Environmental Medicine* 55:126–131.

Ramadoss P, Perdew GH. 2004. Use of 2-azido-3-[125i]iodo-7,8-dibromodibenzo-*p*-dioxin as a probe to determine the relative ligand affinity of human versus mouse aryl hydrocarbon receptor in cultured cells. *Molecular Pharmacology* 66(1):129–136.

Ramlow JM, Spadacene NW, Hoag SR, Stafford BA, Cartmill JB, Lerner PJ. 1996. Mortality in a cohort of pentachlorophenol manufacturing workers, 1940–1989. *American Journal of Industrial Medicine* 30(2):180–194.

Rose MC, Voynow JA. 2006. Respiratory tract mucin genes and mucin glycoproteins in health and disease. *Physiology Reviews* 86:245–278.

Ruder AM, Yiin JH. 2011. Mortality of US pentachlorophenol production workers through 2005. *Chemosphere* 83(6):851–861.

Sawin CT, Castelli WP, Hershman JM, McNamara P, Bacharach P. 1985. The aging thyroid. Thyroid deficiency in the Framingham Study. *Archives of Internal Medicine* 145(8):1386–1388.

Schreinemachers DM. 2010. Perturbation of lipids and glucose metabolism associated with previous 2,4-D exposure: A cross-sectional study of NHANES III data, 1988–1994. *Environmental Health: A Global Access Science Source* 9:11.

Senthilselvan A, McDuffie HH, Dosman JA. 1992. Association of asthma with use of pesticides. Results of a cross-sectional survey of farmers. *The American Review of Respiratory Disease* 146(4):884–887.

Slager RE, Poole JA, LeVan TD, Sandler DP, Alavanja MCR, Hoppin JA. 2009. Rhinitis associated with pesticide exposure among commercial pesticide applicators in the Agricultural Health Study. *Occupational and Environmental Medicine* 66(11):718–724.

Spaulding SW. 2011. The possible roles of environmental factors and the aryl hydrocarbon receptor in the prevalence of thyroid diseases in Vietnam era veterans. *Current Opinion in Endocrinology, Diabetes and Obesity* 18:315–320.

Steenland K, Piacitelli L, Deddens J, Fingerhut M, Chang LI. 1999. Cancer, heart disease, and diabetes in workers exposed to 2,3,7,8-tetrachlorodibenzo-*p*-dioxin. *Journal of the National Cancer Institute* 91(9):779–786.

Sugamo T, Nakamura K, Tamura H. 2009. Effects of cytochrome p450 inducers on the gene expression of ocular xenobiotic metabolizing enzymes in rats. *Journal of Health Science* 55(6):923–929.

Suskind RR, Hertzberg VS. 1984. Human health effects of 2,4,5-T and its toxic contaminants. *Journal of the American Medical Association* 251(18):2372–2380.

Svensson BG, Nilsson A, Jonsson E, Schutz A, Akesson B, Hagmar L. 1995. Fish consumption and exposure to persistent organochlorine compounds, mercury, selenium and methylamines among Swedish fishermen. *Scandinavian Journal of Work, Environment, and Health* 21(2):96–105.

Sweeney MH, Calvert GM, Egeland GA, Fingerhut MA, Halperin WE, Piacitelli LA. 1997/98. Review and update of the results of the NIOSH medical study of workers exposed to chemicals contaminated with 2,3,7,8-tetrachlorodibenzodioxin. *Teratogenesis, Carcinogenesis, and Mutagenesis* 17(4–5):241–247.

't Mannetje A, McLean D, Cheng S, Boffetta P, Colin D, Pearce N. 2005. Mortality in New Zealand workers exposed to phenoxy herbicides and dioxins. *Occupational and Environmental Medicine* 62(1):34–40.

Takeuchi A, Takeuchi M, Oikawa K, Sonoda KH, Usui Y, Okunuki Y, Takeda A, Oshima Y, Yoshida K, Usui M, Goto H, Kuroda M. 2009. Effects of dioxin on vascular endothelial growth factor (VEGF) production in the retina associated with choroidal neovascularization. *Investigative Ophthalmology and Visual Science* 50(7):3410–3416.

Teske S, Bohn AA, Hogaboam JP, Lawrence BP. 2008. Aryl hydrocarbon receptor targets pathways extrinsic to bone marrow cells to enhance neutrophil recruitment during influenza virus infection. *Toxicological Sciences* 102(1):89–99.

Turunen AW, Verkasalo PK, Kiviranta H, Pukkala E, Jula A, Mannisto S, Rasanen R, Marniemi J, Vartiainen T. 2008. Mortality in a cohort with high fish consumption. *International Journal of Epidemiology* 37(5):1008–1017.

Turyk ME, Anderson HA, Persky VW. 2007. Relationships of thyroid hormones with polychlorinated biphenyls, dioxins, furans, and DDE in adults. *Environmental Health Perspectives* 115(8):1197–1203.

Uno S, Dalton TP, Dragin N, Curran CP, Derkenne S, Miller ML, Shertzer HG, Gonzalez FJ, Nebert DW. 2006. Oral benzo[a]pyrene in *Cyp1* knockout mouse lines: CYP1A1 important in detoxication, CYP1B1 metabolism required for immune damage independent of total-body burden and clearance rate. *Molecular Pharmacology* 69(4):1103–1114.

Valcin M, Henneberger PK, Kullman GJ, Umbach DM, London SJ, Alavanja MC, Sandler DP, Hoppin JA. 2007. Chronic bronchitis among nonsmoking farm women in the Agricultural Health Study. *Journal of Occupational and Environmental Medicine* 49(5):574–583.

van den Berg M, Birnbaum LS, Denison M, De Vito M, Farland W, Feeley M, Fiedler H, Hakansson H, Hanberg A, Haws L, Rose M, Safe S, Schrenk D, Tohyama C, Tritscher A, Tuomisto J, Tysklind M, Walker N, Peterson RE. 2006. The 2005 World Health Organization reevaluation of human and Mammalian toxic equivalency factors for dioxins and dioxin-like compounds. *Toxicological Sciences* 93(2):223–241.

Vena J, Boffeta P, Becher H, Benn T, Bueno de Mesquita HB, Coggon D, Colin D, Flesch-Janys D, Green L, Kauppinen T, Littorin M, Lynge E, Mathews JD, Neuberger M, Pearce N, Pesatori AC, Saracci R, Steenland K, Kogevinas M. 1998. Exposure to dioxin and nonneoplastic mortality in the expanded IARC international cohort study of phenoxy herbicide and chlorophenol production workers and sprayers. *Environmental Health Perspectives* 106(Suppl 2):645–653.

Volotinen M, Maenpaa J, Kankuri E, Oksala O, Pelkonen O, Nakajima M, Yokoi T, Hakkola J. 2009. Expression of cytochrome p450 (CYP) enzymes in human nonpigmented ciliary epithelial cells: Induction of CYP1B1 expression by TCDD. *Investigative Ophthalmology and Visual Science* 50(7):3099–3105.

Voynow JA, Gendler SJ, Rose MC. 2006. Regulation of mucin genes in chronic inflammatory airway diseases. *American Journal of Respiratory Cell and Molecular Biology* 34:661–665.

Waggoner JK, Kullman GJ, Henneberger PK, Umbach DM, Blair A, Alavanja MCR, Kamel F, Lynch CF, Knott C, London SJ, Hines CJ, Thomas KW, Sandler DP, Lubin JH, Beane Freeman LE, Hoppin JA. 2011. Mortality in the Agricultural Health Study, 1993–2007. *American Journal of Epidemiology* 173(1):71–83.

Warren TK, Mitchell KA, Lawrence BP. 2000. Exposure to 2,3,7,8-tetrachlorodibenzo-*p*-dioxin (TCDD) suppresses the humoral and cell-mediated immune responses to influenza A virus without affecting cytolytic activity in the lung. *Toxicological Sciences* 56(1):114–123.

Watanabe K, Kang H. 1996. Mortality patterns among Vietnam veterans: A 24-year retrospective analysis. *Journal of Occupational and Environmental Medicine* 38(3):272–278.

Wong PS, Vogel CF, Kokosinski K, Matsumura F. 2010. Arylhydrocarbon receptor activation in NCI-H441 cells and C57b1/6 mice: Possible mechanisms for lung dysfunction. *American Journal of Respiratory Cell and Molecular Biology* 42(2):210–217.

Yan C, Avadhani NG, Iqbal J. 2011. The effects of smoke carcinogens on bone. *Current Osteoporosis Reports* 9:202–209.

Yang JH, Lee YG. 2010. 2,3,7,8-Tetrachlorodibenzo-*p*-dioxin induces apoptosis of articular chondrocytes in culture. *Chemosphere* 79:278–284.

Yang JM, Salmon AG, Marty MA. 2010. Development of TEFs for PCB congeners by using an alternative biomarker—thyroid hormone levels. *Regulatory Toxicology and Pharmacology* 56(2):225–236.

Yoshizawa K, Walker NJ, Nyska A, Kissling GE, Jokinen MP, Brix AE, Sells DM, Wyde ME. 2010. Thyroid follicular lesions induced by oral treatment for 2 years with 2,3,7,8-tetrachlorodibenzo-*p*-dioxin and dioxin-like compounds in female Harlan Sprague-Dawley rats. *Toxicologic Pathology* 38:1037–1050.

Zhang J, Jiang Y, Zhou J, Wu B, Liang Y, Peng Z, Fang D, Liu B, Huang H, He C, Wang C, Lu F. 2010. Elevated body burdens of PBDEs, dioxins, and PCBs on thyroid hormone homeostasis at an electronic waste recycling site in China. *Environmental Science and Technology* 44(10):3956–3962.

Zober A, Ott MG, Messerer P. 1994. Morbidity follow up study of BASF employees exposed to 2,3,7,8-tetrachlorodibenzo-*p*-dioxin (TCDD) after a 1953 chemical reactor incident. *Occupational and Environmental Medicine* 51:479–486.

14

Conclusions and Recommendations

SYNOPSIS OF COMMITTEE CONCLUSIONS

The committee weighed the strengths and limitations of the epidemiologic evidence reviewed in its report and in previous *Veterans and Agent Orange* (VAO) reports. Although the studies published since *Update 2010* are the subject of detailed evaluation here, the committee drew its conclusions in the context of the entire body of literature. The contribution of recent publications to the evidence database was considerable, but the committee did not weigh them more heavily merely because they were new. Epidemiologic methods and analytic capabilities have improved, but many of the recent studies were also particularly useful for the committee's purpose because they produced results in terms of serum 2,3,7,8-tetrachlorodibenzo-*p*-dioxin (TCDD) concentrations or total toxic equivalents (TEQs), which take into account exposure to all dioxin-like chemicals, or because their findings consisted of observations on the aging population of primary concern, Vietnam veterans. The committee also notes that experimental data related to biologic plausibility of health conditions statistically associated with exposure to the components of Agent Orange have gradually emerged since the beginning of this series of VAO reports. The findings now do more to inform decisions about how to categorize the degree of association for individual conditions, so the committee for *Update 2008* added a footnote to this effect to its summary tables. The committee for *Update 2010* added a notation to Table 14-1 indicating the correspondence of the lymphohematopoietic cancers (LHCs) that have been found to have evidence of an association with herbicide exposure to the biologic understanding of the clonal derivation of LHCs that is the basis of the World Health Organization's classification system for these neoplasms. The

TABLE 14-1 Summary of *Ninth Biennial Update* of Findings on Vietnam-Veterans, Occupational, and Environmental Studies Regarding Scientifically Relevant Association[a] Between Exposure to Herbicides and Specific Health Outcomes[b]

Sufficient Evidence of an Association

Epidemiologic evidence is sufficient to conclude that there is a positive association. That is, a positive association has been observed between exposure to herbicides and the outcome in studies in which chance, bias, and confounding could be ruled out with reasonable confidence.[c] For example, if several small studies that are free of bias and confounding show an association that is consistent in magnitude and direction, there could be sufficient evidence of an association. There is sufficient evidence of an association between exposure to the chemicals of interest and the following health outcomes:

Soft-tissue sarcoma (including heart)
* Non-Hodgkin lymphoma
* Chronic lymphocytic leukemia (including hairy cell leukemia and other chronic B-cell leukemias)
* Hodgkin lymphoma
Chloracne

Limited or Suggestive Evidence of an Association

Epidemiologic evidence suggests an association between exposure to herbicides and the outcome, but a firm conclusion is limited because chance, bias, and confounding could not be ruled out with confidence.[b] For example, a well-conducted study with strong findings in accord with less compelling results from studies of populations with similar exposures could constitute such evidence. There is limited or suggestive evidence of an association between exposure to the chemicals of interest and the following health outcomes:

Laryngeal cancer
Cancer of the lung, bronchus, or trachea
Prostate cancer
* Multiple myeloma
* AL amyloidosis
Early-onset peripheral neuropathy
Parkinson disease
Porphyria cutanea tarda
Hypertension
Ischemic heart disease
Stroke (category change from *Update 2010*)
Type 2 diabetes (mellitus)
Spina bifida in offspring of exposed people

Inadequate or Insufficient Evidence to Determine an Association

The available epidemiologic studies are of insufficient quality, consistency, or statistical power to permit a conclusion regarding the presence or absence of an association. For example, studies fail to control for confounding, have inadequate exposure assessment, or fail to address latency. There is inadequate or insufficient evidence to determine association between exposure to the chemicals of interest and the following health outcomes that were explicitly reviewed:

Cancers of the oral cavity (including lips and tongue), pharynx (including tonsils), or nasal cavity (including ears and sinuses)

continued

TABLE 14-1 Continued

- Cancers of the pleura, mediastinum, and other unspecified sites in the respiratory system and intrathoracic organs
- Esophageal cancer
- Stomach cancer
- Colorectal cancer (including small intestine and anus)
- Hepatobiliary cancers (liver, gallbladder, and bile ducts)
- Pancreatic cancer
- Bone and joint cancer
- Melanoma
- Nonmelanoma skin cancer (basal-cell and squamous-cell)
- Breast cancer
- Cancers of reproductive organs (cervix, uterus, ovary, testes, and penis; excluding prostate)
- Urinary bladder cancer
- Renal cancer (kidney and renal pelvis)
- Cancers of brain and nervous system (including eye)
- Endocrine cancers (thyroid, thymus, and other endocrine organs)
- Leukemia (other than chronic B-cell leukemias, including chronic lymphocytic leukemia and hairy cell leukemia)
- Cancers at other and unspecified sites
- Infertility
- Spontaneous abortion (other than after paternal exposure to TCDD, which appears *not* to be associated)
- Neonatal or infant death and stillbirth in offspring of exposed people
- Low birth weight in offspring of exposed people
- Birth defects (other than spina bifida) in offspring of exposed people
- Childhood cancer (including acute myeloid leukemia) in offspring of exposed people
- Neurobehavioral disorders (cognitive and neuropsychiatric)
- Neurodegenerative diseases, excluding Parkinson disease
- Chronic peripheral nervous system disorders
- Hearing loss
- Respiratory disorders (wheeze or asthma, chronic obstructive pulmonary disease, and farmer's lung)
- Gastrointestinal, metabolic, and digestive disorders (changes in hepatic enzymes, lipid abnormalities, and ulcers)
- Immune system disorders (immune suppression, allergy, and autoimmunity)
- Circulatory disorders (other than hypertension, ischemic heart disease, and stroke)
- Endometriosis
- Disruption of thyroid homeostasis
- Eye problems
- Bone conditions

This committee used a classification that spans the full array of cancers. However, reviews for nonmalignant conditions were conducted only if they were found to have been the subjects of epidemiologic investigation or at the request of the Department of Veterans Affairs. *By default, any health outcome on which no epidemiologic information has been found falls into this category.*

Limited or Suggestive Evidence of *No* Association

Several adequate studies, which cover the full range of human exposure, are consistent in not showing a positive association between any magnitude of exposure to a component of the

TABLE 14-1 Continued

herbicides of interest and the outcome. A conclusion of "no association" is inevitably limited to the conditions, exposures, and length of observation covered by the available studies. *In addition, the possibility of a very small increase in risk at the exposure studied can never be excluded.* There is limited or suggestive evidence of *no* association between exposure to the herbicide component of interest and the following health outcome:

Spontaneous abortion after paternal exposure to TCDD

[a]This change in wording was made to emphasize the scientific nature of the VAO task and procedures and reflects no change in the present committee's criteria from those used in previous updates.

[b]*Herbicides* indicates the following chemicals of interest: 2,4-dichlorophenoxyacetic acid (2,4-D), 2,4,5-trichlorophenoxyacetic acid (2,4,5-T) and its contaminant 2,3,7,8-tetrachlorodibenzo-*p*-dioxin (TCDD or dioxin), cacodylic acid, and picloram. The evidence regarding association was drawn from occupational, environmental, and veteran studies in which people were exposed to the herbicides used in Vietnam, to their components, or to their contaminants.

[c]Evidence of an association is strengthened by experimental data supporting biologic plausibility, but its absence would not detract from the epidemiologic evidence.

*The committee notes the consistency of these findings with the biologic understanding of the clonal derivation of lymphohematopoietic cancers that is the basis of the World Health Organization classification system.

current committee did not modify the criteria used by previous VAO committees to assign categories of association to particular health outcomes, but decided to refer to the object of its evaluation as "scientifically relevant association" in the title of Table 14-1 to clarify that the strength of evidence evaluated, based on the quality of the scientific studies reviewed, was a fundamental component of the committee's deliberations to address the imprecisely defined legislative target of "statistical association."

On the basis of its evaluation of Vietnam veterans, occupational, and environmental studies, the committee assigned each health outcome to one of four categories of relative certainty of association with exposure to the herbicides that were used in Vietnam or to any of their components or contaminants (with no intention of specifying particular chemicals). This committee's findings were the same as those of the committee for *Update 2010* with a single exception: the committee voted unanimously to move stroke to the limited and suggestive category because of new evidence showing a statistically significant association of stroke with exposure to dioxin-like chemicals in the well-designed Prospective Investigation of the Vasculature in Uppsala Seniors; evidence of an overall increase in stroke or cerebrovascular disease associated with exposure to the chemicals of interest in Vietnam veteran, occupational, and environmental populations in the most relevant of previously considered studies; demonstrated biologic plausibility in human and animal studies; and the strong connection between stroke and hypertension, cardiovascular disease, and diabetes (three conditions already in the limited and suggestive category). The published data did not permit the committee to distinguish hemorrhagic from ischemic stroke, but given that only a small percentage of strokes are of the hemorrhagic type in Western populations, that was not seen to be an impediment. This change made by the current committee to the categorizations determined by the committee for *Update 2010* (as presented in Table 1-1) is noted in boldface in Table 14-1.

Although the Department of Veterans Affairs (VA) did not find hypertension to be presumptively related to service in Vietnam (VA, 2010), on the basis of the total weight of available evidence the current committee reaffirmed the conclusion of the committees for *Update 2006*, for *Update 2008*, and for *Update 2010* to categorize hypertension as having limited or suggestive evidence of association.

As mandated by Public Law (PL) 102-4, the distinctions among categories are based on statistical association, not on strict causality. The committee was directed to review the scientific data, not to recommend VA policy; therefore, conclusions reported in Table 14-1 are not intended to imply or suggest policy decisions. The conclusions are related to associations between exposure and outcomes in human populations, not to the likelihood that any individual's health problem is associated with or caused by the chemicals in question.

COMMITTEE RECOMMENDATIONS

As part of its charge, the committee was asked to offer recommendations concerning the need, if any, for additional scientific studies to resolve uncertainties concerning the health effects of the chemicals of interest sprayed in Vietnam: 2,4-dichlorophenoxyacetic acid (2,4-D), 2,4,5-trichlorophenoxyacetic acid (2,4,5-T) and its contaminant TCDD, picloram, and cacodylic acid. This chapter summarizes the committee's recommendations.

Although progress continues to be made in understanding the health effects of exposure to the chemicals of interest and in elucidating the mechanisms underlying them, gaps in our knowledge remain. The scope of potential research on the chemicals is far-reaching, and what follows here is not an exhaustive list of future research that might have value. Many additional opportunities for progress in such fields as toxicology, the conduct of continuing or additional epidemiologic studies, and systematic and comprehensive integration of existing data have not been explicitly noted here. The committee for *Update 2010* offered a high-priority recommendation that research be undertaken to address chronic obstructive pulmonary disease (COPD) from a morbidity perspective with appropriate functional diagnosis of COPD and collection of data to permit adjustment for smoking and other relevant confounders; the current committee is pleased to note that VA has started such a study on its Army Chemical Corps (ACC) cohort. Several of the recommendations detailed below were included in previous VAO updates but have been included here to reiterate the committee's conviction that more progress should be made in the research fields noted.

- **VA should evaluate possibilities for studying health outcomes in Vietnam-era veterans by using the existing administrative and health-services databases.**

The original *VAO* committee recommended that the Department of Defense (DOD) and VA identify Vietnam service in the computerized index of records. Linking that information with the VA electronic medical-record and associated administrative databases, such as discharge-diagnosis and pharmacy-use records, should make it possible to assemble epidemiologic information on common health conditions for evaluation of possible associations with military service in Vietnam. Particular attention should be paid to the feasibility of conducting epidemiologic studies of conditions that have been noted to be of special interest but on which the current evidence is inadequate or insufficient to determine whether there is an association with herbicide exposure, such as COPD, brain cancer, tonsil cancer, melanoma (with particular attention given to ocular types), stroke, and Alzheimer disease. For very uncommon health outcomes, a case-control design would probably be most appropriate. Creative analysis of VA's own data resources may well be the most effective way to address those outcomes and to gain a better understanding of the role of herbicide exposure in development of stroke, prostate cancer, and Parkinson disease in Vietnam veterans.

VA could possibly use its medical databases more effectively, particularly if there is concern about a perceived conflict of interest in surveying its own databases, by involving external analysts. For example, an independent panel could be commissioned to identify and assign priorities to database information that would aid future VAO committees in fulfilling their charge from Congress. Alternatively, or in addition, VA could establish an external advisory group that could recommend the most efficient mechanisms for mining the medical database information, which could include issuing requests for proposals for the conduct of analytic studies related to specific health outcomes of interest.

Finally, as noted in previous VAO updates, data related to the distribution of claims that have been filed by Vietnam veterans could be very informative. Although applications for compensation and appeals constitute a nonrepresentative, self-selected sample that is influenced by which conditions are already judged to be service-related, an effort to use existing VA information should include a more systematic review of the distribution of health outcomes in the databases. The information that had accumulated in VA's records clearly generated a signal that motivated VA to ask prior VAO committees to make special evaluations of whether several specific malignancies were associated with herbicide exposure; ancillary information was adequate to enable the committees to conclude that chronic lymphocytic leukemia (CLL) and hairy-cell leukemia belong in the category of sufficient evidence of an association, but perhaps an answer for

Vietnam veterans concerning tonsil cancer will be found only by a case-control study that addresses deployment status and other emerging risk factors, such as viral infection.

In general, it is the committee's conviction that improved data linkage and data-sharing between DOD and VA would greatly enhance the conduct of military epidemiology and the utility of its results. The committee endorses DOD's efforts to improve collection of exposure data during current deployments; the impasses associated with missing exposure information will not impede investigations of health consequences in future veterans, as has been the case for Vietnam veterans. For optimal use, however, such DOD information on a veteran's combat experience needs to be readily connected with future medical events, much of which resides with VA.

- **Available information should be gleaned from existing cohort studies.**

In 2006, the Committee on the Disposition of the Air Force Health Study (AFHS) (IOM, 2006) recommended that all data from the AFHS be retained and suggested mechanisms by which the data could be made available to researchers. Since then, the Institute of Medicine (IOM) Medical Follow-up Agency (MFUA) has become the custodian of the data and biologic specimens (PL 109-364; 120 Stat. 2290); the specimens are held in storage at the Wright-Patterson Air Force Base under MFUA's aegis, and funding has been provided for IOM to maintain and manage the materials and to make them available for research. A strong commitment by the federal government is required to provide sufficient funds to develop the infrastructure necessary to meet the goals of further research that uses these invaluable data and biospecimens. Moreover, dedicated funding is required so that focused analyses can be carried out by independent investigators, especially in relation to the research questions that concern the present committee. The investment would be a small fraction of the $143 million invested to date in the AFHS. Such research could clarify the various issues and would reap substantial benefits in the understanding of health issues of Vietnam veterans exposed to herbicides. Comprehensive longitudinal analyses of the data collected in the six intensive medical examinations—which include data on medical interventions (such as hospitalizations and emergency-department visits), cancer incidence, mortality, and exposures—should be conducted to investigate some or all of the health outcomes that may be associated with the exposures under consideration in the present report. Distillation of existing data could be enhanced by incorporating new results derived from assays of the biologic samples. For example, analysis of banked semen samples for epigenetic markers on sperm DNA and measurement of TCDD in seminal fluid, particularly in comparison with the subjects' serum TCDD concentrations, could provide insight into the likelihood of male Vietnam veterans' transmitting effects to their offspring, as well as supplementing general knowledge on paternal transmission.

In Spring 2012, the Committee on the Management of the Air Force Health

Study Data and Specimens issued a request for proposals to use the AFHS materials (data or specimens) for innovative research. Each submission was subject to an intensive review by the entire committee to ensure that it was scientifically sound and feasible. Seven proposals were approved. The investigations have begun only fairly recently, so no results are available. A second request for proposals was issued in May 2013. The committee enthusiastically supports these new and continuing research efforts.

Members of the ACC constitute the largest cohort of Vietnam veterans exposed directly to herbicides and TCDD. They were involved in the handling and distribution of the chemicals in Vietnam. ACC veterans who reported spraying herbicides as part of their duties have been shown to have increased serum TCDD concentrations; this highly exposed population has also been shown to be at increased risk for several diseases. Previous VAO committees recommended that VA conduct additional studies of ACC veterans because the population presents a unique opportunity to examine the association between health effects of exposure to TCDD and the herbicides used in Vietnam. Recently, VA launched the Army Chemical Corps Vietnam-Era Veterans Health Study to investigate the relationship between herbicide exposure during the Vietnam War and hypertension and COPD in ACC veterans. Information garnered from the study could benefit VA and future VAO committees as potential associations between exposure to the chemicals of interest and respiratory outcomes are evaluated.

Although about 250,000 US women served in the military during the Vietnam War and 5,000–7,000 women served in Vietnam, few data on the health of the deployed and nondeployed female veterans are available. More than a decade ago, Kang et al. (2000a,b) examined the prevalence of gynecologic cancers in female Vietnam veterans and of birth defects in their children. More recently, Cypel and Kang (2008) reported a mortality study of the population, but additional followup of the health status of the group has been lacking. In 2009, VA announced the start of the Health of the Vietnam Era Veteran Women's Study, a 4-year undertaking to investigate the mental and physical health of deployed and nondeployed US women who served during the Vietnam War. Although findings from the study have yet to be published, the committee supports these VA efforts and hopes that the findings will help to elucidate how military service in Vietnam may have affected the health of female veterans who served.

At the direction of Congress, the National Vietnam Veterans Readjustment Study (1986–1988) investigated primarily psychiatric sequelae in a representative cohort of about 1,600 men and women. In 2000, Congress mandated (PL 106-419) that VA assess the current physical and mental well-being of the members of that cohort. In 2001, VA contracted for the work, named the National Vietnam Veterans Longitudinal Study (NVVLS), but progress ceased within 2 years. The VA Office of Inspector General (VAOIG, 2005) ruled that "the Study was not properly planned, procured, or managed" but directed that it be completed and that provisions be made to avoid the previous problems. Because baseline information is available on symptoms and chronic health problems in the original cohort, VAO committees have thought that completion of the NVVLS could generate useful information for future updates. On May 5, 2011, at a hearing of the House Veterans' Affairs Committee, the chair of the VAO committee for *Update 2008* had the privilege of testifying to that effect. In 2010, VA announced that a contractor had been engaged to conduct the study, with an expected completion date of 2013. Unfortunately from the perspective of VAO committees, the questionnaires and interviews are focusing on PTSD and psychologic issues rather than expanding the data-gathering to include the physical health status of this well-defined cohort. Particular attention should be paid to occurrence of conditions that have been noted to be of special interest but on which the current evidence is inadequate or insufficient to determine whether there is an association with herbicide exposure, such as COPD, brain cancer, tonsil cancer, melanoma (with particular attention given to ocular types), and Alzheimer disease. However, if a reliable, up-to-date estimate of overall mortality could be generated by following up this cohort, that presently elusive information would be quite helpful.

In 1978, the National Institute for Occupational Safety and Health (NIOSH) began to study US workers potentially exposed to TCDD. A total of 5,132 workers in 12 large manufacturing companies were included in the NIOSH cohort. The cohort has been a source of data very valuable in assessing the health effects associated with TCDD exposure, such as data from the recent study of PCP workers with and without TCDD exposure (Ruder and Yiin, 2011) that is referred to throughout the present report. The NIOSH studies have included high-quality exposure assessment, and evaluations of a wide array of health outcomes have been published. Given its value as an important source of epidemiologic data, the committee recommends that studies of the NIOSH cohort be extended.

The committee also notes that future analyses of health outcomes in those and other important study populations should be as specific as possible because generic findings, such as those for "all respiratory outcomes," are not useful in addressing the committee's charge to determine associations of herbicide exposures with specific health conditions.

- **Possible health effects in offspring of exposed men merit further investigation.**

The rapidly expanding field of epigenetics is revealing the molecular mechanisms by which environmental agents can modify gene expression without changing DNA sequence long after exposure occurs, even in later generations—at least in the case of maternal exposure to some chemicals. There is a growing body of evidence that TCDD can induce epigenetic changes in animal models, but there are few data that support risk of adverse effects in offspring of men exposed to xenobiotics in general and the VAO chemicals of interest in particular.

VAO committees have been monitoring studies of morphologic birth defects and cancer in the offspring of exposed people. Two major information gaps identified by the committee for *Update 2010* concerning possible association between exposure of male Vietnam veterans to the chemicals of interest and the development of disease in their offspring remain unfilled: a paucity of studies of the endpoints that VAO committees have been monitoring related to paternal exposure in the absence of maternal exposure and a failure to review systematically defined clinical health conditions that are manifested later in the offspring's lives. The few data on toxic contaminants in seminal fluid suggest that fetal exposure due to paternal transmission during later acts of intercourse is highly unlikely, but it now appears more physiologically possible that epigenetic modifications of sperm, including alterations in sperm mRNAs, microRNAs, and DNA after paternal exposure, might lead to changes in the offspring. The last of the few publications on birth defects in the offspring of male Vietnam veterans was published before the report on the children of female Vietnam veterans (Kang et al., 2000b), and none of the epidemiologic studies recently reviewed by the present committee assessed the role of paternal exposure in the occurrence of such effects. Thus, most of the available epidemiologic studies of effects in offspring are not relevant to the primary exposure group of concern: male Vietnam veterans. In addition, the epidemiologic studies of maternal exposure and adverse effects in offspring other than morphologic birth defects and cancer reviewed by this committee did not assess specific diseases in the offspring, but rather measured physiologic biomarkers that might or might not predict the potential for disease development later in life.

On the basis of those information gaps, the present committee favors renewed efforts to conduct epidemiologic studies on all the developmental effects in offspring that may be associated with *paternal exposure*. In addition, new studies should evaluate offspring for *defined clinical health conditions that develop later in life*, focusing on organ systems that have shown the greatest effects after maternal exposure, including neurologic, immune, and endocrine effects. Finally, although the committee recognizes that there is evidence that environmental exposures can affect later generations through fetal and germ line modifications, epidemiologic investigation designed to associate toxicant exposures with health effects manifested in *later generations* will be even more challenging to conduct than is research on adverse effects on the first generation. Thus, the committee recommends development of epidemiologic protocols to address the logistical challenge of determining whether adverse effects are being manifested in later generations as a result of paternal exposure: consideration must be given to the minimum sample size needed to detect changes if present, the most sensitive and reliable outcome measures that should be included, and the need for animal studies to provide mechanistic insight into documented epidemiologic associations. The best cohorts for revealing potential associations would be those with known, well-characterized exposure information. Another approach could be adopting a case-control structure and exploring whether information about Vietnam exposure or specific herbicide exposure could be ascertained in any of the many birth cohorts that have been established in the last several decades. To home in on a paternal effect, however, it will be necessary to establish that the mothers did not have the opportunity for other than background exposure to the chemicals of interest. Epidemiologic studies of the potential for paternally mediated effects on health outcomes in offspring of Vietnam veterans (such as Operation Ranch Hand veterans or ACC) vs nondeployed Vietnam-era veterans are also strongly encouraged by this committee.

- **There is a need for epidemiologic studies of the incidence of COPD.**

As discussed above, VA has initiated a renewed morbidity study of the ACC cohort and may publish findings in time for the next VAO update. The committee would welcome studies in additional populations of COPD diagnosed individuals using appropriate functional tests with adjustment for smoking status and consideration of comorbidities that could contribute to death from COPD.

- **There is a need for new animal models to elucidate mechanisms of diseases and disease progression.**

The committee believes that experimental research in the mechanisms that underlie human health outcomes (particularly cardiovascular disease, B-cell cancers, and paternally mediated effects in offspring) could provide valuable information related to the risk of disease in Vietnam veterans and their children. The development of animal models of neurologic outcomes and various chronic health conditions and their progression would be useful for understanding the possible contributions of the chemicals of interest to compromise the health of aging Vietnam veterans. Specifically, determining the mechanism by which dioxin-like chemicals induce B-cell cancers and how exposure to dioxin-like chemicals alters susceptibility to obesity and components of metabolic syndrome would fill important knowledge gaps. Furthermore, animal models elucidating the effects of paternal exposure on the development of disease in offspring would be very informative, particularly in identifying the timing and duration of exposure that are most critical and the susceptibility of specific organ systems to disease development in offspring later in life. Animal studies of the mechanisms of inhibition of fetal growth, particularly in male offspring, after maternal exposure could help to elucidate findings seen in some epidemiologic studies that examined maternal exposure and birth weight.

The predecessors of this committee have offered similar recommendations of additional research to resolve outstanding questions. This committee remains particularly concerned about stroke, COPD, hypertension, melanoma, tonsil cancer, Alzheimer disease, and paternally transmitted effects on offspring.

REFERENCES[1]

Alavanja MC, Sandler DP, Lynch CF, Knott C, Lubin JH, Tarone R, Thomas K, Dosemeci M, Barker J, Hoppin JA, Blair A. 2005. Cancer incidence in the Agricultural Health Study. *Scandinavian Journal of Work, Environment and Health* 31(Suppl 1):39–45.

Cypel Y, Kang H. 2008. Mortality patterns among women Vietnam-era veterans: Results of a retrospective cohort study. *Annals of Epidemiology* 18(3):244–252.

IOM (Institute of Medicine). 2006. *Disposition of the Air Force Health Study.* Washington, DC. National Academies Press.

Kang HK, Mahan CM, Lee KY, Magee CA, Selvin S. 2000a. Prevalence of gynecologic cancers among female Vietnam veterans. *American Journal of Industrial Medicine* 38(4):447–454.

Kang HK, Mahan CM, Lee KY, Magee CA, Mather SH, Matanoski G. 2000b. Pregnancy outcomes among US women Vietnam veterans. *American Journal of Industrial Medicine* 38(4):447–454.

Ruder AM, Yiin JH. 2011. Mortality of US pentachlorophenol production workers through 2005. *Chemosphere* 83(6):851–861.

VA (Department of Veterans Affairs). 2010. Health effects not associated with exposure to certain herbicide agents. *Federal Register* 75(109):32540–32553.

VAOIG (Department of Veterans Affairs Office of Inspector General). 2005. *Audit of VA Acquisition Practices for the National Vietnam Veterans Longitudinal Study* (Report No. 04-02330-212). Washington, DC.

[1]Throughout this report, the same alphabetic indicator after year of publication is used consistently for a given reference when there are multiple citations by the same first author in a given year. The convention of assigning the alphabetic indicators in order of citation in a given chapter is not followed.

Appendix A

Issues Raised by the Public and Agendas of Public Meetings Held by the Committee to Review the Health Effects in Vietnam Veterans of Exposure to Herbicides (Ninth Biennial Update) and Other Written Submissions to the Committee

ISSUES RAISED BY THE PUBLIC

Following delivery of the committee's charge by a VA representative at the first meeting, the open session continued with brief presentations by other members of the public. It has been the practice of VAO committees to conduct open sessions, not only to gather additional information from people who have particular expertise on points that arise during deliberations but also especially to hear from individual Vietnam veterans and others concerned about aspects of their health experience that may be service-related. Open sessions were held during the first four of the committee's five meetings.

Having solicited input, the committee feels a responsibility to address the concerns raised, even if it is only to the extent of noting that a topic does not fall within the committee's charge. The issues raised by veterans or their advocates during the current updating period fell into five general categories. The following is a summary of the topics raised at the open sessions or in submitted written statements with the committee's responses to them.

- **Veterans exposed to Agent Orange in places other than Vietnam**: Veterans noted several locations or situations (listed below) where they believe they were exposed to Agent Orange and so are entitled to coverage of those diseases recognized as service-related for veterans who had "boots on the ground" in Vietnam. Evaluating data on the basis of *where* veterans may have experienced herbicide exposure is not within the scope of this committee's charge.
    - Thailand

- Guam
- State-side military facilities
- Blue Water Navy
- Post-Vietnam exposure of reservists to residual Agent Orange contamination in C123 aircraft

- **Health problems in children and grandchildren** of Vietnam veterans: Chapter 10 addresses evidence related to the possibility that the herbicide exposure of Vietnam veterans has had adverse consequences for their progeny. It discusses the current paucity of information on the *general phenomenon* of the transmission of adverse effects to offspring following *paternal exposure to toxic agents*.
- **Health outcomes not currently treated as being related to Vietnam service:**
  - **Autoimmune conditions** (such as negative rheumatoid-factor arthritis and fibromyalgia): The paucity of evidence from human studies on herbicide exposure and immunologic responses, despite the substantial toxicologic evidence of TCDD's role in such health problems, motivated the committee for *Update 2010* to address this issue in considerable depth. The current committee endorses the usefulness of its predecessor's discussion of factors that may contribute to this apparent discrepancy (see Chapter 7).
  - **Bladder cancer**: The relevant available epidemiologic evidence remains inadequate and insufficient to support an association. See Chapter 8 for specific discussion.
  - **Squamous-cell cancer of head and neck**: The relevant available epidemiologic evidence remains inadequate and insufficient to support an association, but the committee continues to recommend that VA endeavor to use its own data to determine whether they constitute supportive evidence. See Chapter 8 for specific discussion.
  - **Ocular melanoma** (particularly **choroidal melanoma**): A Vietnam veteran who had choroidal melanoma submitted information received from VA after a Freedom of Information Act (FOIA) request. The data are not adequately explained and labeled, but they suggest that the condition is being treated in VA facilities far more often than expected on the basis of national incidence rates. Without more details on how the statistics were abstracted, it is not possible for the committee to interpret their meaning. The paucity of information on this specific form of malignancy is discussed in Chapter 8. The committee recommends that VA systematically evaluate the information on the condition that is available in its records.
  - **Myelodysplastic syndrome (MDS)**: The relevant available epidemiologic evidence remains inadequate and insufficient to support an association of MDS with exposure to the herbicides constituting the

committee's COIs. See Chapter 9 for specific discussion. Exposure to benzene is recognized as being a risk factor for MDS, and it is a component of the petroleum products used as dispersants with the herbicides. Benzene is so highly volatile that it would no longer be part of the sprayed herbicides as they reached ground level, and so it is not covered under the committee's charge. Several epidemiologic studies addressing risk factors for MDS were identified in the recent update period, but the available evidence remains insufficiently specific with respect to the COIs to provide a basis of a decision concerning association other than the default decision of inadequate or insufficient.

- **Neurologic problems** (delayed-onset peripheral neuropathy, restless leg syndrome, Willis-Ekbom disease or periodic limb-movement disorder, migraines, and anterior ischemic optic neuropathy): VAO committees continue to consider any relevant information concerning possible associations between the COIs and the delayed-onset form of peripheral neuropathy (see Chapter 11). The other neurologic conditions have not been subjects of epidemiologic research identified in VAO literature searches.
- **High blood pressure**: Although VA has not regarded this health outcome as presumptively compensable for Vietnam veterans, the committee continues to endorse the finding of the committee for *Update 2008* that there is limited or suggestive evidence of an association between hypertension and exposure to components of the herbicides used in Vietnam.
- **Peripheral vascular disease**: See Chapter 12.
- **Endocrine effects**: See Chapter 13.

• **Health effects of chemicals other than Agent Orange**: All chemicals in the herbicides used in Vietnam (picloram, cacodylic acid, phenoxy herbicides, TCDD, and dioxin-like compounds) are considered COIs by VAO committees. It should be noted, however, that studies of Vietnam veterans addressing only deployment status, rather than characterizing specific agents of exposure of individual subjects, have always been regarded as contributors to the evidentiary database in keeping with the provision of the Agent Orange Act that veterans serving in Vietnam were presumptively exposed to herbicides.

- Petroleum-based dispersants used in spraying Agent Orange: These dispersants are recognized to contain benzene, which is acknowledged to be a causal agent of AML and MDS; this volatile chemical would not remain present in sprayed herbicides. There is a vast toxicologic literature on petroleum products and their constituents (for example, see *Gulf War and Health: Volume 3—Fuel, Combustion Products, and Propellants* [IOM, 2005]) and on the various

chemical families of insecticides (see also *Gulf War and Health: Volume 2—Insecticides and Solvents* [IOM, 2003]).
    - CS gas: This cyanocarbon was used as the defining component of tear gas during military training and in Vietnam.
    - Vietnam veterans may have experienced **multiple potentially harmful exposures** in addition to herbicide exposure: Addressing interactions or synergies of other substances (such as benzene-containing **petroleum products**, the extensively used **insecticides**, or **CS gas**) with the several components of the herbicides is beyond the scope of the committee's charge. People are continually exposed to many chemicals whose possible adverse effects might be exacerbated by exposure to other agents. The number of pairs that could be addressed is enormous, and it would rise exponentially if triads and larger combinations were considered.
- **Exposure modeling for Agent Orange (AgDrift [Ginevan and Ross] vs Exposure Opportunity Model [Stellmans]**: The merits of these two exposure models and their potential usefulness for resolving outstanding issues are discussed in Chapter 3.
- **Issues with VA procedures**: These topics are not within the scope of the committee's statement of task.
    - Living overseas prevents getting VA medical care.
    - IOM's standard for evaluating health outcomes should not be changed from association to causality by Congress or any other party.
    - VA's claims process takes too long.
    - Judgments made in VA's appeals process for claims of service-related health outcomes are not consistent for a given condition—for example, squamous-cell carcinomas of the head and neck (tonsil cancer), bladder cancer, AML, and MDS.

FIRST PUBLIC MEETING

June 28, 2012
NAS Building, Room 125
2100 C Street, NW
Washington, DC 20418

Presentations

- Welcome; Goals and Conduct of the Public Meeting; Introduction of Committee Members
  Mary Walker, Committee Chair

- Charge to the Committee
  Wendi Dick, MD, US Department of Veterans Affairs

- Similar Health Conditions of Era Veterans with Agent Orange Exposure on Guam
  LeRoy Foster
  Frank Stanton

- Agent Orange Exposure at Fort McClellan, Alabama
  Helena Van Clief, Army Staff Sergeant

- Injustice to Vietnam Veterans
  Placido Salazar

- Vietnam–era Veterans Exposed Outside of Vietnam
  Carlo Albanese

- Herbicide Use in Thailand
  Ken Witkin, President, Airborne Battlefield Command Control Center Association

- Advocate of Vietnam Veterans
  William G. Jeff Davis, Founder and Senior Legislative Advocate, The Veterans Association of Sailors of the Vietnam War, Inc.

- Children of American Vietnam Veterans
  D. Karen Reyes, Co-Founder, Agent Orange Legacy, Children of American Vietnam Veterans

- Speaking on Behalf of Vietnam Veterans
  Rick Weidman, Executive Director for Policy and Government Affairs, Vietnam Veterans of America

Additional written statements received from:

David A. Aswad	Bladder cancer
Thomas Jefferson Barr, Jr.	Delayed peripheral neuropathy and restless leg syndrome
Gary J. Chenett	On behalf of the Order of the Silver Rose, recognize health problems in veterans exposed to Agent Orange outside Vietnam; personally, diagnosed with four cancers

Michael Eckstein	Willis-Ekbom disease/Periodic Limb Movement Disorder
Charles W. Griesler	Migraines daily from 1967 and other neurological problems
Debbie J. Gunn	Husband lost nose to squamous cell carcinoma
Geraldine Hall-Bast	First Vietnam Veteran husband died at 48 of cardiac disease; their daughter has asthma and other respiratory problems; second Vietnam Veteran husband had post-traumatic stress disorder (violent), hepatitis, and died of cancer; third VV husband peripheral numbness due to Parkinson's and post-traumatic stress disorder
Michael P. Hartmaier	All chemicals in herbicides used in Vietnam should be covered, not just Agent Orange
Damiana Hortas-Dowdy	Basic training at Ft. McClellan; now, negative rheumatoid arthritis/ fibromyalgia
Floyd McKinney	Exposed to Agent Orange at Fort Sill, OK; type 2 diabetes and prostate cancer
Mark and Beth Rutz	Veterans Administration responded to their Freedom of Information Act request with information indicating choroidal (type of ocular) melanoma is treated more often than expected among veterans
Larry Sauger	Myelodysplastic syndrome; benzene in petroleum products used to thin Agent Orange
Jim Wallace	Exposed to Agent Orange at several military locations stateside; he and son have Agent Orange-related conditions
Wane Wolcott	Anterior ischemic optic neuropathy, numb toes, high blood pressure, borderline diabetes, autoimmune disorder related to connective tissue; lives overseas so not getting VA medical care

SECOND PUBLIC MEETING

August 9, 2012
Courtyard Marriott
Meeting Room A
300 West Michigan Street
Milwaukee, WI 53203

Presentations

- Welcome; Goals and Conduct of the Public Meeting; Introduction of Committee
  Mary Walker, Committee Chair

- Speaking on Behalf of Wisconsin Vietnam Veterans
  Kim Michalowski, Director of Bureau of Claims, Wisconsin Department of Veterans Affairs

- Veteran Concerned about Effects in Offspring
  John Crespi

- Veteran Concerned about Effects in Offspring
  Mike Demske, Agent Orange Committee of National Vietnam Veterans of America

- Concerns about Congress Changing IOM's Standard from Association to Causality
  Kent Draper

- Veteran with Peripheral Vascular Disease
  Eugene Pogorzelski

- Veteran Speaking on Myelodysplastic Syndromes (MDS)
  Larry Sauger

- Blue Water Navy Veteran with Agent Orange Health Conditions
  James W. Sobotta

Additional written statements received from:

Donald Lund	Concern about exposure to CS gas
James Wachtendonk	K-9 handler in Vietnam

Zachary James Wachtendonk	(deceased at age 30) Son of Vietnam veteran with congenital problems exacerbated by exposure as child to 2,4-D in park
Mary S. Wachtendonk	(wife of Vietnam veteran)

THIRD PUBLIC MEETING

November 27, 2012
Hotel Monteleone
Royal Salon D
214 Royal Street
New Orleans, LA 70130

Presentations

- Welcome; Goals and Conduct of the Public Meeting; Introduction of Committee
  Mary Walker, Committee Chair

- Metabolic and Vascular Diseases *(Invited Speaker)*
  Lisa Cassis, Ph.D., Professor and Chair, University of Kentucky

- Speaking on Behalf of Vietnam Veterans
  Suzanne Moore

- Concerns about Endocrine Effects
  Marc McCabe, Bureau Chief/Regional Director, St. Petersburg Regional Office, Vietnam Veterans of America

- Department of Veterans Affairs—Past and Present Research *(Invited Speaker)*
  Han Kang, Ph.D., retired Director, Environmental Epidemiology Service, Department of Veterans Affairs

Additional written statements received from:

James Tomes	Exposure of Vietnam-era veterans stateside

FOURTH PUBLIC MEETING

January 16, 2013
Arnold and Mabel Beckman Center
National Academies of Sciences & Engineering
100 Academy
Irvine, CA 92612-3002

Presentations

- Welcome; Goals and Conduct of the Public Meeting; Introduction of Committee
  Mary Walker, Committee Chair

- Health Concerns of Vietnam Veterans
  Ken Holybee, Director at Large, Vietnam Veterans of America

- National Health Committee co-chair, Associates of VVA—paternally mediated birth defects
  Elayne Mackey

- Health Issues and Effects in Children
  Conrad T. Gomez

- Health Problems as Daughter of Vietnam Veteran and Data Collection by Children of Vietnam Veterans Health Alliance (COVVHA)
  Jenna Van Leer, COVVHA

- Widow of Vietnam Veteran
  Debra Kraus, artist

- Contamination of C123 Aircraft Used by Reservists
  Wes Carter

Phone conversation (invited speakers)—Paternal transmission of adverse effects to offspring

- *Andy Olshan*, PhD, Chair of Epidemiology, University of North Carolina
- *Kim Boekelheide*, MD, PhD, Professor of Medical Science, Brown University

Additional written statements received from:

Dale Hemrick	Health issues in veterans and their offspring

Nancy McMaa	Oral squamous cell carcinoma of her Vietnam veteran husband
Jim Purtell	Song composed concerning damage from Agent Orange
Martha Sidwell	(wife of Vietnam veteran, Dale Hemrick) Relationship difficulties of returning deployed veterans
Jeanne Stellman, PhD	Response to Ginevan and Ross on exposure opportunity model

REFERENCES

IOM (Institute of Medicine). 2003. *Gulf War and Health: Volume 2—Insecticides and Solvents.* Washington, DC: The National Academies Press.

IOM. 2005. *Gulf War and Health: Volume 3—Fuel, Combustion Products, and Propellants.* Washington, DC: The National Academies Press.

Appendix B

Short-Term Adverse Health Responses

The committee responsible for *Update 2008* advised removal of chloracne, porphyria cutanea tarda (PCT), and early-onset peripheral neuropathy from the body of the Veterans and Agent Orange (VAO) reports, and the committee for *Update 2010* removed them. The three conditions that occur in temporal proximity to exposure have little relevance to new claims from Vietnam veterans, and there has been minimal new evidence since they were classified as having evidence of an association with herbicide exposure.

The three conditions have long been recognized by the Department of Veterans Affairs as presumptively related to service in Vietnam. Consequently, the committee wants to provide easy access to the body of biomedical evidence on which these decisions were made by retaining the information distilled in this appendix, and it recommends their inclusion in the corresponding appendixes of future volumes in the VAO series.

CHLORACNE

Chloracne is a skin disease that is characteristic of exposure to 2,3,7,8-tetrachlorodibenzo-*p*-dioxin (TCDD) and other diaromatic organochlorine chemicals. It shares some pathologic processes (such as the occlusion of the orifice of the sebaceous follicle) with more common forms of acne (such as acne vulgaris), but it can be differentiated by the presence of epidermoid inclusion cysts, which are caused by proliferation and hyperkeratinization (horn-like cornification) of the epidermis and sebaceous gland epithelium. Although chloracne is typically distributed over the eyes, ears, and neck, it can also occur on the trunk, genitalia, and buttocks of chemical-industry workers exposed to TCDD (Neuberger et al., 1998). It is resistant to acne treatments, but it usually regresses.

Chloracne has been used as a marker of exposure in epidemiologic studies of populations exposed to TCDD and related chemicals. It is one of the few findings in humans that are consistently associated with such exposure, and it is a well-validated indicator of high-dose exposure to TCDD and related chemicals (Sweeney et al., 1997/98). If chloracne occurs, it appears shortly after the chemical exposure, not after a long latent period; therefore, new cases of chloracne among Vietnam veterans would not be the result of exposure during the Vietnam War. It should be noted that absence of chloracne does not necessarily indicate absence of substantial exposure to TCDD, as is apparent from studies of people who had documented exposure to TCDD after the Seveso incident in 1976 in Italy (Baccarelli et al., 2005a), nor is there necessarily a correlation between serum TCDD concentration and the occurrence or severity of chloracne. Susceptibility to the development of chloracne varies among individuals.

Conclusions from *VAO* and Previous Updates

The committee responsible for *Veterans and Agent Orange: Health Effects of Herbicides Used in Vietnam* (referred to as *VAO*; IOM, 1994) determined that there was sufficient evidence of an association between exposure to at least one chemical of interest (TCDD) and chloracne. Additional information available to the committees responsible for *Veterans and Agent Orange: Update 1996* (IOM, 1996), *Update 1998* (IOM, 1999), *Update 2000* (IOM, 2001), *Update 2002* (IOM, 2003), *Update 2004* (IOM, 2005), *Update 2006* (IOM, 2007), *Update 2008* (IOM, 2009), and *Update 2010* (IOM, 2011) has not modified that conclusion.

Even in the absence of a full understanding of the cellular and molecular mechanisms that lead to the disease, several notable reviews (Panteleyev and Bickers, 2006; Sweeney and Mocarelli, 2000) have deemed the clinical and epidemiologic evidence of dioxin-induced chloracne to be strong. The occupational epidemiologic literature has many examples of chloracne in workers after reported industrial exposures (Beck et al., 1989; Bond et al., 1987, 1989a,b; Cook et al., 1980; Goldman, 1972; May, 1973, 1982; Oliver, 1975; Pazderova-Vejlupkova et al., 1981; Poland et al., 1971; Suskind and Hertzberg, 1984; Suskind et al., 1953; Zober et al., 1990). With relative-risk estimates as high as 5.5 in exposed workers compared with referent nonexposed workers, Bond et al. (1989a) identified a dose–response relationship between probable exposure to TCDD and chloracne. Not everyone exposed to relatively high doses develops chloracne, and some with lower exposure may acquire it (Beck et al., 1989).

Almost 200 cases of chloracne were recorded in those residing in the vicinity of the accidental industrial release of dioxin in Seveso. Most cases occurred in children, particularly those who lived in the highest-exposure zone, and most cases resolved within 7 years (Assennato et al., 1989a,b; Caramaschi et al., 1981; Mocarelli et al., 1991). No cases of chloracne were identified in conjunction with the nonextreme environmental dioxin contamination at Times Beach, Missouri (Webb et al., 1987).

Exposures of Vietnam veterans were substantially lower than those observed in occupational studies and in environmental disasters, such as the one in Seveso. The long period since the putative exposure has imposed methodologic limitations on studies of Vietnam cohorts for chloracne. Nonetheless, the Vietnam Experience Study (CDC, 1988) found that chloracne was self-reported more often by Vietnam veterans than by Vietnam-era veterans (odds ratio [OR] = 3.9). An excess incidence was also found in Vietnam vs era veterans among subjects who were physically examined (OR = 7.3). In comparison with a nonexposed group, Air Force Ranch Hand personnel potentially exposed to Agent Orange reported a significant excess of acne (OR = 1.6) (Wolfe et al., 1990), but no cases of chloracne or postinflammatory scars were found on physical examination 20 years after possible herbicide exposure (AFHS, 1991b).

Biologic Plausibility

Previous updates have reported that chloracne-like skin lesions have been observed in several animal species in response to exposure to TCDD but not to purified phenoxy herbicides. Data accruing over the last several decades demonstrated that TCDD alters differentiation of human keratinocytes, and more recent studies have illuminated how. Geusau et al. (2005) found that TCDD accelerates the events associated with early differentiation but also obstructs completion of differentiation. Panteleyev and Bickers (2006) proposed that the major mechanism of TCDD induction of chloracne is activation of the stem cells in the basal layer of the skin to differentiate and inhibition of their ability to commit fully to a differentiated status. Ikuta et al. (2010) have investigated the expression of B-lymphocyte maturation protein 1 in epidermal keratinocytes and sebocytes in mice after induction of the aryl hydrocarbon receptor (AHR). Recent work with a constitutively activated form of the AHR implicated additional inflammation-related mechanisms by which TCDD exposure may lead to chloracne (Tauchi et al., 2005). The data support a biologically plausible mechanism for the induction of chloracne by TCDD.

Synthesis

No epidemiologic data in the last decade have refuted the conclusion of prior VAO committees that the evidence of an association between exposure to dioxin and chloracne is sufficient. The 2004 poisoning case of Ukrainian politician Victor Yushchenko has provided a high-profile instance that supports the idea that this condition can be a response to high-level exposure to TCDD, and the careful monitoring of his case has demonstrated the course of chloracne's resolution in conjunction with subsiding serum concentrations (Sorg et al., 2009). The formation of chloracne lesions after administration of TCDD has been observed in some species of laboratory animals.

Conclusion

On the basis of numerous epidemiologic studies of occupationally and environmentally exposed populations and supportive toxicologic information, previous VAO committees have consistently concluded that there is sufficient evidence of an association between exposure to at least one chemical of interest and chloracne. Because TCDD-associated chloracne becomes evident shortly after exposure, there is no risk of new cases long after service in Vietnam. Given the established relationship of an association between TCDD and chloracne and the long period that has elapsed since service in Vietnam, the committee for *Update 2010* concluded that the emergence of additional biologic or epidemiologic evidence that would merit review and deliberation by later VAO committees is unlikely. The current committee found that to be the case.

PORPHYRIA CUTANEA TARDA

Porphyrias are uncommon disorders caused by deficiencies of enzymes involved in the pathway of biosynthesis of heme, the iron-containing nonprotein portion of the hemoglobin molecule. PCT, the most common of the porphyrias, is a heterogeneous group of disorders caused by a deficiency of a specific enzyme, uroporphyrinogen decarboxylase. It can be inherited but usually is acquired. Type I PCT, which accounts for 80–90% of all cases, is an acquired disease that typically becomes evident in adulthood. It can occur spontaneously but usually occurs in conjunction with environmental factors, such as alcohol consumption, exposure to estrogens, or use of some medications.

The most important clinical finding in PCT is cutaneous photosensitivity. Sensitivity to sunlight is thought to result from the excitation of excess porphyrins in the skin by long-wave ultraviolet radiation, which leads to cell damage. Fluid-filled vesicles and bullae develop on sun-exposed areas of the face and on the dorsal surfaces of the hands, feet, forearms, and legs. Other features include hypertrichosis (excess hair) and hyperpigmentation (increased pigment), especially on the face. People with PCT have increased porphyrins in the liver, plasma, urine, and stools. Iron, estrogens, alcohol, viral hepatitis, and chlorinated hydrocarbons can aggravate the disorder. Iron overload is almost always present in people who have PCT.

Conclusions from *VAO* and Previous Updates

On the basis of strong animal studies and case reports demonstrating TCDD-induced PCT and resolution after cessation of exposure, the committee responsible for *VAO* determined that there was sufficient evidence of an association between exposure to TCDD and PCT in genetically susceptible people.

Epidemiologic studies of occupational populations have indicated inconsistent associations between the chemicals of interest and increased urinary uroporphyrin. Bleiberg et al. (1964) reported increased urinary uroporphyrin in 11 of 29 workers in a factory that manufactured 2,4-dichlorophenoxyacetic acid (2,4-D) and 2,4,5-trichlorophenoxyacetic acid (2,4,5-T) and the manifestation of some clinical evidence of PCT in three of them. In a followup study of the same facility 6 years later, no abnormalities in urinary porphyrins were observed (Poland et al., 1971). Calvert et al. (1992) reported no difference in porphyrinuria or the occurrence of PCT between 281 workers in the National Institute for Occupational Safety and Health (NIOSH) cohort who were involved in the production of trichlorophenol and were exposed to TCDD and 260 nonexposed workers. Serum TCDD concentration was not associated with uroporphyrin or coproporphyrin concentrations.

Among people who were exposed to TCDD as a result of the 1976 chemical plant explosion in Seveso, Italy, clinical PCT was observed only in a brother and a sister who had a mutant enzyme that confers susceptibility in the heterozygous state. In 1977, 60 Seveso residents were tested for increased porphyrins, and 13 had secondary coproporphyrinuria; increased concentrations persisted in only three cases that were thought to be due to liver damage and alcohol consumption (Doss et al., 1984). In the Quail Run mobile-home park in Missouri, residents exposed to dioxin as a result of the spraying of waste oil contaminated with TCDD were found to have higher urinary uroporphyrins than did controls, but no cases of clinical PCT were diagnosed (Hoffman et al., 1986; Stehr-Green et al., 1987).

The baseline study of the US Air Force Operation Ranch Hand veterans (AFHS, 1984) showed no difference in uroporphyrin or coproporphyrin concentrations in urine between the Ranch Hand veterans and controls. There were no indications of the clinical appearance of PCT in the Ranch Hand veterans. Followup studies of the Ranch Hand cohort revealed that mean uroporphyrin was greater in the comparison group than in that cohort, whereas mean coproporphyrin was higher in the Ranch Hand cohort. The clinical significance of the small differences between the Ranch Hand veterans and the comparison groups was uncertain.

The committee responsible for *Update 1996* considered three additional nonpositive citations of populations that had substantial exposure to TCDD. Jung et al. (1994) presented porphyrin data on former workers in a German pesticide plant that had manufactured 2,4-D and 2,4,5-T. Of 170 men tested, 27 had present or past chloracne. The study found no difference in porphyrin concentrations between subjects with and without chloracne. There was also no relationship between abnormal results of liver-function tests or porphyrin concentrations and the presence of chloracne. And there was no relationship between porphyrin concentrations in urine, red blood cells, or plasma and TCDD concentrations in adipose tissue. Three cases of chronic hepatic porphyria (none with overt PCT and none with chloracne) were identified—a number that did not exceed the expected prevalence in this population. Von Benner et al. (1994) found no indication of clinical porphyria in self-referred workers in six other German chemical plants. Another report on the NIOSH cohort (Calvert et al., 1994) was negative. On the basis of the cumulative findings, the committee responsible for *Update 1996* concluded that there was only limited or suggestive evidence of an association. The committees for later updates have not changed the revised conclusion.

Because PCT is manifested shortly after exposure to TCDD, new cases of PCT attributable to exposure during the Vietnam War are not expected to occur.

Biologic Plausibility

PCT has not been exactly replicated in animal studies of the effects of TCDD, although other porphyrin abnormalities have been reported. Administration of TCDD to mice results in an accumulation of uroporphyrin that occurs in a manner that requires the AHR, cytochrome P450 1A1 (CYP1A1), and CYP1A2 (Robinson et al., 2002; Smith et al., 2001; Uno et al., 2004), but the underlying mechanism of action has not been fully illuminated (Smith and Chernova, 2009; Smith and Elder, 2010).

Synthesis

No epidemiologic data have emerged in the last decade that refute the conclusion of previous VAO committees that there is limited or suggestive evidence of an association between the chemicals of interest and PCT.

Conclusion

On the basis of the evidence reviewed here and in previous VAO reports, the committee concludes that there is limited or suggestive evidence of an association between exposure to at least one chemical of interest and PCT. PCT is rare, and its occurrence may be influenced by genetic predisposition in people who have low concentrations of protoporphyrinogen decarboxylase. Because TCDD-associated changes in porphyrin excretion become evident shortly after exposure, there is no risk that new cases will occur long after service in Vietnam. Given the recognized association between TCDD and porphyrin excretion and the long period that has elapsed since service in Vietnam, the committee concludes that the emergence of additional biologic and epidemiologic evidence that would merit review and deliberation by later VAO committees is unlikely.

EARLY-ONSET PERIPHERAL NEUROPATHY

Since *Update 1996*, VAO committees have partitioned their consideration of peripheral neuropathy into early-onset (implicitly transient) peripheral neuropathy and chronic peripheral neuropathy. Primarily on the basis of reports of short-term health effects after industrial accidents, the committee responsible for *Update 1996* concluded that there was limited or suggestive evidence of an association between exposure to the chemicals of interest and "acute and subacute" neuropathy, which was redesignated early-onset transient peripheral neuropathy by the committee responsible for *Update 2004*. The committee for *Update 2010* recognized the imprecision in the nomenclature that had been used to characterize the type of peripheral neuropathy that is regarded as service-connected. The diagnosis in question is, in fact, contingent on the *proximity of its occurrence to the time of exposure* rather than on the transitory nature of the adverse outcome. Clinically, in cases of an immediate response of peripheral neuropathy after toxicant exposure, stabilization or improvement is the rule after exposure ends. However, recovery may not be complete; the degree of recovery can depend on the severity of the initial deficits and the particular exposure. Furthermore, there is a possibility of "subclinical" effects, and a person might be unaware of symptoms even though evidence of nerve dysfunction can be found through detailed neurologic examination or electrodiagnostic testing. Thus, the committee chose to delete the word *transient* to recognize that symptoms of early-onset peripheral neuropathy may be protracted and that recovery from them may be incomplete.

The information about peripheral neuropathy presented in this appendix demonstrates that it may occur soon after exposure to extremely high concentrations of dioxin. In addition, this appendix addresses the evidence that some people who experience early-onset peripheral neuropathy (that is, during or shortly after dioxin exposure) may continue to manifest the problem long after exposure has ceased; this would show that early-onset peripheral neuropathy is not necessarily transient.

Conclusions from *VAO* and Previous Updates

Several occupational studies have evaluated whether herbicide exposure or production may lead to early-onset neuropathy. In March 1949, an explosion occurred in a reactor vessel in a chemical plant in Nitro, West Virginia, where 2,4,5-T was being produced. Many workers reported health effects (toxic hepatitis, increased serum lipids, and central nervous system involvement), including a severe acute neuropathy in four workers who had chloracne (Ashe et al., 1949, 1950). Thirty years later, an attempt was made to identify workers who had been exposed during that accident and workers who may have been chronically exposed during 1948–1969 (Suskind and Hertzberg, 1984). Neurologic examination and nerve-conduction studies did not demonstrate abnormalities compared with a cohort of unexposed controls; however, the procedure for obtaining controls did not ensure equivalence. It is unclear whether the four subjects who had acute neuropathy were included in the effort.

In April 1979, chlorinated dibenzo-*p*-dioxin contamination was found in a community in Arkansas that was close to a plant where 2,4,5-T and 2,4-D had been produced since 1957. Fifty-five workers in that plant who had no history of diabetes or alcohol abuse were identified from the total workforce; they underwent neurologic examination and nerve-conduction studies (Singer et al., 1982). Both median motor and calf sensory nerve-conduction studies showed significantly lower conduction velocity in the plant workers than in control subjects.

Other industrial accidents have also suggested a link between chemicals of interest and early-onset neuropathic symptoms, which persisted in some people. Jirasek et al. (1974) studied 55 of 80 workers who complained of a variety of symptoms after chronic exposure to 2,4,5-T in a manufacturing facility in the Czech Republic; of the 55, results of physical examinations of 17 suggested neuropathy that was said to have been confirmed with electromyographic abnormalities. Followup of 44 of the 55 was conducted 10 years after exposure had ceased; about 30% of them were reported to have continued neuropathic symptoms (Pazderova-Vejlupkova et al., 1981). More recently, Urban et al. (2007) evaluated long-term sequelae in subjects who developed neuropathy after the original exposure. Subjects had increased serum TCDD concentrations more than 30 years after exposure, and evidence of continued neuropathy was noted in nine of 15 subjects who were available for study.

Acute neuropathic symptoms were reported after the Seveso accident, and persistent signs were noted. Gilioli et al. (1979) evaluated 35 subjects who had been exposed during the accident and noted abnormalities in a variety of neurophysiologic measures compared with age-matched controls 2 years after the exposure. However, it is unclear how the exposed subjects were selected for study. In a more complete survey, Boeri et al. (1978) studied 470 subjects from two exposure zones about a year after the accident and found a higher incidence of neurophysiologic abnormalities than in nonexposed controls; the residents of the zone of greater exposure were more severely affected than those of the less exposed zone. The same group (Filippini et al., 1981) found increased prevalence of peripheral neuropathy in residents who had indicators of exposure compared with those who did not (relative risk [RR] = 2.6, 95% confidence interval [CI] 1.0–7.2 for those with choracne; RR = 3.6, 95% CI 1.3–10.2, for those with increased hepatic enzymes) when they were evaluated 21 months after the accident. Improvement may have occurred since the accident. Assennato et al. (1989a,b) studied 193 exposed residents of the area 9 years after the accident and did not find neurophysiologic abnormalities. However, the number of residents in the group who originally complained of neuropathic symptoms was not discussed. Similiarly, 6 years after the accident, Barbieri et al. (1988) examined 153 residents who had developed chloracne. World Health Organization critieria for neuropathy were not fulfilled for any subjects, but there was a statistically significant increase in neurophysiologic abnormalities compared with those in nonexposed age-matched controls.

There have been a number of case reports of exposure-associated early-onset neuropathy. Goldstein et al. (1959) reported the cases of three patients seen at the Mayo Clinic who had acute weakness and sensory loss demonstrated to be due to peripheral neuropathy; symptoms occurred within hours of an exposure to 2,4-D that included sufficient skin contact for clothes and skin to be wet. The three patients recovered incompletely: in one, a cerebrospinal fluid (CSF) examination was normal except for minimally increased protein. Todd (1962) reported another case of neuropathy that occurred about 4 days after 2,4-D exposure, again in sufficient quantities to cause large areas of skin to be wet. Clinical examination demonstrated a sensory motor polyneuropathy; CSF examination showed slightly increased protein but was otherwise normal. The patient recovered substantially but not completely over 2 years. Finally, Berkley and Magee (1963) reported a case of a 39-year-old man who had symptoms of acute neuropathy that progressed to inability to walk starting 4 days after 2,4-D exposure; CSF analysis was normal, including normal protein concentrations, and he recovered nearly completely over the course of 8 months.

Case reports do not provide conclusive evidence of causal relationships, but the cases discussed above showed a close temporal relationship between high exposure to 2,4-D and neuropathy. The most likely non–toxicant-related acute neuropathy is Guillain-Barré syndrome; however, this syndrome is associated with characteristic findings on clinical neurophysiologic examination and highly increased protein in CSF. In the three cases above that had CSF evaluation, protein concentrations were either normal or increased to a minimal extent not consistent with Guillain-Barré syndrome. In addition, patients who had clinical neurophysiologic studies also showed abnormalities not consistent with Guillain-Barré. Thus, it seems likely that the cases represent the results of 2,4-D exposure.

Biologic Plausibility

Neuronal cell cultures treated with 2,4-D showed decreased neurite extension associated with intracellular changes, including a decrease in microtubules, inhibition of the polymerization of tubulin, disorganization of the Golgi apparatus, and inhibition of ganglioside synthesis (Rosso et al., 2000a,b). Those mechanisms are important for maintaining synaptic connections between nerve cells and supporting the mechanisms involved in axon regeneration during recovery from peripheral neuropathy. Grahmann et al. (1993) and Grehl et al. (1993) reported observations of electrophysiologic and pathologic abnormalities, respectively, in the peripheral nerves of rats treated with TCDD. When the animals were sacrificed 8 months after exposure, there was pathologic evidence of axonal nerve damage and there were histologic findings typical of toxicant-induced injury.

Those results constitute evidence of the biologic plausibility of an association between exposure to the chemicals of interest and peripheral neuropathy.

Conclusions

On the basis of studies of health effects after industrial accidents and the well-documented cases reported above, VAO committees since the one responsible for *Update 1996* have concluded that there is limited or suggestive evidence of an association between exposure to the chemicals of interest and early-onset peripheral neuropathy. Inasmuch as new data on this subject, especially with regard to Vietnam veterans, are unlikely to emerge, the present committee reaffirms that finding.

REFERENCES[1]

AFHS (Air Force Health Study). 1984. *An Epidemiologic Investigation of Health Effects in Air Force Personnel Following Exposure to Herbicides. Baseline Morbidity Study Results.* Brooks AFB, TX: USAF School of Aerospace Medicine. NTIS AD-A138 340.

AFHS. 1991b. *An Epidemiologic Investigation of Health Effects in Air Force Personnel Following Exposure to Herbicides. Mortality Update: 1991.* Brooks AFB, TX: Armstrong Laboratory.

Ashe WF, Suskind RR. 1949, 1950. *Reports on Chloracne Cases, Monsanto Chemical Co., Nitro, West Virginia, October 1949 and April 1950.* Cincinnati, OH: Department of Environmental Health, College of Medicine, University of Cincinnati (unpublished).

Assennato G, Cervino D, Emmett E, Longo G, Merlo F. 1989a. Follow-up of subjects who developed chloracne following TCDD exposure at Seveso. *American Journal of Industrial Medicine* 16:119–125.

Assennato G, Cannatelli P, Emmett E, Ghezzi I, Merlo F. 1989b. Medical monitoring of dioxin clean-up workers. *American Industrial Hygiene Association Journal* 50:586–592.

Baccarelli A, Pfeiffer R, Consonni D, Pesatori AC, Bonzini M, Patterson DG Jr, Bertazzi PA. Landi MT. 2005a. Handling of dioxin measurement data in the presence of non-detectable values: Overview of available methods and their application in the Seveso chloracne study. *Chemosphere* 60(7):898–906.

Barbieri S, Pirovano C, Scarlato G, Tarchini P, Zappa A, Maranzana M. 1988. Long-term effects of 2,3,7,8-tetrachlorodibenzo-*p*-dioxin on the peripheral nervous system. Clinical and neurophysiological controlled study on subjects with chloracne from the Seveso area. *Neuroepidemiology* 7:29–37.

Beck H, Eckart K, Mathar W, Wittkowski R. 1989. Levels of PCDDs and PCDFs in adipose tissue of occupationally exposed workers. *Chemosphere* 18:507–516.

Berkley MC, Magee KR. 1963. Neuropathy following exposure to a dimethylamine salt of 2,4-D. *Archives of Internal Medicine* 111(3):351–352.

Bleiberg J, Wallen M, Brodkin R, Applebaum IL. 1964. Industrially acquired porphyria. *Archives of Dermatology* 89:793–797.

[1]Throughout this report, the same alphabetic indicator after year of publication is used consistently for a given reference when there are multiple citations by the same first author in a given year. The convention of assigning the alphabetic indicators in order of citation in a given chapter is not followed.

Boeri R, Bordo B, Crenna P, Filippini G, Massetto M, Zecchini A. 1978. Preliminary results of a neurological investigation of the population exposed to TCDD in the Seveso region. *Rivista di Patologia Nervosa e Mentale* 99:111–128.

Bond GG, Cook RR, Brenner FE, McLaren EA. 1987. Evaluation of mortality patterns among chemical workers with chloracne. *Chemosphere* 16:2117–2121.

Bond GG, McLaren EA, Brenner FE, Cook RR. 1989a. Incidence of chloracne among chemical workers potentially exposed to chlorinated dioxins. *Journal of Occupational Medicine* 31:771–774.

Bond GG, McLaren EA, Lipps TE, Cook RR. 1989b. Update of mortality among chemical workers with potential exposure to the higher chlorinated dioxins. *Journal of Occupational Medicine* 31:121–123.

Calvert GM, Hornung RV, Sweeney MH, Fingerhut MA, Halperin WE. 1992. Hepatic and gastrointestinal effects in an occupational cohort exposed to 2,3,7,8-tetrachlorodibenzo-*para*-dioxin. *Journal of the American Medical Association* 267:2209–2214.

Calvert GM, Sweeney MH, Fingerhut MA, Hornung RW, Halperin WE. 1994. Evaluation of porphyria cutanea tarda in US workers exposed to 2,3,7,8-tetrachlorodibenzo-*p*-dioxin. *American Journal of Industrial Medicine* 25(4):559–571.

Caramaschi F, Del CG, Favaretti C, Giambelluca SE, Montesarchio E, Fara GM. 1981. Chloracne following environmental contamination by TCDD in Seveso, Italy. *International Journal of Epidemiology* 10:135–143.

CDC (Centers for Disease Control and Prevention). 1988. Centers for Disease Control Vietnam Experience Study. Health status of Vietnam veterans. II: Physical health. *Journal of the American Medical Association* 259(18):2708–2714.

Cook RR, Townsend JC, Ott MG, Silverstein LG. 1980. Mortality experience of employees exposed to 2,3,7,8-tetrachlorodibenzo-*p*-dioxin (TCDD). *Journal of Occupational Medicine* 22:530–532.

Doss M, Sauer H, von Tiepermann R, Colombi AM. 1984. Development of chronic hepatic porphyria (porphyria cutanea tarda) with inherited uroporphyrinogen decarboxylase deficiency under exposure to dioxin. *International Journal of Biochemistry* 16(4):369–373.

Filippini G, Bordo B, Crenna P, Massetto N, Musicco M, Boeri R. 1981. Relationship between clinical and electrophysiological findings and indicators of heavy exposure to 2,3,7,8-tetrachlorodibenzodioxin. *Scandinavian Journal of Work, Environment, and Health* 7(4):257–262.

Geusau A, Khorchide M, Mildner M, Pammer J, Eckhart L, Tschachler E. 2005. 2,3,7,8-tetrachlorodibenzo-*p*-dioxin impairs differentiation of normal human epidermal keratinocytes in a skin equivalent model. *Journal of Investigative Dermatology* 124(1):275–277.

Gilioli R, Cotroneo L, Bulgheroni C, Genta PA, Rota E, Cannatelli P, Fereari E. 1979. Neurological monitoring of workers exposed to TCDD: Preliminary neurophysiological results. *Activitas Nervosa Superior* 21:288–290.

Goldman P. 1972. Critically acute chloracne caused by trichlorophenol decomposition products. *Arbeitsmedizen Sozialmedizen Arbeitshygiene* 7:12–18.

Goldstein NP, Jones PH, Brown JR. 1959. Peripheral neuropathy after exposure to an ester of dichlorophenoxyacetic acid. *Journal of the American Medical Association* 171:1306–1309.

Grahmann F, Claus D, Grehl H, Neundorfer B. 1993. Electrophysiologic evidence for a toxic polyneuropathy in rats after exposure to 2,3,7,8-tetrachlorodibenzo-*p*-dioxin (TCDD). *Journal of the Neurological Sciences* 115(1):71–75.

Grehl H, Grahmann F, Claus D, Neundorfer B. 1993. Histologic evidence for a toxic polyneuropathy due to exposure to 2,3,7,8-tetrachlorodibenzo-*p*-dioxin (TCDD) in rats. *Acta Neurologica Scandinavica* 88(5):354–357.

Hoffman RE, Stehr-Green PA, Webb KB, Evans RG, Knutsen AP, Schramm WF, Staake JL, Gibson BB, Steinberg KK. 1986. Health effects of long-term exposure to 2,3,7,8-tetrachlorodibenzo-*p*-dioxin. *Journal of the American Medical Association* 255:2031–2038.

Ikuta T, Ohba M, Zouboulis CC, Fujii-Kuriyama Y, Kawajiri K. 2010. B lymphocyte-induced maturation protein 1 is a novel target gene of aryl hydrocarbon receptor. *Journal of Dermatological Science* 58(3):211–216.

IOM (Institute of Medicine). 1994. *Veterans and Agent Orange: Health Effects of Herbicides Used in Vietnam.* Washington, DC: National Academy Press.

IOM. 1996. *Veterans and Agent Orange: Update 1996.* Washington, DC: National Academy Press.

IOM. 1999. *Veterans and Agent Orange: Update 1998.* Washington, DC: National Academy Press.

IOM. 2001. *Veterans and Agent Orange: Update 2000.* Washington, DC: National Academy Press.

IOM. 2003. *Veterans and Agent Orange: Update 2002.* Washington, DC: The National Academies Press.

IOM. 2005. *Veterans and Agent Orange: Update 2004.* Washington, DC: The National Academies Press.

IOM. 2007. *Veterans and Agent Orange: Update 2006.* Washington, DC: The National Academies Press.

IOM. 2009. *Veterans and Agent Orange: Update 2008.* Washington, DC: The National Academies Press.

IOM. 2011. *Veterans and Agent Orange: Update 2010.* Washington, DC: The National Academies Press.

Jirasek L, Kalensky J, Kubec K, Pazderova J, Lukas E. 1974. Chronic poisoning by 2,3,7,8-tetrachlorodibenzo-*p*-dioxin. *Ceskoslovenska Dermatologie* 49:145–157.

Jung D, Konietzko J, Reill-Konietzko G, Muttray A, Zimmermann-Holz HJ, Doss M, Beck H, Edler L, Kopp-Schneider A. 1994. Porphyrin studies in TCDD-exposed workers. *Archives of Toxicology* 68:595–598.

May G. 1973. Chloracne from the accidental production of tetrachlorodibenzodioxin. *British Journal of Industrial Medicine* 30:276–283.

May G. 1982. Tetrachlorodibenzodioxin: A survey of subjects ten years after exposure. *British Journal of Industrial Medicine* 39(2):128–135.

Mocarelli P, Needham LL, Marocchi A, Patterson DG Jr, Brambilla P, Gerthoux PM, Meazza L, Carreri V. 1991. Serum concentrations of 2,3,7,8-tetrachlorodibenzo-*p*-dioxin and test results from selected residents of Seveso, Italy. *Journal of Toxicology and Environmental Health* 32:357–366.

Neuberger M, Kundi M, Jäger R. 1998. Chloracne and morbidity after dioxin exposure (preliminary results). *Toxicology Letters* 96–97:347–350.

Oliver RM. 1975. Toxic effects of 2,3,7,8 tetrachlorodibenzo 1,4-dioxin in laboratory workers. *British Journal of Industrial Medicine* 32:49–53.

Panteleyev AA, Bickers DR. 2006. Dioxin-induced chloracne—Reconstructing the cellular and molecular mechanisms of a classic environmental disease. *Experimental Dermatology* 15(9):705–730.

Pazderova-Vejlupkova J, Lukáš E, Nemcova M, Pickova J, Jirasek L. 1981. The development and prognosis of chronic intoxication by tetrachlorodibenzo-*p*-dioxin in men. *Archives of Environmental Health* 36:5–11.

Poland AP, Smith D, Metter G, Possick P. 1971. A health survey of workers in a 2,4-D and 2,4,5-T plant with special attention to chloracne, porphyria cutanea tarda, and psychologic parameters. *Archives of Environmental Health* 22:316–327.

Robinson SW, Clothier B, Akhtar RA, Yang AL, Latour I, Van Ijperen C, Festing MF, Smith AG. 2002. Non-AhR gene susceptibility Loci for porphyria and liver injury induced by the interaction of 'dioxin' with iron overload in mice. *Molecular Pharmacology* 61(3):674–681.

Rosso SB, Caceres AO, Evangelista de Duffard AM, Duffard RO, Quiroga S. 2000a. 2,4-dichlorophenoxyacetic acid disrupts the cytoskeleton and disorganizes the golgi apparatus of cultured neurons. *Toxicologic Sciences* 56:133–140.

Rosso SB, Garcia GB, Madariaga MJ, De Duffard AME, Duffard RO. 2000b. 2,4-dichlorophenoxyacetic acid in developing rats alters behaviour, myelination and regions brain gangliosides pattern. *NeuroToxicology* 21(1-2):155–164.

Singer R, Moses M, Valciukas J, Lilis R, Selikoff IJ. 1982. Nerve conduction velocity studies of workers employed in the manufacture of phenoxy herbicides. *Environmental Research* 29:297–311.

Smith AG, Chernova T. 2009. Chapter 6 disruption of heme synthesis by polyhalogenated aromatics. *Advances in Molecular Toxicology* 3(C):161–210.

Smith AG, Elder GH. 2010. Complex gene-chemical interactions: Hepatic uroporphyria as a paradigm. *Chemical Research in Toxicology* 23(4):712–723.

Smith AG, Clothier B, Carthew P, Childs NL, Sinclair PR, Nebert DW, Dalton TP. 2001. Protection of the Cyp1a2 (-/-) null mouse against uroporphyria and hepatic injury following exposure to 2,3,7,8-tetrachlorodibenzo-*p*-dioxin. *Toxicology and Applied Pharmacology* 173(2):89–98.

Sorg O, Zennegg M, Schmid P, Fedosyuk R, Valikhnovskyi R, Gaide O, Kniazevych V, Saurat JH. 2009. 2,3,7,8-tetrachlorodibenzo-*p*-dioxin (TCDD) poisoning in victor yushchenko: Identification and measurement of TCDD metabolites. *Lancet* 374(9696):1179–1185.

Stehr-Green P, Hoffman R, Webb K, Evans RG, Knutsen A, Schramm W, Staake J, Gibson B, Steinberg K. 1987. Health effects of long-term exposure to 2,3,7,8-tetrachlorodibenzo-*p*-dioxin. *Chemosphere* 16:2089–2094.

Suskind RR, Hertzberg VS. 1984. Human health effects of 2,4,5-T and its toxic contaminants. *Journal of the American Medical Association* 251(18):2372–2380.

Suskind R, Cholak J, Schater LJ, Yeager D. 1953. *Reports on Clinical and Environmental Surveys at Monsanto Chemical Co., Nitro, West Virginia, 1953.* Cincinnati, OH: Department of Environmental Health, University of Cincinnati (unpublished).

Sweeney MH, Mocarelli P. 2000. Human health effects after exposure to 2,3,7,8-TCDD. *Food Additives and Contaminants* 17(4):303–316.

Sweeney MH, Calvert GM, Egeland GA, Fingerhut MA, Halperin WE, Piacitelli LA. 1997/98. Review and update of the results of the NIOSH medical study of workers exposed to chemicals contaminated with 2,3,7,8-tetrachlorodibenzodioxin. *Teratogenesis, Carcinogenesis, and Mutagenesis* 17(4–5):241–247.

Tauchi M, Hida A, Negishi T, Katsuoka F, Noda S, Mimura J, Hosoya T, Yanaka A, Aburatani H, Fujii-Kuriyama Y, Motohashi H, Yamamoto M. 2005. Constitutive expression of aryl hydrocarbon receptor in keratinocytes causes inflammatory skin lesions. *Molecular and Cellular Biology* 25(21):9360–9368.

Todd RL. 1962. A case of 2,4-D intoxication. *Journal of the Iowa Medical Society* 52:663–664.

Uno S, Dalton TP, Sinclair PR, Gorman N, Wang B, Smith AG, Miller ML, Shertzer HG, Nebert DW. 2004. Cyp1a1(-/-) male mice: Protection against high-dose TCDD-induced lethality and wasting syndrome, and resistance to intrahepatocyte lipid accumulation and uroporphyria. *Toxicology and Applied Pharmacology* 196(3):410–421.

Urban P, Pelclová D, Lukas E, Kupka K, Preiss J, Fenclová Z, Smerhovsky Z. 2007. Neurological and neurophysiological examinations on workers with chronic poisoning by 2,3,7,8-TCDD: Follow-up 35 years after exposure. *European Journal of Neurology* 14(2):213–218.

Von Benner A, Edler L, Mayer K, Zober A. 1994. "Dioxin" investigation program of the chemical industry professional association. *Arbeitsmedizin Sozialmedizin Praventivmedizin* 29:11–16.

Webb K, Evans RG, Stehr P, Ayres SM. 1987. Pilot study on health effects of environmental 2,3,7,8-TCDD in Missouri. *American Journal of Industrial Medicine* 11:685–691.

Wolfe WH, Michalek JE, Miner JC, Rahe A, Silva J, Thomas WF, Grubbs WD, Lustik MB, Karrison TG, Roegner RH, Williams DE. 1990. Health status of Air Force veterans occupationally exposed to herbicides in Vietnam. I. Physical health. *Journal of the American Medical Association* 264:1824–1831.

Zober A, Messerer P, Huber P. 1990. Thirty-four-year mortality follow-up of BASF employees exposed to 2,3,7,8-TCDD after the 1953 accident. *International Archives of Occupational and Environmental Health* 62:139–157.

Appendix C

Clarification of Cancer Groupings Used in Reporting Results, with Correspondence to National Institute for Occupational Safety and Health Cause-of-Death Codes and International Classification of Diseases Codes for Cancers

In response to a request from the Department of Veterans Affairs, the committee responsible for *Update 2006* prepared Table C-1 to demonstrate how conclusions provided for the full range of cancer types and to clarify into which groupings any specific cancer diagnosis falls. The committee for *Update 2010* reframed its overview of lymphohematopoietic neoplasms according to the World Health Organization (WHO) classification system (WHO, 2008), which partitions these disorders first according to the lymphoid or myeloid lineage of the transformed cells rather than as lymphomas or leukemias; this emphasizes the close etiologic relationship of chronic lymphocytic leukemia and hairy-cell leukemia with Hodgkin and non-Hodgkin lymphomas and with the neoplasm multiple myeloma and its related condition AL amyloidosis.

The major portion of evidence compiled for review in the Veterans and Agent Orange (VAO) series comes from cohort studies, primarily of mortality but some of incidence. Other data have been generated by case-control studies, which follow the only design amenable to studying very infrequent or very specific health outcomes. How researchers are able to group, analyze, and report their findings is influenced by the distribution of cases that they observe, so the data that VAO committees have had available for review reflect mortality experience at a level of specificity concordant with statistical analysis.

The *International Classification of Diseases* (ICD) system is used by physicians and researchers around the world to group related diseases and procedures so that morbidity and mortality information can be classified for statistical purposes in a standard form that is amenable to data storage and retrieval. It is a comprehensive hierarchic system that permits great detail but can be collapsed into broad categories. Codes mentioned in VAO reports are stated in terms of

TABLE C-1 Mapping of Groupings of Malignant Neoplasms That Are the Subjects of Conclusions in the Veterans and Agent Orange Series with ICD-9 Codes

NIOSH Category for Cause of Death: Major	Minor	NIOSH Groupings of Cancer Sites	**"VAO Characterization of Grouping"**[a] Subsites	**ICD-9 Codes**
02		Buccal cavity and pharynx	**"Oral, nasal, and pharyngeal"**	
	004	Lip		140
	005	Tongue		141
	006	Other parts of buccal cavity		
			Salivary glands	142
			Floor of mouth	144
			Gum and other mouth	143, 145
	007	Pharynx		
			Oropharynx	146
			Tonsil	146.0–146.2
			Nasopharynx	147
			Hypopharynx	148
			Other buccal cavity and pharynx	149
				(160 = nasal below)
03		Digestive organs and peritoneum		
	008	Esophagus	**"Esophagus"**	150
	009	Stomach	**"Stomach"**	151
	010	Intestine except rectum	**"Colorectal"**	
			Small intestine	152
			Colon (large intestine)	153
	011	Rectum		154
	012	Biliary passages, liver, and gall bladder	**"Hepatobiliary"**	
			Liver and intrahepatic bile ducts	155
			Gallbladder and extrahepatic bile ducts	156
	013	Pancreas		157

	014	Retroperitoneum and other and unspecified digestive organs		158–159
04		Respiratory system	**"Respiratory"**	
	015	Larynx	**"Larynx"**	161
	016	Trachea, bronchus, and lung	**"Lung"**	162
			Trachea	162.0 (there is no ICD 162.1)
			Lung and bronchus	162.2–162.9
	017	Pleura		163
	018	Other respiratory		
			Nasal cavity, middle ear, and accessory sinuses	(160, above with oral and pharyngeal)
			Thymus, heart, and mediastinum	164 (164.0, below with endocrine; 164.1, below with soft tissue sarcoma)
			Other respiratory, unspecified	165 (discontinuity with ICD codes)
05	019	Breast (male and female)	**"Breast"**	174, 175
06		Female genital organs	**"Female reproductive"**	
	020	Cervix uteri		180
	021	Other unspecified parts of uterus		179, 181, 182
			Uterus, parts unspecified	179
			Placenta	181
			Body of uterus	182
	022	Ovary, fallopian tube, and broad ligament		183
			Ovary	183.0 (there is no ICD 183.1)
			Fallopian tube and other uterine adnexa	183.2–183.9
	023	Other female genital organs		184
07		Male genital system		185, 186
	024	Prostate	**"Prostate"**	185
	025	Testis	**"Testicular"**	186
		Penis and other male genital organs	[for NIOSH in minor group 036]	187

continued

TABLE C-1 Continued

NIOSH Category for Cause of Death		NIOSH Groupings of Cancer Sites	"VAO Characterization of Grouping"[a] Subsites	ICD-9 Codes
Major	Minor			
08		Urinary system		
	026	Kidney (including renal pelvis and ureter)	**"Renal"**	189.0–189.2
	027	Bladder and other urinary organs	**"Urinary bladder"**	188, 189.3–189.9
			Bladder	188
			Urethra, paraurethral glands, other and unspecified urinary	189.3–189.9
				(discontinuity with ICD codes)
09		Other and unspecified sites		
	028	Bone ("and articular cartilage" in ICD nomenclature)	**"Bone and joint"**	170
	029	Melanoma	**"Melanoma"**	172
	030	Other malignant skin neoplasm	**"Non-melanoma skin"**	173
	031	Mesothelioma		No codes (new minor code, above with lung)
	032	Connective ("and other soft" in ICD nomenclature) tissue	**"Soft-tissue sarcoma"**	171
			(heart)	(164.1)
	033	Brain and other parts of nervous system (ICD "soft tissue" includes peripheral nerves and autonomic nervous system)	**"Brain"**	191–192
	034	Eye		190
	035	Thyroid		193
			(thymus)	164.0
	036	Other and unspecified sites	Other endocrine cancers	194
			Other and ill-defined sites	195

			Stated or assumed to be secondary of specified sites	196–198
			Site unspecified	199
10		Lymphatic and hematopoietic tissue		
		Lymphoma		
	037	**Hodgkin disease**		201
	038	**Non-Hodgkin lymphoma**		200, 202 (excluding 202.4), 273.3
	039	**Multiple myeloma**		203 (excluding 203.1)
	040	Leukemia and aleukemia	**"Leukemia (other than chronic B-cell leukemias)"**	204–208
		Lymphocytic	primary grouping now with other neoplasms of lymphocytic origin, lymphomas and multiple myeloma	
			Acute lymphocytic	204.0
			"Chronic lymphocytic (including hairy cell leukemia)"	204.1
			Other lymphocytic	202.4, 204.2–204.9
		Myeloid (granulocytic)		
			Acute myeloid	
			Acute	205.0
			Acute erythremia and erythroleukemia	207.0
			Megakaryocytic leukemia	207.2
			Chronic myeloid	205.1
			Other myeloid	205.2–205.3, 205.8–205.9
		Monocytic		
			Acute monocytic	206.0
			Chronic monocytic	206.1
			Other monocytic	206.2–206.9
		Other leukemia		
			Other acute	208.0
			Other chronic	207.1, 208.1
			Aleukemic, subleukemia and "not otherwise specified"	203.1, 207.2, 207.8, 208.2–208.9

[a]**Boldface cancer (sub)site:** most comprehensive grouping for which a conclusion has been drawn.

ICD, Revision 9 (ICD-9). ICD-7, ICD-8, and ICD-9 were in effect for deaths that occurred in 1960–1967, 1968–1978, and 1979–1998, respectively; the differences among them are fairly subtle. Although ICD-10, which went into effect for coding causes of deaths that occurred from 1999 on, appears radically different from the earlier versions, it corresponds in large part to basically the same disease entities (see Table C-2). Most published epidemiologic studies considered in the VAO series have been related to health outcomes that occurred and were encoded before ICD-10 went into effect.

Since 1983, the National Institute for Occupational Safety and Health (NIOSH) has maintained software for generating standardized expectations, as derived from US mortality data assembled by the National Center for Health Statistics, for ICD-encoded mortality datasets. An article by Robinson et al. (2006) discusses revisions to that standard software to incorporate deaths coded according to ICD-10 and includes conversions and equivalences among ICD-7, ICD-8, ICD-9, and ICD-10 for 119 exhaustive categories of cause of death. Codes for malignant neoplasms span the ICD-9 range 140.0–208.9, NIOSH's major categories 02–10, or NIOSH's more specific minor categories 004–040.

The NIOSH death codes for neoplasms provide comprehensive scaffolding for organizing the committee's reviews and conclusions by cancer type that is somewhat simpler than ICD classifications but maps completely to the ICD system as it has evolved. Because the NIOSH system has been used to mediate analysis of many sets of cohort data, its groupings correspond quite closely to the published research findings available for review by VAO committees. In general cohort studies, one is unlikely to encounter results on more specific groupings than NIOSH's minor categories.

As discussed in Chapter 2, the VAO committees have not framed its conclusions strictly in terms of ICD codes, but the ICD system has been a valuable tool for the work of VAO committees. There can be coding errors on hospital records or death certificates, but when researchers present their results labeled with ICD codes, there can be little ambiguity about what they intended. When their most definitive indication is something like "respiratory cancers," however, there can be uncertainty about where the evidence should be considered. In such cases, the committee has done its best to follow the hierarchy laid out in Table C-1.

As indicated above, many of the studies reviewed by the committee use or were written up at a time when ICD-9 was in place. Accordingly, ICD references in this report use that scheme. ICD-10 began to be implemented in the United States in 1999. It differs from ICD-9 in level of detail (about 8,000 categories vs about 5,000 in ICD-9) and nomenclature (alphanumeric vs the numeric codes of ICD-9); additions and modifications were also made with regard to some coding rules and the rules for selecting an underlying cause of death (Anderson et al., 2001). Table C-2 lists the ICD-9 and ICD-10 codes for the various forms of malignant neoplasm addressed in this report. In situ neoplasms, benign neoplasms,

TABLE C-2 Surveillance, Epidemiology, and End Results (SEER) Program Malignant Neoplasm Site Groupings for ICD-9 and ICD-10

Cancer Site	ICD-9 Codes	ICD-10 Codes
Buccal cavity and pharynx		
Lip	140.0–140.9	C00.0–C00.9
Tongue	141.0–141.9	C01, C02.1–C02.9
Salivary glands	142.0–142.9	C07, C08.0–C08.9
Floor of mouth	144.0–144.9	C04.0–C04.9
Gum and other mouth	143.0–143.9, 145.0–145.6, 145.8–145.9	C03.0–C03.9, C05.0–C05.9, C06.0–C06.9
Nasopharynx	147.0–147.9	C11.1–C11.9
Tonsil	146.0–146.2	C09.0–C09.9
Oropharynx	146.3–146.9	C10.1–C10.9
Hypopharynx	148.0–148.9	C12, C13.0–C13.9
Other buccal cavity and pharynx	149.0–149.9	C14.0–C14.9
Digestive system		
Esophagus	150.0–150.9	C15.0–C15.9
Stomach	151.0–151.9	C16.0–C16.9
Small intestine	152.0–152.9	C17.0–C17.9
Colon excluding rectum	153.0–153.9, 159.0	C18.0–C18.9, C26.0
Rectum and rectosigmoid junction	154.0–154.1	C19, C20
Anus, anal canal, and anorectum	154.2–154.3, 154.8	C21.0–C21.9
Liver and intrahepatic bile duct		
Liver	155.0,155.2	C22.0, C22.2–C22.4, C22.7–C22.9
Intrahepatic bile duct	155.1	C22.1
Gallbladder	156.0	C23
Other biliary	156.1–156.9	C24.0–C24.9
Pancreas	157.0–157.9	C25.0–C25.9
Retroperitoneum	158.0	C48.0
Peritoneum, omentum, and mesentery	158.8–158.9	C48.1–C48.2
Other digestive organs	159.8–159.9	C26.8–26.9, C48.8
Respiratory system		
Nasal cavity, middle ear, and accessory sinuses	160.0–160.9	C30.0, C30.1, C31.0–C31.9
Larynx	161.0–161.9	C32.0–C32.9
Lung and bronchus	162.2–162.9	C34.0–C34.9
Pleura	163.0–163.9	C38.4
Trachea, mediastinum, and other respiratory organs	162.0, 164.2–165.9	C33, C38.1–C38.3, C38.8, C39
Bones and joints	170.0–170.9	C40.0–C40.9, C41.0–C41.9
Soft tissue (including heart)	171.0–171.9, 164.1	C38.0, C47.0–C47.9, C49.0–C49.9
Skin		
Malignant melanomas	172.0–172.9	C43.0–C43.9
Other malignant skin neoplasms	173.0–173.9	C44.0–C44.9

continued

TABLE C-2 Continued

Cancer Site	ICD-9 Codes	ICD-10 Codes
Breast (male and female)	174.0–174.9, 175	C50.0–C50.9
Female genital system		
Cervix	180.0–180.9	C53.0–C53.9
Corpus	182.0–182.1, 182.8	C54.0–C54.9
Uterus, not otherwise specified	179	C55
Ovary	183.0	C56.0–C56.9
Vagina	184.0	C52
Vulva	184.1–184.4	C51.0–C51.9
Other female genital organs	181, 183.2–183.9, 184.8, 184.9	C57.0–C57.9, C58
Male genital system		
Prostate	185	C61
Testis	186.0–186.9	C62.0–C62.9
Penis	187.1–187.4	C60.0–C60.9
Other male genital organs	187.5–187.9	C63.0–C63.9
Urinary system		
Urinary bladder	188.0–188.9	C67.0–C67.9
Kidney and renal pelvis	189.0, 189.1	C64.0–C64.9, C65.0–C65.9
Ureter	189.2	C66.0–C66.9
Other urinary organs	189.3–189.4, 189.8–189.9	C68.0–C68.9
Eye and orbit	190.0–190.9	C69.0–C69.9
Brain and other nervous system		
Brain	191.0–191.9	C71.0–C71.9
Meninges	192.1	C70.0–C70.9
Other nervous system[a]	192.0, 192.2–192.9	C72.0–C72.9
Endocrine system		
Thyroid	193	C73
Other endocrine (including thymus)	164.0, 194.0–194.9	C37, C74.00–C74.92, C75.0–C75.9
Lymphomas		
Hodgkin's disease	201.0–201.9	C81.0–81.9
Non-Hodgkin's lymphomas	200.0–200.8, 202.0–202.2, 202.8–202.9	C82.0–C82.9, C83.0–C83.9, C84.0–C84.5, C85.0–C85.9, C96.3
Multiple myeloma	203.0, 238.6	C90.0, C90.2
Leukemias		
Lymphocytic		
Acute lymphocytic	204.0	C91.0
Chronic lymphocytic	204.1	C91.1
Other lymphocytic	202.4, 204.2–204.9	C91.2-C91.4, C91.7, C91.9
Myeloid (granulocytic)		
Acute myeloid	205.0, 207.0, 207.2	C92.0, C92.4–C92.5, C94.0, C94.2

TABLE C-2 Continued

Cancer Site	ICD-9 Codes	ICD-10 Codes
Chronic myeloid	205.1	C92.1
Other myeloid	205.2–205.3, 205.8–205.9	C92.2–C92.3, C92.7, C92.9
Monocytic		
Acute monocytic	206.0	C93.0
Chronic monocytic	206.1	C93.1
Other monocytic	206.2–206.9	C93.2, C93.7, C93.9
Other leukemia		
Other acute	208.0	C94.4, C94.5, C95.0
Other chronic	207.1, 208.1	C94.1, C95.1
Aleukemic, subleukemic and "not otherwise specified"	203.1, 207.2, 207.8, 208.2–208.9	C90.1, C91.5, C94.3, C94.7, C95.2, C95.7, C95.9
Miscellaneous malignant neoplasms	159.1, 195.0–195.8, 196.0–196.9, 199.0–199.1, 202.3, 202.5–202.6, 203.8	C26.1, C76.0–C76.8, C77.0–C77.9, C78.0–C78.8, C79.0–C79.8, C80, C88.0–C88.9, C96.0–C96.2, C96.7, C96.9, C97

[a]Cancers of the peripheral nerves and the autonomic nervous system are classified as "soft tissue" in ICD. Adapted from Ries et al. (2003), Table A-4.

neoplasms of uncertain behavior, and neoplasms of unspecified behavior have separate codes in both schemes.

REFERENCES

Anderson RN, Minino AM, Hoyert DL, Rosenberg HM. 2001. Comparability of cause of death between ICD-9 and ICD-10: preliminary estimates. *National Vital Statistics Reports* 49(2):1–32.

Ries LAG, Eisner MP, Kosary CL, Hankey BF, Miller BA, Clegg L, Mariotto A, Fay MP, Feuer EJ, Edwards BK (eds). 2003. *SEER Cancer Statistics Review, 1975–2000.* Bethesda, MD: National Cancer Institute.

Robinson CF, Schnorr TM, Cassinelli RT, Calvert GM, Steenland K, Gersic CM, Schubauer-Berigan MK. 2006. Tenth revision U.S. mortality rates for use with the NIOSH Life Table Analysis System. *Journal of Occupational and Environmental Medicine* 48(7):662–667.

WHO (World Health Organization). 2008. *WHO Classification of Tumours of Haematopoietic and Lymphoid Tissue* (4th edition). Lyon, France: World Health Organization.

Appendix D

Biographies of Committee to Review the Health Effects in Vietnam Veterans of Exposure to Herbicides (Ninth Biennial Update) and Staff

Mary K. Walker, PhD (*Chair*), is Regents' Professor of Pharmacology/Toxicology in the University of New Mexico College of Pharmacy. Her research focuses on the mechanisms by which various ligands (including dioxin) for the aryl hydrocarbon receptor (AHR) induce excessive or insufficient activation and thereby produce subtle changes in gene expression that lead to an increased risk of cardiovascular disease in adulthood and on the structural, functional, and molecular changes in adult cardiovascular physiology in a genetic mouse model that lacks the AHR gene. Dr. Walker has written numerous peer-reviewed articles and several book chapters. She is a fellow of the American Heart Association, a member of the Society of Toxicology, a panelist on the Environmental Protection Agency's Science Advisory Board, and a reviewer for several journals and study sections. She served on the Institute of Medicine (IOM) Committee on Veterans and Agent Orange for *Update 2006* and chaired the committee for *Update 2010*.

Rebecca A. Betensky, PhD, is professor of biostatistics at the Harvard School of Public Health in Boston. She received her bachelor's degree in mathematics from Harvard and a PhD in statistics from Stanford University. She is a fellow of the American Statistical Association, an elected member of the International Statistical Institute, and the 2005 recipient of American Public Health Association's Mortimer Spiegelman Award for outstanding contributions to health statistics by a statistician under 40 years old. Her current methodologic interests are in latent-class modeling for genomic data and survival analysis under complex sampling and with auxiliary information. The applications of her epidemiologic analyses have primarily been in neurology and oncology. She served on the Institute of

Medicine Committee on Cognitive Rehabilitation Therapy for Traumatic Brain Injury.

Michael J. Carvan, III, PhD, MS, is Shaw Associate Professor at the School of Freshwater Sciences and School of Public Health, both of the University of Wisconsin–Milwaukee. He earned his MS in biologic oceanography at the University of Miami's Rosenstiel School of Marine and Atmospheric Science in Coral Gables and his PhD in veterinary anatomy and public health with a focus in toxicology from Texas A&M University's College of Veterinary Medicine in College Station. After obtaining his doctorate, Dr. Carvan held National Institute of Environmental Health Sciences molecular toxicology fellowships at the University of Cincinnati Medical Center. His research uses zebrafish as a genetic system for identifying genes that influence susceptibility of response to xenobiotics.

Scott Davis, PhD, MS, is a professor in and chair of the department of epidemiology at the University of Washington's School of Public Health and a member of the Division of Public Health Sciences of the Fred Hutchinson Cancer Research Center in Seattle. Dr. Davis is a fellow of the American College of Epidemiology and a member of the Russian Academy of Medical Sciences. He received undergraduate training in biology and chemistry at the University of New Mexico, an MS in community health from the University of Rochester, and his PhD in epidemiology from the University of Washington. Early in his career, he participated in epidemiologic investigations at the Radiation Effects Research Foundation in Hiroshima. He previously served on the National Research Council's Committee on Health Risks from Exposure to Low Levels of Ionizing Radiation (BEIR VII) and recently completed a 4-year term on the National Cancer Institute's Board of Scientific Counselors.

Naihua Duan, PhD, MA, is a professor of biostatistics at Columbia University and director of the Division of Biostatistics of the New York State Psychiatric Institute in New York City. He received a BS in mathematics from National Taiwan University, an MA in mathematical statistics from Columbia University, and a PhD in statistics from Stanford University. His research interests include study design, particularly for investigations that have multilevel data structures. He previously served on the National Academies committees that prepared *Human Exposure Assessment to Airborne Pollutants: Advances and Opportunities*; *Organ Procurement and Transplantation: Assessing Current Policies and the Potential Impact of the DHHS Final Rule*; *Carbon Monoxide Episodes in Meteorological and Topographical Problem Areas*; *Assessing the Medical Risks of Human Oocyte Donation for Stem Cell Research*; *Assessment of Readjustment Needs of Military Personnel, Veterans, and Their Families Phase 2*; *Veterans and Agent Orange: Update 2008*; and *Veterans and Agent Orange: Update 2010*.

Stephanie M. Engel, PhD, MSPH, is an associate professor of epidemiology at the University of North Carolina's Gillings School of Global Public Health. She earned her MSPH and PhD from the University of North Carolina at Chapel Hill. Dr. Engel's research considers the effect of environmental exposures and innate susceptibility factors on adverse pregnancy outcomes and neurodevelopmental impairment in children. She has conducted multiple studies of maternal and child genetic variability in relation to prematurity, growth restriction, pre-eclampsia, and gestational hypertension. Dr. Engel has also conducted studies of prenatal exposure to endocrine-disrupting chemicals and pesticides in relation to neonatal, infant, and child neurodevelopment. She is particularly engaged in efforts to characterize the mechanistic relations between endocrine disrupting exposures and neurodevelopment.

Jennifer R. Grandis, MD, FACS, is professor of otolaryngology and pharmacology at the University of Pittsburgh School of Medicine and director of the Head and Neck Cancer Program of the University of Pittsburgh Cancer Institute. Consistently funded by grants from the National Institute of Health and the National Cancer Institute, Dr. Grandis's research laboratory is devoted to the study of autocrine signaling pathways and genetic alterations in squamous-cell carcinoma of the head and neck. Dr. Grandis completed medical school, residencies in otolaryngology and surgery, and a fellowship in infectious disease at the University of Pittsburgh School of Medicine. She has contributed numerous articles and abstracts to the scientific literature and holds patents for novel concepts pertaining to cancer treatments and diagnostics. She was elected to the IOM, the American Society for Clinical Investigation, and the Association of American Physicians. She is a Fellow of the American College of Surgeons and the American Laryngological, Rhinological and Otological (Triologic) Society.

Karl Kelsey, MD, MOH, is a professor of epidemiology and pathology and of laboratory medicine at Brown University. He received his MD from the University of Minnesota and a master's degree in occupational health from Harvard University. Until 2007, he was on the faculty of the Harvard School of Public Health and Harvard Medical School. He is interested in the application of laboratory-based biomarkers in chronic-disease epidemiology and tumor biology and in characterizing individual susceptibility to cancer. He is an author of more than 200 publications and has served on the National Academies Committees on Toxicity Testing and Assessment of Environmental Agents; on Copper in Drinking Water; on the Evaluation of the Department of Veterans Affairs Uniform Case Assessment Protocol; to Review the Health Consequences of Service During the Persian Gulf War; to Conduct a Study on Curriculum Development in Environmental Medicine; and on the Health Effects of Mustard Gas and Lewisite. He also served on the IOM Committee on Veterans and Agent Orange for *Update 2010*.

Stephen B. Kritchevsky, PhD, MSPH, is a professor of internal medicine and translational science and director of the J. Paul Sticht Center on Aging of Wake Forest University Baptist Medical Center. After receiving both his MSPH and PhD in epidemiology from the University of North Carolina at Chapel Hill, he joined the Departments of Biostatistics and of Epidemiology at the University of Tennessee Health Science Center, where he founded that school's Master's of Clinical Epidemiology Program. Dr. Kritchevsky's research interests are related to conditions that compromise the health of aging populations, particularly inflammation, obesity, metabolic syndrome, and cardiovascular disease. He has published more than 250 articles in peer-reviewed scientific journals. He is a fellow of the Gerontological Society of America and editor-in-chief of the *Journal of Gerontology of Medical Sciences*. He previously served on the IOM Committees on Veterans and Agent Orange for *Update 2008* and for *Update 2010*.

James R. Olson, PhD, MS, is a professor of pharmacology and toxicology at the School of Medicine and Biomedical Sciences of the University at Buffalo, where he also serves as director of the Environmental Health Sciences Division in the School of Public Health and Health Professions. His research focuses on the toxicity and mechanism of action of dioxin and related chemicals in laboratory animals and humans and on human exposure to, metabolism of, and susceptibility to pesticides and polybrominated diphenyl ethers. Dr. Olson is the author or coauthor of numerous articles. He served on the IOM Committee on Veterans and Agent Orange for *Update 2010*.

Gail S. Prins, PhD, is the Michael Reese Professor of Urology and Physiology and director of the University Andrology Laboratory at the University of Illinois at Chicago. She received her PhD in physiology from the University of Illinois Medical Center and completed a National Institutes of Health fellowship at Northwestern University Medical School. Her primary research interest is in prostate growth and function and how developmental reprogramming by natural and environmental estrogens contributes to carcinogenesis with aging. She has done extensive research in tying bisphenol A exposure early in life to later susceptibility to health issues. In 2011, Dr. Prins received the 2011 Researcher of the Year award from the University of Illinois for this research. She previously served on the External Scientific Review Committee for the National Institute of Environmental Health Sciences and was a member of the Integration Panel for the Department of Defense Prostate Cancer Research Program. Dr. Prins is a past president of the American Society of Andrology and currently serves as editor of *Endocrinology* and associate editor of *Andrology*.

Helen H. Suh, ScD, is associate professor of health sciences and an affiliate faculty member of the Department of Civil and Environmental Engineering at Northeastern University. She is also a senior fellow at the National Opinion Research Center at the University of Chicago and an adjunct senior lecturer at the Harvard School of Public Health. Dr. Suh is an expert in air-pollution exposure assessment, measurements, and environmental epidemiology. She has been the principal investigator of numerous exposure and health studies, including those to characterize multipollutant exposures, to examine cardiovascular health effects of air pollution, and to develop GIS-based spatial smoothing models to estimate chronic exposures to particles. She is a member of the Environmental Protection Agency's Clean Air Scientific Advisory Committee and has been a member of previous National Academies committees, including the Committee to Review the Draft IRIS Assessment on Formaldehyde. Dr. Suh is an associate editor of the *Journal of Exposure Science and Environmental Epidemiology*. She has performed advisory work in environmental sciences for numerous international, national, and local organizations. Dr. Suh received a BS in biology from the Massachusetts Institute of Technology and an MS and a ScD in environmental health sciences from the Harvard School of Public Health.

Marc Weisskopf, PhD, ScD, is an associate professor of environmental and occupational epidemiology at the Harvard School of Public Health. Dr. Weisskopf received his PhD in neuroscience from the University of California, San Francisco, and his ScD in epidemiology from the Harvard School of Public Health. His research focuses on how environmental factors affect the nervous system and on the epidemiology of neurologic disorders, such as amyotrophic lateral sclerosis, Parkinson disease, and autism spectrum disorders. He has served on the IOM committee on the long-term neurologic consequences of traumatic brain injury and the external advisory board for the Department of Defense Millennium Cohort Study, and he assisted the Environmental Protection Agency in the section on adult neurological health effects of the National Assessment of Air Quality Standard for Lead.

Lori A. White, PhD, MS, is associate professor in the Department of Biochemistry and Microbiology of the School of Environmental and Biological Sciences of Rutgers, the State University of New Jersey. She received a master's degree in zoology from the University of Maine, earned a PhD in biochemistry from Dartmouth Medical School, and did postdoctoral work at the University of Wisconsin. She has been active in Gordon Conference programs and was the chairperson for the Mechanisms of Toxicology summer session in 2008. Her research interests include elucidation of dioxin's carcinogenic activity and use of the zebrafish as a model for investigating the effects of environmental chemicals on development.

Luoping Zhang, PhD, is an adjunct professor of toxicology in the Division of Environmental Health Sciences of the School of Public Health of the University of California, Berkeley (UC Berkeley). She is also an associate director of the Genes and Environment Laboratory and co-leader and co-principal investigator of the UC Berkeley Superfund Basic Research Program. Dr. Zhang received her PhD in biochemistry and toxicology from Simon Fraser University, British Columbia, Canada, in 1993. Her research has focused on investigating biologic consequences and molecular mechanisms of leukemia and lymphoma associated with exposures to toxic chemicals (such as benzene, formaldehyde, and trichloroethylene). Most recently, Dr. Zhang's group used many high-throughput novel technologies, such as single-cell genetic analysis and array-based omic technologies, including toxicogenomics, proteomics and epigenetics in molecular epidemiology studies, and micro RNA and RNA interference in human cell cultures. A *systems biology* approach is applied in her population studies. Recently, she has turned her attention to studying chemically induced toxicity in hematopoietic stem and progenitor cells. Dr. Zhang was a member of the IOM Committee on Veterans and Agent Orange for *Update 2010*.

Staff Biographies

Mary Burr Paxton, PhD, is a Senior Program Officer in the IOM's Board on the Health of Select Populations. Before joining IOM, she worked as a consultant on the regulation of toxic substances and managed the conduct and analysis of several epidemiologic studies on veterans' health. She received an MS in biostatistics from the Johns Hopkins School of Hygiene and Public Health and a doctorate in genetics from the George Washington University. She is a diplomate of the American Board of Toxicology. Dr. Paxton has worked on several National Academies reports, including *Issues in Risk Assessment*; *Environmental Neurotoxicology*; *Gulf War and Health: Insecticides and Solvents*; *Gulf War and Health: Fuels, Combustion Products, and Propellants*; *Asbestos: Selected Cancers*; *Veterans and Agent Orange: Update 2004*; *Veterans and Agent Orange: Update 2006*; *Veterans and Agent Orange: Update 2008*; and *Veterans and Agent Orange: Update 2010*.

Jennifer A. Cohen, MPH, is a Program Officer in the IOM's Board on the Health of Select Populations. She received her undergraduate degree and her MPH from the University of Maryland. She has been involved with the IOM committees that produced *Organ Procurement and Transplantation*; *Clearing the Air: Asthma and Indoor Air Exposures*; *Veterans and Agent Orange: Herbicide/Dioxin Exposure and Type 2 Diabetes*; *Veterans and Agent Orange: Update 2000*; *Veterans and Agent Orange: Herbicide/Dioxin Exposure and Acute Myelogenous Leukemia in the Children of Vietnam Veterans*; *Veterans and Agent Orange: Update 2004*; *Veterans and Agent Orange: Update 2006*; *Veterans and Agent Orange: Update 2008*; and *Veterans and Agent Orange: Update 2010*. She was also rapporteur for the IOM report *Challenges and Successes in Reducing Health Disparities*.

Tia S. Carter, MS, is a Senior Program Assistant in the IOM's Board on the Health of Select Populations. She earned her master's in health care administration from the University of Maryland University College. She received her undergraduate degree in community health from the University of Maryland, College Park. Before joining IOM, she worked at the Greater Washington Urban League in the Division of Aging and Health Services as the health-promotions coordinator, where she was responsible for health-promotion and disease-prevention education services and activities among the elderly. She has been involved with the IOM committees that produced *Asbestos: Selected Cancers; Provision of Mental Health Counseling Services under TRICARE*; *Climate Change, the Indoor Environment, and Health*; *Veterans and Agent Orange: Update 2004*; *Veterans and Agent Orange: Update 2006*; *Veterans and Agent Orange: Update 2008*; and *Veterans and Agent Orange: Update 2010*.

Frederick (Rick) Erdtmann, MD, MPH, is Director of the IOM's Board on the Health of Select Populations. He earned his MD from Temple University School of Medicine, and he holds an MPH from the University of California, Berkeley. He completed a residency program in general preventive medicine at Walter Reed Army Institute of Research in 1975 and is board-certified in that specialty. Dr. Erdtmann's assignments with the Army Medical Department included being chief of preventive-medicine services at Fitzsimons Army Medical Center, at Frankfurt Army Medical Center in Germany, and at Madigan Army Medical Center. He also served as division surgeon for the Second Infantry Division in Tongduchon, Korea. He later served as Deputy Chief of Staff for Clinical Operations in the Department of Defense's TRICARE Region 1 before assuming hospital command at Walter Reed Army Medical Center in March 1998. After that, he was assigned to the Office of the Surgeon General as the Deputy Assistant Surgeon General for Force Development. In 2001, after 30 years of commissioned military service, Dr. Erdtmann joined the National Academies and assumed his present responsibilities.

Norman Grossblatt, ELS(D), is a senior editor at the National Academies. Before joining the National Research Council Division of Medical Sciences in 1963, he worked as an analyst in information storage and retrieval at Documentation Incorporated and as a technical editor at the Allis-Chalmers Manufacturing Co., Nuclear Power Department, in Washington, DC. He received a BA in English from Haverford College. Mr. Grossblatt is a diplomate editor in the life sciences and was the founding president of the Board of Editors in the Life Sciences. He is a fellow of the American Medical Writers Association and a recipient of its President's Award; a member of the Council of Science Editors and, since 1997, the manuscript editor of its journal, *Science Editor*; and a member of the European Association of Science Editors. At the National Academies, he has edited more than 300 reports.